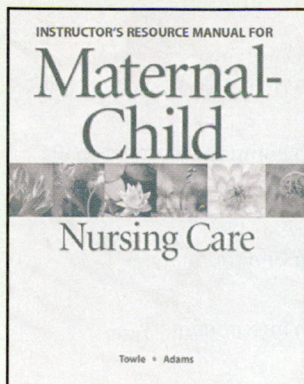
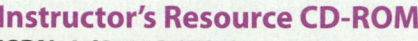
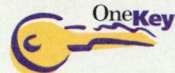
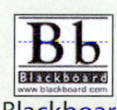

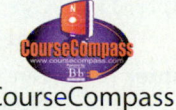
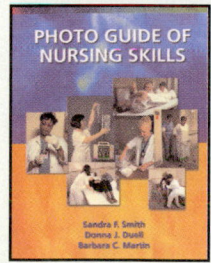
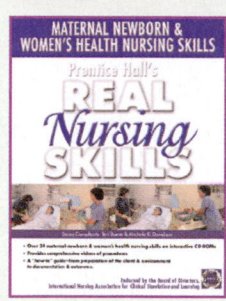
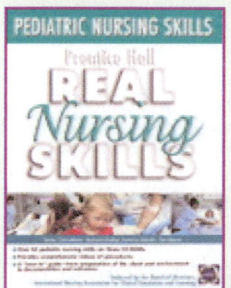

Brief Table of Contents

Maternal-Child

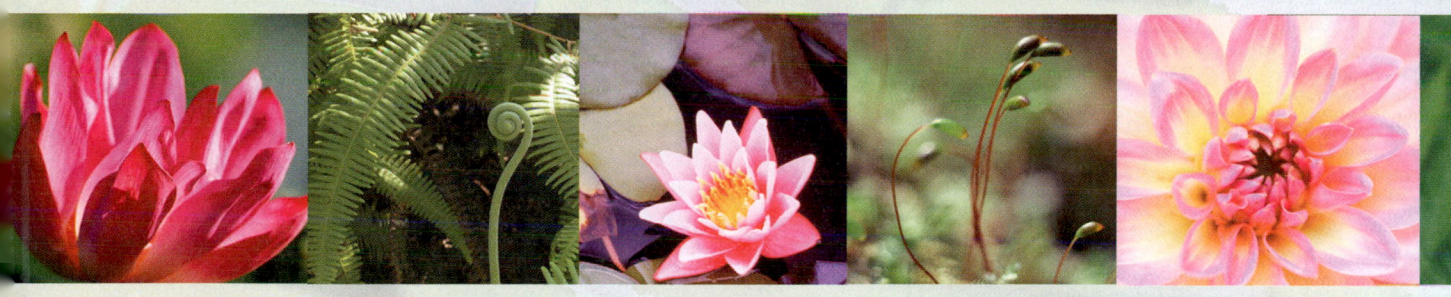

Nursing Care

Mary Ann Towle, RN, MEd, MSN
Faculty
Boise State University
Boise, Idaho

Ellise D. Adams, CNM, MSN, CD (DONA), ICCE
Clinical Assistant Professor
The University of Alabama in Huntsville
Huntsville, Alabama

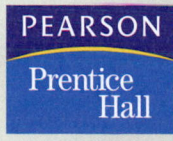

PEARSON
Prentice Hall

Upper Saddle River, New Jersey 07458

Publisher: Julie Levin Alexander
Publisher's Assistant: Regina Bruno
Editor-in-Chief: Maura Connor
Acquisitions Editor: Kelly Trakalo
Editorial Assistant: JulieAnn Oliveros
Development Editor: Rachel Bedard
Managing Editor, Development: Marilyn Meserve
Managing Production Editor: Patrick Walsh
Production Liaison: Yagnesh Jani
Production Editor: Penny Walker, Techbooks
Manufacturing Manager: Ilene Sanford
Manufacturing Buyer: Pat Brown
Design Director and Cover Designer: Mary Siener
Photographer: Patrick Watson
Director of Marketing: Karen Allman
Senior Marketing Manager: Francisco Del Castillo
Marketing Coordinator: Michael Sirinides
Marketing Assistant: Patricia Linard
Associate Editor: Michael Giacobbe
Media Development Editor: John J. Jordan
Media Production Manager: Amy Peltier
New Media Project Manager: Tina Rudowski
Composition: Techbooks
Printer/Binder: Courier Kendallville, Inc.
Cover Printer: Phoenix Color

Pearson Education LTD.
Pearson Education Australia PTY, Limited
Pearson Education Singapore, Pte. Ltd
Pearson Education North Asia Ltd
Pearson Education Canada, Ltd.
Pearson Educación de Mexico, S.A. de C.V.
Pearson Education–Japan
Pearson Education Malaysia, Pte. Ltd
Pearson Education, Upper Saddle River

Fern background & image: Akira Keade/Getty Images, Inc. Lotus lilly: Jeremy Woodhouse/Getty Images, Inc. Fiddlehead: Mary Siener. Lilly pad with bloom: Eyewire/Getty Images, Inc. Plant buds: Photodisc/Getty Images, Inc. Dahlia flower: PNC/Getty Images, Inc. Fern bud: Eyewire/Getty Images, Inc.

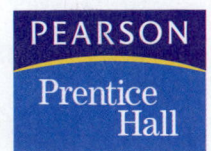

ISBN 0-13-113627-5

Student Success is built in from the start...

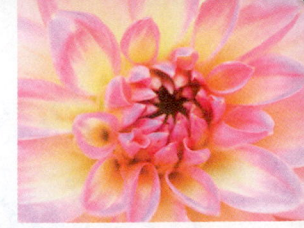

Practical and vocational nurses from around the country told us that they needed two things to succeed as students in order to achieve their LPN/LVN licenses. First, they needed books that explain what the LPN/LVN needs to know and do. Second, they needed a variety of excellent review materials to reinforce their learning. *Maternal Child Nursing Care* contains power-packed, built-in support to ensure your success throughout your LPN/LVN education.

As you start each chapter—

Brief Outlines preview what the chapter will cover for quick access and review.

Learning Outcomes identify what you can expect to learn from each chapter and help you focus your reading.

Chapter 7

Health Promotion During Labor and Delivery

BRIEF Outline

Theories About the Beginning of Labor
Signs of Impending Labor
Admission to the Birthing Facility
Variables Affecting Labor

Pain in Labor
Stages of Labor
Delivery Room Care of the Neonate
Nursing Care

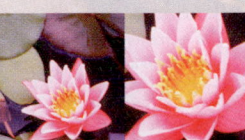

HEALTH PROMOTION ISSUE:
Client Wanting Second Labor to Be Better Than First
NURSING PROCESS CARE PLAN:
Woman in Active Stage One Labor
CRITICAL THINKING CARE MAP:
Caring for a Woman in Transition

LEARNING Outcomes

After completing this chapter, you will be able to:
- Discuss appropriate nursing actions for women who present for admission when in labor.
- Describe variables affecting labor and delivery.
- Identify various methods of pain relief used during labor.
- Differentiate the stages of labor.
- Discuss the mechanisms of labor.
- Identify nursing diagnoses and nursing interventions to assist in the labor process.
- Provide appropriate care for a client during labor and delivery.
- Describe important aspects of nursing care of the neonate immediately after birth.

MediaLinks call your attention to the additional learning tools that are available on the Student CD-ROM and Companion Website that accompany your textbook, including:

Student CD-ROM
- *Learning Outcomes*
- *Audio Glossary*—key terms, definitions, and pronunciations
- *NCLEX-PN® Review Questions*—unique to this CD-ROM
- *Animations & Videos*—difficult concepts brought to life

Companion Website
- *Learning Outcomes*
- *Chapter Outlines*
- *Audio Glossary*
- *NCLEX-PN® Review Questions*—unique to this website
- *Key Term Review*—matching questions and crossword puzzles to help with new terminology and definitions.
- *Case Studies*—scenarios and critical-thinking questions
- *Challenge Your Knowledge*—visual critical thinking questions
- *WebLinks*—content-related hyperlinks
- *Nursing Tools*—handy reference materials

Otitis

Otitis

the *eust*
middle
ing the
eustach
flat for
oral ph
tube in
grows
become
throat
well.

Otitis Media

MediaLink

MediaLink Tabs prompt you to explore videos, animations, and activities on the Student CD-ROM and Companion Website.

Makes need-to-know information easy to find and use!

Medical Child Nursing Care contains color-coded boxes and tables with important information for you to remember.

BOX 14-1   CULTURAL PULSE POINTS

Mexican American Family Support System

The Mexican American family is a strong support system. Although the father is the spokesperson for the family, extended family members may be present during hospitalization. The nurse should include them in explanations about health care.

With every family, it is important for the nurse to try to answer certain questions:

- Who is the decision maker?
- Is the family expressive or stoic about their feelings?
- What kind of physical presence does the family expect or want to have with the hospitalized child?

Cultural Pulse Points boxes provide insight into populations and situations nurses may meet.

BOX 25-3   NUTRITION THERAPY

Foods for a Low-Salt, Low-Protein Diet

Low-Salt Diet

- The health care professional will order the amount of restriction (e.g., a 2-g Na diet). Most foods do contain some sodium, so foods that are lowest in sodium should be selected.
- The nurse reinforces the following guidelines to help the client (or parents) maintain a low-salt diet:
  - Check labels for Na (sodium).
  - Add no salt to foods.
  - Avoid salty snacks (chips, salty popcorn, pretzels with salt).
  - Avoid processed, prepared foods because they tend to contain higher levels of sodium.

Low-Protein Diet

- The health care professional will order the amount of restriction (e.g., a 40-g protein diet).
- The nurse reinforces the following guidelines to help the client (or parents) maintain a low-protein diet:
  - All meats and milk are high in protein (about 3 oz meat = 8 g protein).
  - Cereal/bread and vegetables are moderate to low in protein.
    - ½ cup cereal or 1 slice bread = 2 g protein
    - ½ cup vegetables = 1 g protein
  - Avoid seafood.
  - Limit meat to half of a serving.
  - Use bread and vegetables for food volume.

Nursing Care Checklists provide handy summaries of important nursing interventions.

BOX 20-1   NURSING CARE CHECKLIST

First Aid for Bleeding

- ☑ Obtain assistance from another health care worker.
- ☑ Apply personal protective equipment.
- ☑ Apply direct pressure with sterile gauze to the site of bleeding for at least 15 minutes.
- ☑ If gauze becomes soaked, do not remove. Add additional gauze.
- ☑ Raise the site of bleeding above the heart while applying pressure.
- ☑ Apply ice packs to promote vasoconstriction.
- ☑ If bleeding has not slowed after 15 minutes of these measures, apply additional pressure to the pulse site above the wound.
- ☑ Monitor vital signs closely.
- ☑ If the child does not have venous access, initiate access to administer IV fluid or blood replacement as ordered.
- ☑ Offer emotional support to the child and his or her family.

BOX 11-4   CLIENT TEACHING

Toilet Training

Determining Readiness

Although readiness is individualized, the child must have achieved the following developmental skills:

- Stand and walk
- Pull pants up and down
- Recognize need to "go"
- Can wait to reach bathroom

Helpful Hints

- If child is afraid of toilet, use small chair or small toilet seat insert.
- If using toilet, place sturdy stool in front of toilet for child to stand on to reach the seat.
- Place child on seat upon rising in the morning, before and after naps, before bath, before bed, and at regular intervals through the day.
- Teach hand washing after toileting.
- Praise success. Do not punish accidents.
- If child does not cooperate, wait a few weeks and try again.

BOX 27-4   ASSESSMENT

Manifestations of Abuse

Child's Behavior

- Shows sudden changes in behavior or school performance
- Has not received help for physical or medical problems brought to the parents' attention
- Has learning problems (or difficulty concentrating) that cannot be attributed to specific physical or psychological causes
- Is always watchful, as though preparing for something bad to happen
- Lacks adult supervision
- Is overly compliant, passive, or withdrawn
- Comes to school or other activities early, stays late, and does not want to go home

Parent's Behavior

- Shows little concern for the child
- Denies the existence of—or blames the child for—the child's problems in school or at home
- Asks teachers or other caregivers to use harsh physical discipline if the child misbehaves
- Sees the child as entirely bad, worthless, or burdensome
- Demands a level of physical or academic performance the child cannot achieve
- Looks primarily to the child for care, attention, and satisfaction of emotional needs

---

Client Teaching, and Nutrition Therapy boxes help you prepare for your role as educators in health care settings.

Assessment box summarizes data collected during assessment, common risk factors, and manifestations you might observe.

TABLE 14-4

Pharmacology: Drugs Used for Conscious Sedation

DRUG	USUAL ROUTE/DOSE	CLASSIFICATION	SELECTED SIDE EFFECTS	DON'T GIVE IF
Diazepam (Valium)	IM/IV # 5 years 0.2–0.5 mg slowly every 2–5 minutes up to 5 mg $ 5 years1 mg every 5 minutes up to 10 mg	Anxiolytic, anticonvulsant	Drowsiness, dizziness, hypotension, respiratory distress	Other drugs are being administered; (do not mix)
Midazolam (Versed)	IM 0.08 mg/kg IV 0.15 mg/kg followed by 0.05 mg/kg every 2 minutes × one to three doses	Short-acting benzodiazepine anxiolytic, sedative hypnotic	Retrograde amnesia, respiratory distress, hypotension	Severe organic heart disease; caution with renal or hepatic impairment
Lorazepam (Ativan)	PO, IV, IM 0.05 mg/kg	Benzodiazepine anxiolytic, sedative hypnotic	Drowsiness, sedation, respiratory distress	Child is younger than 12 years

PHARMACOLOGY tables reinforce selected common medications nurses will encounter in practice. Additional boxes and tables offer information on key topics.

HEALTH PROMOTION ISSUE

DEVELOPING A THERAPEUTIC RELATIONSHIP WITH A PEDIATRIC CLIENT

The LPN/LVN working in a pediatrician's office is approached by a recently hired LPN/LVN. Her past nursing experience has been with adult clients in an acute-care setting. She states that she has never worked with children before and is having some difficulty relating to them. She is most distressed that the children seem afraid of her. The children will not open up to her and talk to her about issues related to their health care. She is concerned that these factors will affect the type of nursing care she is able to give and ultimately affect the child's health care. She wants some assistance in performing her nursing tasks without scaring the children.

DISCUSSION

For the nurse to assist the child to become healthy, a positive nurse–client relationship must be established. This relationship develops over time, demonstrates respect and confidentiality, is client focused and not nurse focused, and has respect and mutual trust as its basis.

For the relationship between a child and a nurse to be therapeutic, the nurse must display caring behaviors mixed with a professional attitude that conveys competence. Trust develops when children believe that the nurse cares about them and is capable of helping them through a situation. Trust develops as the nurse:

- Listens attentively to what the child says, even if the child is talking about cartoons or toys.
- Displays empathy. Empathy includes recognizing the child's needs, acknowledging the child as real, and showing the child that the nurse is working diligently to meet expressed needs.
- Is honest with the child. Children can see through dishonesty. They need

straight, simple responses or an honest "I don't know."

- Is genuine. Caring cannot be contrived. Caring for a child requires knowledge of their developmental levels, of their emotional status, and of their social history. The genuine nurse displays spontaneous behaviors that seek to restore and protect the child.

As the nurse communicates with children, she must recognize that this is accomplished both verbally and nonverbally. Although many people think that spoken words convey our message, in actuality nonverbal communication conveys more than 80% of our message. Nonverbal communication includes our personal appearance. It is said that an opinion of us is formed by other individuals within the first 3 seconds of our first encounter. This opinion is developed before we ever say a word and is largely based on our dress, our posture, our facial expressions, and our gait.

Verbal communication is more than the words we say; it is also how we say them. The nurse can communicate a message effectively by speaking with enthusiasm, energy, and at a pace that indicates interest and not anxiety. Verbal communication should be easy to understand, clear, and as brief as possible.

The timing of verbal communication is also important. The message can go unheard if the child is not ready or willing to listen.

Children learn in different ways. Some must hear the information, whereas others must see it. Still others need to use their hands (e.g., write information or handle a stethoscope) before they can learn.

Developmental levels also influence how a child learns. For instance, a pre-

schooler enjoys learning by trial and error. An adolescent needs to learn independently.

The nurse must consider the child's vocabulary, education, psychomotor abilities, emotional status, societal values, and attention span when developing a teaching plan.

It is also important to choose an appropriate teaching strategy. The nurse can use demonstration to teach a skill and then ask the child to return demonstration. The nurse could also model specific behaviors. Teaching aids may assist the nurse in communicating the proper information. Written materials, posters, anatomic models, games, videos, computers, or dolls may be used in both formal teaching and informal teaching.

PLANNING AND IMPLEMENTATION

Development of a Nurse–Client Relationship

Prior to the child's appointment, the nurse reviews the child's chart, noting any medical or social history that would impact the behavior of the child. The nurse should note the child's age and recall information about the appro-

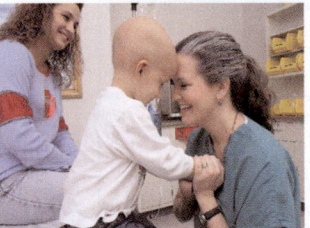

priate developmental age. The nurse should practice pronouncing the child's name and note any special likes or dislikes that are noted in the chart. For example, if the child likes a certain cartoon character, the nurse might be able to find a Band-Aid with that character on it or place the child in an exam room decorated with this character. Be sure to include this documentation in the child's chart and update as needed.

Social interaction at the beginning of the appointment is necessary to help ease the child's anxiety and to develop a trusting relationship. The nurse should be at eye level with the child when speaking directly to him or her (see Figure 13-1). Initially, the nurse should avoid touching the child until trust is established.

As the appointment progresses and the nurse seeks to understand the health care needs of the child, listening becomes vital. Active listening requires much energy and is vital in achieving trust. Listening behaviors include eye contact and body language that suggests a willingness to listen (e.g., relaxed body parts, a face-to-face position, a slight leaning toward the child). Listening also requires silence on the nurse's part. As the child speaks, the nurse must actively consider the child's words and not try to develop a wise or witty comeback while the child is speaking. Only after gathering all subjective and objective data can the nurse develop a plan of action. Plans developed before data collection is complete are likely to be ineffective.

Appropriate Communication Techniques

Pediatric nurses often choose brightcolored uniforms that will appeal to children. Hair should be neat. Makeup should look natural, so as not to distract or frighten the child. Posture should be erect but not tense.

Children can read the thoughts of the nurse through the nurse's facial expressions. It is important for nurses to learn to control feelings of disgust, impatience, or boredom. The nurse's face needs to display interest, enthusiasm, and energy. If a child confides that he or she has been abused by an adult, the nurse must not express horror or anger. The nurse's face should convey interest and concern so the child will continue to share information.

When communicating verbally with children, the nurse should speak to the child in language and terms that they can understand. The nurse should use open-ended questions when trying to obtain information from a child. Questions such as "Tell me how your tummy feels" or "What happened to your leg?" will elicit more information than a question that can simply be answered "yes" or "no."

Appropriate Teaching Methods

The nurse needs to have a variety of teaching aids available in order to conduct formal or informal teaching for the child. A simple drawing of the

body can help the nurse describe a disease, procedure, or surgery. Dolls or puppets appeal to preschoolers.

In school settings, videos are often a way of providing information. If videos are used, the dialogue should be appropriate for the age group. Slides or photographs should also be age appropriate. For example, photographs of genitalia should not be shown in a classroom of mixed genders. The nurse should carefully assess readiness to learn and evaluate learning following the teaching session.

With diligence and continued effort, the nurse should be able to relate to the pediatric client and provide effective care.

SELF-REFLECTION

When a child reacts negatively to you, what feelings do you have? If a child has never acted negatively to you, imagine what the scenario might look like. Be honest about your feelings. When you encounter a strange environment, what factors make you feel more uncomfortable? What factors make you feel more comfortable? What do you need to change in your nursing practice to help develop trust with your clients? To communicate better with your pediatric clients? To be more effective in providing them with teaching as it relates to their health care?

SUGGESTED RESOURCES

For the Nurse

www.ChildbirthGraphics.com The catalog available at this website can provide the nurse with posters, pamphlets, three-dimensional models, and videos to assist in health care teaching.

Blackwell, P., & Baker, B. (2002). Estimating communication competence of infants and toddlers. *Journal of Pediatric Health Care, 16*(1), 19–35.

Humphries, J. (2002). The school health nurse and health education in the classroom. *Nursing Standard, 16*(17), 42–45.

Sydnor-Greenberg, N., & Dokken, D. (2001). Communication in healthcare: Thought on the child's perspective. *Journal of Child and Family Nursing, 4*(3), 225–230.

Health Promotion Issues examine topical issues and show you how to move from problems to solutions as you care for clients.

clinical ALERT

The passage of meconium prior to delivery signals some type of fetal distress.

Clinical Alerts call your attention to clinical roles and responsibilities for heightened awareness, monitoring, and/or reporting.

Learn to prioritize nursing actions and deliver safe, effective nursing care as a part of the health care team!

Nursing Care is presented in the five-step nursing process format, but emphasizing the scope of practice for the LPN/LVN. Rationales after each nursing action explain why the action is important and support the evidence-based nursing process.

NURSING CARE

PRIORITIES IN NURSING CARE

The priorities of nursing care for the high-risk newborn are similar to those for the normal newborn. However, the method in which the needs are met may be different.

- Maintaining the airway, breathing, and circulation
- Maintaining body temperature
- Providing nutrition
- Ensuring elimination
- Teaching parents to provide care for their newborn.

ASSESSING

The high-risk newborn requires a more frequent and in-depth assessment than the normal newborn. The high-risk newborn may have equipment such as a heart monitor, a

Priorities in Nursing Care focuses your thinking on key assessments and interventions.

Critical Thinking in the Nursing Process

1. What are some other topics that should be discussed with Jeremy's parents before surgery?
2. What topics should the nurse plan to discuss with Jeremy's parents before discharge?
3. What is the role of the LPN/LVN in providing care to the NICU patient and family?

Critical Thinking questions allow you to apply your new knowledge to a specific client.

NURSING PROCESS CARE PLAN
Client with Diarrhea

Wesley is a 3-month-old infant who is formula fed. He is typically a pleasant child who has regular bowel habits. His big brother, Mark, has been home from school with a stomach virus this week. Today, after his morning bottle, Wesley has had several loose stools and is irritable when awake. His mother calls the pediatrician's office for advice.

Assessment. The nurse should gather the following data during the phone call:

- Changes in diet by obtaining a 24-hour diet history
- Onset of diarrhea
- Color, consistency, frequency, amount, and odor of stools
- The presence of mucous in the stools
- Associated symptoms such as vomiting, fever, and lethargy.

Nursing Process Care Plans illustrate nursing care in a "real-life" scenario.

PROCEDURE 13-26 — Administering Oxygen to Children

Purpose

- To provide the prescribed concentration of oxygen to the child

Equipment

- Oxygen supply, including a flowmeter
- Device to humidify the oxygen
- Nasal cannula, face masks, or oxygen tent
- Oxygen tubing

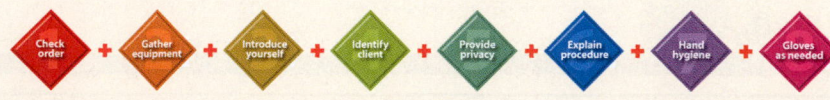

Check order + Gather equipment + Introduce yourself + Identify client + Provide privacy + Explain procedure + Hand hygiene + Gloves as needed

Interventions

- Perform preparatory steps (see icon bar).
- Set up oxygen delivery method, including humidification.
- Turn on oxygen to prescribed flow rate.
- Place the face mask over the bridge of the child's nose to the cleft of the chin (see Figure 13-33). OR
- Place the nasal cannula into the anterior nares and put an elastic band around the child's head. OR
- Surround the child in the hospital bed with the oxygen tent. Secure the edges of the tent to deliver prescribed oxygen dosage and prevent escape of oxygen.

SAMPLE DOCUMENTATION

(date) 0700 *(Note: Oxygenation portion only. This is a focused part of a complete documentation entry.)* O_2 per nasal cannula at 2 L/minute applied. Band secured around head.

_____ K. Coffey, LPN

Procedures give you step-by-step instructions and rationales for nursing actions. Special icons in the procedures reinforce essential preliminary steps in client care. "Live" documentation at the end of each procedure demonstrates samples of good record-keeping.

Comprehensive reviews at the end of the chapter...

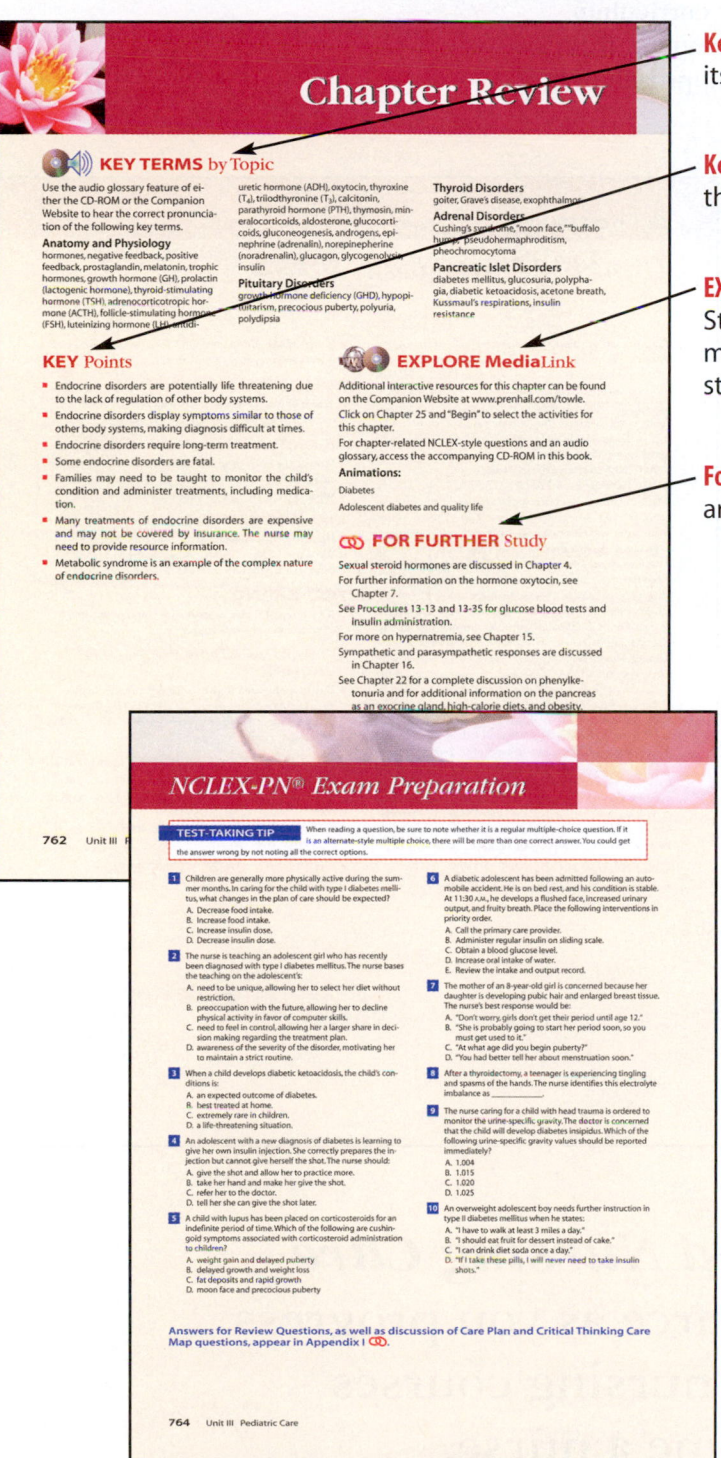

Key Terms by Topic link important new vocabulary to its content area in the chapter.

Key Points summarize need-to-know concepts from the chapter.

EXPLORE MediaLink encourages you to use the Student CD-ROM and Companion Website for a multi-modal review, regardless of your learning style.

For Further Study shows where related content areas are cross-referenced throughout the book.

Critical Thinking Care Map prepares you for success on NCLEX-PN®, in clinical, and on-the-job with a focused review of a client problem, including:

- NCLEX-PN® Focus Area
- Case Study
- Nursing Diagnosis
- Data Collection
- Reporting
- Nursing Care
- Documentation

NCLEX-PN® Exam Preparation includes:

- A **Test-Taking Tip** with a focused study hint
- **NCLEX-PN®** style questions for review and test practice, with questions in both traditional and alternative formats. Answers are found in Appendix I.

Prepare for your career as an LPN/LVN...

After each unit in this book, use the **Thinking Strategically About...** pages as an opportunity to reflect on the topics you have just read in the context of important themes across the LPN/LVN curriculum. Short scenarios and project ideas spotlight the unit's content from a variety of angles. Review of concepts enables you to approach unit topics from a more integrated perspective.

Critical Thinking questions highlight specific challenges you will face as a new nurse and assist you to provide the best possible care.

Collaborative Care challenges you to think about the different health care settings and to envision the many health care workers who may participate in a client's care.

Delegating helps you determine which nursing interventions may be delegated to assistive personnel.

Management of Care highlights specific nursing interventions appropriate to the care of the client.

Communication and **Client Teaching** focus on communication methods and educational strategies necessary to teach the client and the family.

Time Management and **Priorities in Nursing Care** help you organize care and focus on the most important aspects of care first.

Documenting and Reporting helps you practice what and how to document and when to report your findings.

Cultural Care Strategies build your confidence by providing information and scenarios to familiarize you with cultural patterns and differences.

UNIT II WRAP-UP

Thinking Strategically About...

You are a new graduate LPN, employed in a small hospital obstetric unit. The unit is staffed with one RN and one LPN per 8-hour shift. In report, you learn that a gravida 4, para 3 woman is laboring rapidly and is currently 8 cm dilated. The RN will need to remain with this client and assist in the delivery. You will be assigned to the other clients. There is an RN in another part of the hospital who can assist you if necessary.

At 0700, you receive the following report:

Mrs. Jessie Owens, a 22-year-old gravida 2, para 2, had a 7-lb 2-oz boy at 1300 yesterday by spontaneous vaginal delivery. She had no episiotomy or lacerations. She has had no postpartum complications. She is breastfeeding and plans to go home late this afternoon. Her baby, Philip, is nursing 8 minutes per breast. He has voided and stooled. Jessie has blood type B−, rubella positive. Philip has blood type A+. He is to be circumcised before discharge.

Miss Monica McQuire, a 19-year-old, gravida 1, para 1, delivered an 8-lb 10-oz girl at 0130 this morning by primary cesarean section for failure to progress in labor. Prior to delivery, Monica had pregnancy-induced hypertension with a blood pressure of 154/92. She had 2+ pitting edema in her ankles. Her reflexes were brisk without clonus. She has an IV of lactated Ringer's solution with magnesium sulfate and a Foley catheter that can be discontinued this morning. Her baby, Amanda, has voided but not stooled. Monica has only tried to breastfeed once since delivery, with poor results.

Mrs. Chung, a 24-year-old, gravida 7, para 6, is scheduled for admission and Pitocin induction of labor because she is overdue. She has just arrived at the hospital with her husband. They have only been in the United States for 4 months. They need to return to the China as soon as possible after the baby is born because Mr. Chung's mother is extremely ill.

CRITICAL THINKING
- At what point do you become concerned that baby Amanda has not stooled?

- Is baby Philip nursing enough? What would indicate he is not obtaining enough nutrition?

COLLABORATIVE CARE
- Which of your assigned clients may need referral to an outside agency for follow-up care? Why?

PRIORITIES IN NURSING CARE
- Identify the order in which you will assess these assigned clients.
- What is your rationale for your prioritization of care?

MANAGEMENT OF CARE
- How frequently should you monitor Miss McQuire?
- What part of Mrs. Chung's induction can you begin before the RN returns from the delivery room?

DELEGATING
- If a CNA is available to assist with your assignment, what care would you delegate?

COMMUNICATION AND CLIENT TEACHING
- Due to your responsibilities with postpartum clients, what communication should be given to Mrs. Chung?
- What teaching should be provided to Mrs. Owens before she is discharged?

DOCUMENTING AND REPORTING
- What changes in Miss McQuire would indicate a decline in her condition? How and to whom would you report them?
- Document the teaching provided to Mrs. Owens regarding circumcision care.

CULTURAL CARE STRATEGIES
- What cultural strategies should be incorporated into the care of Mrs. Chung?

330　Unit II　Maternal-Newborn Care

Maternal-Child Nursing Care
will be a key resource as you progress
through your nursing courses
and become a nurse.

The nature of nursing—grow with it!

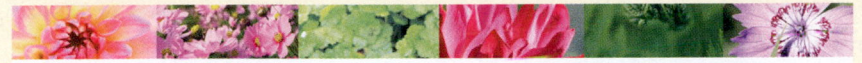

To my family: my children, Wendy and Mariah; my grandchildren, Kenya, Olivia and Leia; and my sister, Kathleen, whose love and support have helped me to stay focused through life's journey.

Mary Ann

To Freeda Vest, Ruby Adams, Gertrude Brockway, and Lila Darnell, the strong women in my life who taught me to love, nurture, and pursue excellence with grace.

Ellise

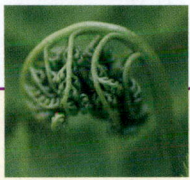

Preface

Maternal-Child Nursing Care is written to provide you, the LPN/LVN student, with a foundation for providing safe, effective nursing care of mother and child within the community. The basic premise of the book is that the community is made up of families working and living within a given set of boundaries, and the child-bearing family is best cared for within the community. While the traditional role of the LPN/LVN has been in acute and long-term care, nursing practice is moving out of the hospital and into a variety of settings within the community. This shift has resulted in a more interdisciplinary approach to client care. The task of defining the role of the LPN/LVN in community-based nursing practice is in its early stages. The themes of the book have been developed to provide a basic understanding of community-based nursing practice and care of the childbearing family in a variety of settings within the community. A strong emphasis is placed on understanding the role of the LPN/LVN and helping the student learn to make appropriate decisions within that role.

Organization

Maternal-Child Nursing Care is divided into three units. Unit One focuses on community-based nursing practice. This unit helps you make decisions, delegate activities, and provide care within the legal scope of practice for an LPN/LVN. You will learn how to assist the Registered Nurse in health promotion activities, in working with families, and in client teaching in a variety of client settings, including the home.

Unit Two focuses on the care of the mother and infant during pregnancy, childbirth, and the postpartum period. Also provided is a review of the reproductive system and disorders that affect reproduction. Emphasis is placed on health promotion during this time of transition. You will learn to care for the mother and infant during an uncomplicated pregnancy as well as to assist the Registered Nurse when common complications occur. You will learn about potential complications and warning signs.

Unit Three focuses on the care of the child in a variety of settings. While most texts present growth and development as a basis for nursing assessment, many end with the adolescent. To complete a family assessment and promote family health, the nurse must have an understanding of growth and development of all family members, including the adult and older adult. Therefore, growth and development across the life span is presented in its entirety.

Disorders are discussed by body system. You will learn health promotion activities, care of the child when illness occurs, and specific ways of adapting nursing interventions to children and adolescents.

Features

Throughout each chapter you will find consistent features to facilitate and reinforce your learning.

- Each chapter begins with **Learning Outcomes** to help you focus your learning.
- A **Nursing Care** section demonstrates the nursing process format and includes references to the role of the LPN/LVN in a variety of settings. Because time management and prioritizing tasks are such an important part of your day, this section begins with **Priorities in Nursing Care,** a summary of the areas in which you must focus in order to provide quality nursing care. Nursing interventions are followed by rationales, to reinforce your understanding of why selected nursing actions are performed.
- **Case Studies** and **Critical Thinking** exercises are designed to bring the concepts to life and to engage you in problem-solving in situations you might encounter at work.
- **Health Promotion Issues** explore current issues in healthcare and provide a step-by-step solution for managing them.
- **Pharmacology** tables occur within clinical chapters to reinforce some of the most common medications you will administer.
- **Key Terms** and **Key Points** are reviewed at the end of each chapter.
- **NCLEX-PN® Review Questions** help you practice your test-taking skills.
- **Appendices** contain invaluable reference material including growth and development charts, normal laboratory values, and answers to Critical Thinking and NCLEX-PN® Review Questions.

Acknowledgments

A project such as this could not be accomplished without the contributions of many people. Without LPN/LVN students, there would not be a need for this book. Our students have been our inspiration and our motivation. Their enthusiasm for learning stimulates and challenges us to provide a quality textbook. It is our hope that this text will enhance students' knowledge and understanding of the care of mother and child, and prepare them for success. We want to thank our students, past, present, and future, from whom we have learned so much.

Many nursing professionals gave invaluable time and expertise to this project. Our contributors provided knowledge and writing skill in selected chapters and features of the book. Reviewers used their skill as educators to help maintain quality. They gave us ongoing assistance in deciding what students need to know and how to express our ideas for optimal learning. Contributors and reviewers for *Maternal-Child Nursing Care* are shown in a listing that follows this preface.

Healthcare is a team effort. This textbook is no different. Many intelligent individuals contributed their expertise to this work. Kelly Trakalo, Senior Acquisitions Editor, took up this project midstream but quickly made it her own by meticulous review of materials, quality cross-checks, and active support to reach our goals and deadlines. Our Development Editor, Rachel Bedard, was our visionary, our sounding board, our cheerleader, and most importantly, our nurse. When we were energy depleted, she gave us encouragement to just keep writing. This textbook is what it is because of Rachel. Her knowledge and endless attention to detail have kept us on track. Through our weekly conversations she helped us remain focused and not let the day-to-day issues of life prevent us from accomplishing our goal. Other important people in the production of this book were Yagnesh Jani (production editor); Marilyn Meserve (managing editor); Patrick Walsh (managing production editor); Ilene Sanford and Pat Brown (manufacturing managers); Patrick Watson (art coordinator), Kristin Lynch (copy editor); editorial assistant Teresa Himpsl; photographer Molly Schlachter; Penny Walker (TechBooks project manager) and the TechBooks staff; Mary Siener, design; John Jordan, Amy Peltier, and Dorothy Cook in media; and Francisco Del Castillo and Michael Sirinides in marketing. Our thanks to all of you!

Finally, we want to thank our nursing colleagues, our friends, and our families for their support and encouragement. To all of you we are most grateful!

Nursing is an exciting, ever-changing profession. Advances in the medical management of clients have resulted in shorter length of stay in acute care hospitals and more clients being cared for in the home. Providing care in the home is a new challenge for many nurses and a new role for the LPN/LVN. To meet this challenge, the LPN/LVN must be more knowledgeable than ever before and be able to think critically in a variety of situations. With this text, we hope to prepare the LPN/LVN for these challenges.

About the Authors

Mary Ann Towle, RN, MEd, MSN

Mary Ann Towle "always wanted to be a nurse," but teaching science in high school also seemed appealing. After graduating from Idaho State University with a Baccalaureate Degree in Nursing, she moved to Boise, Idaho, where she accepted a position at St. Luke's Medical Center. Mary Ann felt confident with her entry-level knowledge but was unsure of herself when it came to performing nursing procedures. Several LPNs helped her gain the necessary skills and confidence. Within a few months, she was working in the Coronary Intensive Care Unit as the evening charge nurse.

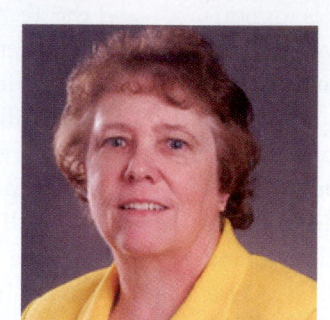

While Mary Ann enjoyed the direct client care of the CCU, she felt something was missing in her career. She taught a few in-service programs and workshops to nurses as well as to Respiratory Therapy students from Boise State University. After three years, an opportunity became available to teach in the LPN program at Boise State University. Mary Ann jumped at the chance to combine her love for nursing with her desire to teach.

All faculty in the Vocational-Technical Education programs were required to take education classes in order to improve their teaching performance. With a husband and two young children to care for and while teaching full time, Mary Ann attended classes two or three nights a week. In 1983, she completed a Master of Education degree with a specialty in Vocational Education. A proponent of lifelong learning, Mary Ann returned to school once her family was grown and completed a Master of Science degree in Nursing in 1998. Having taught the entire curriculum, Mary Ann sees herself as a generalist with experience in maternity, pediatrics, medical-surgical nursing, and geriatrics.

It has been 30 years since Mary Ann began her career as a nursing instructor at Boise State University. She has been recognized by the American Vocational association as vocational Teacher of the Year at the state and regional levels, and as first runner-up at the national level. Mary Ann's students have received state and national recognition by Vocational Industrial Clubs of America (VICA). Mary Ann is a strong advocate for the LPN. She works to advance their education and scope of practice within the health care community. Mary Ann feels that by reducing the stress involved in learning, providing positive feedback, and role modeling, she can help all students develop into quality nurses who can think critically and function in any situation.

Ellise D. Adams, CNM, MSN, CD (DONA), ICCE

Ellise D. Adams, is an instructor of nursing at the University of Alabama in Huntsville where she serves as Clinical Assistant Professor. She enjoys lecturing, counseling students, and watching them learn and grow in the clinical setting. Ellise has been affiliated with Prentice Hall Publishers since 2000. The publication of this textbook fulfills a primary career goal.

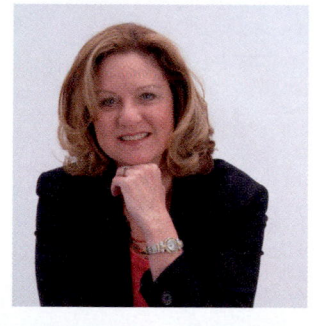

Ellise is a member of the Association of Women's Health, Obstetric, and Neonatal Nurses (AWHONN) and serves as Alabama's co-chair for programs. She is an invited presenter to the national conventions, consultant to special projects, research grant recipient, and contributor to publications. In 2000, she was awarded the AWHONN Johnson and Johnson Pediatric Institute Marshal Klaus Award along with her colleague Ann L. Bianchi for their research entitled "Intrapartum Nurses as Doulas: Increasing Training in Supportive Behaviors to Aid in the Reduction of Cesarean Rates, Length of Labor, and Anesthesia and Analgesia Use."

Ellise obtained her Bachelor of Science in Nursing from the University of Alabama in Huntsville. Because her first son was born during her tenure in nursing school, she is especially sensitive to the concerns of students who attempt to balance school, children, and a marriage. She received her Master of Science in Nursing from Case Western Reserve University in Cleveland, Ohio, and her Certificate of Nurse-Midwifery from Frontier School of Midwifery and Family Nursing in Hyden, Kentucky. She feels especially privileged to have had the opportunity to learn nurse-midwifery in the hills of Kentucky where Mary Breckenridge left an amazing legacy.

Ellise views nursing as one of the noblest of professions. Someone once asked her why she did not just become a doctor. Her response was, "Because I want to be a nurse. I want to spend time with patients in their hour of need. I want to provide nursing care, not make medical decisions." Nursing also provides diversity. There are so many opportunities in nursing that the nurse can always find professional fulfillment.

Ellise has been married to her husband Tom for 26 years. They have two sons, David and Jonathan. She is proud that her daughter-in-law Karla is studying nursing. Ellise enjoys volunteering in a variety of capacities at her church, including serving as a short-term missionary to Mexico City, Mexico; Vienna, Austria; and Cuzco, Peru. She also enjoys leisure travel, especially tailgating on the campus of her favorite SEC team, the University of Alabama.

Contributor Team

Chapter Contributors

Ann L. Bianchi, RN, MSN, ICCE, ICD
Faculty
Calhoun Community College
Huntsville, AL

Jeanne Hately, RN, MSN, PhD
President, Professional Nurse Consultants, LLC
Aurora, CO

Supplement Contributors

Student CD-ROM

Ann Bianchi (info as above)

Companion Website (www.prenhall.com/towle)

Ann Bianchi (info as above)

Virginia Lester, RN, MSN
Assistant Professor
Angelo State University
San Angelo, TX

Student Study Guide

Janice Ankenmann-Hill, RN, MSN, CCRN, FNP
Faculty
Napa Valley College
Napa, CA

Kim Cooper, RN, MSN
Instructor
Ivy Tech Community College
Terre Haute, IN

Jan Weust, RN, MSN
Instructor
Ivy Tech Community College
Terre Haute, IN

Julie Anne Will, RN, MSN
Instructor
Ivy Tech Community College
Terre Haute, IN

Instructor's Resource Manual and Instructor's Resource CD-ROM

Laura L. Brown, RN, MSN, CPN
Nursing Instructor
Asheville-Buncombe Technical Community College
Asheville, NC

Test Bank

Cheryl DeGraw, RN, MSN, CRNP
Faculty/Course Coordinator
Florence-Darlington Technical College
Florence, SC

Jane Headland, RNC, MSN
Nursing Instructor
Asheville-Buncombe Technical Community College
Asheville, NC

Reviewer Panel

Priscilla Anderson, RN, MSN
Assistant Professor of Nursing
New Hampshire Technical Institute
Concord, NH

Janice Ankenmann-Hill, RN, MSN, CCRN, FNP
Faculty
Napa Valley College
Napa, CA

Marjorie L. Archer, MS, RNC, WHCNP
Vocational Nursing Coordinator
North Central Texas College
Gainesville, TX

Margaret Batson, RN-cMSN
Nursing Instructor
San Joaquin Delta College
Stockton, CA

Nancy Bradley, RN, BSN
Instructor, Practical Nursing Program
Carl Sandburg College
Galesburg, IL

Laura L. Brown, RN, MSN, CPN
Nursing Instructor
Asheville Buncombe Technical Community College
Asheville, NC

Marti Burton, RN, BS
Instructor and Curriculum Designer/Developer
Canadian Valley Technology Center
El Reno, OK

Rebecca Cappo, RN, MSN
Coordinator
Lenape LPN Program
Ford City, PA

Traudel Cline, RN, MSN
Nursing Instructor
Milwaukee Area Technical College
Milwaukee, WI

Kathy Cochran, RN, MSN
Director of Practical Nursing
Coosa Valley Technical College
Rome, GA

Kim Cooper, RN, MSN
Instructor
Ivey Tech Community College
Terre Haute, IN

Mary Davis, RN, MSN
Nursing Faculty
Valdosta Technical College
Valdosta, GA

Patricia M. Demers, RN, MS/MPH, CNA, BC
Associate Professor
Northern Essex Community College
Lawrence, MA

Gail Finney, MSN, RN
Nursing Education Specialist
Concorde Career College, Inc.
Mission, KS

Shari Gholson, MSN, RN
Associate Professor
West Kentucky Community and Technical College
Paducah, KY

Julie Hansen, RN, BSN, MA
LPN Program Instructor
Southeast Technical Institute
Sioux Falls, SD

Jeanne Hately, RN, MSN, PhD
President, Professional Nurse Consultants, LLC
Aurora, CO

Michelle Helderman, RN, MSN
Nursing Instructor
Ivey Tech Community College
Terre Haute, IN

Susie Huyer, MSN, RN
Nursing Education Consultants
Chantilly, VA

Julie Kay, RN, BSN, MSN
Nursing Instructor
San Joaquin Delta College
Stockton, CA

Kimberly McDonnell, RN
NICU Nurse
Lancaster General Hospital
Respiratory Home Care Nurse
Lancaster, PA

Debra S. McKinney, MBA/HCM, MSN
Instructor
TESST College of Technology
Alexandria, VA

Jeffrey C. McManemy, PhD, APRN, BC
Professor of Nursing/Chairperson
St. Louis Community College
St. Louis, MO

Mary Pat Norrell, RNC, BSN, MS
Professor, Nursing Department
Ivy Tech Community College of Indiana
Seymour, IN

Deborah Andreas Ostdiek, RNC, BSN
PN Instructor
Western Nebraska Community College
Scottsbluff, NE

Colleen Quinn, RN, MS
Assistant Professor of Nursing
Broward Community College
Pembroke Pines, FL

Carolyn Reese, MSN, RN
Nursing Instructor
Blinn College, Bryan Campus
Bryan, TX

LuAnn Reicks, RNC, BS, MSN
Professor/PN Coordinator
Iowa Central Community College
Fort Dodge, IA

Betty Kehl Richardson, PhD, RN CS
Psych-MH, BC
Professor Emeritus
Austin Community College
Private Practice Marriage and Family Therapy
Austin, TX

Russlyn St. John, RN, MSN
Coordinator, Practical Nursing
St. Charles Community College
St. Peters, MO

Patricia Schrull, RN, MSN, MBA, MEd
Assistant Professor and Program Director
Lorain County Community College
Elyria, OH

Marcia Scherer, RN, BSN, PHN, LSN
Nursing Faculty
Hennepin Technical College
Eden Prairie, MN

Molly Showalter, BS, RN
Vocational Nursing Program Coordinator
North Central Texas College
Gainesville, TX

Sue Smith, RN, MSN, MEd
Assistant Professor
Iowa Western Community College
Harlan, IA

Carlotta South, RN
Licensed Vocational Nursing Instructor
San Jacinto College North
Houston, TX

Cindy Steury Lattz, MSN, APRN, BC
Professor of Nursing
Kankakee Community College
Kankakee, IL

Angie Sutherland, RN, BSN, CPN
Faculty
Spencerian College
Louisville, KY

Elaine Tobias, RN, BSN, IBCLC
Maternity Nurse, Lactation Specialist
Heart of Lancaster Hospital
Lancaster, PA

Laura Travis, RN, BSN
Health Careers Coordinator
Tennessee Technology Center at Dickson
Dickson, TN

Cheryl S. Weidman, RN, BSN
PN Administrator
Brown Mackie College
Findlay, OH

Julie Anne Will, RN, MSN
Instructor
Ivey Tech Community College
Terre Haute, IN

Janice Wimbish, RN, CCRN
Instructor, Practical Nursing Program
Forsyth Technical Community College
Winston-Salem, NC

Contents

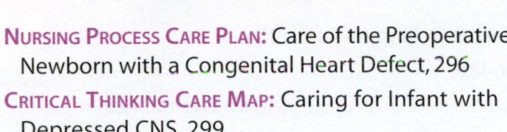

Introduction to Community-Based Nursing Practice

UNIT I

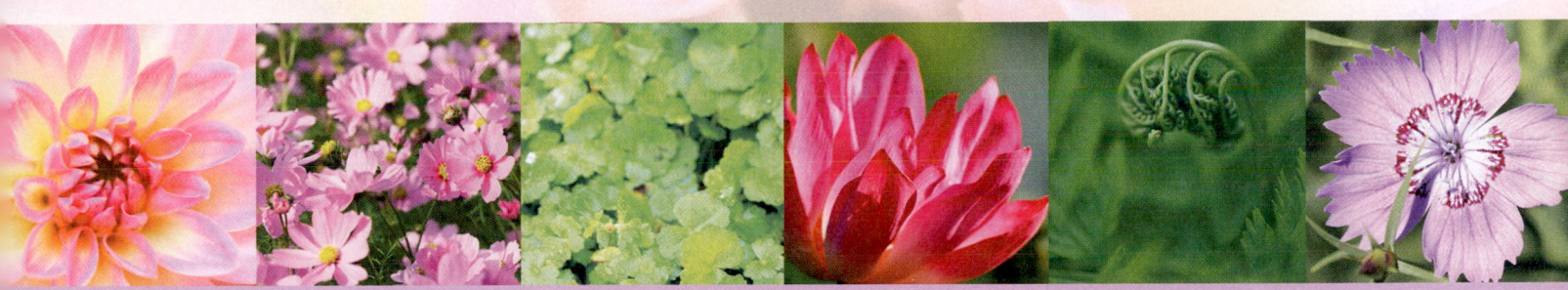

Chapter 1

The LPN/LVN in Maternal-Child, Community-Based Nursing

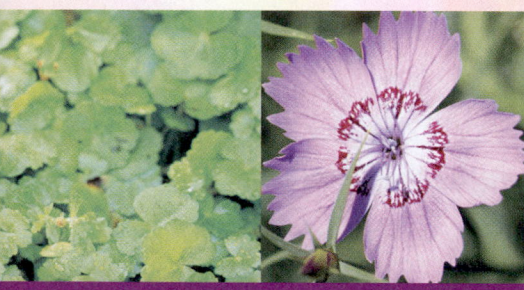

NURSING PROCESS CARE PLAN:
Caring for a Family That Desires Alternative Therapies

HEALTH PROMOTION ISSUE:
Male Circumcision Without Anesthesia

CRITICAL THINKING CARE MAP:
Caring for a Client with Hyperbilirubinemia

BRIEF Outline

History of Maternity Nursing

History of Pediatrics

Changes in Nursing

Review of the Nursing Process

Research-Based Nursing Practice

Community-Based Nursing Practice

Roles of the LPN/LVN

LEARNING Outcomes

After completing this chapter, you will be able to:

- Describe the historical changes in maternity care and pediatrics.
- Describe the steps of the nursing process.
- Describe the benefit of research for nursing practice.
- Describe community-based nursing practice.
- Describe LPN/LVN roles in maternal–child nursing.
- Describe decision making and prioritizing as they relate to nursing scope of practice.
- Describe the delegation process related to nursing scope of practice.

What is **maternal-child nursing**? Maternal-child nursing is the care of women through pregnancy, childbirth, and postpartum; it is also care of the child from birth through the teenage years. This simple answer arises from a long and complex history.

History of Maternity Nursing

Throughout history, women have learned about pregnancy from interactions with female family members in the home. In the early 1900s in the United States, more than 90% of births were in the home. These births were attended by female family or close friends, and sometimes by midwives without formal training.

From 1900 to the early 1940s, medical science made dramatic changes (Table 1-1 ■). The standard for childbirth shifted from care provided by untrained personnel to care provided by physicians. Hospitals were built, and health care increasingly moved from the home environment to the hospital setting. Improvements in anesthesia led to more common use of spinal blocks and inhaled medications that produced a "twilight sleep" for painless deliveries. This was seen as a tremendous advancement in the care of women in labor.

TABLE 1-1		
Interesting Names and Events in Maternal-Child Care		
DATE	**NAME AND/OR EVENT**	**IMPORTANCE TO OR EFFECT ON MATERNAL-CHILD CARE**
2nd Century AD	Soranus	Known as the father of obstetrics. Developed the Podalic version procedure in which the fetus is rotating to a breeched position (was important in delivering the second twin).
16th Century AD	Fallopius	Fallopius, an Italian anatomist, identified the tubes that carry eggs from the ovary to the uterus, hence, fallopian tubes.
1796	Edward Jenner	His experiments mark the beginning of immunology. He infected people with cowpox to make them immune to small pox. This procedure involves injecting harmless microbes to stimulate immunity to a more dangerous microbe. His contribution both enabled control of this dreaded disease and established the science of immunization.
1802	Pediatric hospitals	The first children's hospital was established in Paris, France. In 1855, the United States established its first children's hospital, known as The Children's Hospital of Philadelphia (still in existence today).
1807	Samuel Bard	Wrote the first American textbook for midwives.
1842	Oliver Wendell Holmes	Published a paper on the contagious nature of puerperal fever, which increased the survival rate of the mother and child during childbirth.
1853	New York City Children's Aid Society	This society was the first founded in the United States to care for homeless children.
1861	Ignaz Semmelweis	Pioneer in the use of antisepsis, he required medical students to wash their hands with chlorinated lime solution between examinations. He also proved puerperal fever is a form of septicemia. He theorized that the relationship between the incidences of puerperal fever was higher when examination of the new mother was done by doctors working on cadavers. This was not an accepted theory until 1890. He wrote *The Causes, Understanding and Prevention of Childbed Fever.*
1860s	Louis Pasteur	He confirmed that puerperal fever was caused by bacteria, the "germ theory of disease." Established that simple handwashing is an important means of preventing the spread of infection.
1867	Joseph Lister	He adopted the use of carbolic acid as an antiseptic agent in the prevention of infections. This form of sterilization introduced the era of antiseptic surgery and dramatically reduced mortality rate following surgery.

(continued)

TABLE 1-1

Interesting Names and Events in Maternal-Child Care (continued)

DATE	NAME AND/OR EVENT	IMPORTANCE TO OR EFFECT ON MATERNAL-CHILD CARE
1884	Karl Sigismund Franz Credé	Developed the method of placing drops of an antiseptic solution of silver nitrate in the eyes of the newborn to prevent blindness caused by gonorrhea.
1888	Arthur Jacobi	Recognized as the "Father of Pediatrics." He established pediatric units in several New York hospitals and was instrumental in the formation of the American Pediatric Society. He also initiated the boiling of milk to lower the incidence of diarrhea in children.
1896	Incubators	These were first developed in 1896 by a German physician. In 1903, the incubator was brought to the United States by Dr. Martin A. Couney, the "incubator doctor." He set up incubators at Coney Island as part of the carnival's exhibition. He also toured the country with his display, showing it at the World's Fair in 1933. He reportedly saved 6,500 of the 8,000 babies who used his incubators. However, it was not until the 1940s that incubators were used in hospitals.
1912	Children's Bureau	Creation of this bureau marked the beginning of modern child welfare programs and public recognition of children's special needs. Focused on infant and maternal mortality. Mandated birth registration in all states. It established the hot lunch school program in 1930.
1920	"Twilight sleep"	This form of anesthesia was a major influence in a woman's choice to deliver in a hospital. Morphine and scopolamine were used to ease the pain; it also gave physicians more control over the birthing process. This in turn led to an increase in hospital births.
1921	Sheppard Tower Act	Provides funds for state-managed programs for maternity care. It also provides federal grants-in-aid to states to promote better care for mothers and dependent children.
1930	White House Conference on Children and Youth White House Conference on Children and Youth Protection charter	Issues statements related to the needs of children in the areas of education health, welfare, and protection.
1930	American Academy of Pediatrics	Dr. Clifford Grulee, Dr. Isaac Abt, and Dr. William Lucas were key figures in the founding of the American Academy of *Pediatrics,* whose goals are to develop the scope and field of pediatrics, and to have a positive influence on the life and health of its clients.
1931	School of the Association for the Promotion and Standardization of Midwifery	Provided formal education for midwives.
1932–1970	Neonate stimulation or maternal deprivation	Joseph Brennamen was the first to recognize the relationship between an infant's poor health and the lack of stimulation the infant received in the maternity ward. Over the years, many physicians have studied mother–infant bonding and the effects of a long-term hospital stay on children. Today, hospitals have modified their policies of visitation to reflect these findings.
1939	Mary Breckinridge	Opened the Frontier School of Midwifery. After a family nursing curriculum was added to the school's program in 1970, the name was changed to the Frontier School of Midwifery and Family Nursing.

DATE	NAME AND/OR EVENT	IMPORTANCE TO OR EFFECT ON MATERNAL-CHILD CARE
1955	American College of Nurse-Midwifery (later renamed the American College of Nurse-Midwives)	Instituted to develop and support educational programs, sponsor research, develop professional relationships, and participate in the international organization of midwives.
1956	La Leche League (LLL)	Breastfeeding rates in the United States had dropped close to 20% when the first meeting of LLL was held. Their first publication was a loose-leaf edition of *The Womanly Art of Breastfeeding*.
1960	Lamaze childbirth method	The Lamaze organization, currently known as Lamaze International, Inc., promoted the philosophy that childbirth is a natural event for which women are equipped. They consider the ideal birthing experience to be awake, aware, supported by family and friends, and with no maternal–infant separation.
1962	Child Protection Laws	Laws that require the reporting of incidents of child abuse. All states are required to have such laws.
1974	Women, Infants, and Children (WIC)	Program provides supplemental food and education to lower-income children younger than the age of 5, and women who are pregnant, postpartum, or breastfeeding.
1975	Amniocentesis	Test that allows physicians to diagnose congenital or inherited diseases before childbirth. A new, less invasive procedure (called *chorionic villi sampling*) is now available for genetic screening.
1979	International Year of the Child	Focused attention to the critical needs of the world's children. Its stated mission was to consider how to provide food globally to children in need.
1980s	Artificial insemination	Initiated as a means of fertilization. Many couples now resort to various methods of *in vitro* fertilization ("test tube" babies) or transplantation of fertilized ova from one womb to another.
1992	Office of Alternative Medicine (OAM) within the National Department of Health	Agency developed to promote research and publicize information on complementary and alternative therapies. Emphasizes prevention, wellness, and a holistic approach to health care.
1996	Newborns' and Mothers' Health Protection Act	Provides for a postpartum stay of 48 hours following a vaginal birth and 96 hours for a cesarean birth.
2002	Best Pharmaceutical for Children Act (BPCA)	Established a drug program that identifies drugs and clinical studies that are needed for children.
2003	Human Genome Map	Completion of 99% of human genome map has led to enhanced diagnosis of genetic disorders. The use of gene transfer therapy in curing some genetic conditions is a promising and expanding field.

However, in the 1960s through the 1980s, data were gathered showing some negative effects of this type of anesthesia. Mothers under anesthesia were unable to push effectively, leading to the use of forceps to deliver the infant. Large doses of medication caused respiratory distress in the neonate. The number of caesarean deliveries in some hospitals increased dramatically. Eventually, questions were raised about whether births were occurring at the convenience of physicians or mothers.

The result of research was that women began taking charge of the birthing process again as much as possible. Prenatal classes formed to teach women about pregnancy, nutrition, and natural childbirth. In an attempt to have the safety of hospital deliveries in a "homelike" environment, birthing suites have been built to allow the woman to labor, deliver, and recover in the same room. The husband, and sometimes other family members, may be present at the birth. Epidural anesthesia has replaced spinal block anesthesia, allowing for a painless delivery with fewer adverse effects.

As hospitals became the main setting for childbirth, maternity nursing emerged as a specialty. The Nurses Association of the American College of Obstetricians and

Gynecologists, later renamed the Association of Women's Health, Obstetrics and Neonatal Nurses (AWHONN), was formed to improve the health of women and newborn infants. Together with the American Nurses Association (ANA), AWHONN works to improve the education of nurses engaged in obstetric-gynecologic care.

Today, many couples are postponing childbirth to pursue a career. As a result, they may come to parenting with greater risk of complications or fetal anomalies than they would have had if they had gotten pregnant in early adulthood. For example, the risk of having a child with Down syndrome is increased when parents are older than 40. Although they may be highly motivated to have a child, the changes and discomforts of pregnancy may place a greater strain on overall wellness than would have been the case a decade or two earlier in their lives. At the same time, changes in the health care system have resulted in shorter hospital stays than previous generations of women experienced. Instead of having a week of bed rest after delivery, women are now expected to return to the home 2 or 3 days after the birth.

Nurses in this type of environment must be knowledgeable about the physiology of pregnancy and about family dynamics. They must be alert to potential difficulties as the pregnancy progresses. They must be prepared to provide client teaching at every available opportunity. They must be able to recognize and work with a variety of family dynamics in order to promote the health of both mother and child.

Parents of today are involved in every aspect of the birthing process. They are less likely to be viewed as **patients** (with its suggestion of people who are ill, who need care, and who may have others make decisions for them). They are more often seen as **consumers** (purchasers of a service) and as **clients** (active participants in a process who obtain assistance from specialists). We use the word "clients" throughout this book.

History of Pediatrics

Pediatrics is the medical science related to the diagnosis and treatment of childhood illness. This medical specialty has been in existence only a short time in relation to all medical science. In the Middle Ages, health care focused on meeting the immediate needs of adults. "Infancy" lasted until age 7, when the child entered adulthood and was expected to work and assist with the family income. The average life span was 30 years. (In some areas of the world today, this is still the case.)

As infants survived longer, parents and society took more interest in the health of children (see Table 1-1). Through the work of child development specialists such as Erikson,

Piaget, and others (see Chapter 4 🔗), society has accepted childhood as a separate stage of development. Over the years, laws have been passed to protect children's rights, including the right to health care. For example, Aid to Families with Dependent Children was established by the Social Security Act of 1935 to provide money for needy children without fathers. In 1965, Medicaid was established to reduce the financial barriers to health care for the poor. (The Child Health Assessment Program is a major part of the Medicaid program.) In 1974, the Women, Infants, and Children (WIC) program was started to provide nutritious foods and education to low-income pregnant, postpartum, and lactating women and to infants and children up to age 5.

Changes in Nursing

Like maternal-child care, nursing care has changed dramatically. In Florence Nightingale's time, nursing involved providing for the sick person's activities of daily living. Nurses would do cooking, cleaning, stoking the coal stove, and trimming the wicks on the kerosene lamps. The nurse was an assistant to the doctor, helping only when requested.

Today, nursing is described as a knowledge-based process discipline where the licensed nurse's specialized education, professional judgment, and discretion are essential for quality nursing care (National Council of State Boards of Nursing [NCSBN], 1995). The ANA defines nursing practice as "the nursing diagnosis and treatment of human response to actual or potential health problems" (ANA, 1980, p. 9). The ANA (1991) further identifies four essential features of nursing practice.

- Attention to the full range of human experiences and responses to health and illness without restriction to a problem-focused orientation.
- Integration of **objective data** (data that can be observed and measured by the senses or by mechanical instruments) with **subjective data** (knowledge gained from an understanding of the client or group's subjective or personal experience).
- Application of scientific knowledge to the process of diagnosis and treatment.
- Provision of a caring relationship that facilitates health and healing.

Until the mid-twentieth century, nursing care followed the medical model, focusing on the treatment of illness. The nurse worked "for" and was dependent on the doctor's orders. It was quite common for nurses and hospital staff to refer to "the appendectomy in room 225" or "the C-section in room 20." Medical advances, such as the development of antibiotics and laparoscopic surgery, had a tremendous impact on the medical care of individuals, but they did little to change nursing practice.

Many areas of medicine have continued to become narrower and more specialized. Nursing, though, has become **holistic** (inclusive of the physical, psychological, and spiritual aspects of the person). Through the work of nursing theorists such as Jean Watson, Martha Rogers, and others, nursing has come to recognize that health and illness are more than simple physical states. Instead, they reflect the whole person, the person's level of development, mental status, physical health, coping ability, and more.

Furthermore, especially in maternal–child nursing, the client is no longer just an individual. Instead, "client" refers to the entire family. The nurse who takes vital signs from an infant is also actively involved in helping the parent promote the infant's health. This is done by observing parenting skills and by providing teaching to the parent to positively affect the child.

Review of the Nursing Process

The nurse must use a systematic approach (the nursing process) when planning and implementing nursing care. The practical or vocational nurse participates in every aspect of the nursing process. The depth of involvement depends on:

1. The particular state's nurse practice acts
2. The policies of the facility where the nurse works
3. The nurse's skills and experience.

ASSESSING

The nursing process is a continuous, unbroken process (Figure 1-1 ■). During assessment, the licensed practical nurse (LPN) or licensed vocational nurse (LVN) collects and analyzes data from the client and family. The LPN/LVN is not required to analyze and synthesize data as much as the registered nurse does. Still, it is the LPN/LVN at the bedside who monitors changes in the client, compares the data with given normal ranges, and decides whether findings should be reported.

DIAGNOSING AND PLANNING

In defining nursing as a distinct profession, it was important to identify actions the nurse performs independently of physicians or other members of the health care team. Names for client conditions that nurses are qualified and trained to treat independently (called **nursing diagnoses**) have been defined and developed by the North American Nursing Diagnosis Association (NANDA). When a NANDA label such as Pain is identified, an experienced nurse immediately knows the desired **outcome** (the client goal that relates to a specific nursing diagnosis). When Pain is identified as the nursing diagnosis, the desired outcome for the client would be reduction in pain to tolerable levels.

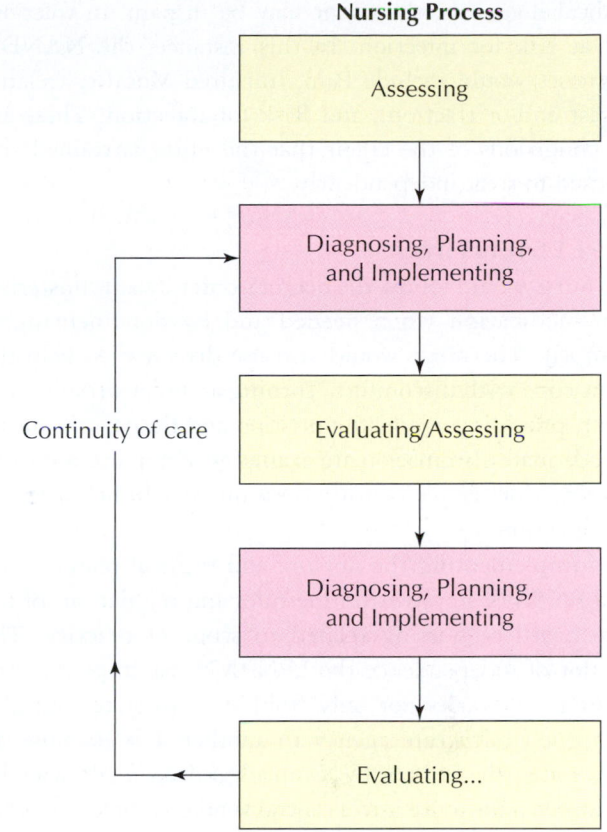

Nursing Process

- Assessing
- Diagnosing, Planning, and Implementing
- Evaluating/Assessing
- Diagnosing, Planning, and Implementing
- Evaluating...

Continuity of care

Figure 1-1. ■ Nursing process model.

The experienced nurse can also name several possible nursing actions to assist the client toward an improvement in health. These nursing actions (called **interventions**) include administration of prescribed analgesics, nonpharmacologic comfort measures such as a bath or a backrub, or distractions such as soft music or a favorite TV program.

In some states, the LPN/LVN assists the registered nurse in writing and updating the nursing diagnoses and nursing **care plan.** The care plan—an organized, prioritized plan—addresses the nursing diagnoses and helps the client reach measurable, identified outcomes (or *goals*). For example, for a client with pain measuring 9 on a scale of 1 to 10, a client outcome might be to reduce the client's sensation of pain to 5 or lower to allow rest.

Regardless of whether planning is a shared role with the registered nurse, the LPN/LVN must understand the difference between the nursing diagnoses and the medical diagnoses and follow both the nursing and the medical plan of care.

Nursing Versus Medical Diagnoses

Medical diagnoses are statements about a disease process or disorder. For example, a client may have a medical diagnosis of left compound tibial fracture. Because of this medical diagnosis, the client may be in pain, in traction, and at risk for infection. In this instance, the NANDA diagnoses would include Pain, Impaired Mobility (related to cast and/or traction), and Risk for Infection. These are the conditions of the client that the nurse is trained and licensed to treat independently.

IMPLEMENTING

The nurse would follow the doctor's order by administering pain medication when needed and by documenting it promptly. The nurse would also use diversion to help the client cope with discomfort. Turning and repositioning the client, providing adequate nutrition and fluids, and ensuring adequate elimination are examples of nursing orders in this situation. Implementing these orders will help prevent complications.

In implementing the nursing and medical plan of care, the LPN/LVN stays within the rules and regulations of the state board of nursing related to scope of practice. The amount of independence the LPN/LVN has in performing nursing care varies not only from state to state, but also from one health care agency to another. For example, in some states, the LPN or LVN can administer medication by the intravenous route into a central venous catheter. In other states, this route of medication administration is reserved for the registered nurse. In a large, acute-care hospital, the LPN/LVN may be expected to provide direct client care to a few or many clients, depending on the institution. In a long-term care facility, this same nurse might assume the responsibility of "charge nurse" for an entire care unit. (Ideally, in the charge nurse role, the LPN/LVN would supervise the care, instead of providing the care.)

EVALUATING

Once nursing actions have been carried out, the responsibility of the nurse is to evaluate those actions and determine whether they are moving the client toward identified goals. Data collected from ongoing assessments are compared with expected outcomes and with decisions made regarding care. In the case mentioned above, the nurse would return to evaluate (and document) how well the medication has worked. If the client says the pain is reduced to 4 and he feels sleepy, the goal has been met. If the client is moaning and still reports pain at 9, the goal has not been met. The LPN/LVN would report this to the RN team leader or charge nurse. This report could lead to a change in medication (medical solution) or to a change in the nursing care plan (increased use of nonpharmacologic methods to help reduce pain).

LPNs and LVNs will work with a variety of care plans and care pathways, depending on the facility. This text illustrates Nursing Process Care Plans in each chapter to provide realistic examples of situations in which LPNs and LVNs must make decisions. Questions following the care plans will help students practice necessary thought processes that will be part of everyday nursing practice. The following is a sample.

NURSING PROCESS CARE PLAN
Caring for a Family That Desires Alternative Therapies

Two young parents bring their 8-week-old son to the pediatrician's office. The child is gaining weight appropriately. He is breastfed and has adequate output. The nurse discusses immunizations with the family. The mother and father express concern about the safety of immunizations. They have done some reading on the Internet that led them to believe that a child could be healthy without immunizations. There are no other children in the home. The mother reports allergies, and the father smokes regularly in the home.

Assessment
- Believe child could be healthy without immunizations
- Stated resource is the Internet
- Unaware of the need for immunizations, especially in a high-risk environment (family history of allergies and smoking in the home)

Nursing Diagnosis. The following important nursing diagnosis (among others) is established for this client:
- Deficient Knowledge related to misinterpretation of information

Expected Outcomes
- Parents will demonstrate adequate knowledge about immunizations prior to giving informed consent.

Planning and Implementation
- Assess the parents' ability to learn. *If the parents had learning disabilities, it would be important for the nurse to know prior to developing a teaching plan.*
- Clarify the knowledge the parents have about immunizations. *The nurse needs to understand what information should be confirmed and what should be corrected.*
- Collaborate with the registered nurse and the physician prior to developing a teaching plan for these clients. *This situation will be best handled with a team approach.*
- Design an environment conducive to learning to present the teaching plan. *To maximize learning, the family should be comfortable and the area should be free of distractions.*

■ Present information about the effects of the diseases for which immunizations are available. *It is important for the parents to understand the symptoms, treatments, and long-term effects of the diseases.*

■ Present information about methods of immunizations and the side effects related to each. Include rates of occurrence. *Clear, concise, accurate information about the immunizations will give the parents an understanding of immunizations.*

■ Encourage feedback and document understanding. *The nurse can assess learning better when the parents provide verbal feedback.*

■ Provide the parents with printed literature. *This provides a way to reinforce the teaching the nurse has given.*

Evaluation. Verbal and written information provided to family. Father expressed surprise that item on Internet might not be reliable. Internet address to Centers for Disease Control and Prevention (CDC) site offered, so parents could pursue reliable sources and statistics. Mother had wondered whether her allergies might affect her child. Both agreed to consider immunizing child at 6-month visit.

Critical Thinking in the Nursing Process

1. Describe the alternative thinking of those who do not want to immunize their children.
2. Review the history of the polio vaccine.
3. How might you show support to a family who chooses not to immunize their child?

Note: Discussion of Critical Thinking questions appears in Appendix I.

Research-Based Nursing Practice

Nurses are trained to ask questions and to observe. Observations that begin to form a pattern are often the basis for nursing research. Research gives direction to nursing practice. When research indicates a need for change in current practice, the prudent nurse changes the way care is provided. Over time, these changes can have a great impact on the quality of health.

MORTALITY

The health of mothers, infants, and children is of critical importance in assessing the current health status of a population and in predicting the health of the next generation. **Mortality** describes the number of deaths over a given period of time for a given population. For example, infant mortality rate is the number of deaths per 1,000 lives births during the first year of life. The disparity in mortality rates among different races, areas of the country, or parts of the world is significant in reflecting the general health of the population. The infant mortality rate of 5.7 for White infants and 13.5 for Black infants, as well as other data regarding the circumstances of the mother, serve to document the lower health status of Black families in the United States. This information can be used when seeking funding to provide prenatal care to Black women in poverty-stricken areas or when identifying target groups for prenatal teaching. Infant mortality rates for the United States are illustrated in Table 1-2 ■.

Maternal mortality in the United States has declined from 363.9 in 100,000 live births in 1940, to 7 or 8 in 100,000 live births in 2003, according to the CDC (Reuters, 2003). The incidence stands at 7 to 8 deaths per 100,000

TABLE 1-2							
Infant, Neonatal, and Postneonatal Deaths and Mortality Rates by Origin of Mother: United States, 2003							
HISPANIC ORIGIN AND RACE OF MOTHER		NUMBER OF DEATHS			MORTALITY RATE PER 1,000 LIVE BIRTHS		
	LIVE BIRTHS	INFANT	NEONATAL	POSTNEONATAL	INFANT	NEONATAL	POSTNEONATAL
All origins[1]	4,090,007	27,995	18,938	9,060	6.84	4.63	2.22
Total Hispanic	912,331	5,151	3,573	1,579	5.65	3.92	1.73
Nonhispanic White	2,321,921	13,228	8,797	4,431	5.70	3.79	1.91
Nonhispanic Black	576,047	7,836	5,335	2,501	13.60	9.26	4.34
Not stated	28,609	448	368	80	N/A	N/A	N/A

[1]Origin of mother not stated included in "All origins" but not distributed among origins.
N/A: Category not applicable.
Notes: Infant deaths are weighted so numbers may not exactly add to totals due to rounding. Neonatal is less than 28 days and postneonatal is 28 days to less than 1 year.
Source: National Vital Statistics Report, Vol. 54, No. 16, May 3, 2006.

TABLE 1-3

Maternal Mortality for Complications of Pregnancy, Childbirth, and the Puerperium, According to Race and Age: United States, Selected Years 1950–1999

RACE, HISPANIC ORIGIN, AND AGE	1950[1]	1960[1]	1970	1980	1990	1995	1996	1997	1998	1999[2]
NUMBER OF DEATHS										
All persons	2,960	1,579	803	334	343	277	294	327	281	391
White	1,873	936	445	193	177	129	159	179	158	214
Black	1,041	624	342	127	153	133	121	125	104	154
American Indian or Alaska Native	N/A	N/A	N/A	3	4	1	6	2	2	5
Asian or Pacific Islander	N/A	N/A	N/A	11	9	14	8	21	17	18
Hispanic[3]	N/A	N/A	N/A	N/A	47	43	39	57	42	67
White, non-Hispanic[3]	N/A	N/A	N/A	N/A	125	84	114	121	116	149
DEATHS PER 100,000 LIVE BIRTHS										
All ages, age adjusted	73.7	32.1	21.5	9.4	7.6	6.3	6.4	7.6	6.1	8.3
All ages, crude	83.3	37.1	21.5	9.2	8.2	7.1	7.6	8.4	7.1	9.9
Younger than 20 years	70.7	22.7	18.9	7.6	7.5	3.9	N/A	5.7	N/A	6.6
20–24 years	47.6	20.7	13.0	5.8	6.1	5.7	5.0	6.6	5.0	6.2
25–29 years	63.5	29.8	17.0	7.7	6.0	6.0	6.6	7.9	6.7	8.2
30–34 years	107.7	50.3	31.6	13.6	9.5	7.3	7.6	8.3	7.5	10.1
35 years and older[4]	222.0	104.3	81.9	36.3	20.7	15.9	19.0	16.1	14.5	23.0

N/A: Data not available.
*Based on fewer than 20 deaths.
[1] Includes deaths of persons who were not residents of the 50 states and the District of Columbia.
[2] Starting with 1999 data, changes have been made in the classification and coding of maternal deaths under ICD-10. The large increase in the number of maternal deaths between 1998 and 1999 is due to changes associated with ICD-10.
[3] Excludes data from states lacking an Hispanic origin item on their death and birth certificates.
[4] Rates computed by relating deaths of women 35 years and older to live births to women 35 to 49 years.
Source: Data are based on National Center for Health Statistics. Health, *United States 1950–1999.* (2002). Hyattsville, MD: Author.

live births, a 98% decline from 1940 (Table 1-3 ■). It is estimated that perhaps half these deaths would be preventable with improved prenatal care. Some factors that may interfere with reduction in the maternal death rate are access to and use of health care services, differences in pregnancy-related morbidity, and the content and quality of care.

SUDDEN INFANT DEATH SYNDROME

The leading causes of infant mortality are congenital anomalies, sudden infant death syndrome (SIDS), and low birth weight. Research into causes and prevention of these problems impacts the nursing care provided to infants, parents, families, and communities. For example, until the mid-1990s, parents were taught to position infants on their abdomens to sleep. It was believed that if an infant vomited during sleep, this position would enable the infant to clear the airway and prevent aspiration. Through research led by the American Academy of Pediatrics, it was determined that infants positioned on the side or back during sleep had fewer incidents of SIDS. This information has changed not only the nursing care of infants, but also the teaching that nurses provide to parents (see Chapter 18 ⬭).

MORBIDITY

Morbidity is the prevalence of a specific disease or disorder in the population at a specific period of time. Data are collected from physician office visits, hospital admissions, and interviews. The data may not reflect the general population, but they do reflect those who are accessing health care in a given area. It is important, therefore, to look at trends rather than one-time numbers.

Childhood morbidity rate varies according to the age of the child. By studying the common causes of childhood illness or injury, plans for prevention can be made. For example, at one time polio was a leading cause of illness, disability, and death. However, through immunization against polio, this illness is being eradicated.

Falls from playground equipment are a leading cause of injury in the preschool child. Knowing this, nurses can focus parent teaching toward prevention. They can try to influence the design and selection of playground equipment, and can assist community leaders in providing safe places for children to play.

The nurse must use every opportunity to improve health care. This is done through client and family teaching, conducting research to document quality of care (either via formal study or informal data collecting), and assisting in the revision of facility standards-of-practice policies. The Health Promotion Issue on pages 12 and 13 shows how observations and information gathered during the nursing process can lead to improvements in care of the mother or the child. This issue is presented here as an example of how data can be used to initiate change. Further information regarding circumcision is presented in Chapter 9 ⬭.

Community-Based Nursing Practice

Community-based nursing is a response to the changes in health care. The philosophy of community-based nursing is that care should be provided to individuals, families, and groups wherever they are, including where they live, work, play, pray, or attend school (Zotti et al., 1996).

In recent years, there has been a tremendous debate over health care reform. Policy makers have pressed for a cost-effective health care system. This cost consciousness has resulted in decreases in the average length of stay for inpatient care. Along with clients being discharged "sicker," there has been greater emphasis on the impact of lifestyle choices on individual health and illness prevention.

Community-based care is vital to bringing health promotion initiatives to underserved populations. The "Issues and Trends" portion of *Healthy People 2010* indicates that effective community-based programs would have the following characteristics (U.S. Department of Health and Human Services [USDHHS], 2000):

- *Community participation* with representation from at least three of the following areas:
  - Government
  - Education
  - Business
  - Faith organizations
  - Health care
  - Media
  - Voluntary organizations
  - The public.
- *Community assessment* of the community's health problems, resources, perceptions, and priorities for action. (The community decides together what problem areas should be addressed. It is not told what its problems are by an outside agency.)
- *Measurable objectives* addressing at least one of the following:
  - Health outcomes
  - Risk factors
  - Public awareness
  - Services and protection.
- *Monitoring and evaluation processes* to determine whether goals have been reached.
- *Interventions that target several areas for change* and that are culturally relevant. Interventions would address the community at several levels:
  - Individual (e.g., racial or ethnic, age, or socioeconomic group)
  - Organizational (e.g., schools, workplaces, faith communities)
  - Environmental (e.g., local policies and regulations).

AND

- Interventions would include multiple approaches to change:
  - Education
  - Community organization
  - Regulatory and environmental reform.

In an effort to implement these guidelines, neighborhood health care clinics have become common. Educational programs are being produced to teach children the effect of lifestyle choices on their health. Greater effort is being placed on providing care to those with limited financial resources. These advances have caused a necessary change in the way nursing care is provided.

In response to political debates, the American Nurses Association and the National League for Nurses composed *Nursing's Agenda for Health Care Reform* (also known as

(Text continues on p. 14.)

HEALTH PROMOTION ISSUE

MALE CIRCUMCISION WITHOUT ANESTHESIA

The staff in the newborn nursery has become increasingly concerned that their male clients are not given anesthesia during circumcision because they have observed painful reactions to the procedure. Parents are questioning more frequently why their children are not given anything for pain relief. Also, two of the nurses attended a national nursing convention where they learned that providing anesthesia during circumcision is common practice in many hospitals nationwide. At the monthly unit meeting, these nurses address their concerns to the unit manager.

DISCUSSION

The debate lingers: Is there pain associated with newborn circumcision? If so, how can we be sure? Pain can be assessed by looking at behavioral parameters and physiologic parameters. Several assessment tools have been developed to assist health care practitioners in assessing pain in the newborn. These include the Neonatal Infant Pain Scale (NIPS); the CRying, Increased vital signs, Expression, and Sleeplessness scale (CRIES); and Pain

Assessment in Neonates (PAIN). Each scale measures criteria associated with pain and awards a score indicating pain or lack of pain.

Behavioral parameters associated with pain in the newborn include furrowing of the brow, tightly closed eyes, a quivering chin, a high-pitched cry, increased motor movements, and withdrawal from painful stimulus. Physiologic symptoms indicating pain include tachycardia, tachypnea, hypertension, and sweating of the palms.

Pain Relief Options for Newborns

The American Academy of Pediatrics suggests that health care practitioners provide pain relief in the newborn during circumcision in the form of environmental, nonpharmacologic, or pharmacologic measures.

- Environmental measures would include decreasing the stimuli in the setting where the circumcision is performed. Music, increased room temperature, a soft surface, and dimmed lighting are environmental measures of pain relief.
- Nonpharmacologic measures include nonnutritive sucking on either a pacifier or the breast of the mother who has not begun to lactate. Nonnutritive sucking provides analgesia only during the period of sucking. Nutritive sucking in the form of breastfeeding has also been found to provide pain relief to the newborn. Nutritive sucking or ingestion of sucrose has been found to provide analgesia. Sucrose can be supplied to the infant via a specially designed pacifier, nasogas-

tric tube, or drops placed directly on the tongue.
- Pharmacologic measures for pain relief in the newborn include administration of acetaminophen preoperatively and postoperatively. Application of eutectic mixture of local anesthetic (EMLA) cream administered 60 minutes before the circumcision will give the newborn up to 3 hours of pain relief. Nerve blocks can also provide the newborn with pain relief during circumcision.

What Is Evidenced-Based Practice (EBP)?

EBP can be defined as use of current research to make decisions about client care. If a clinical procedure is not based on research, it is based on a commonly accepted tradition. Health care practitioners have the responsibility of providing the best care possible. This care must be based on scientific data. Evidenced-based care provides benefits to the nurse, physician, client, and administration.

Implementing Research into Practice

These eight steps have been suggested by Gennaro et al. (2001).

1. Review the current literature related to the clinical issue.
2. Resolve to move forward only when you have gathered enough data to provide a rationale for the proposed change in practice.
3. Present your findings creatively. Use graphs, charts, posters, etc.
4. Include in your presentation a detailed clinical practice guideline. Develop a timeline for implementation.

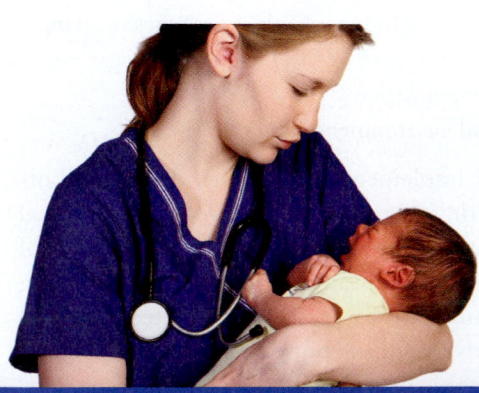

(Source: Jaimie Duplass/Shutterstock)

5. Present a plan for evaluating client outcomes as they relate to the change in practice. Include how and when data will be reported.

6. Invite to the presentation each practitioner and administrator who might be affected by this change in practice. Discussing the idea with the opposition as well as with supporters is crucial for the plan to succeed.

7. Realize that small measures may need to be implemented prior to a full-blown change in policy.

8. Publish positive client outcomes and successful changes in practice in order to inspire others.

PLANNING AND IMPLEMENTATION

During the unit meeting, the nursing supervisor selected staff members and formed a committee to research the issue of pain relief during circumcision. The committee consisted of the two staff members who had recently attended the convention (one LPN and one RN), one pediatrician, one obstetrician, the nursing supervisor, and a parent who volunteers regularly in the nursery. Following is an outline of the committee's work.

1. They performed a literature search using the databases Cumulative Index to Nursing and Allied Health Literature (CINAHL) and MedLine. Key words used in the search were *pain, analgesia, anesthesia, newborn,* and *circumcision.*

2. Each committee member was responsible for outlining several research articles. Once in summary form, each article was reviewed by each member of the committee.

3. The information was developed into a PowerPoint presentation depicting the risks and benefits of using pain relief for newborn circumcision.

4. The committee also contacted several hospitals who had policies for using analgesia and anesthesia for newborn circumcision. After reviewing these policies, the committee developed a proposed policy for their own institution based on the literature review.

5. The committee also developed a cost analysis and client outcome evaluation method for implementing this change in practice.

6. All nursing staff, pediatricians and family physicians, obstetricians, nursing administration, and hospital administration were invited to hear the presentation of the literature review and proposed policy change.

7. After the presentation, it was decided that nonpharmacologic pain relief methods would be implemented immediately. Pharmacologic pain relief methods would be reviewed carefully by each obstetrician. Obstetricians would meet with the committee in 6 months to discuss which pharmacologic method they would implement.

8. The committee planned to compare CRIES pain assessment scores in three situations:
   a. Prior to implementation of pain relief during circumcision
   b. Following implementation of non-pharmacologic pain relief methods
   c. Following implementation of pharmacologic pain relief methods.

They planned to publish the results of this research.

SELF-REFLECTION

Have you ever heard this rationale for a procedure: "because we've always done it that way?" What procedures or nursing interventions do you perform routinely without considering whether there is adequate research to support it? Could client safety be compromised because of your belief? Develop an action plan to review the literature as it relates to this procedure. Develop a plan, if necessary, for changing your unit's policy and procedure for this procedure.

SUGGESTED RESOURCES

Brady-Fryer, B., Wiebe, N., & Lander, J. (2004). Pain relief for neonatal circumcision. *The Cochrane Library, 4.*

Clifford, P. A., String, M., Christensen, H., & Mountain, D. (2004). Pain assessment and intervention for term newborns. *Journal of Midwifery and Women's Health, 49*(6), 514–519.

Gennaro, S., Hodnett, E., & Kearney, M. (2001). Making evidence-based practice a reality in your institution: Evaluating the evidence and using the evidence to change clinical practice. *The American Journal of Maternal/Child Nursing, 26*(5), 236–250.

Henry, P. R., Haubold, K., & Dobrzykowski, T. (2004). Pain in the healthy full-term neonate: Efficacy and safety of interventions. *Newborn Infant Nursing Review, 4*(2), 126–130.

Razmus, I., Dalton, M., & Wilson, D. (2004). Practice applications of research. Pain management for newborn circumcision. *Pediatric Nursing, 30*(5), 414–417.

Nursing's Agenda). Nursing's Agenda for reform is "to provide primary health care services to households, and individuals in convenient, familiar places" (ANA, 1991, p. 1). The "convenient, familiar places" are homes, schools, work sites, churches, and neighborhood clinics.

LEVELS OF CARE

Community-based nursing encompasses primary, secondary, and tertiary care.

- **Primary care** includes prevention activities such as immunizations, well-child checkups, routine physical examinations, and use of infant car seats. Its purpose is to maintain health and prevent illness or injury from occurring.
- **Secondary care** refers to relatively serious or complicated care. Historically, this care was provided in acute-care hospitals. However, with new techniques and procedures, much of it has moved to community settings, including outpatient centers and home care. The purpose of secondary care is to help the client return to health after an acute disorder or disease. An example of this level of care would be care of a client after an appendectomy.
- **Tertiary care** is the management of chronic, terminal, complicated, long-term health care problems such as osteoporosis or chronic obstructive pulmonary disease (COPD). This level of care is frequently delivered in hospitals and community settings, including rehabilitation centers and home care. Its purpose is to help the client return to or maintain the highest possible level of functioning, and to adapt as necessary to the changes the condition requires.

CULTURALLY PROFICIENT CARE

For over three decades, nurses have placed increased emphasis on understanding and responding to unique aspects of diverse groups of clients. At first, ethnicity was equated with culture and identified on the admission paperwork. Slowly, the term "cultural awareness" became used to describe knowledge of the similarities and differences among cultures. Unfortunately, many nurses focused on clients' differences instead of their similarities. The quality of nursing care did not change.

Since the 1990s, the nursing profession has been talking about **cultural competence,** or a set of skills, knowledge, and attitudes that includes:

- Awareness and acceptance of differences
- Awareness of one's own cultural values
- Understanding of the dynamics of difference
- Development of cultural knowledge
- Ability to adapt practice skills to fit the cultural context of the client or patient.

BOX 1-1	CULTURAL PULSE POINTS

Ways Institutions Can Respond to Cultural Diversity

- Hiring interpreters when there is a sizable non–English-speaking population in an area
- Posting "Se habla español" signs at hospitals and clinics where Spanish is spoken
- Providing teaching materials that are visual, not just written
- Offering options on hospital menus for special diets (kosher, vegetarian, etc.)
- Opening neighborhood clinics that cater directly to non–English-speaking populations
- Purchasing toys for children's hospitals that reflect a variety of racial and ethnic backgrounds

When these components become second nature to the nurse, **cultural proficiency** has been obtained (Leininger, McFarland, & McFarland, 2002).

The United States as a nation is becoming more supportive of its variety of cultures. Colleges and universities are requiring that educational programs provide courses addressing cultural differences. Health care institutions are adapting to provide a better environment for people from many different backgrounds. Being bilingual or multilingual is becoming a requirement for employment in some areas. Box 1-1 ■ illustrates some ways that health care institutions are working to provide culturally proficient care. Each chapter of this text contains further information about culture and culturally proficient nursing care.

Roles of the LPN/LVN

COLLABORATING WITH THE INTERDISCIPLINARY TEAM

For children and families to receive quality health care, nurses cannot practice in isolation. As health care moves from the acute-care setting into many places in the community, the members of the health care team must have a better understanding of how each role affects the quality of care provided. Collaboration and consultation with members of the health care team, in partnership with the child and family, are essential (Figure 1-2 ■). The health care team is composed of physicians, social workers, psychologists, respiratory care professionals, physical therapy professionals, dietitians, and pharmacists, as well as nurses with a variety of educational backgrounds. Auxiliary workers or unlicensed assistive personnel and family members may be trained to perform selected tasks. As a result,

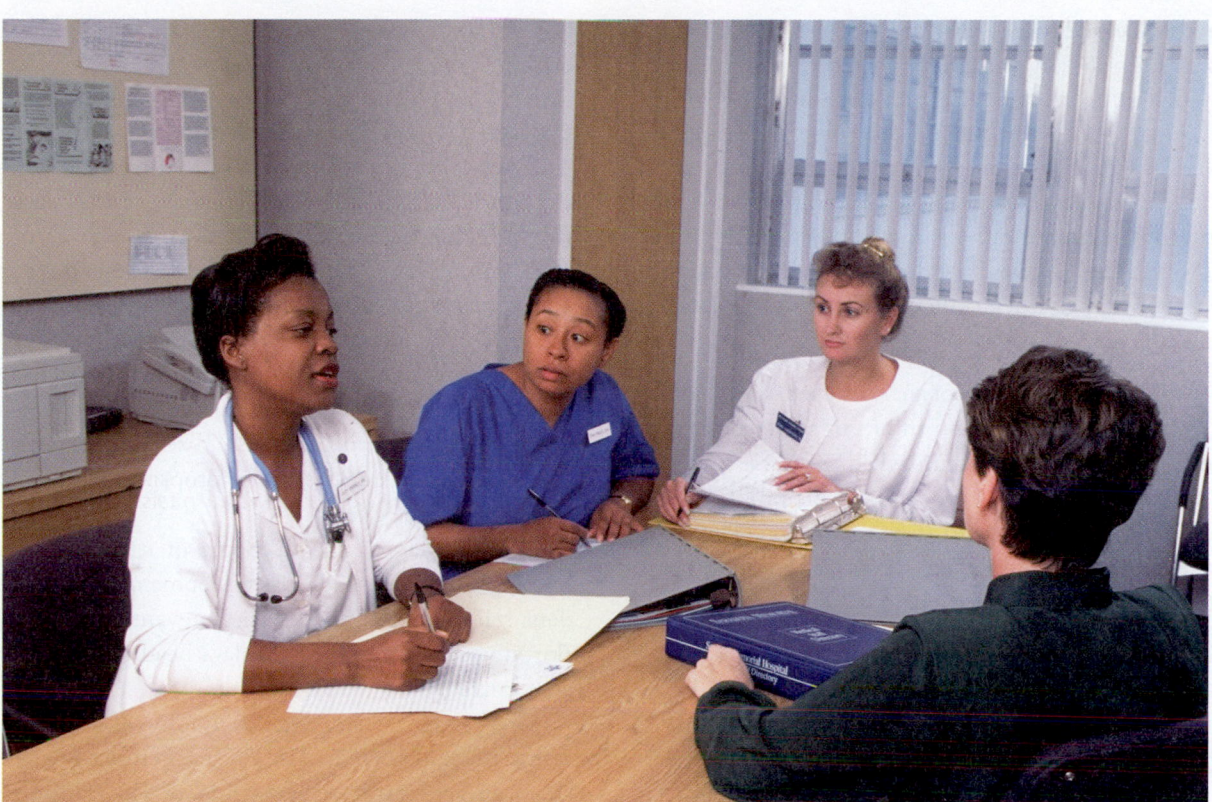

Figure 1-2. ■ Interdisciplinary team with LPN/LVN.
(Source: Michal Heron\Pearson Education/PH College)

nurses collaborate with a wide variety of individuals in delivering professional care.

To provide nursing care outside the acute-care setting, nurses used to need a bachelor's degree. Today, though, there are many opportunities for LPNs and LVNs in community-based nursing practice. With the move to community-based nursing practice, nursing roles are being redefined. The role of the LPN/LVN is no exception. Because the scope of practice for the LPN/LVN is more varied from state to state than that of the registered nurse, the role of this nurse in community-based nursing is varied as well. Collaborative efforts with other health team workers are always based on the state's nurse practice acts, facility policy, and the individual's capabilities.

UTILIZING THE NURSING PROCESS

In an acute-care setting, the LPN/LVN assists the registered nurse and physician to provide direct client care. In most cases, this involves assisting in all aspects of the nursing process.

In community-based nursing practice, the LPN/LVN performs the same functions as in the acute-care facility. In this case, though, the client and the client's family are the recipients of care. The LPN/LVN is responsible for keeping the registered nurse informed of changes in the client or family.

Communication and collaboration with other nurses and health care team members might be by telephone or electronic devices instead of face to face. For example, the LPN/LVN providing care to a child in the home may notice a wound has become red and inflamed and is draining purulent fluid. The child's temperature is elevated. The LPN/LVN would instruct the parents in the care of the wound and in the disposal of contaminated dressings. The nurse would then contact the nursing supervisor and provide input to revise the plan of care to include more frequent nursing assessments and dressing changes. The physician would be notified and appropriate medications obtained. The pharmacist might provide instructions about medication use and side effects.

PROBLEM SOLVING

Problem solving is a complex process that is at the heart of nursing. The LPN/LVN must collect data, evaluate the importance of the information to the safety of the client, and take appropriate action. The nurse uses a variety of cognitive skills in the problem-solving process and two different types of reasoning.

Inductive reasoning is the process of making generalized statements from a limited set of facts. For example, if a client has dry skin, poor skin turgor, and dry mucous membranes, the nurse can *induce* that the client is dehydrated.

Deductive reasoning is the opposite process: taking a generalized idea and figuring out what specifics to expect from it. For example, the nurse may hear in report that a client is being treated for dehydration after vomiting and having diarrhea for 2 days. From the generalized information that the client is dehydrated, the nurse can *deduce* that the client's mucous membranes will be dry, the urinary output will be low, and the urine will be dark amber. The nurse will look for these findings when collecting data on the client.

CRITICAL THINKING

Critical thinking is the process of analyzing one's own thinking and improving how a person thinks or solves problems. In nursing, critical thinking occurs when the nurse uses specialized nursing knowledge to identify client problems and to make decisions about what to do in a situation. The nurse considers a variety of related issues when making judgments in the decision-making process. The nurse considers:

- *The purpose of thinking.* The purpose might be to decide what data to collect, to determine the cause and effect of some action, or to identify possible solutions to a problem.
- *The bias or prejudice the nurse has about the client or situation.* Everyone learns some biases in the process of growing up. To think about situations clearly and professionally, nurses must recognize their underlying or "automatic" responses to different types of people. For example, a nurse might believe all people who are elderly are confused and unable to care for themselves, or that all people who are poor are dirty and uneducated. These biases can affect the judgments the nurse makes. A nurse who thinks all people who are elderly get confused may miss signs of urinary tract infection, which can also cause confusion in clients who are elderly.
- *Knowledge and past experiences.* If the nurse made a decision in a similar situation that had a positive effect, the nurse might make the same decision again. However, if the nurse's past decision had a negative effect, the nurse might consider other options and avoid making that choice.
- *Need for further information.* The nurse might need to collect more data from the client, confer with other staff members, or read articles on the subject in order to have current information about the client's condition.

Critical thinking takes practice. The nurse uses critical thinking to sort out facts from opinions, to evaluate the validity of information, and to obtain information from the client history or progress notes.

By discussing situations and answering questions in a nonclinical setting, the student can learn to process clinical information and make decisions in a safe environment. This practice allows the student to process thoughts more rapidly and accurately when a similar situation occurs in the clinical environment.

Critical Thinking Care Maps

This text provides an interactive tool for practicing critical thinking. At the end of each chapter of this book, critical thinking exercises are presented in the form of a Critical Thinking Care Map. The care map presents a clinical situation related to the content of the chapter. It identifies the NCLEX-PN® focus area related to the case study to help the student think in terms of the categories needed for licensure. An **NCLEX-PN® focus area** is 1 of 11 areas of Client Needs around which the NCLEX-PN® test is constructed. The care map then identifies one appropriate NANDA nursing diagnosis for the client.

A list of data is shown. Some of it is irrelevant to the nursing diagnosis that is given. Some of it is not. The student selects and organizes the relevant information under the subjective and objective data headings. Irrelevant data are omitted.

The student then decides if any of the information needs to be reported. Are any ranges outside normal? Is there an acceptable explanation for the data outside the normal range? For example, if a client is receiving an IV infusion to correct hypercalcemia, the nurse would see calcium balance outside normal range until the problem was corrected. It would not be necessary to report the calcium imbalance unless the condition was not improving with therapy, or unless it appeared that the client's calcium level was decreasing.

The student needs to decide who should get the report. For example, the nurse might report to the team leader or charge nurse if a postsurgical client complains that pain medications are not effective. However, if the client complains of pain 4 days after surgery and the client also has bright red bleeding from the wound site, the nurse would immediately inform the surgeon of the possibility of *wound dehiscence* (separation of the wound).

The next step in the care map is for the student to select relevant interventions. Again, the student would select *only* those interventions that relate to the nursing diagnosis identified for this exercise. Other interventions, even though they might be suitable for the client, would not be chosen from the list provided.

Finally, the student practices documenting the pertinent information. The date, the time, the pertinent data, the interventions performed, the results of the nursing actions, and the nurse's signature are all essential elements of narrative notes in the client chart. Sample documentations for the Critical Thinking Care Maps and answers to the questions posed in the exercise are provided in Appendix I . A sample Critical Thinking Care Map is provided on page 17.

This line provides an appropriate nursing diagnosis.

This line provides the appropriate NCLEX-PN® focus area.

This information is provided to give you basic information about the client.

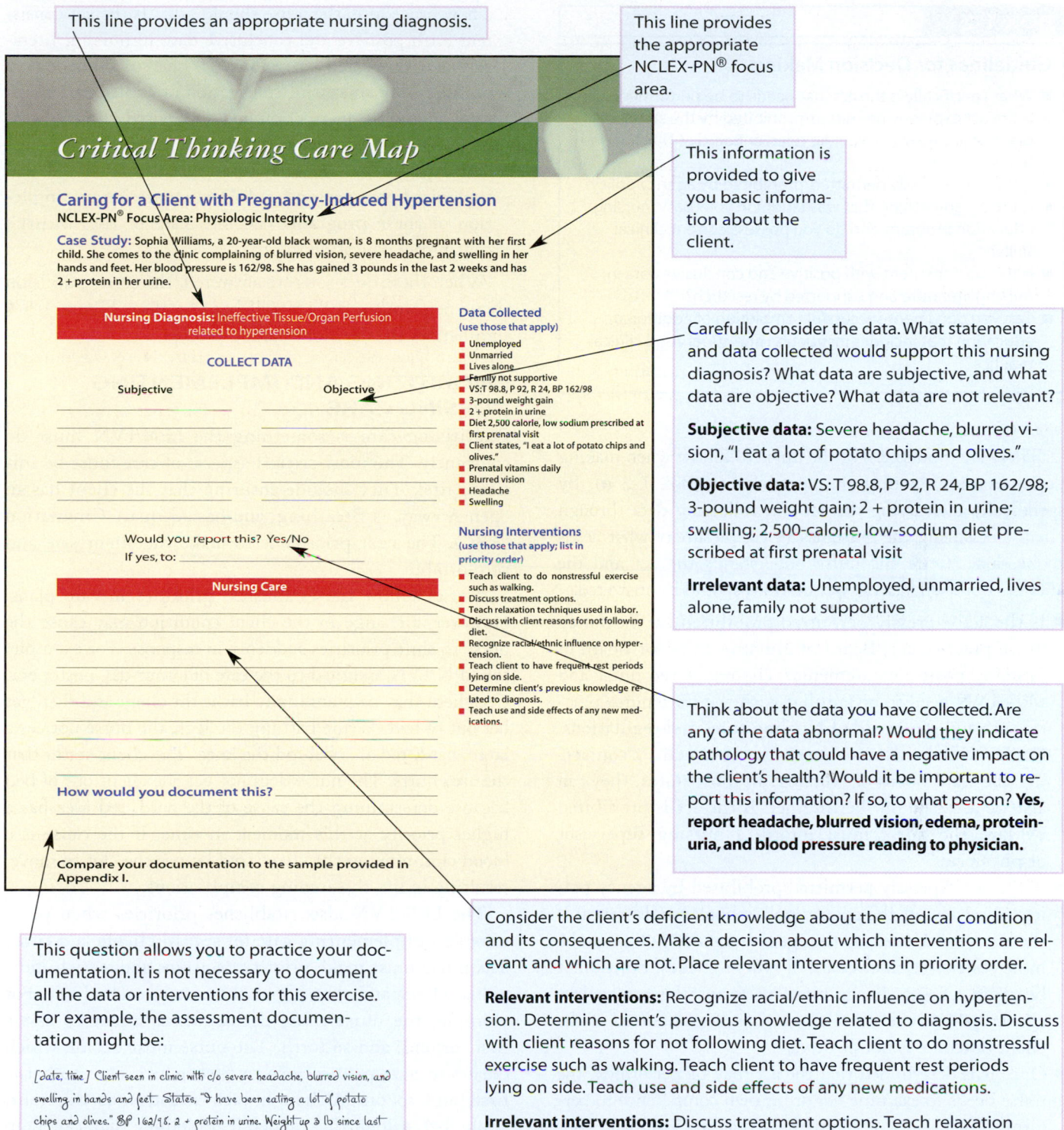

Critical Thinking Care Map

Caring for a Client with Pregnancy-Induced Hypertension
NCLEX-PN® Focus Area: Physiologic Integrity

Case Study: Sophia Williams, a 20-year-old black woman, is 8 months pregnant with her first child. She comes to the clinic complaining of blurred vision, severe headache, and swelling in her hands and feet. Her blood pressure is 162/98. She has gained 3 pounds in the last 2 weeks and has 2 + protein in her urine.

Nursing Diagnosis: Ineffective Tissue/Organ Perfusion related to hypertension

COLLECT DATA

Subjective   Objective

Would you report this? Yes/No
If yes, to: _____

Nursing Care

How would you document this?

Compare your documentation to the sample provided in Appendix I.

Data Collected
(use those that apply)
- Unemployed
- Unmarried
- Lives alone
- Family not supportive
- VS: T 98.8, P 92, R 24, BP 162/98
- 3-pound weight gain
- 2 + protein in urine
- Diet 2,500 calorie, low sodium prescribed at first prenatal visit
- Client states, "I eat a lot of potato chips and olives."
- Prenatal vitamins daily
- Blurred vision
- Headache
- Swelling

Nursing Interventions
(use those that apply; list in priority order)
- Teach client to do nonstressful exercise such as walking.
- Discuss treatment options.
- Teach relaxation techniques used in labor.
- Discuss with client reasons for not following diet.
- Recognize racial/ethnic influence on hypertension.
- Teach client to have frequent rest periods lying on side.
- Determine client's previous knowledge related to diagnosis.
- Teach use and side effects of any new medications.

Carefully consider the data. What statements and data collected would support this nursing diagnosis? What data are subjective, and what data are objective? What data are not relevant?

Subjective data: Severe headache, blurred vision, "I eat a lot of potato chips and olives."

Objective data: VS: T 98.8, P 92, R 24, BP 162/98; 3-pound weight gain; 2 + protein in urine; swelling; 2,500-calorie, low-sodium diet prescribed at first prenatal visit

Irrelevant data: Unemployed, unmarried, lives alone, family not supportive

Think about the data you have collected. Are any of the data abnormal? Would they indicate pathology that could have a negative impact on the client's health? Would it be important to report this information? If so, to what person? **Yes, report headache, blurred vision, edema, proteinuria, and blood pressure reading to physician.**

This question allows you to practice your documentation. It is not necessary to document all the data or interventions for this exercise. For example, the assessment documentation might be:

[date, time] Client seen in clinic with c/o severe headache, blurred vision, and swelling in hands and feet. States, "I have been eating a lot of potato chips and olives." BP 162/98. 2 + protein in urine. Weight up 3 lb since last visit. M. Fowler, LPN

Consider the client's deficient knowledge about the medical condition and its consequences. Make a decision about which interventions are relevant and which are not. Place relevant interventions in priority order.

Relevant interventions: Recognize racial/ethnic influence on hypertension. Determine client's previous knowledge related to diagnosis. Discuss with client reasons for not following diet. Teach client to do nonstressful exercise such as walking. Teach client to have frequent rest periods lying on side. Teach use and side effects of any new medications.

Irrelevant interventions: Discuss treatment options. Teach relaxation techniques used in labor.

DECISION MAKING

On a daily basis, nurses are faced with decisions about performing specific acts. Sometimes the nurse will be asked to perform a task outside the routine and must make a decision about whether to perform it. The new graduate or inexperienced nurse who is learning the routine might find decision making challenging. The nurse working in an environment as structured as an acute care or long-term care agency may not be faced with the same kind of decisions as the nurse working in other community agencies. In all cases, however, nurses are held to the standard of reasonable and prudent care (see more in Chapter 2 ⬭).

BOX 1-2

Guidelines for Decision Making

- What specifically is the act that needs to be performed?
- Is the act expressly permitted/prohibited by the state's nurse practice act, Board of Nursing rules, or Board of Nursing position statements?
- Is the act expressly permitted/prohibited by agency policy?
- Is the act something that was taught in your basic nursing education program, and do you possess current clinical skills?
- Is the act consistent with positive and conclusive data in nursing literature and supported by research?
- Can you document successful completion of additional education that includes instruction and supervised clinical practice?

There are guidelines for the nurse to follow when making decisions about performing specific acts (Box 1-2 ■). By specifically identifying the act and collecting data through client assessment, the nurse has a clear picture of what needs to be done. Once the nurse understands the act and the client's condition, a series of questions should be answered.

- Is the act expressly permitted/prohibited by the state's nurse practice act, Board of Nursing rules, or Board of Nursing position statements? The registered nurse and LPN/LVN need to be familiar with the state nurse practice act and the Board of Nursing rules and regulations. Copies of these documents can be obtained by contacting the state Board of Nursing. In most states, they can also be accessed on the Internet. If the act is prohibited by law, the nurse must inform a nursing supervisor or physician.

- Is the act expressly permitted/prohibited by agency policy? A review of the agency policy book would reveal if the act is sanctioned by the agency. Agency policy can be more restrictive than Board of Nursing rules, but cannot be more lenient. If the nurse performs the act against agency policy, the nurse might not be supported if the client outcome is not positive.

- Once it is determined that the act may be performed, the nurse needs to examine her or his own competence to perform the act. Is the act something that was taught in your basic nursing education program, and do you possess current clinical skills? Even if the act was taught in the basic nursing education program, it may be unwise to proceed unassisted or unsupervised if you have not performed the act for a long time. (Even experienced nurses need assistance when confronted with an unfamiliar act.)

- As advances are made in health care, new techniques will be found and new equipment produced. Before performing a new procedure, the nurse should ask: "Is the act consistent with positive and conclusive data in nursing literature and supported by research? Is there documentation on file of my successful completion of additional education, including instruction and supervised clinical practice?" (Most agencies provide in-service programs where new equipment and techniques are demonstrated and supervised practice is offered. Documentation of completion of these programs becomes part of the facility's continuing education file.)

When these questions are answered, the correct decision about performing the act will become clear. Figure 1-3 ■ summarizes the decision-making process.

PRIORITIZING AND IMPLEMENTING NURSING CARE

Prioritizing care is something the LPN/LVN must do constantly. The most critical aspects of care must be initiated first. They include ensuring that the client has an open Airway, is Breathing, and has adequate Circulation (ABC). The next priority is to make the client safe and comfortable.

Nurses follow the established priorities in care plans. However, a change in the client condition may cause the nurse to shift priorities suddenly in response. For example, the LPN/LVN assigned to the care of a first-day postoperative client may be planning to bathe the client and then get her out of bed. While bathing the legs, the nurse notices a large, hard, red area behind the knee. The client states that the area hurts. The nurse does not get the client out of bed because determining the cause of the hard, red area has a higher priority at this moment in time. If the cause is a blood clot, moving the client could cause the clot to move, resulting in life-threatening complications.

The LPN/LVN also establishes priorities when planning and implementing care for several clients at a time. The nurse must make priority decisions about each individual client and then about the care of each client. For example, the nurse must decide which client to assess first, second, and so forth. The nurse must decide which clients to give medications to first, which ones to bathe first, and so on. Although each situation is different, Table 1-4 ■ identifies general guidelines that can help with priority setting.

DELEGATING

Delegation is transferring to a competent individual the authority or right to perform selected nursing tasks in a selected situation. The nurse retains the accountability for the delegation. In today's health care environment, nurses have increasing responsibility to provide care to

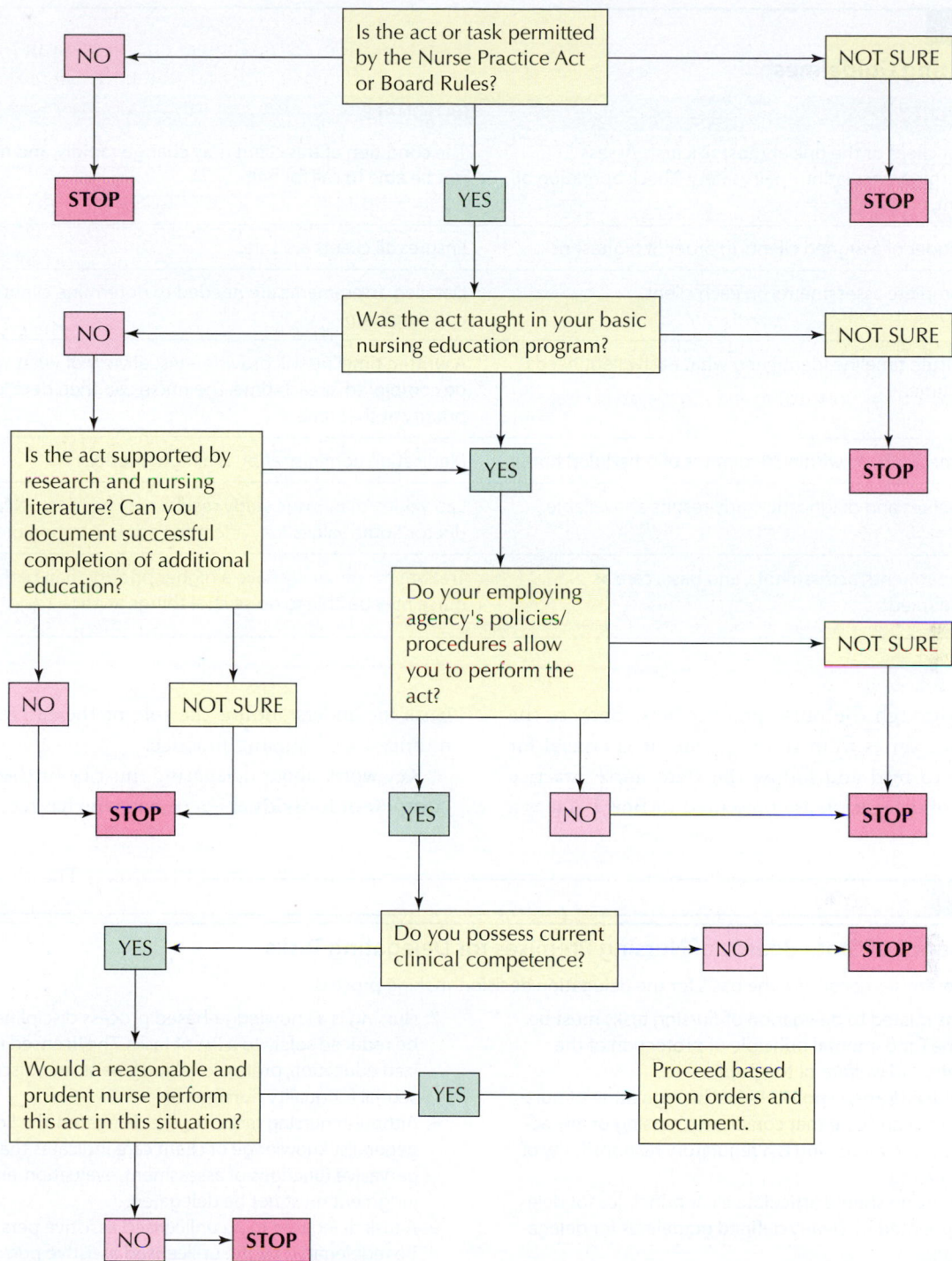

Figure 1-3. ■ Decision-making model.

the individual client, to support the family, to develop health promotion activities, and to work to improve the health of entire communities. As a result, there is increasing use of unlicensed assistive personnel (UAP) in direct client care activities. To maintain quality care, it is critical for the nurse to understand the delegation process. To help the nurse make wise decisions in delegating tasks,

the National Council of State Boards of Nursing published a list of premises or explanatory statements. These premises are listed in Box 1-3 ■.

"All decisions related to delegation of nursing tasks must be based on the fundamental principle of protection of health, safety, and welfare of the public" (NCSBN, 1995, p. 2). State Boards of Nursing have established standards

TABLE 1-4

Priority-Setting Guidelines

PRIORITY ACTIVITY	RATIONALE
1. Check sickest client or the one at most risk first. Assess ABC (airway/breathing/circulation), pain/safety. Check operation of all equipment.	The condition of this client may change rapidly, and he or she may not be able to call for help.
2. Check remainder of assigned clients in order of highest risk.	Ensures all clients are safe.
3. Return to complete assessments on each client.	Detailed assessments are needed to determine client problems and condition.
4. Update a written timeline identifying what each client needs and at what time.	A written timeline will provide a visual view of what will need to be completed at each time. The nurse can then decide what has priority at that time.
5. Administer medications within 30 minutes of scheduled time.	Medication administration is a high priority.
6. Review lab values and diagnostic study results as available.	Lab values/diagnostic study results may need to be called to the doctor. Some values may affect the administration of medication.
7. Provide all treatments, assessments, and basic care as ordered/scheduled.	Treatments generally have a higher priority than bathing, but the nurse may be able to do several things at once.

of delegation through the nurse practice acts. Because the scope of practice varies from state to state, it is crucial for the LPN/LVN to read and follow the state nurse practice act. Five rules of delegation are presented in Box 1-4 ■ as a basis for understanding the role of the LPN/LVN in community-based nursing practice.

Key words about delegating must be further described. A **competent individual** is a person who has received training,

BOX 1-3

National Council of State Boards of Nursing Premises for Delegating Tasks

The following premises constitute the basis for the delegation decision-making process.

1. All decisions related to delegation of nursing tasks must be based on the fundamental principle of protection of the health, safety, and welfare of the public.
2. Boards of Nursing are responsible for the regulation of nursing. Provision of any care that constitutes nursing or any activity represented as nursing is a regulatory responsibility of Boards of Nursing.
3. Boards of Nursing should articulate clear principles for delegation, augmented by clearly defined guidelines for delegation decisions.
4. A licensed nurse must have ultimate responsibility and accountability for the management and provision of nursing.
5. A licensed nurse must be actively involved in and be accountable for all managerial decisions, policy making, and practices related to the delegation of nursing care.
6. There is a need and a place for competent, appropriately supervised, unlicensed assistive personnel in the delivery of affordable, quality health care. However, it must be remembered that unlicensed assistive personnel are equipped to assist—not replace—the nurse.
7. Nursing is a knowledge-based process discipline and cannot be reduced solely to a list of tasks. The licensed nurse's specialized education, professional judgment, and discretion are essential for quality nursing care.
8. Although nursing tasks may be delegated, the licensed nurse's generalist knowledge of client care indicates that the practice-pervasive functions of assessment, evaluation, and nursing judgment must not be delegated.
9. A task delegated to an unlicensed assistive personnel cannot be redelegated by the unlicensed assistive person.
10. Consumers have a right to health care that meets legal standards of care. Thus, when a nursing task is delegated, the task must be performed in accord with established standards of practice, policies, and procedures.
11. The licensed nurse determines and is accountable for the appropriateness of delegated nursing tasks. Inappropriate delegation by the nurse and/or unauthorized performance of nursing tasks by unlicensed assistive personnel may lead to legal action against the licensed nurse and/or unlicensed assistive personnel.

Source: National Council of State Boards of Nursing, Inc. (1995). *Delegation: Concepts and decision-making process.* Chicago: Author.

> **BOX 1-4**
>
> ### Five Rules of Delegation
>
> - **RIGHT TASK:** One that is delegated for a specific client
> - **RIGHT CIRCUMSTANCES:** Appropriate client setting, available resources, and other relevant factors considered
> - **RIGHT PERSON:** *Right person* delegating the right task to the *right person* to be performed on the *right person*
> - **RIGHT DIRECTION/COMMUNICATION:** Clear, concise description of the task, including its objective, limits, and expectations
> - **RIGHT SUPERVISION:** Appropriate monitoring, evaluation, intervention as needed, and feedback

including instruction and clinical practice, to perform certain tasks and who can demonstrate safe performance. Before care is delegated to an unlicensed assistive person, the nurse must verify that the unlicensed person is competent to perform the task. Many health care agencies hire only unlicensed assistive personnel who have completed a certified nursing assistant course and are listed on the state registry. In this case, the nurse needs to observe the Certified Nursing Assistant perform the desired tasks in order to evaluate competence. If the unlicensed assistive person has not completed formal instruction, the nurse must provide instruction and clinical supervision prior to allowing the unlicensed person to provide care independently. In either case, periodic evaluation of the unlicensed person's competence is necessary to ensure the health and safety of the client.

The nursing task being delegated must be selected based on client assessment, the individual situation, and the skill of the individual unlicensed person. For example, an activity such as ambulating might be delegated if the client's condition is stable. If the client is unstable, has been in bed for some time, or has just had surgery, it would probably not be wise to delegate this task to an unlicensed person.

The National Council of State Boards of Nursing (1995, p. 3) states, "While nursing tasks may be delegated, the licensed nurse's generalist knowledge of client care indicates that the practice-pervasive functions of assessment, evaluation, and nursing judgment must not be delegated." If the purpose of the task is to assess the client's stability or progress, the task should not be delegated. If the client's strength needs to be evaluated to determine readiness for discharge or ability to provide self-care, the ambulation should not be delegated.

Once the nurse decides to delegate specific tasks to a competent unlicensed person, the nurse must give specific directions. Directions should include the following:

- What is to be done
- Expected outcome of the task
- Possible complications
- What the unlicensed person should do if complications occur.

In circumstances such as acute care, where the licensed nurse is readily available, these directions may be given verbally with frequent supervision by the licensed nurse. In circumstances such as home care, where the licensed nurse is not readily available but may be reached by telephone, both verbal and written directions should be given. For example, if the unlicensed person will be assisting the home-bound elderly client with administering ear drops, the licensed nurse should provide the unlicensed person with written directions on how to administer the ear drops, the name of the medication, the reason for the medication, the dose, the side effects, and the actions to take in case of emergency. The licensed nurse should visit the client with the unlicensed person and observe the unlicensed person administering the medication.

REDELEGATION

An unlicensed person who has accepted a delegated task may *not* redelegate the task to someone else. For example, if the licensed nurse delegates a blood sugar measurement by finger stick and the unlicensed assistive person cannot complete the task, the unlicensed assistive person should inform the licensed nurse. The unlicensed assistive person should not ask another UAP to do the task. Because it is the responsibility of the licensed nurse to determine the competence of the individual performing delegated tasks, the unlicensed assistive person is not qualified to delegate nursing care.

Licensed nurses are accountable for the outcome of the tasks they delegate. Therefore, it is essential for the licensed nurse to provide supervision for the unlicensed assistive personnel to whom the tasks have been delegated. **Supervision** means to give directions to workers and to inspect the tasks performed.

The licensed nurse must provide appropriate monitoring of the unlicensed assistive person's work to evaluate the performance and provide feedback as needed. If the unlicensed assistive person is not performing to acceptable standard of care, the licensed nurse needs to provide for review of instructions, further education, clinical practice, and re-evaluation. This process might involve other licensed nurses, such as agency nurse educators, or it might be the responsibility of the individual licensed nurse. In either case, documentation of the evaluation, education, clinical practice, and re-evaluation must become part of the UAP's employment file. Inappropriate delegation by the nurse or unauthorized performance of nursing tasks by the UAP may lead to legal action. Figure 1-4 ■ provides a flowchart for delegation.

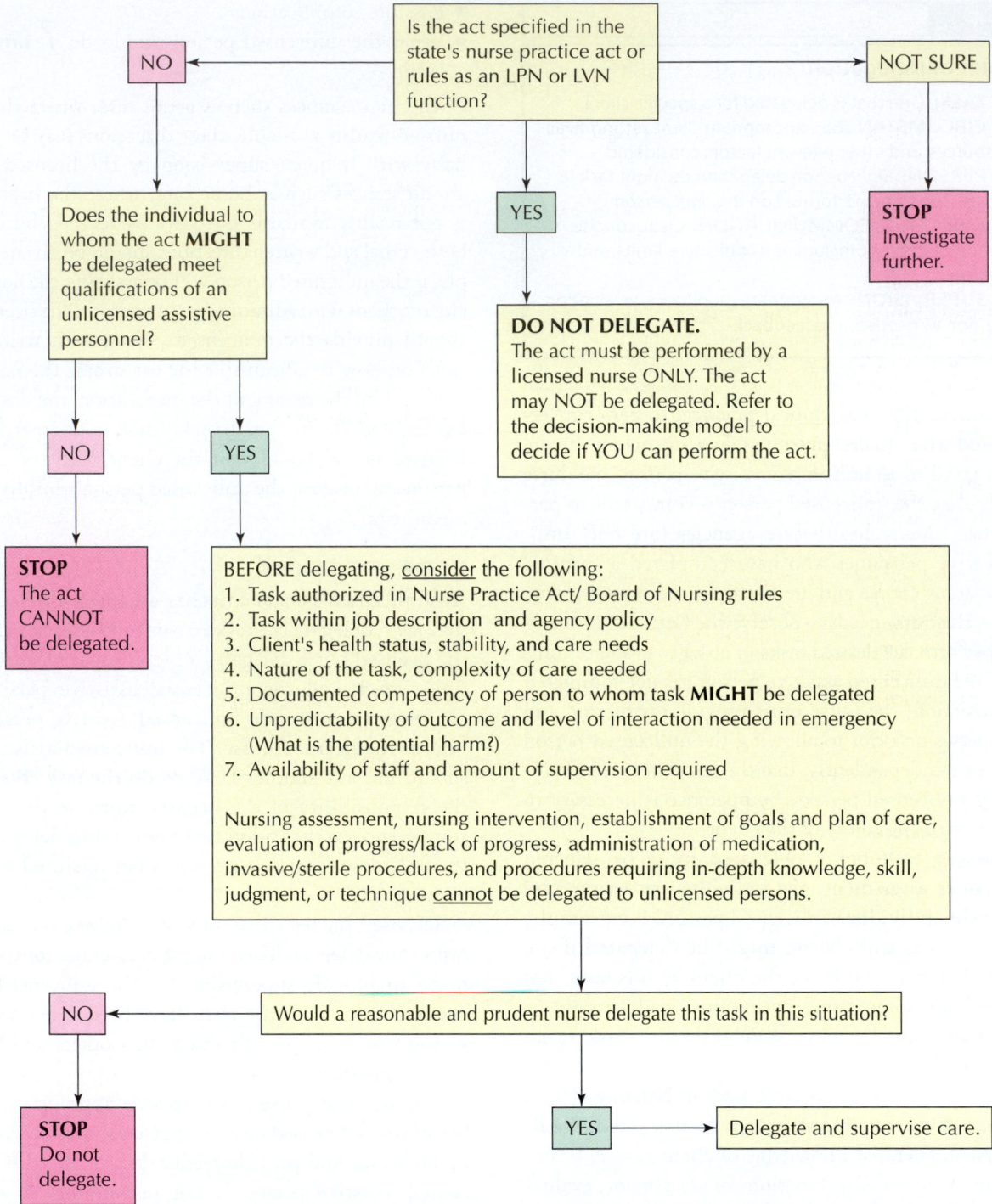

Figure 1-4. ■ Delegation model.

HEALTH PROMOTION TEACHING

A major role of practical and vocational nurses is client teaching. The U.S. Department of Health and Human Services (1991) developed a systematic approach to health with its set of goals called *Healthy People 2000*. In this publication, goals and objectives were identified to assist individuals, communities, and the nation to move toward improved health. Its update, *Healthy People 2010* (USDHHS, 2000), continues the effort to educate the public about ways they can positively affect their own health.

More and more people are recognizing the benefits of staying healthy. Health promotion activities emphasize nutrition, exercise, and stress reduction. Nurses often provide information about complementary or alternative therapies that can support a client's efforts to achieve or maintain health. Box 1-5 ■ lists some complementary

| **BOX 1-5** | **COMPLEMENTARY THERAPIES** |

Selected Complementary and Alternative Therapies

- **Homeopathy**   A healing system that uses a small amount of a substance to produce the same symptom as the disorder. It stimulates the body's system to increase its immune response.
- **Naturopathy**   Natural medicines are used in the prevention and treatment of a disease. Naturopathy often employs a variety of approaches to solve a problem (e.g., changes in diet, increased ingestion of some vitamins, changes in activity).
- **Traditional Chinese Medicine**   Trigger points in acupressure and acupuncture, and breathing exercises and body movements in T'ai chi or Qi Gong, are used to achieve a balance of energy and promote well-being and harmony throughout the body.
- **Reiki (ray-key)**   Japanese energy healing employs a light laying on of hands from head to throat, heart, abdomen, knees, and feet. It is often used with people who have cancer or chronic health problems.
- **Mind-Based Therapies**   Guided imagery, hypnosis, visualization, biofeedback, music therapy, meditation, prayer, and chanting all help in the reduction of stress and can be helpful in the relief of chronic pain and some addictions. These therapies can also be combined with exercise forms of therapies such as yoga that use meditation, exercise, and diaphragmatic breathing to induce a relaxation response.

- **Massage Therapy and Therapeutic Touch**   Touch in the form of massage and reflexology is used to relax muscles, improve blood flow, and stimulate the immune system.
- **Chiropractic**   Manipulation to correct misalignment of the vertebrae can reduce the stress of pregnancy on the lower back. Clients should be cautioned to use a fully qualified chiropractor.
- **Hydrotherapy**   Relaxation is achieved through the use of water. It is often used during labor and delivery in the form of a relaxing shower or to deliver the baby underwater. Cold compresses, hot compresses, and sweat baths are also types of hydrotherapy.
- **Herbal Therapies**   Plants have been used for medicinal purposes for thousands of years. Herbal therapies are often used to treat specific symptoms, such as to reduce menopausal symptoms. However, it is very important to teach the pregnant client that certain herbs can cause a miscarriage or have other toxic effects (see Box 6-4 🔗).
- **Aromatherapy**   Aromatherapy uses scented oils for relaxation and a psychological response. It is believed that different aromas can influence heart rate and blood pressure. They can also be used on the skin during massage therapy. *Note*: Because of little or no regulation of essential oils, pregnant women should be advised not to use them during pregnancy.

therapies that are commonly seen today. Related topics (such as immunizations, infection control, and identifying risk factors) are directed toward illness prevention. Nurses are instrumental in health promotion and illness prevention because they provide health teaching to individuals and groups. Teaching is an important role of the LPN or

LVN. Health promotion activities are presented throughout the text.

Note: The references and resources for this and all chapters have been compiled at the back of the book.

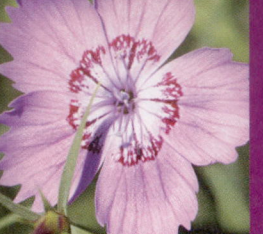

Chapter Review

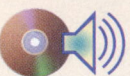 **KEY TERMS** by Topic

Use the audio glossary feature of either the CD-ROM or the Companion Website to hear the correct pronunciation of the following key terms.

Introduction
maternal-child nursing

History of Maternity Nursing
patients, consumers, clients

History of Pediatrics
pediatrics

Changes in Nursing
objective data, subjective data, holistic

Review of the Nursing Process
nursing diagnoses, outcome, interventions, care plan, medical diagnoses

Research-Based Nursing Practice
mortality, morbidity

Community-Based Nursing Practice
community-based nursing, primary care, secondary care, tertiary care, cultural competence, cultural proficiency

Roles of the LPN/LVN
inductive reasoning, deductive reasoning, critical thinking, NCLEX-PN® focus area, delegation, competent individual, supervision

KEY Points

- The nursing care of mothers and children as a specialty is evolving to include the entire family.

- The nursing process guides the care planning process.

- Community-based nursing practice is the provision of nursing care wherever the client lives, works, plays, or prays.

- Nursing includes health promotion and illness prevention activities, as well as assistance in the medical management of illness.

- The terms "client," "patient," and "consumer" all refer to the recipient of health care services. The term "client" indicates the person is actively involved in health care decisions.

- Being able to set priorities is essential in providing safe care.

- The state nurse practice act governs nursing practice. Facility policy regulates nursing practice within the specific clinical setting.

- Delegating care is within the LPN/LVN scope of practice. The nurse retains accountability for all tasks delegated to unlicensed personnel.

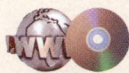 **EXPLORE Media**Link

NCLEX-PN® review and other interactive resources for this chapter can be found on the Companion Website at www.prenhall.com/towle.

For additional NCLEX-PN® questions, an audio glossary, animations and videos go to the accompanying CD-ROM in this book.

FOR FURTHER Study

Cultural issues and competency are addressed in each chapter in Cultural Care boxes.

Standards of care and other legal and ethical issues are discussed in Chapter 2.

For a full discussion on child development, see Chapter 4.

Circumcision is discussed in Chapter 9.

See discussion of SIDS in Chapter 18.

For discussion of hyperbilirubinemia, see Chapter 22.

Critical Thinking Care Map

Caring for a Client with Hyperbilirubinemia*

NCLEX-PN® Focus Area: Physiologic Integrity

Case Study: Andrew, a 4-day-old infant, was discharged from the hospital following a diagnosis of hyperbilirubinemia (physiologic jaundice). His pediatrician ordered that he spend time each day wrapped in a *biliblanket* (a fiber-optic phototherapy blanket designed to provide light therapy and to keep the baby warm). An LPN was assigned to make a home visit to reassess the infant. On the first home visit, the LPN found that the parents were accurately using the biliblanket. The baby's urine output was only four wet diapers a day. She also noted that his mucous membranes were dry and that he was lethargic. The mother stated that Andrew was rarely hungry and drank about 5 ounces of formula every 5 to 6 hours.

Nursing Diagnosis: Deficient Fluid Volume

COLLECT DATA

Subjective	Objective
____________________	____________________
____________________	____________________
____________________	____________________
____________________	____________________
____________________	____________________
____________________	____________________
____________________	____________________

Would you report this? Yes/No

If yes, to: ____________________

Nursing Care

____

____

____

____

____

____

____

How would you document this? ____________________

____

____

____

Compare your documentation to the sample provided in Appendix I.

Data Collected
(use those that apply)

- Decreased urine output (four diapers daily when typical should be six to eight)
- Dry mucous membranes
- Father states Andrew smiled yesterday
- Umbilical cord drying
- Lethargy
- Decreased oral intake
- Mother states infant rarely hungry
- Intake of 5 ounces every 5 to 6 hours

Nursing Interventions
(use those that apply; list in priority order)

- Contact the registered nurse to report findings.
- Encourage parents to also place infant in the sunlight several times a day.
- Teach parents the importance of adequate fluid intake during the use of the biliblanket.
- Teach parents the symptoms of dehydration.
- Obtain vital signs every 1 to 2 hours.
- Closely monitor vital signs.
- Obtain a daily electroencephalogram (EEG).
- Provide fluid replacement per order.
- Teach parents to obtain and record vital signs.

**This care map gives students the chance to apply critical thinking concepts and prior knowledge in a real situation. Hyperbilirubinemia is discussed in detail in Chapter 22.*

NCLEX-PN® Exam Preparation

TEST-TAKING TIP   Cover the answers and read the question. Try to answer the question without looking at the answers. Trust your first instinct, and do not try to rationalize why another given response might also be correct by reading into the question.

1 The nurse understands that primary nursing care is best identified as:
1. providing a pregnant woman who is at risk for gestational diabetes with nutritional counseling.
2. administering magnesium sulfate for treatment of preterm labor.
3. monitoring fetal heart rate during active labor.
4. management of a child recently diagnosed with cerebral palsy.

2 The nurse understands that tertiary nursing care is best identified as:
1. obtaining a sterile urinary specimen for the purpose of determining the effectiveness of antibiotic therapy.
2. immunizing a 3-year-old child for influenza.
3. monitoring hematocrit each trimester during pregnancy.
4. administering tracheotomy care to a 4-year-old with a permanent tracheostomy.

3 The LPN/LVN has many roles in the acute-care setting. Choose all of the following that apply to these roles:
1. administering PO medications
2. supervising unlicensed assistive personnel
3. collecting data
4. administering blood products intravenously
5. developing a nursing diagnosis based on assessment of data

4 The LPN has recently graduated from nursing school and has her first job in labor and delivery. She is alone in a client's room when the physician asks her to apply a fetal scalp electrode. Which decision below is appropriate for the LPN to make?
1. Apply the fetal scalp electrode as she had seen the RN do yesterday.
2. Read the policy and procedure for applying a fetal scalp electrode and then go ahead with the procedure.
3. Contact the RN and ask her to complete the physician's order.
4. Tell the physician that she does not know how to do that and that he should ask someone else.

5 The LPN is working in a long-term nursing care facility. She is responsible for the supervision of five unlicensed assistive personnel. She assigns one UAP to bathe a resident. Later in the morning, the resident is found on the floor of her room. Ultimate responsibility for the nursing care provided, and for the incident, rests with _____.

6 The LPN appropriately applies the Five Rules of Delegation. When she or he evaluates the care given by the unlicensed assistive personnel, which of the following rules is being applied?
1. right task
2. right circumstances
3. right person
4. right direction
5. right supervision

7 The LPN needs to delegate a finger-stick blood sugar (FSBS) on a client who is hospitalized for management of diabetes mellitus. Which of the following is an appropriate individual to perform this skill?
1. unlicensed assistive personnel in his first week on the job
2. the unit secretary who is also a diabetic
3. the client's husband
4. a certified nursing assistant with 5 years' experience

8 The LPN delegated the skill of blood glucose testing. The client's blood sugar is found to be elevated. Which of the following scenarios is appropriate nursing care?
1. Ask the client's husband to administer the insulin.
2. The UAP gives the insulin and then notifies the LPN.
3. The LPN notifies the RN and works collaboratively to administer the insulin.
4. The UAP notifies the physician about the client's blood sugar.

9 The LPN determines that the CNA instructed the client, who is to obtain a 24-hour urine specimen to begin @ 8:00 A.M., to include the first voided urine in the container. Which nursing action, in a supervisory role, is appropriate?
1. Praise the CNA.
2. Review the procedure with the CNA.
3. Recommend that the CNA be reassigned to another unit.
4. Recommend that the CNA receive a raise.

10 The LPN and RN are determining who should be included in the health care team of a client. Which of the following individuals are appropriate to include in the collaborative team? Choose all that apply.
1. physician
2. social worker
3. psychologist
4. respiratory care therapist
5. physical therapist
6. dietitian
7. pharmacist
8. beautician

Answers for Review Questions, as well as discussion of Care Plan and Critical Thinking Care Map questions, appear in Appendix I.

Chapter 2

Legal and Ethical Issues in Maternal-Child Nursing

BRIEF Outline

Federal Programs Affecting
Children

Legal and Ethical Issues Affecting
Children

Legal and Ethical Issues Affecting
the Mother

Role of the LPN/LVN
Nursing Care

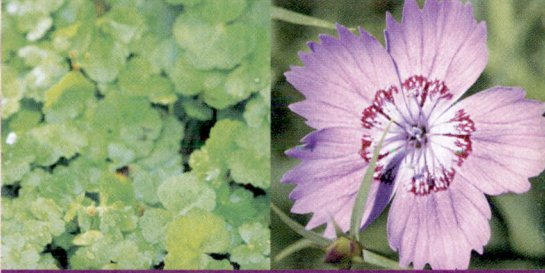

LEARNING Outcomes

After completing this chapter, you will be able to:

- Describe federal initiatives to protect children.
- Describe parents' rights as they relate to the care of children.
- Describe client rights as they relate to children.
- Name situations in which the nurse must legally report to public agencies.
- Describe the difference between legal and ethical issues.
- Describe common legal and ethical issues that can affect the mother, child, and family.
- Describe the LPN/LVN role in legal/ethical issues.

HEALTH PROMOTION ISSUE:
Sexually Transmitted Infection
Education

**NURSING PROCESS CARE
PLAN:** Client with Hodgkin's
Lymphoma

CRITICAL THINKING CARE MAP:
Caring for a Client Desiring
Pregnancy Termination

Maternal or pediatric care, like other areas of nursing, may sometimes present nurses with challenges to their worldview and their values. Nurses may disagree with laws or policies but still be required to uphold them. They may also disagree with a client's **ethics** (system of values and ideas that shape a sense of right and wrong). In fact, it is certain that every nurse will someday face a situation in which his or her personal standards of right and wrong are challenged. The challenge may come from a client, a supervisor, a facility regulation, or a state or federal law. Also, the nurse may encounter situations in which there is no "right" decision because all solutions involve some negative outcomes. At these times, the nurse will need to act professionally and without bias to support the client and family and help them make a decision.

Federal Programs Affecting Children

Since the early 1900s, groups called the White House Conference on Children and Youth have met at the federal level to discuss the health care of children. Following these meetings, recommendations and some federal laws have been passed to improve children's care. The U.S. government established programs like Medicaid's Early and Periodic Screening, Diagnosis, and Treatment (EPSDT); the Women, Infants, and Children (WIC) program; and the National School Lunch Program (NSLP) to assist low-income families (Table 2-1 ■).

TABLE 2-1	
Federal Programs Affecting Children	
ACRONYM OF FEDERAL PROGRAM	**FULL NAME OF FEDERAL PROGRAM**
EPSDT	Early and Periodic Screening, Diagnosis, and Treatment
NCLB	No Child Left Behind
NSLP	National School Lunch Program
SCHIP	State Children's Health Insurance Program
SFSBP	Summer Food Service Breakfast Program
SF/SC	Strong Families/Safe Children
TANF (Idaho)	Temporary Assistance for Needy Families
VFC	Vaccination Funding for Children
WIC	Women, Infants and Children

HEALTHY PEOPLE 2000 AND *HEALTHY PEOPLE 2010*

In 1990, the U.S. Department of Health and Human Services (USDHHS) released *Healthy People 2000: National Health Promotion and Disease Prevention Objectives.* This document presented an opportunity for Americans to take responsibility for their health. It recommended access to health care for all, particularly the most vulnerable. Figure 2-1 ■ illustrates factors from the more recent *Healthy People 2010* that determine an individual's health (U.S. Department of Health and Human Services [USDHHS], 2000).

Some of the objectives in the *Healthy People 2000* document that related to maternal health included the following:

- Reducing disparities in key maternal, infant, and child health indicators so all could have access to quality care
- Understanding issues related to preconception, prenatal, and obstetric care
- Preventing birth defects and developmental disabilities.

Some of the objectives in the *Healthy People 2000* document that related specifically to children included the following:

- Increased participation in school physical education programs
- Reduced use of drugs, alcohol, and tobacco by children
- Reduced teen pregnancy
- Reduced prevalence of dental cavities.

In 2000, the U.S. Department of Health and Human Services updated goals and objectives for health care for the next 10 years. *Healthy People 2010* contains 467 objectives divided into 28 focus areas. One of these is Maternal, Infant, and

Healthy People 2010 Leading Health Indicators

- Physical Activity
- Overweight and Obesity
- Tobacco Use
- Substance Abuse
- Responsible Sexual Behavior
- Mental Health
- Injury and Violence
- Environmental Quality
- Immunization
- Access to Health Care

Figure 2-1. ■ *Healthy People 2010* identifies objectives for each indicator (USDHHS, 2000).

Child Health. Important topics within the Maternal–Child focus area are:

- Reducing infant, child, and maternal mortality
- Increasing the proportion of women who receive early and adequate prenatal care
- Increasing the percentage of healthy full-term infants who are put down to sleep on their backs
- Reducing the occurrence of developmental disabilities
- Increasing abstinence from alcohol, cigarettes, and illicit drugs among pregnant women. (USDHHS, 2000)

Achieving Maternal–Child objectives involves both research and teaching. The government publishes weekly reports on various topic areas of *Healthy People 2010.* Current information about *Healthy People 2010* is available on the Internet.

Legal and Ethical Issues Affecting Children

Even when laws and programs ensure health care for children, legal and ethical issues will still exist. For example, a 16-year-old girl is pregnant and wants an abortion. Because she is a minor, does she need parental consent? If she delivers, can she make decisions about the health care of the infant? At what age can a minor make decisions to accept or refuse treatment? Although answers to these questions might differ from state to state, the nurse should understand the general guiding principles and obtain legal advice for complex family issues.

PARENTS' RIGHTS

In most situations, parents or legal guardians have the authority to make decisions for their minor children. There are a few exceptions.

- If the parent(s) is (are) incapacitated and cannot make a decision
- If there is actual or suspected child abuse or neglect
- If the parent's choice does not permit lifesaving procedures for the child

Even though the nurse may not agree with the parent's decision about treatment, nursing care must be provided in an unbiased manner. The LPN/LVN should report all concerns to the supervising RN. Legal counsel might be necessary to settle disputes.

Usually it is the parent or legal guardian who gives **informed consent** (written approval for a treatment or procedure, following explanation of pros and cons by the physician or other professional who is performing the procedure). Procedure 2-1 ■ reviews important steps and rationales for witnessing informed consent.

CHILD'S RIGHTS

There are some exceptions to parents giving informed consent. Some states have a **mature minor act** (an act that permits adolescents age 14 or 15 to make decisions about their treatment). In some cases, self-supporting adolescents are emancipated by court decision. Such minors, including minors who marry, are called **emancipated minors.** They are responsible for their own health care decisions and expenses.

The "Patient's Bill of Rights," a fundamental document of health care, is illustrated in Box 2-1 ■. These rights, with some modifications, apply to both the pediatric client and adults. For example, young children may not be able to understand the diagnosis and treatment of a disorder in order to provide an informed consent, yet they should still be included in the process. Explanations in age-appropriate language should be given, and every attempt should be made to acquire their cooperation. It is important to give children as much control as possible over what happens to them by including them in decisions about their welfare. (However, do not attempt to give them a choice when there is really no option.) It is reasonable to expect parents and older children to participate in health care in the following ways:

- By providing accurate and complete information about health issues
- By increasing their knowledge about diagnosis and treatment
- By being responsible for their own actions
- By reporting changes in client condition
- By keeping appointments
- By meeting financial obligations for health care.

It is the responsibility of the nurse to help the client and family understand how to participate in their care.

PRIVACY AND CONFIDENTIALITY

The child has as much right to privacy and confidentiality as an adult. On the physical level, privacy means screening from view: closing curtains and draping the client to prevent a third party from seeing the body or body parts. At the legal level, privacy also means keeping the client's chart screened from a third party. **Confidentiality** means keeping secret any privileged information.

For a young child, this right may not pose a problem. The nurse protects the infant's privacy by screening him or her from view during procedures and by keeping the medical record secure. The parent's confidentiality is also maintained.

In an older child or adolescent, maintaining confidentiality may cause some conflict for the nurse. For example, an adolescent may request treatment for a sexually transmitted disease, birth control, pregnancy, or drug and alcohol treatment without notifying the parents. If the nurse breeches confidentiality and informs the parents, the client may lose

(*Text continues on p. 32.*)

MediaLink Healthy People 2010

PROCEDURE 2-1   # Witnessing Informed Consent

Purpose

- To document informed consent (agreement by a client or client's parent/guardian to accept a course of treatment or procedure after complete information has been provided by the health care provider).

Equipment

- Copy of the agency informed consent form
- Black pen

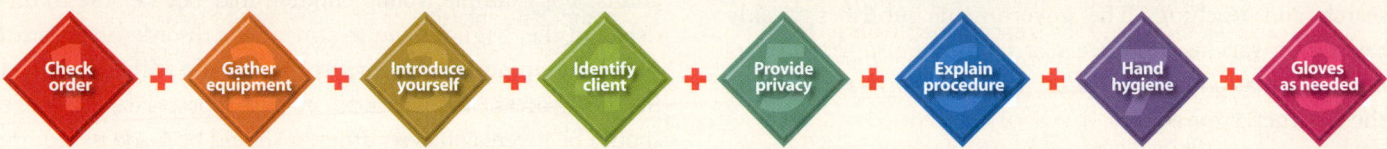

Check order + Gather equipment + Introduce yourself + Identify client + Provide privacy + Explain procedure + Hand hygiene + Gloves as needed

INTERVENTIONS

1. Stamp the agency informed consent form with the client's addressograph plate. *The addressograph information identifies the form as part of the client's legal record.*

2. Complete all information requested on the form. **Note:** The informed consent form may be computer generated in some facilities. Complete the information requested before printing out the form. *Ensures complete, accurate information is obtained.*

3. Write the procedure for which consent is being given in the space provided. Use proper medical terminology with no abbreviations. Include "right" or "left" as appropriate (For example, "Right inguinal herniorrhaphy" not "fix R inguinal hernia). *For accuracy in communication, the legal record must contain appropriate medical terminology and identification of appropriate body part when more than one exists.*

4. Listen to the information the primary care provider gives to the client or client's parent/guardian. *When you witness an informed consent, you are witnessing the exchange between the primary care provider and the client, client's parent, or guardian. You are establishing that they really did understand (were informed).*

5. Have the client or client's parent/guardian sign the form. The nurse should sign as a witness. **Note:** Some schools of nursing do not allow student nurses to serve as witnesses for informed consent. *Signatures document that information was provided and the client, client's parent, or guardian understood and agreed to the procedure.*

6. If the primary care provider is not present and you did not hear the information provided, ask the client or client's parent/guardian to tell you what they were told. Ask if they have any questions. If they have accurate information and no questions, have them sign the consent from. Sign on the witness line with the statement "witnessing signature only" written under your signature. *Because you did not hear the information provided by the physician, you cannot witness that interaction. If they have accurate information and no questions, you can be reasonably assured they have been informed. When you write "witnessing signature only," you are not held accountable for the information.*

7. If the information they tell you is incorrect or they have questions, do not have the consent signed. Instead, notify the primary care provider. *It is the responsibility of the primary care provider to obtain informed consent. If more teaching is needed, the primary care provider should provide it.*

8. Place the signed informed consent form in the client's chart. *The informed consent form is part of the legal record and should be kept with the client's chart.*

SAMPLE DOCUMENTATION

(date/time)   Dr. R. Jones talked with parents regarding need to repair R inguinal hernia, including benefits, risks, and possible complications. Informed consent form for right inguinal herniorrhaphy signed and witnessed. _____
L. Lopez, LPN

BOX 2-1

Patient's Bill of Rights

A Patient's* Bill of Rights was first adopted by the American Hospital Association (AHA) in 1973. The Bill of Rights below incorporates the AHA update as well as Bill of Rights information from the American Academy of Pain Management and the National Institutes of Health.

Bill of Rights

These rights can be exercised on the client's behalf by a designated surrogate or proxy decision maker if the client* lacks decision-making capacity, is legally incompetent, or is a minor.

1. The client has the right to considerate and respectful care.
2. The client has the right to and is encouraged to obtain from physicians and other direct care givers relevant, current, and understandable information about diagnosis, treatment, and prognosis. Except in emergencies, when the client lacks decision-making capacity and the need for treatment is urgent, the client is entitled to the opportunity to discuss and request information related to specific procedures and treatments, the risks involved, the possible length of recuperation, and the medically reasonable alternatives and their accompanying risks and benefits.

    Clients have the right to know the identity of physicians, nurses, and others involved in their care, as well as when those involved are students, residents, or other trainees. The client also has the right to know the immediate and long-term financial implications of treatment choices insofar as they are known.
3. The client has the right to make decisions about the plan of care prior to and during the course of treatment and to refuse recommended treatment or plan of care to the extent permitted by law and hospital policy and to be informed of the medical consequences of this action. In case of such refusal, the client is entitled to other appropriate care and services that the hospital provides or transfers to another hospital. The hospital should notify the client of any policy that might affect client choice within the institution.
4. The client has the right to have an advance directive (such as a living will, health care proxy, or durable power of attorney for health care) concerning treatment or designating a surrogate decision maker with the expectation that the hospital will honor the intent of that directive to the extent permitted by law and hospital policy.

    Health care institutions must advise clients of their rights under state law and hospital policy to make informal medical choices, ask if the client has an advance directive, and include that information in client records. The client has the right to timely information about hospital policy that may limit its ability to implement fully a legally valid advance directive.
5. The client has the right to have every consideration of privacy. Case discussion, consultation, examination, and treatment should be conducted as to protect each client's privacy.
6. The client has the right to expect that all communications and records pertaining to his/her care will be treated as confidential by the hospital, except in cases of suspected abuse or public health hazard when reporting is permitted or required by law. The client has the right to expect that the hospital will empha-

size the confidentiality of this information when it releases it to any other parties entitled to review information in these records.

7. The client has the right to review the records pertaining to his/her medical care and have information explained or interpreted as necessary, except when restricted by law.
8. The client has the right to expect that, within its capacity and policies, a hospital will make reasonable response to request of a client for appropriate and medically indicated cares and services. The hospital must provide evaluation, services, and/or referral, as indicated by the urgency of the case. When medically appropriate and legally permissible, or when a client has so requested, a client may be transferred to another facility. The institution to which the client is to be transferred must first have accepted the client for transfer. The client must also have the benefit of complete information and explanation concerning the need for, risks, benefits, and alternatives to such a transfer.
9. The client has the right to ask and be informed of the existence of business relationships among the hospital facility, educational institutions, other health care providers, or payers that may influence the client's treatment and care.
10. The client has the right to consent to or decline to participate in proposed research studies or human experimentation affecting care and treatment or requiring direct client involvement, and to have those studies fully explained prior to consent. A client who declines to participate in research or experimentation is entitled to the most effective care that the hospital can otherwise provide. The client has the right to know in advance what appointment times and physicians are available and where to go for continuity of care provided by the Clinical Center when such care is required under the study for which the client was admitted.
11. The client has the right to expect reasonable continuity of care when appropriate and to be informed by physicians and other caregivers of available and realistic client care options when hospital care is no longer appropriate.
12. The client has the right to be informed of hospital policies and practices that related to client care, treatment, and responsibilities. The client has the right to be informed of available resources for resolving disputes, grievances, and conflicts such as ethics committees, client representatives, or other mechanisms available in the institution. The client has the right to be informed of the hospital's charges for services and available payment methods.
13. The client has the privilege to examine and receive an explanation of the bill.
14. The client has the right to expect that medical information about him or her discovered at the Clinical Center, as well as an account of his or her medical program here, will be communicated to the referring physician.
15. The client has the right, at any time during the medical program, to designate additional physicians or organizations to receive medical updates. The client should inform the Outpatient Department staff of these additions.

*Note: This book uses the word "client" instead of "patient" to indicate that the person is an active participant in the process of achieving or maintaining health.
Data from: American Hospital Association, Chicago, IL; American Academy of Pain Management, Sonora, CA; National Institutes of Health, Washington, DC.

trust in the nurse and possibly in the entire health care system. However, if the parents learn about the health problem from another source, they may accuse the nurse of withholding information from them. As parents, they may have the right to access their dependent child's medical record.

REPORTABLE SITUATIONS

In certain instances, the decision about reporting the health concern of a child is made by law.

- If the child has a **reportable disease** (a disease that poses a public health hazard), the health care provider must file a report with the appropriate agency (usually the public health department). See more about this topic in Chapters 26 and 27 ⃝⃝.
- Suspected cases of child abuse or neglect must be reported to state law enforcement officers (local police, child protection services, and the Department of Health and Human Services).
- Threats to injure oneself must be reported to the supervisor in charge. This must be done even if a child asks the nurse to "promise" not to tell anyone. In this case, the nurse would tell the child that the nurse's job requires him or her to report anything that might cause harm to a client.

It is important for the nurse to be clear with clients about the limits of confidentiality and the mandatory reporting requirements.

Reportable diseases may include, but are not limited to, sexually transmitted infections, some foodborne infections, and some viral or airborne infections such as measles, whooping cough, and tuberculosis. (Information about these illnesses—including pathology, signs and symptoms, and treatment—is included in other chapters of this book. See Chapter 11 ⃝⃝ and appropriate chapters by body system.) The LPN/LVN might contact the health care provider or report the condition directly to the local health department. Infections must be reported immediately so investigation, diagnosis, and treatment of others can be made in a timely manner. The nurse would be provided with reporting forms either from the employing agency or from the health department. Documentation should also be included in the client chart.

Suspicion of Abuse

Every state has child abuse laws that define different types of abuse and the agency to which abuse issues should be directed. Any professional who reasonably suspects that abuse has occurred is required to report the suspicion to the local authorities. When suspicion of abuse occurs, the LPN/LVN should follow facility policy and always be careful to ensure privacy during the interview. Questions should be referred to the registered nurse.

Reports of suspected abuse that are made in good faith are not liable for countersuits. However, professionals who fail to report suspicions may be held responsible by the courts.

Signs of abuse and related nursing care issues are discussed in Chapter 27 ⃝⃝ of this text. The nurse must record detailed information in the client's chart and complete any report forms provided by the investigating agency.

PATIENT SELF-DETERMINATION ACT

The federal Patient Self-Determination Act requires health care institutions to inform clients of their rights to treatment, including advanced directives or "living wills" (Figure 2-2 ■). Nurses frequently discuss these issues with adult clients and families. They also discuss them with minor children and their parents.

When it becomes apparent a child will not recover, an open discussion about treatment and terminal care should take place. This discussion should involve key decision makers in the family. It should also involve the child.

"Do not resuscitate" orders for a child can raise a more emotional response than the same order for an older adult. Also, conflict can arise when the child wants to stop treatment, but the parent(s) is (are) not ready to allow the child to die. It is important for the nurse to use effective therapeutic communication in all situations, including group meetings, to help resolve the conflict. (Care of the dying child is discussed in Chapter 28 ⃝⃝ of this text.)

Legal and Ethical Issues Affecting the Mother

Although a few ethical and legal issues that affect the child have been introduced, there are some ethical and legal issues that affect the mother as well. There are no easy answers to these issues, and they are addressed here for discussion purposes only. Each person's situation will be different, and at times, the courts will make the final decisions. The nurse must be able to look at each situation with an open mind, and provide the necessary care for the mother, child, and family. Box 2-2 ■ reviews steps in making ethical decisions. Nurses who frequently work with these families must become familiar with the state and federal laws governing these situations.

ASSISTED REPRODUCTION

For a variety of reasons, some couples who try to have children are unable to conceive. Some of these couples use their ova and sperm for *in vitro* fertilization. Others use the ova

POWER OF ATTORNEY FOR HEALTH CARE
(1) **DESIGNATION OF AGENT:** I designate the following individual as my agent to make health care decisions for me: _____

(Name of individual you choose as agent)

(address) (city) (state) (zip code)

(home phone) (work phone)

OPTIONAL: If I revoke my agent's authority or if my agent is not willing, able, or reasonably available to make a health-care decision for me, I designate as my first alternate agent:

(Name of individual you choose as first alternate agent)

(address) (city) (state) (zip code)

(home phone) (work phone)

OPTIONAL: If I revoke the authority of my agent and first alternate agent or if neither is willing, able, or reasonably available to make a health care decision for me, I designate as my second alternate agent:

(Name of individual you choose as second alternate agent)

(address) (city) (state) (zip code)

(home phone) (work phone)

(2) **AGENT'S AUTHORITY:** My agent is authorized to make all health care decisions for me, including decisions to provide, withhold, or withdraw artificial nutrition and hydration, and all other forms of health care to keep me alive, **except** as I state here:

(3) **WHEN AGENT'S AUTHORITY BECOMES EFFECTIVE:** My agent's authority becomes effective when my primary physician determines that I am unable to make my own health care decisions unless I mark the following box. If I mark this box [ ], my agent's authority to make health care decisions for me takes effect immediately.

(4) **AGENT'S OBLIGATION:** My agent shall make health care decisions for me in accordance with this power of attorney for health care, any instructions I give below, and my other wishes to the extent known to my agent. To the extent my wishes are unknown, my agent shall make health care decisions for me in accordance with what my agent determines to be in my best interest. In determining my best interest, my agent shall consider my personal values to the extent known to my agent.

(5) **AGENT'S POSTDEATH AUTHORITY:** My agent is authorized to make anatomical gifts, authorize an autopsy, and direct disposition of my remains, except as I state here or elsewhere in this form:

INSTRUCTIONS FOR HEALTH CARE
Strike any wording you do not want.

(6) **END-OF-LIFE DECISIONS:** I direct that my health care providers and others involved in my care provide, withhold, or withdraw treatment in accordance with the choice I have marked below: **(Initial only one box)**
[ ] (a) **Choice NOT To Prolong Life**
I do not want my life to be prolonged if (1) I have an incurable and irreversible condition that will result in my death within a relatively short time, (2) I become unconscious and, to a reasonable degree of medical certainty, I will not regain consciousness, or (3) the likely risks and burdens of treatment would outweigh the expected benefits, **OR**
[ ] (b) **Choice To Prolong Life**
I want my life to be prolonged as long as possible within the limits of generally accepted health care standards.

(7) **RELIEF FROM PAIN:** Except as I state in the following space, I direct that treatment for alleviation of pain or discomfort should be provided at all times even if it hastens my death:

DONATION OF ORGANS AT DEATH
(8) Upon my death: (mark applicable box)
[ ] (a) I give any needed organs, tissues, or parts,
OR
[ ] (b) I give the following organs, tissues, or parts only: _____
[ ] (c) My gift is for the following purposes:
(strike any of the following you do not want)
(1) Transplant
(2) Therapy
(3) Research
(4) Education

(9) **EFFECT OF COPY:** A copy of this form has the same effect as the original.

(10) **SIGNATURE:** Sign and date the form here:

(date)	(sign your name)
(address)	(print your name)
(city)	(state)

(11) **WITNESSES:** This advance health care directive will not be valid for making health care decisions unless it is either: (1) signed by two (2) qualified adult witnesses who are personally known to you and who are present when you sign or acknowledge your signature; or (2) acknowledged before a notary public.

Figure 2-2. ■ A sample power of attorney for health care plus organ donor form.

BOX 2-2	NURSING CARE CHECKLIST

Steps in Making Ethical Decisions

Collect information.

☑ What decisions are needed?

☑ Who are the key people involved?

☑ What information will help make the situation more clear?

☑ Are there any legal constraints?

Identify the ethical issues or concerns of the situation.

☑ What historic, religious, or philosophic roots can be identified in this situation?

☑ What are current societal views of the issue or issues involved?

Define personal and professional moral positions on the issues.

☑ Are any personal constraints raised by this issue?

☑ What guidance does the professional code of ethics provide?

☑ Are there any conflicting loyalties or obligations?

☑ What are the moral positions of the key individuals involved?

Identify any value conflicts.

☑ What is the basis for the conflict?

☑ What are possible ways of resolving the conflict?

Identify factors in decision making.

☑ Who should make the decision?

☑ What are the possible actions and their anticipated outcomes?

☑ What is the moral justification for each action?

☑ Which action fits the criteria for this situation?

☑ Decide on a course of action and carry it out.

Evaluate the results of the decision or action.

☑ Did the expected outcome occur?

☑ Is a new decision needed?

☑ Is the decision process complete?

Source: Adapted from Thompson, J. B., & Thompson, H. O. (1981). *Ethics in nursing.* New York: Macmillan. Copyright Joyce Thompson. Used with permission.

and/or sperm from donors. Some couples adopt infants from other mothers or choose to have a surrogate mother carry the fetus and give the infant to the couple after delivery.

Many ethical and legal questions arise from situations seen today. What are the rights and responsibilities of the ova/sperm donors? What are the rights and responsibilities of the surrogate mother? What if the surrogate mother chooses not to give the infant to the couple after birth? If more than one infant is produced, must the couple assume responsibility of all infants? If the infant born from ova/sperm donation or surrogacy has birth defects, who is financially responsible for this child? Does the child have the right to know the birth mother and father and to develop a relationship with them?

NONTRADITIONAL PARENTS

Regulations that placed adopted children only in traditional family settings no longer apply. Blended families (see Chapter 3 ⚭) can adopt. Single parents who show they have the means to support a child may also adopt.

It is becoming more common for same-sex couples to want to marry and raise children. Gay men might request to adopt a child or donate sperm to have a child carried by a surrogate mother. Gay women could have one (or both) partners inseminated and carry the pregnancy. Because few states recognize same-sex marriages, which partner is legally responsible for the child? If the partners separate, who retains legal custody of the child?

PREGNANCY AFTER RAPE

Many women are sexually assaulted every year. The rapist could be a stranger, a friend, or a relative. At times, pregnancy results from these crimes. If the woman seeks health care immediately, measures may be taken to prevent pregnancy. However, even with medical care, pregnancy could result. The woman could choose to abort the pregnancy, adopt the child to another person, or keep the infant. Regardless of whether she chooses to keep the child, some ethical and legal questions exist. For example, if she keeps the child and the rapist is identified by DNA testing, can he be forced to pay child support? What rights would he have as the biologic father?

BARRIER-BREAKING TECHNOLOGIES

Increased capability with DNA testing and therapy has raised a host of ethical issues. Stem cell therapy can be viewed as a huge medical breakthrough, similar to the discovery of penicillin in the last century. It may have potential to correct heart defects, cure inherited diseases such as sickle cell anemia, and prevent degenerative diseases such as Parkinson's. However, it can also be viewed as the intrusion of humans into the very process of life. When more genes and gene markers are identified, it may be possible to know with near certainty that a child will be born with a crippling condition. What effect will it have if insurance companies refuse to cover the needs of this child? What controls will there be to ensure quality of life for those who cannot afford advanced and expensive gene therapy?

Parents are now presented with the option of "banking" their child's umbilical cord blood after birth. The frozen stem cells from the cord could be used in later years if the child needed therapy, such as for leukemia. However, it is not clear who owns the blood. Would the parent have the right to sell this cord blood for cash? Would the hospital have the right to keep the blood and use it to help others who have an immediate need for it? Could a child sue a parent or a facility because his or her cord blood was disposed of without his or her consent?

Fetal research is another broad area of ethical conflict. Some believe that unused embryos from *in vitro* fertilization should be used to aid research. Others believe equally strongly that these embryos are alive and that no human has the right to terminate that life. Advances in neonatal care and equipment only further the controversy, as neonates survive from increasingly premature stages of development.

Medical advances can also raise ethical issues from the maternal side. Consider the case of the pregnant dying woman who asked to be maintained on life support to bring her child to term. Is it right to maintain life support on someone who is brain dead? Does the family have the right to demand life support? Is it right to stop life support, knowing that the fetus will not survive? What might the effects be on an infant if most of its development has occurred inside a cadaver? These and other questions will become more common as technology continues to advance.

Role of the LPN/LVN

LPNs and LVNs are not ultimately responsible for resolving legal or ethical issues. However, they need to have a basic understanding of the issues in order to be supportive of the client, the family, and other health care professionals. The LPN/LVN's Code of Ethics is shown in Box 2-3 ■.

FOLLOWING SCOPE AND STANDARDS OF PRACTICE

In maternal–child nursing, as in any other area, the nurse must know and abide by the scope and standards of practice. Familiarity with a procedure does not give the nurse the right to perform it. State practice acts and facility policies provide the framework for nursing practice. The facility's policies can be more restrictive than state nurse practice acts; however, they cannot be more lenient. If an unintended incident occurs (such as a client fall), it must be fully reported (Figure 2-3 ■).

PROVIDING TESTIMONY

When the courts decide legal issues, the LPN/LVN may be required to provide documentation or testimony. Therefore, it is critical for the nurse to provide accurate and complete documentation of the care provided, the client response,

---

BOX 2-3

Code of Ethics for the Licensed Practical/ Vocational Nurse

The Licensed Practical and Licensed Vocational Nurse shall:

- Consider as a basic obligation the conservation of life and the prevention of disease.
- Promote and protect the physical, mental, emotional, and spiritual health of the client and his/her family.
- Fulfill all duties faithfully and efficiently.
- Function within established legal guidelines.
- Accept personal responsibility for his/her acts, and seek to merit the respect and confidence of all members of the health team.
- Hold in confidence all matters coming to his/her knowledge, in the practice of his/her profession, and in no way at no time violate this confidence.
- Give conscientious service and charge just remuneration.
- Learn and respect the religious and cultural beliefs of his/her client and of all people.
- Meet the obligation to the client by keeping abreast of current trends in health care through reading and continuing education.
- As a citizen of the United States of America, uphold the laws of the land and seek to promote legislation that will meet the health needs of its people.

Source: Reprinted by permission of the National Association of Practical Nurse Education and Service.

---

and family interactions. Box 2-4 ■ illustrates the principles and importance of accurate documentation.

DO NO HARM

Practical and vocational nurses often witness parents struggling with treatment options. Because children are often not capable of making decisions that affect them, ethical issues in pediatrics are more complex. Ethical decisions are based on respect for the child and his or her ability to make decisions independently. The underlying principle is to "do no harm." Sometimes consultation with other health care professionals is necessary to determine whether responsibility is limited to care of the child or includes the desires of the parents.

ETHICS COMMITTEES

Health care institutions generally have ethics committees that make treatment recommendations or decisions. LPNs and LVNs may be asked to serve on these committees (see Health Promotion Issue on pages 38 and 39). Work on ethics committees would require the nurse to increase her or his knowledge in several areas such as:

- The specific health care problem
- The makeup of the family
- The religious and cultural beliefs of the family
- State and local statutes that relate to the legal and ethical choice of the client.

CONFIDENTIAL REPORT OF UNUSUAL OCCURRENCE
NOT a part of the Medical Record - Please forward to RISK MANAGEMENT

I. (COMPLETE IF ADDRESSOGRAPH UNAVAILABLE)

CLIENT/VISITOR _____ PHYSICIAN _____

MEDICAL RECORD # _____ DATE OF BIRTH _____

ADDRESSOGRAPH

II. DATE OF OCCURRENCE _____ TIME OF OCCURRENCE _____ LOCATION (ROOM OR FLOOR) _____

NAME OF M.D. NOTIFIED _____ CLIENT AWARE OF OCCURRENCE: YES___NO___ FAMILY AWARE OF OCCURRENCE: YES___NO___

REPORT COMPLETED BY _____ OTHERS FAMILIAR WITH OCCURRENCE _____

III. ADMITTING DIAGNOSIS _____

CLIENT CONDITION PRIOR TO OCCURRENCE: ALERT _____ ASLEEP _____ ANESTHETIZED _____ DISORIENTED _____ OTHER _____

IF SEDATIVE/NARCOTICS/DIURETICS GIVEN IN LAST 12 HOURS (WHERE APPLICABLE) PLEASE COMPLETE: (MED, DOSE, TIME)

IV. EVENT

FALLS
- 100 Unobserved Fall
- 101 Assisted to Floor
- 102 Fell from Bed
- 103 Fell from Table/Equipment
- 104 Fell in Bathroom
- 105 Walking/Standing/Slip & Fall
- 106 Sitting Commode/Wheelchair
- 107 Restrained Prior to Fall
- 108 Restrained After Fall
- 109 Bed Rails Up (1 2 3 4)
- 110 Bed Rails Down (1 2 3 4)
- 112 Visitor Fall
- 113 Outpatient Fall
- 119 Other_____

BURNS
- 120 Electrical/Chemical Burn
- 121 Spill
- 122 Fire
- 129 Other_____

ALTERCATION/COMPLAINTS
- 130 Pt/Family/Employee/Visitor
- 131 Complaint-Waiting Time
- 132 Complaint-Billing Services
- 133 Complaint-Food Services
- 134 Complaint-Housekeeping/Ancillary
- 135 Complaint-Nursing
- 136 Complaint-Medical Staff
- 137 Complaint-Security
- 139 Other_____

MISCELLANEOUS
- 140 Suicide/Attempt
- 141 Left AMA/Elopement
- 142 Equipment-Struck/Failure
- 143 Property Loss/Damage
- 144 Unexpected Death
- 145 Non-Compliant Smoking
- 148 Development of Pressure Ulcer
- 149 Other_____

MEDICATIONS Drug_____
- 150 Order (Computer Entry)
- 151 Wrong Time
- 152 Wrong Dosage
- 153 Wrong Route
- 154 Wrong Drug
- 155 Wrong Patient
- 156 Omission
- 157 Adverse Drug Reaction
- 158 Prescribing Error
- 159 Other_____

INTRAVENOUS Sol._____
- 160 Infiltration
- 161 Wrong Rate
- 162 Wrong Solution
- 163 Wrong Time
- 164 Order (Computer Entry)
- 165 Infected Site/Phlebitis
- 169 Other_____

BLOOD TRANSFUSION
- 170 Allergic/Adverse Reaction
- 171 Delay in Administration
- 172 Incorrect Flow Rate
- 173 Infiltration
- 174 Omitted/Client Refusal
- 175 Wrong Amount
- 176 Wrong/Omitted Filter
- 177 Wrong Component
- 178 Biological Product Deviation
- 179 Other_____

PATHOLOGY
- 180 Reference Laboratory Error
- 181 Lost/Mishandled Specimen
- 182 Specimen Collection Error
- 183 Cytology/Biopsy Discrepancy
- 184 Biopsy/Resection Discrepancy
- 185 Autopsy Suggests Serious Clinical Discrepancy
- 186 Frozen Section/Pathological Discrepancy
- 187 Error Performing Test/Error Reporting Results
- 188 Delayed Draw
- 189 Hematoma Following Draw
- 190 Other_____

OR/PACU/OPS/WOR
- 200 Removal Foreign Body
- 210 Incorrect Count-Sponge/Needle/Instr
- 202 X-rays Taken/Deferred
- 203 Arrest
- 204 Wrong Pt/Side/Site/Procedure
- 205 OPS Pt Admitted Post-Op
- 206 Unplanned Organ Repair/Removal
- 207 Lac/Tear/Puncture-Organ/Body Part
- 208 Canceled Surg-Prep/Equipment Problem
- 209 Unplanned Return to OR
- 210 Surgery Delayed
- 211 Consent Incorrect/Incomplete/Not Done
- 212 Reddened Area
- 213 Unsterile Situation
- 214 Specimen Problem
- 215 Eye Irritation/Injury
- 216 Post Arterial Hematoma
- 217 Improper Discharge
- 219 Other_____

ANESTHESIA
- 220 Unexpected Arrest
- 221 Canceled Surgery After Induction
- 222 Injury/Death Post Induction
- 223 Tooth/Face/Lip/Mandible Damage
- 224 CNS Injury/Brain Damage
- 225 Unplanned Transfer to Special Care Unit
- 226 Aspiration
- 229 Other_____

EMERGENCY DEPARTMENT
- 230 Arrives DOA After Discharge/Seen in ED within Past 7 Days
- 231 Seen for Complication Post Treatment/Procedure from Prev. Hospitalization
- 232 Left AMA
- 239 Other_____

OB/GYN/INFANT CARE
- 240 Delivery Occurred Outside L&D Area
- 241 Mother Transferred to ICU
- 241 Unplanned Return to Surgery
- 243 Stirrup Related Injury
- 244 Delivery Unattended by any Physician
- 245 Blood Loss > 1500 cc
- 246 Cord Blood Gas pH <7.0
- 247 Cardiac/Respiratory Arrest
- 248 Infant Seizures in Delivery Room
- 249 Apgar Score 5 or Less at 5 Minutes
- 250 Unusual Condition - Child
- 251 Infant Injury-skull fx/paralysis/palsy
- 252 Transfer From NB Nursery to ISC/NICU
- 253 Instrumented Delivery-Injury
- 259 Other_____

ADULT/PEDIATRIC CARE
- 260 Unexpected Tx – Higher Care Level
- 261 Significant Neurosensory/Functional Deficit/Intractable Pain not Present upon Admit
- 262 Acute MI/CVA within 48 hours of Surgery/Procedure
- 263 Death within 48 hours of Surgery/Procedure
- 264 Nosocomial Infection Prolonging Stay or Complicating Pt's Condition > 5 days
- 265 Client Found Unresponsive
- 266 Self Extubation
- 267 Arrest – Code Team Activation
- 268 Soft Tissue Injury
- 269 Other_____

TESTS/TREATMENTS
- 270 Wrong Client
- 271 Wrong Test/Treatment
- 272 Treatment Delayed
- 273 MD Ordered-Not Done
- 274 Complication Resulting in Injury
- 275 Computer Entry
- 276 Infection Control issue
- 279 Other_____

RADIOLOGY/RAD ONC/IMAGING
- 280 Complication Requiring Surgical Correction
- 281 New Onset Nerve Deficit
- 282 Reaction to Contrast Agent
- 283 Overexposure to Radiation
- 284 Cardiac/Respiratory Arrest
- 285 Treatment Delayed Worsening Condition
- 286 Unplanned Repeat Diagnostic Procedure
- 287 Monitored Inadequately
- 288 X-ray Inaccurately Read
- 289 Equipment Failure
- 290 Lack of Prep-Cancel Procedure
- 291 Wrong Pt/Side/Site/Prodedure
- 299 Other_____

V. OUTCOME

SEVERITY OF OUTCOME
- 350 **No Injury/Unaffected**
- *351 **Minor Injury**
- *352 **Major Injury/Consequential**

*_SPECIFY INJURY BELOW –

GENERAL
- 300 Delay in Therapy
- 301 Embolism
- 302 Reaction/Toxic Effect
- 303 Death
- 304 Prolonged Hospital Stay
- 305 Neurological Sensory
- 306 Decubitus
- 307 Arrest/CPR
- 309 Other_____

OBSTETRICAL
- 310 Unusually Low Apgar
- 311 Fetal Injury
- 312 Fetal Death
- 313 Maternal Injury
- 314 Maternal Death
- 319 Other_____

SKELETAL
- 320 Fracture
- 321 Dislocation
- 322 Teeth
- 323 Sprain
- 329 Other_____

TISSUE
- 330 Hematoma/Contusion
- 331 Necrosis
- 332 Laceration
- 333 Fistula
- 334 Dehiscence
- 335 Abrasion/Blister
- 336 Swelling
- 337 Reddened Area/Ecchymosis
- 338 Skin Tear
- 339 Other_____

VI. BRIEF COMMENTS IF NECESSARY _____

_____

_____

_____

Figure 2-3. ■ An incident report form.

BOX 2-4   **NURSING CARE CHECKLIST**

Accurate Documentation

When documenting, remember the following guidelines:

- ☑ Make documentations correct and accurate.
- ☑ Show the timing and the sequence of actions.
- ☑ Identify the dose, route, and time of medications.
- ☑ Indicate equipment or materials used.
- ☑ Use accepted terminology and abbreviations.
- ☑ Label late entries and continued notes on charts.
- ☑ Provide facts, not opinions.

Note the following two examples. The underlined portions of Example 2 make the second documentation much more accurate and measurable than the first.

Example 1

(date) On admission ulcerated area noted on lower, inner aspect of right leg. No apparent dressing. Moderate

amount of drainage observed. Foul odor noted. Pedal pulses present but weak, foot slightly cyanotic with edema. Wound edges red, surrounding skin hot. Charge nurse notified. Wound cleansed, dressing applied. Acetaminophen 500 mg given PO per physician's order. Teaching done. M. Penn, LVN

Example 2

(date) <u>0830</u> On admission ulcerated area noted on lower, inner aspect of right leg. No apparent dressing. Moderate amount of <u>thick yellow-green</u> drainage observed. Foul odor noted. <u>Area 15 cm long, 6 cm wide, 1.5 cm deep</u>. Pedal pulses present but weak, foot slightly cyanotic with <u>+2</u> edema. Wound edges red, surrounding skin hot. <u>States wound has "stinging pain."</u> Charge nurse notified. Wound cleansed <u>with sterile normal saline, wet-to-dry</u> dressing applied. <u>Foot placed in dependent position, with blanket for warmth.</u> Acetaminophen 500 mg given PO per physician's order. Teaching <u>about wound contamination</u> done. M. Penn, LVN

Through group decision by nonfamily members, an unbiased, objective decision can be made.

REFERRAL TO SUPPORT GROUPS

There are also many community agencies and groups to support the family. Some of these agencies are federally funded, while others are privately funded. The practical or vocational nurse should be aware of community support groups that can help families cope with pediatric issues. For example, local churches or hospice may be the site of support groups for parents of terminally ill children. Schools may offer evening seminars on health topics that affect school-age children.

SUPPORT GROUPS FOR STAFF

Many facilities have staff support groups to assist nurses and other health care workers to adjust to difficult situations in pediatric care. For example, when a chronically ill child has received care at the same hospital for several years, the staff may become attached to both client and family. If the child dies, the staff may need time and a safe place away from work to share their feelings of loss. They may also experience feelings of failure because the child died despite their care.

NURSING CARE

PRIORITIES IN NURSING CARE

When providing nursing care to a client who has legal or ethical issues, the priorities are therapeutic listening, critical thinking, and awareness of the law. Using skills such as reflecting, open-ended questions, and silence, the nurse can

support the client and family to explore their reactions to the situation, whether it is a first pregnancy or the death of a child. The nurse can practice critical thinking by teaching the family about treatment options and by helping them to shape questions to ask the care provider. In situations such as suspected child abuse, the nurse will also know that the law requires a report to social services.

ASSESSING

The data the nurse gathers in legal and ethical situations will likely relate to psychosocial factors. Does the 2-year-old flinch when the mother suddenly turns toward her? Does the family argue in the visitors' lounge about treatment decisions for their boy with leukemia? Has the teenager been yelling at the staff since he heard the diagnosis of cancer? The nurse would document these findings in objective, nonjudgmental terms. In situations that have legal or ethical difficulties, the LPN/LVN would collaborate with other members of the health care team to see that client needs were met.

DIAGNOSING, PLANNING, AND IMPLEMENTING

Some common nursing diagnoses in legal and ethical client situations are:

- Deficient Knowledge related to [details, such as beginning pregnancy]
- Altered Family Processes related to [details, such as learning a child was born with cerebral palsy]
- Anticipatory Grieving related to [details of terminally ill child]

(Text continues on p. 40.)

HEALTH PROMOTION ISSUE

SEXUALLY TRANSMITTED INFECTION EDUCATION

The nurse works for a family planning clinic and has provided sex education in the public school system for 11th graders for the past 5 years. Recently, the state regulations for sex education have changed and her curriculum needs to be revised. She now needs to promote abstinence and provide information about contraception. She will also need to include detailed information about sexually transmitted infections (STIs). She needs to understand her state laws, as well as neighboring state laws, related to consent to care in pregnancy, contraception, abortion, and STI treatment. She seeks the assistance of her nurse manager on this project.

DISCUSSION

There is a great need to approach the issue of teenage pregnancy and teenage

STI prevalence. In the United States, more than 800,000 women younger than the age of 20 become pregnant every year. Nine million teenagers will acquire an STI each year. Although these rates seem staggering, they are down for the first time in many years. Data seem to support the use of abstinence in sex education and the increased use of condoms as effective in this decline.

Although the decline is encouraging within our own nation, when compared to other nations, American teens still get pregnant more often, have more abortions, and get more STIs. Data from the Alan Guttmacher Institute suggests that American teens do not have more sex than teens in other nations, but they are less likely to use effective contraception

and have more sexual partners. The other countries with lower pregnancy, abortion, and STI rates are more accepting of teenage sex but strongly condemn teenage parenthood. These countries also provide greater access to contraception and have more developed sex education programs, including STI prevention.

Sex education curricula should include comprehensive information about physical and emotional changes of adolescence, pregnancy, and conception; the emotional effects of sexual intercourse; decision making related to sexual intercourse; the risks of sexual intercourse to include pregnancy and STIs; and contraception control methods, including abstinence. Each state has particular regulations that must be followed related to the content taught in sex education programs.

States regulate whether sex education and HIV/STI prevention is mandated in the school setting. The content is also regulated. For sex education and HIV/STI prevention alike, abstinence and contraception may be stressed, covered, or not allowed. Each state also regulates the parental role in sex education as it relates to consent. The regulation may require consent, not require consent, or allow the parent who is religiously or morally opposed to sex education for their children to ask

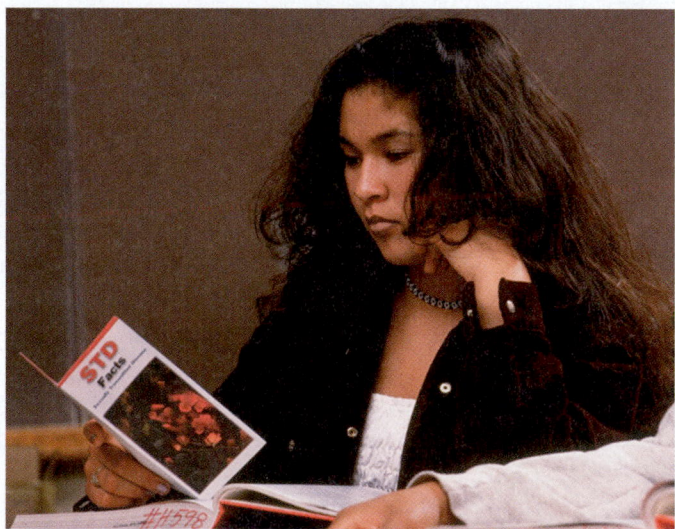

Source: Will Hart

that their children be placed in another class.

PLANNING AND IMPLEMENTATION

The LPN and her nurse manager decide that a committee needs to be developed to redesign this curriculum. The committee members are a teacher in the public school system, a physician, a certified nurse-midwife, the LPN and her nurse manager, and several parents from the community.

The community carefully reviews the existing curriculum for age and development appropriateness. They also review the teaching methods for applicability to all learning styles. They take care to include the state regulations for abstinence. It is decided that all content should be presented in a nonjudgmental, risk–benefit manner. The nature of this content requires students to make life decisions that may be at times life altering. Therefore, a course will be presented prior to this one on how to make sound decisions. The LPN can then incorporate those methods into the content on sex education and HIV/STI prevention.

Audiovisual (AV) aids are discussed in the committee. All posters, videos, and slides are reviewed for age appropriateness and content. AV aids chosen include images of teenagers of this era that are simple and easy to understand. There was much discussion about the use of graphic, realistic images of STIs. Some committee members were concerned that the images would be ignored due to the graphic nature. Other committee members rationalized that these images presented a reality that discussion alone could not afford. The committee decided that the benefits of these slides were important and that the LPN should use her judgment regarding the appropriateness from class to class.

There also was some discussion among the committee members about whether the class should include males and females or should separate them into different sections. There was also discussion about whether the female LPN would be as effective with the male students. It was decided that separate classes would be best and that they would hire a male nurse to teach the male students. These decisions were made to encourage students to discuss the issues presented.

The committee was pleased with the final product. They have expanded the curriculum and added a section with a new male instructor. Long-term evaluations will be conducted to determine the effectiveness of this program.

SELF-REFLECTION

What are your personal beliefs about teenage sexuality and pregnancy? Where did you learn information regarding sex during your teenage years? What information do you wish you had during that time frame? Was there any education or support system that would have influenced your sexual behavior during adolescence?

Why do you think the rates of teenage sexuality and pregnancy in America are so high? Do you think the promotion of abstinence in sex education is a good idea? Why or why not? Should school clinics distribute contraceptive devices to students? What is the parent's responsibility? Devise a plan you believe would be effective in decreasing the teenage pregnancy rate. Approach a school system and offer to present this program in the school system.

SUGGESTED RESOURCES

For the Nurse

- **www.guttmacher.org** This website provides information concerning state policies and requirements for minors related to pregnancy, contraception, abortion, and STIs.

- **www.cdc.gov** This website, sponsored by the Centers for Disease Control and Prevention, offers several downloads related to STI prevention, including slides containing realistic images of STIs.

- Risk for Injury related to physical abuse
- Risk for Violence (parent) related to inability to manage anger.

The expected outcomes for these clients and their families might include:

- Client/family will express a clearer understanding of the condition and treatment options.
- Client/family will confer with social services to establish a plan of care and obtain referrals.

Nursing interventions for clients with legal and ethical issues are based on the particular situation. The following interventions may apply:

- Always practice within the limits of the nurse practice acts of your state and the guidelines of your facility. *It is your responsibility to learn the laws of the state in which you practice and the guidelines (which may be more strict) of your workplace.*
- Become familiar with the laws of your state as they relate to health care. *It will be useful for you as a professional to know more about the legal or ethical situations you may encounter in your job.*
- Think about your own values, and imagine positive ways of responding to those whose values are different from your own. Never advise clients to choose one option over another. *Your job is to provide quality care, regardless of what the client decides. Your own decisions and choices must be left aside.*
- Uphold client confidentiality. *Violation of HIPAA regulations can lead to severe penalties. Your standing as a professional and the trust of your clients and colleagues depends on your integrity.*
- Use other members of the health care team as a resource when you are unsure of an answer or correct action. Do not try to answer what you do not know. *Your facility will have a person or persons trained to answer difficult legal questions or will have referrals to qualified people in the community.*
- Practice culturally sensitive nursing care (Box 2-5 ■). *Most communication occurs through nonverbal "language." By paying attention to cues and showing genuine concern for clients, nurses can provide culturally proficient, individualized care.*
- Always provide quality nursing care using the "five rights and three checks" (Box 2-6 ■). *The most common reason for lawsuits is improper administration of medications. Be careful and consistent to ensure client safety.*
- Be prompt and accurate in reporting any incidents. Remember that the nurse who delegates a task is responsible for the successful completion of that task. Figure 2-3 shows an incident report form. *Prompt reporting can prevent further problems from occurring and supports quality care for the client.*

BOX 2-5	CULTURAL PULSE POINTS

ETHICAL ISSUES

The following situations relate to cultural issues and ethical issues. They all have the potential to affect the nurse–client relationship.

- A woman from the Middle East might not want to have a male nurse do postpartum care because of the cultural rule that no one but her husband see her unclothed.
- A Korean mother may be upset when she must consent to emergency surgery without discussing the decision with her husband.
- An African American woman may be offended by being asked to be quiet during a visit with friends who come to celebrate her new baby.
- A Hispanic woman may avoid breastfeeding in the hospital because of the chance of being seen with her breasts exposed.
- A young Vietnamese mother may be reluctant to ask for pain medication after a cesarean delivery.
- An Irish Catholic family may reject therapeutic abortion, even if the pregnancy puts the mother's life at risk.

Think about your own reactions to these situations. What are some of the ways you could help clients make decisions without expressing your personal point of view?

EVALUATING

In evaluating legal and ethical issues, the nurse would collect data about whether the specific interventions were effective. For example, the client's questions have been answered sufficiently for the time. The parents state that they have met with social workers. The nurse would ensure that reports and referrals have been made, and that written materials have been provided if possible. The nurse would also note any conclusions about treatment the family has reached.

BOX 2-6	

Five Rights and Three Checks of Medication Administration

The most common reason for legal action against a nurse can be avoided by remembering and practicing these safety measures:

Five Rights	Three Checks
Right Client	Compare the drug to the Medication Administration Record (MAR) when removing the drug from the drawer.
Right Drug	
Right Dose	
Right Route	Compare the drug to the MAR when pouring it into the cup.
Right Time	
	Compare the drug to the MAR when returning the container to the drawer.

Source: Adapted from Ramont, R. P., Niedringhaus, D. M., & Towle, M. A. (2006). Comprehensive nursing care. Upper Saddle River, NJ: Prentice Hall, p. 399.

NURSING PROCESS CARE PLAN
Client with Hodgkin's Lymphoma

Jean, a 16-year-old girl, is admitted to a pediatric unit with a diagnosis of recurrent Hodgkin's lymphoma. Jean has been fighting this disease for 4 years. She has been in remission three times, each one shorter than the time before. This time she was in remission only 3 months. During the admission process, Jean tells the nurse she does not want any more treatments. She says, "They make me so sick. They are not working anyway, I just want to die and get it over with."

Jean's parents are sure the treatments will "work this time and she will get well." Jean is requesting all treatment be stopped.

Assessment. The following data should be collected as soon as possible after admission:

- Strength of marital relationships
- Character of parent-child relationship
- Knowledge of illness and treatments
- Jean's feeling about illness and treatment
- Parents' feelings about illness and treatment.

Nursing Diagnosis. The following important nursing diagnosis (among others) is established for this client:

- Dysfunctional Family Processes related to terminal illness of a child

Expected Outcomes. The family will:

- Develop methods of communication and problem solving related to terminal illness of the child.
- Come to an agreement concerning Jean's treatment that is satisfying for both parties.

Planning and Implementation

- Provide opportunities for the family and the client to express fears and expectations both privately and collectively. *Therapeutic communication will enhance family dynamics and facilitate decision making.*
- Promote understanding and empathy among family members and client. *Understanding of feelings, concerns, and viewpoints will promote respect and trust.*
- Encourage family members to set appropriate goals as they work through the decision-making process. *Goal establishment assists the family with organization and provides a framework for decision making.*

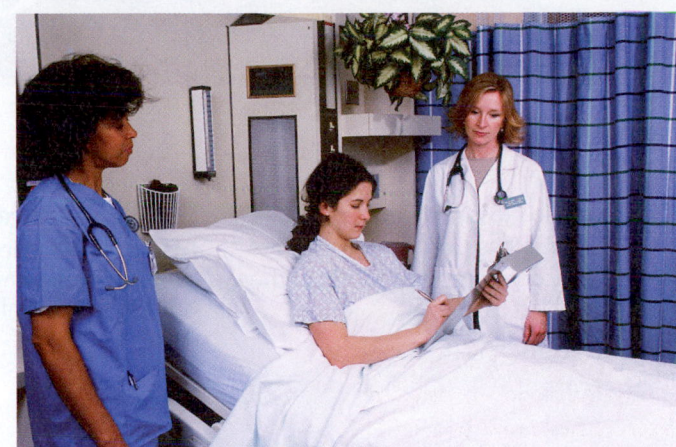

Figure 2-4 ■ Obtaining informed consent is the responsibility of the person performing the procedure. The nurse may be asked to witness the consent signature.

- Ask questions to be sure client and family understand procedures for which they must give written consent. Obtain answers to questions if necessary, or report the need for more information. Witness informed consent (Figure 2-4 ■). *If they cannot answer questions, they might not really be informed. By asking questions, the nurse can document that they are informed about the procedure.*
- Provide referrals as necessary. *Provides the family with information and assistance as they work through the issues.*

Evaluation. The nurse would review client outcomes to determine whether they have been met. The nurse might also assess the following: Have the client and family members verbalized their fears? Do client and family members verbalize appropriate goals for health care? Have client and family members been in contact with support groups/agencies?

Critical Thinking in the Nursing Process

1. Explore Jean's legal right in your state to refuse treatment.
2. If Jean's parents are unaware of her desires to stop treatment, what should the nurse do?
3. What type of resources would be helpful to Jean and her family?

Note: Discussion of Critical Thinking questions appears in Appendix I.

Note: The references and resources for this and all chapters have been compiled at the back of the book.

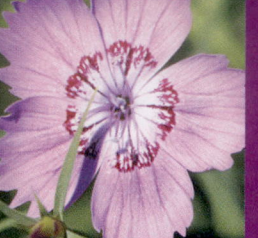

Chapter Review

 **KEY TERMS** by Topic

Use the audio glossary feature of either the CD-ROM or the Companion Website to hear the correct pronunciation of the following key terms.

Introduction
ethics

Legal and Ethical Issues Affecting Children
informed consent, mature minor act, emancipated minors, confidentiality, reportable disease

KEY Points

- Nurses should be familiar with the agencies and groups in their community.

- The pediatric client is guaranteed the same rights as any other client, but it is often the parent(s) who will make decisions about treatment(s).

- Conflicts may arise when the desires of the child are different from those of the parent(s). LPNs and LVNs may seek assistance from the shift supervisor or from legal counsel.

- If any client has a health problem that puts the community at risk, or if child abuse or neglect is suspected, the nurse must notify the appropriate public health or law enforcement agency.

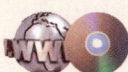 **EXPLORE Media**Link

Additional interactive resources for this chapter can be found on the Companion Website at www.prenhall.com/towle.

Click on Chapter 2 and "Begin" to select the activities for this chapter.

For chapter-related NCLEX-style questions and an audio glossary, access the accompanying CD-ROM in this book.

FOR FURTHER Study

Reportable sexually transmitted diseases are discussed in Chapter 11.

Reportable infectious diseases are discussed in Chapter 26.

Signs of abuse, reportable concerns, and related nursing care are discussed in Chapter 27.

Care of the dying child is discussed in Chapter 28.

Critical Thinking Care Map

Caring for a Client Desiring Pregnancy Termination

NCLEX-PN® Focus Area: Safe and Effective Care Environment: Coordinated Care

Case Study: SV is a 15-year-old female who is 12 weeks pregnant. Her parents are unaware of her pregnancy. SV states she just doesn't know what to do. There is no way she can raise a baby, but she doesn't think abortion is right for her either. She is crying inconsolably.

Nursing Diagnosis: Hopelessness

COLLECT DATA

Subjective

_____
_____
_____
_____
_____
_____
_____

Objective

_____
_____
_____
_____
_____
_____
_____

Would you report this? Yes/No

If yes, to: _____

Nursing Care

_____
_____
_____
_____
_____
_____
_____
_____

How would you document this? _____
_____
_____
_____

Data Collected
(use those that apply)

- Crying
- States lack of sleep times 3 days
- LMP (date/month/year)
- Reports breast tenderness and nausea
- 24-Hour diet recall: six soft drinks
- No eye contact with nurse
- Current weight: 135 pounds
- States unable to care for a baby
- States family incapable of financially supporting another family member
- Urine dipstick negative for protein and glucose
- Reproductive history: no previous pregnancies
- "My boyfriend says I have to abort the baby or he won't have anything to do with me."
- Concerned father will be physically abusive if he finds out she is pregnant

Nursing Interventions
(use those that apply; list in priority order)

- Explore options available to this client and the pros and cons of each.
- Encourage client to express feelings and concerns openly.
- Discuss importance of prenatal care.
- Teach client about signs and symptoms of early pregnancy.
- Encourage client to explore personal strengths.
- Encourage client to engage parents in decision-making process.
- Encourage client to register for childbirth classes and a tour of the birth facility.
- Address client in a nonjudgmental fashion.
- Explore client's past successes in difficult circumstances.

Compare your documentation to the sample provided in Appendix I.

NCLEX-PN® Exam Preparation

1 Mary, a 4-year-old girl, is seen in the clinic with complaints of burning on urination. The nurse notices two large bruises on Mary's inner thigh. Mary's stepfather states she fell on the bar of her brother's bicycle. The LPN/LVN should:

1. believe the stepfather.
2. call the police.
3. keep the stepfather's comment confidential.
4. report the information to the RN.

2 Jeremy, a 10-year-old boy, is diagnosed with acute leukemia and requires a blood transfusion. His mother agrees, but his father refuses because of religious beliefs. The nurse should:

1. side with the mother to save Jeremy's life.
2. side with the father because the man is the head of the household.
3. provide care for Jeremy without taking sides.
4. refuse to provide care for Jeremy until the parents resolve the conflict.

3 Which of the following is NOT a breech of confidentiality?

1. The nurse talks with her neighbor about Jeremy, his condition, and his parents' conflict.
2. The nurse leaves the client chart open on the counter in the hall.
3. The nurse talks with the hospital chaplain about Jeremy's parents' conflict.
4. An off-duty nurse from the adult unit, a friend of Jeremy's mother, reads Jeremy's chart.

4 Alyce, a 14-year-old girl, confides in the nurse that she is sexually active with several partners who are 15 to 17 years old and states she does not want her parents to know. She states she cannot get pregnant because she only has sex during her menstrual period. The most appropriate nursing response would be to:

1. call her parents.
2. provide instruction on use of condoms and contraceptives.
3. tell her she is breaking the law and you will not help her.
4. ask her the names of her partners so you can call the authorities.

5 John, age 12, is in the final stage of muscular dystrophy. His family asks the nurse what to do in planning for John's death. The best nursing response would be:

1. "It would be best to keep John from knowing he is in the final stages."
2. "I will notify the charge nurse and set up a meeting with John, the entire family, and the doctor."
3. "John is not old enough to have a "Do not resuscitate" order so we must put him on life support."
4. "We will let you know when it is time to make funeral arrangements."

6 Patty, a 3-year-old, is scheduled to have a myringotomy. Her mother signed the consent for surgery. When providing preoperative care, the nurse should ask Patty:

1. "Do you want an IV in your right arm?"
2. "Is it OK if I start your IV?"
3. "Do you want your ears to feel better?"
4. "Do you want to take your doll with you?"

7 Mrs. Cross states: "I understand this hospital does lots of research. I don't want you experimenting on my daughter or giving her experimental drugs." The best nursing response should be:

1. "I don't know which drugs are experimental and which are sugar."
2. "You must sign a consent to participate in research studies, so you can be assured no experimental treatment would be done without your knowledge and permission."
3. "Only the doctor knows when experiments are being done. You need to talk with him."
4. "You are wrong; only prisoners are used for experiments."

8 The nurse understands that which of the following are appropriate expectations for clients and families regarding their participation in health care decisions? Choose all that apply.

1. Complete and accurate health information will be provided by health care personnel.
2. Families and clients have a responsibility to seek information regarding their medical condition and required treatments.
3. Health care personnel have the sole responsibility to ensure that families and clients understand their medical condition and required treatments.
4. Health care personnel are responsible to ensure that families and clients keep all appointments.
5. Families and clients are financially responsible for health care.

9 A 23-year-old woman comes to the emergency department after she fell on the sidewalk outside a local bar. She appears intoxicated. She insists she can drive home. What is the legally correct response?

10 The newborn nursery nurse is concerned about privacy issues in the nursery. Which of the following would be of most concern to her?

1. Crib cards visible to the public through the nursery windows.
2. Client charts stay in the nursery instead of on the crib when infant is taken to mother's room.
3. Procedures such as circumcisions are performed in a closed procedure room.
4. Consent forms are signed by parents prior to releasing information to hospital website.

Answers for Review Questions, as well as discussion of Care Plan and Critical Thinking Care Map questions, appear in Appendix I.

Chapter 3

Nursing Care of the Family

BRIEF Outline

The Family Unit

Theoretical Framework for Working with Families

Roles and Functions of the Family

Family Assessment Techniques and Tools

LPN/LVN Role in Family Care

Family Under Stress

Nursing Care

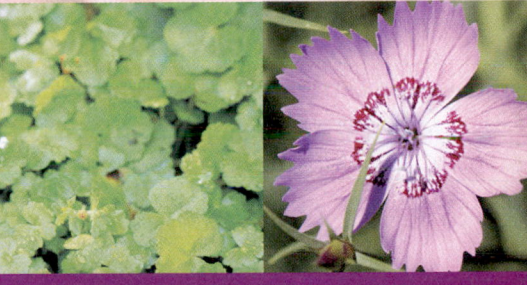

HEALTH PROMOTION ISSUE: Woman at Risk for Premature Labor

NURSING PROCESS CARE PLAN: Stressful Family Situation

CRITICAL THINKING CARE MAP: Caring for a Child Following Divorce of His Parents

LEARNING Outcomes

After completing this chapter, you will be able to:

- Describe family assessment techniques such as genogram and ecomap.
- Describe the effect of cultural and religious beliefs on family functioning.
- Describe the characteristics of family systems.
- Describe the normal changes a family undergoes over time.
- Describe the characteristics of a family under stress.
- Identify the role of the LPN/LVN in family assessment and care.
- Apply the nursing process to care of the family.

When planning care for the individual client, it is also important to consider the needs of the family. This is most obvious in the areas of maternal/infant care, pediatrics, geriatrics, and mental health. **Family-centered care** is treatment to a designated client with recognition that the family system or unit may also need intervention. The LPN/LVN must have a basic understanding of how a family functions and how to assess that functioning. The LPN/LVN must be able to identify characteristics of families under stress and understand when to seek assistance and guidance from the supervising registered nurse.

The Family Unit

What is a **family**? The classic definition of family is two or more people related by blood or marriage who reside together. In recent years, the definition has been broadened to two or more individuals who come together for the purpose of nurturing. The structure of families traditionally is linked to the relationship between parent and child, between spouses, or both.

NUCLEAR FAMILY

The traditional family type is the **nuclear family**, consisting of parents and biologic offspring. At one time, the majority of nuclear families in America were made up of a married father and mother with two to four children. The father was the breadwinner, working 9:00 A.M. to 5:00 P.M. to provide for his family. The mother remained at home, caring for the children and completing the household chores.

EXTENDED FAMILY

The **extended family** was traditionally described as a network of relatives including grandparents, aunts, uncles, and cousins who lived within a 50-mile radius and took an active role in the emotional support of the family. Some families now include close friends as part of their extended family unit. Individuals may even consider pets as vital family members. It is important to remember that the family, not the nurse or society, identifies its members (Figure 3-1 ■).

Today, the makeup of the family is changing. For reasons of employment, income, or living conditions, nuclear families have moved away from extended families. This dividing of the family structure is believed by many social scientists to be the cause of the breakdown of American society. This book does not address global issues of family functioning. Instead, the functioning of the family in neighborhoods or communities is the focus.

SINGLE-PARENT FAMILY

Today, we see many types of families. With the high divorce rate and an increasing number of unwed mothers, single-parent families are becoming more commonplace. In a **single-parent family**, either a mother or a father raises the children alone. There may be support from extended family, but the second parent does not play an active role.

OTHER FRAMEWORKS FOR FAMILY

The rise in the divorce rate since the mid-1950s has meant that a majority of children do not spend their developing years in nuclear families. Some divorced parents maintain shared custody of children, essentially splitting the child's time between two homes and parents.

When parents remarry, they find themselves in a stepfamily situation, or blended family. The term **blended family** describes a situation in which one or both spouses have had a previous marriage and children from that marriage (Figure 3-2 ■). Blending of families can cause major changes for children in the midst of other developmental challenges. Often, the blending of families brings greater financial and emotional stability to a family, as well as "ready-made" siblings. The struggle to become a larger functioning family can encourage tolerance and understanding. Occasionally, however, the blending of families results in child abuse (when new parents and children clash) or in sexual abuse (by the new parent or a stepbrother or stepsister). The nurse needs to be aware of the potential for these situations.

There is an increase in the number of families in which grandparents are raising their grandchildren. Guardians, foster care, and adoptions provide a family for almost 2 million children in this country.

Interracial families are an ever-growing part of family groupings. In 2000, nearly 7 million Americans of all ages were identified as more than one race.

Unmarried partners with or without children form a large number of families. In the 2000 census in the United States, the number of these families had increased 72% in the previous decade (including same-sex and heterosexual couples).

The final family type is the **communal family.** This family includes adults and children who may or may not be related. In this type of family, family decisions and responsibilities are shared. A communal family should not be confused with a **cult family**, a group in which a leader makes all decisions and controls the actions of those who live there.

Theoretical Framework for Working with Families

As stated in Chapter 1 ⚭ of this book, theory guides nursing practice. As part of community-based nursing practice, family theories and culture theories are used to determine the health of the family unit. This section briefly examines several theories that are beneficial in understanding and assessing the family functioning.

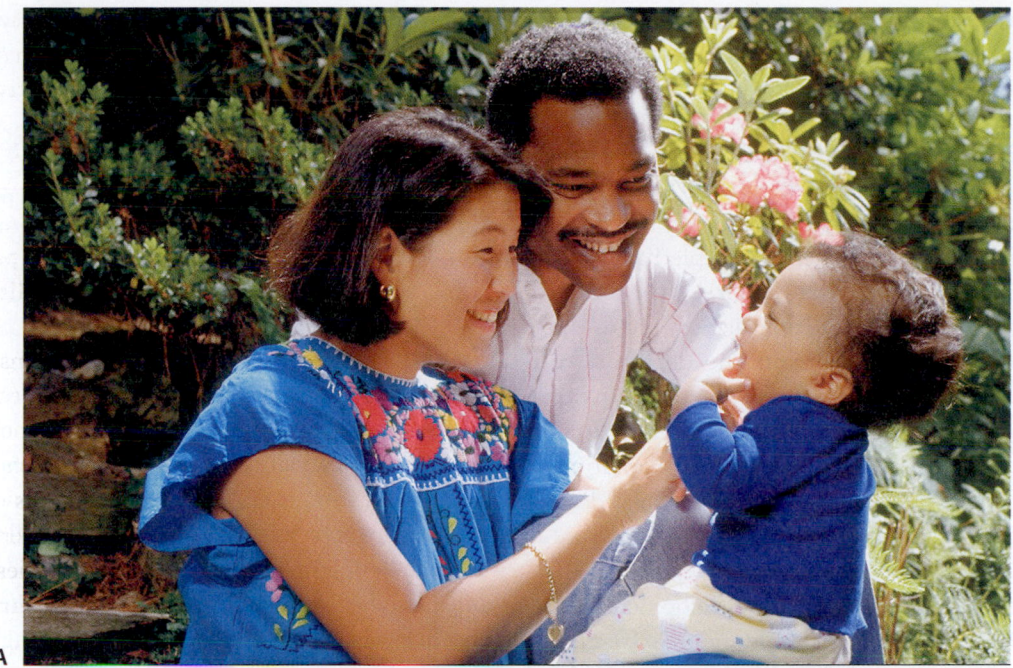

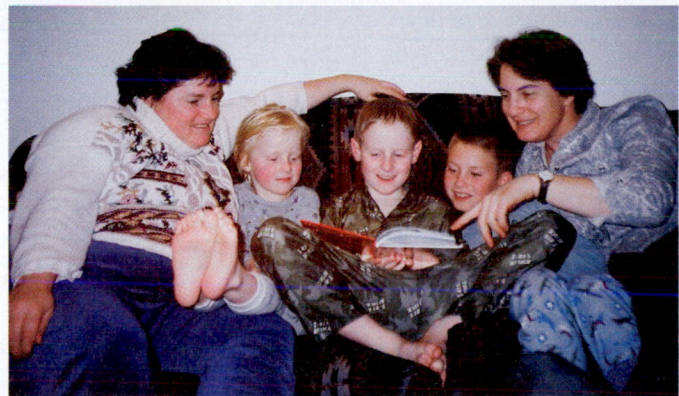

Figure 3-1. ■ (A) Families come in many different sizes, racial or gender mixtures, and types. (B) Evidence indicates that children raised in a homosexual family are at no greater developmental or dysfunctional risk than children raised in a heterosexual family (Ariel and McPherson, 2000). (Source: A. Lawrence Migdale/ Lawrence Migdale/Pix.)

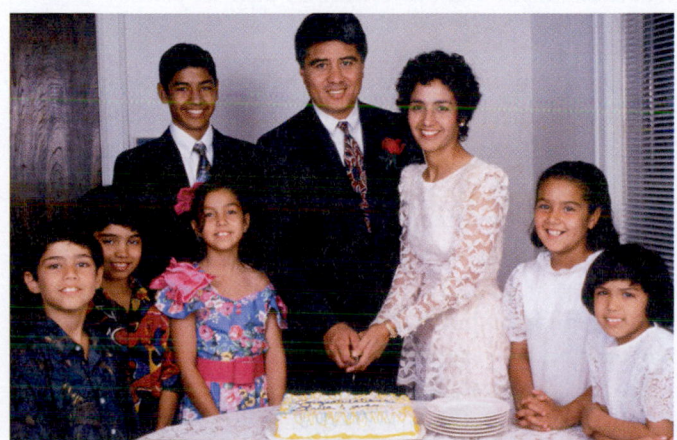

Figure 3-2. ■ Blended families are a regular part of U.S. culture in the 21st century. (Source: M. Bridwell\PhotoEdit Inc.)

FAMILY SYSTEMS THEORY

In **family systems theory,** the family system maintains a flexible boundary with the world. Boundary maintenance is healthy when the family can adjust the boundary to the needs of its members. For example, at times the family allows friends to visit, have dinner, and interact with the family members. At other times, friends are not allowed to participate in family business. The family chooses when to allow friends into the interaction and when to keep them out.

How well the family changes when faced with problems is called **adaptability.** A family that has an open boundary is able to adapt to problems by accepting new ideas. It can reach out for help from available resources. The family that has a closed boundary resists input and has more difficulty adapting to change. When illness occurs, a closed family's stress increases because it is forced to allow health care providers to participate in family decisions. Even when the family as a whole is not closed, the nurse needs to understand that some family members may need time to adjust to help from an "outsider."

FAMILY DEVELOPMENT THEORY

Family development theory describes the changes the family undergoes over time. Family restructuring will occur several times over the parents' life span. People have children and form a family knowing that, in time, the children will leave the home. With the addition of each child, the death of grandparents or parents, and the departure of grown children, the family unit changes. The flexibility of boundaries here, although stressful, is expected. The maturing of the family unit brings strength through adaptation. The mature family may be better prepared to make decisions than the young family; therefore, it may need less assistance from the nurse.

For the individual to have a healthy development, the family must progress through predictable stages of a family life cycle. Table 3-1 ■ provides a snapshot of stages in the family life cycle. By being familiar with each stage of development, the practical or vocational nurse can assess the family more accurately and report areas of concern.

CULTURE THEORY

Culture theory describes factors of culture that should be considered when working with families. These factors include:

- Communication
- Space
- Time
- Role.

Communication

Communication can be problematic when the nurse is working with families of a different cultural background. We know that communication includes verbal language and dialect. Yet, more of what we "mean" is expressed nonverbally through touch, gestures, eye contact, and volume of speech than through words themselves. (Consider the rolled-up eyes and sarcastic tone a teenager might use with the words "thanks a lot!" when a parent will not let him use the family car.)

Expression and interpretation of communication vary from culture to culture. For example, a person who is raised in a family with Japanese ancestry might not be comfortable speaking loudly or requesting more analgesics, even when in pain. In contrast, a person from a Mediterranean culture might be quite vocal, both about the pain and about the need for more medication. The nurse who cares for these clients must be able to perceive the differences in the ways they communicate. Otherwise, the nurse might

miss the needs of the first client and feel "yelled at" by the second.

clinical ALERT

Nursing measures that comfort one person may seem intrusive or wrong to another. The best way for you to know what the client wants is to ask.

Space

Personal space and feelings of territory are developed in a cultural setting. Although the environment can have an impact on personal space, the need to have some personal space is consistent. For example, the person living in a two-room apartment with 10 other people still has a need for a small area in which to keep belongings. Personal space also includes the area around the individual. Invading personal space or moving someone's personal belongings decreases a sense of security and causes stress.

Time

The element of time varies greatly among cultures. Members of a cultural group may be past, present, or future oriented. Those who focus on the past generally work to maintain traditions. They may have difficulty setting goals. Those who focus on the present may also have difficulty setting goals and may not save for the future. Those who focus on the future will put off rewards and work today to accomplish future goals.

The importance each member of the family places on time can have a great effect on health care decisions. For example, the family who is focused on the past may not bring a child to the clinic for immunizations to prevent future illness. The family who is focused on the present may be late to an office visit because a good friend dropped by. The family who is working for future goals may have difficulty dealing with a family crisis that causes them to move away from their set plans.

Role

The family **role** (expectations or behaviors associated with position in the family, e.g., mother, father, grandparent, child) is affected by the family's culture. Distinct roles based on gender may be stressed by the culture and are taught to the children. For example, in some cultures the husband makes all decisions for each family member. When pregnancy occurs, the husband would decide between breastfeeding or bottle feeding. These roles may conflict with the health care provider's expectation that clients will make decisions for themselves.

Cultural family groups are also an important consideration in planning and implementing family-centered care. In the United States, there are four main cultural groups:

TABLE 3-1

Stages of Family Development

STAGE	FAMILY TASKS	FAMILY ROLES	PARENTAL TASKS AND CLIENT TEACHING
I. Beginning family (no children)	■ Learning to live together ■ Relating harmoniously to three families (families of origin and newly established family) ■ Family planning (whether to have children) ■ Satisfactory sexual and marital role adjustment	Husband Wife Parent of adults In-laws	**Tasks:** Partners establish patterns of communication and problem solving. Roles at work and home are set. **Teaching:** Nurses should use every opportunity to encourage open, healthy communication techniques. For example, this formula can be used for discussing conflicts: "When _____ [something happens], I feel _____ because _____." It is much easier to problem solve with a statement like, "When the kitchen counter gets left messy, I feel frustrated because I have to clear a place to make my sandwich," than with a blaming statement like this, "You always leave messes around so that I'll have to clean them up!"
II. Early childbearing (birth of first child until infant reaches 30 months of age)	■ Develop a stable family unit with new parent roles ■ Reconciling conflicting developmental tasks of family members ■ Facilitating development needs of family members to strengthen the family unit ■ Accepting new child (children's) personality	Husband Wife Parent Child In-law Parent of adults Grandparent	**Tasks:** Bonding with the child. Learning to understand the child's cues. Supervising safety and development. Adjusting roles to fit new responsibilities. **Teaching:** Teach all caregivers (parents, siblings, grandparents) methods of holding, feeding, cleaning, and dressing. Identify actions, reflexes, appearance, and behavior that can be expected at each stage. Encourage a calm but watchful response to exploration.
III. Families with preschool children (first born 2½ to 5 years)	■ Child explores environment ■ Establish privacy, housing, and adequate space ■ Husband-father more involved in household responsibilities ■ Preschooler assumes responsibilities of self-care ■ Socialization of children ■ Integration of new family members ■ Separation from children as they enter school	Husband Wife Parent Child In-law Parent of adult Grandparent Sibling	**Tasks:** Accepting child's beginning independence. Supporting learning. Establishing behavioral norms. **Teaching:** Provide information about limit setting, "time-out" sessions, usual attention span of children (e.g., some suggest 1 minute of time-out per year of life as a guide). Stress the value of consistent expectations. Encourage "play groups" that can provide support for both the child and the parent. Support the parents as primary decision makers for their children.
IV. Family with school-age children (first born 6 to 13 years)	■ Promote school achievement of children ■ Maintain satisfying marital relationship ■ Promote open communication in family ■ Accept approaching adolescence	Husband Wife Parent Child In-law Parent of adult Grandparent Sibling	**Tasks:** Letting children participate consistently in group settings for education and socialization. **Teaching:** Teach that children need to learn from positive and negative experiences. The parents' role is not to ensure that the child always "feels good," but to help the child learn how to deal with life's ups and downs. The parent should guide

(continued)

TABLE 3-1

Stages of Family Development (continued)

STAGE	FAMILY TASKS	FAMILY ROLES	PARENTAL TASKS AND CLIENT TEACHING
			but should not make all decisions for the child. Grandparents can often provide useful support and perspective.
V. Families with teenagers	■ Maintain satisfying marital relationships while handling parental responsibilities ■ Maintain family ethical and moral standards while teens are searching for their own beliefs and values ■ Allow children to experiment with independence ■ Begin to become involved in care of aging parents	Husband Wife Parent Child In-law Parent of adult Grandparent Sibling Adolescent	**Tasks:** Recognizing the importance of peers. Allowing the child to make independent decisions and to accept the consequences of his or her actions. **Teaching:** Humor and empathy may be valuable when discussing changes in teens. Emphasize that teens are beginning to view the world through their own eyes, not as they have been taught to see it. Teach that some rejection of parental habits or life choices is normal and not always permanent.
VI. Launching center families (first child through last child leaving home)	■ Expand the family circle to include new members by marriage ■ Accept new couple's own lifestyle and values ■ Devote time to activities and relationships other than with children ■ Re-establish the wife-husband roles as children achieve independence ■ Assist aging and ill parents of husband and/or wife	Husband Wife Parent Child In-law Parent of adult Grandparent Sibling Young adult	**Tasks:** Assisting children to leave the parental home. Adapting to and incorporating people children choose as mates. Readjusting life in the home to fewer people. Parents beginning to take on some care of older generation. **Teaching:** Support parents to consider life problems in a broader perspective and to begin to plan for their future without children in the home and with needier parents.
VII. Families of middle years ("empty nest" period through retirement)	■ Maintain a sense of well-being psychologically and physiologically by living in a healthy environment ■ Attain and enjoy a career or other creative accomplishments by cultivating leisure time activities and interests ■ Sustain satisfying and meaningful relationships with aging parents and children ■ Adopt new role of grandparent ■ Sometimes provide housing and/or support for a grown child who returns home	Husband Wife Parent Child In-law Parent of adult Grandparent Grandchild Sibling Young adult Great-grandparent	**Tasks:** Finding mutually acceptable ways to keep connected with grown children. Being caring listeners while respecting that children will solve their own problems. Assisting grandparents to adapt to changes of old age or to death of spouse. **Teaching:** Support parents to separate from grown children and to explore their own interests. Encourage parents to seek information about activities they can enjoy independently of their children.
VIII. Families in retirement and old age (begins with retirement of one or both spouses, continues through loss of one spouse to death, and terminates with death of other spouse)	■ Maintain satisfying living and extended family relationships ■ Maintain marital relationship ■ Adjust to reduced income ■ Adjust to loss of spouse, family member, or friend	Husband Wife Parent Child In-law Parent of adult Grandparent of adult Grandchild Sibling Great-grandparent	**Tasks:** Welcoming grandchildren. Accepting children's lifestyle and choices. Accepting the loss of loved ones. **Teaching:** Encourage participation to create a bond with grandchildren. Encourage acceptance of differences and a focus on positive aspects of child or situation. Provide information on activities and support groups to keep the survivor from becoming isolated in his or her loss.

Rasa Latina, Asian Pacific, American Black, and Caucasian. Box 3-1 ■ provides some insight into these cultural groups. Detailed descriptions of all cultural and religious beliefs is not possible due to variance in different areas of the country. However, it is important for the nurse to become familiar with the cultural and religious beliefs of families in their immediate community. Family roles, views, and expectations may vary widely among these groups.

Cultural and religious beliefs have an impact on the interaction of family members. It is vital for the nurse to have an understanding of these beliefs and the importance the family places on them. **Culture** is a style of behavior patterns, beliefs, and *products of human work* (e.g., art, music, literature, architecture) within a given community or population. Patterns of behavior include dress, language, and patterns of person-to-person interaction. Beliefs include **religion,** the

---

BOX 3-1	CULTURAL PULSE POINTS

Major Cultural Groups and Traits

Rasa Latina Group

Rasa Latina families are those whose native language is Spanish and whose religion, most commonly, is Catholic. The family is led by a male head of the household, who is strong but distant, especially with father–son relationships. Mothers and daughters have a very close relationship. In the traditional family, the mother's role is to care for the home and children and to teach daughters to do the same. The Rasa-Latina family functions in the here and now. Customs, ethnic foods, and music are important, and they are passed on, especially during celebrations. The family may follow native health care practices rather than seeking medical care. This is frequently related to lack of access to medical care. Health care professionals frequently become frustrated with Rasa-Latina mothers who are reluctant to make health care decisions, especially for their children. Before she can make a decision, the Rasa-Latina woman must often discuss it with the head of the household. (Note: Modern Rasa Latina women are changing. Many are seeking education and job training. Attempts to increase their independence may cause resentment and family disruptions.)

Asian Pacific (or Pacific Rim) Group

The Asian Pacific or Pacific Rim group includes Japanese, Chinese, Vietnamese, Filipinos, Pacific Islanders, etc. These cultures do not have a common language or religion. The one common thread with this culture is the fact that they are not time limited. When Asian Pacific individuals speak of family, they are including many generations of ancestors. The family is a continuation of those who have gone before. An individual who brings shame upon him- or herself brings shame on the entire family. Many times a young Asian female who becomes pregnant prior to marriage may be reluctant to confide in her family because of the disgrace she perceives she has brought upon her family. When young people marry, they do not form a new family. Instead, the young wife is absorbed into the family of the new husband. Although the westernization of young Asian individuals has precipitated change, many families continue to arrange marriages. Health practices may involve Eastern medical treatment, with the acceptance of some alternative medical practices in this country. Asians are more comfortable using Western medicine along with their native health care practices. In the Asian Pacific family, the father is the head of the household. His main responsibility is providing for the family. Traditionally, he leaves all household and childrearing responsibilities to the wife. An Asian Pacific mother would seek medical care for the children and herself, and make decisions in this area independently.

American Black Group

The American Black (or African American) family is traditionally a matriarchal family. This is a result of husbands and fathers being separated from the family during the slavery period in the United States. Today there continues to be an alarming number of fatherless Black American families. This is especially true in lower socioeconomic areas. Middle-class Black American families are frequently two-parent families. Many of them also are two-income families. Black American children often have the advantage of care by extended family members. Children contribute to the household early on by learning to do chores. They often seek employment as soon as they are of age. Family, as well as the church, is the center of the Black American family social support system. Health-seeking behaviors in the lower socioeconomic area continue to be a problem. Access is difficult, and many Black American children are without a primary health care provider. In many urban areas, hospital emergency rooms have become the primary provider for Black children. This fact is frightening when it is noted that the highest infant mortality rates in this country are in three of our largest urban areas (Philadelphia, Detroit, and Washington, DC).

Caucasian Group

The Caucasian family in the United States has changed dramatically since the mid-1970s. Once the middle-class family was provided for by the husband and father, and the mother was the homemaker and primary caregiver for the children. Now, a second income is often required, and child care is provided outside the home. Caucasian women are better educated than other groups and often seek a career. Women are no longer completely dependent on the status of their husbands. For Caucasians, the "American dream" not only includes a house and one or more cars, but also health care. Good health care is viewed as a right by middle-class White families. They also believe that health care should be paid for by their employer and that they should have a choice in who delivers the care. Caucasian workers may turn down a career opportunity because of benefits that do not equal those of the present job. The white American family differs from other family groups in that individual needs frequently take precedence over the needs of the family.

Source: Ramont, R. R., Niedringhaus, D. M., & Towle, M. A. (2006). *Comprehensive nursing care.* Upper Saddle River, NJ: Prentice Hall.

belief in a superhuman power recognized as creator or governor of the universe, and other ideas accepted as true or factual.

An understanding of cultural background can give clues to assessment and implementation of care. The nurse must be careful not to engage in **stereotyping** (expectation that all members of a group will think and behave the same). This kind of generalized thinking is not appropriate.

Ethnicity is identity based on common ancestry, race, religion, and culture. Ethnicity is deeply rooted in the family and is transmitted by family values. For example, food preparation and family recipes are handed down from generation to generation. Religious beliefs influence food preparation and avoidance. The specific combination of seasoning, cooking, and presenting the food is part of the family's ethnicity.

Race should not be confused with ethnicity. **Race** is defined by biologic deviations shown in physical features, such as skin color, hair texture, and facial features. People of one race can have different cultures and ethnicity. For example, the Black race living in the African rain forest differs in culture and ethnicity from the Black race living in the southern United States.

The LPN/LVN must be observant of the family's environment, take clues offered by family interactions, and ask direct questions to identify specific aspects of the family's culture and religious beliefs. By being aware of the family's culture and religion, care planning and implementation can better meet the needs of the client and the family.

Roles and Functions of the Family

The functions of the family are to:

- Provide economic support for other family members.
- Satisfy emotional needs for love and security.
- Provide a sense of place and position in society.

Roles play an important part in healthy family functioning. Clear family roles within a family are directly connected to the family's ability to deal with day-to-day life.

Individual members occupy specific roles. As family members mature, they take on new roles. Children grow, mature, leave home, marry, and become parents. Parents become grandparents. A person's role is always expanding or changing, depending on age and family stage. Family expectations are closely connected to roles. Parents are expected to teach, discipline, and provide for their children. Children are expected to cooperate with and respect their parents.

Parenting styles play an important part in family expectations. There are two important factors to consider when analyzing parenting styles.

- **Demandingness,** which relates to the demands that parents make on the children, their expectations for mature

TABLE 3-2			
Parenting Styles			
STYLE	CONTROL	WARMTH	DESCRIPTION
Authoritative	High	High	Give-and-take communication; clear expectations for behavior. Children are mature, resilient, and achievement oriented. "We can talk about it."
Authoritarian	High	Low	Highly directive, value obedience. Children show lower internalization of prosocial values and ego development. "Because I said so."
Permissive	Low	High	Parents make few demands, allow children to regulate self, and avoid confrontation of behavior. "Do whatever you want."

Source: Ramont, R. R., Niedringhaus, D. M., & Towle, M. A. (2006). *Comprehensive nursing care.* Upper Saddle River, NJ: Prentice Hall.

behavior, the discipline and supervision they provide, and their willingness to confront behavioral problems

- **Responsiveness,** which relates to how much parents foster individuality, self-assertion, and self-regulation, and how responsive they are to special needs and demands

Table 3-2 ■ lists types and descriptions of some parenting styles.

Family Assessment Techniques and Tools

ASSESSMENT OF RELATIONSHIPS

As described in Chapter 4 ⊙⊙ of this book, each family member is continually growing and developing. The stage of growth and development of these members needs to be identified and recorded so appropriate care can be given.

Family assessment is an ongoing process of examining the relationships and functioning of family members. These relationships need to be identified in order to understand the individual family.

The first step in family assessment is to ask the client to identify the members of the family and their relationships to each other. To do this, a genogram is often used. A **genogram** is a diagram of relationships among family members. Figure 3-3 ■ illustrates an uncomplicated genogram. Symbols are used to represent family members. For example, a square is used for males, and a circle is used for females. The client is identified by a double circle or square. Small marks inside the circle or square represent deceased members. Straight lines are used to identify the relationships. Slash marks represent broken relationships, such as separation and divorce. A dotted line is drawn around all members living in the same household. As more information is learned about the family members, it is added to the genogram.

The second step in family assessment is to develop an **ecomap.** An ecomap provides a diagram of family member interactions with the immediate environment. Figure 3-4 ■ shows an uncomplicated ecomap. The family is located in the center with significant people, organizations, and agencies placed in circles around the family. Different lines are used to show relationships between family members and those outside influences. Straight lines represent strong relationships, dotted lines represent tenuous relationships, and slashed lines represent stressful or conflicted relationships.

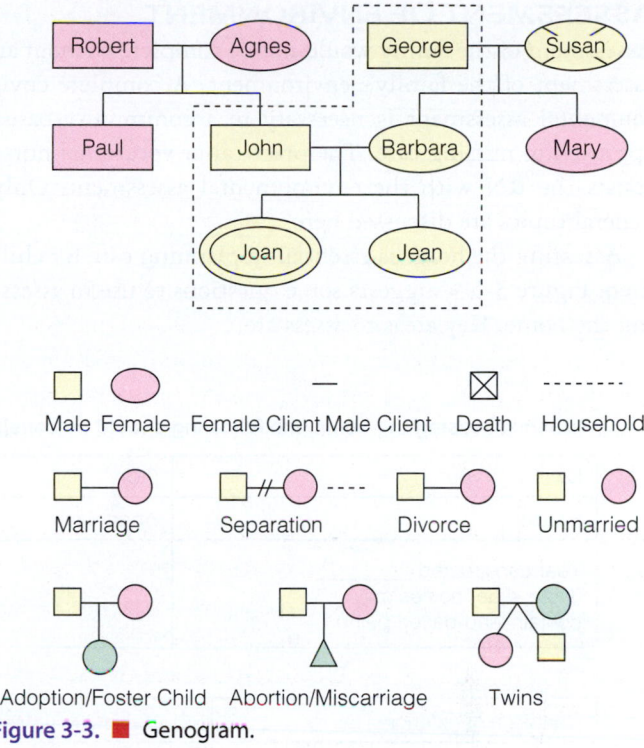

Figure 3-3. ■ Genogram.

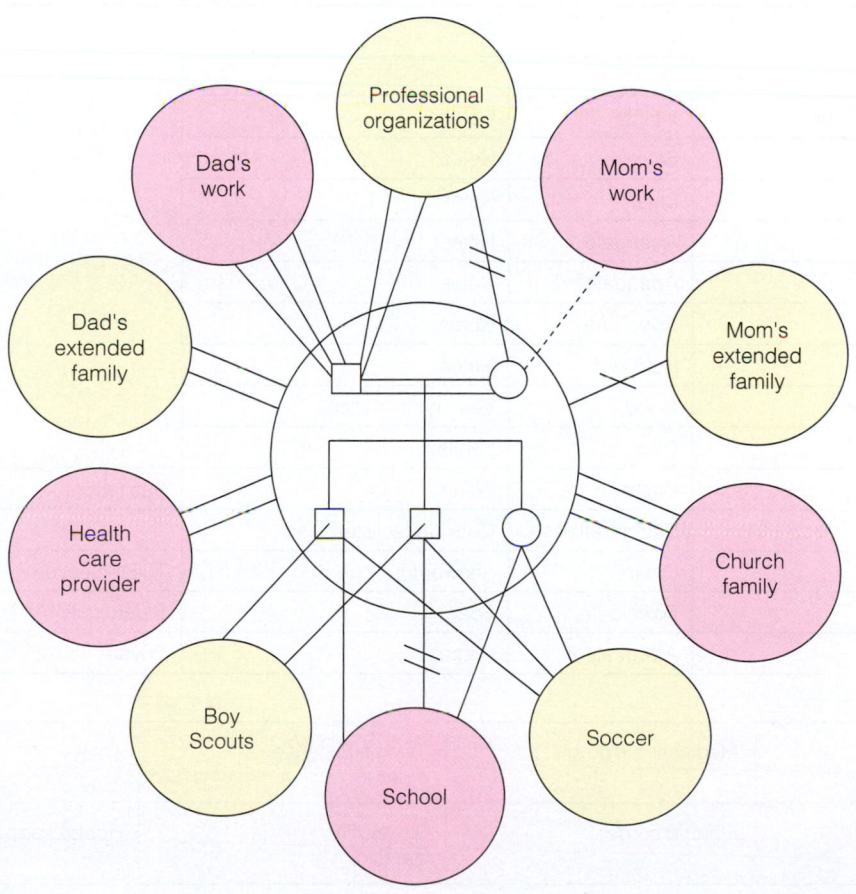

Figure 3-4. ■ Ecomap.

ASSESSMENT OF ENVIRONMENT

Assessment of the family would not be complete without an assessment of the family's environment. A complete environmental assessment is necessary in a community-based approach to nursing care. The practical or vocational nurse assists the RN with the environmental assessment. Only general topics are discussed here.

Assessing the home is essential in planning care for children. Figure 3-5 ■ suggests some questions to use in assessing the home. Key areas to assess are:

- Condition of housing, both inside and outside
- Availability of sanitary conditions, running water, toilet facilities, and garbage disposal
- Kitchen area, including cooking and refrigeration facilities
- Sleeping arrangements for each member of the family
- Presence or absence of safety hazards.

Certain aspects of the neighborhood or community must also be assessed. Figure 3-6 ■ offers sample questions used to assess the neighborhood. The major topics to examine here are:

When assessing the home, the following should be considered.

Dwelling Type	Own:		Rent:	
House	Apartment		# Bedrooms	
Year constructed _____ (Note: older homes may contain lead-based paint)				

Condition of Exterior				
Paint/Siding	Intact	Detached	Flaking/peeling
Yard	Clean/trimmed	Unkempt	Fenced
Hazards	Sand box	Play equipment	Swimming pool

Condition of Interior			
Paint	Intact	Flaking	
Furnishings	Safe	Notes:	
Floors/stairs/railing	Safe	Notes:	
Heating/cooling	Adequate	Notes:	
Lighting	Adequate	Notes:	
Telephone access	Adequate	Notes:	
Water supply	Hot/Cold	Notes:	
Cleanliness/sanitation	Good	Vermin infestation	
Pets	Clean	Sanitation	
Kitchen	Clean	Water	Sanitation
	Refrigeration	Cooking facilities	
Bathroom	Clean	Shower/tub	Toilet function
	Towels	Soap	Safety rails
Bedrooms	Adequate #	Clean	Private

SAFETY ISSUES	Medication storage	Toxic substance storage	Toys
	Electric cords	Smoke/fire detector	Hobby supplies

Figure 3-5. ■ Home assessment.

In assessing the neighborhood or community, the following should be considered.

Type of neighborhood	Rural	Suburban	Urban	Inner-city
Types of buildings	Residential	Agrarian	Industrial	Combined
Condition of buildings	Excellent	Good	Poor	Unsafe
Condition of streets	Paved Unpaved	Curbs	Sidewalks	Kept up Deteriorating
Traffic	Congested	Stop signs/ lights	Public transportation	
Environmental hazards	Soil	Air	Water	Noise
Population	Young families	Older families	Sparsely populated	Densely populated
Facilities available	Market Shopping	Church	School	Parks & playgrounds
Health care facilities	Doctor office Clinics	Hospital Long-term care	Home health	Other
Distance from home to health care facility				

Figure 3-6. ■ Neighborhood or community assessment.

- Availability of shopping for clothes and groceries
- Location of schools and churches
- Availability of health care, including doctors' offices, clinics, and hospitals
- Opportunities for employment.

The gathering of data in family assessment is quite time consuming. Relationships between family members and the environment change. Although the nurse might think the family is stable with working, healthy relationships, outside stressors can threaten the stability of the relationships.

The nurse will use active listening and therapeutic communication to obtain assessment data. At times, the nurse talks with individual members. At other times, group meetings are best in order to see family interaction. The nurse must always keep an open mind and a nonjudgmental attitude. The nurse's role is not to take sides or show preference to individuals, but rather to facilitate a move toward healthy relationships.

ASSESSMENT OF POTENTIAL ABUSE

The nurse, working with families, must be alert for signs of possible family violence. Family violence includes spousal abuse, child abuse and neglect, and elder abuse. While in the home, children learn behaviors they will practice as adults.

In homes where spousal or child abuse occurs, children grow up believing that this behavior is acceptable, and the cycle continues. Abusive parents may have a knowledge deficit about the needs of their children and how to meet these needs best. Abusive parents are often without a support system. They may be alone, angry, in crisis, or have unrealistic expectations.

Indicators of abuse may include:

- Changes in appointments with health care provider (increased appointments with vague somatic complaints or missed appointments)
- Depression, attempted suicide, self-directed abuse
- Severe anxiety, insomnia, violent nightmares
- Alcohol and/or drug abuse
- Unexplained bruising or other injuries.

Sample questions that need to be addressed during family assessment are included in Box 3-2 ■ on page 58. As you recall (see Chapter 2 ⚭), if the nurse suspects abuse or neglect, a report must be filed with law enforcement agencies. The LPN/LVN must also notify the supervising RN or health care provider. Complete documentation of the nurse's observations must be made in the client record. A more detailed description of child abuse is included in Chapter 27 ⚭.

HEALTH PROMOTION ISSUE

WOMAN AT RISK FOR PREMATURE LABOR

Peggy James, a 26-year-old African American, gravida 2, para 1, is seen in the obstetrician's office for her initial obstetric assessment. Ms. James' obstetric history reveals her last child was born 3 years ago at 32 weeks. This child was low birth weight and had difficulty with respiratory distress syndrome. He was hospitalized for 6 weeks. Peggy wants to avoid a premature baby this time if possible.

Ms. James' assessment further reveals the client is married. She did not finish high school and works 50 to 60 mandatory hours each week in a local factory where she stands on her feet for most of the day. She smokes one pack of cigarettes per day and does not drink alcohol or use illegal substances. Her prepregnancy weight is appropriate for her height. Her 24-hour diet recall reveals protein and calcium deficits.

DISCUSSION

What Is Prematurity?

Prematurity is a live birth prior to the completion of 37 weeks of pregnancy. When considering prematurity, low birth weight must also be considered. Low birth weight is defined as an infant who weighs less than 2,500 grams regardless of gestational age. The extremely low-birth-weight infant (ELBW) weighs less than 800 grams at birth regardless of gestational age.

In the United States, more than 476,000 infants (one in eight babies) are born prematurely each year. Approximately 10% of these infants die and about 25% will have a significant health problem. These health problems include respiratory distress syndrome (RDS), intraventricular hemorrhage (IVH), and necrotizing enterocolitis (NEC). The babies may also deal with lifelong complications such as respiratory illnesses, poor vision, poor hearing, cerebral palsy, and a host of developmental deficits.

Why Does Prematurity Occur?

According to Moos (2004), 25% of the cases of prematurity are due to iatrogenic causes. For, example, elective inductions may be performed based on inaccurate dating of the pregnancy. Twenty-five percent of the cases are due to premature rupture of membranes. The remaining 50% are due to idiopathic causes or spontaneous labor.

Researchers have studied this problem and have determined two methods for predicting preterm birth. These methods are fetal fibronectin (fFN) testing and transvaginal ultrasonographic assessment of cervical length. These tests have proven to be effective in determining which clients are unlikely to deliver prematurely, not which clients will deliver prematurely.

The fFN test measures the presence of fFN in a cervical mucous specimen. The fFN, a glycoprotein, is found between gestational weeks 16 and 20 and then again prior to birth. To obtain the appropriate specimen, a sterile speculum examination is performed, and a sample of vaginal and cervical fluids is obtained. The rapid fFN test provides results in 1 hour; the standard test pro-

vides results in 24 hours. This test is not used in a woman whose cervix is dilated more than 3 centimeters, has rupture of membranes, has had a vaginal examination in the last 24 hours, has a cervical cerclage, has placenta previa, has vaginal bleeding, or has had sexual intercourse in the last 24 hours.

Transvaginal ultrasonographic assessment of cervical length measures cervical length and width as well as the funneling or dilatation of the internal cervical os. Between 30% and 40% of clients with a shortened cervix give birth prematurely.

Who is at Risk for Premature Labor and Birth?

The following factors place a client at great risk for giving birth prematurely:

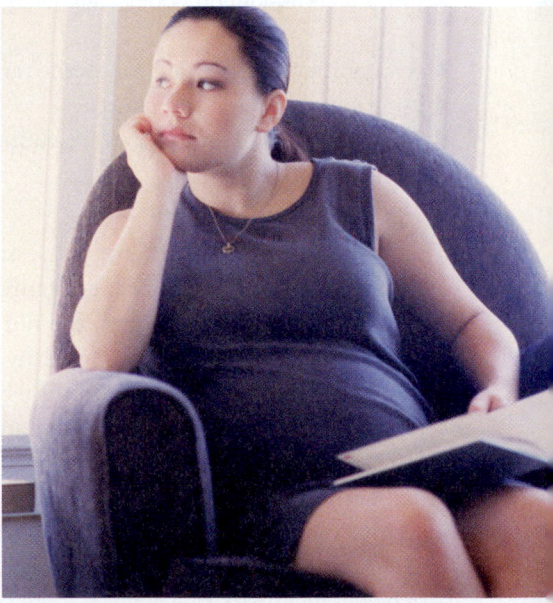

(Source: Geoff Manasse/Photodisc/Getty Images)

LPN/LVN Role in Family Care

The LPN's or LVN's role is to assist with data collection, report findings, and implement the written plan of care. For example, the practical or vocational nurse can assist in collecting information about family members and can diagram relationships on a genogram and ecomap. When interacting with family members, the nurse identifies healthy functioning patterns as well as characteristics of stress, documents this information, and reports observations to the registered nurse.

Medialink

Premature labor & birth

- African American ethnicity
- Age less than 17 or more than 34 years
- Low socioeconomic status
- Single-parent status
- Low educational level
- History of premature labor or birth
- Multiple abortions
- Parity 0 or more than 4
- Pre-existing diabetes or hypertension
- Multiple gestation
- Infections
- Incompetent cervix
- Placental irregularities such as placenta previa or placenta abruptio
- Anemia
- Premature rupture of membranes
- Exposure to toxins such as cigarette smoking, diethylstilbestrol, alcohol, other illicit drugs, or air pollution
- Poor nutritional status
- Domestic violence
- Lack of prenatal care
- Stress
- Long work hours. (Moos, 2004)

Premature labor can be prevented through prenatal education, smoking and alcohol cessation programs, assessment for domestic violence, continuous prenatal care, improved nutritional status, avoiding the use of illicit drugs, stress reduction, and prompt notification of signs and symptoms of premature labor.

PLANNING AND IMPLEMENTATION

It is important for the nurse to identify Ms. James' risks for prematurity. These would include her race, her history of a premature birth, low educational level, long work hours, stress, smoking, and poor nutritional status.

Ms. James most likely understands the risk of prematurity to her unborn child, but she may not understand how she can prevent it from recurring. The nurse can assist her in developing a plan for stress reduction. They should explore the option of changing her work assignment so it is not as physically taxing. If possible, she should reduce her hours or break them up and implement rest periods throughout the day.

The nurse should discuss with Ms. James the importance of smoking cessation. Referral to a program with identified success and regular follow-up would be of assistance.

The nurse can assist Ms. James in improving her nutritional status. Discuss with her sources of protein and calcium. She can assist her in meal and snack planning. If she needs financial assistance, the nurse should make the appropriate referrals.

Finally, the nurse must ensure that Ms. James is familiar with the symptoms of premature labor and understands the importance of seeking prompt medical attention if the symptoms occur. These symptoms include uterine contractions occurring every 10 minutes or more frequently, a low dull backache, stomach cramps that may or may not be accompanied by diarrhea, pelvic pressure, and increased vaginal discharge or fluid leaking from the vagina.

SELF-REFLECTION

Carefully consider your knowledge of the effects of prematurity. Do you consider this to be a problem related to only a specific population? Do you recognize the need to provide all pregnant women with teaching about the effects of prematurity and ways to prevent it? What type of community education could you provide for the nonpregnant woman to increase awareness of the problem of prematurity?

SUGGESTED RESOURCES

For the Nurse

Moos, M. (2004). Understanding prematurity: Sorting fact from fiction. *Lifelines, 8*(1), 33–37.

Bernhardt, J., & Dorman, K. (2004). Pre-term birth risk assessment tools: Exploring fetal fibronectin and cervical length for validating risk. *Lifelines, 8*(1), 38–45.

Preventing Premature Babies Chart Collection. Waco, TX: Childbirth Graphics. Retrieved June 29, 2006, from www.childbirthgraphics.com.

For the Client

- **www.marchofdimes.com** There are several client documents about premature labor and birth on the March of Dimes website.

- Sears, J., Sears, M., Sears, R. et al. (2004). The premature baby book: Everything you need to know about your premature baby from birth to age one. New York : Little, Brown.

Family Under Stress

Many factors can put stress on the family unit. Financial problems, drug and alcohol use, extramarital relationships, and chronic illness of family members are but a few. Dealing with stress can strengthen family ties and promote a healthy family unit, or it can cause additional stress and lead to a breakdown in family unity. The LPN/LVN helps identify signs of the unhealthy family unit and communicates this information to the caregiver in charge.

BOX 3-2 ASSESSMENT

Abuse in Women or Children

Actions Suggestive of Abuse in Adults

1. Inappropriate laughing
2. Crying
3. No eye contact (may be usual in some cultures)
4. Searching eye contact (look of "fear")
5. Comments about emotional abuse (of self or of "friend")

Questions for Pregnant Women

1. Are you in a relationship with a person who hurts you?
2. Does the person threaten to abuse you?
3. Has the person hit, slapped, kicked, or hurt you since you have been pregnant?
4. If yes, has the abuse increased since you became pregnant?
5. Do you know where you can go for help?

Actions Suggestive of Abuse in Children

1. Failure to thrive
2. Poor hygiene, unclean, inappropriate dress
3. Frequent injuries, unexplained injuries and bruising
4. Dull, inactive, passive behavior
5. Begging or stealing food
6. Frequent absences from school, poor or declining grades
7. Drug and/or alcohol abuse
8. Vandalism, shoplifting

Questions for Children

1. Has someone hurt you?
2. Did they hit, slap, kick, or hurt you in some other way?
3. Are you left alone?
4. Has someone touched you in your "private parts"?
5. How did your get this bruise (and other injuries)?

In most instances, parents use the same or similar strategies to reduce stress that their parents used. Healthy families tend to work together to reduce stress, whereas unhealthy families tend to become defensive and blame others for their problems. If individuals learn healthy strategies, they will use effective communication and problem-solving techniques to reduce stress and promote emotional stability. Unhealthy families, using ineffective communication and problem solving, place blame on others for their problems, causing those individuals to feel unwanted, unloved, and worthless. These negative feelings tend to block communication and lead to additional stress. Box 3-3 ■ lists some signs of an unhealthy family that should be reported to the charge nurse.

BOX 3-3 ASSESSMENT

Signs of an Unhealthy Family

The following signs of an unhealthy family should be reported to the registered nurse:

- Denial of problem(s)
- Active overt exploitation/scapegoating
- Use of threat
- Abandonment
- Drug or alcohol abuse
- Violence including
  - Spouse abuse
  - Child abuse
  - Sibling abuse
  - Elder abuse
  - Parent abuse
  - Gay/lesbian abuse

NURSING CARE

PRIORITIES IN NURSING CARE

When caring for individuals, remember to include family members as well. Focus your care on establishing a therapeutic relationship based on trust. Be careful to develop a nonthreatening, nonjudgmental attitude when family values and behaviors differ from yours. Use positive, supportive words of encouragement and provide a list of resources for family support.

ASSESSING

The practical or vocational nurse follows state nurse practice acts and facility policies to help the RN or care provider collect the individual's data and identify signs of healthy and unhealthy family units. LPNs and LVNs document and report findings to the registered nurse. They implement the plan of care to help the family achieve a healthier level of functioning.

DIAGNOSING, PLANNING, AND IMPLEMENTING

Families cope with health events together throughout their lives. They may be excitedly awaiting the birth of their first child. They may be trying to decide whether a family member should have surgery, chemotherapy, and/or radiation for cancer. They may be exhausted from years of caring for a chronically ill child or spouse.

Certain NANDA diagnoses that relate particularly to families are the following:

- Caregiver Role Strain
- Coping: Family (Compromised, Disabled, or Readiness for Enhanced)

- Family Process (Interrupted, Readiness for Enhanced)
- Parenting (Impaired, Readiness for Enhanced)
- Role Conflict, Parental
- Therapeutic Regimen Management: Family, Ineffective

Client outcomes for these diagnoses would address the particulars of the family situation. For example, a family with a chronically ill child with a worsening condition of cystic fibrosis may have a nursing diagnosis of Caregiver Role Strain. The nurse would be sure to inform the family of all groups and services that might be able to provide some support for the primary caregivers. In a new family in which the mother has just had a cesarean delivery, the nursing plan might indicate that the father is eager to learn to help (Readiness for Enhanced Parenting). The nurse could demonstrate diaper care and burping techniques to the father so the mother could get more rest.

Situations with Compromised Family Coping are more challenging for the nurse because they often involve working with family members who are in conflict. The movement from unhealthy to healthy functioning takes time and patience. Once the plan of care is established, all health care providers must be consistent in their approach to individual family members. For example, the nurse may observe a mother who continually tells a child he is "a brat" and "nothing but trouble." The nurse could suggest that the child might listen better if the parent focused on his good attributes and if the parent was specific and matter of fact when correcting undesirable behaviors. The practical/vocational nurse, working with families in the care of the maternal or pediatric client, has the opportunity and responsibility to promote a healthier family unit.

Nursing interventions could include the following.

- Provide instructions (on topics specific to the situation). *An important role of LPNs and LVNs is teaching. In stressful situations such as health crises, it is useful to repeat or explain information that has been given. This may allow the family to ask questions about the disorder or about treatment options. If nurses do not know the answer, they can either obtain it and tell the family or refer the family to the appropriate professional.*
- Provide a list of support groups and agencies. *Continuity of care includes having information about follow-up after leaving the facility.*
- Support the family in decision-making processes. *The nurse provides information, answers questions, encourages the family to explore options, and shows respect for family processes and decisions.*
- Observe family relationships, watching for signs of abuse. *Thankfully, abuse is not common. However, the nurse must be vigilant in noting injuries or actions that suggest abuse may have occurred.*

clinical ALERT

Signs of abuse or neglect must be reported to law enforcement agencies.

EVALUATING

Working from the care plan laid out for the family, the LPN/LVN would ask questions to determine whether desired outcomes had been met. Progress and unmet outcomes are documented and reported as necessary. The nurse would report any suspicions of abuse to the appropriate agency (see Chapter 2 ⬭).

DISCHARGE CONSIDERATIONS

The nurse should ensure the client and family are prepared for discharge. The new mother must be given instruction in both self-care and infant care. The parents (or care providers) will need home care instructions specific to the care of the individual child. Printed information should include:

- Use, action, and side effects of medication
- Use and care of any equipment
- Signs of complications that need to be reported to the health care provider
- The date and time of follow-up appointments
- Name, address, and phone number of any referral agency (WIC, abuse shelters, counseling services, etc.).

Documentation of client's and family's understanding of instructions should be included in the client chart.

NURSING PROCESS CARE PLAN
Stressful Family Situation

Jean, a 5-year-old girl, was injured in a motor vehicle crash on June 10. She sustained a ruptured spleen, a compound fracture of her left arm, and a traumatic amputation of the left leg. Her parents and baby sister were also in the crash but received only minor injuries. The nurse is preparing the client for discharge.

Assessment.   The following data should be collected:

- Family knowledge of extent of traumatic event
- Family knowledge of care necessary for family member
- Coping mechanisms used by the family
- Support systems available to the family
- Resources available to the family.

Nursing Diagnosis.   The following important nursing diagnosis (among others) is established for this client:

- Compromised Family Coping related to traumatic event

Expected Outcome.   Family members will identify the effect of the traumatic event on the family unit and identify resources to assist with coping.

Planning and Implementation

- Assess past family coping to include strengths and weaknesses. *Past coping is a predictor of future coping.*

- Identify symptoms of family stress to include fatigue, insomnia, and depression. *Stress symptoms would further compromise family coping.*
- Identify support system and outside resources available to the family. *Support and resources assist with coping. Lack of support and resources compromise family coping.*
- Assist the family in developing a plan for coping with the traumatic event. *The nurse provides suggestions and resources, and then supports the family's decisions in coping with the traumatic event.*
- Offer assistance in contacting resources if accepted by the family. *Following periods of illness or trauma, families usually require outside assistance in managing these events.*

Evaluation. Parents were instructed in care of the wound and given written information about signs of infection or other reasons to contact the physician. Follow-up visits were scheduled. Parents were provided with referrals for physical therapy, occupational therapy, and an amputees' support group. Parents reported that their church would provide dinners for the family for the first 2 weeks.

Critical Thinking in the Nursing Process

1. What information would be important to include in an ecomap for this family?
2. In assessing the family home, what areas would be most important?
3. What community or neighborhood resources should be assessed and included in Jean's care?

Note: Discussion of Critical Thinking questions appears in Appendix I.

Note: The references and resources for this and all chapters have been compiled at the back of the book.

Chapter Review

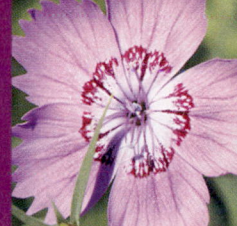

 **KEY TERMS** by Topic

Use the audio glossary feature of either the CD-ROM or the Companion Website to hear the correct pronunciation of the following key terms.

Introduction
family-centered care

The Family Unit
family, nuclear family, extended family, single-parent family, blended family, communal family, cult family

Theoretical Framework for Working with Families
family systems theory, adaptability, family development theory, culture theory, role, culture, religion, stereotyping, ethnicity, race

Roles and Functions of the Family
demandingness, responsiveness

Family Assessment Techniques and Tools
family assessment, genogram, ecomap

KEY Points

- The LPN or LVN who works with families in an acute-care setting or home/community setting must be alert for signs of healthy and unhealthy family functioning.

- Tools such as a genogram and ecomap are useful in assessing the family.

- Cultural and religious beliefs affect the functioning of the family members.

- By understanding the characteristics of family systems, the nurse can more accurately assess family functioning.

- The family develops and changes over time.

- Identifying the characteristics of the family under stress enables the nurse to make appropriate referrals.

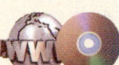 **EXPLORE MediaLink**

Additional interactive resources for this chapter can be found on the Companion Website at www.prenhall.com/towle.

Click on Chapter 3 and "Begin" to select the activities for this chapter.

For chapter-related NCLEX-style questions and an audio glossary, access the accompanying CD-ROM in this book.

Animations

Defining family

What is cultural competence?

FOR FURTHER Study

For a complete discussion on community-based nursing practice, see Chapter 1.

For information about reporting abuse, see Chapter 2.

Growth and development of the family is described in Chapter 4.

For signs of abuse, see Chapter 27.

Critical Thinking Care Map

Caring for a Child Following Divorce of His Parents
NCLEX-PN® Focus Area: Health Promotion and Maintenance

Case Study: Ms. Jacobs brings her 7-year-old son, Sam, to the pediatrician's office. She reports that he is not eating, sleeps frequently, complains of a stomachache daily, and refuses to go to school. Ms. Jacobs reports that she and her husband have recently finalized their divorce. She and her ex-husband are finding it difficult to be civil to one another. Sam is living with her but seeing his father weekly, sometimes spending several nights at his father's house. His father has a girlfriend who also spends the night.

Nursing Diagnosis: Interrupted Family Processes related to divorce

COLLECT DATA

Subjective	Objective
_____	_____
_____	_____
_____	_____
_____	_____
_____	_____
_____	_____

Would you report this? Yes/No

If yes, to: _____

Nursing Care

_____
_____
_____
_____
_____
_____
_____
_____
_____
_____

How would you document this? _____
_____
_____
_____

Compare your documentation to the sample provided in Appendix I.

Data Collected
(use those that apply)

- Weight 35 pounds
- Bowel sounds active in all four quadrants
- No masses or tenderness noted following light abdominal palpation
- Complaint of daily stomachache
- Sleeping 10 hours plus a 2.5-hour nap daily
- Refuses to go to school
- Parents recently divorced
- Parental relationship strained
- Some days spent with mother, some spent with father
- Father has new female relationship
- Pulse 55 bpm
- Sam's responses barely audible
- Dark circles under eyes

Nursing Interventions
(use those that apply; list in priority order)

- Assist the family in setting realistic goals
- Encourage the use of stimulation to keep Sam awake during the day
- Refer to community resources as needed
- Encourage Sam and his mother to express concerns and fears
- Explore negative feelings of anger, worry, sorrow, etc.
- Evaluate family strengths and weaknesses
- Administer antidepressant as ordered
- Encourage each family member to try to understand the other's feelings

NCLEX-PN® Exam Preparation

1 John's and Denise's 6-month-old son has been diagnosed with cystic fibrosis. In assessing the dynamic of this family, the nurse completes a genogram. This assessment tool is useful in:

1. understanding the family member's relationships in the community.
2. understanding the relationships of family members.
3. identifying the genetic link for cystic fibrosis.
4. identifying the physical characteristics of family members.

2 The Gilbert family of five is new to the area. They have come to the health clinic for an introductory visit. To understand each family member's relationship to the community, the nurse would complete the assessment tool called a

_____.

3 A Chinese family is in the United States as tourists when their 10-year-old daughter develops appendicitis and requires emergency surgery. The emergency room nurse notes that the child's mother never makes eye contact with the doctor. The nurse should:

1. request that the woman look at the doctor when spoken to.
2. understand the behavior is consistent with her culture.
3. ignore the mother and ask the doctor to speak with the father.
4. determine that this behavior could indicate guilt over child abuse and contact social services.

4 A pediatric client is discharged following an acute episode of muscular dystrophy. You have been asked by the RN to make a home visit and collect data for an environmental assessment. Choose the assessments that would be appropriate.

1. lawn maintenance
2. condition of the floors
3. exterior color
4. number of televisions and their locations
5. availability of hot and cold water

5 Jana Ricketts has leukemia. Mrs. Ricketts says to you, "I just need to pray with my minister in order to make Jana well." The most appropriate response would be:

1. "The medicine ordered by the doctor will make Jana well."
2. "Why do you think only prayer will make her well?"
3. "May I call her minister for you?"
4. "When Jana goes home, you can take her to church."

6 It is important to be aware of a family's religion and culture because:

1. differences in care should not be based on culture or religion.
2. aspects of care might be adapted to meet cultural and religious beliefs.
3. reimbursement is based on cultural and religious beliefs.
4. some cultures and religious groups are more numerous than others.

7 Which of the following statements would indicate the family is coping well and does not need additional help?

1. "People tell us we need help since the death of our children, but we are fine."
2. "It is nice having Aunt Sue and Uncle Ben living so close. We talk with them daily, and they have been so supportive."
3. "If my wife had been home like a good wife should be, the house would not have burned down! It is her fault!"
4. "Look missy, you might be 16, but I'm your dad and if you try sneaking out again, you won't live to be 17. Do you hear me?"

8 If the LPN/LVN suspects the family is under undue stress, he or she should:

1. set up a meeting with a family counselor.
2. meet with the family as a group to solve the problem.
3. tell the supervising RN.
4. ignore the problem; it is not an LPN/LVN concern.

9 A mother and father ask the nurse why she is so interested in how their family functions. The nurse responds:

1. "I'm very interested in the differences among families. I like to compare notes."
2. "I have a responsibility to identify factors that might affect the health of a child."
3. "I have a legal responsibility to search out illegal behavior and alert the police."
4. "I am the only person trained to search out wrongdoing."

10 An LPN/LVN, caring for a child with a progressive terminal illness, is looking for local resources to help a family that needs financial support. Choose the interventions that would be appropriate.

1. Perform a web search.
2. Look in the local yellow pages.
3. Contact social services.
4. Take a quick survey of other patients.
5. Consult with the registered nurse.

Answers for Review Questions, as well as discussion of Care Plan and Critical Thinking Care Map questions, appear in Appendix I.

Thinking Strategically About...

You are an LPN/LVN employed by a home health agency. At 0800, you arrive at the office to receive your assignment. You are expected to visit the clients on your assignment and report to the supervising RN by telephone. You can organize your time as you choose. The clients are all within a 3-mile radius from the home health agency office.

The first client, Jenny, is a 3-year-old who suffered a near drowning 6 months ago. She has severe neurologic damage and is in a persistent vegetative state. Her family provides all necessary care in their home with the help of a certified nursing assistant (CNA). A nurse visits on a weekly basis to evaluate the child's condition and make any necessary changes in the care plan.

Your second client is 18-year-old Marie. She delivered her first baby, Jason, 3 days ago. She is not married, has limited financial resources, and has few close friends. She was discharged from the hospital yesterday. She requested a visit from the home health nurse because she has never taken care of a baby and is unsure of herself.

Your third client is Juan, a 13-year-old who received a spinal cord injury in a car crash. Juan is being transferred from the hospital's surgical unit to the rehabilitation unit. The plan is for Juan to go home in approximately 6 weeks. The home health agency where you are employed will be providing home visits at that time. In preparation for Juan's discharge, the house and yard need to be assessed for safety and accommodation for Juan's wheelchair and other equipment necessary for his care. You are to go to Juan's home and complete a home assessment that will be used in a planning session this afternoon with Juan's family, rehabilitation personnel, and the home health supervisor.

CRITICAL THINKING

- What is the main focus in assessing Juan's home prior to his arrival from the rehabilitation unit?
- When visiting Marie, what questions should be asked to determine the risk of her abusing the infant?

COLLABORATIVE CARE

- What agency should Marie be referred to that will provide support and monitoring of this young family?

MANAGEMENT OF CARE AND PRIORITIES IN NURSING CARE

- In what order will you visit these clients?
- What is your rationale for prioritizing care?

DELEGATING

- When visiting Jenny, how would you determine the care delegated to the CNA has been performed appropriately?

COMMUNICATION AND CLIENT TEACHING

- How would you identify what instruction and supervision needs to be provided to the CNA caring for Jenny?
- What instruction should be given to Juan's family regarding environmental safety?

DOCUMENTING AND REPORTING

- After you have assessed Marie and her baby, if you believe she is at a high risk for neglecting him, what should you do?

CULTURAL CARE STRATEGIES

- If Juan is of Hispanic origin, what aspects of his culture should be taken into consideration when planning care for him?

Maternal-Newborn Care

UNIT II

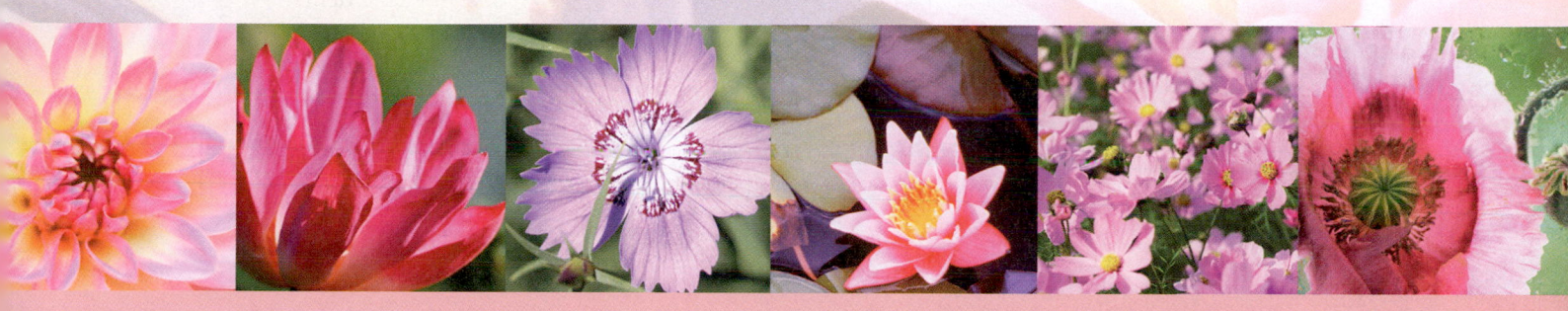

Chapter 4

Reproductive Anatomy and Physiology

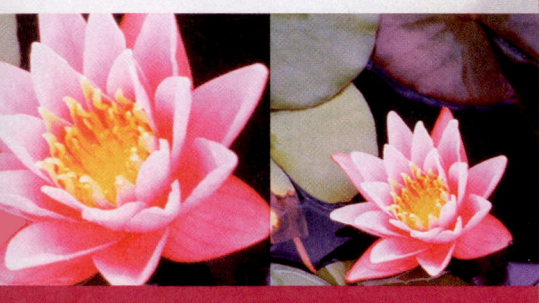

NURSING PROCESS CARE PLAN:
Client with Ovarian Cyst

HEALTH PROMOTION ISSUE:
Genetic Testing

CRITICAL THINKING CARE MAP:
Caring for a Client with Epididymitis

BRIEF Outline

Chromosomes and Genes
Male Reproductive System

Female Reproductive System
Nursing Care

LEARNING Outcomes

After completing this chapter, you will be able to:

- Explain the developmental steps of spermatogenesis and oogenesis.
- Describe basic information about genes in relation to reproduction.
- List the essential and accessory organs of the male and female reproductive systems.
- Describe the general function of each organ of the male and female reproductive systems.
- Discuss the primary functions of the sex hormones.
- Discuss the phases of the menstrual cycle, and correlate each with physical changes during a 28-day cycle.
- Explain the process of lactation.

New human life results from the equal contribution of two parent cells, one from the father and the other from the mother. In both men and women, the reproductive systems have adapted to the specific functions of **gamete** (sex cell) formation and fertilization. (Sex cell formation, or **gametogenesis,** is illustrated in Figure 4-1 ■ .) The female body also has mechanisms for fetal (infant) development and birth.

Male and female infants are not equipped at birth for reproduction. Instead, at about 12 years in females and about 14 years in males, they enter a period of transition and sexual maturation called **puberty.** At puberty, hormonal changes occur that cause the reproductive organs to begin functioning. The external changes of puberty signal that maturation is occurring. Some of these changes are addressed in the Assessing section of the chapter.

This chapter reviews the normal anatomy and physiology of the male and female reproductive systems.

Chromosomes and Genes

The genetic makeup of each parent plays a critical role in reproduction. The genetic coding carried by gametes from the father and mother creates a unique combination in each fertilized egg. The results can be seen in the variety of individuals who are born from one set of parents. Genetic coding is determined by a person's chromosomes. **Chromosomes** are structures made of DNA and protein that govern

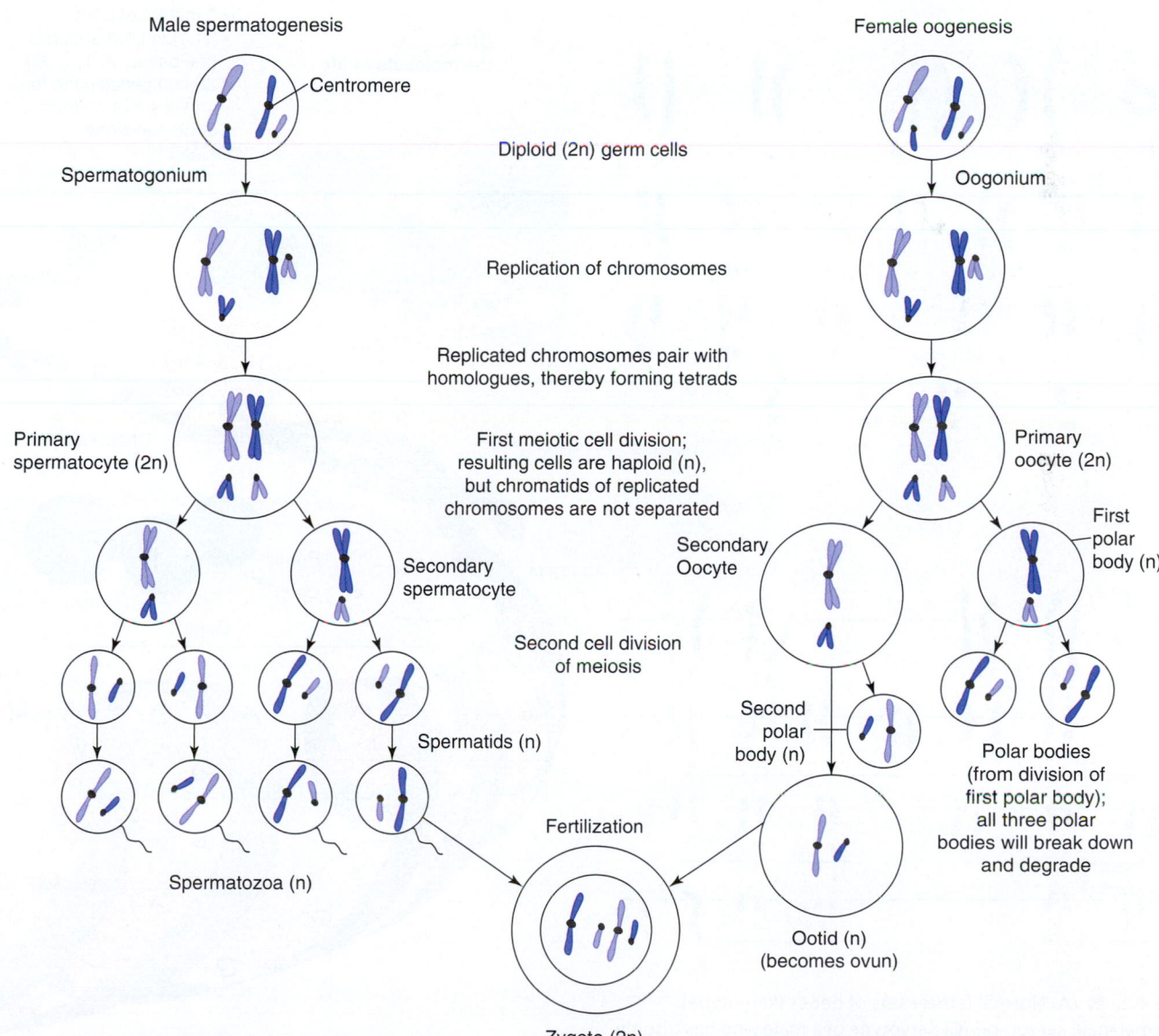

Figure 4-1. ■ Gametogenesis involves meiosis within the ovaries and testicles. (Female) During meiosis, each oogonium produces a single haploid ovum, once cytoplasm moves into the polar bodies. The three polar bodies that remain once the egg is formed are broken down. (Male) Each spermatogonium, in contrast, produces four haploid spermatozoa. When fertilization occurs, they form a zygote. (Pearson Education/PH College.)

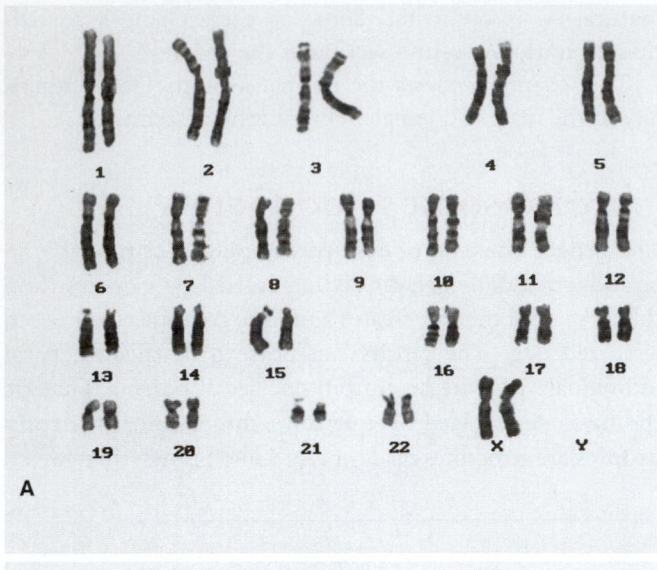

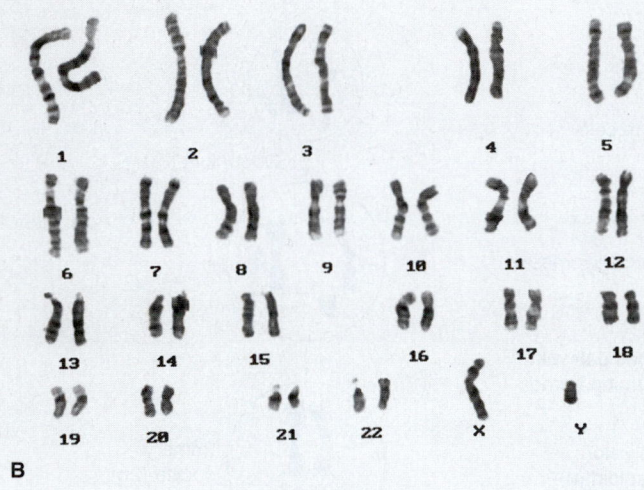

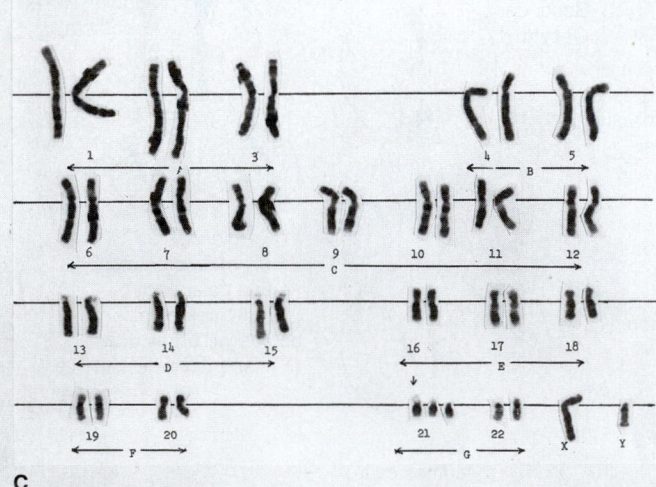

Figure 4-2. ■ (**A**) Normal female sets of genes (karyotype). (**B**) Normal male karyotype. (**C**) Karyotype of a male who has trisomy 21, Down syndrome. Note that position 21 has one extra chromosome. (**A, B**: Courtesy of David Peakman, Reproductive Genetic Center, Denver, CO. **C**: Courtesy of Dr. Arthur Robinson, National Jewish Hospital and Research Center, Denver, CO.)

development of an organism. Figure 4-2A and B ■ show a normal set of female and male chromosomes. Abnormalities in the genetic structure of chromosomes can cause lifelong conditions such as Down syndrome (Figure 4-2C ■). In humans, there are 23 sets with 2 chromosomes in each set, for a total of 46 chromosomes.

Genetic information is contained in DNA's pairs of chemical components (bases). These four proteins (adenine and thymine; guanine and cytosine) form pairs creating the "twisted ladder" appearance associated with DNA. Figure 4-3 ■ illustrates structures from chromosomes down to base pairs of protein in DNA.

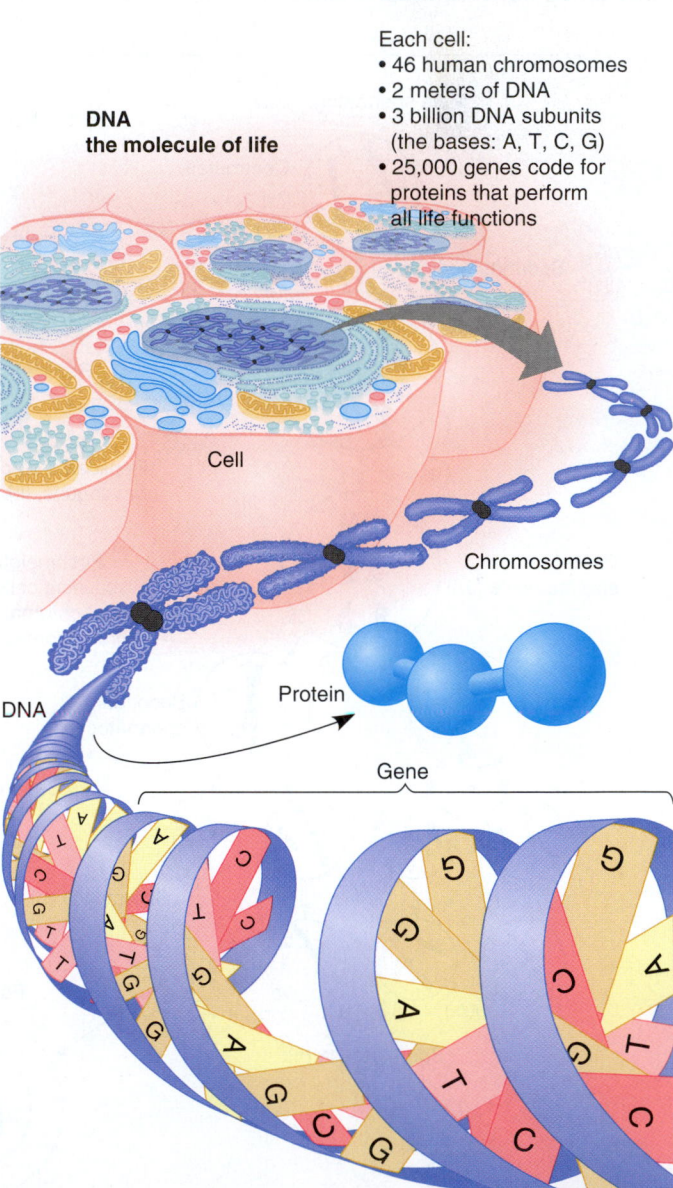

Trillions of cells

Each cell:
- 46 human chromosomes
- 2 meters of DNA
- 3 billion DNA subunits (the bases: A, T, C, G)
- 25,000 genes code for proteins that perform all life functions

DNA the molecule of life

Cell

Chromosomes

Protein

DNA

Gene

Figure 4-3. ■ Expanding view from DNA strand to chromosome. Each cell nucleus throughout the body contains the genes, DNA, and chromosomes that make up the majority of an individual's genome. The remaining portion of the human genome is in the mitochondria.

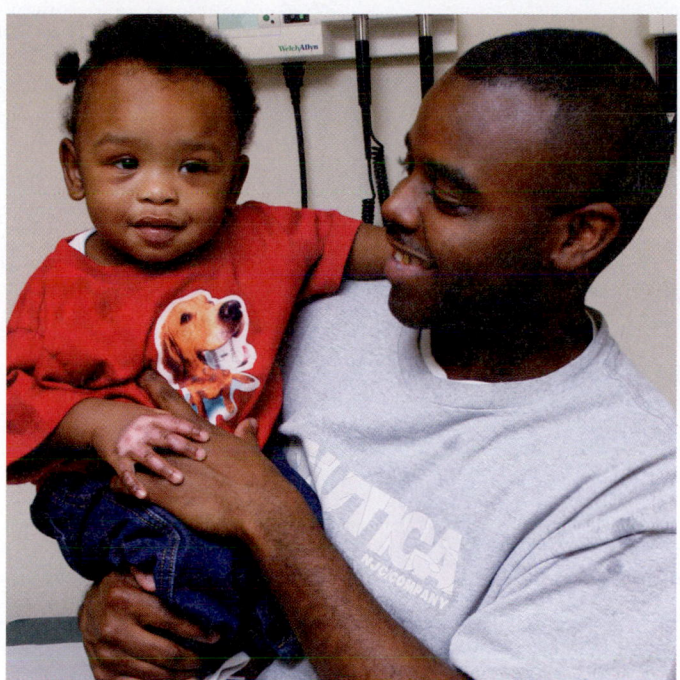

Figure 4-4. ■ Transmission of traits. Children manifest physical characteristics related to their racial or ethnic groups.

The DNA sequence is the unique side-by-side arrangement of bases along the DNA strand. The pattern created by the DNA sequence determines the development of each organism with its own special traits. The DNA se-

quence determines both the physical traits of a person (Figure 4-4 ■) and the person's basic state of health or disease. Figure 4-5 ■ shows how disease can be passed through a person's genes.

U.S. HUMAN GENOME PROJECT

In 2003, the U.S. Human Genome Project, a long-term project to create the first complete human genetic map, was completed. The human **genome** (our organism's complete set of DNA) contains approximately 3 billion base pairs. (In contrast, the smallest known genome for a free-living organism, the genome for bacteria, contains about 600,000 DNA base pairs.) All organisms are related through similarities in DNA sequences. Therefore, insights gained from nonhuman genomes often lead to new knowledge about human biology.

Some stretches of DNA are unstable and "transposable" (i.e., they can move around on and between chromosomes). In fact, nearly half of the human genome is composed of transposable elements (**transposons** or jumping DNA). Scientists now believe that transposons may be linked to some genetic disorders such as hemophilia, leukemia, and breast cancer (U.S. Department of Energy, 2004).

The U.S. Human Genome Project has fueled hope that many inherited diseases may some day be cured. As mentioned in Chapter 2 ⊂⊃, it has also raised some ethical

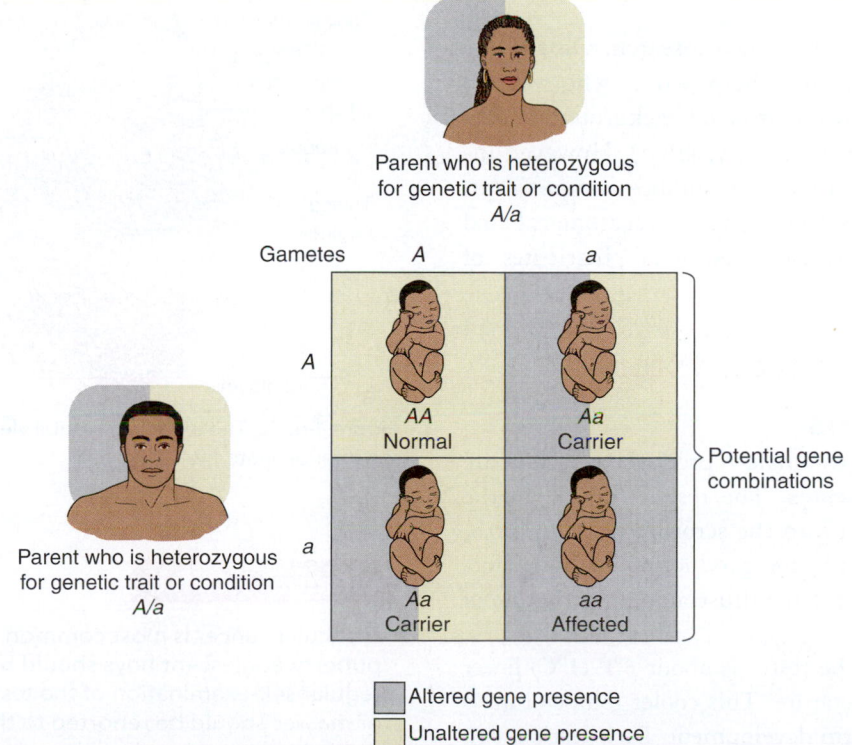

Figure 4-5. ■ Example of transmission of disease. Punnett square shows potential gene combinations (genotypes) and resulting phenotypes of children from parent genotypes with an autosomal recessive altered gene. These are possible genotypes/phenotypes for each pregnancy. Phenotypes are expressed (affected) when a male or female has two copies of the gene alteration.

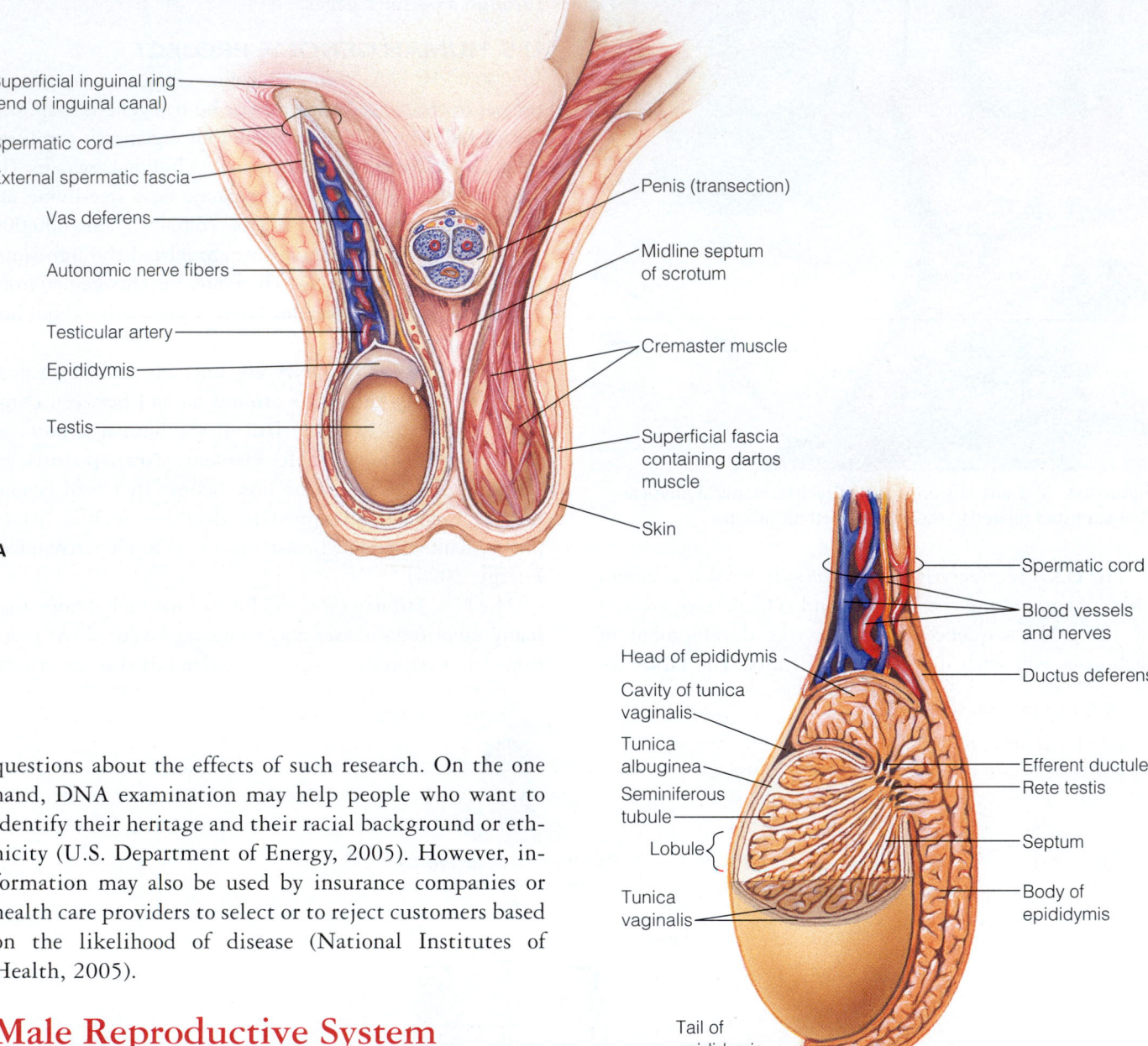

Figure 4-6. ■ The testes. (**A**) Frontal view. (**B**) Sagittal view showing interior anatomy.

questions about the effects of such research. On the one hand, DNA examination may help people who want to identify their heritage and their racial background or ethnicity (U.S. Department of Energy, 2005). However, information may also be used by insurance companies or health care providers to select or to reject customers based on the likelihood of disease (National Institutes of Health, 2005).

Male Reproductive System

ESSENTIAL ORGANS

The essential organs of the male reproductive system are the pair of gonads or **testes.** The testes, formed in the lower abdomen, descend into the scrotum prior to birth. The testes are responsible for production of male hormones and sperm. Figure 4-6 ■ illustrates the structure of the testes.

The environment of the testes is about 3°F (1°C) lower than normal body temperature. This cooler temperature is necessary for normal sperm development. Each testis is egg shaped, approximately 1½ in. long by 1 in. wide (3 cm × 2.5 cm or about the size of a walnut).

clinical ALERT

Testicular cancer is most common in young men. At puberty, adolescent boys should be taught to perform regular self-examination of the testes. Any enlargement or masses should be reported to the care provider. Procedure 4-1 ■ describes steps in performing a testicular self-examination (TSE).

PROCEDURE 4-1 Testicular Self-Examination

Purpose

- To provide instruction in monthly self-examination of the testes
- To identify abnormalities in the testicular tissue

Equipment

- Hand mirror

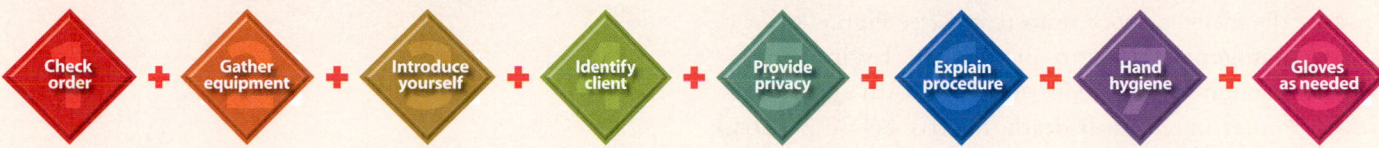

Check order + Gather equipment + Introduce yourself + Identify client + Provide privacy + Explain procedure + Hand hygiene + Gloves as needed

Interventions

1. Instruction is provided by demonstration, return demonstration, and written material. *Showing the client what to do and then watching him return the demonstration ensures proper technique. Written material is a useful reference when at home.*

2. Stand in front of a mirror in good light with genitals exposed. *Using a hand mirror with good light provides the opportunity to inspect all areas of the genitals.*

3. Observe the scrotum and penis for lumps, edema, sores, or discharge. *The scrotum and penis should be free of lumps, swelling, sores, and discharge.*

4. While standing in the shower, support the scrotum with one hand. Place the fingers of the other hand under one testicle and the thumb on top. *Soap and water make the skin slick and decrease discomfort.*

5. Gently roll each testicle between the thumb and fingers feeling for lumps, thickening, or hardening of the tissue (Figure 4-7 ■). *The testes should feel smooth.*

6. Palpate the epididymis, a cordlike structure on top and back of the testicle. The epididymis feels soft but not as smooth as the testicle. *Feel for firm masses in the epididymis.*

7. Palpate the vas deferens (spermatic cord), which extends upward toward the base of the penis. The vas deferens should feel firm and smooth. *Feel for hard masses in the vas deferens.*

8. Use a calendar to record when TSE was performed. TSE should be performed on the same day of each month. *Recording when TSE was performed is a useful reminder of when to do the next TSE as well as providing documentation should abnormalities occur.*

9. Report any lumps, dimpling, asymmetry, or discharge to the primary health care provider.

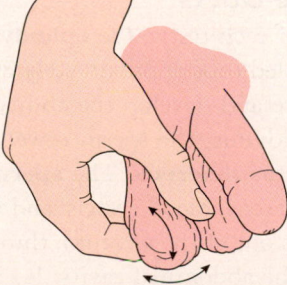

Figure 4-7. ■ Self-examination of the testes should be done monthly to check for the possibility of testicular cancer. Young men are at higher risk for this than other groups.

SAMPLE DOCUMENTATION

(date/time) Instruction in TSE provided. Return demonstration indicates appropriate technique. Written material provided. W. Clark, LPN

Covering the front and sides of the testes and epididymis is the **tunica vaginalis testis.** This serous membrane is composed of the *parietal* (outer) layer and the *visceral* (inner) layer). Underneath the visceral layer is the tunica albuginea. The **tunica albuginea** covers the outside of the testes and forms the septum between the many sections or lobules. Each lobule consists of long narrow coiled tubes called **seminiferous tubules.** Sperm are produced in the walls of the seminiferous tubules and are released into the lumen to begin their journey to the outside. Specialized interstitial cells located between the septum and seminiferous tubules produce the male hormone testosterone (see Figure 4-6).

Spermatogenesis, sperm production, begins at puberty. Although sperm production slows with age, it continues uninterrupted until death. Shortly before puberty, **spermatogonia** (sperm precursor or stem cells) increase in number by the process of mitosis. As you can see in Figure 4-1, mitosis results in two "daughter cells" identical to the "parent" cell, each containing 46 chromosomes (23 pair).

When the boy enters puberty, the anterior pituitary gland releases **follicle-stimulating hormone (FSH).** Spermatogonia that undergo cell division under the influence of FSH produce two "daughter" cells—each containing 46 chromosomes. One daughter cell remains a spermatogonium; the other develops into a specialized **primary spermatocyte.** The primary spermatocyte divides once by mitosis and then by meiosis. You will recall that in meiosis, the DNA is not replicated; the cells resulting from that division contain 23 chromosomes (one-half of each pair). The result of the meiotic division is four **spermatids** that will develop into sperm.

Of the 46 chromosomes in humans, 22 pair (44 chromosomes) are **autosomes** (alike in males and females), and 1 pair consists of sex chromosomes. Males have an Xy pair, and females have an XX pair. During sperm formation, two spermatids will have the X chromosome, and two will have the y chromosome.

Mature **spermatozoa** (sperm cells) are among the smallest and most highly specialized cells in the body (Figure 4-8 ▪). The characteristics the infant will inherit from the father are condensed in the genetic material located in the head of the sperm. The genetic material from both father and mother will fuse if successful fertilization occurs.

For fertilization to occur, sperm deposited in the vagina during ejaculation must move through the female reproductive system and penetrate the outer membrane of the ovum (egg). Note in Figure 4-8 that the head of the sperm is covered by the **acrosome,** a specialized structure containing enzymes that can break down the covering of the ovum. Each sperm also has a midpiece with mitochondria to provide energy for the sperm. A tail moves, propelling the sperm in a "swimming" motion through the female reproductive ducts.

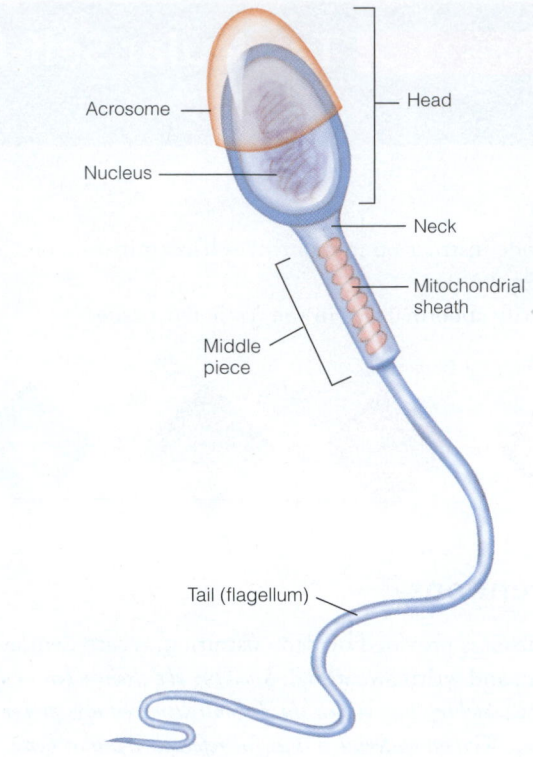

Figure 4-8. ▪ Structure of a mature sperm cell.

In addition to sperm production, the testes are responsible for the production of testosterone. **Testosterone,** produced in the interstitial cells, is a hormone that causes:

- Development of male accessory organs
- Greater muscle mass and strength
- Masculine characteristics such as a deep voice and body hair.

ACCESSORY ORGANS

The male accessory organs consist of a series of ducts, supportive glands, and external genitalia (Figure 4-9 ▪). Each component is discussed separately.

Reproductive Ducts

Located on top of each testis, the **epididymis** consists of a single tightly coiled tube approximately 20 feet long. Here the sperm mature and develop the ability to move. Upon leaving the epididymis, the sperm travel through the **vas deferens** or **ductus deferens.** The **spermatic cord** comprises the vas deferens, blood vessels, and nerves. The spermatic cord passes out of the scrotum, through the inguinal canal, and into the abdominal cavity. It circles the urinary bladder and joins the duct from the seminal vesicle to form the **ejaculatory duct.** The ejaculatory duct passes through the substance of the prostate gland, allowing sperm to empty into the **urethra** and pass through the penis to the exterior at the external urinary meatus.

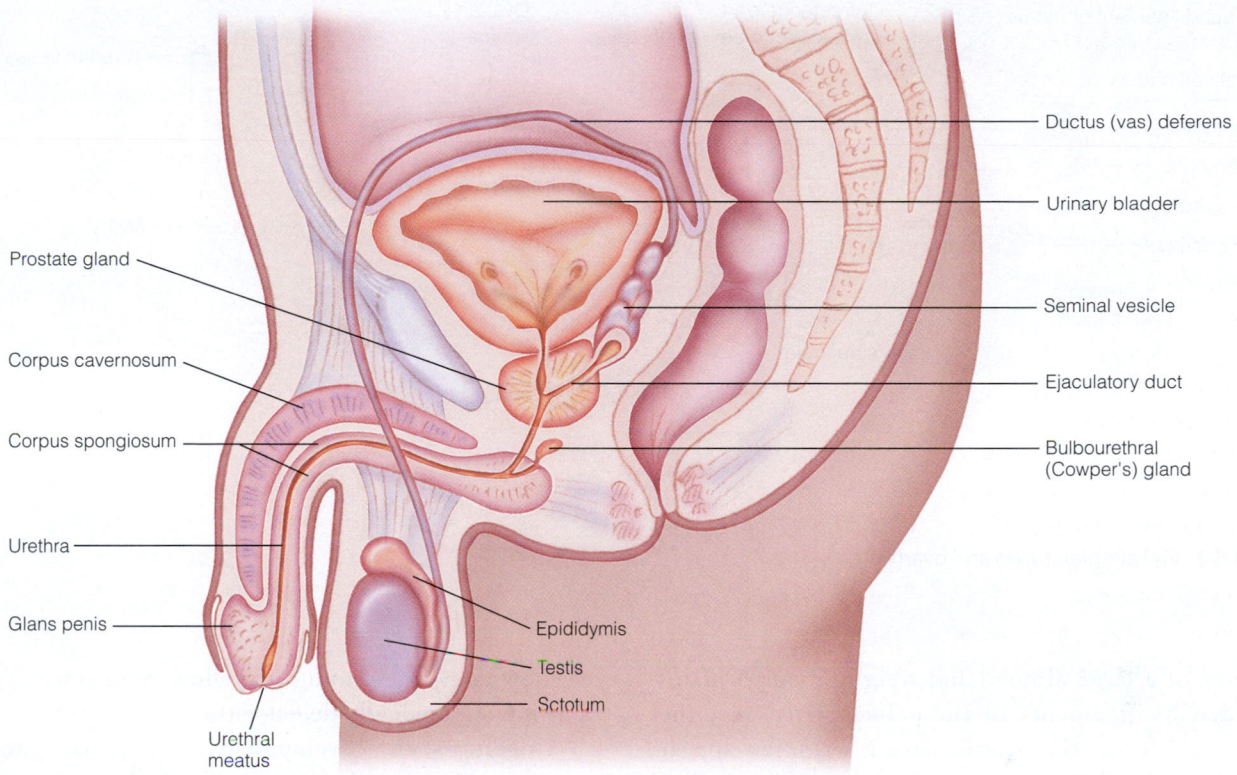

Figure 4-9. ■ Male reproductive organs.

Labels, clockwise from top right: Ductus (vas) deferens · Urinary bladder · Seminal vesicle · Ejaculatory duct · Bulbourethral (Cowper's) gland · Epididymis · Testis · Scrotum · Urethral meatus · Glans penis · Urethra · Corpus spongiosum · Corpus cavernosum · Prostate gland

Infection or inflammation of these structures is described as the gland + -*itis* (e.g., epididymitis or prostatitis).

Accessory Reproductive Glands

Semen or **seminal fluid** is the term used to describe the mixture of sperm and fluid from the reproductive glands. The two **seminal vesicles** are located under and behind the urinary bladder. The seminal vesicles produce a thick, yellowish fluid rich in fructose. This part of the seminal fluid helps provide a source of energy for the highly mobile sperm. The **prostate** gland is a doughnut-shaped gland located just below the urinary bladder (see Figure 4-9). The urethra passes through the center of prostate gland. The prostate produces a thin milky fluid that helps activate the sperm and maintain their motility.

<div class="clinical-alert">

clinical ALERT

Adult men are encouraged to have regular prostate examination, including a test for prostate-specific antigen (PSA). They should report any urinary or sexual difficulty to their care provider.

</div>

The two **bulbourethral glands** or **Cowper's glands** are located below the prostate. These glands secrete a mucus-like fluid into the penile section of the urethra. This alkaline fluid helps neutralize the acid environment of the urethra and lubricate the end of the penis. Review Figure 4-9 to view the location of these accessory glands.

External Genitalia

The external male genitalia consists of the penis and scrotum. The **penis** is the male organ of copulation or sexual intercourse. The shaft of the penis comprises three separate columns of erectile tissue: one corpus spongiosum, which surrounds the urethra, and two corpora cavernosa, which are along the anterior surface of the penis. During sexual arousal, this tissue engorges with blood, causing the penis to become erect.

The distal end of the penis is the enlarged **glans.** It is encased by loose-fitting, retractable skin called the **foreskin** or **prepuce.** The urethra opens in the center of the glans. Surgical removal of the foreskin is called **circumcision** (see discussion in Chapter 9 ⬤⬤).

The **scrotum** is a skin-covered pouch suspended from the groin. Internally, the scrotum is divided by a septum. The scrotum contains the testes, epididymis, and lower end of the vas deferens at the beginning of the spermatic cords.

Female Reproductive System

ESSENTIAL ORGANS

The essential organs of the female reproductive system are the two ovaries (Figure 4-10 ■). Each ovary is the size

MediaLink Oogenesis

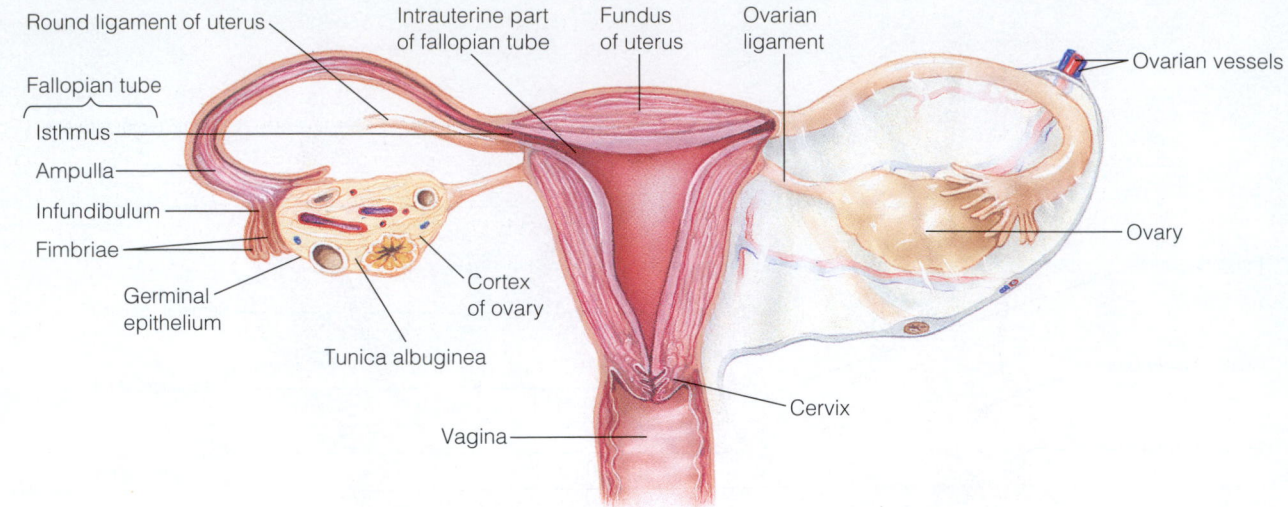

Figure 4-10. ■ Fallopian tubes and ovaries.

and shape of a large almond and weighs about 3 grams. Suspended by ligaments in the pelvic cavity on either side of the uterus, the ovaries have a wrinkled appearance. About 1 million **ovarian follicles** are embedded under the surface of each ovary of a newborn girl. Each ovarian follicle contains an **oocyte,** or immature sex cell. By the time the girl reaches puberty, the number of follicles has reduced to about 400,000 primary follicles. During her reproductive lifetime, 350 to 500 of the primary follicles develop into **Graafian follicles** (mature follicles) and release a ripened **ovum** (egg). The follicles that do not mature degenerate and are absorbed by the ovarian tissue.

The progression of development from a primary follicle to ovulation is illustrated in Figure 4-11 ■. Each primary follicle has a layer of cells surrounding the oocyte (**granulosa cells**). Under the influence of follicle-stimulating hormone (FSH) from the anterior pituitary gland, the layer of granulosa cells thickens, forming a hollow chamber called an **antrum.** The follicle, called a *secondary follicle*, continues to enlarge and move closer to the surface of the ovary until the follicle ruptures and releases the ovum. The ruptured follicle transforms into a glandular structure called the **corpus luteum.** The corpus luteum is also called

"yellow body," describing its yellow appearance. The corpus luteum gradually degenerates.

Oogenesis, the development of the female gamete or ovum, results from the process of meiosis (see Figure 4-1). Although spermatogenesis begins at puberty, oogenesis occurs during fetal development of the female infant. As a result of meiosis, the number of chromosomes is reduced equally to 23, one of which will be an X chromosome. However, the cytoplasm does not divide equally in each daughter cell. The result is one large ovum and small **polar bodies** that degenerate. After fertilization, the large

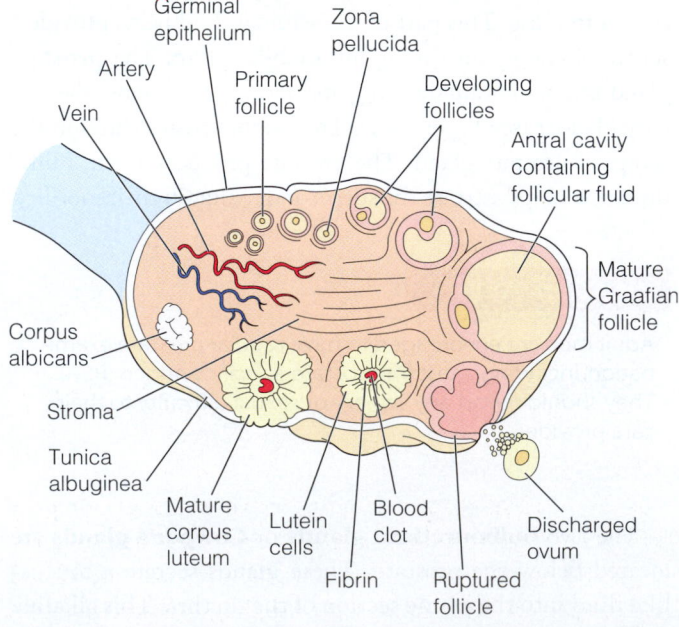

Figure 4-11. ■ Various stages of development of the ovarian follicles.

clinical ALERT

At times a sac containing serous fluid or blood forms in the ovary, resulting in an ovarian cyst. The cyst frequently forms in the area of the corpus luteum. The cyst is benign but may cause pain, may rupture into the pelvic cavity, and may need medical or surgical intervention.

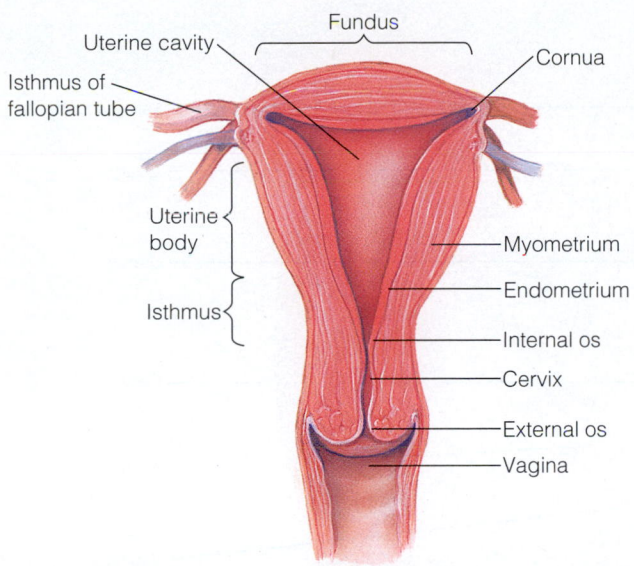

Figure 4-12. ■ Structures of the uterus.

actually opens into the pelvic cavity, the female reproductive system is called an *open system*. The outer end of each fallopian tube is a funnel-shaped structure with finger-like projections called **fimbriae** along the edge (see Figure 4-10). The lumen of the fallopian tube is lined with **cilia**, or minute hairlike structures. Although the fimbriae are not attached to the ovary, the sweeping movements of these finger-like projections, as well as the movement of the cilia, cause the ovum to move into the lumen of the fallopian tube. Fertilization usually occurs in the outer third of the fallopian tube (the third closest to the ovaries).

clinical ALERT

If the fertilized egg implants into the wall of the fallopian tube, the developing embryo enlarges and eventually ruptures the fallopian tube. This results in a surgical emergency (discussed in Chapter 8 ⚭) to stop internal bleeding.

supply of cytoplasm will be necessary for nutrition until the developing embryo implants in the uterus.

Besides oogenesis, another function of the ovary is the production and secretion of the two hormones, estrogen and progesterone. Hormone production begins at puberty with the development and maturation of the Graafian follicle. The granulosa cells around the ovum produce estrogen. After ovulation, the corpus luteum produces progesterone and some estrogen. **Estrogen** is the hormone responsible for the development and maintenance of the secondary sex characteristics and growth of the **endometrium,** the inner lining of the uterus (Figure 4-12 ■). Progesterone is produced for approximately 11 days after ovulation. **Progesterone** is the hormone that stimulates thickening and vascularization of the endometrium. A decrease in progesterone causes the endometrium to slough off, resulting in **menses.**

ACCESSORY ORGANS

The accessory organs in the female consist of a series of ducts, glands, and external genitalia. Each component is discussed separately. Figure 4-13 ■ illustrates the organization of the female reproductive organs and the ligaments that support them. It also depicts their relationship to surrounding organs and structures.

Reproductive Ducts

The two **fallopian tubes** (also called **uterine tubes** or **oviducts**) serve to transport the ovum from the ovary toward the uterus. However, the structures are not closed and connected (e.g., the way the esophagus is connected to the stomach). Because the distal end of the fallopian tube

The **uterus** (see Figure 4-12) is a small organ about the size of a pear. The uterus consists almost entirely of muscle (**myometrium**), with a small cavity in the center. The endometrium (inner lining) is a vascular mucous membrane that responds to hormone influence as described earlier in this chapter. The uterus is suspended in the pelvic cavity between the urinary bladder and the rectum.

The uterus is divided into two parts: the upper portion is the **body,** and the lower region is the **cervix.** Just above the attachment of the fallopian tubes, the uterus forms a round dome called the **fundus.** Except during pregnancy, the normal uterus is tipped forward over the urinary bladder. In some women, atypical uterine positions occur (Figure 4-14 ■). They may make implantation of the embryo more difficult. During pregnancy, the uterus straightens and rises into the abdominal cavity, pressing the intestines backward and the stomach and liver up against the diaphragm.

The **vagina** is a 4-inch-long tube that connects the cervix to the vaginal opening. Composed mainly of smooth muscle, the vagina is lined with mucous membrane. The mucous membrane lies in folds (**rugae**), which allow for stretching of the vagina during delivery. The vagina is the site of deposition of sperm and the passageway for the delivery of the infant. The vaginal orifice is partially covered by a thin membrane called the **hymen.** The hymen usually tears with the first sexual intercourse. It could also tear during insertion of a tampon or from pelvic trauma such as falling on the center bar of a bicycle.

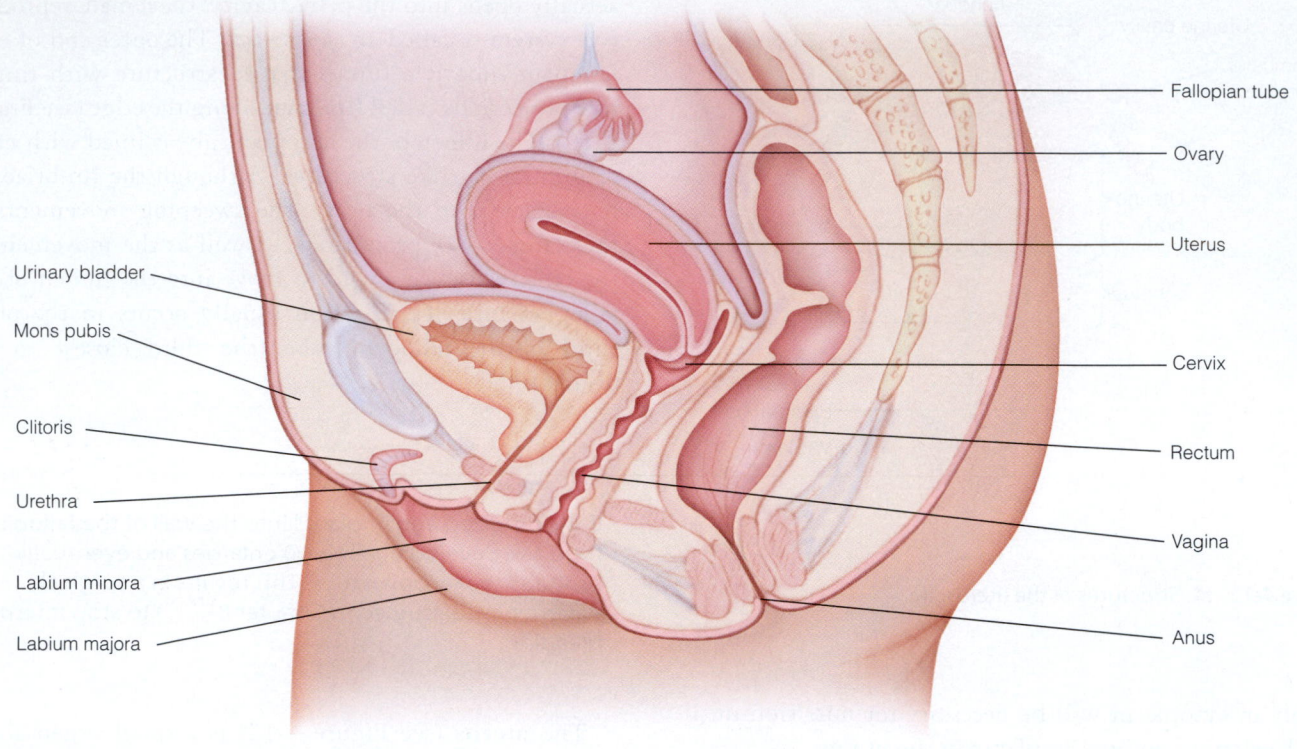

A

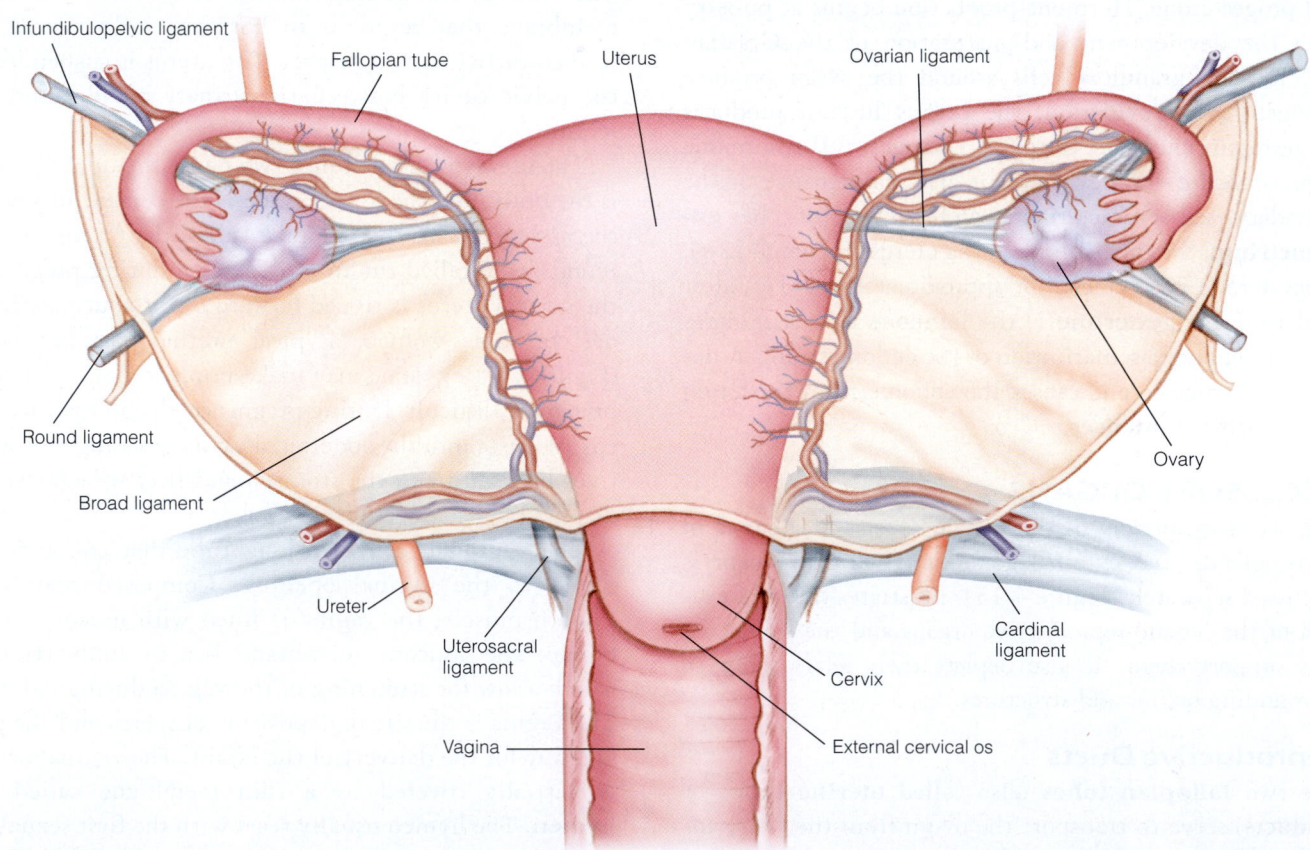

B

Figure 4-13. ■ **(A)** Internal female reproductive organs. **(B)** Uterine ligaments that support reproductive structures.

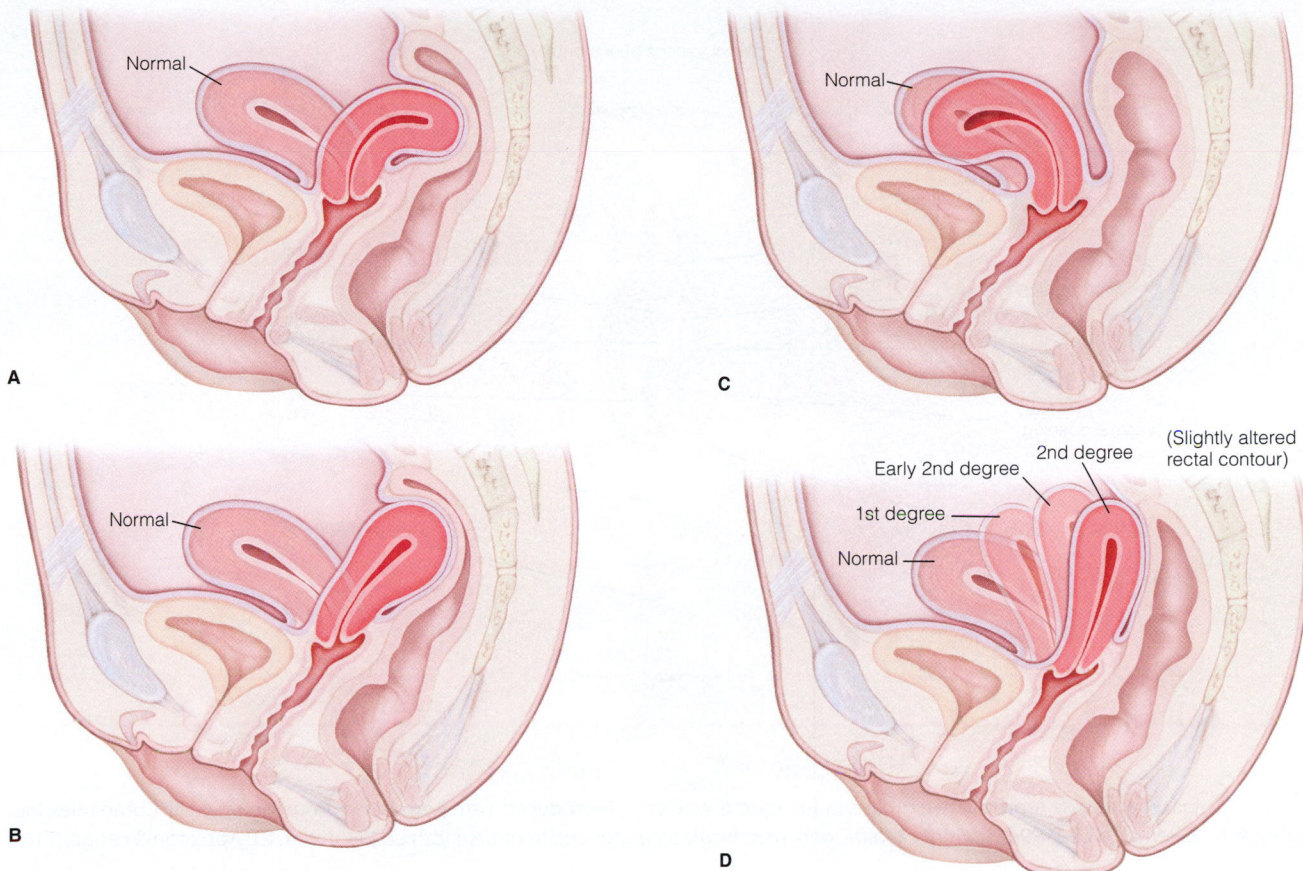

Figure 4-14. ■ Variations in uterine position. (**A**) Retroflexion. (**B**) Retrocession. (**C**) Anteflexion. (**D**) Retroversion. (Reproduced, with permission, from McGraw-Hill Companies, Inc. DeCherney, A. H., & Pernoll, M. L. [1994]. *Current obstetric and gynecologic diagnosis and treatment* [8th ed.]. Norwalk, CT: Appleton & Lange, p. 16.)

External Genitalia

Figure 4-15 ■ illustrates the external structures of the female reproductive system. The skin-covered fat pad over the symphysis pubis is called the **mons pubis.** This area is covered with course hair beginning at puberty and continuing throughout life. Extended downward from the mons pubis are two large folds of skin, the **labia majora.** The **labia minora,** or small folds of tissue, are located inside the labia majora. These folds of tissue join anteriorly at the midline. Located just behind the junction of the labia is erectile tissue called the **clitoris.** The purpose of the clitoris is sexual arousal and pleasure. The area between the labia minora is the **vestibule.** Opening onto the vestibule are the **urinary meatus,** the vagina, and the orifice of several small glands. The **true perineum** is the area between the vaginal opening and the anus.

CULTURAL CONSIDERATIONS. The nurse must be aware of and sensitive to practices by non-Western cultures related to female genitalia. Box 4-1 ■ discusses some of these practices.

BOX 4-1	CULTURAL PULSE POINTS

Female Circumcision and Infibulation

Female circumcision and infibulation are practiced in many African countries and by some groups in Malaysia and India. **Female circumcision** is a partial or complete removal of the clitoris, generally performed before puberty. The result is a loss of pleasure during sexual intercourse. **Infibulation** is the removal of the labia majora and labia minora. The excised edges are then sewn together to prevent or limit sexual intercourse. Complications of both procedures include infection, hemorrhage, painful intercourse (**dyspareunia**), difficult childbirth, anxiety, and depression.

Although the international political community has denounced these practices, they are still being performed. The nurse must respect the culture, while creating an environment in which the client is free to discuss the condition, complications, and possible surgical reconstruction.

ACCESSORY SEX GLANDS

On each side of the vagina is a small **Bartholin's gland** or **greater vestibular gland.** The ducts of these glands open

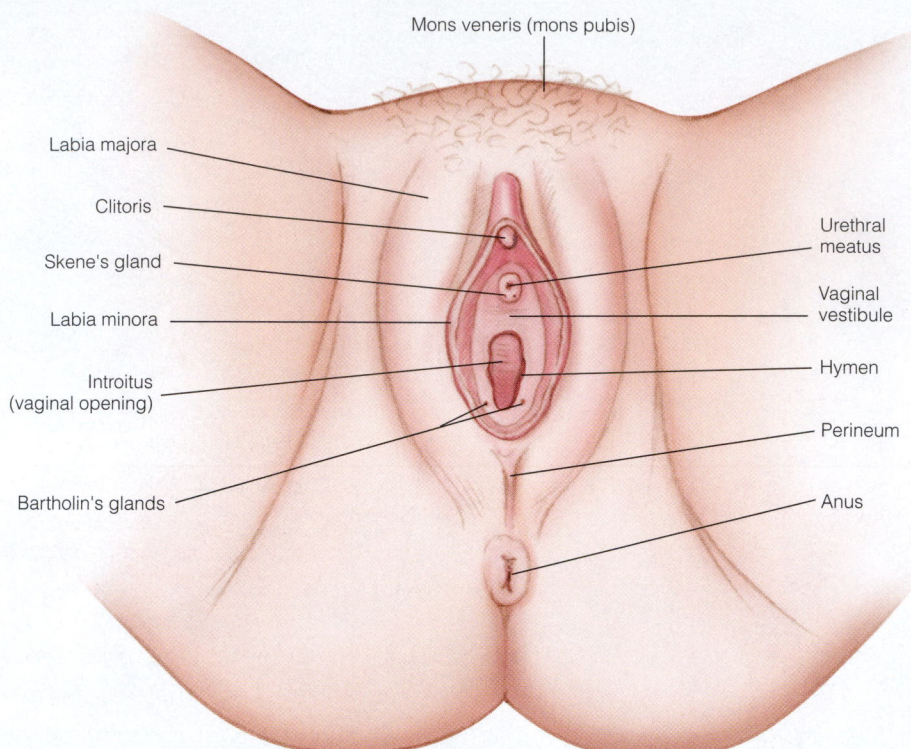

Mons veneris (mons pubis)

Labia majora

Clitoris

Skene's gland

Labia minora

Introitus
(vaginal opening)

Bartholin's glands

Urethral
meatus

Vaginal
vestibule

Hymen

Perineum

Anus

Figure 4-15. ■ External female reproductive organs (adult parous woman). (Reproduced, with permission, from McGraw-Hill Companies, Inc. DeCherney, A. H., & Pernoll, M. L. [1994]. *Current obstetric and gynecologic diagnosis and treatment* [8th ed.]. Norwalk, CT: Appleton & Lange, p. 16.)

onto the vestibule. They secrete a thin, mucus-like substance that provides lubrication during sexual intercourse.

The breasts are located on the anterior chest and are attached to the pectoralis muscles by ligaments. (Figure 4-16 ■ illustrates the structure of the breast.) The mammary glands within the breasts are surrounded by fat tissue. The amount of fat tissue generally determines the size of the breast. The breast consists of 15 to 20 lobes arranged in a circle. Each lobe has several lobules, which contain milk-secreting glandular cells. These glandular cells are arranged in grapelike clusters called **alveoli**. **Lactiferous ducts** drain each alveoli and converge toward the nipple. Only one lactiferous duct from each lobe drains into the lactiferous sinus located under the colored area around the nipple (the **areola**). The lactiferous sinus drains through a pore on the nipple.

MILK PRODUCTION

Lactogenesis (milk production) begins in pregnancy due to the sustained levels of estrogen and progesterone. The first fluid to be produced by the mammary glands is colostrum. **Colostrum** is a translucent yellow fluid rich in protein, antibodies, and other substances to meet the needs of the newborn. Stimulation of the nipple causes the pituitary gland to secrete pitocin (Figure 4-17 ■). Pitocin causes the milk-ejecting cells in the lactiferous sinus to contract, forcing the

colostrum and later the milk from the nipple. (It also stimulates contraction of the uterus, helping it return to its prepregnant size.)

About 1 week after delivery, the level of estrogen and progesterone decreases, causing the mammary glands to change from producing colostrum to producing mature milk. As soon as milk is removed from the breast during feeding, synthesis of more milk begins. If the breast is left full, milk production is limited. (Milk production is discussed further in Chapter 9 ⚭.)

clinical ALERT

Beginning at puberty, adolescent girls should be taught to perform breast self-examination (BSE) on a monthly basis. Procedure 4-2 ■ shows steps in BSE.

FEMALE PELVIC STRUCTURE

Although the pelvis is not part of the female reproductive system, it is important in carrying and delivering an infant. The pelvic structures, their shapes, and their measurements are discussed in Chapter 7 ⚭. Figure 7-4 illustrates the female pelvis and shows typical measurements that can affect the labor and birth process.

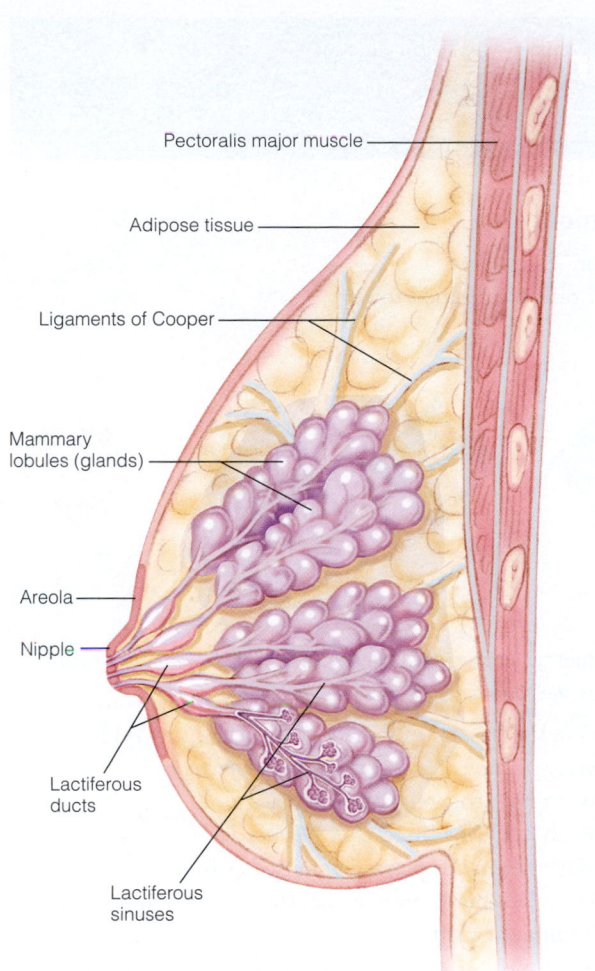

Figure 4-16 ■ Structures of the breast.

MENSTRUAL CYCLE

A review of the female reproductive system would not be complete without discussing the menstrual cycle. Refer often to Figure 4-21 ■ as you review this information.

For most women, the events of the menstrual cycle occur with almost precise regularity from their onset (**menarche**) until the cycle ends (**menopause**). Although the length of the cycle varies among women, the average is 28 days. Each cycle can be divided into three phases: menses, proliferative phase, and secretory phase.

The menstrual phase, or menses, begins with menstrual bleeding or flow. The first day of flow is considered the first day of the menstrual cycle; this would be the date listed on the client record as "last menstrual period" (LMP). Menses typically lasts 5 days, with a range of 2 to 10 days.

The **proliferative phase** begins around day 3 when FSH secretion from the anterior pituitary gland begins to increase. You may recall that FHS begins to change the primary follicle into a secondary follicle. The secondary follicle begins to secrete estrogen around day 8. Estrogen helps heal the endometrium and stimulates the production of luteinizing hormone (LH) from the anterior pituitary gland. LH levels increase and cause ripening of one or more Graafian follicles by day 11 and ovulation on day 14.

The **secretory phase** begins with ovulation. Following ovulation, FSH and LH levels decrease. The corpus luteum (see Figure 4-11) produces progesterone until day

(Text continues on p. 82.)

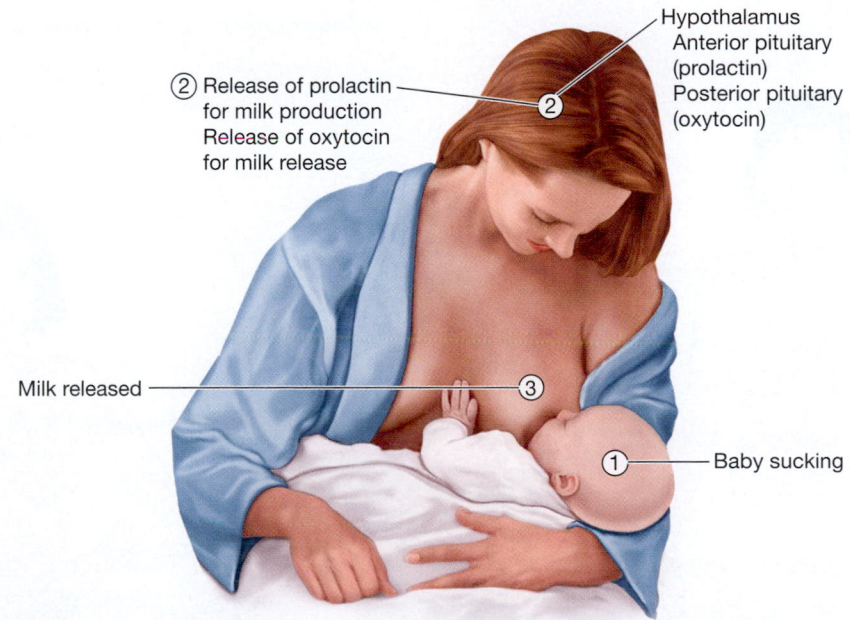

Figure 4-17. ■ Relationship between the pituitary gland and milk production. Sucking of the nipple triggers endocrine release of prolactin (which stimulates new milk production). It also triggers oxytocin (which allows milk to be released from the breast). Oxytocin also stimulates uterine contractions, which help the organ return to its smaller size.

PROCEDURE 4-2 Breast Self-Examination

Purpose

- To provide instruction in monthly self-examination of the breasts
- To identify abnormalities in the breast tissue

Equipment

- Mirror
- Small pillow or folded towel

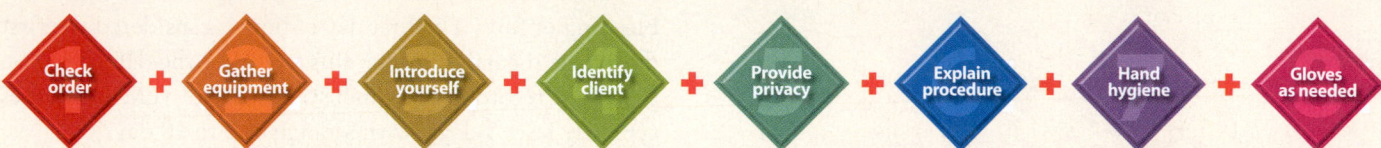

Check order **+** Gather equipment **+** Introduce yourself **+** Identify client **+** Provide privacy **+** Explain procedure **+** Hand hygiene **+** Gloves as needed

Interventions

1. Instruction is provided by demonstration, return demonstration, and written material. *Showing the client what to do and then watching her return the demonstration ensures proper technique. Written material is a useful reference when at home.*

2. Stand in front of a mirror in good light with both breasts exposed. *Standing in front of a mirror with good light provides the opportunity to visually inspect all areas of the breast.*

3. Observe the breasts individually for lumps, dimpling, deviation, recent nipple retraction, irregular shape, edema, or discharge. Compare the right and left breast for symmetry. *Tissue should be consistent throughout the breast. Inconsistent tissue could indicate abnormalities.*

4. Observe the breasts in these positions (Figure 4-18 ■). *Changing position allows for adequate inspection.*
   - With her arms relaxed at her sides
   - With her arms lifted over her head
   - With her hands pressed against her hips
   - With her hands pressed together at her waist and leaning forward

5. While sitting or standing in the shower, place one hand behind the head. Use the finger pads of the other hand to palpate the breast, moving in small, dime-sized circles. *Soap and water make the skin slick and decrease discomfort.*

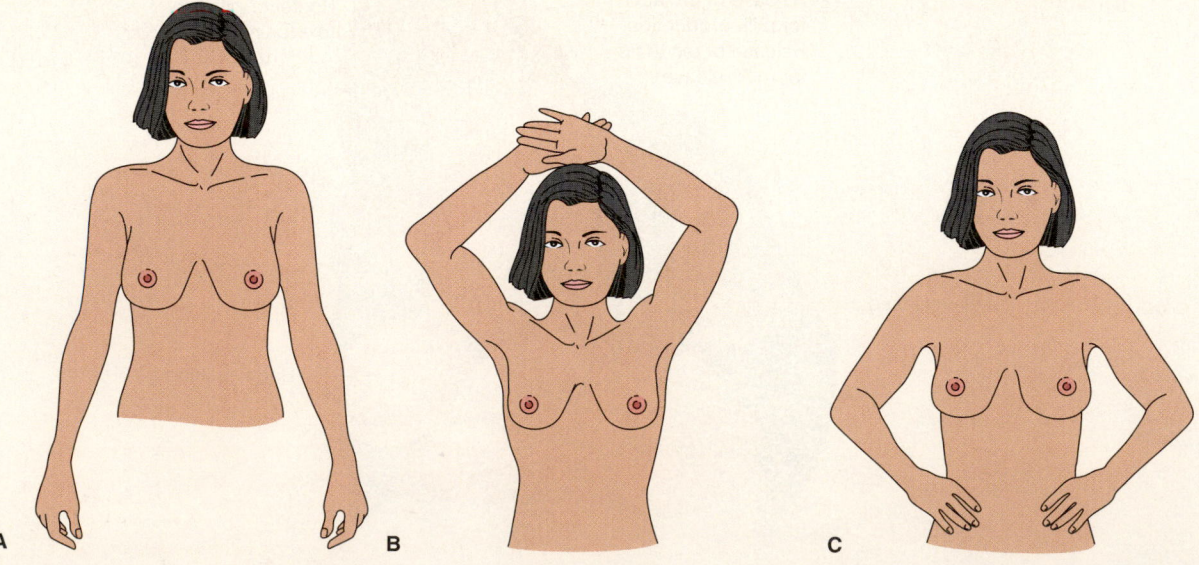

Figure 4-18. ■ Some positions for inspection of the breast. (**A**) Both arms relaxed at sides. (**B**) Both arms above the head. (**C**) Both hands on hips while leaning forward. (Data from National Breast Cancer Foundation, Inc.®; *Breast Health Access for Women with Disabilities,* produced by The Susan G. Komen Breast Cancer Foundation of San Francisco; and American Cancer Society.)

6. Palpate the area from the collarbone to below the breasts, and from the middle of the armpit to the breastbone. Gently press the breast tissue against the chest wall, feeling for lumps or thickening of the tissue. *This pattern ensures all areas of the breast are examined.*

7. Repeat on the other side.

8. Position supine with a small pillow or folded towel under one shoulder. Place the arm on that side under the head (Figure 4-19 ■). *In this position, gravity pulls the breast into a different position, allowing for more complete examination.*

9. Using the pads of the fingers, palpate the breast again as in step 6. Move down and up across the breast, starting at the axilla (see Figure 4-19A).

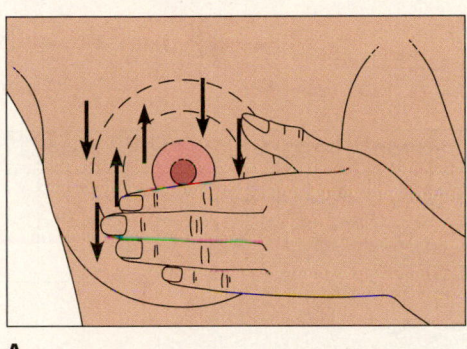

Move the hand vertically down and up across the breasts, starting at the axilla and working toward the center of the body. Press with the finger-pads in small, dime-sized circles to feel the chest wall.

A

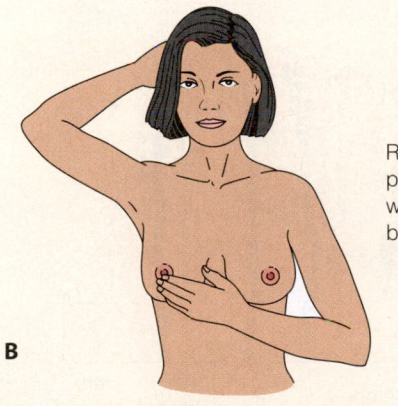

Repeat the same procedure sitting up with your hand still behind your head.

B

Figure 4-19. ■ (**A**) Check each breast using the pads of the fingers, feeling all parts of the breast. (**B**) While holding one hand behind your head, palpate your breast. (Data from National Breast Cancer Foundation, Inc.®; *Breast Health Access for Women with Disabilities,* produced by The Susan G. Komen Breast Cancer Foundation of San Francisco; and American Cancer Society.)

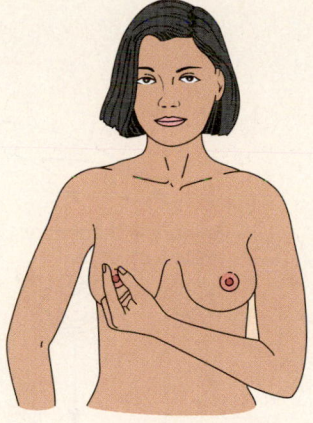

Squeeze your nipple between your thumb and forefinger; look for any clear or bloody discharge.

Figure 4-20. ■ Squeeze the nipple and look for any drainage. (Data from National Breast Cancer Foundation, Inc®; *Breast Health Access for Women with Disabilities,* produced by The Susan G. Komen Breast Cancer Foundation of San Francisco; and American Cancer Society.)

10. Repeat on the other side.

11. Palpate the areola and the nipple. Compress the nipple between the thumb and finger to check for discharge (Figure 4-20 ■). *Gently compressing the nipple forces any drainage from the lactiferous duct.*

12. Use a calendar to record when BSE was performed. BSE should be performed once a month, usually on the fifth day after onset of menses. *Recording when BSE was performed is a useful reminder of when to do the next BSE as well as providing documentation should abnormalities occur. On the fifth day after menses begins, the breast tissue has the least hormonal influence.*

13. Report any lumps, dimpling, asymmetry, or discharge to the primary health care provider.

SAMPLE DOCUMENTATION

(date/time)   Instruction in BSE provided. Return demonstration indicates appropriate technique. Written material provided. _____
C. Downey, LPN

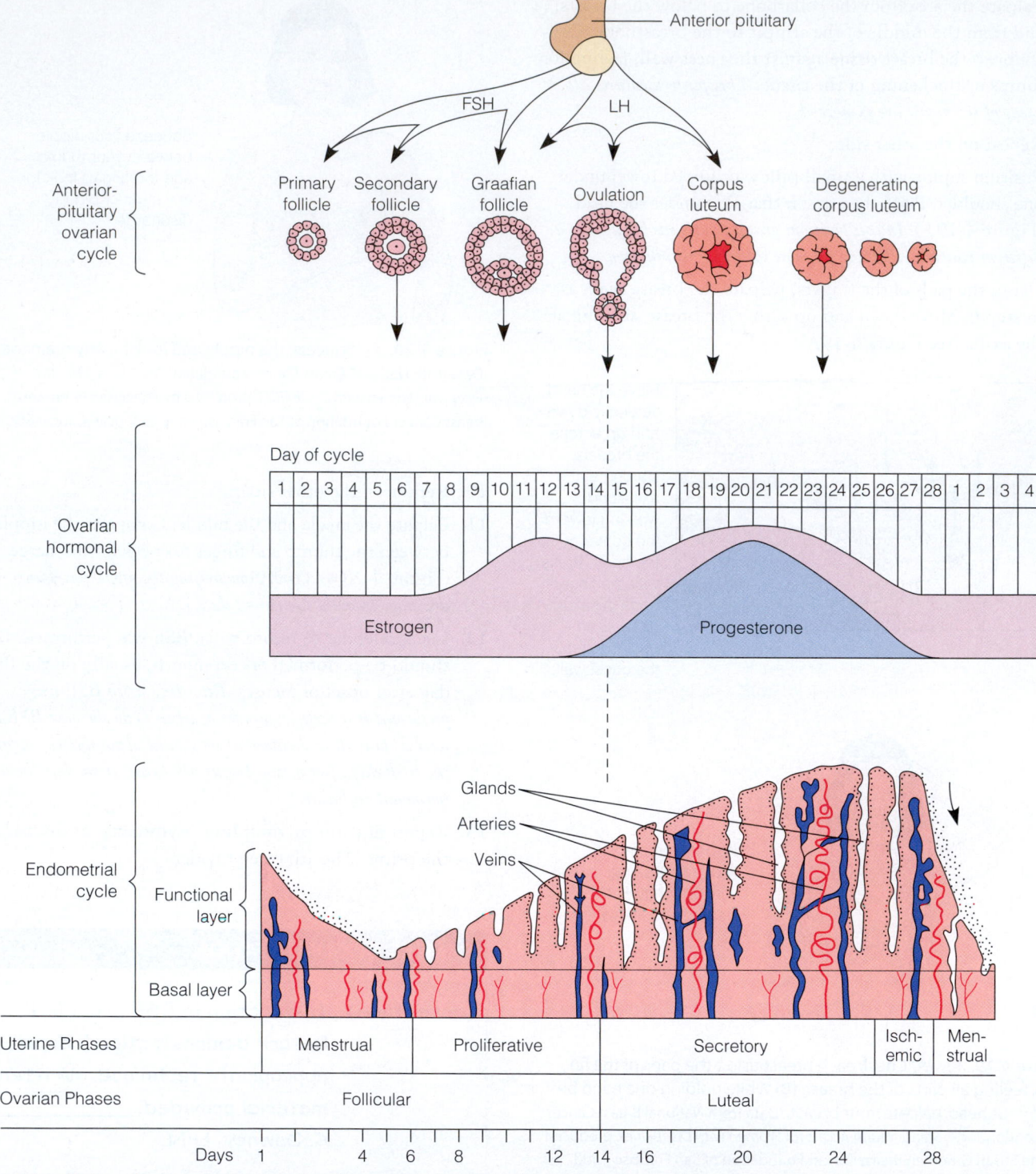

Figure 4-21. ■ Female reproductive cycle showing interrelationships of hormones, phases of the ovarian cycle, and phases of the uterine cycle.

25 or 26. Progesterone stimulates the endometrium to become more vascular in preparation for a pregnancy. If pregnancy does not occur, the decrease in progesterone causes menses and stimulates the anterior pituitary gland to again release FSH. If pregnancy does occur, the developing embryo secretes hormones to maintain the endometrium. This process is discussed in more detail in Chapter 6 ○○ of this text.

SEXUAL RESPONSE

As anatomic and physiologic development occurs in both genders, sexual responses become more common. When sexual responses become stronger, sexual activity may begin.

In both genders, there is a pattern to sexual response. Masters and Johnson (1966) described phases of sexual response that are still commonly used: excitement, plateau, orgasm, and resolution. Table 4-1 ■ summarizes these changes.

TABLE 4-1

Physiologic Changes in the Sexual Response Cycle

PHASE OF THE SEXUAL RESPONSE CYCLE	SIGNS PRESENT IN BOTH GENDERS	SIGNS PRESENT IN MALES ONLY	SIGNS PRESENT IN FEMALES ONLY
Excitement	Increased muscle tension Moderate increase in heart rate, respirations, and blood pressure Sex flush (less prevalent in men than in women; present in 75% of women) Nipple erection (60% of men and most women)	Penile erection Tensing, thickening, and elevation of the scrotum Partial elevation and increase in size of testicles	Enlargement of the clitoral glans Vaginal lubrication Widening and lengthening of vaginal barrel Separation and flattening of the labia majora Reddening of the labia minora and vaginal wall Breast tumescence (enlargement) and enlarged areolae
Plateau	Increased voluntary and involuntary myotonia Abdominal, intercostal, anal, and facial muscle contraction Accelerated heart rate and respiratory rate, and increased blood pressure Sex flush (appearance in some men late in the phase; spread over the entire body in women)	Increase in penile circumference at the coronal ridge (base of the prepuce) and deepening of color 50% increase in testicular size and elevation close to the perineum Appearance of a few drops of mucoid secretions from the bulbourethral glands at tip of penis; may contain sperm	Retraction of the clitoris under the hood Appearance of the orgasmic platform (increase in the size of the outer one-third of the vagina and the labia minora) Slight increase in the width and depth of the inner two-thirds of the vagina Further reddening of the labia minora Appearance of a few drops of mucoid secretion from the Bartholin's glands to lubricate inner labia Further increase in breast size and areolar enlargement
Orgasm	Involuntary spasms of muscle groups throughout the body Diminished sensory awareness Involuntary contractions of the anal sphincter Peak heart rate (110–180 bpm), respiratory rate (40/min or greater), and blood pressure (systolic 30–80 mm Hg and diastolic 20–50 mm Hg above normal)	Rhythmic, expulsive contractions of the penis at 0.8-sec intervals Emission of seminal fluid into the prostatic urethra from contraction of the vas deferens and accessory organs (stage 1 of the expulsive process) Closing of the internal bladder sphincter just before ejaculation to prevent retrograde ejaculation into bladder Orgasm may occur without ejaculation Ejaculation of semen through the penile urethra and expulsion from the urethral meatus; the force of ejaculation varies from man to man and at different times but diminishes after the first two to three contractions (stage 2 of the expulsive process)	Approximately 5–12 contractions in the orgasmic platform at 0.8-sec intervals Contraction of the muscles of the pelvic floor and the uterine muscles Varied pattern of orgasms, including minor surges and contractions, multiple orgasms, or a simple intense orgasm similar to that of the male

(continued)

TABLE 4-1

Physiologic Changes in the Sexual Response Cycle (continued)

PHASE OF THE SEXUAL RESPONSE CYCLE	SIGNS PRESENT IN BOTH GENDERS	SIGNS PRESENT IN MALES ONLY	SIGNS PRESENT IN FEMALES ONLY
Resolution	Reversal of vasocongestion in 10–30 min; disappearance of all signs of myotonia within 5 min Genitals and breasts return to their pre-excitement states Sex flush disappears in reverse order of appearance Heart rate, respiratory rate, and blood pressure return to normal Other reactions include sleepiness, relaxation, and emotional outbursts such as crying or laughing	A refractory period during which the body will not respond to sexual stimulation; varies, depending on age and other factors, from a few moments to hours or days	N/A

NURSING CARE

PRIORITIES IN NURSING CARE

When assessing and caring for clients with reproductive system disorders, keep in mind that many men and women place a high value on their ability to reproduce. Focus your care on being supportive through active listening. Obtaining a comprehensive sexual history is a high priority for the client with pelvic or reproductive system symptoms. A nonjudgmental nurse in a nonthreatening environment is critical in obtaining complete, accurate data. Maintaining confidentiality is also a high priority. Be sensitive to sexual concerns of people from non-Western cultures. Open-ended questions are generally less threatening. Also, spend time promoting sexual health through teaching safe sex practices.

ASSESSING

Reproductive assessment includes recording data of the client's past and present sexual history, and risk factors. Any presenting signs and symptoms are recorded. Observation of the stage of physical maturation is also noted (Figure 4-22A and B ■). The client's understanding of the medical condition is important for the nurse to assess. Because of the close proximity of the urinary system to the reproductive system, the nurse should assess for urinary symptoms.

DIAGNOSING, PLANNING, AND IMPLEMENTING

Nursing diagnoses are made specifically for the individual client. However, they might include:

- Sexual dysfunction reacted to (specific problem)
- Pain related to (specific problem)
- Disturbed Body Image related to (specific problem)
- Risk for Infection related to (specific problem)
- Rape Trauma Syndrome.

Client outcomes might include:

- Expresses understanding of the cause and treatments of sexual dysfunction
- Achieves adequate pain relief
- Expresses acceptance of change in body image
- Maintains infection-free status
- Expresses feelings and initiates positive measures to deal with feelings.

To achieve these outcomes, the nurse provides various interventions.

- Assist with screening and diagnostic examinations. *The primary care provider will need to perform a series of diagnostic exams to determine the exact medical diagnosis. The nurse may need to set up equipment, assist with specimen collection, and provide instructions to the client.*
- Teach clients about specific problems. *The primary care provider will provide information to the client about the specific problem. Often, the nurse needs to reinforce teaching and answer questions.*
- Provide pharmacologic and nonpharmacologic pain relief methods. *The care provider will often prescribe medication to relieve pain. The nurse must provide information about the administration, use, and side effects of medication. Other pain relief methods may also be helpful, including heat/cold, positioning, and relaxation techniques.*

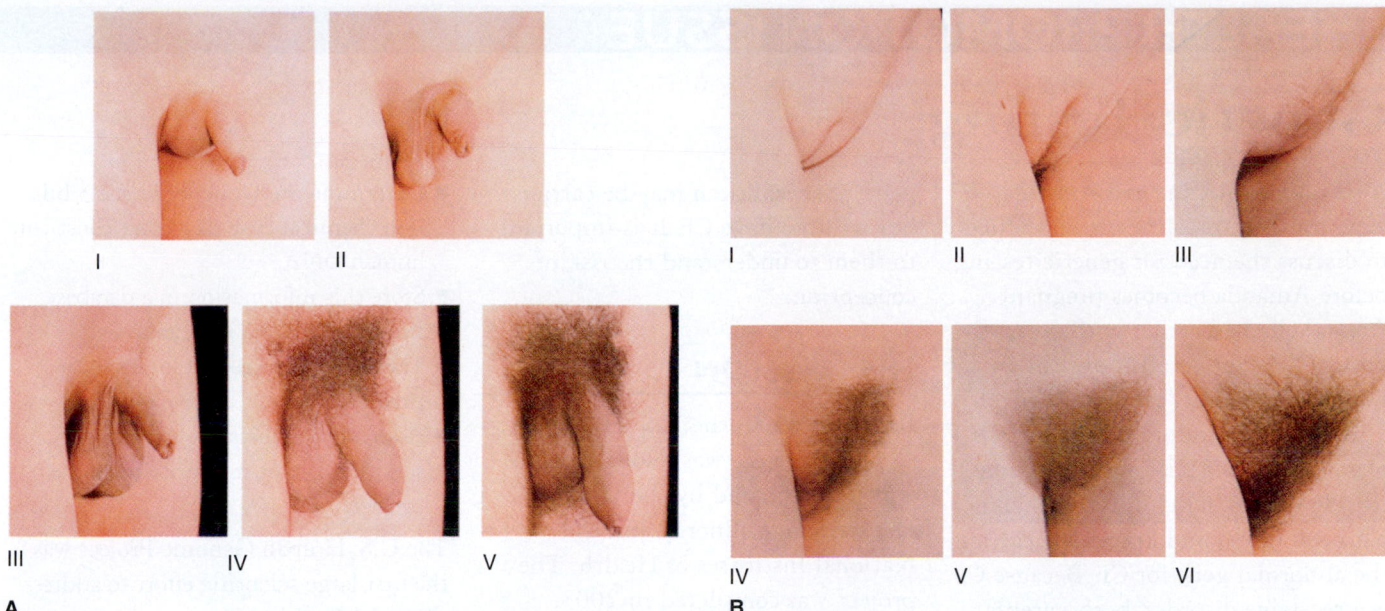

Figure 4-22. ■ (**A**) Stages of male pubic hair and external genital development. (**B**) Stages of female pubic hair development. From Ven Wieringen et al. (1971). *Growth diagrams 1965 Netherlands.* Groningen: Walters-Noardhof.

■ Monitor surgical sites for signs of complications. *Any surgical sites should be observed for signs of bleeding and infection.*

■ Refer clients to local support groups as appropriate. *Knowing you are not alone with a medical problem is helpful for emotional support. Many health care facilities have established groups of clients with similar problems. These support groups meet to discuss feelings and solutions for common concerns.*

EVALUATING

The nurse modifies care until expected outcomes are achieved. For example, if vital signs after a complication are altered, the nurse would modify the care plan to take vital signs more frequently.

NURSING PROCESS CARE PLAN
Client with Ovarian Cyst

Janice, 17 years old, was admitted to the postsurgical unit following laparoscopic surgery for a left ovarian cyst. The operative report states that the ovarian cyst was removed with minimal damage to the ovary. The client's mother is at the bedside.

Assessment. VS: T 98.4, P 96, R 24, BP 130/72. Janice states that the nursing assistant just helped her to the bathroom and now she has right upper quadrant pain radiating to right shoulder. She states the pain is a 6 on a 1 to 10 scale. Denies nausea. Abdominal dressings are dry.

Nursing Diagnosis. The following important nursing diagnosis (among others) is established for this client:

■ Acute Pain (pelvic) related to laparoscopic surgery for left ovarian cyst

Expected Outcomes

■ Client will verbalize pain as 3 or less on a scale of 1 to 10.

Planning and Implementation

■ Teach Janice that she may experience pain in the right upper quadrant and the right shoulder for 24 to 48 hours after laparoscopic surgery. *This teaching will help Janice understand that her pain is normal and should subside in a few days.*

■ Teach Janice relaxation techniques to lessen pain and ease breathing. *Diaphragmatic pain can lead to hypoventilation, which could lead to pneumonia. It is important for the client to relax and breathe normally.*

■ Teach Janice to lie flat, turning side to side, for most of the day. *Lying flat and turning from side to side will facilitate the absorption of the carbon dioxide gas used in surgery.*

■ Teach Janice the use and side effects of prescribed medication. *Taking medication as prescribed can help in the recovery process by allowing Janice to turn, move, and deep breathe. Side effects should be reported and documented.*

Evaluation. Janice's pain level was evaluated 30 minutes after medication and every 2 hours for 24 hours. Her respirations

(*Text continues on p. 88.*)

HEALTH PROMOTION ISSUE

Genetic Testing

A young couple, Joe and Amanda, have come to the obstetrician's office to discuss the need for genetic testing before Amanda becomes pregnant. Amanda had a brother with cystic fibrosis (CF). She recalls how difficult it was for her and her parents to watch him die of respiratory complications. She is concerned that she could give this disease to her children. Amanda has been tested and knows she carries the abnormal gene for CF. Because CF is a recessive disorder, both parents must pass on the defective gene in order for the child to have the disease. If Joe is not a carrier of the defective gene, their children may be carriers but will not have CF. It is important to them to understand the risk of conception.

DISCUSSION

Begun in 1990, the U.S. Human Genome Project was a long-term effort coordinated by the U.S. Department of Energy and the National Institutes of Health. The project was completed in 2003. The project goals were to:

- Identify the approximately 20,000 to 25,000 genes in human DNA.

- Determine the sequence of the 3 billion chemical base pairs that constitute human DNA.
- Store this information in a database.
- Improve tools for data analysis.
- Transfer related technologies to the private sector.
- Address the ethical, legal, and social issues (ELSI) that may arise from the project.

The U.S. Human Genome Project was the first large scientific effort to address potential ELSI implications resulting from project data.

Another important aspect of the U.S. Human Genome Project was the federal government's dedication to transferring the technology learned through this study to the private sector. By licensing private companies and awarding grants for continued research, the project could become the catalyst for developing new knowledge.

DNA Structure and Disease

A chromosome is made up of numerous segments called genes. A single gene or genome contains the DNA of the organism. Genes carry the information the organism needs for all life processes. DNA is made of four similar chemicals: adenine (A), thymine (T), guanine (G), and cytosine (C). The order of these chemicals underlies all life's diversity, even determining whether the organism

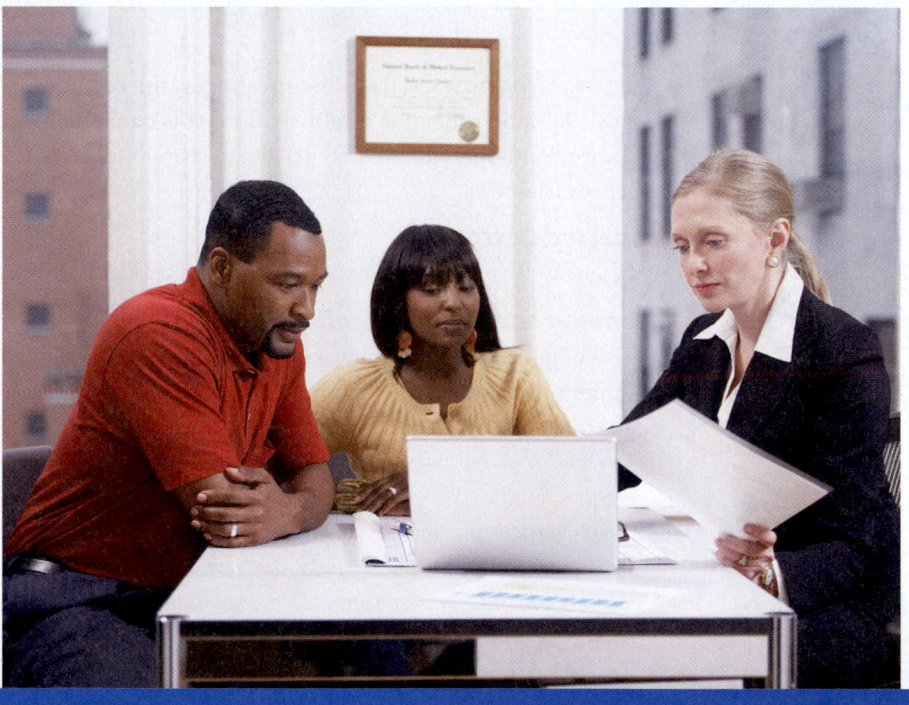

is human or another species, such as fruit fly or yeast. Identifying and recording the order of these chemicals is the basis of genetic research. Alteration or mutation in the order of A, T, G, and C results in disease. The cause of some disorders has been identified through genetic research.

Prenatal (during pregnancy) genetic testing of the mother and fetus may be recommended if abnormalities are suspected. Although any baby could end up with a genetic disorder caused by a new mutation, babies who have a family history of genetic disorders are at increased risk. In this case, genetic testing before conception is recommended so the parents have an understanding of the risks involved in pregnancy. Once research has identified the exact location of disease-causing genes, it is easier and faster to identify whether parents are carriers of these abnormal genes. If there is a risk that the fetus will inherit a particular genetic disorder, such as cystic fibrosis, genetic counselors can discuss options with the couple.

PLANNING AND IMPLEMENTATION

Although there is never a pregnancy without risk, parents who participate in family planning are requesting information to reduce the risk of abnormalities as much as possible. Genetic testing may be the first in a long line of choices facing the couple. For example, if Joe tests negative for cystic fibrosis, the couple has only a slim chance of having a child with this disorder. However, if Joe tests positive, there is a 50% chance the child will have cystic fibrosis. The couple will need to decide whether to go ahead and have a baby, whether to have artificial insemination with donor sperm, whether to adopt a child, or whether not to have children. If the couple decides to have a baby, they may choose to test the fetus for cystic fibrosis and possibly abort the pregnancy if the disease is present. Before these choices are made, the couple will need accurate, up-to-date information. The best person to help with such decision making is a genetic counselor.

The nurse in the obstetrician's office may need to reinforce information that is presented by the doctor, such as why genetic testing is needed, how specimens are obtained, and what laboratory results mean. The nurse should prepare a list of genetic counselors in the area. When genetic testing is complete, referral to these counselors can be made in a timely manner. If pregnancy does occur, the nurse will need to provide emotional support for the family. Genetic testing is becoming more financially affordable, but finances may prevent many couples from seeking testing before pregnancy. The nurse may be able to suggest financial resources, including research studies, that may be able to perform the tests free of charge.

SELF-REFLECTION

Have you ever had a strong desire to do something, and when you finally had the opportunity, something went wrong and someone was hurt? Do you recall how badly you felt? These are the same feelings parents experience when they have a child with a genetic disorder. They feel guilty. They might blame each other. They tell themselves, "If only I had been tested...." By recalling similar feelings, the nurse can be more empathetic in supporting the parents and helping them work through their feelings.

SUGGESTED RESOURCES

- **www.ornl.gov/sci/techresources/Human_Genome** This large government site provides information about genetic disorders and testing.
- **www.nsgc.org** National Society of Genetic Counselors.
- **www.beyonddiscovery.org** National Academy of Sciences website.

and lung sounds were also evaluated every 2 hours and remained clear. Pain gradually reduced to 3 out of 10 within 12 hours of surgery.

Critical Thinking in the Nursing Process

1. What complications to the ovary might occur because of the ovarian cyst and surgery?
2. Why would diaphragmatic pain be common after laparoscopic abdominal surgery?

3. What are some possible treatments to prevent future ovarian cysts?

Note: Discussion of Critical Thinking questions appears in Appendix I.

Note: The references and resources for this and all chapters have been compiled at the back of the book.

Chapter Review

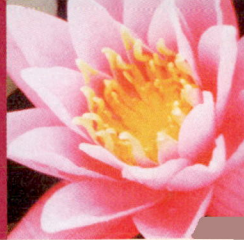

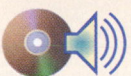 **KEY TERMS** by Topic

Use the audio glossary feature of either the CD-ROM or the Companion Website to hear the correct pronunciation of the following key terms.

Introduction
gamete, gametogenesis, puberty

Chromosomes and Genes
chromosomes, genome, transposons

Male Reproductive System
testes, tunica vaginalis testis, tunica albuginea, seminiferous tubules, spermatogenesis, spermatogonia, follicle-stimulating hormone (FSH), primary spermatocyte, spermatids, autosomes, spermatozoa, acrosome, testosterone, epididymis, vas deferens, ductus deferens, spermatic cord, ejaculatory duct, urethra, semen, seminal fluid, seminal vesicles, prostate, bulbourethral glands, Cowper's glands, penis, glans, foreskin, prepuce, circumcision, scrotum

Female Reproductive System
ovarian follicles, oocyte, Graafian follicles, ovum, granulosa cells, antrum, corpus luteum, oogenesis, polar bodies, estrogen, endometrium, progesterone, menses, fallopian tubes, uterine tubes, oviducts, fimbriae, cilia, uterus, myometrium, body, cervix, fundus, vagina, rugae, hymen, mons pubis, labia majora, labia minora, clitoris, vestibule, urinary meatus, true perineum, female circumcision, infibulation, dyspareunia, Bartholin's glands, greater vestibular gland, alveoli, lactiferous ducts, areola, lactogenesis, colostrum, menarche, menopause, proliferative phase, secretory phase

KEY Points

- The unique combination of traits a person has results from that person's genetic makeup. Chromosomal abnormalities and genetically inherited illnesses affect a person's physical being and health.

- It is important for the nurse to consider the anatomy and physiology of the male or female reproductive system each time a history or physical is taken.

- The nurse needs to understand the process of sperm and ovum production in order to answer a couple's fertility questions.

- The nurse should understand the function of sex hormones in order to explain the signs of puberty.

- The nurse uses knowledge of the process of lactation when helping the new mother with breastfeeding techniques.

- The nurse must be able to explain the phases of the menstrual cycle and correlate each with physical changes during a 28-day cycle. This information is important when teaching clients about signs of menstrual problems, hormone replacement therapy, and birth control measures.

- The nurse uses knowledge of the sexual response when teaching clients about their own and their partner's sexual responses, and when identifying sexual dysfunction.

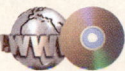 **EXPLORE Media**Link

Additional interactive resources for this chapter can be found on the Companion Website at www.prenhall.com/towle.

Click on Chapter 4 and "Begin" to select the activities for this chapter.

For chapter-related NCLEX-style questions and an audio glossary, access the accompanying CD-ROM in this book.

Animations

Oogenesis

Spermatogenesis

Ovulation

Conception

FOR FURTHER Study

For a complete discussion of ethical questions concerning the U.S. Human Genome Project, see Chapter 2.

See Chapter 6 for an in-depth discussion on pregnancy and the developing embryo.

The pelvic structures, their shapes, and their measurements are discussed in Chapter 7 and Figure 7-4.

For additional information on the surgical treatments for reproductive problems, see Chapter 8.

Circumcision and milk production are discussed further in Chapter 9.

Critical Thinking Care Map

Caring for a Client with Epididymitis

NCLEX-PN® Focus Area: Psychosocial Integrity

Case Study: Juan Martinez, a 24-year-old man, comes to the health clinic with pain and swelling in the scrotum. He admits to burning with urination and a purulent discharge from the penis. He states that he has had unprotected sexual intercourse with several women over the past few weeks. He states, "I hope this will not affect my being able to get an erection."

Nursing Diagnosis: Disturbed Body Image related to infection of the epididymis

COLLECT DATA

Subjective	Objective
_____	_____
_____	_____
_____	_____
_____	_____
_____	_____
_____	_____

Would you report this? Yes/No

If yes, to: _____

Nursing Care

_____
_____
_____
_____
_____
_____
_____
_____
_____
_____
_____
_____

How would you document this? _____
_____
_____
_____

Data Collected
(use those that apply)

- 24-year-old male
- Pain and swelling in the scrotum
- Burning with urination
- Voice shaky, avoids eye contact
- Purulent discharge from the penis
- States unprotected sexual intercourse with several women over the past few weeks
- "I hope this will not affect my being able to get an erection."

Nursing Interventions
(use those that apply; list in priority order)

- Teach client about the need for protection from infection during sexual intercourse.
- Obtain a urine specimen for culture and sensitivity.
- Teach client about normal physiology of erection and infection of reproductive system.
- Teach client use and side effects of medication.
- Encourage client to discuss sexuality.
- Obtain a specimen from the penile drainage for culture and sensitivity.

Compare your documentation to the sample provided in Appendix I.

1 When teaching clients about the fertilization process, the nurse explains that fertilization usually occurs:

1. in the ovary.
2. in the distal end of the fallopian tube.
3. in the upper uterus.
4. in the vagina.

2 What structure should men check monthly in self-examination? Mark an X over the area in the figure below.

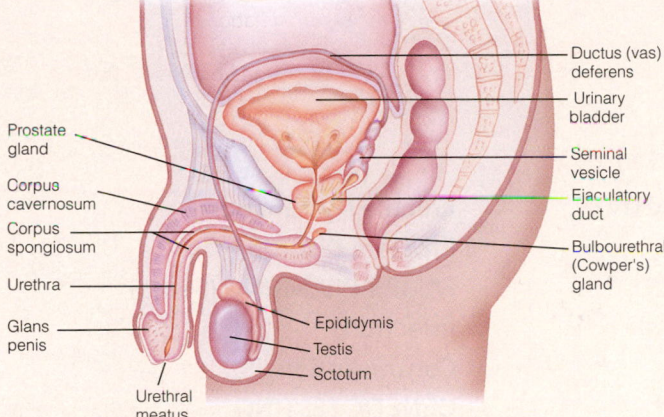

Prostate gland
Corpus cavernosum
Corpus spongiosum
Urethra
Glans penis
Urethral meatus
Ductus (vas) deferens
Urinary bladder
Seminal vesicle
Ejaculatory duct
Bulbourethral (Cowper's) gland
Epididymis
Testis
Scrotum

3 When teaching parents-to-be about the development of their baby, the nurse includes the fact that:

1. the gender of the baby is determined by the father's sperm.
2. the gender of the baby is determined by the mother's ovum.
3. the gender of the baby is determined by maternal hormones.
4. the gender of the baby is determined by paternal hormones.

4 The female reproductive system is sometimes described as an open system because:

1. the vagina opens to the outside of the body.
2. the cervix opens to allow the baby to leave the uterus.
3. the distal end of the fallopian tubes open into the pelvic cavity.
4. the Graafian follicle opens to release the ovum.

5 In the woman with a 30-day menstrual cycle, ovulation would probably occur on:

1. day 1.
2. day 13.
3. day 15.
4. day 30.

6 When teaching a new mother to breastfeed her baby, the nurse stresses that at least one breast should be emptied at each feeding. What is the reason for this?

1. Emptying the breast stimulates more milk production.
2. The infant will not get enough nutrition if he or she does not drink all of the milk.
3. If milk is allowed to remain in the breast, the breast can get infected.
4. Emptying the breast will prevent leaking of milk.

7 When are ova formed in the ovary?

1. continuously after puberty
2. during fetal development
3. just prior to puberty
4. monthly following puberty

8 When assessing a 21-year-old female who comes to the clinic with yellow, odorous vaginal discharge, the nurse should ask which of the following questions? (Select all that apply.)

1. When was your last menstrual period?
2. Are you sexually active?
3. What method of contraception do you use?
4. When was your last bowel movement?
5. Does you sexual partner use condoms?
6. How many children have you had?

9 Following a prostatectomy, the man is generally considered unable to father children. What is the reason for this statement? (Select all that apply.)

1. The urethra is destroyed and sperm cannot leave the body.
2. The vas deferens is cut and the sperm cannot leave the epididymus.
3. The ejaculatory duct is altered.
4. Lack of prostatic fluid makes sperm less mobile.
5. Swelling from the procedure permanently closes the vas deferens.

10 A young client asks the nurse, "Why do I have a period every 26 days and my friend has hers every 29 days?" The nurse's best response would be:

1. "Your menstrual cycle is controlled by hormones from the pituitary gland and uterus."
2. "Your menstrual cycle is controlled by hormones from the ovaries and uterus."
3. "Your menstrual cycle is controlled by hormones from the ovaries and pituitary gland."
4. "Your menstrual cycle is controlled by hormones from the uterus."

Answers for Review Questions, as well as discussion of Care Plan and Critical Thinking Care Map questions, appear in Appendix I.

Chapter 5

Reproductive Issues

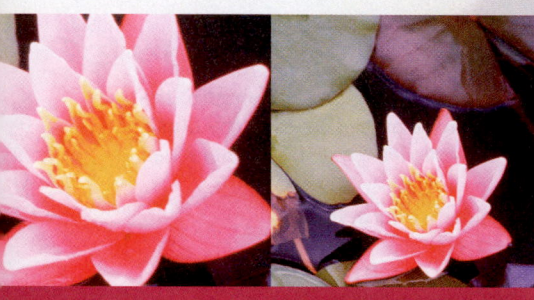

HEALTH PROMOTION ISSUE:
Teaching About Sex

NURSING PROCESS CARE PLAN:
Care of the Client with Rape Trauma Syndrome

CRITICAL THINKING CARE MAP:
Caring for a Client with Genital Warts

BRIEF Outline

WOMAN'S REPRODUCTIVE HEALTH ISSUES

Breast Disorders

Uterine Disorders

Ovarian Disorders

Pelvic Floor Disorders

Rape Trauma Syndrome

MEN'S REPRODUCTIVE HEALTH ISSUES

Testicular and Epididymal Disorders

Erectile Dysfunction

Prostate Disorders

FAMILY PLANNING ISSUES

Infections

Contraception

GENETIC TESTING

Infertility Issues

Future Issues

Nursing Care

LEARNING Outcomes

After completing this chapter, you will be able to:

• Describe possible causes of reproductive issues.

• Discuss the medical and surgical interventions used to treat the client with reproductive issues.

• Identify nursing diagnoses and nursing interventions to assist the couple with reproductive issues.

• Provide appropriate care for the couple with reproductive issues.

Since the mid-1960s, more emphasis and support have been placed on reproductive issues than at any other time in recent history. Many of these issues carry with them emotional, moral, and ethical concerns. This chapter presents common reproductive issues and currently accepted interventions. For a more in-depth study of specific disorders, pathology, and medical treatment, the reader should refer to a medical-surgical textbook.

WOMAN'S REPRODUCTIVE HEALTH ISSUES

Throughout her life, a woman faces many reproductive system issues. Some are minor, easily treatable conditions. Others are major life-threatening disorders. Some disorders affect the woman's ability to conceive, carry a pregnancy to term, or to breastfeed the infant. Some disorders may occur early in life but have an impact on the woman's ability to reproduce years later.

Breast Disorders

Breast disorders may be detected by the woman during a monthly BSE, during a physical examination by the primary care provider, or by **mammography** (diagnostic x-ray of the breast). Because early detection is critical to the treatment of malignancy, women should be taught the BSE technique (see Chapter 4, Procedure 4-2) and encouraged to seek annual physical examination and mammogram.

NONMALIGNANT BREAST DISORDERS

Fibrosis is the replacement of inflamed or damaged tissue with connective or scar tissue. In the breast, the result is a painless encapsulated tumor or fibroid. Frequently the fibroid degenerates, accumulating fluid in the process. This fluid-filled mass or **fibrocyst** puts pressure on surrounding tissue and becomes painful. Commonly, more that one fibrocyst forms in each breast, resulting in breast irregularities or "lumpiness." Occasionally, the cyst will drain into the nipple. Table 5-1 ■ describes

TABLE 5-1			
Breast Disorders: Symptoms and Treatment			
DISORDER	**SYMPTOMS**	**DIAGNOSIS/TREATMENT**	**NURSING INTERVENTIONS**
Fibrocystic breast disease	Fluid-filled movable mass Drainage from nipple Localized pain No skin retraction	Diagnosed by history, mammography, aspiration Medication to suppress estrogen and stimulate progesterone Mild analgesic	Teach BSE. Encourage to limit caffeine in diet. Provide emotional support.
Fibroadenoma	Freely movable mass with well-defined edges Rubbery in texture Nontender mass Most common in teens and early twenties	Fine-needle biopsy Excision with caution to prevent structural damage	Teach postoperative wound care. Provide emotional support.
Intraductal papillomas	Small ball-like nonpalpable mass May have nipple drainage of serosanguineous or brownish-green fluid	Found on mammogram Potential for malignancy Surgical removal	Reinforce teaching by health care provider. Provide emotional support. Provide referral to support group as appropriate.
Breast cancer	Small, hard painless lump, change in the size or shape of the breast, nipple Discharge, dimpling, pulling, or retraction of the skin of the breast resembling an orange peel	BSE, mammography, biopsy Surgical removal, chemotherapy, radiation Long-term therapy with tamoxifen	Reinforce teaching by health care provider. Teach postoperative care. Teach medication use and side effects. Provide emotional support. Provide referral to support group as appropriate.

symptoms and treatment of fibrocystic and other breast disorders.

Fibrocystic breast disease is most common in women between 30 and 50 years of age. Fibrocystic changes in the breast are an excessive response to cyclic hormonal changes. After menopause, these breast changes usually decrease. If cell growth occurs in conjunction with cyst formation, the woman is at a greater risk for breast cancer. Oral intake of caffeine found in coffee, tea, cola, and chocolate may contribute to fibrocystic breast disease. Medical management of fibrocystic breast disease focuses on diagnosis, screening for malignancy, and suppressing estrogen while stimulating progesterone. Aspirated fluid from the cysts is used for diagnosis as well as for relieving pressure and discomfort. There is no evidence that fibrocystic breast disease prevents breastfeeding.

Fibroadenoma is a freely movable, rounded mass with well-defined borders and a solid rubbery texture. These nontender masses are most common in women in their teens and early twenties. Diagnosis is by history and fine-needle biopsy. Excision may be indicated, but caution is exercised to prevent damage to the developing breast structure. Fibroadenomas are not associated with breast cancer.

Intraductal papillomas are tumors growing in a mammary duct. They most commonly occur during menopause. Although they are not malignant, they have the potential of becoming cancerous. These small ball-like tumors are often not palpable but are found on mammography. If they occur near the nipple, a serosanguineous or brownish-green discharge may be present. Because of the risk for malignancy, papillomas are usually removed surgically.

BREAST CANCER

Breast cancer is the second leading cause of cancer-related deaths among women. The most significant risk factor is the woman's age, with most breast cancer occurring after 50. Box 5-1 ■ describes breast cancer risk factors.

BOX 5-1	ASSESSMENT

Breast Cancer Risk Factors

- *Personal Data:* Female, over 50
- *Race:* White
- *Family History:* Mother or sister with breast cancer
- *Genetic History:* Defective genes BRCA1 and BRCA2
- *Medical History:* Cancer of breast, endometrial cancer, proliferative fibrocystic breast changes
- *Menstrual/Reproductive History:* Early menarche (before age 12), late menopause (after age 50), first birth after age 30, use of estrogen replacement therapy more than 5 years
- *Radiation Exposure:* Multiple chest x-rays or fluoroscopic exams, particularly before age 30
- *Lifestyle:* More than two alcoholic drinks daily, obesity, smoking, high economic status, breast trauma

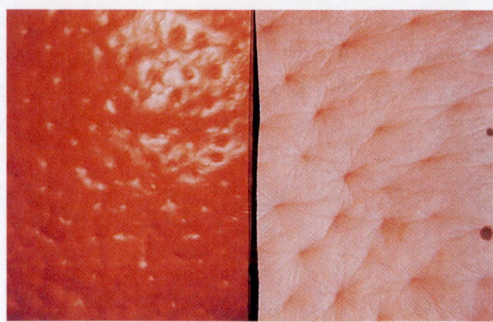

Figure 5-1. ■ *Left,* orange peel; *right,* peau d'orange cancerous changes in a breast.

Breast cancer is an uncontrolled growth of abnormal cells in the breast. Women who have never had functioning ovaries and who have never had estrogen replacement do not develop breast cancer. Most cancerous tumors occur in the ductal areas of the breast.

Noninvasive (also called *in situ*) malignancies develop within the ducts or lobes of the breast without invading the surrounding tissue. Diagnosis of these tumors, which often lie under the areola and nipple, is usually made by mammography rather than palpation.

Invasive tumors grow from the intermediate ducts of the breast. Tumors are classified by cell type. However, prognosis and treatment depend on the progression of the disease (stage of development). Symptoms of breast cancer include a small, hard painless lump; change in the size or shape of the breast; nipple discharge; dimpling; or pulling or retraction of the skin of the breast resembling an orange peel (Figure 5-1 ■).

Breast cancer can metastasize to the ribs, sternum, or lungs. In this case, the woman may also exhibit pain, spontaneous bone fractures, and respiratory symptoms such as labored breathing, cough, and **hemoptysis** (bloody sputum).

Treatment of breast cancer depends on the stage of cancer progression. Surgical intervention may include a **lumpectomy** (removal of the lump), breast-conserving surgery (removal of the tumor, a disease-free margin surrounding the tumor, and adjacent lymph nodes), simple **mastectomy** (removal of the breast), or radical mastectomy with removal of the breast, surrounding lymph nodes, and underlying muscle structure. Radiation and chemotherapy may also be used to shrink and destroy the cancer cells. Long-term treatment with tamoxifen (Nalvadex) is usually recommended (see Table 5-2 ■).

BREAST SURGERY

Surgery on the breast can be done for several reasons. As mentioned, surgery can be performed to remove a tumor or the entire breast and surrounding tissue due to a malignancy. Breast reconstruction (**mammoplasty**) may be performed

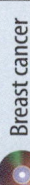

TABLE 5-2

Pharmacology: Common Drug for Clients with Breast Cancer

DRUG	USUAL ROUTE/DOSE	CLASSIFICATION	SELECTED SIDE EFFECTS	DON'T GIVE IF (CALL HEALTH CARE PROVIDER IF)
Tamoxifen (Tamofen, Tamone)	10–20 mg once or twice a day for 5 years	Antiestrogen, antineoplastic	Bone pain, blood clot formation, alteration in CBC, GI upset	Suspected blood clots, signs of thrombophlebitis, or pulmonary embolism

at the time of the mastectomy or at a later date if extensive therapy is required. (This information is covered in depth in medical-surgical courses.)

Some women have breasts that are large and heavy, putting strain on the shoulders and upper back. These women sometimes request that a **reduction mammoplasty** be performed. In women of childbearing age, the size of the breast will be reduced by removing fat tissue with an attempt to leave the mammary glands intact. This would allow the woman to breastfeed if she desires. In older women, the breast may be reduced by removing mammary glands and fat tissue.

Some women have smaller breasts. The ability to breastfeed is not related to the size of the breast. However, breast augmentation or implants may help these women improve their self-image. Implants contain either saline or silicone. In recent years, there has been controversy over the safety of silicone implants. Continued research should resolve this controversy.

Postoperatively, the woman may have drains leading away from the surgical site. The dressings are usually large and may be cumbersome. It will take 1 week or more for the swelling and bruising to subside. Before discharge, the woman should be taught to care for the incision, apply dressings, and empty the drainage container. During this time, she should be encouraged to look at the breast with a mirror and to begin to adjust to her new image. If a mastectomy has been performed, the woman will need to perform arm exercises on the affected side in order to facilitate lymphatic drainage and achieve full range of motion (Figure 5-2 ■). Due to the change in body image, she may need additional emotional support and referral to a mastectomy support group.

Uterine Disorders

MENSTRUAL DISORDERS

Most women experience minor discomforts just prior to and during menstruation. These include bloating, breast tenderness, cramping, and backache. Other effects can be symptoms of more serious disorders.

Premenstrual syndrome (PMS) is a group of symptoms resulting from an imbalance of estrogen and progesterone, as well as increased prolactin and aldosterone levels. Rising aldosterone causes sodium and water retention. The neurotransmitters monoamine oxidase (MAO) and serotonin may also play a role in PMS. Symptoms, including irritability, depression, edema, and breast tenderness, begin 7 to 10 days before menses and stop with the beginning of the menstrual flow. The manifestations of multisystem effects of PMS (shown in Figure 5-3 ■) vary for each client and each month.

Management of PMS focuses on diet, exercise, and relaxation techniques to reduce stress. A diet high in complex carbohydrates with limited simple sugars and alcohol is recommended. Restricting caffeine may reduce irritability. Limiting salt intake is useful in reducing fluid retention. An increased intake of calcium, magnesium, and vitamin B_6 may be helpful. A balance between exercise and rest can also help reduce irritability. Relaxation techniques and stress management include muscle relaxation, deep abdominal breathing, guided imagery, and meditation.

Other common conditions associated with menses include **menorrhalgia** (painful menses, also known as **dysmenorrhea**), **menorrhagia** (excessive menstruation in volume or number of days), **metrorrhagia** (bleeding between periods), and **amenorrhea** (absence of periods). These conditions are signs of underlying pathology and should be investigated by a health care provider.

Menopause (**climacteric**), the permanent cessation of menstruation, occurs between 35 and 58 years of age. Menses may stop suddenly or may decrease in volume until cessation occurs, or the time between periods becomes longer. Women who have short menstrual cycles or who smoke usually experience menopause 1 to 2 years sooner than women with longer menstrual cycles or women who do not smoke.

Symptoms of menopause begin shortly after the ovaries stop functioning whether menopause occurs naturally or due to surgical removal of the ovaries (**oophorectomy**). Symptoms include hot flashes, irritability, fatigue, apathy, depression, crying episodes, palpitations, vertigo, and vaginal dryness. Decalcification of bones occurs more commonly after menopause. Hormone replacement therapy

MediaLink   Premenstrual syndrome

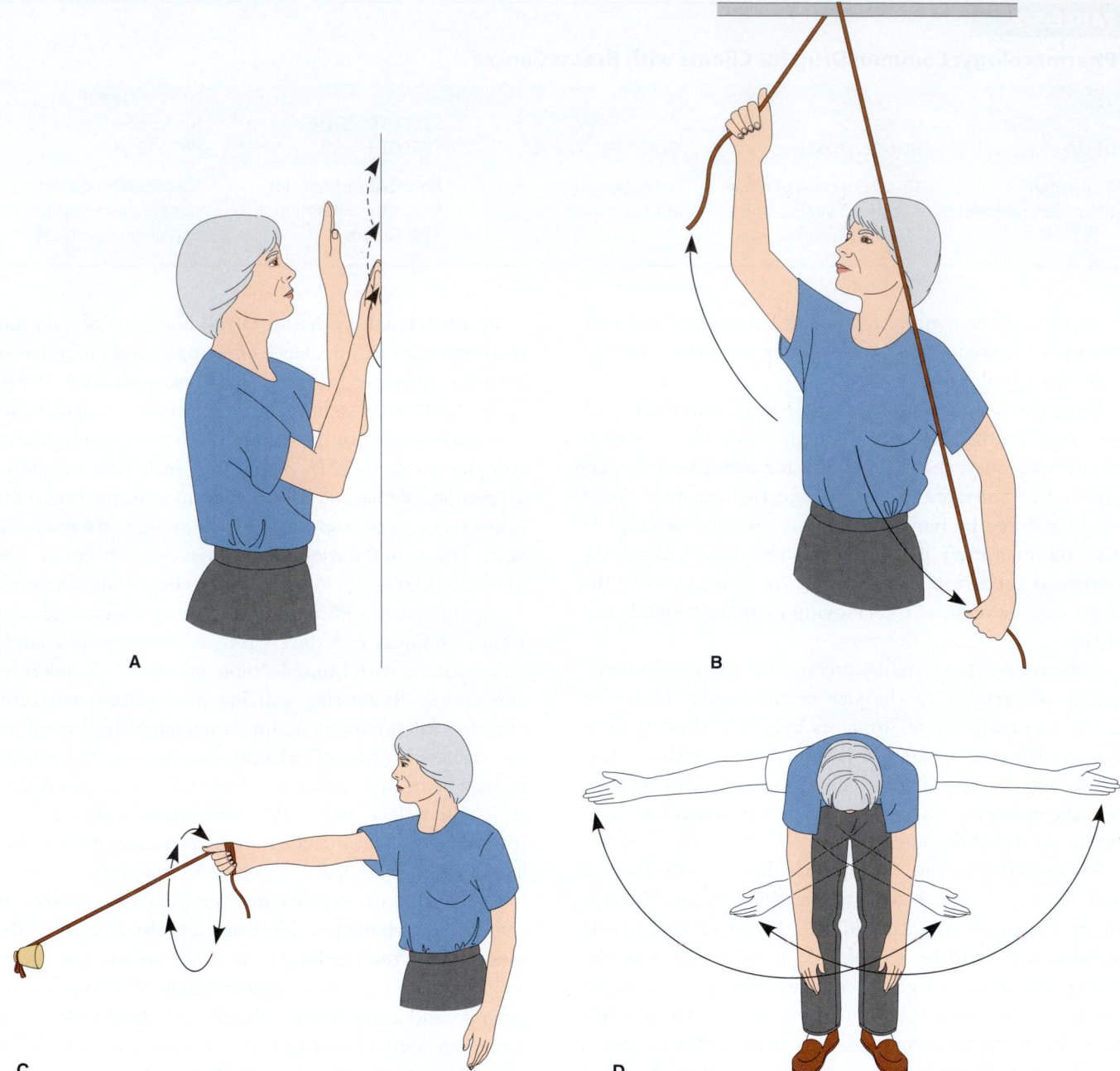

Figure 5-2. ■ Postmastectomy exercises. (**A**) Wall climbing: Stand facing wall with toes 6 to 12 inches from wall. Bend elbow and place palms against wall at shoulder level. Gradually move both hands up the wall parallel to each other until incisional pulling or pain occurs. (Mark that spot on wall to measure progress.) Work down to shoulder level. Move closer to wall as height of reach improves. (**B**) Overhead pulley: Using operated arm, toss 6-foot rope over shower curtain rod (or over top of a door that has a nail in the top to hold the rope in place for exercise). Grasp one end of rope in each hand. Slowly raise operated arm as far as comfortable by pulling down on the rope on opposite side. Keep raised arm close to your head. Reverse to raise unoperated arm by lowering the operated arm. Repeat. (**C**) Rope turning: Tie rope to door handle. Hold rope in hand of operated side. Back away from door until arm is extended away from body, parallel to floor. Swing rope in as wide a circle as possible. Increase size of circle as mobility returns. (**D**) Arm swings: Stand with feet 8 inches apart. Bend forward from waist, allowing arms to hang toward floor. Swing both arms up to sides to reach shoulder level. Swing back to center, then cross arms at center. Do not bend elbows. If possible, do this and other exercises in front of a mirror to ensure even posture and correct motion.

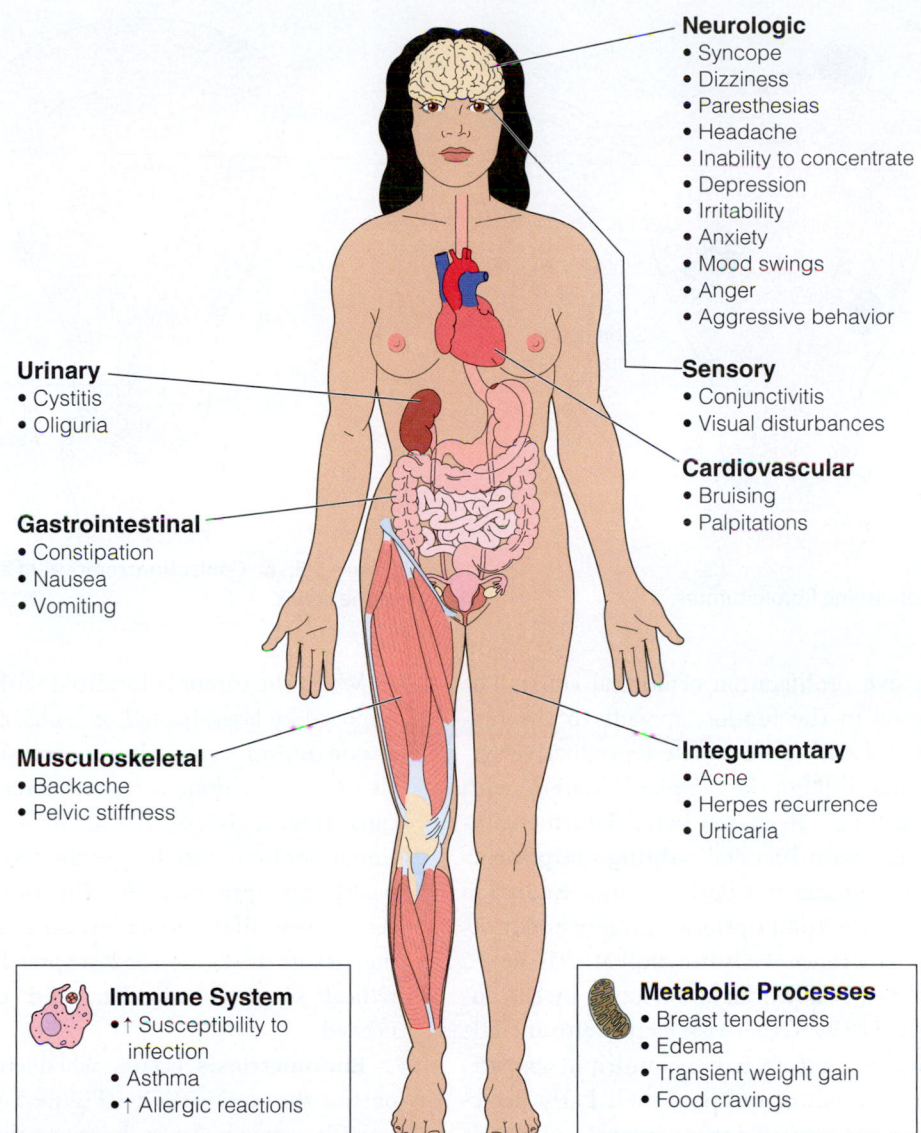

Neurologic
- Syncope
- Dizziness
- Paresthesias
- Headache
- Inability to concentrate
- Depression
- Irritability
- Anxiety
- Mood swings
- Anger
- Aggressive behavior

Sensory
- Conjunctivitis
- Visual disturbances

Cardiovascular
- Bruising
- Palpitations

Integumentary
- Acne
- Herpes recurrence
- Urticaria

Urinary
- Cystitis
- Oliguria

Gastrointestinal
- Constipation
- Nausea
- Vomiting

Musculoskeletal
- Backache
- Pelvic stiffness

Immune System
- ↑ Susceptibility to infection
- Asthma
- ↑ Allergic reactions

Metabolic Processes
- Breast tenderness
- Edema
- Transient weight gain
- Food cravings

Figure 5-3. ■ The multisystem effects of premenstrual syndrome.

(HRT) is recommended for many women to ease the menopausal symptoms and promote bone health. Some women choose herbal or food-based supplements instead of HRT (Box 5-2 ■).

UTERINE TUMORS

Common uterine tumors include nonmalignant fibroids, endometrial cancer, and cervical cancer. Fibroid tumors of

---

BOX 5-2   **COMPLEMENTARY THERAPIES**

Herbal Therapy

Black cohosh (*Cimicifuga racemosa*) is popular in the treatment of PMS and menopausal symptoms. No interaction with other drugs has been reported. Recommended doses may cause gastrointestinal upset. Black cohosh is contraindicated in pregnancy and lactation.

---

the uterus, common among women of all ages, are classified by their location within the uterus (Figure 5-4 ■). Although the exact cause of fibroid uterine tumor is unclear, they are probably related to estrogen secretion. Small tumors may go unnoticed for some time. Large tumors can enlarge the uterus, cause menorrhagia, put pressure on surrounding tissues, and cause lower abdominal and pelvic pain. In asymptomatic women who want to bear children, the fibroid tumors are monitored. In some cases, a laparoscopic **myomectomy** (removal of tumor and surrounding myometrium) may be performed. If tumors are large, a **hysterectomy** (removal of the uterus) may be necessary.

Endometrial cancer is common, affecting women between 50 and 70 years of age. Risk factors include an early menarche, late menopause, use of estrogen preparations without progestin for prolonged periods, obesity, and diabetes. These slow-growing tumors begin with endometrial

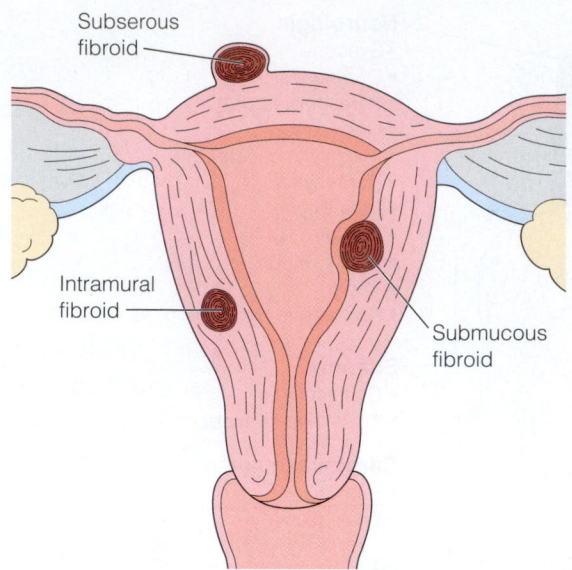

Figure 5-4. ■ Sites of uterine fibroid tumors.

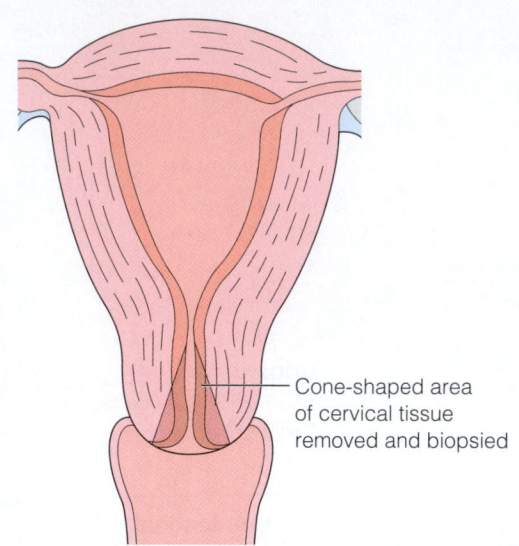

Figure 5-5. ■ Conization: removal of a cone-shaped section of the cervix.

hyperplasia (excessive proliferation of normal cells). The tumor usually begins in the fundus, spreads to the myometrium, and invades the entire female reproductive system. Metastasis occurs through the lymphatic system, with common sites being lungs, liver, and bone. Treatment includes a hysterectomy with bilateral **salpingo-oophorectomy** (removal of the uterus and both ovaries). Radiation may be used to shrink the tumor prior to surgery and postoperatively to eliminate cancer cells in lymphatic tissue.

Most cervical cancers result from an infection by the human papillomavirus (HPV). Other risk factors also include early sexual intercourse, unprotected sex, multiple sex partners, HIV infection, smoking, and poor diet. Early detection and intervention have reduced the incidence of invasive cervical carcinoma.

Most cervical cancers begin as **cervical dysplasia** (abnormal changes in the tissue of the cervix) or cervical intraepithelial neoplasia (CIN), including changes in the squamous cells of the cervix. Over time these cellular changes develop into carcinoma *in situ*, a localized cancer that becomes invasive if not treated. Cervical cancer invades the surrounding tissue, including the vagina, urethra, bladder, and rectum.

In the early stages, cervical cancer is asymptomatic. Once invasion occurs, bleeding, back and thigh pain, hematuria, bloody stools, and anemia are common. Diagnosis is made by a "thin prep" or a Papanicolaou (Pap) smear. In these tests, cells and secretions from the cervix are collected and sent to the laboratory for examination. If cancerous cells are identified, magnetic resonance imaging (MRI) or a computed tomography (CT) scan of the pelvis, abdomen, and bones may be ordered to determine the extent of invasion.

When the tumor is localized within the cervix, it may be removed by laser, heated or cooled probes, or cauterization. A **conization** (removal of a cone-shaped wedge of cervical tissue) may be done if lesions extend into the endocervical canal (Figure 5-5 ■). If the client becomes pregnant, it is important for her to discuss the cervical conization with her health care provider. As the pregnancy progresses, the cervix may dilate under pressure, and premature delivery may result. If the cancer has spread to surrounding organs, radical surgery, radiation, and chemotherapy may be needed.

Endometriosis occurs when endometrial tissue grows outside the uterine cavity (Figure 5-6 ■). Although the exact cause is unknown, it is theorized that endometrial cells migrate to deeper uterine tissue (myometrium) during fetal development or are washed through the fallopian tubes during menstruation. Endometrial cells can also be picked up in the lymph vessels and transported throughout the body. Endometrial cells that are **ectopic** (outside the uterus) respond to cyclic hormone influence just as uterine endometrium does. The cyclic bleeding results in inflammation, scar tissue formation, adhesions, and occlusions. Endometriosis may lead to infertility.

No single symptom is diagnostic of endometriosis. Often the client will complain of dysmenorrhea with pelvic pain or premenstrual **dyspareunia** (painful intercourse). Dysuria may indicate involvement of the urinary bladder. Premenstrual **tenesmus** (painful straining to defecate) and diarrhea may indicate colon involvement. Diagnosis is made by laparoscopic examination and biopsy of suspected tissue.

The goal of treatment is to preserve fertility for as long as possible. The woman who wants to have children is

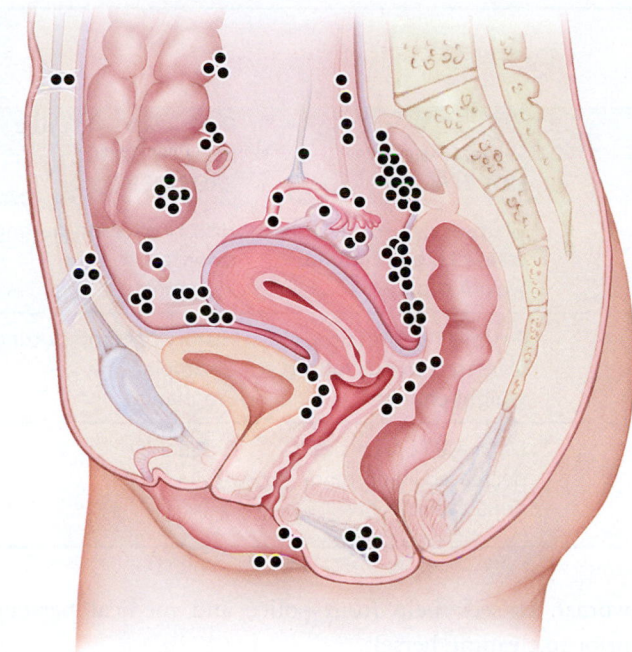

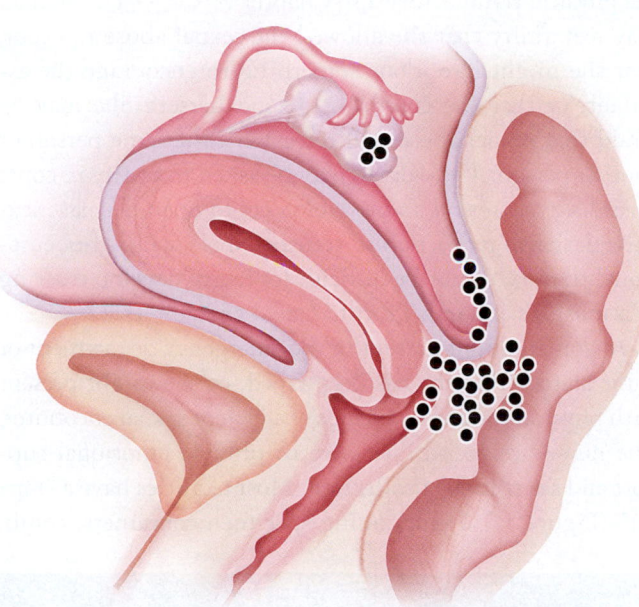

Figure 5-6. ■ Common sites for endometriosis. (Reproduced, with permission, from McGraw-Hill Companies, Inc. Way, L. W. [Ed.]. [1994]. *Current surgical diagnosis and treatment* [10th ed.]. Norwalk, CT: Appleton & Lange, p. 985.)

encouraged to become pregnant as soon as she can. Hormones may be prescribed to cause endometrial atrophy. Table 5-3 ■ identifies common medications used to treat endometriosis.

Surgical treatment may include endometrial obliteration with a laser or electrocautery via a laparoscope. If adequate symptom relief is not achieved, a hysterectomy with bilateral salpingo-oophorectomy may be required.

Ovarian Disorders

Cysts (fluid-filled sacs) commonly form in the ovary, whether from the Graafian follicle or from the corpus luteum. Most cysts regress spontaneously in two to three menstrual cycles. Some cysts become so large that they rupture and drain into the pelvis. Bleeding and a surgical emergency could occur.

Polycystic ovary syndrome (PCOS) results from numerous follicular cysts. This endocrine disorder is characterized by higher than normal LH, estrogen, and androgen levels, and low FSH levels. This hormone imbalance results in irregular menstrual cycles, **hirsutism** (excessive hair growth), acne, obesity, and infertility. The woman may develop type 2 diabetes mellitus and has an increased risk for endometrial cancer, hypertension, and high cholesterol.

Diagnosis of ovarian cysts is made by pelvic ultrasound. Hormone levels are evaluated to diagnose PCOS. Laparoscopic surgery may be necessary to drain large cysts or control bleeding. Hormone therapy may be useful to prevent cyst formation.

Ovarian cancer is the most lethal of female reproductive cancers. Ovarian cancer is asymptomatic until the cancer has spread to surrounding tissue or has been transported by the lymphatic system to other parts of the body. Risk factors for ovarian cancer include older age, early menarche, late menopause, history of infertility, treatment of infertility with Colomid (clomiphene), and a history of breast or ovarian cancer.

Diagnosis of ovarian cancer is made by pelvic ultrasound and laparoscopic biopsy. The treatment of choice is abdominal hysterectomy with bilateral salpingo-oophorectomy. The pelvic organs are examined for metastasis. Radiation and chemotherapy are used to destroy remaining malignant cells.

Pelvic Floor Disorders

Relaxation or damage of the pelvic muscles may result in prolapse or displacement of pelvic organs, including the urinary bladder, uterus, and rectum. A **cystocele** is prolapse of the urinary bladder into the vagina. It develops when the ligaments supporting the bladder are stretched, thinned with aging, or damaged during delivery. The client may experience stress incontinence, urgency, and difficulty emptying the bladder. Frequent bladder infections may develop.

A **rectocele** develops when the anterior rectal wall protrudes into the vagina. This condition may be caused by childbirth trauma or chronic constipation with straining to defecate. Symptoms include pelvic pressure and difficulty defecating. The woman may need to push up on the perineum or press against the back wall of the vagina to assist proper bowel alignment for defecation.

TABLE 5-3

Pharmacology: Drugs Used to Treat Endometriosis

DRUG	USUAL ROUTE/DOSE	CLASSIFICATION	SELECTED SIDE EFFECTS	DON'T GIVE IF (CALL HEALTH CARE PROVIDER IF)
Oral contraceptives	mg/tab depends on specific drug, one tablet daily	Contraceptive hormone	GI upset, depression, increased blood clotting, weight change	History of blood clotting disorders Pregnancy
Progesterone	Individual	Hormone	GI upset, depression, increased blood clotting, weight change	History of blood clotting disorders Pregnancy
Danozol (andro-gen hormone)	100–400 mg twice daily	Androgen hormone	Decreased breast size, decreased libido, emotional lability	Pregnancy

Uterine prolapse develops when the ligaments supporting the uterus in the pelvic cavity are stretched or damaged. The result is a slipping of the uterus into the vagina. The woman may notice a heavy or dragging sensation in the pelvis. She may also experience stress incontinence, constipation, and dyspareunia. She may be able to feel or see the cervix or entire uterus protrude from the vagina, especially after bearing down or heavy lifting.

Kegel exercises may be ordered to strengthen the pelvic muscles (see Figure 6-20 ⚭). Pelvic organ prolapse is often treated with surgery to shorten the muscle and supportive ligaments, and resuspend the pelvic organs in their natural position. In postmenopausal women, a hysterectomy is the preferred treatment for significant uterine prolapse. When surgery is contraindicated, the uterus and bladder may be supported with a vaginal pessary. The pessary must be removed, cleaned, and reinserted at regular intervals.

Rape Trauma Syndrome

Rape is forced sexual intercourse that involves vaginal, anal, or oral penetration. The rape can be forced by physical or psychological coercion, and drug or alcohol ingestion may be used to decrease the woman's awareness of the situation. The rapist can be a stranger, friend, or relative. **Incest** is sexual intercourse between close blood relatives and may or may not be consensual.

Sexual abuse affects the woman physically and mentally. Rape can cause trauma to the reproductive organs and lead to infection and scarring. Scarring may result in painful intercourse and may prevent future pregnancy. Following a rape, many women have a strong urge to shower and "wash away" all traces of the experience. Showering can actually destroy vital evidence the police will need to apprehend and prosecute the offender. It is, therefore, important for the woman to seek help from police and medical personnel prior to cleaning herself.

The psychological trauma is as great as or greater than the physical trauma. (See also Chapter 27 ⚭.) The woman may feel guilty that she allowed the sexual abuse to occur, that she might have done something to encourage the assailant, or that she could not defend herself. She may be afraid that sexual abuse will recur with the same person or another person. The woman may be asked to testify in court regarding the sexual abuse, which could open her past sexual relationships to public scrutiny. Following this emotional trauma, it may be difficult for her to develop trusting relationships and enjoy future sexual encounters.

A woman might present in the emergency department or clinic stating that she has been raped, or she might present with physical trauma suspicious of a violent sexual encounter. The nurse's responsibilities are to provide emotional support and assist in data collection. Most facilities have a "rape kit" (Figure 5-7 ■) containing specimen containers, comb,

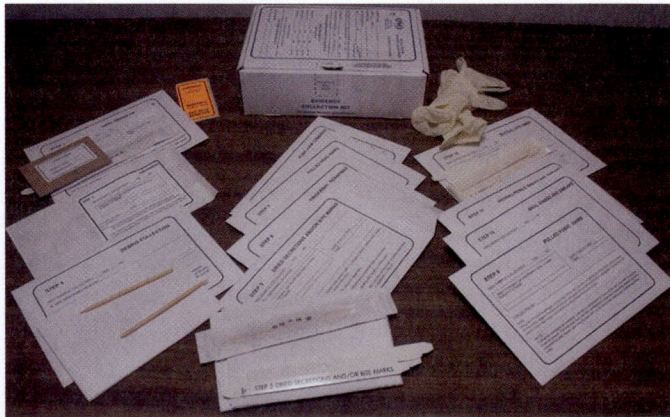

Figure 5-7. ■ Rape evidence collection kit contains a step-by-step system to gather samples for evidence. (Courtesy of Family Services of New York.)

slides, and other supplies necessary to collect evidence. It is important that all evidence be collected and secured according to legal standards. Guidelines and procedures for collecting this evidence should be outlined in a facility's policy and procedure manual.

Before collecting data, the woman needs to sign an informed consent form (see Chapter 2 ⊂⊃ for legal responsibilities of the nurse). A detailed history is obtained using the woman's own words to describe the events. The caregiver should use a nonjudgmental approach and must avoid coaching or leading the woman. The collecting of physical evidence serves the purpose of:

- Confirming recent sexual contact
- Showing that force or coercion was used
- Identifying the assailant
- Collaborating the woman's story.

The woman will be asked to remove all her clothing, and each item will be placed in a separate paper bag and labeled. Samples of stains and body fluids will be obtained for sperm analysis. The absence of sperm does not indicate that a rape did not occur because the assailant could have used a condom or might not have ejaculated. Hair samples will be pulled from the woman's head and pubic area to compare with other hair found on her body. The pubic hair will be combed to check for loose hairs that may have been transferred from the assailant. Debris will be collected from under her fingernails to check for blood or tissue from the assailant. Photographs should be taken of any injuries. A colposcope with photographic capability can be used to photograph intravaginal injury. All evidence must be labeled, placed in a paper bag, and remain in the possession of a professional until it is turned over to the police.

Because the psychological trauma during a rape is so great, the woman should receive counseling immediately. Many areas have rape crisis centers and personnel trained to provide the psychological support and counseling required in this situation. The psychological response to rape can be described in a series of overlapping phases. The acute phase begins during the rape and can last for a few days or longer. The woman feels fear, shock, disbelief, powerlessness, or helplessness. She may feel angry, humiliated, and unclean. She may suppress her feelings or exhibit an outward response in the form of crying or being tense and restless. She may experience alterations in sleep patterns such as insomnia or nightmares.

Within a few weeks, the woman may appear calm and composed as though she has adjusted to the situation. Frequently, however, these are outward signs of denial. She may go about her daily activities and return to work or school. This resumption of routine is important for her to regain a sense of control over her life. She may seek some forms of self-protection such as installing extra locks on her doors, taking a self-defense course, or buying a weapon. These activities do not resolve the emotional trauma. Instead, they give the impression to her support system that she is "over it." The support system may then withdraw.

However, denial does not last long. She may become depressed and anxious. She may want to talk about the rape. She may develop phobias, especially to situations similar to those in which the rape occurred. For example, if she was attacked at night, she may fear leaving her home after dark. If the rape occurred in her home, she may fear returning to an empty house. If her attacker was a stranger, she may fear crowds. She may continue to have nightmares in which she relives the rape. She may replay the incident repeatedly until she finally resolves that the attack was out of her control. It is important for the nurse to be a good, nonjudgmental listener and to make appropriate referrals to the registered nurse, physician, or counselor.

MEN'S REPRODUCTIVE HEALTH ISSUES

A discussion of reproductive issues would not be complete without reviewing male reproductive conditions. Only common conditions are discussed here. For more detailed information, pathology, medical treatment, and nursing interventions, refer to a medical-surgical textbook.

Testicular and Epididymal Disorders

Testicular cancer is the most common cancer of men between 15 and 35 years of age. Fortunately, testicular cancer has a greater than 90% cure rate. Most men with testicular cancer have no risk factors. Therefore, beginning at 15 years of age, all men should perform testicular self-exam. (See Chapter 4 ⊂⊃, Procedure 4-1.)

Testicular cancer grows within the testicle, eventually replacing all normal tissue. Normal tissue will feel soft, while the tumor will be a hard painless mass. Most commonly, only one testicle is affected. Testicular cancer spreads rapidly through the lymph vessels into the retroperitoneal lymph nodes (located behind the peritoneum but outside the abdominal/pelvic cavity). Enlarged lymph nodes may be palpated in the groin. If the cancer cells reach the vascular system, they commonly metastasize to the lungs, liver, and bone.

Treatment usually involves a radical **orchiectomy** (removal of one testis and spermatic cord) with removal of the retroperitoneal lymph nodes. The surgery is accomplished through an inguinal incision, taking care not to damage the nerves needed for ejaculation. Following surgery, radiation and chemotherapy are used to destroy any remaining cancer cells. If only one testicle is removed, reproduction may still be possible. However, the banking of sperm prior to surgery, radiation, and chemotherapy should be discussed with the client and his partner. If the client is a minor, teaching and support must also be provided to the parents.

An infection of the male reproductive system may result in **epididymitis** (inflammation of the epididymis) and **orchitis** (inflammation of the testes). In young men, the infection is most commonly caused by sexually transmitted infections (STIs) such as chlamydia or gonorrhea. (Sexually transmitted infections will be discussed later in this chapter.) In older men, epididymitis is associated with urinary tract infection or **prostatitis** (inflammation of the prostate).

Manifestations of epididymitis include pain and swelling of the scrotum, at times interfering with ambulation. Medical treatment includes antibiotics and analgesics. Nursing care focuses on relieving symptoms with ice packs and scrotal support. Epididymitis can cause infertility and should be evaluated after the infection is resolved.

Orchitis may be caused by the same organisms as epididymitis, as well as by a mumps virus that is excreted in the urine, or by trauma. Manifestations include severe testicular pain and swelling. Complications include **hydrocele** (fluid in the scrotal sac) and abscess. These complications can result in infertility and erectile dysfunction.

Erectile Dysfunction

Erectile dysfunction (ED, or impotence) is the inability to achieve or maintain an erection that allows for satisfactory sexual intercourse. Most commonly, this disorder affects men over 65 years of age. Any disorder that impairs circulation (e.g., atherosclerosis) or interrupts nerve or hormone intervention (e.g., diabetes and multiple sclerosis), or trauma that results in scar tissue (e.g., chronic infection or prostate surgery), may cause ED. Drugs that also alter circulation (e.g., antihypertensives) depress the central and peripheral nervous system (e.g., antidepressants), and some hormones may also have side effects of ED.

Diagnostic exams include:

- Blood tests for chemistry, testosterone, prolactin, thyroxine, and prostate-specific antigen (PSA)
- Nocturnal penile tumescence and rigidity monitoring. This test monitors the number and firmness of erections during sleep. It is useful in determining if ED is physical or psychological.

Medical or surgical treatment may influence the degree of erection but have little effect on fertility. ED can be treated with drugs such as Viagra (sildenafil), which enhances natural response to sexual stimuli. Testosterone replacement may be used if blood levels are low. Aldostadil (prostaglandin E_1) pellets may be inserted into the urethra or injected into the penis. This drug stimulates an erection but may be an unacceptable option for many men (Table 5-4 ■).

TABLE 5-4

Pharmacology: Drugs Used to Treat Erectile Dysfunction

DRUG	USUAL ROUTE/DOSE	CLASSIFICATION	SELECTED SIDE EFFECTS	DON'T GIVE IF (CALL HEALTH CARE PROVIDER IF)
Viagra (sildenafil)	50 mg taken 1 hr before sexual activity; not more than once daily	Anti-impotence agent	GI upset, headache, cardiovascular collapse	There are numerous drug–drug interactions that could result in death. Teach client to contact health care provider if erection lasts longer than 4 hours.
Alprostadil (prostaglandin E_1)	5–20 mcg injected into penis or urethral pellets; not more than one dose three times a week with 24 hr between doses	Tissue hormone	Dizziness, low blood pressure, drug allergy including redness at site, and respiratory distress	Teach client to contact health care provider if erection lasts longer than 4 hours.

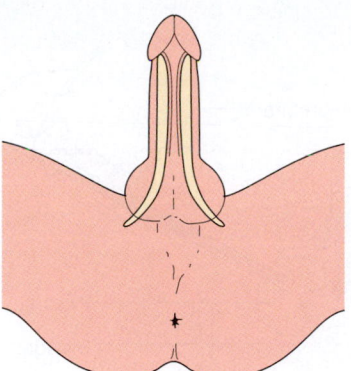

A Semirigid

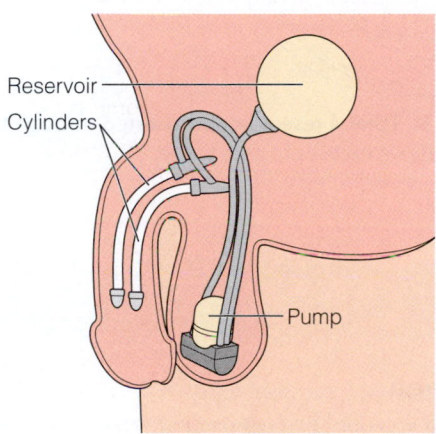

Reservoir
Cylinders
Pump

B Inflatable

Figure 5-8. ■ Types of penile implants. **(A)** Semirigid rods implanted in the corpora cavernosa keep the penis in a constant state of semierection. **(B)** With an inflatable penile implant, the client compresses a pump in the scrotum to fill cylinders in the corpora cavernosa and achieve an erection. Pressing a release valve returns the fluids to a reservoir.

When ED does not respond to less invasive treatment, penile implants may be surgically inserted into the penis. Two types of penile implants are available (Figure 5-8 ■). The semirigid implant maintains a constant state of partial erection. The inflatable penile implant has a fluid-filled reservoir that is inserted in the lower abdominal cavity, cylinders are inserted in the penis, and a pump is inserted in the scrotum. Erection is obtained when the pump is compressed, filling the cylinders with fluid. A release valve returns the fluid to the reservoir.

Prostate Disorders

Benign prostatic hyperplasia (BPH) most commonly affects men over the age of 50. Normally testosterone is converted to dihydrotestosterone (DHT) in the prostate.

DHT, along with estrogen (normally found in small amounts in men), may contribute to the growth of the prostate gland. The prostate gland enlarges in the center, compressing surrounding tissue and narrowing the urethra.

The primary symptoms include **nocturia** (the need to void frequently at night), difficulty getting the stream of urine started, a narrow stream of urine, dribbling after voiding, incomplete emptying of the bladder, frequency, and urgency. Diagnostic exams include:

■ Digital rectal exam (DRE) to assess the size and consistency of the prostate.

■ PSA—this chemical produced by the prostate gland indicates prostate cancer when elevated. Note that incidence of prostate cancer is affected by race (Box 5-3 ■).

■ Routine urinalysis and urine culture to determine if a urinary tract infection is present.

■ Uroflowmeter to determine the degree of urinary obstruction.

Treatment includes medication to shrink the prostate or relax the smooth muscles of the prostate, urethra, and bladder neck. Some of these drugs can cause a decrease in **libido** (the sexual drive). The herbal remedy saw palmetto reduces the symptoms of BPH and has few side effects. Often, surgery to remove the prostate will be required. The most common surgical approach is through the urethra or transurethral resection of the prostate (TURP; Figure 5-9 ■). Following surgery, a large three-lumen catheter is left in the urethra, and a continuous bladder infusion is instituted to prevent blood clots from obstructing the flow of urine. Following surgery, retrograde ejaculation (discharge of seminal fluid into the bladder instead of the urethra) may occur,

MediaLink

Conception

resulting in a low sperm count. However, it should not be assumed that the man is sterile.

Prostate cancer is a leading type of cancer in men. Prostate cancer rarely occurs before the age of 40. When diagnosed early and confined to the prostate, the 5-year cure rate is 100%. The cancerous tumor usually begins in the posterior region of the prostate and may spread into the seminiferous tubules or bladder. If metastasis occurs in the lymph nodes, tumors may also involve the lung, liver, and bone, especially the pelvis and spine. Besides a DRE and PSA, other diagnostic tests include transurethral ultrasound to help differentiate BPH from prostate cancer. Tissue biopsy is done to confirm diagnosis. A bone scan, MRI, or CT is done to identify possible metastasis.

Treatment includes drugs to block the effects of testosterone, radiation, and surgery. If the tumor is isolated in the prostate, a TURP may be performed. If metastasis has occurred, a radical prostatectomy is done through a different approach.

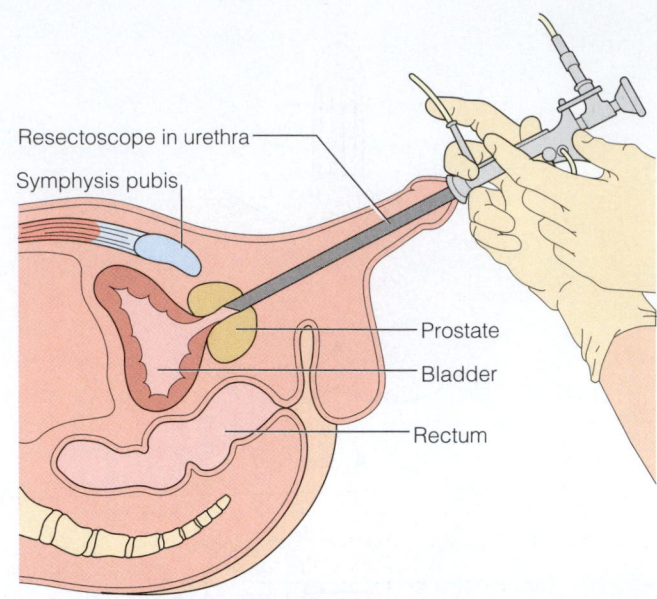

Figure 5-9. ■ TURP. A resectoscope inserted through the urethra is used to remove excess prostate tissue.

FAMILY PLANNING ISSUES

Infections

SEXUALLY TRANSMITTED INFECTIONS

STIs result from sexual contact with an infected person. Many people believe that only sexual intercourse can result in STIs. The reality is that infection can occur not only through sexual intercourse, but also through genital-genital, oral-genital, or rectal-genital contact. The most common STIs are chlamydia, genital herpes, gonorrhea, genital warts, trichomoniasis, and syphilis. Table 5-5 ■ lists these common infections, their manifestations, and their medical treatment.

COMMON SEXUALLY TRANSMITTED INFECTIONS

Chlamydia

Chlamydia is caused by *Chlamydia trachomatis*. In males, chlamydia is the major cause of nongonorrhea urethritis. In females, it infects the vagina, cervix, uterus, fallopian tubes, and urethra. The infection can be passed to the newborn during the birth process, resulting in eye infection and pneumonia. Complications include pelvic inflammatory disease, scarring of the fallopian tubes, and ectopic pregnancy. The newborn of an infected, untreated woman is at risk for developing ophthalmia neonatorum (an infection of the eye that can result in blindness; see Chapter 9 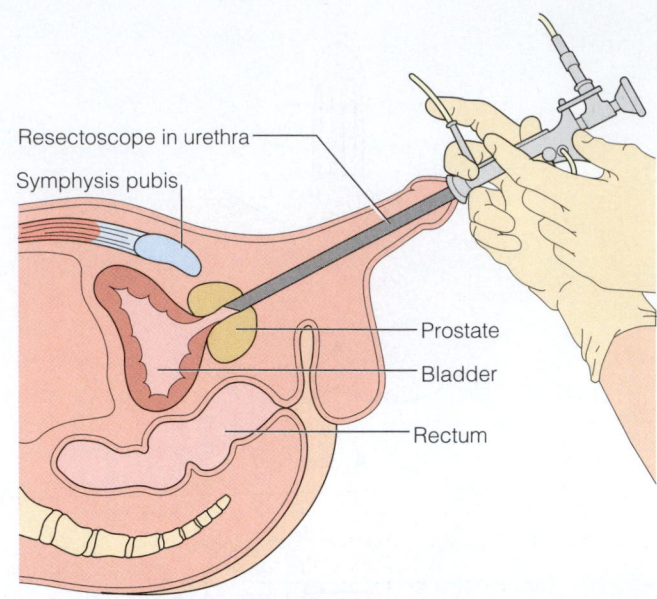). In men, chlamydia can cause scarring of the urethral mucosa.

Gonorrhea

Gonorrhea is caused by *Neisseria gonorrhoeae*. In males, gonorrhea is associated with urethritis, purulent urethral drainage, and burning on urination. Females are usually asymptomatic. Prior to pregnancy, gonorrhea can ascend through the cervix and infect the uterus, fallopian tubes, and pelvis. After the third month of pregnancy, the cervical mucous plug prevents gonorrhea from ascending into these organs. When the fetal membranes rupture during the birth process, gonorrhea can infect the infant's eyes and respiratory tract.

Like chlamydia, gonorrheal infection of the reproductive organs can lead to permanent scarring of the fallopian tubes and seminiferous tubules. The scarring may result in infertility.

Chlamydia and gonorrhea are commonly found together. Adequate treatment of both partners is essential to cure the infections. Abstinence or condom use is needed to prevent reinfection until cure is achieved. Further cultures must be taken to verify that treatment was successful.

Syphilis

Syphilis is an infection by the bacteria *Treponema pallidum*. Syphilis is divided into three stages with different symptoms at each stage.

■ Primary syphilis: Initially, a **chancre** (painless open sore) forms at the entry site (Figure 5-10A ■). General signs of infection, including slight fever and malaise,

TABLE 5-5

Summary of Sexually Transmitted Infections

DISEASE	ORGANISM	MANIFESTATIONS	MEDICAL TREATMENT
Chlamydia	*Chlamydia trachomatis*	Males: urethritis Females: permanent scarring	Erythromycin Amoxicillin
Genital herpes	Herpes simplex virus (HSV-2)	Burning, itching sensation prior to blister formation; blisters break, resulting in painful open lesions	Acyclovir
Gonorrhea	*Neisseria gonorrhoeae*	Females: asymptomatic, permanent scarring Males: urethritis, purulent urethral drainage, burning on urination	Ceftriaxone Cefixime with erythromycin or amoxicillin
Genital warts (condylomata acuminata)	Human papillomavirus (HPV)	Grayish-pink cauliflower-like lesions appear on the vulva or penis approximately 3 weeks after exposure	Cryotherapy Trichloroacetic acid
Trichomoniasis	*Trichomonas vaginalis*	Inflammation of the vagina and cervix, yellow-green, frothy, odorous discharge	*Note:* Metronidazole (Flagyl) is *contraindicated* in the first trimester of pregnancy due to its effects on the fetus (can cause birth defects).
Syphilis	*Treponema pallidum*	Stage 1: painless open sore, chancre, slight fever, and malaise Stage 2: fine red rash over the body, palms, and soles Stage 3: damage to heart, nervous system, bone, and skin Aneurysm, gait disturbances, blindness, dementia	Benzathine Penicillin G

may occur. If left untreated, the chancre disappears in 3 to 4 weeks.

- Secondary syphilis: Several months later, the symptoms of secondary syphilis appear. These include a fine red rash over the body, palms, and soles of the feet. Highly infectious moist papules may appear on the perineum. If untreated, these symptoms will also disappear in a few weeks. Symptoms of infection may not recur for many years.
- Tertiary syphilis: In the tertiary stage, damage to the heart, nervous system, bone, and skin become apparent. Aneurysm, gait disturbances, blindness, and dementia are a few disorders that can result from untreated syphilis.

Genital Herpes
Herpes is caused by one of two types of herpes simplex virus (HSV). HSV-1 causes cold sores and typically occurs above the waist. HSV-1 is not sexually transmitted. HSV-2 is associated with sexual contact. The symptoms include a

burning, itching sensation prior to blister formation (Figure 5-10B ■). The blisters break and result in painful open lesions. Many viruses are shed at this time, and an infection is highly contagious. Lesions heal spontaneously in several weeks.

Genital herpes also results in lifelong health problems that will affect infected people and their partners. Therefore, during an acute outbreak, the couple should abstain from sexual intercourse. If a pregnant woman has an acute outbreak and goes into labor, a cesarean section delivery should be performed to prevent infection of the infant.

Genital Warts
Genital warts (or condylomata acuminata) are caused by HPV. The grayish-pink cauliflower-like lesions appear on the vulva (Figure 5-10C ■) or penis approximately 3 weeks after exposure. Because genital warts resemble other lesions and can undergo malignant transformation, they should be biopsied and treated. Some strains of HPV, for

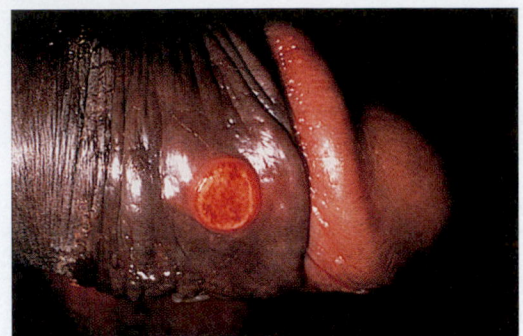

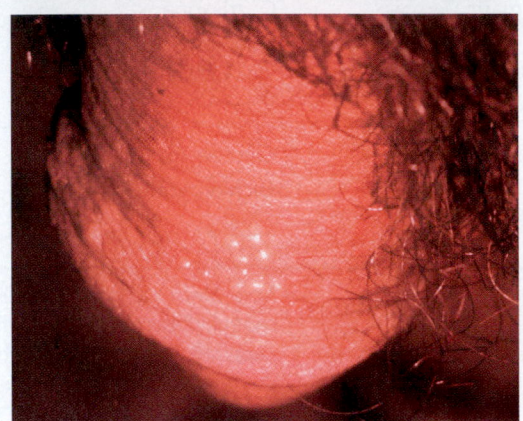

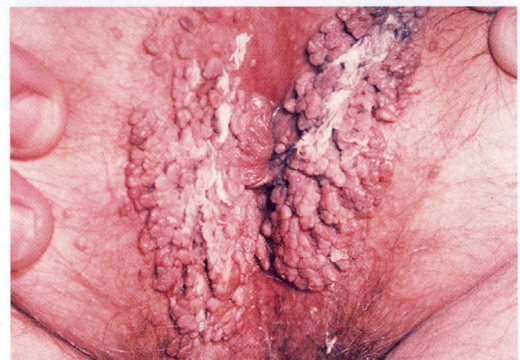

Figure 5-10. ■ Some sexually transmitted infections. (**A**) Primary syphilis. The entry point of syphilis develops a chancre. (**B**) Genital herpes blisters on the penile shaft signal the infectious phase. (**C**) Condylomata acuminata (genital warts) on the labia. (**A.** Custom Medical Stock Photo. **B.** Camera MD Studios, Carroll Weiss, Director, 8290 NW 26th Place, Sunrise, FL 33322. **C.** Ken Greer Visuals Unlimited.)

which a vaccine is available, are associated with cancer of the cervix.

Trichomoniasis

Trichomoniasis, caused by the protozoa *Trichomonas vaginalis,* is most commonly transmitted through sexual contact. It can also be transmitted through shared bath facilities, wet towels, and wet swimwear. Symptoms in women include inflammation of the vagina and cervix as well as a yellow-green, frothy, odorous discharge. In men, trichomoniasis

causes burning on urination due to urethral irritation. The treatment consists of administration of metronidazole (Flagyl) to all partners. Flagyl is contraindicated in the first trimester of pregnancy because it acts as a **teratogen** (a chemical that can cause abnormal fetal development). Clotrimazole vaginal suppositories are used to provide symptomatic relief during the first 12 weeks of pregnancy, and then Flagyl can be given.

HIV and AIDS

Human immunodeficiency virus (HIV) is a retrovirus that attacks and destroys the body's immune system. The method of transmission is by direct contact with body fluids. **Acquired immunodeficiency syndrome (AIDS)** is life-threatening, end-stage infection with HIV. Although HIV is being treated with increased success, HIV infection is still considered fatal. The main HIV/AIDS discussion is in Chapter 21 ⬤ of this book. Refer to an adult medical-surgical textbook for further information.

CANDIDIASIS

Candidiasis (**monilia** or **yeast infection**) is a common organism causing vaginitis. Characteristics of a yeast infection are thick white patches resembling cottage cheese adhering to the cervix, vaginal wall, and labia. There is intense itching of the vulva and vagina. The mucous membrane is red and inflamed. When a specimen is viewed under the microscope, *hyphae* (threadlike filaments) and spores may be seen.

Treatment includes medicated creams, vaginal tablets, or suppositories. The sexual partner should also be treated because *Candida* can grow on the foreskin, glans, and outer skin of the penis.

Contraception

Contraception is the prevention of pregnancy. Although several methods are addressed here, it is important to encourage teens and others to discuss methods of contraception with their health care provider (Figure 5-11 ■). Some methods may not be recommended with certain physical disorders. Table 5-6 ■ lists facts about conception and contraception.

FERTILITY AWARENESS

Fertility awareness is based on the assumption that ovulation occurs at the same time each month. By collecting data regarding physical changes that take place throughout the menstrual cycle, the time of ovulation can be identified. The couple then abstains from intercourse or uses other methods of contraception during ovulation. Objective data to identify ovulation include a **basal body**

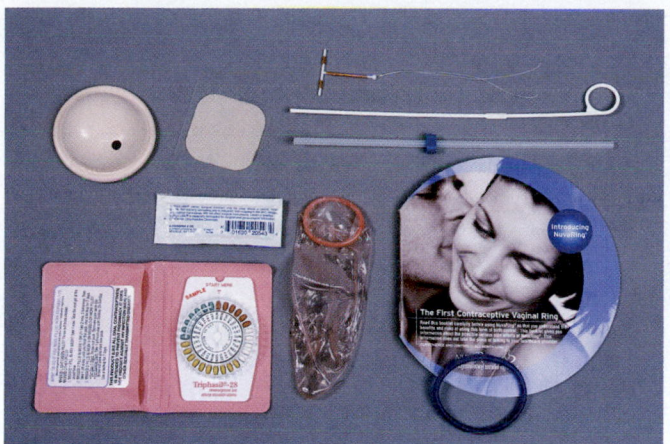

Figure 5-11. ■ Methods of contraception (from top right): Mirena intrauterine device (IUD), applicator for female condom, delivery catheter, Norplant subcutaneous contraceptive, vaginal ring, male condom, "the pill," diaphragm, and contraceptive patch.

temperature taken every morning before activity and assessment of cervical mucus (*spinnbarkeit*) (Figure 5-12 ■). Subjective data include increased libido, bloating, and breast changes. Some women may also experience *mit-*

telschmerz (abdominal pain with ovulation). Once the data are collected for several months, patterns can be identified. Abstinence is generally recommended for several days prior to ovulation and until 3 days after ovulation. The calendar method is the least effective method of contraception.

SPERMICIDES

Spermicides are chemicals in the form of creams, foams, jellies, or suppositories that are inserted into the vagina prior to sexual intercourse. They destroy the sperm or prevent sperm mobility. The chemical must be inserted deep in the vagina and come in contact with the cervix. Suppositories may take up to 30 minutes to dissolve, and they will not offer protection until then. The spermicide must be inserted before each ejaculation.

> **clinical ALERT**
>
> It is important to teach clients that spermicides do not prevent STIs.

TABLE 5-6		
Facts about Conception and Contraception		
1500 BC	First record of vaginal contraception	One of the earliest mentions of contraceptive vaginal suppositories appears in the Ebers Medical Papyrus. The guide suggests that a fiber tampon moistened with an herbal mixture of acacia, dates, colocynth, and honey would prevent pregnancy. The fermentation of this mixture can result in the production of lactic acid, which today is recognized as a spermicide.
16th Century	Male condom	The condom was first created out of sheep intestines by a physician in the court of King Charles II of England. The condom became widely used as a birth control device after the vulcanization of rubber in 1844.
1838	Barrier methods of contraception—female; diaphragm and cervical cap	The modern diaphragm was invented by a German physician. The cervical cap was invented in 1860, but it did not receive the approval of the U.S. Food and Drug Administration for use in the United States until the late 1980s, despite its widespread use in Europe.
1921	Margaret Sanger	An advocate for birth control in the United States, she founded the American Birth Control League, which became the Planned Parenthood Federation of America in 1942.
1960	Gregory Pincus	Developed an oral contraceptive.
1965	Birth control pills or oral contraceptives	First approved for use in the United States. These early pills, known as combination pills, contained both estrogen and progestin (a synthetic form of progesterone). In 1973, progestin-only pills also became available.
1980s	Artificial insemination	Initiated as a means of fertilization. Many couples now resort to various methods of *in vitro* fertilization ("test tube" babies) or transplantation of fertilized ova from one womb to another.

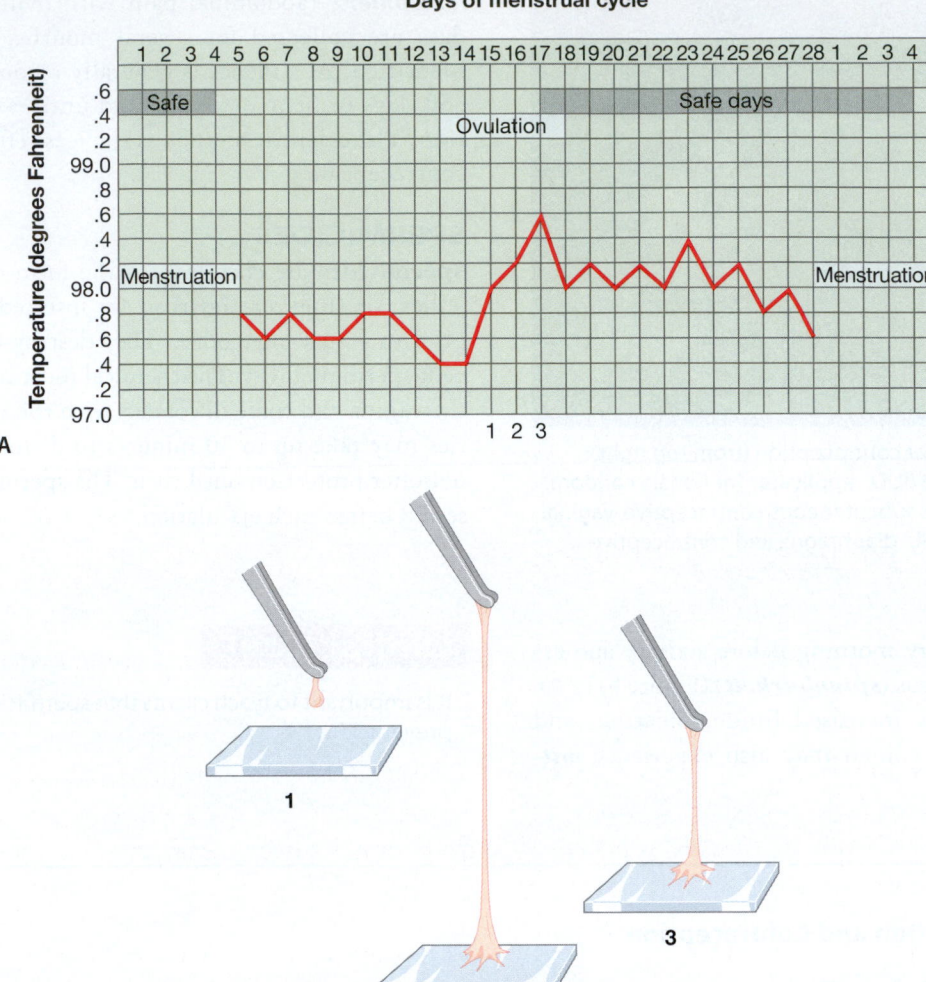

Figure 5-12. ■ (A) Basal body temperature chart with ovulation indicated. If this method is used for contraception, some sources recommend abstaining from intercourse for an additional day prior to ovulation and an additional day after ovulation (end of the fourth day). (B) Determining elasticity of cervical mucus (*spinnbarkeit*) to predict day of ovulation: 1. Three days before ovulation. 2. Day of ovulation. 3. Day after ovulation.

BARRIERS

Barriers, including male and female condoms, vaginal diaphragms, and cervical caps, are devices placed in the vagina or over the penis to prevent sperm from entering the cervix. To be effective, these devices must be correctly applied. The use of spermicide increases their effectiveness.

The male condom is applied to the erect penis before contact with the vulva or vagina. A small space must be available at the end of the condom to contain the ejaculate. After ejaculation, the man should withdraw the penis from the vagina while it is still erect and hold the rim of the condom to prevent spillage. Figure 5-13 ■ illustrates correct male condom use.

The female condom contains a ring at the closed end. It is inserted into the vagina so the ring rests around the cervix. The open end extends from the vagina and partially covers the vulva. The female condom can be inserted up to 8 hours prior to intercourse. A fresh condom must be used with each sexual episode. Figure 5-14 ■ illustrates application of a female condom.

The vaginal diaphragm consists of a metal ring covered with rubber. When inserted high in the vagina, the rubber covers the cervix (Figure 5-15 ■). The cervical cap is a similar device: a small ring covered with rubber that fits over the cervix. Both the vaginal diaphragm and cervical cap are most effective when spermicide is applied to the inner surface and rim before being placed next to the cervix. The devices should be left in place for 6 hours after intercourse in order to ensure that sperm do not enter the cervix. If intercourse is desired again within 6 hours, the diaphragm or cervical cap should remain in place and another method of contraception should also be used.

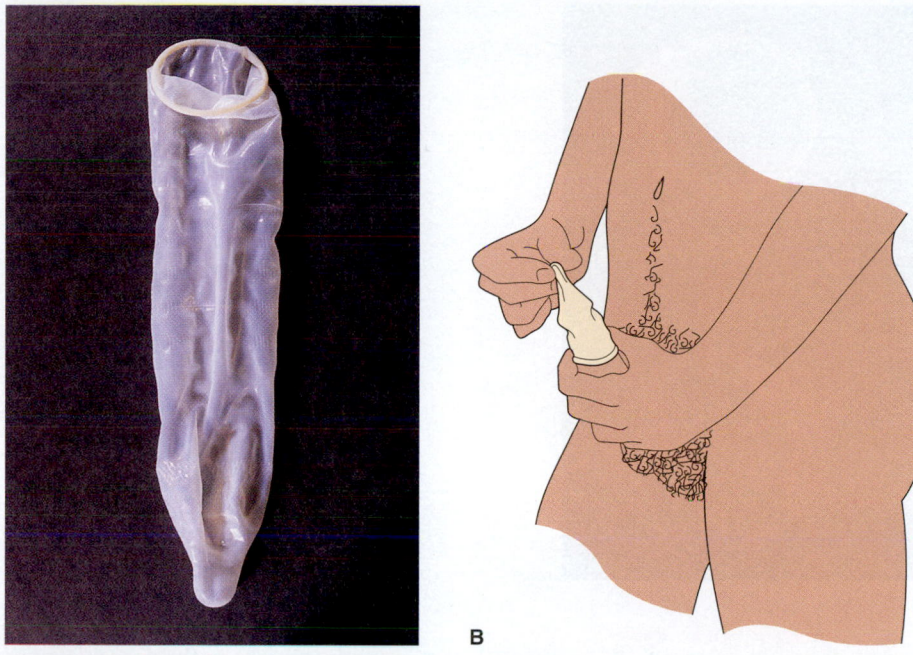

Figure 5-13. ■ The male condom. (**A**) Unrolled condom with reservoir tip. (**B**) Correct application of a condom. After use, it is crucial for the man to keep the condom in place until it is fully removed from the vagina.

INTRAUTERINE DEVICE

The **intrauterine device (IUD)** is a small T-shaped piece of metal covered with copper or levonorgestrel (see Figure 5-11). The exact mechanism of action of an IUD is unclear. It is believed that the copper or levonorgestrel either kills the sperm or alters its motility to prevent conception. The IUD also disrupts the normal turbulence inside the uterus and may prevent implantation of the fertilized egg. The IUD is inserted into the uterus by a qualified health professional so that a string attached to the lower end of the "T" protrudes from the cervix. The woman is instructed to feel the string once a week for the first month and then after each menses to be sure it is in the proper position. If she develops signs of infection or pregnancy, she should consult her health care provider immediately. In case of pregnancy, the IUD is generally removed, but its removal could cause a spontaneous abortion.

HORMONAL CONTRACEPTIVES

Hormonal contraceptives are usually a combination of estrogen and progestin. They may be supplied in oral pill form taken once a day for 21 days (followed by 7 days "off"), a dermal patch applied weekly (see Figure 5-11), an intramuscular injection given every 3 months, or a capsule inserted into the subcutaneous fat of the upper arm that lasts for up to 5 years (Figure 5-16 ■). Women who smoke or who have a history of clotting disorders, liver disease, hyperlipidemia, hypertension, or diabetes should not take oral contraceptives. For further information, please refer to a pharmacology text.

In August 2006, the Food and Drug Administration approved "Plan B", an *emergency contraceptive* formulation of progestin (levonorgestrel). Available over the counter to 18-year-olds and by prescription to girls 17 and younger, the drug acts by delaying ovulation and perhaps preventing fertilization and implantation. (It is not effective if an embryo is already implanted; the pregnancy would continue.) One dose of 0.75 mg is taken as soon as possible after unprotected vaginal intercourse, with a second dose of 0.75 mg taken 12 hours later (FDA, 2006). Although it was dubbed the "morning-after" pill, it is effective up to 72 hours after intercourse. As with all hormonal contraceptives, Plan B does not provide protection against STIs.

SURGICAL STERILIZATION

Surgical sterilization—vasectomy or tubal ligation—is the tying and cutting of the vas deferens or fallopian tubes (Figure 5-17 ■). In rare instances, the procedure can be reversed. However, the couple should understand that the procedure is usually permanent. Following a vasectomy, it might take six or more ejaculations to clear the vas deferens of sperm. The couple must use other methods of birth control until negative sperm counts are obtained.

A tubal ligation might be performed at the time of a cesarean section delivery, through a laparoscopy following delivery or at another time. The woman is encouraged to abstain from sexual intercourse until her healing is complete. She can then engage in unprotected intercourse.

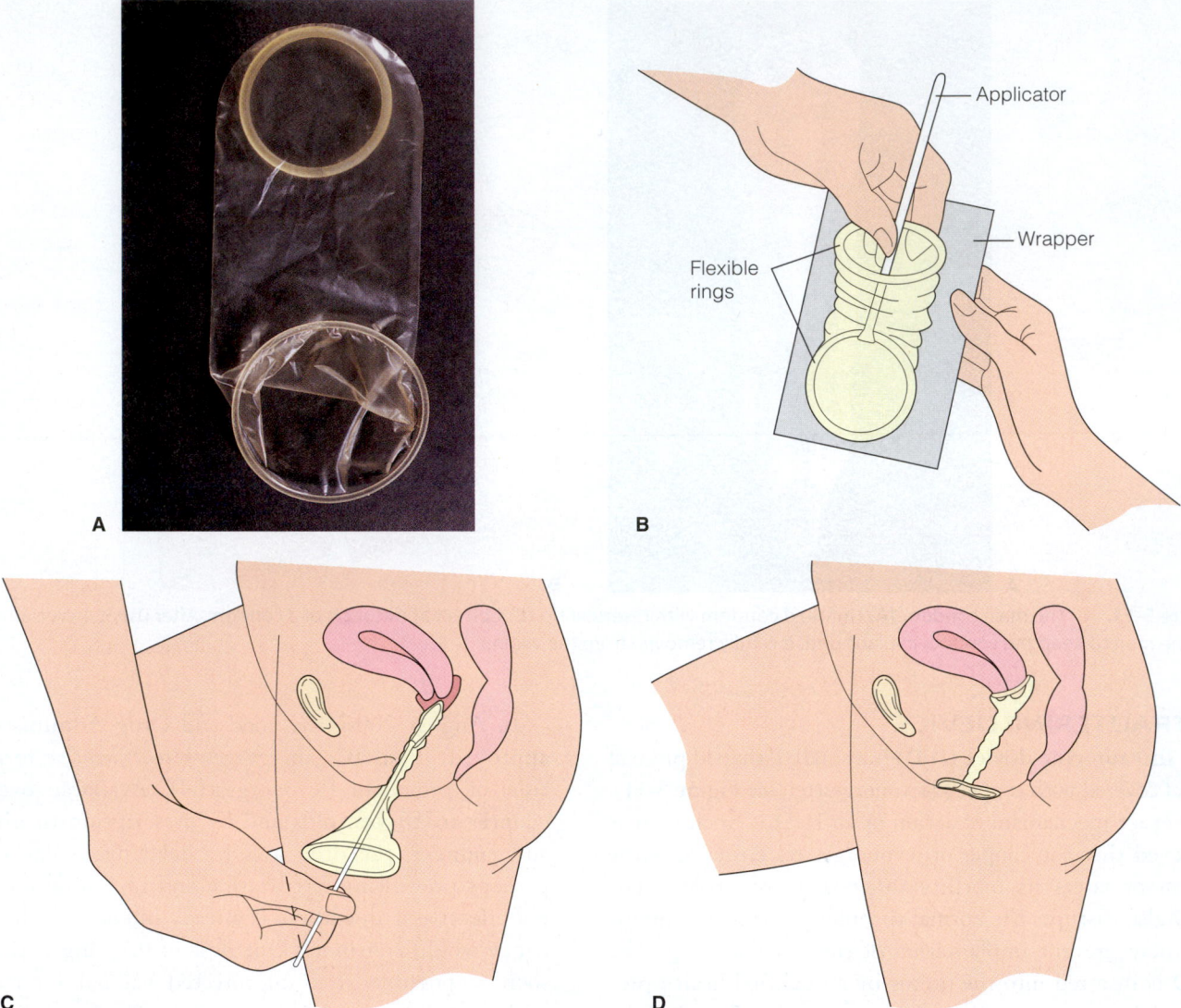

A

B

Applicator

Wrapper

Flexible rings

C

D

Figure 5-14. ■ (**A**) The female condom. To insert the condom: (**B**) Remove condom and application from wrapper by pulling up on the ring. (**C**) Insert condom slowly by gently pushing the applicator toward the small of the back. (**D**) When properly inserted, the outer ring should rest on the folds of skin around the vaginal opening, and the inner ring (closed end) should fit loosely against the cervix.

GENETIC TESTING

Infertility Issues

INFERTILITY

Infertility is the inability to achieve pregnancy after 1 year or more of unprotected intercourse. There are several causes of infertility. The simplest and least invasive diagnostic exam is to obtain a semen sample and analyze the number and quality of sperm. If the sperm count is low, the testes may not be producing enough sperm or there may be occlusion of the seminiferous tubules or vas deferens, preventing the transport of sperm. Some occlusions of the vas deferens may be correctable with surgery. Spermatogenesis may be

stimulated by hormone therapy with varying degrees of success. If the quality of sperm is poor, little can be done to correct the problem.

Infertility in women is generally easier to treat. Diagnostic tests, including hormone levels and ultrasound of the reproductive organs, are used to determine the exact cause. Hormone therapy may be used to stimulate ovulation. Narrow fallopian tubes can sometimes be enlarged, and pregnancy may then be obtained by natural means.

If the couple remains infertile, other methods may be used to become pregnant. The man's sperm can be obtained, stored, and concentrated to obtain a high sperm count. The

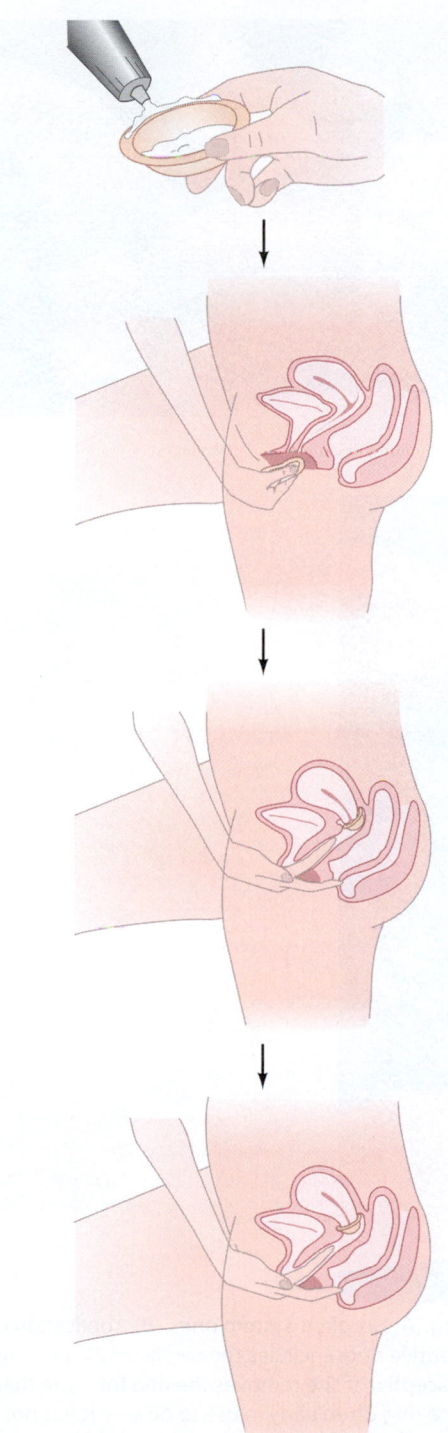

Figure 5-15. ■ Application of spermicide and placement of vaginal diaphragm. Apply gel to the rim and center of the diaphragm. Fold and insert the diaphragm. Check placement; the cervix should be felt through the diaphragm. Push the rim of the diaphragm up under the symphysis pubis.

semen can then be instilled by **artificial insemination.** The eggs can be obtained through a laparoscopic procedure (see Figure 5-17C), fertilized in the laboratory, and then implanted into the uterus. This process is known as *in vitro* **fertilization.** When pregnancy takes place by *in vitro*

fertilization, several fertilized eggs are instilled in an attempt to have at least one embryo implant in the uterus. Hormone therapy, used to stimulate ovulation, frequently results in more than one egg being released from the ovary. Therefore, there is an increased risk of a **multifetal pregnancy.**

Nursing Considerations

The nursing responsibilities include emotional support and teaching. When the couple desiring a child learns that one partner is infertile, feelings of sadness, guilt, and blame put strain on the relationship. Counseling may be needed to help the couple explore these feelings and keep lines of communication open. The nurse, working with the obstetrician, can be helpful in clarifying medical and surgical options. The treatment of infertility can be quite costly, and the couple may need assistance in exploring financial resources.

MULTIPLE PREGNANCY

Multiple pregnancy, also knows as multifetal pregnancy, is the carrying of more than one fetus at a time. Twins, the most common naturally occurring multifetal pregnancy, occur in approximately 1 of 250 births. Dizygotic or **fraternal twins** occur from two eggs fertilized by two sperm (Figure 5-18 ■). These twins could be the same gender or different genders. Dizygotic twins generally have two separate placentas, amnions, and chorions. The placentas may implant close together in the uterus, increasing the risk of complications with the placenta. (See discussion of high-risk pregnancies in Chapter 8 ◑.) **Monozygotic (or identical) twins** occur when one fertilized egg divides into two separate zygotes. These twins will always be the same gender. If the division occurs without complete separation or cleavage, the result will be **conjoined twins** or "Siamese" twins. Monozygotic twins could result in two separate placentas and fetal membranes, but more commonly there is one placenta, one chorion, and two separate amnions. (See more about placental layers in Chapter 6, ◑ Figure 6-4.) When this is the case, one twin may receive more nutrients and grow at a different rate than its sibling.

Triplets occur in about 1 of 7,600 pregnancies. **Triplets** can occur from fertilization of three separate eggs, from fertilization of two eggs and division of one, or from one egg that divides into three embryos. Quadruplets, quintuplets, sextuplets, and so forth occur in a similar manner. Naturally occurring quadruplets, quintuplets, and sextuplets are extremely rare. Multifetal pregnancies, other than twins, occur most commonly from the use of fertility drugs or *in vitro* fertilization.

There are additional risks involved with multifetal pregnancies. Complications such as preterm labor, pregnancy-induced hypertension (see Chapter 8 ◑), and gestational

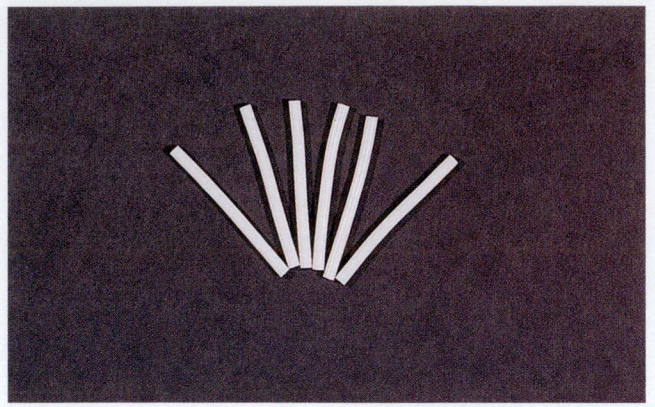

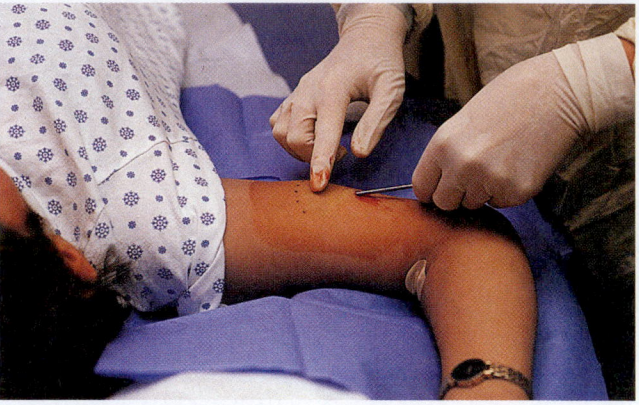

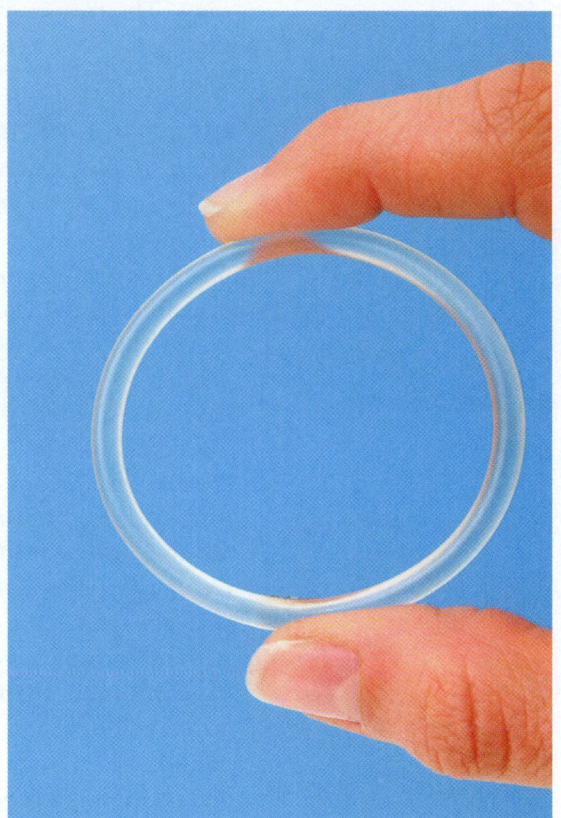

Figure 5-16. ■ Longer-term contraceptive devices include Norplant and the vaginal ring. (**A**) Norplant system units. (**B**) Application of Norplant implant in a woman's upper arm. (**C**) The Nuvaring, a flexible hormonal contraceptive ring, encircles the cervix for 21 days and is removed. A new ring is placed 1 week later. The woman is advised to use a backup contraceptive if she removes the ring for more than 3 hours during the 21-day period. A woman with marked vaginal prolapse should check the ring often early in use to be sure it has not been expelled (Source: vario images GmbH & Co.KG/Alamy.)

diabetes are more common. As the uterus enlarges to accommodate the fetuses, there is an increased risk of rupturing. Cesarean birth may be indicated due to prematurity or malpresentation of one or more of the infants.

CHROMOSOMAL ABNORMALITIES

Young teenage girls, women over 30, and couples who have a family history of genetic anomalies are at a higher risk for developing a fetus with chromosomal abnormalities than other couples. The **karyotype,** a picture analysis of the chromosomes, is usually obtained from stained cells (see Figure 4-2 ⬭). Samples of placental tissue can also be used to determine the karyotype of the fetus. The chromosome pairs are numbered 1 through 22 and XX or Xy. Couples with a family history of genetic disorders may choose to have genetic testing done before they become pregnant. An

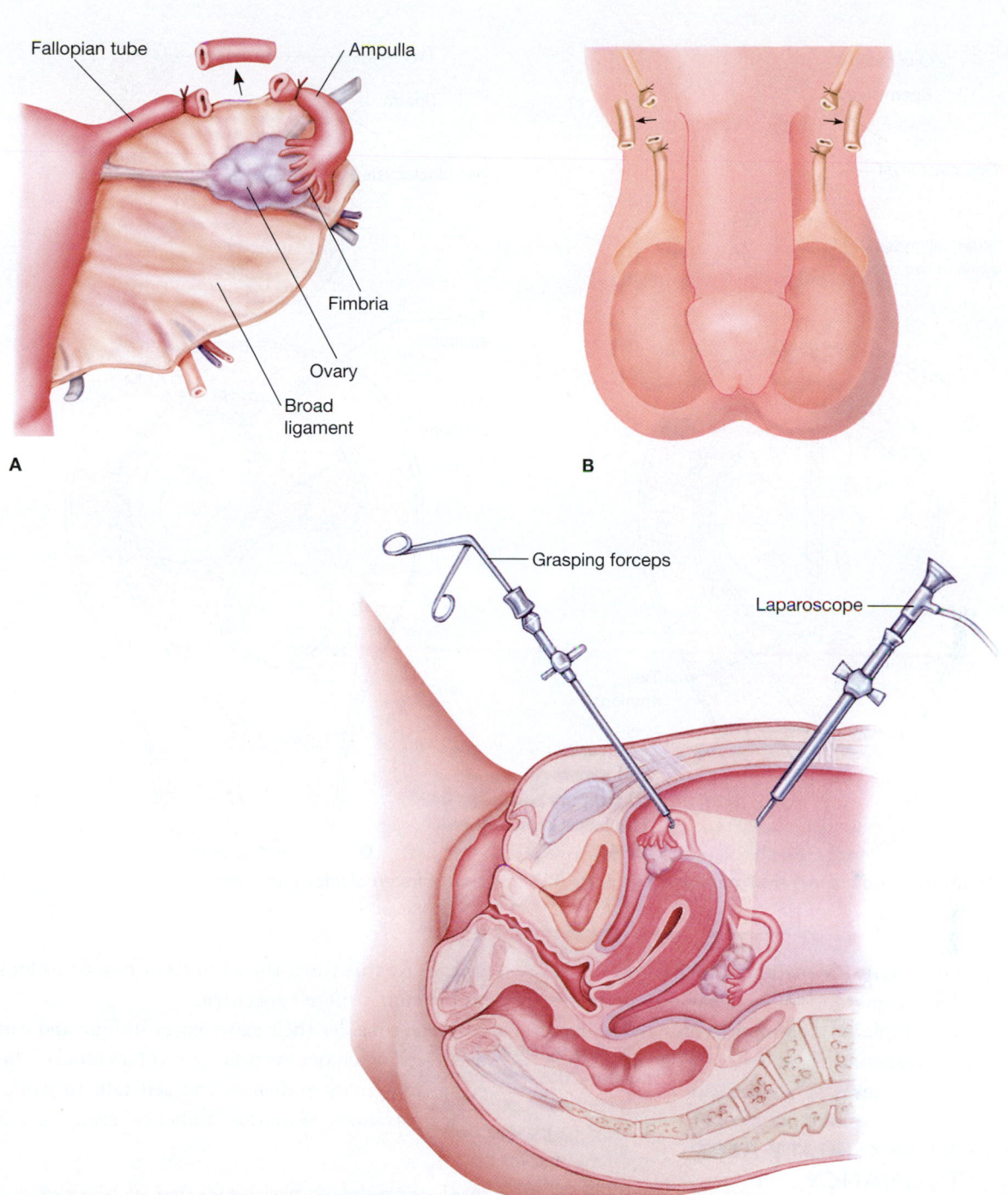

Figure 5-17. ■ Permanent sterilization. (**A**) Tubal ligation. (**B**) Vasectomy. (**C**) Laparoscopy. The laparoscope is used to visualize tubal sterilization accomplished through minilaparotomy incision at level of pubic hair line. (C: Redrawn, with permission, from Hatcher, R. A. et al. [1994]. *Contraceptive technology* [16th rev. ed.]. New York: Irvington.)

informed decision regarding parenting can then be made. Women at risk may have placenta tissue sampling completed to determine the presence of genetic disorders. Informed decisions can then be made regarding termination or continuation of the pregnancy.

Chromosomal defects result from an altered number of chromosomes (one chromosome or three chromosomes—

called **trisomy**) or abnormalities of structure (deletion of one part of the chromosome). Common chromosomal (genetic) anomalies include Down syndrome (trisomy 21), trisomy 18, trisomy 13, and Klinefelter syndrome (extra X chromosome in male XXy).

Chromosomal defects result in a variety of physical anomalies, including malformations and underdeveloped

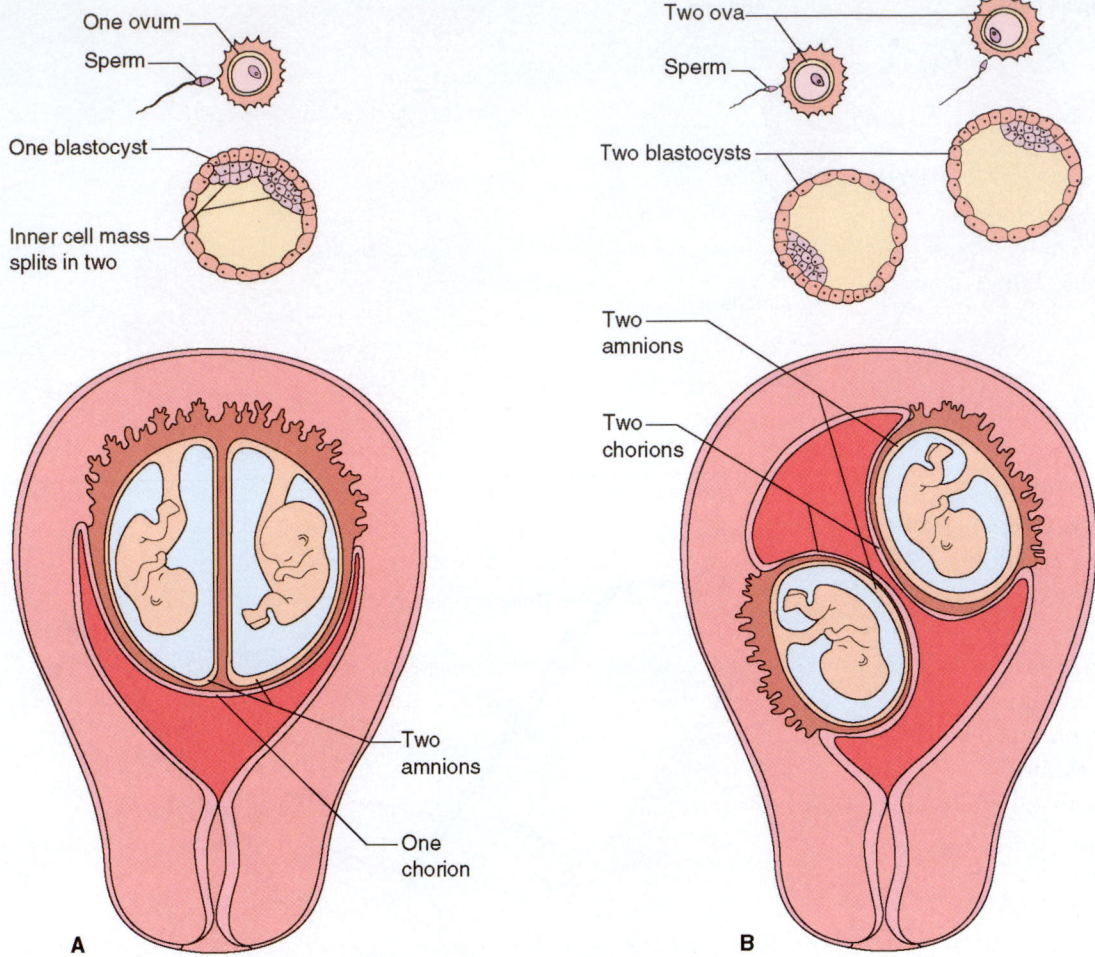

Figure 5-18. ■ (A) Formation of identical (monozygotic) twins. (B) Formation of fraternal (dizygotic) twins.

structures or body systems. Many chromosomal defects result in mental delays, retardation, or behavioral problems. When testing is completed before delivery, and genetic abnormalities are diagnosed, the parents can be better prepared to care for the infant.

ADOLESCENT SEXUALITY AND TEENAGE PREGNANCY

Over 50% of adolescent girls and 75% of adolescent boys report engaging in sexual intercourse before the age of 18. This high-risk behavior not only increases the incidence of teenage pregnancy, but also exposes the teens to STIs. Decreasing the incidence of adolescent pregnancy and STIs is an objective of the U.S. Department of Health and Human Services and many school systems (Figure 5-19 ■).

As we explore this issue, a review of growth and development of the adolescent (see Chapter 11 ⟲⟳) may be necessary. The initial development of secondary sex characteristics (see Figure 4-22 ⟲⟳), occurring between 9 and 14 years of age, marks the beginning of puberty. These body changes affect the adolescent's new body

image. At this time, the adolescent begins to look inward and becomes more egocentric.

Teens consider their experiences unique and can become frustrated when not everything revolves around them. They create imaginary audiences and self-talk to work through their frustrations. With this "audience" always in attendance,

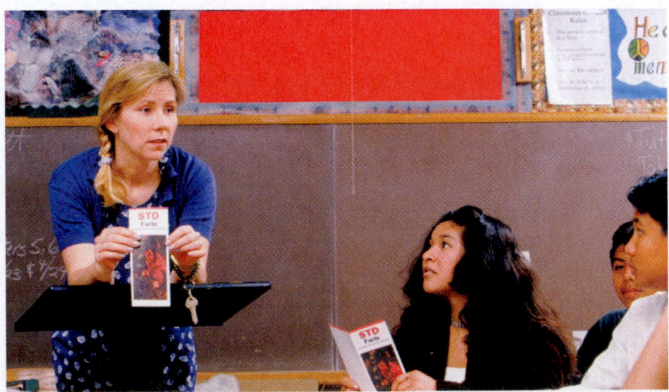

Figure 5-19. ■ Adolescents require age-appropriate teaching about sexuality and sexually transmitted infections.

they believe that people are constantly watching them. This explains the feelings of self-consciousness experienced by many teens.

According to Piaget (1969), the teen who exhibits a high degree of egocentrism has not yet developed the formal operational thought patterns of adulthood. (Piaget's theory is discussed in Chapter 11 .) Continuing to use concrete operational thought, these adolescents cannot imagine the future consequences of their actions. They feel invincible and have the "it can't happen to me" attitude.

As cognitive development matures, so does moral reasoning. The adolescent begins to think more abstractly and questions values of parents and others. Social events expose them to various ethical issues and force them to examine their own beliefs. Over time they gain experience in right and wrong. They also develop their own moral code.

Although teens strive to achieve individuality, they doubt their abilities and seek approval from peers. **Peer pressure** (influencing a person to follow the desire of another person or group) can lead the adolescent to experiment in high-risk activities. This combination of peer pressure, feelings of invincibility, and elevation in sex hormones and sex drive may lead adolescents to engage in premarital sexual intercourse. Some begin to develop a monogamous relationship, at least for a while. Other teens fail to develop a close relationship with one person and move from partner to partner in a short period of time or have multiple partners at one time. Nearly one-half of all high school seniors report having had sexual intercourse. As mentioned, this frequent sexual contact with multiple partners increases the exposure to STIs and the likelihood of pregnancy.

Teens in lower socioeconomic levels engage in sexual relations at nearly the same rate as other teens. However, they have a disproportionate number of teen pregnancies. The lower socioeconomic level adolescent may not have the same access to birth control measures as their counterparts in higher socioeconomic levels. They may not believe that higher education and career development are realistic goals. Instead, they may transition into adulthood by engaging in sexual intercourse and becoming parents. In contrast, teens in higher socioeconomic levels often have ready access to various forms of contraception. They may have been raised with the expectation that they will go on to college or a career before parenting. These teens may be more likely to use contraceptive methods or to terminate pregnancy if it occurs.

UNINTENDED PREGNANCY

The second issue that develops from sexual relationships among adolescents is unintended pregnancy. Pregnancy, occurring while the adolescent girl is in a period of rapid growth and physical maturation, puts additional stress on her body and increases the risk to her and the infant. Teen mothers have a higher incidence of complications such as pregnancy-induced hypertension, gestational diabetes, and preterm labor (see Chapter 8), so early prenatal care is essential to their health. However, the teen mother may deny or try to cover up the pregnancy and not seek help.

Once pregnant, the mother and father have some difficult decisions to make. How should they tell their parents? Should they get married? Should the pregnancy be continued or terminated? Will the child be raised in the family? Will the child be adopted by another family? Some parents provide emotional and financial support when they discover their teen is pregnant. Other parents refuse any form of support because they believe the teen has committed a "terrible sin."

If there were several sexual partners, the teen may not know the identity of the father. Even if she knows the father, he may or may not accept responsibility and offer support. The teen mother may not have the cognitive and emotional resources to make objective decisions for her own well-being or the well-being of her child.

Nursing Considerations

The role of the nurse in helping the pregnant adolescent is twofold. First, the nurse must encourage early and continued prenatal care. This care is outlined in Chapter 6 . Second, the nurse must refer the adolescent to appropriate social services. The professional staff can assist the teen mother, father, and their families in the decision-making process. With early and appropriate care, the health of both the mother and the infant can be protected. This increases the likelihood of a positive outcome for the pregnancy and the family unit.

Teaching is another role of the nurse related to adolescent sexuality (see Health Promotion Issue box on pages 116 and 117.). Many parents are uncomfortable or unknowledgeable about adolescent sexuality, STIs, and teen pregnancy. It can be difficult for adolescents to discuss their feelings with their parents. Some parents fear that discussing sex will encourage the teenager to engage in sexual intercourse. The nurse can be instrumental in opening the lines of communication between parents and their adolescent children. By working with teachers, school counselors, and administrators, the nurse can help develop programs to provide accurate information for adolescents.

ABORTION

Abortion is the termination of a pregnancy before the fetus is viable (see Chapter 6). Abortions may be a spontaneous, naturally occurring event; a therapeutic event due to the medical condition of the mother or fetus; or an elective event for a variety of personal reasons on the part of the

(Text continues on p. 118.)

HEALTH PROMOTION ISSUE

TEACHING ABOUT SEX

The LPN/LVN works at a family practice clinic. During the weekly staff meeting, client cases were reviewed and two issues were noted. The teenage pregnancy rate for their practice had increased slightly over last year's rates, and several mothers of prepubescent girls had asked for help in discussing issues of puberty with their daughters. The staff, consisting of an RN, two LPN/LVNs, a family nurse practitioner, and a family practice physician, discussed how they might address these issues. It was decided that young girls and mothers needed more information, as well as tools to manage the changes that occur before, during, and after puberty. One nurse noted that the challenges of puberty also impact young boys. However, it was decided to develop a plan to address the female issues first. The first task was to look more specifically at the issues.

DISCUSSION

According to the 2004 annual survey of adults and teens conducted by the National Campaign to Prevent Teen Pregnancy, teens state that parents greatly influence their decisions about sexual behavior. Yet, in 2002, the National Survey of Family Growth reports that 14.5% of females and 17.4% of males ages 15 to 19 had no formal education on methods of avoiding sexual behavior. Parents also reported difficulty in communicating with their teens about sex, love, and relationships. They also report being unsure of when to approach these topics with their teens.

Teens report that their personal morals and values influence decisions about delaying sexual behavior and preventing teen pregnancy. Both teenagers and parents state that more help from their religious institutions would be appreciated. In 2002, the National Survey of Family Growth reported that 13% of females and 10.7% of males had taken a vow or pledge to remain a virgin until they married. Teaching surrounding these vows or pledges is usually provided by religious or faith institutions.

IMPLEMENTATION

After reviewing growth and development tasks for the school-age child and the adolescent, the staff decided that they would need to develop two community-based education programs. The first class would be for prepubescent girls, ages 8 to 11, and their moms.

School-age children are interested in how things work; therefore, the class should contain a detailed description of the physical changes occurring during the puberty process. They enjoy books, games, and interactive learning. The staff decided to plan fun activities to learn more about how to care for yourself during puberty. They would purchase age-appropriate books for the girls to read. Posters and graphics would need to be colorful and cartoon-like, and contain correct terms.

Mothers attending the class would be seated with their daughters. Tables that would seat several families would be used. This would encourage friends to attend together. Nutritious snacks would be served to assist in teaching nutritional concepts. Because young girls enjoy thinking about growing older, the staff would provide a gift bag containing items they would need as puberty approaches. These items would include different types of feminine protection with a decorative zippered pouch, deodorant, a safety razor, shampoo, soap, and a pocket calendar.

The tone of the class needed to be fun, energetic, celebratory, and encouraging.

Attention would also need to be given to protecting the privacy of the girls so they would feel free to discuss the issues. The agenda needed to be light enough to allow for variation and discussion. The staff agreed that girls this age were sure to giggle during these discussions. Giggling would be allowed, if not encouraged, to release feelings of embarrassment. The young LPN/LVN was chosen as the instructor for this course because she relates well to school-age children.

The proposed agenda for this class is as follows:

- *Opening question:* Name the one thing that excites you most about growing up.
- *What is puberty?*
- *Physical changes during puberty:* What is it, and what do I do about it?
  - Growth spurts
  - Body shape changes
  - Fatigue
  - Growing pains
  - Perspiration and body odor
  - Pimples and acne
  - Body hair
  - Breast changes
  - Vulva changes
  - Changes to internal organs: vagina, ovaries, fallopian tubes, uterus, and cervix
  - Menstruation.

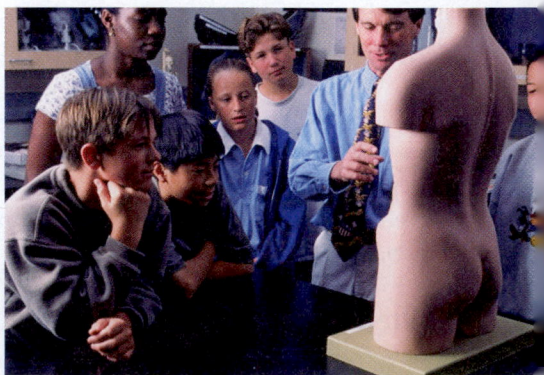

(Source: Jonathan Nourok\PhotoEdit Inc.)

■ *Emotional changes during puberty:* What is it, and what do I do about it?
- Emotions come and go.
- Feelings can be unreliable.
- Desire for independence increases.

The next class that the staff decided to offer to the community was a class for 12- to 15-year-olds discussing age-appropriate topics related to puberty and sexuality. Adolescents are more comfortable with their peers, so the staff decided that mothers would not attend this class. Adolescent thinking is concrete, and abstract thinking is beginning to develop. So, a mix of frank discussions with true-to-life visual aids would be mixed with scenarios for the class to consider.

The instructor for this class should be credible, knowledgeable, and between the ages of 25 and 35 so she is not quite as old as their mothers. It was also suggested that they attempt to find a young teen who had experienced a teenage pregnancy to give her testimony. This teen should describe the experience in her own words. She should

be encouraged to be frank and honest about the positive and negative aspects of her situation. The staff decided that it would be too distracting for the infant to attend the class with this teenage mom, although assistance with child care would be offered.

The proposed agenda for this class is as follows:

■ *Opening:* "You have the right to say 'I pass' to anything tonight. You can be bored by any topic or grossed out by anything I say. You may ask any and all questions that come to mind, and I promise to answer honestly. Please realize that what is said in this room is confidential and private."

■ *Maturity*
- Definition
- Physical maturity
- Emotional maturity
■ Self-esteem
■ Peer pressure
■ Dating and sex
- Emotional differences of males and females

- Emotional consequences of early sex
- Creative dating
- Setting standards
- Physical consequences of early sex
  - Conception control
  - Pregnancy
  - Sexually transmitted infections
  - Abortion
■ Other issues
- Smoking
- Alcohol
- Drugs
- Eating disorders

MediaLink Teen pregnancy

SELF-REFLECTION

Were you raised in a family that discussed reproductive issues openly or where such topics were not directly discussed? What aspect of reproduction or sexuality would be most awkward for you to discuss? How could you respond nonjudgmentally to a teenager who is worried that he might be homosexual?

SUGGESTED RESOURCES

For the Nurse

These community-based classes would be easy to implement in any setting. The following resources would assist the nurse in personalizing the class to fit specific populations.

■ **www.teenpregnancy.org** This is the official website of the National Campaign to Prevent Teen Pregnancy. National and state statistics of teenage pregnancy can be accessed from this site. A number of effective teenage pregnancy prevention programs are reviewed and are available for downloading. There is also a class format for parents interested in ways to effectively discuss teenage pregnancy prevention with their children.

■ **www.cdc.gov** This is the official website of the Centers for Disease Control and Prevention. Presentations and slides depicting sexually transmitted infections can be downloaded from this website.

■ **www.marchofdimes.com** The March of Dimes offers an informative fact sheet about teenage pregnancy. Available in a printable form, the fact sheet could be used as a class handout.

■ **www.contraceptiononline.org** Contraception Online is a resource available to clinicians and educators. Up-to-date information about contraception methods is available.

■ **www.health.org** Girl Power! is the national public education campaign sponsored by the U.S. Department of Health and Human Services to help encourage and motivate 9- to 13-year-old girls to make the most of their lives. Topics include healthy lifestyle suggestions and ways to avoid hazardous behaviors.

Butts, J., & Hartman, S. (2002). Project BART: Effectiveness of a behavioral intervention to reduce HIV risk in adolescents. *The American Journal of Maternal/Child Nursing, 27*, 163–170.

Hershberger, P. (1998). Smoking and pregnant teens: What nurses can do to help. *Lifelines, 2*, 26–31.

For the Client

The nursing staff wanted to have resources available to offer mothers, young girls, and teenagers who wanted to continue learning following the classes. Below is a list of several of their suggestions:

Gravelle, K., & J. *The Period Book.* (2006). New York: Walker & Company.

Kitzinger, S., & Nillsson, L. *Being Born.* (1986). New York: Grosset and Dunlap.

Madaras, L., Madaras, A., Sullivan, S., & Aher, J. *What's Happening to My Body? Book for Girls.* (3rd ed.). (2001). New York: Newmarket Press.

McDowell, J., & Hostetler, B. *Don't Check Your Brains at the Door. How to Help Your Child Say "No" to Sexual Pressure.* (1992). Word Publishing. Available on the internet.

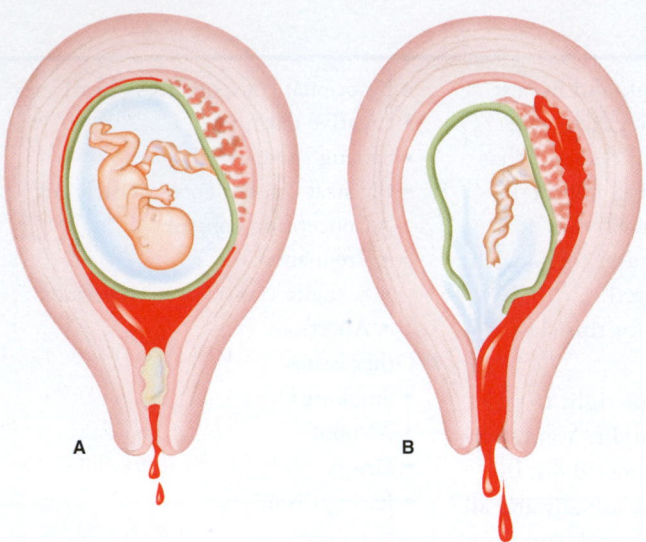

Figure 5-20. ■ Spontaneous abortion (or miscarriage). (**A**) Threatened abortion. (**B**) Incomplete abortion.

mother. A **spontaneous abortion** (or **miscarriage**) occurs most commonly during the first trimester (Figure 5-20 ■). The cause may be a genetic abnormality in the embryo or a hormonal problem, infection, drug problem, or systemic disorder in the mother. Spontaneous abortions later in the pregnancy usually result from a maternal abnormality such as incompetent cervix. Little can be done to correct or prevent genetic causes of abortion, but some maternal causes can be corrected with medication or surgical procedures.

Spontaneous Abortion

Five types of spontaneous abortion are discussed here.

- In a **threatened abortion,** vaginal spotting is noted with a closed cervix. Mild uterine cramping may be noted. Medical management involves bed rest and avoidance of stress and sexual orgasm.
- An **inevitable abortion** occurs when the cervix dilates and part of the placenta detaches from the uterus, resulting in moderate to heavy bleeding.
- If the fetus is passed, but the placenta is retained in the uterus, the condition is termed **incomplete abortion** (see Figure 5-20B). Inevitable and incomplete abortions usually require prompt curettage to control the bleeding.
- A **complete abortion** results when all fetal tissue is passed, the cervix closes, and minimal bleeding occurs. Usually, no medical treatment is required.
- When the fetus dies, but spontaneous abortion does not occur, the condition is termed **missed abortion.** The doctor may wait a reasonable length of time for spontaneous abortion to occur or perform a dilatation and curettage (D&C) to remove the tissue so as to prevent infection and sepsis.

Nursing care during any type of abortion includes monitoring for signs of hemorrhage and providing emotional support to the mother, father, and family members. Although the medical term "abortion" is used in these situations, it may be preferable to use the term "miscarriage" to prevent the emotional and potentially judgmental behavior associated with "abortion."

clinical ALERT

The nurse must be alert for signs of hemorrhaging in women who have had abortions. Monitor and immediately report any pronounced increase in bleeding.

Therapeutic Abortion

A **therapeutic abortion (TAB)** is the termination of the pregnancy when needed to save the life and preserve the health of the mother or when the fetus has a serious developmental or hereditary disorder. A therapeutic abortion may also be performed when the pregnancy is the result of rape or incest.

Elective Abortion

Elective abortion (EAB) is abortion performed at the request of the mother but not for reason of maternal risk or fetal disease. The condition of the mother and the gestational age and size of the fetus determine the method used in performing the abortion. In 1973, the U.S. Supreme Court ruled that first-trimester abortions were permissible. Second-trimester abortions were left to the discretion of the individual states. The nurse must know the laws of the state regarding abortion prior to offering abortion counseling or teaching.

The physical care of the mother before and after an abortion is similar to the physical care of other pregnant women before and after delivery. The emotional care is different. The mother, father, and entire family need support and grief counseling similar to the family that has experienced a stillbirth or other death of a child. Prior to and following a therapeutic or elective abortion, the mother and father will need assistance to make the best-informed decision. The values and moral convictions of the mother and father, their families, and the nurse are involved in the planning and implementing of care. Conflicts and doubts can be communicated.

Health care professionals need assistance in identifying and accepting their own feelings prior to helping the mother and her family. The nurse who objects to abortion for ethical or religious reasons may refuse to care for a woman having an abortion as long as the woman's life is not in danger.

ADOPTION

Adoption is the legal transfer of the responsibility for raising a child from the birth mother to the adoptive parent(s). State laws determine the procedure of adoption. The birth mother may choose an adoption agency or a private attorney to handle the arrangements. In a *closed adoption,* the birth mother does not share identifying information with the adoptive parents and there is no future contact. In an *open adoption,* the birth mother shares information, holds the baby, and may have frequent contact with the adoptive parents and the child.

The nurse has a responsibility to assist the birth mother in decision making, make appropriate referrals, and provide emotional support during the separation process. Even in an open adoption, the birth mother will experience grief over the loss of her child. She needs to be encouraged to share her feelings in order to make positive adjustments. A referral to a professional counselor may be needed.

PREGNANCY AFTER 35

Two groups of women are becoming pregnant after 35. One group consists of women who have other children and now find themselves pregnant again. The older multiparous woman may be one who has never used birth control methods due to personal choice or lack of knowledge or one who chooses to have another baby at this time in her life. The second group consists of women who have postponed pregnancy until their late thirties or early forties. The older nulliparous woman may have delayed pregnancy in order to complete her education or establish a career. She may believe that "time is running out," and that if she does not have a child now, she never will.

Some of the possible negative consequences of having children later in life include:

- Higher risk of fetal anomalies
- Difficulty in changing from a child-free lifestyle to a child-rearing lifestyle
- Feelings of anger and resentment toward the parents or infant about having a "second" family later in life
- Feelings of isolation if parents feel "tied down" and adult friends withdraw.

Due to these consequences, older parents have special needs that should be addressed (before pregnancy occurs if possible). Because the risk for fetal anomalies is greater, an amniocentesis will generally be performed at approximately 16 weeks' gestation. If anomalies are found, decisions about continuing or terminating the pregnancy must be made. In either case, the parents will need emotional support and teaching.

The couple may need assistance in discussing the lifestyle changes required by the raising of an infant. Some couples, excited to have a child later in life, may believe that the ability to bear children indicates that they are still young. Others may be upset by the pregnancy, feeling they will be tied down for the next 18 years. They should be encouraged to express their feelings and develop positive coping skills. Referral to social services may be needed.

Future Issues

Although common reproductive issues are discussed here, stem cell research is also worth mentioning. Many believe that stem cells, harvested from embryos, may be useful in treating and curing a variety of disorders. Others believe that harvesting of stem cells from embryos for research purposes is unethical. Questions about stem cell research and government funding of such research will undoubtedly continue to be debated on many levels in the future. It is important for the public to receive accurate information about the procurement of embryos, the harvesting process, and the use of the harvested stem cells. The nurse can be a key player in obtaining and disseminating accurate and useful information.

NURSING CARE

PRIORITIES IN NURSING CARE

The priority of nursing care for a client with a reproductive system disorder is to identify the nature of the disorder, provide emotional support, and teach clients to care for themselves and prevent complications.

ASSESSING

When assessing men and women for reproductive issues, the nurse must use a nonjudgmental attitude and open communication. Many clients are uncomfortable discussing their sexuality and sexual activity. The nurse must approach the topic in a matter-of-fact manner, with reassurance of confidentiality within the law. Some questions are the same for both genders.

- Ask about history of sexual activity, including the age at first sexual intercourse.
- Ask about the number of sexual partners, currently and in the past.
- Ask about the use of contraceptives.
- Ask about the use of barriers to prevent STIs.
- Ask about a history of sexual trauma, including abuse, rape, or incest.

Women

- Ask about risk factors for breast cancer, including family history.
- Ask about breast self-exam, how often they do it, and any abnormal findings.
- Perform a breast examination, palpating the breast for masses, irregularities in contour, and drainage, if warranted.
- Ask about menstrual history, including onset of menstruation, the date of the last menses, and any irregularities.

Men

- Ask about testicular self-examination, how often they do it, and any abnormal findings.
- Perform a testicular examination, palpating for masses and inspecting the genitals for lesions and drainage, if warranted.
- Ask about difficulty voiding, including difficulty starting or stopping and the size of the stream. Include symptoms of burning, frequency, urgency, or nocturia.
- Ask about sexual functioning, including premature ejaculation, impotence, or other sexual problems.

DIAGNOSING, PLANNING, AND IMPLEMENTING

Possible nursing diagnoses include the following.

Risk for Disturbed Body Image

- Encourage verbalization of feelings. *Alterations in sexual functioning from surgery or disease can change body image. Verbalizing helps the client cope with feelings of loss and change.*
- Provide resources (pamphlets, books, tapes, referrals to support groups and counselors) as appropriate. *Referrals and resources assist with coping and adaptation.*
- Encourage client (and significant other if appropriate) to look at physical changes in body. *Often, the imagined alteration of physical characteristics is worse than the real changes.*

Sexual Dysfunction

- Encourage discussion of sexual function among client, partner, and health care provider. *Open discussion assists with decision making about diagnosis and treatment.*
- Reinforce information given by the health care provider regarding treatment options. *The health care provider is responsible for discussing treatment options with the client. The nurse must reinforce teaching and answer questions. The client can then make an informed decision about treatment.*
- Encourage the client to discuss concerns of sexuality with a therapist or counselor. *The therapist or counselor may be able to offer alternatives for expressing sexuality.*

Deficient Knowledge Related to Risk Factors, Disease Prevention, and Treatment, Including Medications

- Teach clients about risk factors for reproductive dysfunction. For example, STIs increase the risk of infertility. *By understanding risk factors for reproductive dysfunction, clients can make better choices.*
- Teach clients about disease prevention. For example, teach about use of contraceptives and application of condoms. *By understanding disease prevention, clients can take measures to protect themselves.*
- Teach clients (and significant others if appropriate) about their specific disease and prescribed treatment. *When*

clients and significant others understand the specific condition, prescribed treatment, and possible complications, they are more compliant and make healthier choices.

EVALUATING

To evaluate the effectiveness of nursing interventions, collect data such as the following:

- Makes informed decisions about treatment based on the extent of the disorder and individual choice
- Verbalizes understanding of information presented
- Expresses feelings openly.

NURSING PROCESS CARE PLAN
Care of the Client with Rape Trauma Syndrome

Ms. Kelly is an 18-year-old college student living in a coed dorm. She is an average student, a member of the marching band, and a participant in a weekly campus religious organization. While walking home alone after band practice, she was attacked and raped. At the urging of her roommate and resident assistant, she contacted the campus health organization.

Assessment. VS: T 98.3, P 110, R 22 and labored, BP 122/78. Ms. Kelly reports intense perineal and back pain. Weight 110 pounds. Height 5′ 6″. Skin is moist and pink with bruising noted on the upper arms, buttocks, and back. She also has a small 2-cm gash on her forehead. She is alert, yet easily distracted. She is crying frequently. She asks the nurse to call her parents for her. A cervical specimen is obtained for sperm analysis. Hair specimens are obtained. Debris is removed from under Ms. Kelly's fingernails and from her back. A blood sample is obtained for screening of other STIs, including HIV and pregnancy testing. X-rays are taken to determine fractures.

Nursing Diagnosis. The following important nursing diagnoses (among others) have been established for this client:

- Acute Pain related to injuries received during the rape
- Anxiety related to status of physical health and the act of violence experienced
- Fear related to future violence and concern for personal safety.

Expected Outcomes. The expected outcomes for the plan of care are that Ms. Kelly will:

- Demonstrate a decrease in pain within 48 hours of initiating treatment as evidenced by lower rating on pain scale and less facial grimacing.
- Demonstrate decreased symptoms of anxiety in 2 weeks as evidenced by pulse and respirations within normal limits

(WNL) and statement of supportive social interactions with family members.

■ Demonstrate decreased fear in 2 weeks as evidenced by a report of safety measures implemented to provide personal protection.

Planning and Implementation. The following nursing interventions are implemented for Ms. Kelly:

■ Reassess perineal and back pain by telephone follow-up call within 48 hours of initiating treatment.

■ Have Ms. Kelly apply moist heat to the perineum and back. *Moist heat provides comfort and aids healing.*

■ Encourage Ms. Kelly to self-administer analgesics prior to pain levels of 5 or above.

■ Reassess anxiety levels at follow-up clinic visit. *Feelings of anxiety may emerge slowly or be longlasting.*

■ Encourage Ms. Kelly to express her feelings, anxieties, and fears related to her diagnosis. *Verbalization allows appropriate follow-up.*

■ Encourage and support effective coping behaviors.

■ Refer Ms. Kelly to a rape counselor. *Psychological effects of the rape may surface over time and are sometimes difficult to overcome.*

■ Include Ms. Kelly's parents in counseling if Ms. Kelly agrees.

Evaluation. At the follow-up visit, Ms. Kelly's vital signs are T 98.6, BP 120/80, P 66, R 16. She has seen the rape counselor daily and is dealing with her fears and anxiety. She has decided to take a leave of absence from her coursework and return to her hometown. Her back and perineal pain have subsided, and STI and pregnancy tests remain negative. The criminal investigation into the rape continues.

Critical Thinking in the Nursing Process

1. List conditions and procedures for collecting data regarding the specific events of the rape.
2. What types of personal protection should be recommended to Ms. Kelly and why?
3. Describe the psychological support necessary for Ms. Kelly.

Note: Discussion of Critical Thinking questions appears in Appendix I.

Note: The references and resources for this and all chapters have been compiled at the back of the book.

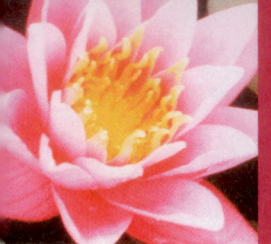

Chapter Review

KEY TERMS by Topic

Use the audio glossary feature of either the CD-ROM or the Companion Website to hear the correct pronunciation of the following key terms.

Breast Disorders
mammography, fibrosis, fibrocyst, fibroadenoma, intraductal papillomas, hemoptysis, lumpectomy, mastectomy, mammoplasty, reduction mammoplasty

Uterine Disorders
premenstrual syndrome (PMS), menorrhalgia, dysmenorrhea, menorrhagia, metrorrhagia, amenorrhea, climacteric, oophorectomy, myomectomy, hysterectomy, hyperplasia, salpingo-oophorectomy, cervical dysplasia, conization, endometriosis, ectopic, dyspareunia, tenesmus

Ovarian Disorders
cysts, polycystic ovary syndrome, hirsutism, ovarian cancer, cystocele, rectocele, uterine prolapse

Rape Trauma Syndrome
rape, incest

Testicular and Epididymal Disorders
testicular cancer, orchiectomy, epididymitis, orchitis, prostatitis, hydrocele

Erectile Dysfunction
erectile dysfunction

Prostate Disorders
benign prostatic hyperplasia (BPH), nocturia, libido, prostate cancer

Infections
chlamydia, gonorrhea, syphilis, chancre, genital warts, trichomoniasis, teratogen, human immunodeficiency virus (HIV), acquired immunodeficiency syndrome (AIDS), candidiasis (monilia or yeast infection)

Contraception
contraception, fertility awareness, basal body temperature, *spinnbarkeit, mittelschmerz,* spermicides, barriers, intrauterine device (IUD), hormonal contraceptives, surgical sterilization

Infertility Issues
infertility, artificial insemination, *in vitro* fertilization, multifetal pregnancy, multiple pregnancy, fraternal twins, monozygotic (or identical) twins, conjoined twins, triplets, karyotype, trisomy, peer pressure, abortion, spontaneous abortion (or miscarriage), threatened abortion, inevitable abortion, incomplete abortion, complete abortion, missed abortion, therapeutic abortion (TAB), elective abortion (EAB), adoption

KEY Points

- Reproductive issues involve physical disorders that can have an impact on psychological health.

- Physical disorders, including infection, hormonal imbalance, and structural defects, may be treated medically or, at times, surgically.

- Some disorders cannot be treated and result in infertility.

- Couples wanting to postpone pregnancy need information about contraception.

- The couple experiencing psychological and emotional problems about reproductive issues may require long-term support and professional counseling.

- Discussing the personal subject of sexual relations can be uncomfortable for the client, the partner, and the nurse. It is important for the nurse to express compassion and understanding, and to be open-minded and nonjudgmental.

Animations
Spermatogenesis
Oogenesis
Conception
H.I.V.
HIV/AIDS
Erectile dysfunction
Vasectomy
Breast cancer
Gonorrhea
Premenstrual syndrome

FOR FURTHER Study

Review Chapter 2 for legal responsibilities of the nurse.

For initial development of secondary sex characteristics, see Figure 4-22; for breast and testicular self-examination, see Procedures 4-1 and 4-2.

See more about pregnancy in Chapter 6; see placental layers in Figure 6-4; see muscles strengthened by Kegel exercises in Figure 6-20.

See discussion of high-risk pregnancies in Chapter 8.

For a discussion of ophthalmia neonatorum, see Chapter 9.

See Chapter 11 for a review of growth and development of the adolescent and a discussion of Piaget's theory.

The main HIV/AIDS discussion is in Chapter 21 of this book.

For further discussion of the effects of trauma, see Chapter 27.

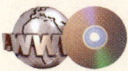

EXPLORE MediaLink

Additional interactive resources for this chapter can be found on the Companion Website at www.prenhall.com/towle.

Click on Chapter 5 and "Begin" to select the activities for this chapter.

For chapter-related NCLEX-style questions and an audio glossary, access the accompanying CD-ROM in this book.

Critical Thinking Care Map

Caring for a Client with Genital Warts

NCLEX-PN® Focus Area: Physiologic Integrity

Case Study: Claire presents to the family planning clinic for her Pap smear with complaints of vaginal spotting and a slight headache. Upon cervical examination, gray-pink lesions are identified. The tissue culture of the lesion reveals condylomata acuminata.

Nursing Diagnosis: Tissue Integrity, Impaired

COLLECT DATA

Subjective
_____
_____
_____
_____
_____

Objective
_____
_____
_____
_____
_____

Would you report this? Yes/No

If yes, to: _____

Nursing Care
_____
_____
_____
_____
_____
_____
_____
_____
_____
_____

How would you document this? _____
_____
_____
_____

Compare your documentation to the sample provided in Appendix I.

Data Collected
(use those that apply)

- Headache pain level 4
- Diet high in fat and calories
- States vaginal spotting has occurred for 4 days
- LMP (month/day/year)
- Exercises two times a week
- Small amount of dark red vaginal discharge noted
- Multiple cervical lesions measuring ½ to 1 cm in diameter
- Labia with diffuse redness
- Breasts without tenderness
- States has had three sexual partners in 3 months

Nursing Interventions
(use those that apply; list in priority order)

- Teach the importance of regular Pap smears.
- Teach the client about cryotherapy treatment.
- Teach the importance of informing all sexual partners.
- Assess characteristics of the lesion.
- Discuss importance of low-fat, high-fiber diet.
- Assess fears and anxieties related to sexual activity.

NCLEX-PN® Exam Preparation

1. As the nursing staff explores options for preventing teenage pregnancy, they review adolescent cognitive development and reasons for increased sexual behavior among teens. The issues considered include:
   1. desire to follow parental teaching.
   2. feelings of invincibility.
   3. low levels of sex hormones.
   4. sex drive equal to middle-age adults.

2. When collecting data related to the client's sexual history, which of the following sexual practices would put the client at risk for contracting HIV? Choose all that apply.
   1. heterosexual intercourse
   2. homosexual activity
   3. oral sex
   4. French kissing
   5. rectal sex
   6. a monogamous relationship

3. The nurse is teaching a client the proper use of an IUD. Which of the following teaching points would the nurse include in her teaching? Choose all that apply.
   1. Feel for the string weekly for the first month.
   2. Feel for the string monthly after menses.
   3. Report fever and chills to the physician immediately.
   4. Report symptoms of pregnancy immediately.
   5. Use a spermicide with each act of intercourse.
   6. This is a permanent form of contraception.

4. The nurse is assisting with the prenatal care of a 36-year-old client. Which of the following statements would the nurse need to explore further?
   1. "I would like to have an amniocentesis."
   2. "The child might have a fetal anomaly."
   3. "I blame my husband for this pregnancy."
   4. "I hope to spend time with my neighbor who is pregnant."

5. Which of the following clients might the nurse expect the physician to diagnose as infertile? The couple that is unable to achieve pregnancy after:
   1. discontinuing oral contraception 4 months ago.
   2. an episode of intercourse where the condom broke.
   3. a year or more of unprotected intercourse.
   4. 6 months of *in vitro* fertilization.

6. The client has just been diagnosed with a multifetal pregnancy of monozygotic twins. She asks the nurse to explain what this means. Which of the following statements made by the nurse would be an appropriate response? The twins:
   1. "occurred from one egg that divided into two embryos; will be identical."
   2. "occurred from two eggs fertilized by two sperm; will be fraternal."
   3. "occurred from one egg that divided into two embryos; will be dizygotic."
   4. "occurred from two eggs fertilized by two sperm; will be monozygotic."

7. The nurse understands that a client who has passed the fetus but retained the placenta is said to have which type of abortion?
   1. complete abortion
   2. incomplete abortion
   3. inevitable abortion
   4. threatened abortion

8. Which of the following nursing interventions are appropriate for the client giving her child up for adoption?
   1. caring for the mother and infant in the same postpartum room
   2. separating the mother and infant and not allowing visitation
   3. withholding information about the baby's physical characteristics from the client
   4. providing opportunities for the client to express her true feelings

9. The nurse works in the emergency department. She is caring for a woman admitted following a rape. Which option is the most appropriate for providing hygiene for this client?
   1. Help the woman immediately with a shower.
   2. Wash only her face and hands.
   3. Avoid washing the perineum.
   4. Avoid showering and bathing at this time.

10. Termination of the pregnancy to save the life of the mother is called:
    1. therapeutic abortion.
    2. elective abortion.
    3. spontaneous abortion.
    4. missed abortion.

Answers for Review Questions, as well as discussion of Care Plan and Critical Thinking Care Map questions, appear in Appendix I.

Chapter 6

Health Promotion During Pregnancy

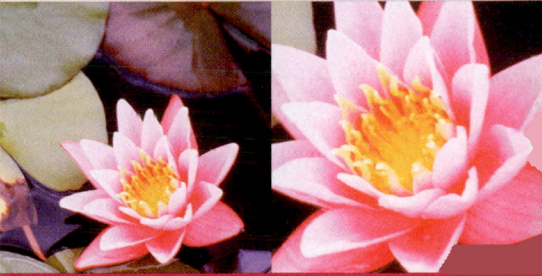

BRIEF Outline

LEARNING Outcomes

After completing this chapter, you will be able to:

- Describe factors that influence prenatal development.
- Describe fetal development.
- Identify signs of pregnancy and maternal changes throughout pregnancy.
- Discuss nutritional requirements during pregnancy.
- Discuss common maternal discomforts during pregnancy and their treatment.
- Discuss prenatal care and client teaching related to prenatal care.

Pregnancy is a powerful and complex time in a woman's life. She may be happily looking forward to the birth of a long-awaited first child. She may be wondering how to make adjustments for another of many children. She may be waiting fearfully through the period of pregnancy to give the baby up for adoption. In any case, she will face physical changes and processes that are unique and life altering. The role of the nurse in caring for pregnant women involves a great deal of emotional support and client education.

PRENATAL DEVELOPMENT

Preconception

For many years, health professionals have recognized that a healthy pregnancy begins before conception with good health habits. The focus of preconception care is to help the couple identify their pregnancy risk and prepare for conception. Unhealthy habits can affect the fetus before the mother knows she is pregnant. Likewise, good eating patterns and regular exercise can promote early fetal health. Box 6-1 ■ provides a list of foods that are high in nutrients required by pregnant women.

MALE CONTRIBUTION

The health of the fetus is not just related to the mother. For example, smoking decreases sperm production and motility. Men who have been exposed to industrial chemicals father more stillborn and small-for-gestational-age infants. They are also involved in more pregnancies that end in preterm labor or spontaneous abortion. Because production of sperm (*spermatogenesis*) is a continuous process, men can decrease these risks by avoiding smoking and industrial chemicals for 3 to 4 months prior to conception.

FEMALE CONTRIBUTION

To carry a pregnancy with minimal risk, the mother should develop a healthy lifestyle well before conception. A healthy lifestyle includes eating a low-fat, high-fiber diet; exercising at least three times per week; and being within 15 pounds of one's ideal weight. Because pregnancies are not always planned, avoiding unhealthy or risk-taking behavior will help ensure a healthy infant.

NUTRITIONAL DEFICITS AND HARMFUL CHEMICALS

Smoking, alcohol, and illicit drug use can have negative effects on pregnancy. Smoking during pregnancy can cause low birth weight and spontaneous abortion. Alcohol, even in moderate amounts, may cause fetal alcohol syndrome (discussed in Chapters 8 and 27 ⬭), including **craniofacial** (head and face) malformation and central nervous system dysfunction. Illicit drugs can cause a variety of **anomalies** (abnormal development of organs or structures). Clients should be encouraged to stop using these substances prior to and during pregnancy. Medications, both prescription and over the counter, may interfere with normal pregnancy and should be discussed with the health care provider.

Because fetal development occurs on a strict timeline, the lack of a certain nutrient at specific times can have a profound effect on the developing organism. For example, a deficiency of folic acid between weeks 3 and 4 is the cause of spina bifida, a very serious birth defect (Figure 6-1 ■).

Addition of drugs or chemicals can have similarly profound effects. Drugs or other agents that cause abnormal fetal development are called **teratogens.** In the 20th century, women were sometimes prescribed the tranquillizer called thalidimide until it was realized that the drug interfered with normal limb development.

BOX 6-1	NUTRITION THERAPY

Food Sources of Iron, Vitamin B$_{12}$, and Folic Acid
Iron-Rich Foods
>   Beef, chicken, pork loin, turkey, veal, egg yolk
>   Bran flakes, oatmeal, brown rice, whole-grain breads
>   Clams, oysters
>   Dried beans
>   Dried fruits
>   Greens

Folic Acid Food Sources
>   Asparagus, broccoli, green leafy vegetables
>   Eggs, liver, milk, organ meats
>   Kidney beans
>   Wheat germ
>   Yeast

Vitamin B$_{12}$ Food Sources
>   Eggs, cheese, milk
>   Fresh shrimp and oysters
>   Meats, organ meats (liver, kidney)

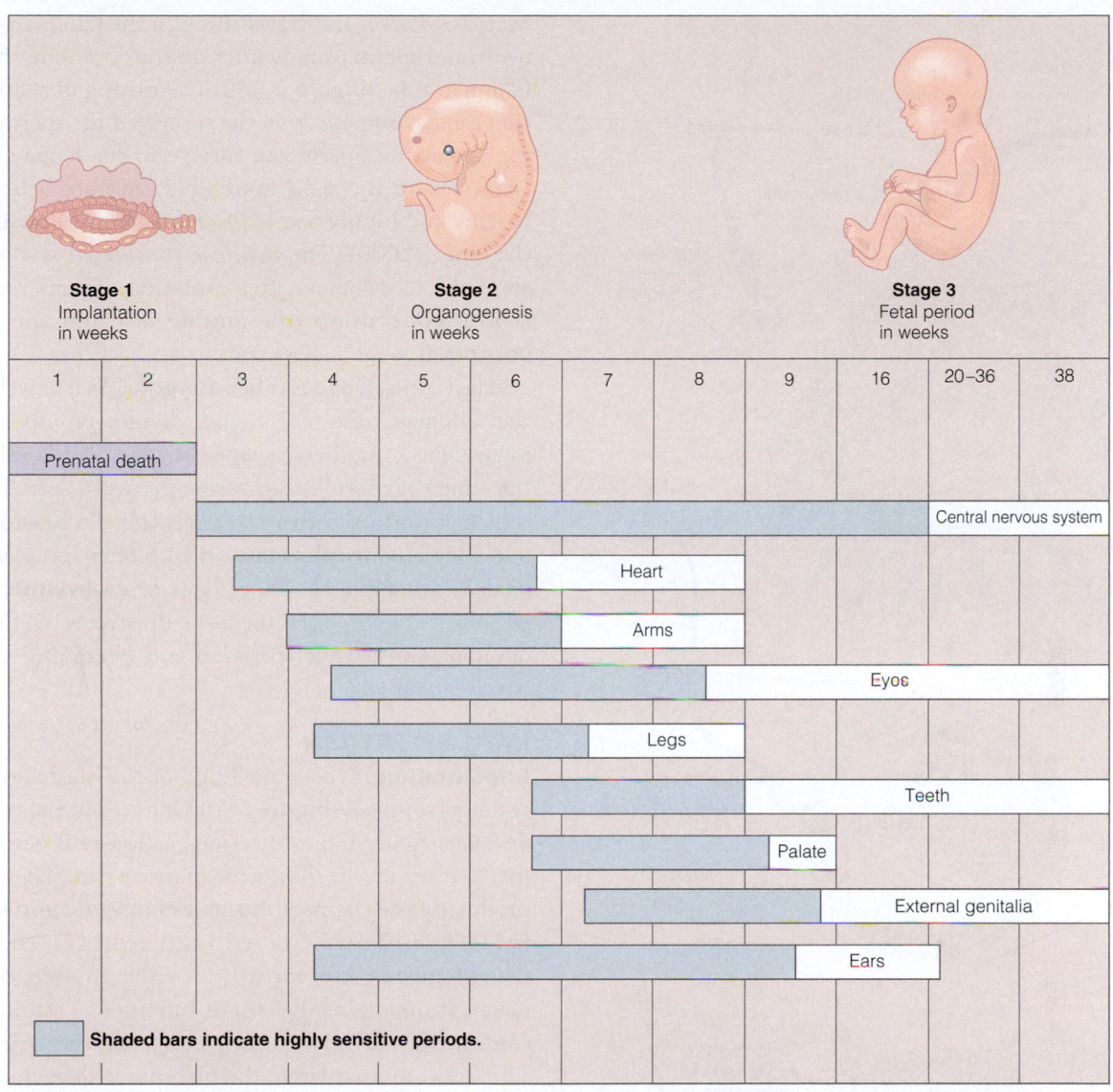

Figure 6-1. ■ Highly sensitive periods during the embryonic stage. For the first 2 weeks after contraception, exposure to a teratogen has an all-or-nothing effect. It either disrupts implantation and causes spontaneous abortion or leaves the embryo unharmed. From about the third through the eighth week of pregnancy (when organs form), exposure to a hazardous agent may cause serious anomalies. After organ formation and for the remainder of the pregnancy, exposure to fetal toxins will not cause malformation but can interfere with maturation of the central nervous system and retard intrauterine growth. It may also cause cognitive or behavioral abnormalities. (Data from Conover, E. [1994]. Guarding against fetal toxins. *Registered Nurse* [July, 31]).

Children born to these mothers had only partially developed limbs.

INFECTIOUS DISEASE COMPLICATIONS

Infectious diseases and other disorders can have a negative impact on pregnancy. Routine testing should be done for infections such as syphilis, gonorrhea, chlamydia, and group B streptococcus. Testing may also be done for HPV, HSV, and HIV. (See Chapter 5 ⬭ for a full discussion.) If the client tests positive, treatment should begin as soon as possible. Infection of the fallopian tubes (**salpingitis**) can cause scarring and narrowing of the lumen. A narrow fallopian tube can lead to infertility or tubal pregnancy. See Chapter 5 ⬭ for disorders of the female reproductive system and Chapter 8 ⬭ for high-risk pregnancy.

Fertilization

Fertilization is the process of uniting two sex cells into one (Figure 6-2 ■). **Pregnancy** is the carrying of the resulting offspring in the uterus. Pregnancy can be described by the events that occur throughout the 40 weeks of development.

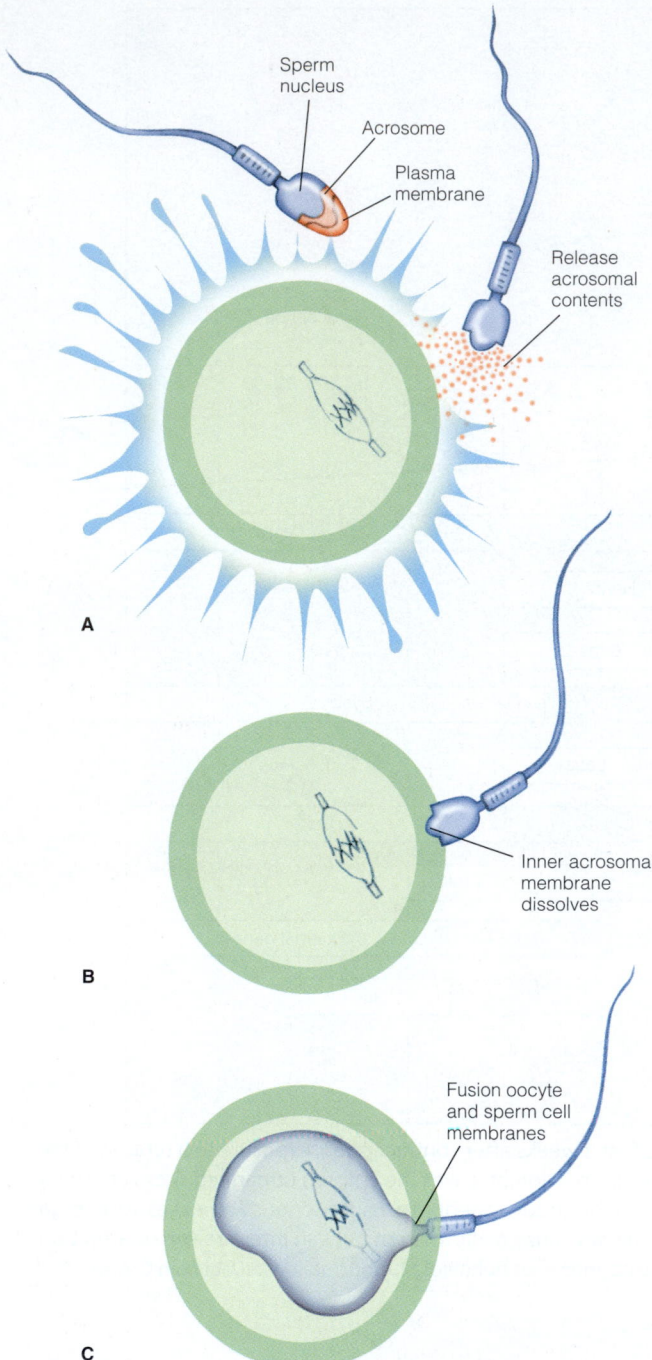

Figure 6-2. ■ At fertilization, the following sequence (called an *acrosome reaction*) occurs: (**A**) Perforations in the acrosome release chemicals onto the cell membrane of the ovum. (**B**) The acrosomal membrane continues to dissolve as the sperm penetrates the ovum. (**C**) The membranes of the sperm and oocyte cell fuse.

For pregnancy to occur, sperm from the male must be deposited near the cervix of the female. Although this most commonly occurs with coitus or copulation, sperm can also be deposited by artificial means (see Chapter 5 ⬭). Once deposited, sperm must "swim" through the mucus inside the cervix, through the uterus, and down the fallopian tube. At the same time, the egg (*ovum*) must leave the

ovary (*ovulation*) and travel through the fallopian tube. The ovum and sperm usually unite in the outer one-third of the fallopian tube (Figure 6-3 ■). The timing of sperm deposition can have an effect on the success of the sperm in reaching the ovum. Sperm can survive in the female reproductive tract for up to 72 hours, but they are believed to be healthy and highly fertile for only about the first 24 hours (DeJonge, 2000). The ovum is considered fertile for only about 12 to 24 hours after ovulation. Therefore, fertilization or **conception** (the uniting of ovum and sperm) is only possible for a short time.

The fertilized egg is called a **zygote.** As it travels through the fallopian tube, the zygote divides rapidly to form a many-celled, mulberry-shaped mass called a **morula.** By the time the morula reaches the uterus in 4 to 5 days, the cells have formed a two-layer ball called a **blastocyst.** The outer layer or **trophoblast** will become the placenta and fetal membranes. The inner layer or **embryonic disc** will become the embryo. Figure 6-4 ■ illustrates the first days of development after fertilization and beginning embryonic development.

IMPLANTATION

Implantation is the embedding of the blastocyst into the endometrium (see Figure 6-3). One area of the trophoblast develops finger-like projections called **villi** (singular, villus) that secure the blastocyst to the uterus. The villi begin producing the chemical **human chorionic gonadotropin (hCG)** 8 to 10 days after fertilization; hCG is the chemical that pregnancy kits identify in order to determine pregnancy. It maintains the corpus luteum and stimulates it to continue producing estrogen and progesterone until 11 to 12 weeks. By that time, the placenta is developed enough to produce estrogen and progesterone to maintain the pregnancy.

Development of Support Structures

FETAL MEMBRANES

The chorionic villi develop into the placenta. The remainder of the trophoblast becomes the outer layer of the membranes called the **chorion** (see Figure 6-4). The inner layer of the placenta, the **amnion,** originates from inside the blastocyst. The amnion grows as the fetus grows until it comes in contact with the chorion. Together the two layers form the **fetal membranes,** also called the **"bag of waters."**

AMNIOTIC FLUID

The **amniotic fluid** is formed by the amnion (see Figure 6-4). Amniotic fluid consists of about 98% water. It also contains glucose, proteins, urea, **lanugo** (fine fetal hair), and **vernix**

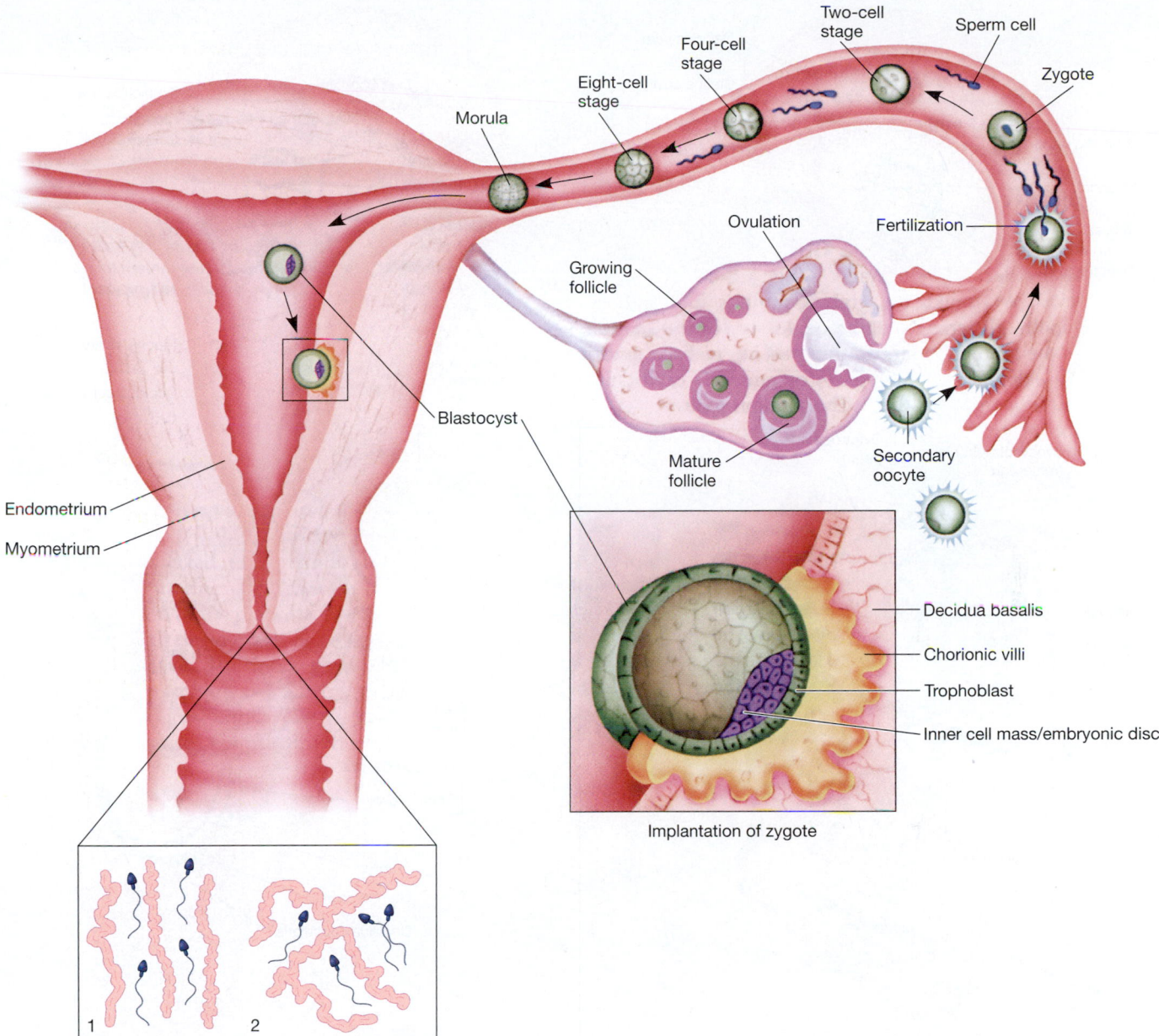

Figure 6-3. ■ Ovulation, fertilization, and implantation. During ovulation, the ovum leaves the ovary and enters the fallopian tube. Fertilization generally occurs in the outer third of the fallopian tube. Subsequent changes in the fertilized ovum from conception to implantation are shown. *(Left inset)* Sperm passage through cervical mucus. (1) During ovulation the mucoid strands become more parallel, allowing sperm to pass through easily. (2) When the client is not ovulating, tangled mucus strands prevent many sperm from passing. *(Right inset)* Implanted zygote. *(Left inset*: Data from Corson, S. [1990]. *Conquering infertility: A guide for couples* [4th ed.]. Vancouver, BC, Canada: EMIS-Canada, p. 16.)

caseosa (white, cheesy covering of the fetus' skin). The fetus drinks the amniotic fluid and urinates into it. Amniotic fluid is reabsorbed and replaced every 3 hours. The amniotic fluid has the following important functions for the developing fetus:

■ Maintains constant temperature
■ Equalizes pressure around the fetus to allow for growth
■ Cushions the fetus from injury and the umbilical cord from compression
■ Prevents the fetal membranes from adhering to the fetus

■ Allows the fetus to move freely
■ Provides the fetus with fluid to swallow.

PLACENTA

By the third week post fertilization, the placenta has formed, but it is not fully functional until the 12th week. The **placenta** is a highly vascular organ connecting the mother and the fetus. The maternal side of the placenta is divided into irregular sections called **cotyledons.** Both the color and the texture are like liver. *Note:* Expulsion of the placenta with

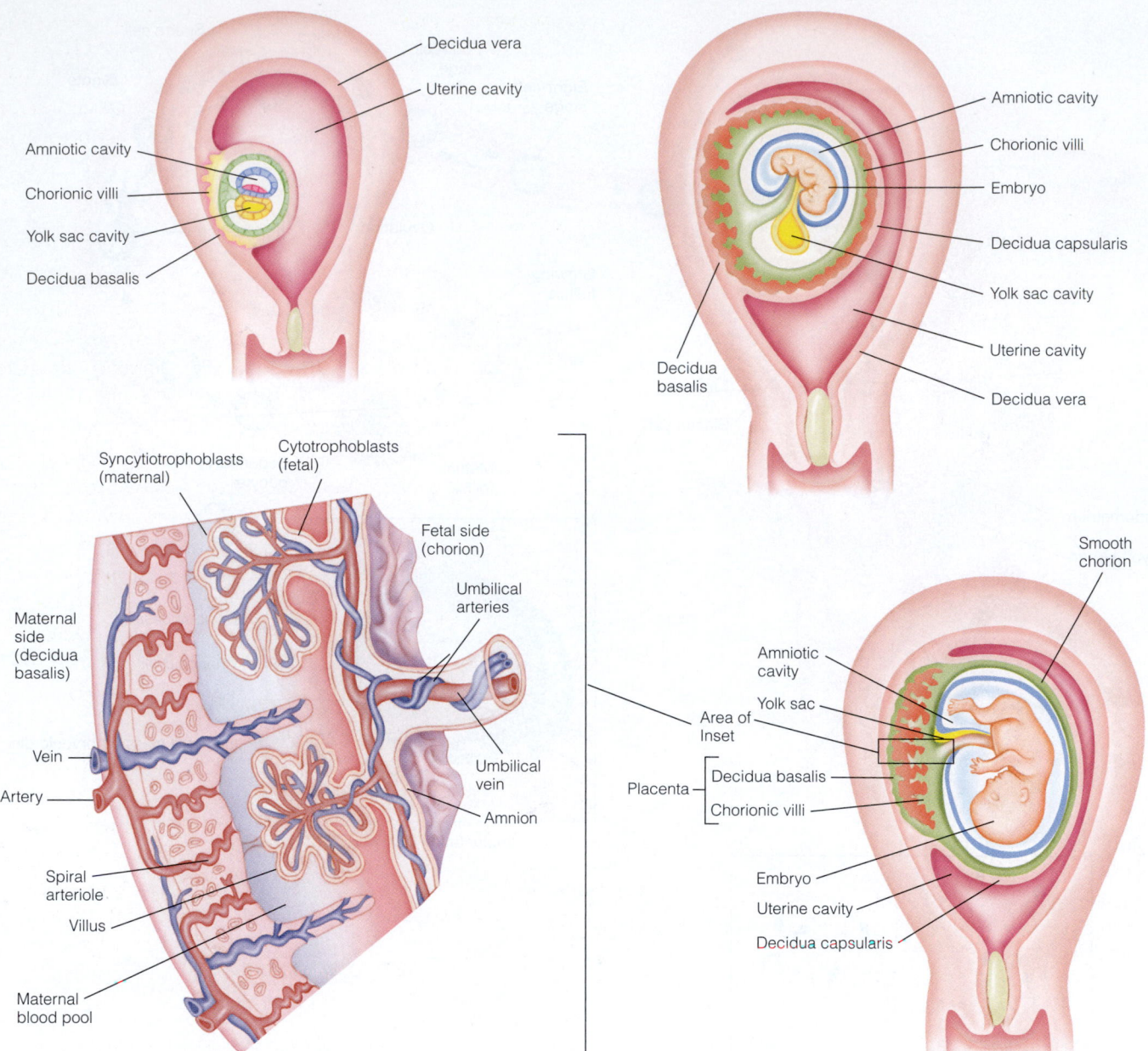

Figure 6-4. ■ Sequence of development of the embryo from primary germ layers. The stages show the implanted blastocyst and development of the embryo, fetal membranes, and yolk sac during the preplacental phase. The inset illustrates vascularization of the placenta.

the maternal side out is called the Duncan mechanism (think *Dirty Duncan*). The fetal side of the placenta is white and shiny, with the large blood vessels leading to the umbilical cord visible. *Note:* Expulsion of the placenta with the fetal side out is called the Schultze mechanism (think *Shiny Schultze*). Figure 6-5 ■ illustrates the inner and outer surfaces of the placenta. At time of delivery, the placenta is about 8 inches in diameter and weighs approximately 1 pound.

The placenta has three main functions:

1. The placenta's first function is transport. Oxygen, glucose, amino acids, electrolytes, and vitamins are transported from the mother's blood to the infant's blood. At the same time, carbon dioxide, urea, creatinine, and

other fetal waste are transported from the infant's blood to the mother's blood. Many drugs entering the maternal blood will also be transported to the infant's blood. Even though chemicals are transported between mother and infant, the blood cells do not cross the placenta.

2. The second function of the placenta is to produce hormones.
   - hCG, the basis for pregnancy tests, has already been discussed.
   - **Human placental lactogen (hPL)** stimulates changes in maternal metabolism. This change makes protein, glucose, and minerals more readily available to the fetus. The hPL is an *insulin antagonist* (it decreases the woman's metabolism of glucose). The mother's body

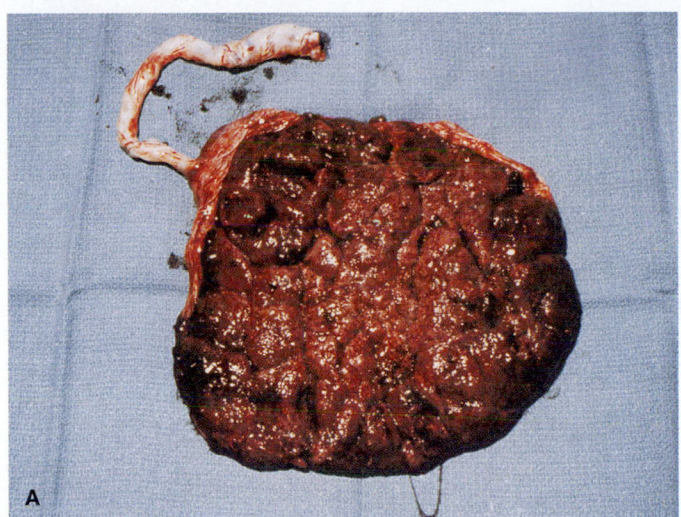

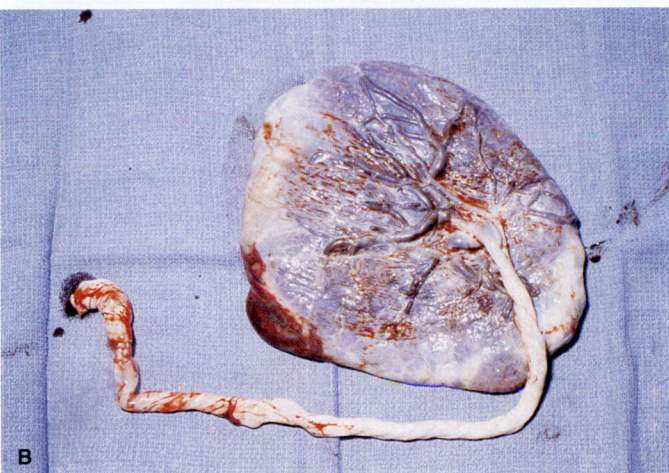

Figure 6-5. ■ Placenta. (**A**) Maternal side of the placenta ("Dirty Duncan"). (**B**) Fetal side ("Shiny Schultze"). (Courtesy of Marcia London, RNC, MSN, NNP.)

prepares for lactation because of an increase in hPL. The placenta also produces estrogen and progesterone to maintain the endometrium, stimulate breast development, and prevent uterine contractions.

- **Relaxin** is a hormone produced by the placenta that causes softening in the collagen connective tissue of the symphysis pubis and sacroiliac joints. In late pregnancy, these joints become moveable, making a larger passageway for the delivery.

3. The third function of the placenta is production of fatty acids, glycogen, and cholesterol for fetal use. Enzymes that are necessary for the transport of nutrients to the fetus are also produced by the placenta.

UMBILICAL CORD

The **umbilical cord** connects the fetus to the placenta. The umbilical cord consists of a white gelatinous tissue called **Wharton's jelly.** Wharton's jelly protects and supports the two umbilical arteries and one umbilical vein. At term, the umbilical cord is 22 to 24 inches long. When the Wharton's jelly comes in contact with air following delivery, it contracts, clamping the blood vessels to prevent bleeding.

Stages of Fetal Development

Fetal development, or **gestation,** is marked in weeks following conception. Fetal development takes place in three stages.

- Stage I, the **pre-embryonic stage,** is from fertilization through 14 days or 2 weeks. This is the time when the fertilized ovum travels through the fallopian tube, differentiates into trophoblast and embryonic disc, and attaches to the endometrium.
- Stage II, the **embryonic stage,** is from weeks 3 through 8. During this stage, all body systems are formed. Developing cells are at greatest risk to environmental teratogens, infections, and drugs at this time.
- Stage III, the **fetal stage,** is from weeks 9 through 38 to 40. During this stage, all body systems are refined and begin to function. Some body systems will take several years to reach their maximum functioning.

Development of Fetal Body Systems

The embryonic disc forms three germ layers from which all body systems develop. Table 6-1 ■ identifies the three germ layers and the body systems derived from each. Figure 6-6 ■ illustrates stages of fetal development through week 30.

TABLE 6-1	
Germ Layers and Body System Development	
EMBRYONIC (GERM) LAYER	**BODY SYSTEM INTO WHICH LAYER DEVELOPS**
Endoderm (inner layer)	Respiratory system Gastrointestinal system, liver, pancreas Bladder and urethra
Mesoderm (middle layer)	Muscular system Skeletal system Heart, blood, and blood vessels Spleen Urinary (renal) system Reproductive system
Ectoderm (outer layer)	Skin Nervous system Sense organs Mouth and anus

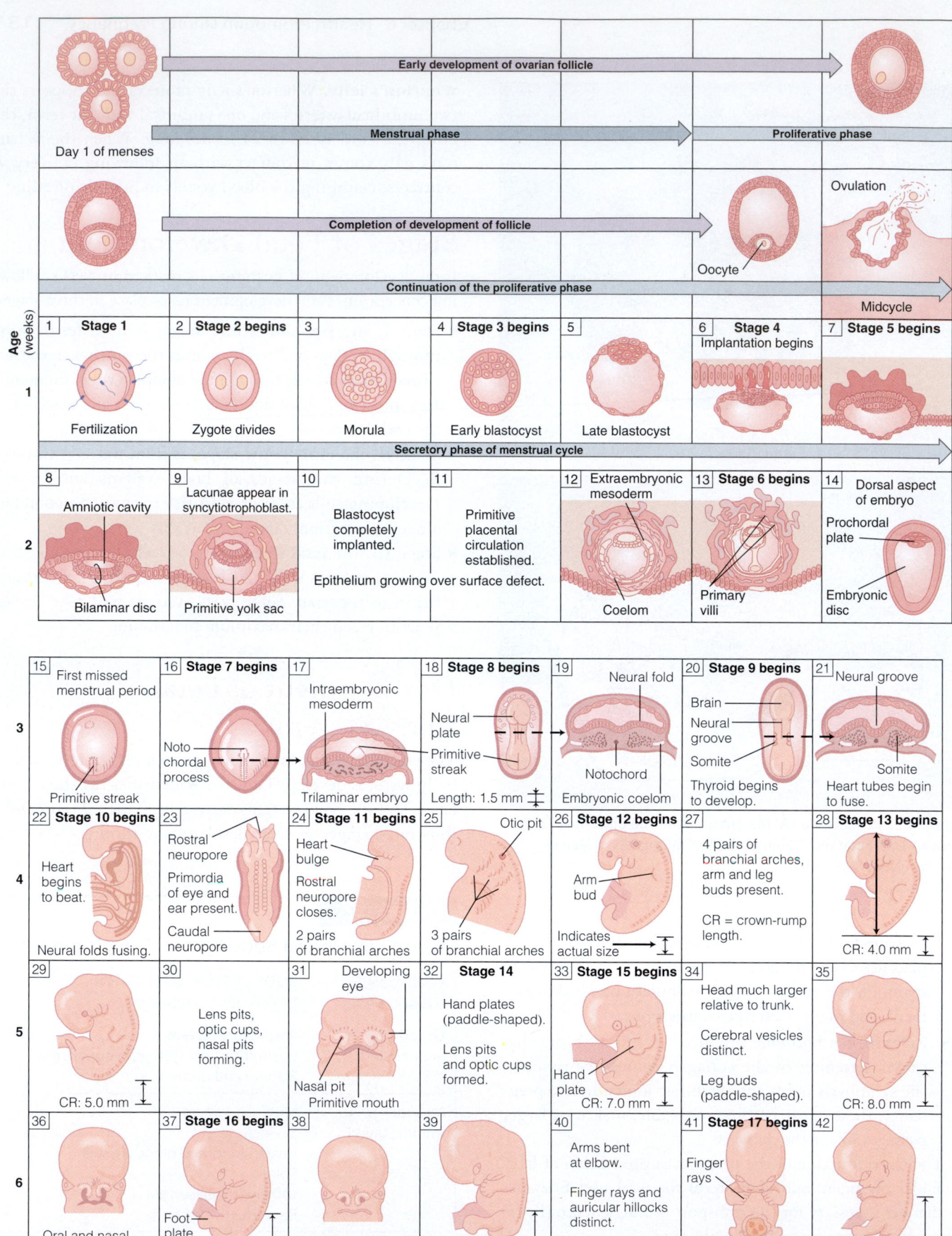

Figure 6-6. ■ (**A**) Human prenatal development from conception to 10 weeks. (**B**) Human fetal development: 12 weeks, 20 weeks, 24 weeks, and 30 weeks. (**A:** Reprinted from Moore, K. L. [1989]. *The developing human: Clinically oriented embryology* [3rd ed.]. Philadelphia: WB Saunders, pp. 2–4, with permission from Elsevier, Inc.)

A (*continued*)

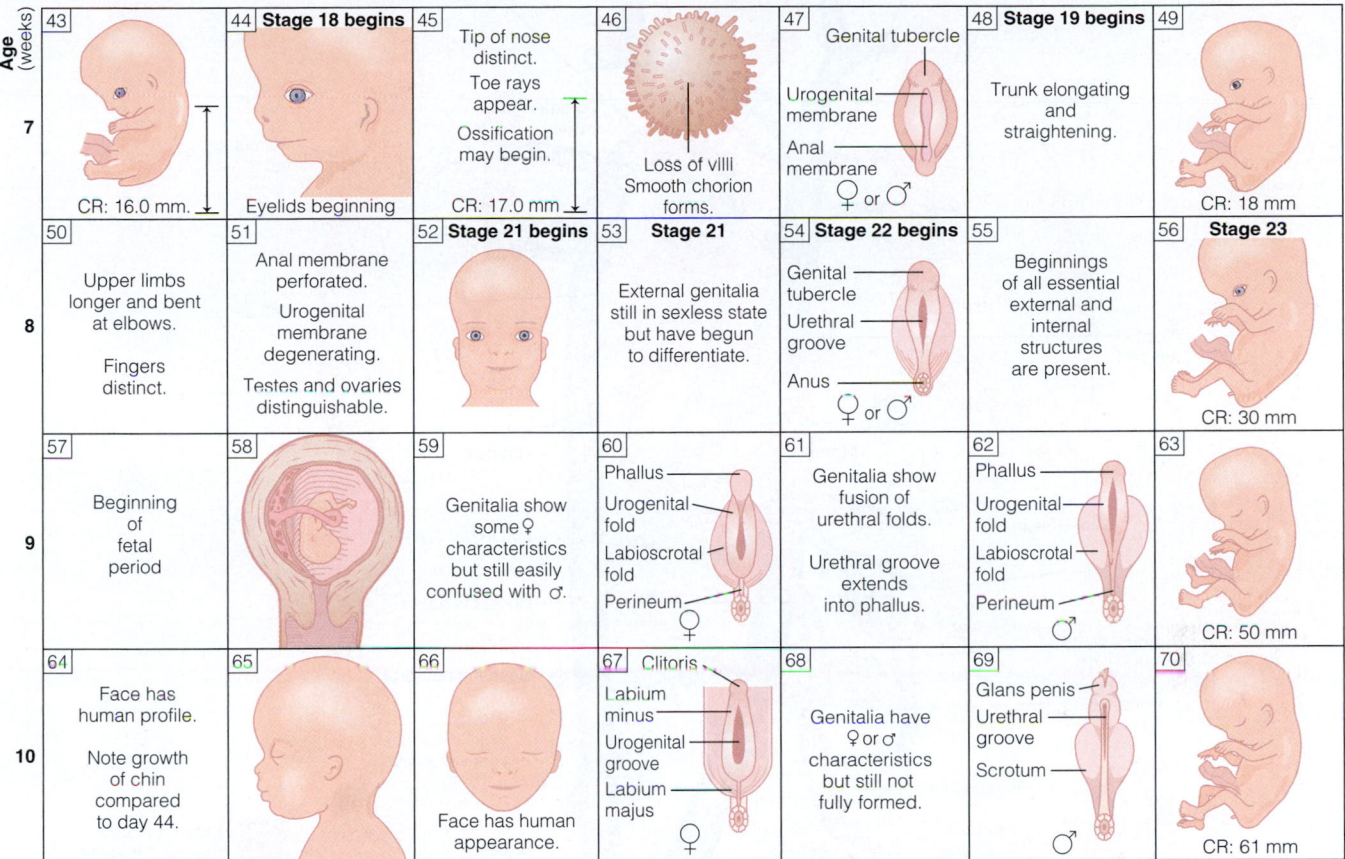

B

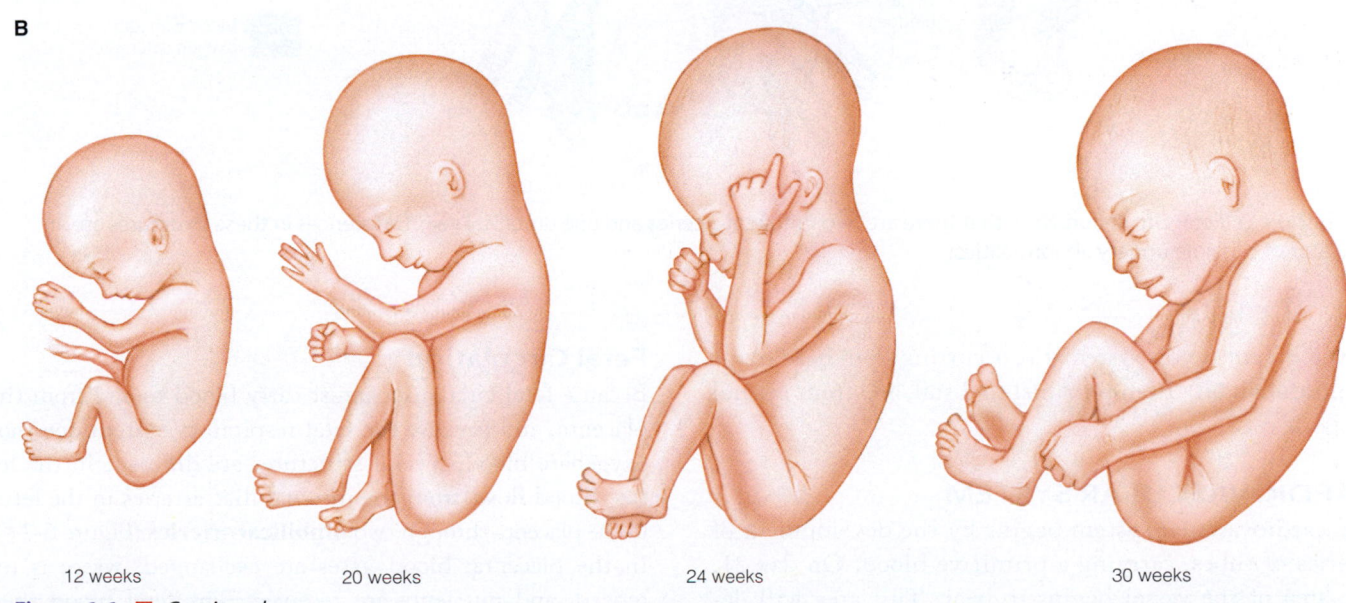

12 weeks   20 weeks   24 weeks   30 weeks

Figure 6-6. ■ *Continued.*

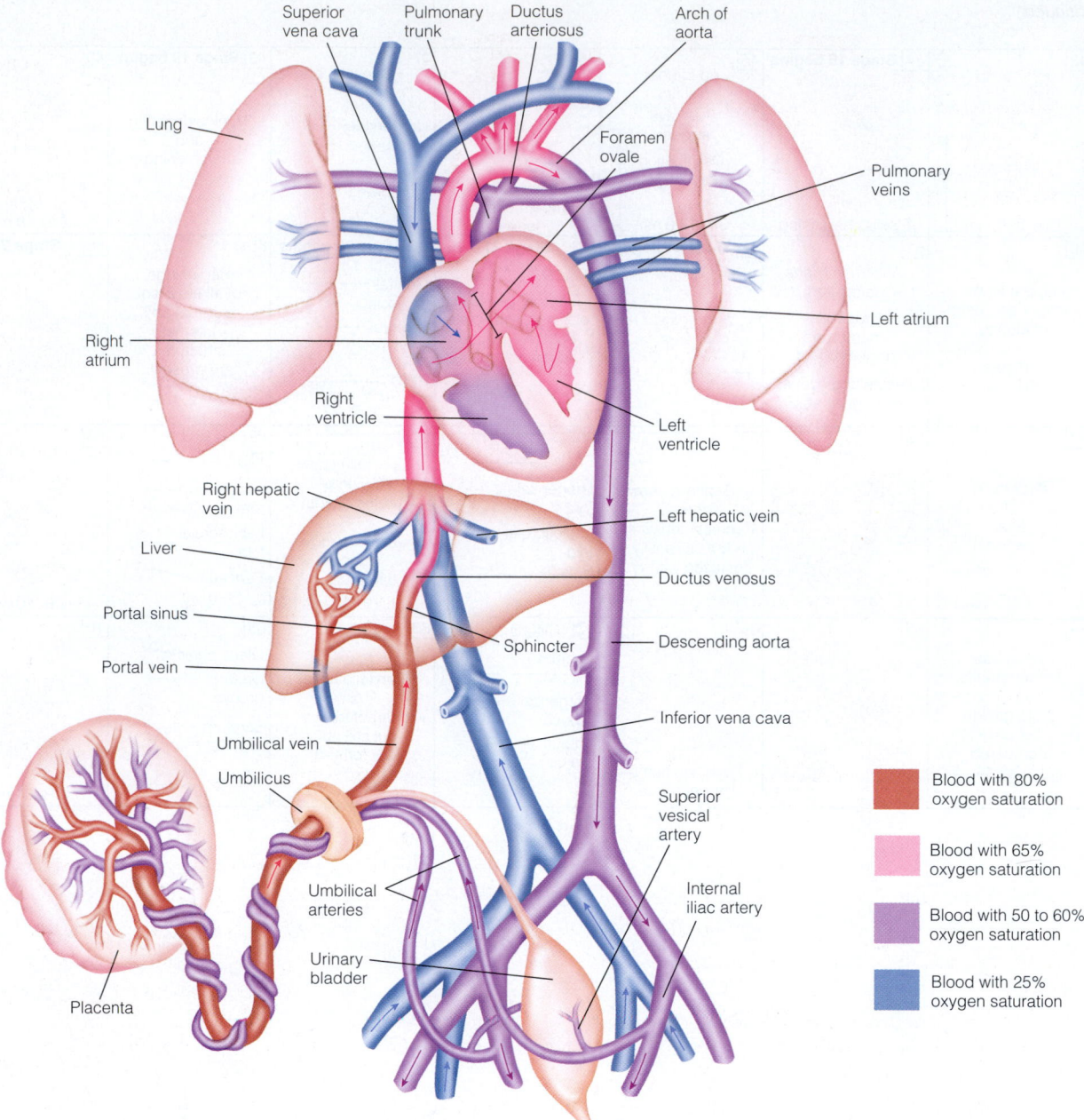

Figure 6-7. ■ Fetal circulation. Note that there are two umbilical arteries and one umbilical vein. Differences in these structures are an indicator of possible urinary abnormalities.

Development is very systematic, occurring from head to toe (**cephalocaudal**), from proximal to distal, and from general to specific.

CARDIOVASCULAR SYSTEM

The cardiovascular system begins by the development of a series of tubes, carrying a primitive blood. On day 21, one area of the vessel begins to beat. This area will develop into the heart through a series of foldings, openings, and closings. Most heart anomalies occur during weeks 6 to 8.

Fetal Circulation

Because fetal circulation must carry blood to and from the placenta, and because the fetal respiratory system does not oxygenate blood, several structures are different in the fetus. Blood flows from the internal iliac arteries in the fetus to the placenta through two **umbilical arteries** (Figure 6-7 ■). In the placenta, blood gases are exchanged, waste is removed, and nutrients are received. The fetal blood then flows back to the fetus through one **umbilical vein.** After entering the fetal abdomen, the umbilical vein divides into two branches. The umbilical vein carries blood to the fetal liver. The other branch, the **ductus venosus**, carries blood to the inferior vena cava.

Two structures limit the amount of blood going to the fetal lungs. Inside the fetal heart, the **foramen ovale** is an opening in the septum between the right atrium and the left atrium. The higher pressure in the right atrium pushes some blood through the foramen ovale into the left atrium. Outside the fetal heart, the **ductus arteriosus** connects the main pulmonary artery to the aorta. Some blood flows from the pulmonary artery to the aorta, thus bypassing the lungs. The small amount of blood actually reaching the lungs is necessary for the development of the respiratory system (see Figure 6-7). Usually, shortly after birth, these fetal structures close, and the cardiovascular system adjusts to normal functioning (see Figure 19-1 ⬭).

Fetal blood is initially formed on day 14 in the **yolk sac**, a structure inside the ovum. The liver will not be able to make blood cells until the fifth week, and the bone marrow will not function until the 10th week. Fetal hemoglobin (HgbF) has a greater attraction for oxygen than maternal hemoglobin does. This helps ensure that the fetus receives an adequate supply of oxygen. The blood type is determined at the time of conception.

Multifetal Circulation

Circulation for multifetal pregnancy with twins may take two different paths, as was shown in the illustration of fraternal and identical twins in Chapter 5, Figure 5-18 ⬭. Two blastocysts may develop into two distinct chorions with two amnions; these are *fraternal twins*. If the inner cell mass of one blastocyst splits in two, *identical twins* are formed, with two amnions within one chorion.

RESPIRATORY SYSTEM

The respiratory system begins as lung buds during the 6th week of development and is formed by the 23rd week, but there are not enough alveoli to maintain gas exchange outside the uterus. By weeks 20 to 23, the primitive lungs begin to produce surfactant. **Surfactant** is a substance that decreases the surface tension of fluid inside the alveoli, allowing the lungs to expand. By the 24th week, the lungs are capable of borderline support outside the uterus. Therefore, the age of **viability** (the ability to live outside the uterus) is 24 weeks. An infant born at this time would require intensive nursing care, including ventilation support. Surfactant production matures by the 35th week, making the prognosis more favorable. The lungs will continue to add alveoli until adulthood.

NERVOUS SYSTEM

The head and brain develop rapidly in the fetus. By the fourth week, the brain has differentiated into lobes. A week later, the cranial nerves are present and function. By the

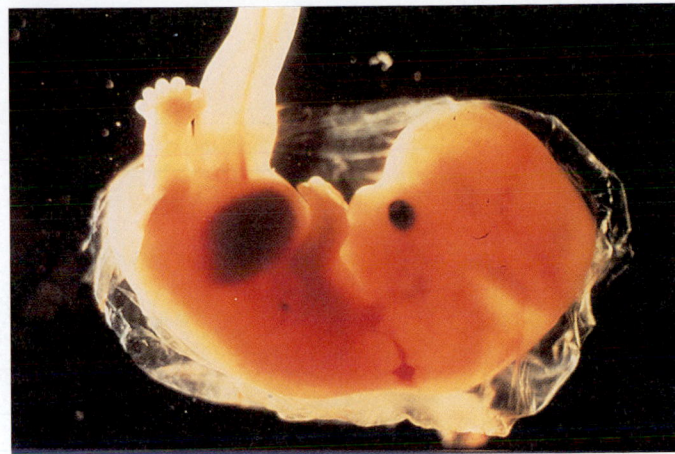

Figure 6-8. ■ The embryo at 7 weeks. The head is round and nearly erect. The eyes have shifted forward and are closer together. The eyelids begin to form. (Used with permission from Petit Format/Nestle/Science Source/Photo Researchers, Inc.)

sixth week, the entire central nervous system is present. The peripheral nervous system, however, will not be functioning completely for another 7 to 10 years.

Special Senses

The ears begin to appear in the 3rd week, low on the head, in the region of the lower jaw. They gradually move upward to their designated place on the head by the 8th week. The infant can hear and respond to sound by the 12th week.

In the 3rd week, the eyes can be seen as large dark discs on the side of the developing head. By the 7th week, eyelids form and seal to protect the developing retina (Figure 6-8 ■). A week later, the eyes have moved to the front of the face. The eyelids will remain closed until the 28th week of development.

GASTROINTESTINAL SYSTEM

The gastrointestinal system begins formation in the fourth week. The esophagus, stomach, small intestines, liver, pancreas, and most of the colon are developed from the same germ layer, the endoderm. (Refer to Table 6-1.) The oral cavity, pharynx, and anus are formed from the ectoderm. Occasionally, there is incomplete development in the area where the germ layers meet, resulting in congenital anomalies.

By the 12th week, the fetus swallows amniotic fluid, and the liver is making bile. In the 16th week, **meconium** (the first fetal stool) is made from amniotic fluid, bile, and epithelial cells. Meconium should remain in the colon until after delivery.

clinical ALERT

The passage of meconium prior to delivery signals some type of fetal distress.

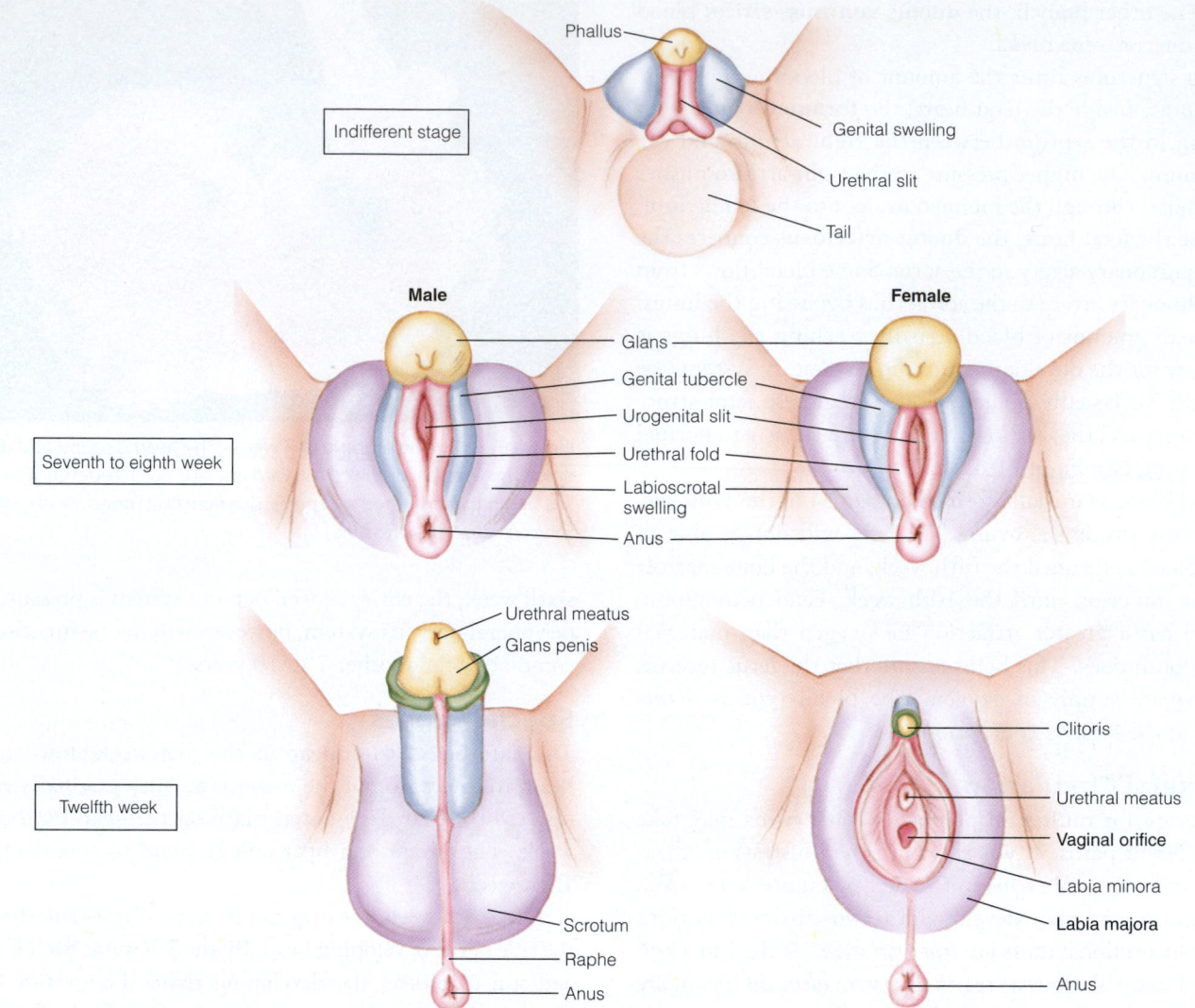

Indifferent stage — Phallus, Genital swelling, Urethral slit, Tail

Male / Female — Glans, Genital tubercle, Urogenital slit, Urethral fold, Labioscrotal swelling, Anus (Seventh to eighth week)

Twelfth week — Urethral meatus, Glans penis, Scrotum, Raphe, Anus / Clitoris, Urethral meatus, Vaginal orifice, Labia minora, Labia majora, Anus

Figure 6-9. ■ Development of the external reproductive structures. (Reproduced, with permission, from McGraw-Hill Companies, Inc. Ganong, W. F. [1995]. *Review of medical physiology* [17th ed.]. Norwalk, CT: Appleton & Lange, p. 384.)

RENAL SYSTEM

The urinary system is another body system that develops from more than one germ layer. (See Table 6-1.) The kidneys, ureters, and *trigone*, or lower section of the bladder, come from the mesoderm. The remainder of the bladder, female urethra, and proximal male urethra come from the endoderm. The distal male urethra develops from the ectoderm. Any disruption in development results in complex anomalies. (Renal disorders are discussed in Chapter 23 ⊙.)

The kidneys develop in several stages in the pelvis and ascend to their normal location. The kidneys begin producing urine in the 10th week, and the fetus urinates into the amniotic fluid by the 11th week of development.

REPRODUCTIVE SYSTEM

The gender of the fetus is determined at conception (see Chapter 4 ⊙). The fetus develops undifferentiated go-

nads until the 7th week. In the presence of the Y chromosome, testosterone stimulates the gonads to differentiate into testes. Sperm will not be produced until puberty. Testosterone will also stimulate the development of male genitalia. Without testosterone, the gonads develop into ovaries, and female genitalia form internally. Ova will be produced and will remain in the ovary until puberty. External male and female genitalia can be identified in the 12th week of development (Figure 6-9 ■).

MUSCULOSKELETAL SYSTEM

Limb buds appear in the 4th week. Cartilage forms a primitive skeleton covered by muscles by the 6th week. A week later, fetal movement can be seen on ultrasound. However, *quickening* (the first fetal movements felt by the mother) will not occur until the 16th to 20th weeks. By the end of the 8th week (Figure 6-10 ■), **ossification** in the bones begins, marking the transition from embryo to fetus.

INTEGUMENTARY SYSTEM

The skin of the fetus is thin and pink. Because the skin lacks fat until the last 4 to 6 weeks of gestation, the blood vessels can readily be seen. Fingernails and toenails reach the end of the digit by the 36th week. Lanugo begins to disappear in the 28th week, leaving only hair on the scalp and, at times, the shoulders and upper back at birth. Vernix caseosa covers the skin to protect it from the amniotic fluid. The white cheesy substance is gradually absorbed by the skin, leaving a small amount in the body folds and the lower back. Skin color is determined at conception.

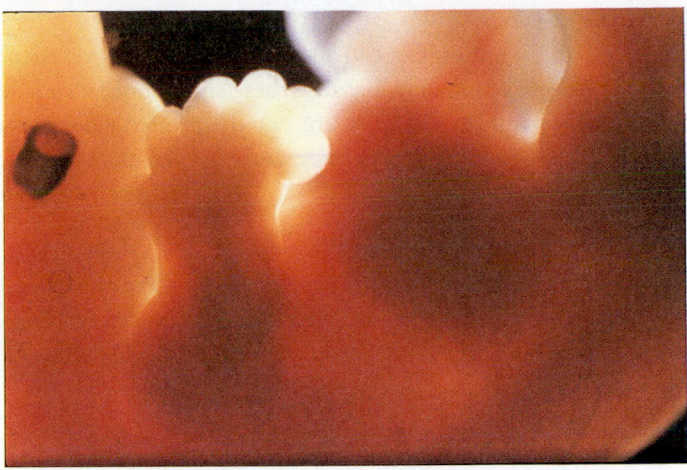

Figure 6-10. ■ The embryo at 8 weeks. Although only 3 centimeter in crown-to-rump (C-R) length, the embryo clearly resembles a human. Facial features continue to develop.

PREGNANCY

Signs of Pregnancy

During pregnancy, many physiologic changes will be reported by the mother or observed by the health care provider. These changes can be categorized as presumptive, probable, and positive signs of pregnancy, fatigue, abdominal enlargement, and quickening.

PRESUMPTIVE SIGNS

The subjective signs the mother experiences during pregnancy are **presumptive signs.** They may be indicators of other conditions besides pregnancy, so are not diagnostic in nature. Presumptive signs include amenorrhea, nausea and vomiting, breast changes, urinary frequency, fatigue, abdominal enlargement, and quickening.

Amenorrhea

Amenorrhea, or the absence of menses, is usually the first sign a woman notices that may cause her to think she is pregnant. Although pregnancy is the most common cause of amenorrhea, other causes could be hormone imbalance, stress, menopause, or tumors.

Nausea and Vomiting

Nausea and vomiting usually occur in the morning, but could occur at any time. Sometimes called morning sickness, these symptoms are commonly experienced during early pregnancy. However, nausea and vomiting are also associated with many other conditions.

Breast Changes

Breast changes, such as tenderness, tingling, and enlargement of the breast, occur in early pregnancy. Many women also experience these changes with the monthly period.

Urinary Frequency

Urinary frequency occurs because the enlarging uterus presses on the bladder, giving the woman the feeling of needing to urinate often. Other disorders, including urinary infection and abdominal tumor, could also elicit this sensation.

Fatigue

Fatigue is most often noted in the first few months of pregnancy, but many other conditions result in fatigue as well.

Abdominal Enlargement

Abdominal enlargement is noted by the 12th week, but may be evident earlier in the very thin woman or later in the large woman. Abdominal enlargement may also be noted when tumors are present.

Quickening

Quickening is a fluttering sensation felt as the fetus moves. The sensation begins between 16 and 22 weeks and gradually becomes stronger and more frequent. Other causes, such as muscle twitch or intestinal gas, can mimic this sensation. Because the mother is experiencing this subjective sensation, quickening is a presumptive sign.

Pregnancy is usually diagnosed before the woman experiences all presumptive signs. Denial of pregnancy could keep the woman from noticing the presumptive signs. False pregnancy, also known as **pseudopregnancy,** occurs when the nonpregnant woman so strongly wants to be pregnant that she experiences the presumptive signs. Treatment of pseudopregnancy is by psychiatric means.

PROBABLE SIGNS

The health care provider can identify objective signs that could indicate pregnancy. Because these signs could also indicate other conditions, they are not diagnostic. Probable signs include positive pregnancy tests, ballottement, and uterine changes.

Positive Pregnancy Tests

Pregnancy tests screen for the presence of hCG in the urine or blood. Most home tests are based on the amount of hCG in the urine. A test may be positive 8 to 14 days after conception. Some medications, the timing and accuracy of specimen collection, and the presence of hormone-producing tumors can affect the accuracy of the test.

Ballottement

Ballottement is a test for pregnancy in which the examiner puts two fingers into the vagina and pushes upward on the uterus. If the woman is pregnant, the fetus will rebound against the fingers.

> ### clinical ALERT
>
> A false-positive result for pregnancy can be obtained with ballottement. It is possible for a tumor in the uterus to elicit the same response.

Uterine Changes

There are physical signs that can be checked to assess the probability of pregnancy (Figure 6-11 ■): **Hegar's sign** (a softening of the lower uterine segment), **Goodell's sign** (a softening of the cervix), and **Chadwick's sign** (a bluish-purple discoloration of the cervix and vagina) can be observed in the first few weeks of pregnancy. The fundus of the uterus can be palpated just above the pubis at 12 weeks. Tumors can also cause uterine enlargement.

When probable signs are combined with presumptive signs, there is a strong indication of pregnancy.

POSITIVE SIGNS

Positive signs are diagnostic of pregnancy. No other condition can cause these signs. Positive signs of pregnancy include hearing fetal heart tones, visualization of the fetus, and fetal movement felt by examiner.

Hearing Fetal Heart Tones

Fetal heart tones (FHT), or the fetal heartbeat, can be heard with a Doppler by 10 to 12 weeks. The normal FHR is 120 to 150 bpm. It is important to distinguish the FHR from the maternal heart rate. When auscultating the abdomen, a soft blowing sound can be heard. The sound occurring at the same rate as the maternal pulse is called **uterine soufflé** and is caused by increased maternal blood flow to the uterus. The sound occurring at the FHR is called **funic soufflé** and is caused by fetal blood flowing through the umbilical cord.

Visualization of the Fetus

An abdominal ultrasound can detect a viable pregnancy by the 6th week. A transvaginal ultrasound can detect a trophoblast by the 10th day after conception. X-ray examination of the pelvis is rarely done due to the risk of radiation exposure to the fetus and maternal reproductive organs.

Fetal Movement Felt by Examiner

The fetus usually does not kick strongly enough for the examiner to feel the movement until the 20th week.

Diagnostic tests to determine fetal status are discussed later in this chapter.

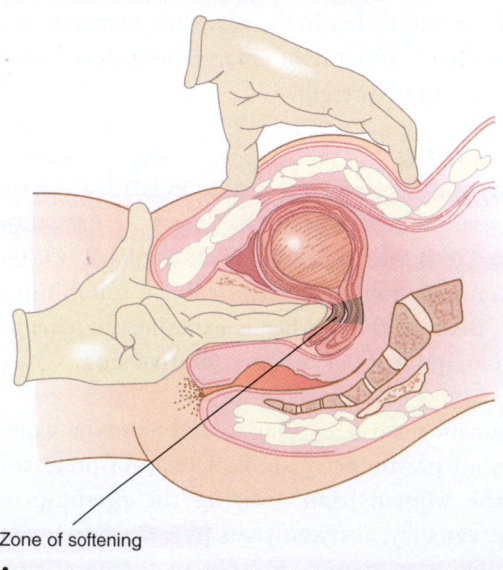

Zone of softening

A

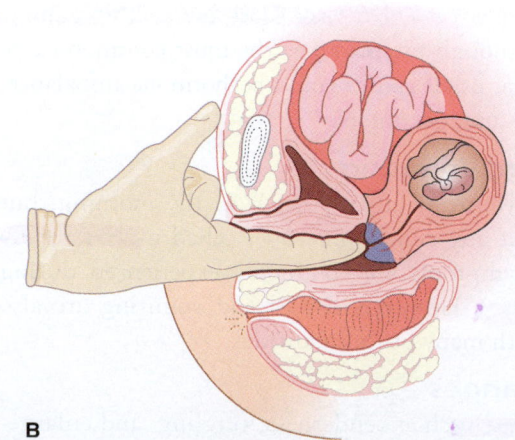

B

Figure 6-11. ■ **(A)** Hegar's sign. **(B)** Goodell's and Chadwick's signs. (Reproduced, with permission, from McGraw-Hill Companies, Inc. DeCherney, A. H., & Pernoll, M. L. [1994]. *Current obstetric and gynecologic diagnosis and treatment* [8th ed.]. Norwalk, CT: Appleton & Lange, p. 187.)

Maternal Changes During Pregnancy

Typically, the progression of the pregnancy is described in 3-month blocks of time called **trimesters.** This might seem confusing when fetal development is described by weeks. A normal pregnancy takes three trimesters equaling 9 calendar months, or 40 weeks equaling 10 lunar months.

Pregnancy causes many changes in a woman's body and additional work in each body system that increases the need for oxygen (Figure 6-12 ■). A healthy woman's body can tolerate the additional work. However, if disease is present, the additional stress may be harmful or life threatening to the mother.

REPRODUCTIVE SYSTEM

The most obvious changes occur in the reproductive system. Prior to pregnancy, the uterus (see Figure 4-12 ⬤⬤) is a small, pear-shaped, thick-walled organ weighing 2 oz (60 g) with a capacity of 10 mL. By the end of pregnancy, the uterus is a large, thin-walled organ weighing 2 lb and having a capacity of 5 L. The structure of the three muscle layers of the uterus allows the uterus to expand evenly in all directions. Painless contractions called **Braxton Hicks contractions** occur throughout the pregnancy but become more noticeable after the 20th week and during periods of rapid fetal growth.

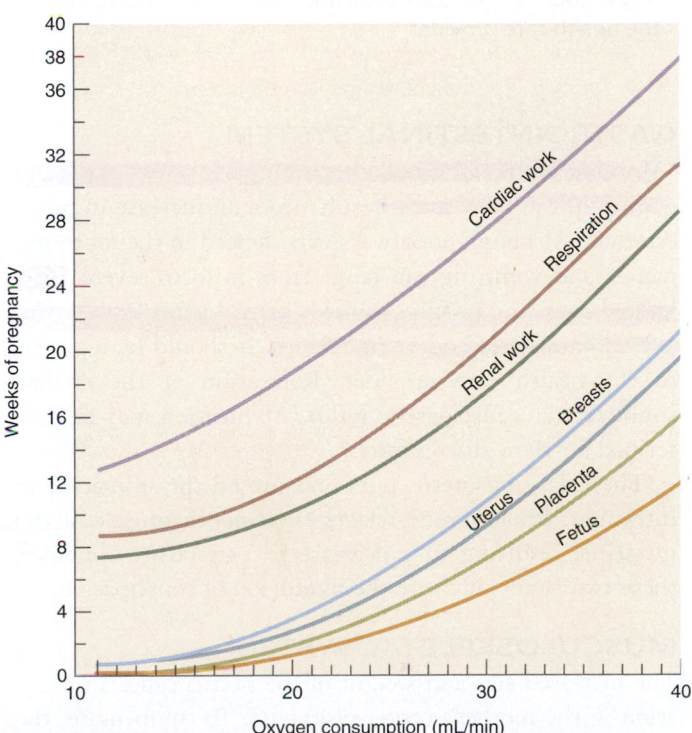

Figure 6-12. ■ Increase in oxygen consumption among body organs during pregnancy.

The fundus should enlarge 1 cm/wk. If the fundus is not enlarging at this rate, the fetus is not growing at a normal rate. Enlargement of more than 1 centimeter each week would indicate the fetus is growing too rapidly or that a multiple pregnancy may exist.

clinical ALERT

From 20 to 36 weeks, the fundal measurement is normally 2 centimeter plus or minus the number of weeks' gestation. So, for example, at 24 weeks' gestation, fundal measurement is typically 22 to 26 centimeter.

The cervix secretes thick, sticky mucus that plugs the os to prevent micro-organisms from entering the uterus. When the cervix dilates, the mucus plug is expelled. Certain changes that occur in the presence of estrogen are present by the 8th week. These signs (Hegar's sign, Goodell's sign, and Chadwick's sign) were described previously under Signs of Pregnancy.

The ovaries do not release ova during pregnancy. The corpus luteum produces estrogen and progesterone for approximately 12 weeks until the placenta takes over this function. Ovulation usually returns within 3 months following delivery.

The breasts enlarge due to hormonal influence. The areolae darken, and the nipple becomes more erect. **Colostrum,** a yellowish fluid rich in antibodies, is secreted in the last trimester and the first few days following delivery. The colostrum is then replaced with milk.

CARDIOVASCULAR SYSTEM

The female's pulse rate increases by 10 to 15 bpm by the end of pregnancy. Cardiac output also increases, and there is an increased blood flow to the uterus and kidneys. The blood pressure decreases slightly in the second trimester due to the influence of progesterone on the smooth muscles of blood vessels, but it returns to normal during the third trimester.

clinical ALERT

Any increase in blood pressure above the normal range should be monitored and reported to the health care provider.

Supine Hypotensive Syndrome

The enlarging uterus puts pressure on the deep veins of the pelvis, resulting in venous stasis in the lower extremities. Venous stasis leads to dependent edema and varicose veins of the legs, vulva, and rectum. **Supine hypotensive syndrome**

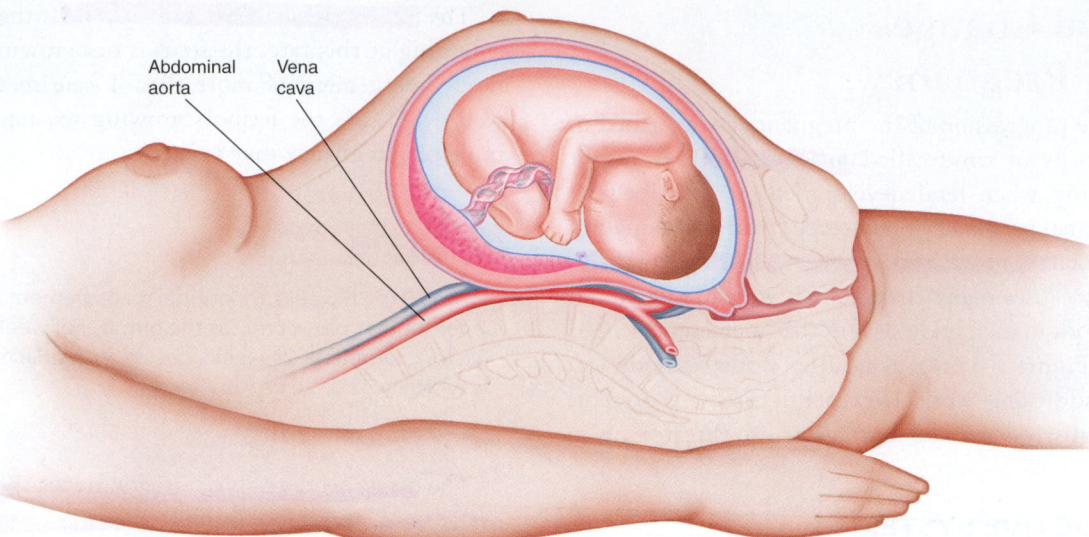

Abdominal aorta   Vena cava

Figure 6-13. ■ Supine hypotensive syndrome. When the woman lies on her back, the large, heavy uterus compresses the vena cava and abdominal aorta against the spinal column, interfering with circulation.

occurs after the 20th week when the mother lies supine (Figure 6-13 ■). The heavy uterus presses on the inferior vena cava, resulting in reduced blood flow back to the right atrium. The mother will experience low blood pressure, dizziness, and pale skin. The mother should be encouraged to sleep on her side to prevent hypotension. Positioning on the left side allows greater blood return than the right.

Physiologic Anemia of Pregnancy

There is an increase in blood volume during pregnancy. The red blood cell count is only slightly elevated, but there is a considerable increase in plasma volume. **Physiologic anemia of pregnancy** occurs between 26 and 32 weeks' gestation. It results from this hemodilution, as evidenced by a hematocrit of 34% to 40%. The number of white blood cells increases beginning in the second trimester. An increase in platelets, fibrin, fibrinogen, and other coagulation factors coupled with venous stasis increases the risk of thrombus formation.

RESPIRATORY SYSTEM

The enlarging uterus presses upward on the diaphragm. The ribs move outward, and the diameter of the chest increases. Progesterone relaxes smooth muscles, decreasing airway resistance and allowing more oxygen into the lungs. Estrogen may cause swelling of the nasal mucosa. As shown in Figure 6-12, oxygen demand is greatly increased during pregnancy.

RENAL SYSTEM

In the first trimester, urinary frequency is caused by the enlarging uterus that presses on the bladder. During the second trimester, the uterus has elevated out of the pelvis and the

pressure is relieved. In the third trimester, the infant descends into the pelvis, again pressing on the bladder.

Glomerular infiltration and tubular reabsorption increase to remove the added waste products from the fetus. If the kidneys are unable to reabsorb the glucose, glucosuria will result.

> ### clinical ALERT
>
> Any amount of glucose over a trace should be reported to the health care provider.

GASTROINTESTINAL SYSTEM

"Morning sickness," usually beginning in the 6th week and ending in the 12th week, results from an increase in progesterone. Although not always experienced in the morning, nausea and vomiting can range from mild to severe. Prolonged vomiting or **hyperemesis gravidarum** leads to dehydration and electrolyte imbalance. It should be reported to the health care provider. Relaxation of the cardiac sphincter can cause gastric reflux. Medication may be prescribed for these discomforts.

The enlarging uterus puts pressure on the stomach and intestines. Progesterone relaxes the smooth muscle of the intestine, resulting in a decrease in peristalsis. Together, these two factors increase the likelihood of constipation.

MUSCULOSKELETAL SYSTEM

The increased size and weight of the uterus cause an alteration in the mother's center of gravity. To compensate, the mother increases the lumbar curve (*lordosis*) and widens her

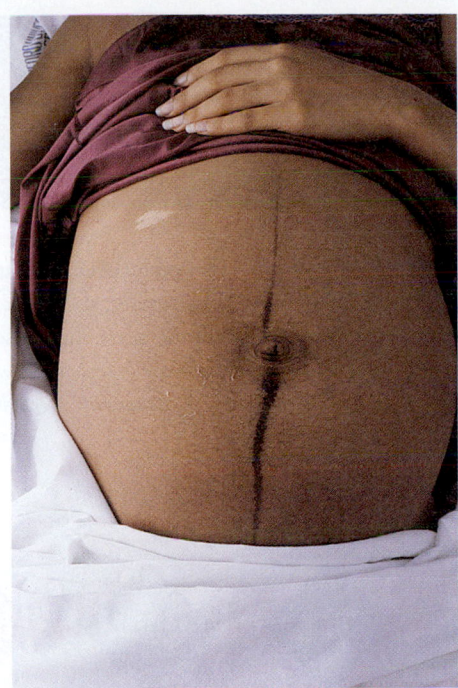

Figure 6-14. ■ Linea nigra.

stance. The pelvic joints become more relaxed in preparation for childbirth. These factors result in low backache and waddling gait.

Muscle cramps, especially in the lower legs, result from venous stasis and possible electrolyte imbalance. Low calcium and phosphorus levels are the most common cause. The mother should be encouraged to consume adequate amounts of milk products to prevent muscle cramps.

INTEGUMENTARY SYSTEM

Changes in skin color result from an increase in maternal hormones. The areolae, nipples, and vulva darken. **Linea nigra** (Figure 6-14 ■) is a dark line on the abdomen, from the umbilicus to the pubis. **Chloasma,** or "mask of pregnancy," is a darkening of the forehead, cheeks, and area around the eyes. Both are more obvious in later pregnancy.

Striae gravidarum, or "stretch marks," occur when the underlying connective tissue separates during periods of rapid growth. Following pregnancy, these dark red streaks gradually lighten and become white, but they never disappear.

ENDOCRINE SYSTEM

Prolactin, from the anterior pituitary gland, stimulates the production of milk by the mammary glands (see Figure 4-17). **Oxytocin,** a hormone produced by the posterior pituitary gland, stimulates uterine contractions, and the **"let-down reflex,"** or release of milk after delivery.

The placenta hormones are insulin antagonists, which means they counteract insulin. As a result, the pancreas needs to produce more insulin to meet the mother's requirements. If the mother is marginal in meeting the need for more insulin, gestational diabetes results. Gestational diabetes is discussed in detail in Chapter 8 .

Hormonal increases affecting the reproductive system are discussed under that system.

Diagnostic Tests of Fetal Status

A variety of tests can be used to assess fetal well-being.

ULTRASOUND

Ultrasound is used to outline the shape and determine the consistency of various organs. Not only is ultrasound used to diagnose pregnancy, but it can also be used to determine the exact position, size, and gender of the fetus and to identify some developmental anomalies. Ultrasound is used in conjunction with other diagnostic tests throughout pregnancy.

AMNIOCENTESIS

Amniocentesis, the withdrawal of amniotic fluid through a needle inserted into the abdomen and the uterus, is a means of gathering data about the developing fetus. It is usually performed between 15 to 18 weeks' gestation. The amniotic fluid and fetal cells contained in the fluid are studied to determine genetic abnormalities, maternal–fetal blood incompatibilities, and the maturity of the fetal lungs. Procedure 6-1 ■ describes the nurse's role in assisting with amniocentesis and similar tests (Figure 6-15 A–C ■).

PERCUTANEOUS UMBILICAL CORD SAMPLING

Percutaneous umbilical cord sampling is also similar to amniocentesis; it is done in the second and third trimesters. The physician locates the fetal parts, and identifies the placenta and umbilical cord by ultrasound. A needle is then inserted through the maternal abdomen into an umbilical vessel in the umbilical cord, approximately 1 to 2 inches (2.5–5 centimeters) from the placenta (see Figure 6-15B). Fetal blood is aspirated and analyzed for chemical content. The test is useful in diagnosing inherited blood disorders, detecting fetal infection, and determining acid–base balance. It is used for diagnosing **erythroblastosis fetalis** (a serious anemia, usually resulting from maternal antibodies to Rh-positive fetal blood), as well as *thrombocytopenia* (a lack of platelets in circulating blood). If necessary, a blood transfusion can be completed.

Assisting with Amniocentesis, Umbilical Cord Sampling, or Chorionic Villus Sampling

Purpose

- To provide information about the genetic makeup of the fetus
- To provide information about the status of the fetus

Equipment

- Ultrasound equipment
- Ultrasonic gel

- Amniocentesis kit containing skin prep (Betadine), sterile drapes, 22-gauge spinal needle with stylet, and amber-colored test tubes. If a kit is not available, the nurse must assemble the supplies from stock. *Amniotic fluid must be protected from light. If amber-colored test tubes are not available, place tape over the test tube to protect the specimen.*
- Sterile gloves
- Local anesthetic (1% Lidocaine)

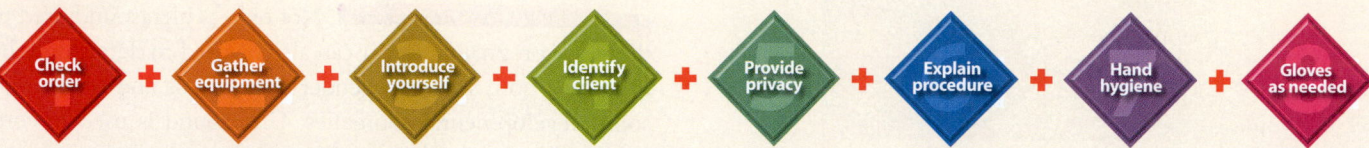

Interventions

1. Ensure that a signed informed consent form is in the chart. If not, inform the care provider. *This procedure requires an informed consent signature.*

2. Obtain the woman's vital signs and the FHR. Monitor maternal vital signs and FHR every 15 minutes during the procedure, and for a minimum of 30 minutes after the procedure. *The first vital signs and FHR readings provide a baseline. Later readings give information about the status of the mother and the fetus. Changes can signal complications.*

3. Position the woman on her back, with a wedge placed under her right hip to displace the weight to the left side. External fetal monitor may be used during the exam to monitor the fetus. *This position will promote better blood flow and prevent supine hypotension.*

4. The physician uses ultrasound to locate the placenta and fetus. Provide ultrasound gel and assist as needed. *Gel creates a seal between the monitor and the woman's skin and improves the quality of the ultrasound reading.*

5. The physician dons sterile gloves and cleanses the woman's abdomen. *Cleansing the abdomen prior to needle insertion helps prevent infection.*

CHORIONIC VILLUS SAMPLING

Chorionic villus sampling is similar to amniocentesis. Using ultrasound to locate the baby, a needle is inserted through the mother's abdomen into the uterus and the placenta. A sample of placental tissue is aspirated through the needle (see Figure 6-15C). The tissue, formed from the zygote, reflects the genetic makeup of the fetus. The procedure, done between the 10th and 12th weeks of gestation, identifies chromosomal anomalies early in the pregnancy. The parents can then make an informed decision regarding the welfare of the baby or possible termination of the pregnancy.

RISKS OF INVASIVE TESTING

Amniocentesis, chorionic villus sampling, and percutaneous umbilical blood sampling do carry some risk to the mother and infant. Complications could include premature rupture of the fetal membranes, placental detachment, hemorrhage (for both mother and infant), and infection. The mother and fetus are monitored closely for an hour or more after the procedure. Follow-up ultrasound may be used to ensure that bleeding or hematoma formation has not occurred. If complications do arise, all efforts will be made to protect both mother and infant. However, in the case of fetal hemorrhage, death may not be preventable.

NURSING CONSIDERATIONS

Parents need emotional support when an amniocentesis or other invasive tests are performed. They will be concerned not only about the welfare of the infant during the test, but also about the possibility of a life-altering diagnosis such as Down syndrome (see Chapter 16 ⚭). Test results may not be obtained for several days or weeks, and the period of waiting may

6. The physician applies sterile drapes, then inserts the needle into the uterus and withdraws a sample of amniotic fluid, umbilical cord blood, or chorionic villi (see Figure 6-15A, B, or C, respectively). *Note*: If a sample of the placenta is obtained for chorionic villus sampling or blood is obtained from an umbilical vessel, other specimen containers may be needed. The nurse may be required to assist with continuous ultrasound monitoring. *Sterile technique is essential to prevent infection of the mother and fetus.*

7. Obtain specimen containers from physician, attach proper labels, and send to lab with appropriate lab slips. *It is the nurse's responsibility to be sure materials are labeled properly. Prompt delivery to the lab helps ensure accurate results.*

8. Assist physician to apply a small dressing over puncture site.

9. Monitor the woman and fetus for 30 minutes, paying close attention to the mother's vital signs, FHR, and any contractions she may be having. *Changes from normal may indicate complications that would need to be reported.*

10. Assess the woman's blood type and determine if Rh immune globulin (RhoGAM) is needed and administer if necessary (see Chapter 8 ⚭). *To prevent Rh sensitization of an Rh-negative woman during the procedure, Rh immune globulin is administered.*

11. Instruct the woman to report any of the following changes immediately to her primary care provider:
    a. Unusual increase in fetal activity or lack of fetal movement
    b. Vaginal discharge, either clear fluid or bloody drainage
    c. Uterine contractions or abdominal cramping
    d. Fever or chills.

    These are signs of complications that will require further medical investigation and treatment.

12. Encourage the woman to engage in only light activity for 24 hours and to increase her fluid intake. *Light activity will decrease uterine irritability. Fluid is needed to replace the amniotic fluid.*

13. Complete the client record. *Full documentation includes date and time, vital signs, type of procedure, name of provider who performed the procedure, number of specimens obtained and disposition of specimens, repeat VS and client status, record of discharge teaching, and follow-up care.*

SAMPLE DOCUMENTATION

(date)	0800 T 98.2, P 82, R 24, BP 136/72, FHR 150. No uterine contractions noted at this time. Dr. Lopez here. Amniocentesis completed without incident. 3 specimens sent to lab.
0830	Vital signs have remained stable since amniocentesis P 78, R 22, BP 130/70, FHR 144–150. No contractions noted on monitor. Written instructions provided and reviewed regarding home care, activity, and warning signs to report to the physician. Instructed to return to clinic in 1 week for follow-up. _____ J. Sole, LPN

---

seem unbearable. If a life-altering diagnosis is made, the parents may decide to keep the pregnancy and accept responsibility for a sick infant, or they may decide to terminate the pregnancy. Either decision brings tremendous emotional strain requiring support, understanding, and nonjudgmental care.

MANUAL READING OF FETAL HEART RATE

In a low-risk pregnancy with no unusual concerns, the nurse may perform manual FHR monitoring at most prenatal visits. Procedure 6-2 ■ provides steps in obtaining a manual FHR. Internal fetal heart monitoring is another method and is discussed in Chapter 8 ⚭.

NONSTRESS TEST

A **nonstress test (NST)** is used to assess fetal movement and FHR. External fetal monitoring equipment is attached to the client's abdomen, and the FHR is recorded. The client identifies episodes of fetal movement. Fetal movement can be stimulated with a low-frequency vibrator. Each episode consists of a FHR increase of 15 bpm, lasting 15 seconds. The test is reactive or normal if two episodes occur in a 20-minute period.

BIOPHYSICAL PROFILE

Biophysical profile is a test that assesses five variables: fetal breathing, fetal movement, fetal tone, amniotic fluid volume, and fetal reaction. To complete a biophysical profile, a combination of ultrasound and nonstress test are used. The LPN/LVN is sometimes taught to collect the data; the trained registered nurse, certified nurse midwife, or physician interprets the data. A score of 8 or more indicates positive fetal well-being.

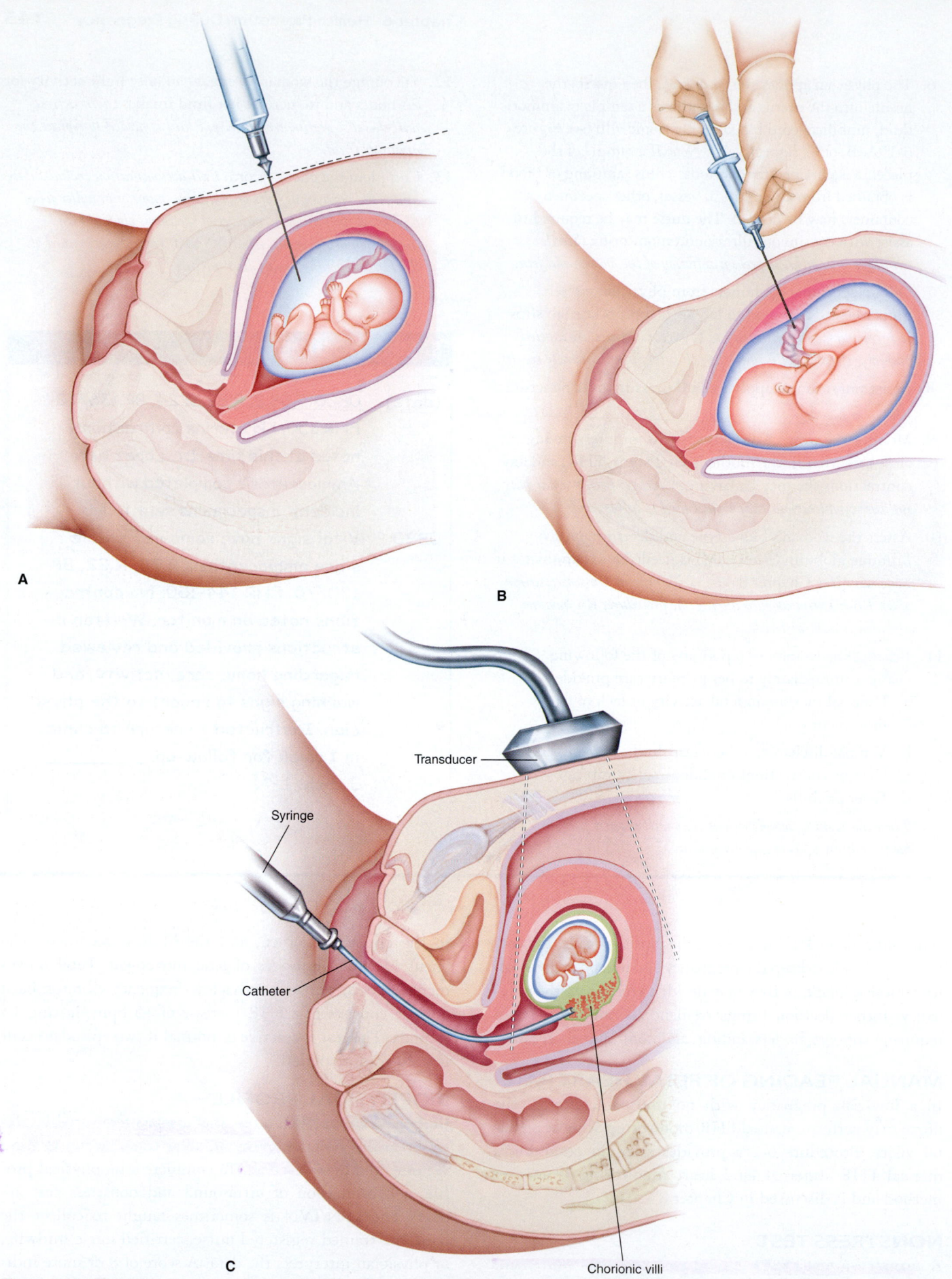

Figure 6-15. ■ (**A**) Amniocentesis. (**B**) Umbilical blood sampling. (**C**) Chorionic villus sampling using transcervical approach.

Transducer

Syringe

Catheter

Chorionic villi

| PROCEDURE 6-2 | **Assessing the Fetal Heart Rate with Doppler** |

Purpose

- To provide information about the status of the fetus
- To monitor the status of the fetus

Equipment

- Doppler device
- Ultrasonic gel

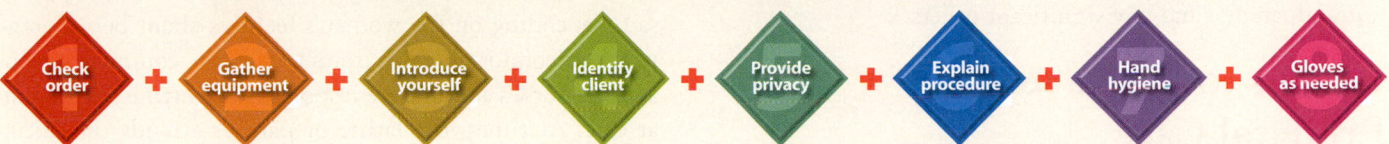

Check order + Gather equipment + Introduce yourself + Identify client + Provide privacy + Explain procedure + Hand hygiene + Gloves as needed

Interventions

1. Apply gel to the diaphragm of the Doppler. *Gel aids sound transmission and helps maintain contact between the Doppler diaphragm and the abdomen.*

2. Uncover the woman's abdomen. Position the diaphragm in the midline of the woman's abdomen halfway between the umbilicus and the symphysis pubis (Figure 6-16 ■). *This is the most likely position in which to hear the fetal heartbeat.*

3. When pulse is heard, check it against the woman's pulse. If they are the same, reposition the Doppler diaphragm. If the pulse is not heard, move the diaphragm laterally. *If the rates are the same, they are probably both the mother's pulse.*

4. If the rates are not the same, count the beats for 1 minute. Count each double rhythm as one beat. *The fetal heart sound has a double rhythm. The beats per minute are the FHR.*

5. Auscultate the FHR at each office visit during pregnancy. FHR is also assessed before, during, and for 30 seconds after a uterine contraction during labor. *This can provide information about fetal health or distress.*

6. Follow recommendations for frequency of auscultation and documentation. *The health and risk status of the woman will determine the usual frequency of auscultation.*

    a. FHR should be assessed at each office visit.
    b. FHR should be assessed anytime the mother accesses health care for any reason during the pregnancy.
    c. FHR should be assessed if the woman believes she is in labor. Fetal assessment during labor is discussed in Chapter 7 ⚭.

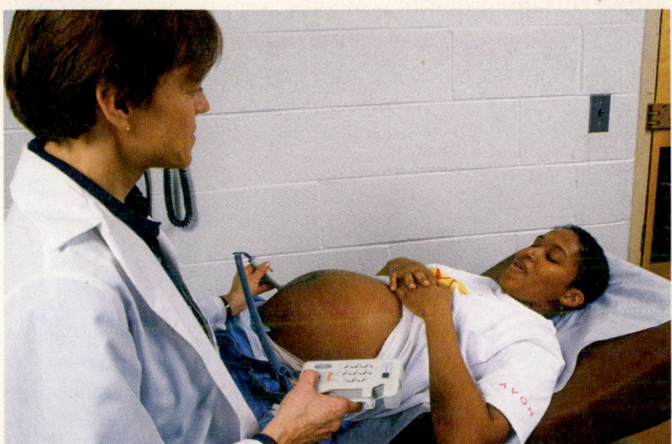

Figure 6-16. ■ Data on the fetal heart rate is collected regularly throughout the woman's pregnancy.
(Source: Pearson Education/PH College)

SAMPLE DOCUMENTATION

(date)   0800 FHR 144. Mother reports increase in fetal activity over the past 2 weeks, especially after periods of maternal activity. Reassured that this is usual during the sixth month of pregnancy. _____
K. Doss, LPN

PRENATAL CARE

Research has shown that prenatal care, beginning as soon as possible, has a dramatic effect on the outcome of the pregnancy. The goals of prenatal care include:

- A healthy, prepared mother who has minimal discomforts during the pregnancy
- The safe delivery of a healthy fetus
- A prepared family, including father or partner, siblings, grandparents, and any significant others.

Access to and Use of Prenatal Care

Although prenatal care is the best way to ensure a healthy child, it does not universally occur. *Healthy People 2010* (U.S. Department of Health and Human Services, 2000) has identified a real shortfall of prenatal care in certain populations. For example, Black Americans are generally less likely to obtain early and regular prenatal care. Certain other cultures may look to sources outside the Western health care establishment for prenatal information and care. Box 6-2 ■ provides more information on this topic.

| **BOX 6-2** | **CULTURAL PULSE POINTS** |

Views on Prenatal Care

A frequent complaint of labor and delivery nurses is the lack of prenatal care by many mothers-to-be from other cultures. Western medicine places a high value on prenatal care. Many Americans view pregnancy and childbirth as a medical condition and are followed by a physician almost from the day they discover that they are pregnant.

Women from other cultures, such as many Hispanic women, view pregnancy as a normal condition. They do not believe that consultation with a physician is necessary. Instead, they depend on older women to supply them with the information and support they need. If the woman does seek prenatal care, it is important to stress the need to continue to see the physician, especially if the mother is considered to be a high-risk client.

Studies show that Black American women do not obtain early, regular prenatal care as often as other cultures. In fact, a study of White (including Hispanic) women from 1940 to 1990 showed that White women consistently received three to four times more prenatal care than Black women. These trends have continued into the 21st century. It is interesting to note, however, that in women in the military—who have unrestricted access to prenatal care—differences between Black and White women virtually disappeared.

Source: Data from Centers for Disease Control and Prevention, Division of Reproductive Health, National Center for Chronic Disease Prevention and Health Promotion; Division of Vital Statistics, National Center for Health Statistics. Washington, DC: U.S. Government Printing Office.

Figure 6-17 ■ illustrates the U.S. infant mortality rate by race and ethnicity from 1995 to 2002. It is clear from this illustration that there is more work to be done in finding and eliminating the causes of infant mortality.

Initial Visit

The initial visit to a health care provider can be happy or sad, depending on the woman's feelings about being pregnant. A comfortable environment, open communication, and the nurse's attitude are important in putting the woman at ease. At times, the father or partner attends the initial visit, and the nurse assesses the degree of support the woman receives from this person.

The initial visit is generally longer than subsequent visits. Unless a health history has been obtained prior to pregnancy, it must be done at this time. The health history includes identifying all past medical issues that could have an impact on the pregnancy. A menstrual history will be obtained, including any past pregnancies. (Table 6-2 ■ provides key terms used to refer to pregnancy.) The woman's **gravida** (G—number of pregnancies), **para** (P—number of deliveries after 24 weeks' gestation), and the outcome of past pregnancies will be recorded. Possible outcomes include **abortion** (A—the loss of pregnancy before the 24th week), **preterm** delivery (P—delivery after the 24th week but before the 38th week), **term** delivery (T—delivery between 38 and 42 weeks), **postterm** delivery (delivery after 42 weeks' gestation), and whether the infant lived (L—live birth). It is important to remember that the word *abortion* is used medically to describe the loss of a pregnancy, whether

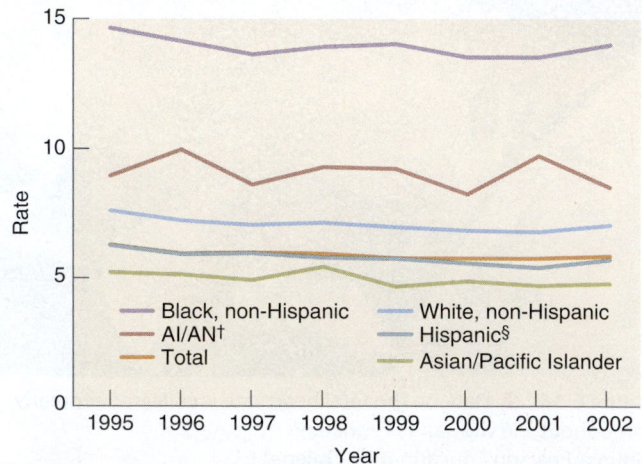

Figure 6-17. ■ U.S. infant mortality rate* by race and ethnicity, 1995–2002. (Courtesy of Centers for Disease Control and Prevention, Rockville, MD.)

*Per 1,000 live birth.
†American Indian/Alaska Native.
§Hispanic mothers might be of any race.

TABLE 6-2

Common Terms Describing Pregnancy

KEY TERM	DEFINITION
Abortion (A)	Loss of pregnancy prior to viable age (usually 24 weeks)
Gravida (G)	Number of pregnancies, including present pregnancy
Para (P)	Number of deliveries after a viable age, including infants born alive and stillborn infants
Term (T)	A pregnancy between 38 and 42 weeks' gestation
Preterm (P)	A delivery after 24 weeks but before 38 weeks' gestation
Postterm	A delivery after 42 weeks' gestation
Nulligravida	Never pregnant
Nullipara	Never delivered an infant after 24 weeks' gestation
Primagravida	First pregnancy
Primapara	First delivery after 24 weeks' gestation
Multigravida	Pregnant two or more times
Multipara	Delivered two or more times after 24 weeks' gestation
GP/TPAL	Gravida, para/term, preterm, abortion, live birth

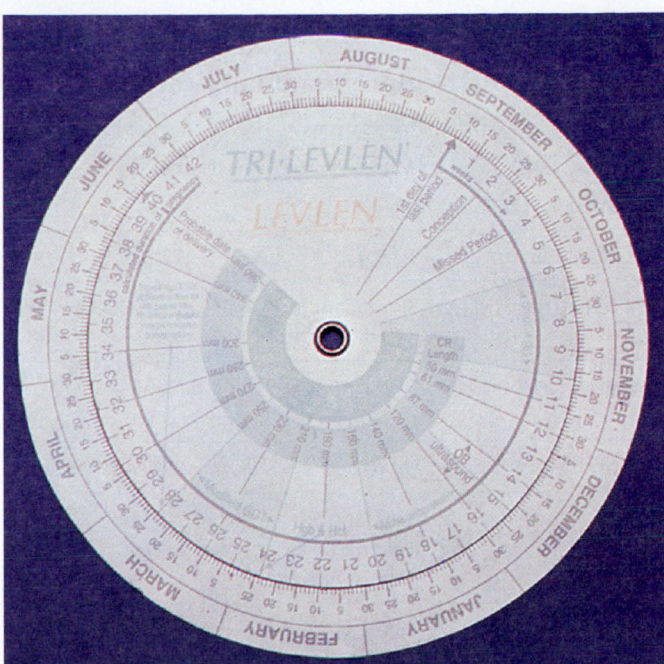

Figure 6-18. ■ The gestational wheel can be used to calculate the EDB (estimated date of birth). To use it, place the "last menses began" arrow on the date of the woman's last menstrual period (LMP). Then read the "EDB date" at the arrow labeled 40. In this case, the LMP is September 8 and the EDB is June 17.

that is a planned, elective event or a spontaneous occurrence (**miscarriage**). A woman who has been pregnant three times, had one abortion at 8 weeks, and had two live births at term would be designated G-3P2/T2A1.

A physical assessment, done by the health care provider, will include a detailed assessment of the reproductive organs. An ultrasound may be performed to diagnose pregnancy. Blood may be drawn to determine a baseline for future reference.

NAEGELE'S RULE

If pregnancy is diagnosed, the duration of pregnancy will be determined. Terms used to refer to the expected delivery date are:

- Estimated date of birth (EDB)
- Estimated date of delivery (EDD)
- Estimated date of confinement (EDC).

The EDB can be determined by several methods. **Naegele's rule** is the most common. To apply the rule, take the first day of the LMP, subtract 3 months, and add 7 days. For example, if the LMP was on January 18; the EDB would be October 25. Adjustments to the rule have to be made if

the LMP falls at the end of a month, for example, on July 29. Subtracting 3 months would be April, and adding 7 days would be April 36. April has only 30 days, so the EDB would be advanced to May 6. A gestational wheel or chart can be used for quick reference. Figure 6-18 ■ illustrates a gestational wheel that provides expected dates for the EDB and other pregnancy landmarks.

Follow-up Visits

The pregnant woman should return to the clinic for follow-up care on the following schedule:

- Every 4 weeks for the first 28 weeks
- Every 2 weeks during weeks 29 to 36
- Every week after 36 weeks until delivery.

LABORATORY TESTS RELATED TO PREGNANCY

Laboratory blood values often change while a woman is pregnant. Laboratory tests (Table 6-3 ■) compare pregnant and nonpregnant values. It can provide valuable data for assessing a woman's health. Nurses should be familiar with values that are normal for women during pregnancy.

MEDICATIONS DURING PREGNANCY

The use of any medication—prescription, nonprescription, or herbal—during pregnancy carries a risk to the fetus. A *teratogen* is any chemical that can cause abnormal development

TABLE 6-3

Pregnant and Nonpregnant Laboratory Values

TEST	PREGNANT VALUES	NONPREGNANT VALUES
Hematocrit (%)	32–42	37–47
Hemoglobin (g/dL)	10–14	12–16
Platelets (mm³)	Significant increase 3–5 days after birth	150,000–350,000
White blood cells (mm³)	5,000–15,000	4,500–10,000
Fibrinogen (mg/dL)	Up to 600	175–400
Serum glucose (mg/dL)	65 (fasting) less than 140 (2 hour PP)	70–80
Sodium (mEq/L)	135–145	135–145
Potassium (mEq/L)	3.5–5.1	3.5–5.1
Chloride (mEq/L)	100–108	100–108
Bicarbonate (mEq/L)	22–26	22–26
Calcium (mg/dL)	Falls 10% by term	8.5–10.5

in the fetus. Drugs are one form of teratogen. To prevent teratogenic effects, the U.S. Food and Drug Administration (FDA) has established five categories of potential risk for the development of birth defects. Box 6-3 ■ identifies these categories. It is important to recall that herbal medicines are categorized as dietary supplements rather than drugs. Therefore, the testing, regulation, and standardization of herbs may not be as strict.

Although the first trimester is the most critical for teratogenic effects of drugs, some drugs can be harmful in the second and third trimesters as well. If medications must be taken during pregnancy, it is wisest to use the lowest dose for the shortest period of time. It is usually safer to select well-known medications than to choose newer medication whose teratogenic effect may be unknown. Pregnant women should be advised to avoid all herbs during the first trimester. During the second and third trimesters, whole plant extracts are safer than concentrated extracts. Certain categories of herbs should be avoided throughout the pregnancy including **abortifacients** (abortion-inducing herbs that induce menstruation), nervous system stimulants, stimulant laxatives, and others. Box 6-4 ■ lists common herbs to avoid during pregnancy because they are considered abortifacients.

Most care providers prescribe a prenatal multivitamin with iron to be taken once a day. This nutritional supplement will help ensure that adequate amounts of vitamins and iron are ingested for the developing fetus. Some women may want to omit the vitamin due to nausea in the early weeks of pregnancy. However, at this time, the woman may not be consuming adequate amounts of nutritious foods. She should be encouraged to adjust the time of day the medication is taken instead of omitting a dose.

Pregnant women may develop headache, respiratory infections, allergies, or flu as often as the nonpregnant woman. Commonly, over-the-counter medications are used to treat these conditions. Many physicians, nurse midwives, and nurse practitioners provide their clients with a list of over-the-counter medications that are acceptable to use during pregnancy. If the client wants to use another medication or herbal supplement, she should contact her health care provider. It is important for the client to communicate to

BOX 6-3

Pregnancy Categories for Medications

Category A
- Studies do not show a risk to the fetus in the first trimester of pregnancy.
- There is no evidence of risk in the second and third trimesters.

Category B
- Animal studies have not proven a risk to the fetus, but there are no adequate studies in pregnant women.
- Animal studies show adverse effects, but adequate studies on pregnant women have not shown risk to the human fetus.

Category C
- Animal studies show an adverse effect on the fetus, but there are no adequate studies in humans.

- There are no animal reproduction studies, and no adequate studies have been performed in humans.
- The drug may be used during pregnancy if the benefits of the drug outweigh its possible risks.

Category D
- Evidence shows a risk to the human fetus.
- The potential benefits from the use of the drug may outweigh the risk to the fetus.

Category X
- Studies in animals and humans prove fetal abnormalities, or reports indicate evidence of fetal risk.
- The risks of using these drugs clearly outweigh any possible benefits.

BOX 6-4   NUTRITION THERAPIES

Common Herbs to Avoid in Pregnancy*

Aloe spp.	Licorice
Angelica	Ma huang
Basil oil	Passion flower
Black cohosh	Pennyroyal
Buckthorn	Rue
Cascara sagrada	Sage
Chamomile, Roman	Senna
Chaste tree berry	St. John's Wort
Dong quai	Stinging nettle
Ephedra (used orally)	Tansy
Feverfew	Wormwood
Goldenseal	Yarrow
Gotu kola	**Use with caution**
Guggul	Garlic
Horehound	Ginger
Horseradish (fresh)	Turmeric
Juniper	
Kava kava	

*Avoid excessive consumption relative to usual and customary food use.

Data from Hardy, M. (2000). Herbs of special interest to women. *Journal of the American Pharmaceutical Association, 40(2),* 234–242; American Pregnancy Association. (2000–2006). Natural herbs & vitamins and pregnancy.

any health care provider that she is pregnant (or suspects pregnancy) before she takes any prescribed medication. For example, a woman who is 6 months pregnant could be taken to an emergency room for treatment following an automobile accident. Because the pregnancy may not be obvious, it is important for her to communicate to the nurses, doctor, and x-ray technician that she is pregnant. When getting a new prescription medication filled at the drug store, the pregnant woman should inform the pharmacist that she is pregnant and question the safety of the drug at this time.

DISCOMFORTS OF PREGNANCY

Numerous changes occur in a woman's body during pregnancy. Initially, there may be feelings of "fullness" or morning sickness, heavier breasts, and a slight sensation of bloating. Later changes affect the woman's center of gravity and her circulation. They alter how a woman stands, walks, and rests, and many of these changes involve some level of discomfort. It is helpful for women to be prepared for these changes ahead of time. Table 6-4 ■ identifies common discomforts and possible interventions to alleviate or decrease the discomforts of pregnancy.

MediaLink Herbs in pregnancy

TABLE 6-4

Common Discomforts of Pregnancy and Treatment

DISCOMFORT	CAUSE	INTERVENTION
Nausea and/or vomiting	Increased hormones Enlarged uterus pushing on stomach	Limit fluids upon waking Eat dry toast or crackers Eat small amounts frequently Avoid fried or spicy foods
Heartburn	Gastric reflux due to relaxed cardiac sphincter from effects of progesterone and pressure from enlarged uterus	Avoid fried or spicy foods Eat small amounts, avoid overeating Sit up for 30 minutes after eating Take antacids ONLY with care provider's approval
Flatulence	Slowing of GI motility due to progesterone and pressure from enlarged uterus	Omit gas-forming foods Increase bulk in diet Have regular bowel movement
Constipation	Slowing of GI motility due to progesterone and pressure from enlarged uterus Decreased activity Inadequate fiber and fluids in diet Iron supplements	Increase fiber from fruits and vegetables (raisins, prunes, apples) Daily activity (walking) Increase fluids
Hemorrhoids	Straining to have bowel movement Pressure from enlarged uterus on rectal veins	Prevent constipation Cool compresses Warm sitz bath Topical analgesic ointment

(continued)

TABLE 6-4

Common Discomforts of Pregnancy and Treatment (continued)

DISCOMFORT	CAUSE	INTERVENTION
Varicose veins	Pressure from enlarged uterus on deep pelvic veins Relaxation of vessel walls due to progesterone Inactivity, long periods of sitting or standing	Rest with feet elevated Avoid restrictive clothing, crossing legs Wear support hose Daily activity (walking)
Ankle edema	Inactivity, long periods of sitting or standing Sodium retention	Daily activity (walking) Rest with feet elevated Avoid salty foods If edema increases or is routinely present upon arising, contact health care provider
Leg cramps	Calcium/phosphorus imbalance Muscle fatigue/strain Restricted circulation	Increase calcium in diet Frequent rest periods with legs elevated
Backache	Relaxation of pelvic joints Exaggerated lordosis due to change in center of gravity Fatigue Poor body mechanics	Rest lying on side Wear low-heeled shoes Use proper body mechanics
Urinary frequency	Pressure of enlarging uterus on bladder Urinary tract infection	Empty bladder frequently Do NOT limit fluids Contact health care provider if other signs of urinary infection are present
Dyspnea	Decreased lung capacity due to pressure of enlarged uterus on diaphragm	Lie on side or semi-Fowler's position
Vaginal discharge	Increased vaginal secretions due to estrogen Vaginal infection	Practice good hygiene If other signs of vaginal infection are present, contact health care provider
Itchy skin	Dehydration Stretching skin	Increase fluids Avoid drying soaps Apply lotion
Mood swings	Hormonal change Fatigue Inadequate diet	Express fears, concerns Adequate diet and fluids Adequate rest periods

NUTRITION

Nutrition is a vital part of prenatal care. Good nutrition provides crucial ingredients to supply the developing fetus. It also provides energy for the extra demands being made on the mother's body.

If the woman is already eating a well-balanced diet, little change needs to be made during pregnancy. During pregnancy, the woman should add 300 kcalories a day to her diet. (This compares to an additional 500 kcalories a day she will need if she breastfeeds; see Chapter 9 .) The addition of two milk servings and one meat serving will meet the need for increased calories as well as calcium and protein. Many women, however, do not eat a well-balanced diet prior to pregnancy. Also, some women are vegetarians and need to seek other alternatives for protein (see Health Promotion Issue box on pages 152 and 153). The nurse must provide these women with more in-depth information or refer them to a dietitian. Many health care providers prescribe a daily multiple vitamin with calcium and iron. Table 6-5 ■ identifies a food guide to meet the nutritional needs of both the woman and the developing fetus.

TABLE 6-5

Food Guide During Pregnancy and Lactation

FOOD GROUP	SERVING SIZE	SUGGESTED SERVINGS PER DAY	
		DURING PREGNANCY	DURING LACTATION
Grain products (whole-grain breads, cereals, pasta, rice)	1 slice bread ½ bun, bagel ½ cup cereal	6–11	6–11
Vegetables (dark green leafy, deep yellow, dry beans/peas)	1 cup leafy greens ½ cup all others	3–5 Eat dry beans and peas often	3–5
Fruits (citrus fruits and others)	1 medium apple, banana, orange, etc. ½ cup canned ¾ cup juice	2–4	2–4
Meat/poultry/fish Beans/nuts/eggs (limit peanut butter and nuts due to fat content) Trim fat, remove skin from poultry	½ cup cooked dry beans 1 egg, 1½ tbsp peanut butter = 1 oz meat	Up to 6 oz total	Up to 6 oz total
Milk and milk products	1 cup milk or yogurt 1½ oz cheese	3 or more	4 or more

Adequate fluid intake is important for the pregnant woman. Drinking 1.5 to 2 L of water, milk, or juice every 24 hours is recommended. It is best to limit caffeine-containing beverages. Women in low socioeconomic levels may have difficulty buying adequate amounts of milk and high protein foods. These women should be referred for aid. Programs such as WIC may provide help (see Table 2-1 ⭕).

EXERCISE

Exercise is increasingly recognized as an important part of a health maintenance program. Healthy, active women are more likely to have healthy infants. Women who are overweight and sedentary are more likely to encounter problems in themselves, such as gestational diabetes, and in their children (see Chapter 9 ⭕). It is important to maintain activity throughout pregnancy. However, modifications should be made to adapt exercise to the physical changes pregnancy causes and the demands it makes on the body. Figure 6-19 ■ illustrates some simple exercises that help relax muscles and prepare the body for childbirth.

Kegel Exercises

Kegel exercises are promoted during the prenatal period. These exercises help women identify muscles groups that are affected by delivery and that need conditioning after birth. Figure 6-20 ■ shows the effect of Kegel exercise on the pubococcygeus muscle; it also shows the muscles of the pelvic floor. To identify the muscles of the pelvic floor, some nurses

suggest stopping urination in midstream. However, it is not recommended to perform the exercise while urinating.

The woman is asked to visualize the pelvic floor muscles as an elevator. In relaxed position, the muscles are on the "ground floor." Then the woman draws the muscles in and up, raising the "elevator" to the first, second, third, and fourth "floor." She holds the muscles in that position, then gradually allows them to return to starting position.

Kegel exercises can be done while standing, sitting, or lying down. Some women use visual cues (e.g., standing in a grocery line, stopping for a red light) to remind them to do Kegel exercises. If properly done, the exercise does not engage the muscles of the thigh or buttocks. It is important to emphasize the importance of full, smooth breaths during the exercise.

Avoiding Hyperthermia

The pregnant woman, in part due to increased blood volume, has an increased tendency toward hyperthermia. Although women generally may continue the types of exercise they did before pregnancy, they will need to make adjustments in the intensity and duration of exercise. Many women are advised to avoid sports such as jogging and tennis that can put excessive strain on joints. Walking and swimming are often recommended to promote circulation and muscle tone. Swimming is especially good because water provides support while the aerobic workout occurs.

(Text continues on p. 155.)

HEALTH PROMOTION ISSUE

PREGNANCY AND VEGETARIANISM

The nurse is taking an initial history of a G2 P1, 29-year-old, married client who is 12 weeks pregnant. Her weight today is 135 pounds, and her height is 5′ 8″. The client works full-time as an accountant. She is concerned about her diet and reports taking her prenatal vitamins faithfully. She states that she does not have time to eat right, eats out frequently because her 3-year-old son loves fast food, and claims that she really cannot cook too well. She also states that she is a vegetarian, although her husband and her son are not. The nurse understands that there are several issues that need to be addressed with this client. She needs help with food choices and food preparation. She needs to be advised of the hazards of poor nutrition during pregnancy and its effect on her children's health. It would also be helpful if she had some sample menus after which to model her diet.

DISCUSSION

Increasing the protein content to 60 to 80 g/day can be especially challenging for the pregnant vegetarian client. Added protein is essential to support the increased metabolic needs of pregnancy and to aid the growth of maternal and fetal tissues. Protein also aids increased energy levels, muscular contractions, and immunity. Lack of protein in the diet of a pregnant woman has been linked to increased incidence of low-birth-weight infants, pregnancy-induced hypertension, and poor fetal brain development.

Nonanimal proteins are said to be incomplete proteins. Incomplete proteins do not contain all essential amino acids. However, the vegetarian can get these essential amino acids in her diet by combining complementary plant proteins. Examples of these combinations are beans and grains or dairy and grains. Many nonanimal foods provide good sources of protein such as chick peas, baked beans, tofu, cow or soy milk, cereals such as muesli, peanuts or peanut butter, and breads. Some vegetarians are not opposed to eggs in their diet.

The pregnant vegetarian woman also needs to be sure to get enough calcium and vitamin D in her diet. Choosing soy milk that is fortified with vitamin D will aid in meeting these needs. Prenatal vitamins should contain iron, vitamin B_{12}, zinc, and vitamin D.

Proper parental food choices and dietary restraint have been found to have a direct effect on childhood obesity. Fast-food meals are typically high in calories and have a high fat content. Parents who are intent on preventing obesity should avoid prepackaged foods, as well as foods high in sugar and fat. A child's diet should contain less than 30% of calories from fat.

PLANNING AND IMPLEMENTATION

The nurse should help the client understand that proper planning and advanced preparation will aid in making proper food choices and, in the long run, will save time and energy. Encouraging her to create a detailed weekly menu and shopping list will prevent her from making unhealthy purchases. Explain to the pregnant client that her weekly food preparation will be aided if upon returning from the grocery store she prepares the food by slicing meats and cheeses, washing and cutting fruits and vegetables, and boiling eggs.

Mornings are typically difficult for working mothers of young children. Time demands rarely allow for meal planning and preparation. The nurse could encourage the client to fix lunches and begin the next night's dinner preparation before bedtime. Following are several choices of easy-to-prepare vegetarian meals.

Because it is virtually impossible to avoid eating out in the fast-paced American society, the nurse should assist the client in making healthy choices

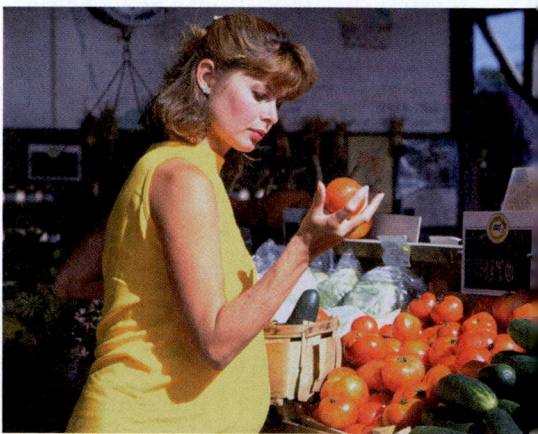

Source: (Ed Malitsky/Index Stock Imagery, Inc.)

	MENU 1	MENU 2	MENU 3
Breakfast	One orange, whole wheat toast with peanut butter, 1 cup low-fat yogurt, 20 oz water	Scrambled egg, cream of wheat with raisins, 1 cup soy milk	Whole wheat waffles with pureed fruit spread, low-fat cream cheese, and peanut butter; 1 cup soy milk
Snack	Trail mix of raisins and almonds, 20 oz water	Frozen low-fat yogurt with fresh blueberries and granola with walnuts, 20 oz water	Whole wheat English muffin toasted with Swiss cheese and tomato, handful of pecans, 20 oz water
Lunch	Spinach salad with tomatoes, feta cheese, and sunflower seeds; five whole wheat crackers; 1 cup of noncaffeinated tea	Steamed broccoli and asparagus with cheese, baked beans, two slices whole wheat bread, 1 cup noncaffeinated tea	Lettuce wraps with black bean spread, onions, and shredded cheddar cheese; baked tortilla chips with salsa, 20 oz water
Snack	Carrots and celery with cottage cheese	Apple slices with peanut butter, crackers, 20 oz water	Whole wheat cereal such as Cheerios, cheese cubes, flax seeds, 20 oz water
Dinner	Veggie burger on whole wheat bun with cheese, lettuce, and tomato; serving of brown rice, 1 cup soy milk	Stir fry of squash, zucchini, slivered almonds, and tofu; serving of brown rice; one plum; 1 cup soy milk	Mushrooms, green pepper, and onions, sautéed, and served over whole wheat pasta with cream sauce made with soy milk and mozzarella cheese; 1 cup herbal tea
Snack	Banana, bran muffin, 1 cup herbal tea	Mixed fruit cup, 10 oz water	Pure fruit sorbet with graham crackers

when dining out. Fortunately, the majority of fast-food restaurants offer healthy, low-fat menu choices. Many restaurants offer a wide range of salads containing fresh vegetables, cheeses, and nuts. Combined with a low-fat salad dressing, this option makes a smart choice for the vegetarian. Some fast-food restaurants offer fruit cups, cole slaw, and yogurt parfaits. For the nonvegetarian, there are grilled chicken sandwiches and deli sandwiches on whole wheat breads.

SELF-REFLECTION

Carefully assess your own nutritional habits. Record your intake for a 24-hour period. Determine excesses and deficiencies in your dietary and fluid intake. What is your weight? Is it appropriate for your height? What poor nutritional habits are you role modeling to your clients? Actions often speak louder than words.

MediaLink Vegetarian pregnancy

SUGGESTED RESOURCES

For the Nurse

Fowles, E. (2004). Prenatal nutrition and birth outcomes. *Journal of Obstetric, Gynecologic, and Neonatal Nursing, 33*(6), 809–822.

Hood, M. Y., Moore, L. L., Sundarajan-Ramamurti, A., Singer, M., Cupples, L. A., & Ellison, R. C. (2004). Parental eating attitudes and the development of obesity in children. The Framingham Children's Study. *International Journal of Obesity Related Metabolic Disorder, 24*(10): 1319–1325.

Moran, R. (1999). Evaluation and treatment of childhood obesity. *American Family Physician, 59*(4): 861–877.

For the Client

Eisenberg, A., Murkoff, H., & Hathaway, S. (1986). *What to eat when you're expecting.* New York: Workman Publishing.

Somer, Elizabeth. (2002). *Nutrition for a healthy pregnancy: The complete guide to eating before, during and after your pregnancy.* New York: Owl Books. Henry Holt and Company, LLC.

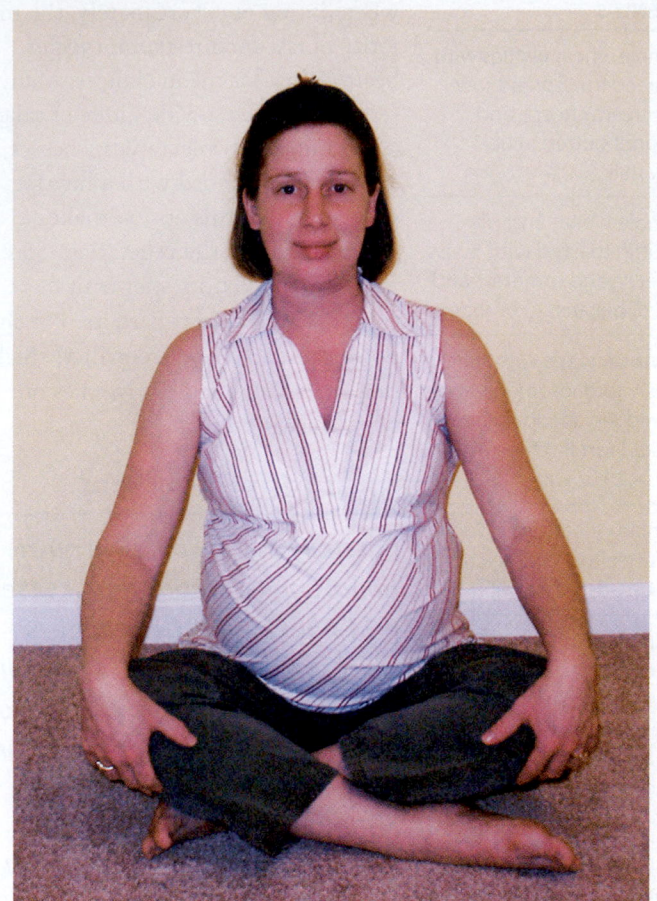

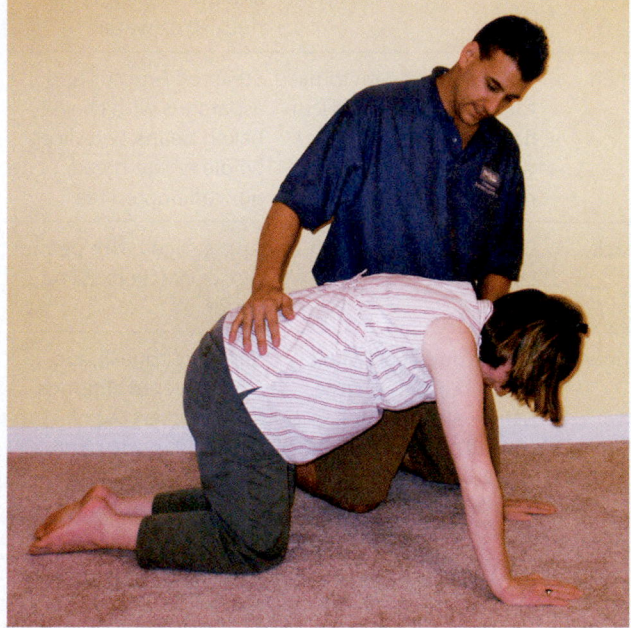

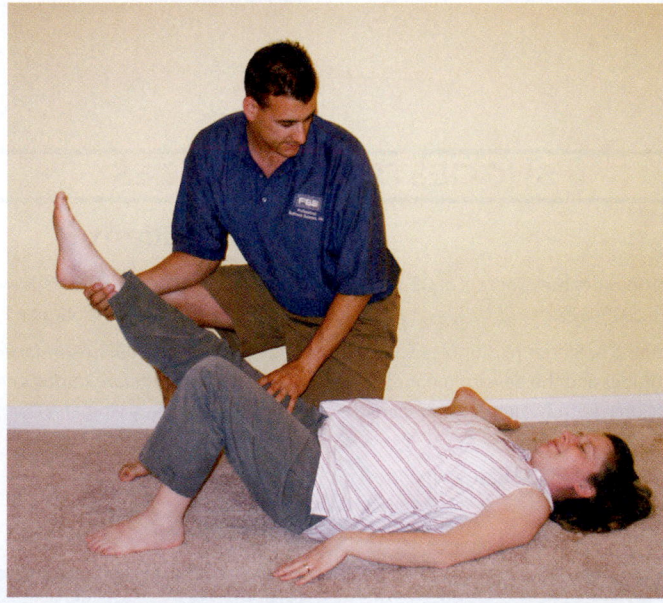

Figure 6-19. ■ Prenatal exercises. (**A**) Tailor sitting. (**B**) Pelvic tilt on hands and knees: The woman arches her lower back and then relaxes it to a flat position. (**C**) Leg raises: To strengthen abdominal muscles, a pregnant woman may be taught to alternately raise one leg, then the other, from a bent position straight up off the floor as shown here. (Source: Courtesy of J. Harro)

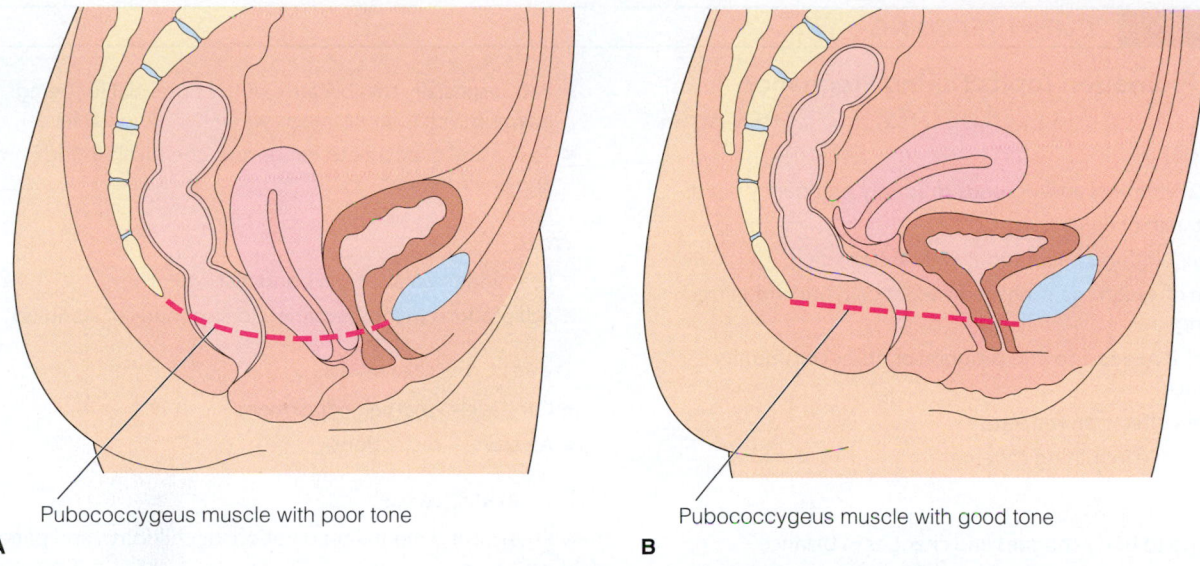

Pubococcygeus muscle with poor tone

A

Pubococcygeus muscle with good tone

B

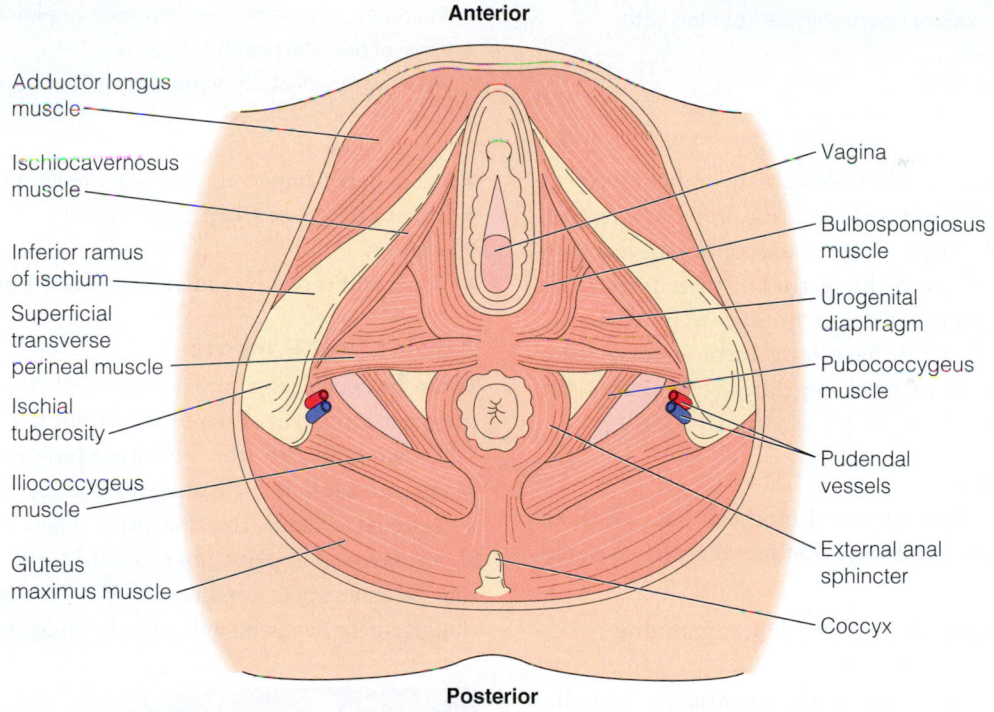

Anterior

Adductor longus muscle

Ischiocavernosus muscle

Inferior ramus of ischium

Superficial transverse perineal muscle

Ischial tuberosity

Iliococcygeus muscle

Gluteus maximus muscle

Vagina

Bulbospongiosus muscle

Urogenital diaphragm

Pubococcygeus muscle

Pudendal vessels

External anal sphincter

Coccyx

Posterior

C

Figure 6-20. ■ Kegel exercises are often taught during pregnancy. They help the woman become familiar with muscles that support the pelvic floor. After birth, these exercises will be useful in regaining muscle tone. (**A**) Pubococcygeus muscle with poor tone. (**B**) Pubococcygeus muscle with good tone. (**C**) Muscles of the pelvic floor. (The puborectalis, pubovaginalis, and coccygeal muscles cannot be seen from this view.)

SAFETY CONCERNS

The home and work environment must be safe for the pregnant client. In late pregnancy, the woman is at risk for falls because her center of gravity has shifted. The home should be inspected for hazards, and any corrections should be made. Chemicals (including cleaning supplies, insecticides, and weed control agents) can harm the fetus. These chemicals should be avoided if possible. If the woman must use these chemicals, she should avoid skin

contact and inhalation of fumes. Excessive heat from hot tubs, saunas, or hot humid weather should be avoided because water of 106°F can cause maternal hyperthermia (Rogers & Davis, 1995).

PRENATAL TEACHING

Every clinical visit is an opportunity for the nurse to provide prenatal teaching. The nurse can answer questions, offer new information, and reassure parents-to-be of things

BOX 6-5	CLIENT TEACHING

Health Promotion Topics During Pregnancy

Nutrition, Diet, and Exercise (affecting both mother and fetus)

- Prenatal vitamins and/or foods to supply pregnancy needs
- Importance of fluids
- Hygiene, clothing adaptations, dental care
- Pattern of weight gain, desired weight gain (individualized teaching)
- Referral, if needed, to WIC program or other community assistance
- Alcohol's effects on the fetus
- Limiting or eliminating caffeine

Safety

- Adapting to body changes and changes in balance
  - Techniques for relieving physical stresses of pregnancy
- Checking all medications (even over-the-counter) with physician before use
- Smoking cessation

- Pets (especially cats because of the potential for being infected with toxoplasmosis when handling cat feces)
- Toxins and exposure to dangerous chemicals in the home and environment

Work

- Learning to balance work and rest
- Adaptations to jobs requiring long periods of standing

Travel Considerations

- Car travel—seatbelt adjustment
- Air travel—restrictions

Prenatal Classes

- Physical and mental preparation for childbirth and parenting
- Effects of pregnancy on sexuality
- Awareness of possible complications requiring medical aid
- Value of prenatal health care visits
- Planning for effects of pregnancy on home life

they are doing right. Office visits are an opportunity to review the importance of good nutrition, regular exercise, and adequate rest. Most women are open to learning about health promotion in this period of their lives. This gives the nurse the chance to encourage steps toward a healthier lifestyle that can have long-term effects. Some important areas of client teaching during pregnancy are listed in Box 6-5 ■.

Prenatal Classes

Prenatal classes are advisable for all mothers, not just those in their first pregnancies. Topics that are generally covered in these classes are:

- Health considerations during pregnancy, including:
  - Nutrition, diet, and exercise
  - Pets (especially cats because of the potential for being infected with toxoplasmosis when handling cat feces)
- Overview of the labor process
- Signs that labor is beginning
- Contraction patterns and timing
- Breathing techniques to assist the woman through contractions
- Chemical and nonchemical methods of providing pain relief during labor
- Possible complications in the mother and their warning signs
- Possible complications of labor, including emergency cesarean delivery and fetal anomaly or death
- Infant feeding (breast or bottle, positions, burping; see Chapter 9)

- Infant care (diapering, dressing, bathing)
- Infant safety (see Chapter 12)
- Siblings
- Work and travel considerations during pregnancy.

Adolescent Parents

It can be beneficial to provide prenatal classes specifically for pregnant teens. An all-teens class (Figure 6-21 ■) can offer a safe environment in which to discuss impending parenthood. Issues such as altered self-image can be much more difficult for adolescents to handle than for adults. There may be resentment about having life plans interrupted by the pregnancy. There may be issues about parental criticism that need to be aired, or disagreement over who will raise the child after birth. In a peer

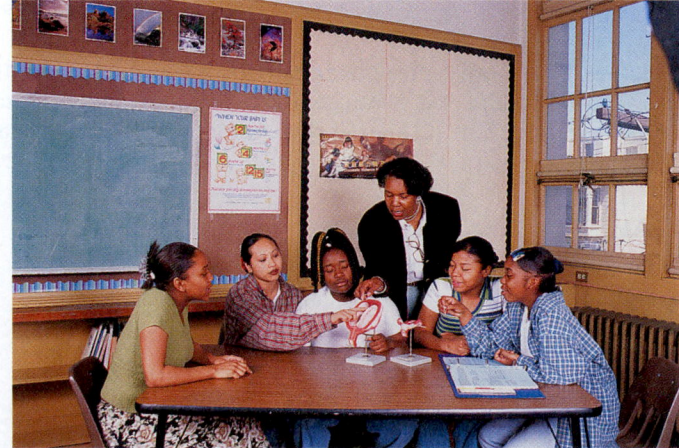

Figure 6-21. ■ Providing prenatal classes specifically for teens can improve the learning environment for young mothers.

TABLE 6-6

Warning Signs During Pregnancy

WARNING SIGN (Need immediate medical evaluation)	POSSIBLE CAUSE
Vaginal bleeding (any)	Spontaneous abortion, placenta previa, abruptio placenta
Fluid gushing or leaking from vagina	Rupture of membranes (leaking urine may appear similar)
Persistent vomiting	Hyperemesis gravidarium
Swelling of hands, face, legs, feet	Pregnancy-induced hypertension (PIH), pre-eclampsia
Visual disturbance: blurred vision, double vision, seeing spots or flashes of light	PIH, pre-eclampsia
Dizziness, fainting, persistent headache	PIH, pre-eclampsia
Fever over 100°F (37.8°C) and chills	Infection
Abdominal pain, cramping	Ectopic pregnancy, spontaneous abortion, abruptio placenta, labor
Thick, white/yellow, irritating vaginal discharge	Vaginal infection
Dysuria	Urinary infection
Oliguria	Dehydration, PIH
Notable decrease or absence of fetal movement	Fetal distress, fetal death

environment, teens can express their views more openly and can receive support from others who share their situation.

MONITORING FOR COMPLICATIONS

The client should be taught warning signs of possible complications. Usually, the sooner interventions are begun, the better the outcome. Signs of impending labor should be discussed with the client in the mid-second to third trimester of pregnancy. Table 6-6 ■ identifies warning signs.

Complications and high-risk pregnancy are discussed in Chapter 8 ∞.

Birthing Facilities and Staff

The settings in which women give birth are varied. Women may go to a local hospital and deliver the baby in a delivery room. They may choose a maternity center where labor and birth occur in a homelike atmosphere. A few elect to deliver their babies at home.

As care providers, women may have a physician, a nurse midwife, or a **doula** (a supportive companion who accompanies the woman through birth, providing physical and emotional support and information, and advocating for the woman and the family). The obstetrician, although no longer the sole person assisting births, is on call to other caregivers in case of emergency.

NURSING CARE

PRIORITIES IN NURSING CARE

The highest priority in providing prenatal care is monitoring the mother and fetus for signs of complications. Any such signs must be reported immediately. Teaching the mother, father, and significant others what to expect during pregnancy is important in health maintenance and preparation for childbirth. The nurse must be prepared to provide instruction at every client contact.

ASSESSING

The assessment of the pregnant family includes collecting physical data, determining the psychological response to pregnancy, and evaluating family functioning. An important piece of data to collect is information about the woman's culture and cultural expectations related to pregnancy.

Cultural Considerations

Families are influenced by their cultures, perhaps especially during times of great change, such as marriage, death, and birth. The nurse must be open to and respectful of their beliefs. Language barriers may pose a challenge in providing client and family teaching. Therefore, it is important to have an interpreter available when possible. Printed material should also be available in the woman's language. Table 6-7 ■ presents activities encouraged or avoided by some cultures.

Initial Visit

■ Provide a pleasant environment and therapeutic listening skills. Use open-ended questions when inquiring about the effect of the pregnancy on the woman's life. *The pregnant woman will have positive or negative feelings about the pregnancy. For her to feel safe about expressing them, the nurse's feeling about pregnancy must not affect the interview. The client and her needs are the focus. There may be a difference of opinion between the woman and her partner. The nurse assists by providing a place in which issues can be raised. In the case of difficult*

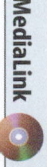

MediaLink

Pre-eclampsia

TABLE 6-7

Activities Encouraged or Avoided by Some Cultures During Pregnancy

TOPIC	BELIEF	NURSING CONSIDERATIONS
Nutrition	**Italian descent:** Desire for certain foods must be satisfied to prevent congenital anomalies. Also, they must smell the food to prevent miscarriage. (Spector, 2000) **African descent:** Eat clay, dirt, or starch to benefit mother and fetus. (Spector, 2000) **Korean descent:** Practice Tae Kyo, rules for safe childbirth, which lists food taboos. (Choi, 1995)	Obtain a diet history. Discuss need for well-balanced diet during pregnancy. If the dietary practice is not harmful, there is no reason to ask the client to discontinue the practice.
Exercise	**Italian descent:** Fear that moving in certain ways can cause fetal anomalies. (Spector, 2000) **Southeast Asian descent:** Inactivity during pregnancy results in difficult labor. (Mattson, 1995) **European, African, Mexican descent:** Reaching over head during pregnancy can harm the baby.	Obtain exercise history. Ask client if there are activities she is afraid to do because of the pregnancy. Assure her that reaching over her head will not harm the baby. Help her identify safe forms of activity. Teach need for activity related to general health and weight control.
Home remedies	**Native American descent:** May use herbal remedies (milky juice from dandelion to increase breast milk). (Spector, 2000) **Chinese descent:** Drink ginseng tea for faintness. Adding bamboo leaves will have sedative effect. **African descent:** Self-medicate for common discomforts of pregnancy (take laxatives to prevent/treat constipation).	Many clients fail to report use of home remedies for fear of being judged unfavorably. When obtaining a health history, ask about home remedies. Teach that some herbs can be harmful when taken with prescribed medication.
Spirituality	**Native American descent:** May use the "medicine man" to ensure safe birth and healthy baby. Tribal spiritual leaders may be invited by family to attend birth, pray, and perform "ceremonies." Many cultures pay attention to spirituality to lessen fear.	Encourage the use of support systems. Be sensitive to "tribal ceremonies" as long as they do not disrupt others.
Alternate health care providers	Women of many cultures may choose to use alternate health care providers. **Mexican descent:** May seek care from a partera (midwife). The partera can speak their language, understands the culture, and may deliver the infant in the home or possibly at a birthing center. (Spector, 2000)	Discuss a variety of health care provider choices. Help the client explore the risks and benefits of different prenatal care and delivery settings. Provide reassurance that the goal is a healthy mother and the delivery of a healthy baby with respect for the client's beliefs. *Note:* Some midwives are RNs with advanced education and certification, whereas others are lay midwives with little or no formal education. During a home delivery, equipment may not be available during an emergency.

family issues, the nurse would bring in a qualified social worker or counselor.

■ A health history will be obtained (in depth, if necessary), including menstrual history and history of past pregnancies. The LPN/LVN will assist the RN in collecting data. *A complete health history is needed to identify any past medical issues that might affect the pregnancy. A history of past pregnancies is important because labor time is usually significantly reduced after the first delivery (see Chapter 7 ⦾). History of abortion, whether elective or spontaneous, is recorded at this time. Important precautions would be instituted for a woman wanting*

children who has had spontaneous abortion in the past (see Chapter 8 ⦾). Review Table 6-2 for the proper terms to use in describing a woman's parous state.

■ Assist with an in-depth physical assessment. *The health care provider will perform a detailed assessment of the reproductive organs. An ultrasound may be done to diagnose pregnancy. Blood may be drawn to determine a baseline for future reference.*

Follow-up Visits

■ Collect data on the woman's vital signs and changes related to pregnancy. Ask about any current concerns or discomforts. Inquire about how the woman and the family are coping with the pregnancy. Provide client teaching related to gestational changes and ways of monitoring the fetus between visits. *Data must be monitored throughout the woman's pregnancy. Client teaching is a regular part of each prenatal visit. Open-ended questions about how the woman and family are responding to the pregnancy allow the woman to bring issues forward for discussion.*

- Assist RN or collect data on the FHR (see Figure 6-16). *Once audible, the FHR is a useful indicator of fetal health.*
- Inquire about any medications, over-the-counter drugs, herbal remedies, or recreational drugs the woman may be using. Encourage the woman to take prenatal vita-

mins as prescribed. *The nurse should collect information about all types of drugs and preparations and should report any unusual or potentially harmful drugs to the care provider. Client teaching should include information about safe and unsafe chemicals. (Review Box 6-3.) Prenatal vitamins help ensure a healthy fetus.*

- Report a blood pressure increase of 30 mm Hg systolic and 20 mm Hg diastolic over previous measurement to the health care provider. If a previous blood pressure measurement is not available, report a recording of 140/90. *A rise in BP could indicate pregnancy-induced hypertension.*
- Track the woman's weight from visit to visit (Figure 6-22 ■). A total weight gain should be 25 to 35 pounds,

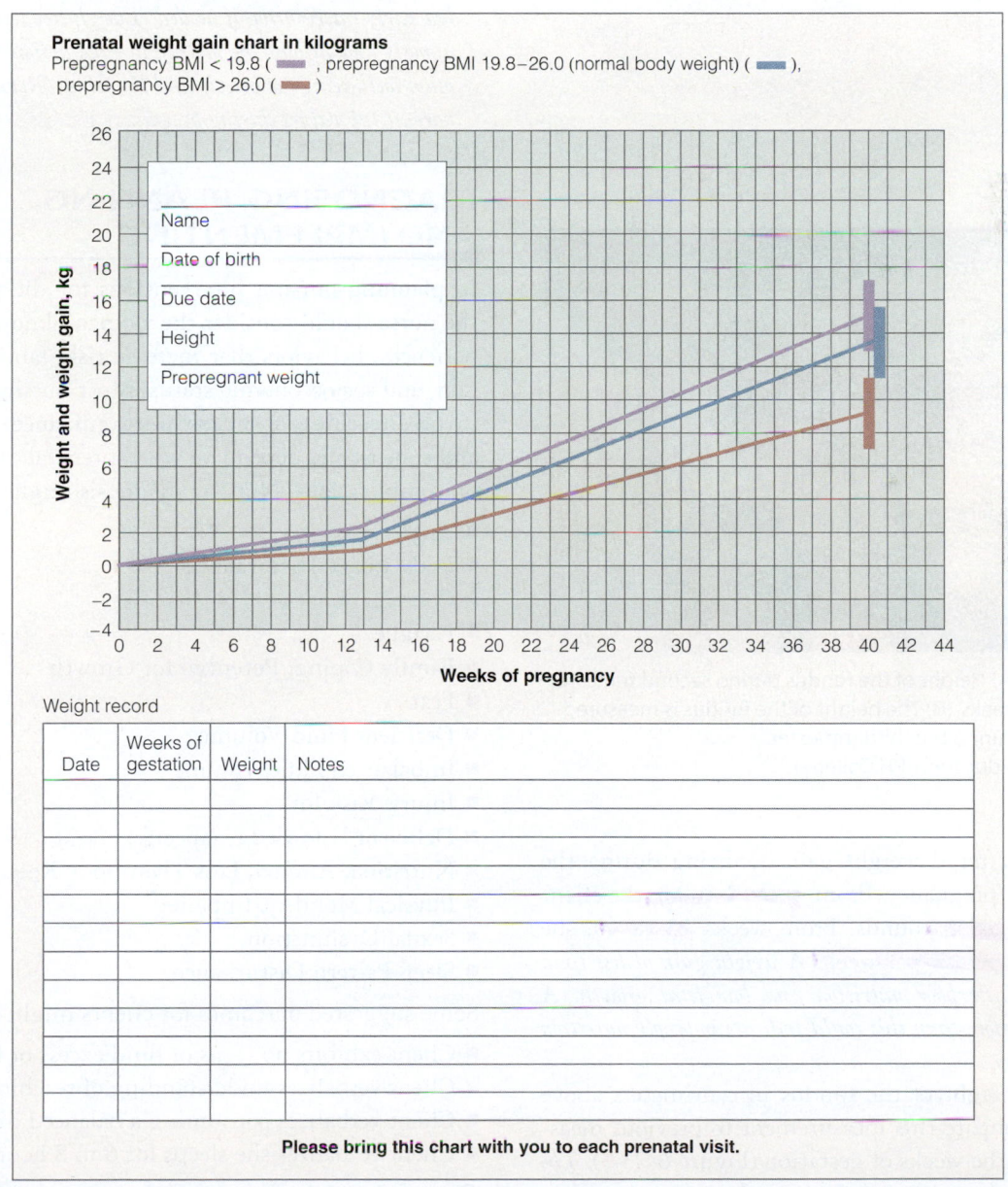

Figure 6-22. ■ Weight gain form shows the typical pattern of weight gain in pregnancy. (From the National Academy of Sciences Institute of Medicine, Subcommittee of Nutritional Status and Weight Gain During Pregnancy. [1992]. *Supplemental materials on nutrition during pregnancy and lactation: An implementation guide.* Washington, DC: National Academy Press.)

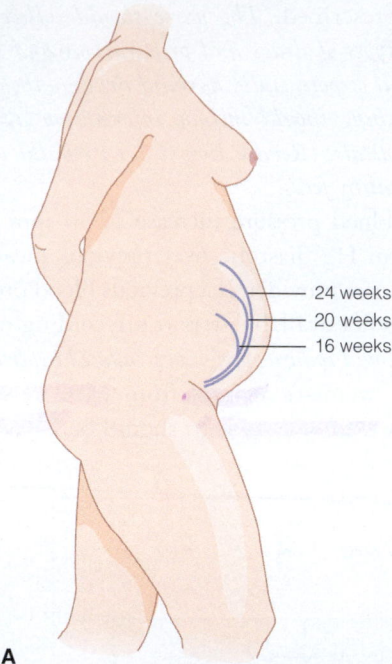

A

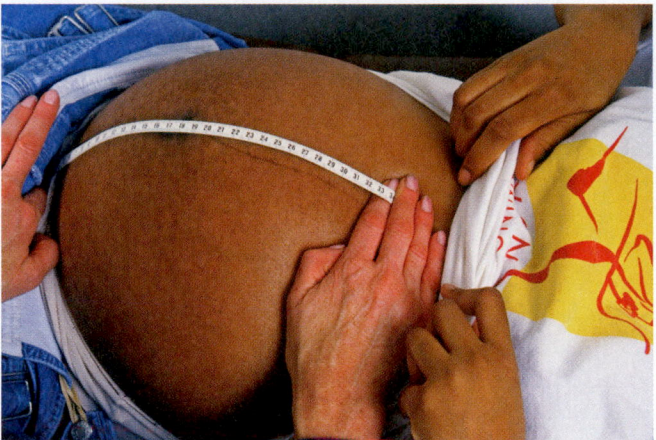

Figure 6-23. ■ (**A**) Height of the fundus during second trimester at 16, 20, and 24 weeks. (**B**) The height of the fundus is measured at prenatal visits during the third trimester.
Source: (Pearson Education/PH College)

with the most rapid weight gain occurring during the last half of the pregnancy. From weeks 1 to 12, the client should gain 3 to 4 pounds. From weeks 13 to 40, she should gain 1 pound per week. *A weight gain of less than this could indicate poor nutrition and low fetal growth. A weight gain of more than this could indicate improper nutrition or fluid retention.*

■ Measure the height of the fundus in centimeters above the pubis. Compare this measurement to previous measurements and the weeks of gestation (Figure 6-23 ■). *The fundus should enlarge 1 cm/wk. If the fundus is not enlarging at this rate, the fetus is not growing at a normal rate. The fundus*

enlarging more than this rate would indicate that the fetus is growing too rapidly or that a multiple pregnancy is suspected. From 20 to 36 weeks, the fundal measurement is normally 2 centimeter +/− the number of weeks gestation. So, for example, at 24 weeks' gestation, fundal measurement should be 22 to 26 centimeter.

■ Monitor for edema. *A small amount of dependent edema is often present in the last few weeks of pregnancy. A large amount of edema in the feet, or edema of the calves, thighs, hands, and face, should be reported to the health care provider.*

■ Collect a urine sample at each visit and perform a dipstick tested for glucose, protein, and ketone bodies. A glucose screening test is ordered in weeks 24 to 28 to determine the presence of gestational diabetes. *The urine test will allow early intervention if needed. The glucose test establishes a diagnosis and allows the mother to take action to promote maximum well-being for herself and the fetus. (Review Table 6-3 for normal lab values during pregnancy.)*

DIAGNOSING, PLANNING, AND IMPLEMENTING

In planning nursing interventions for the prenatal client, the nurse should consider the woman's knowledge, past experiences, behaviors that increase risk, family support system, and socioeconomic status. Most nursing interventions involve teaching or anticipatory guidance. Specific topics and time frames depend on when prenatal care is begun and on complications. Nursing diagnosis might include:

■ Anxiety
■ Body Image Disturbance
■ Constipation
■ Fatigue
■ Family Coping: Potential for Growth
■ Fear
■ Deficient Fluid Volume
■ Imbalanced Fluid Volume
■ Injury, Risk for
■ Deficient Knowledge (specify)
■ Nutrition: Altered, Less Than Body Requirements
■ Physical Mobility, Impaired
■ Sexual Dysfunction
■ Sleep Pattern Disturbance

Some suggested outcomes for clients might include:

■ Client exhibits no signs of fluid excess or fluid deficit.
■ Client verbalizes understanding of teaching.
■ Client verbalizes consuming a balanced diet.
■ Client verbalizes she sleeps for 6 to 8 hours every night.

One of the main functions of the nurse is educating the client and her family about the pregnancy process and

| BOX 6-6 | COMPLEMENTARY THERAPIES |

Physical Modalities for Relief of Backache and Other Pregnancy-Related Muscle Pain

Massage Therapy for Low Back Pain

Massage often helps relieve the low back pain associated with pregnancy. During the first 4 months of pregnancy, the body should be massaged with a gentle, soft touch. The best position for lumbar massage is with the women sitting on a stool, resting her arms on a table, and leaning her forehead against her arms. The person doing the message kneels on the floor behind her, which enhances the masseuse's ability to apply an effective amount of pressure to the back muscles.

Yoga

Many women find that the regular practice of yoga builds and tones muscles, increases flexibility, improves endurance, and promotes a state of relaxation. One of the many applications of yoga is in pregnancy and childbirth. In fact, many of the techniques taught in childbirth classes, such as focus, relaxation, and systematic breathing, have their roots in yoga. The gentle stretching of the poses helps ease the muscle aches of pregnancy and strengthens the muscles that will be used during childbirth. The breathing techniques may lessen the shortness of breath that often accompanies advanced pregnancy.

Yoga practiced while pregnant is slightly different from regular yoga in that some poses are contraindicated. These poses are the extreme stretching positions and any position that puts pressure on the uterus. Full forward bends will probably be uncomfortable for both woman and baby. A woman's center of balance has shifted completely, and thus she must be careful with balance poses. Pregnant women should never lie on the stomach for any pose. In fact, if any pose is uncomfortable, the women should stop at once. If she experiences dizziness, sudden swelling, extreme shortness of breath, or vaginal bleeding, she should see her midwife or doctor immediately.

Reflexology for Sciatica

Reflexology is a field of therapy that uses specific touch techniques to stimulate "reflex points and areas" on the feet, hands, and ears. Reflexologists believe that each point corresponds to a specific part of the body. For example, the growing baby can put pressure on the large sciatic nerve. This pressure inflames the nerve, causing severe low back pain that radiates into the legs. Reflexology may help this condition. The reflex points for the sciatic nerve are on the heel. A woman in her second or third trimester can press gently and release with her thumbs to stimulate first one whole heel, and then the other. Each heel can be worked for 1 to 2 minutes twice a day until the pain is gone.

Women who are in the first trimester of pregnancy should not have reflexology that stimulates the uterine points on the hands, feet, or ears. In general, it is best for pregnant women to receive reflexology that uses light, gentle pressure (Gottlieb, 2000).

Source: Olds, S. B., London, M. L., Ladewig, P. A. W., & Davidson, M. R. (2004). *Maternal-newborn nursing & women's health care* (7th ed.). Upper Saddle River, NJ: Prentice Hall, p. 387.

---

prenatal care. Topics for client and family teaching are included here.

- Encourage the taking of prenatal multivitamins once a day, even if the client is nauseous. Suggest that she adjust the time of day she takes the vitamin so she will be able to continue taking the supplement. If she is unable or unwilling to use prenatal vitamins, provide a list of foods that are high in nutrients that pregnant women need (see Box 6-1). *Most care providers prescribe a prenatal multivitamin with iron to be taken once a day. This nutritional supplement will help ensure that adequate amounts of vitamins and iron are ingested for the developing fetus.*

- Encourage good nutrition and moderate, regular exercise. Remind the woman to drink plenty of fluids. Provide suggestions for discomforts associated with pregnancy (Box 6-6 ■; review Table 6-4). *Good nutrition and regular exercise can help the woman overcome some of the discomforts of pregnancy. It is recommended that pregnant women drink 1.5 to 2 liters of fluid per day and that caffeine intake be limited.*

- If necessary, refer the woman to programs that can supply milk and protein. *Some women may not be able to afford the extra high-calcium and high-protein foods that are useful when pregnant. Assistance programs are available to help provide these nutrients.*

- Remind the woman to consult a physician before taking cold, headache, allergy, flu, or other medications or supplements. *Many physicians, nurse midwives, and nurse practitioners provide their clients with a list of over-the-counter medications that are acceptable for use during pregnancy.*

- Review safety hazards for pregnant women and encourage them to take them seriously. *Women in late pregnancy are at risk for falls. Exposure to chemicals may harm the fetus. Excessive heat can cause maternal hyperthermia.*

- Encourage the client to make and keep regularly scheduled appointments throughout the prenatal period. *The pregnant woman should return every 4 weeks for the first 28 weeks, every 2 weeks during weeks 29 to 36, and every week thereafter until delivery.*

- Teach the client warning signs of possible complications (see Table 6-6). Discuss signs of impending labor with the client in the third trimester. *Usually, the sooner interventions are begun, the better. Giving the woman information allows her to relax when there are no warning signs and to report them promptly if they should occur. Prompt attention may prevent complications.*

Client Self-Care

Self-care generally involves a minimal adjustment of normal habits.

- Teach the client the importance of personal hygiene during pregnancy. *Bathing daily is important due to an increase in perspiration and vaginal secretions. Either a tub bath or shower may be used with warm water. In late pregnancy, the woman may have difficulty rising from a sitting position in the bathtub. Care should be taken to prevent falls in the tub or shower. Douching should be avoided.*

- Teach the client to clean the breasts with water, rub the nipple with a washcloth, and air-dry the breast. Leakage of fluid from the nipple is common. This fluid should be rubbed into the nipple to lubricate the skin and promote breast health. Clients may benefit from wearing a maternity bra. *Prenatal washing and air-drying will toughen breast tissue prior to breastfeeding. A properly fitting maternity bra promotes comfort, supports the enlarged heavy breast, and prevents back strain.*

- Encourage continued activity and periods of rest: The pregnant woman should have regular activity. *Activities routinely practiced before pregnancy can generally be continued as long as there are no complications and the woman can safely participate. Walking and swimming are best, and overly strenuous activity should be avoided. Fatigue should also be avoided. Periods of rest, with the legs elevated to promote venous return, should be scheduled throughout the day.*

- Discuss the importance of clothing for the self-image and comfort during pregnancy. Clothing that is attractive, loose fitting, and easy to care for should be selected. Teach client to steer away from stockings that constrict at knees or thighs and to choose low-heeled shoes for everyday wear. *Because maternity clothing is only worn for a short time, clothing may be shared among friends, or second-hand clothing may be purchased at reasonable prices. Knee-high or thigh-high stockings can interfere with circulation. Low-heeled shoes are generally recommended due to the difficulty of maintaining balance in high-heeled shoes.*

- Advise women to continue dental care on a regular schedule, but not to have x-rays during pregnancy. *The woman should inform her dentist that she is pregnant. Dental care is necessary for ongoing good health. X-ray examinations should be postponed until after the pregnancy because of the risk of radiation to the fetus.*

- Teach that sexual activities may continue throughout the pregnancy unless there are complications. *There may be a change in desire for sexual activity during pregnancy. After the sixth month, the woman should not lie flat on her back due to hypotensive syndrome. A pillow can be placed under her right hip, or an alternative position can be used.*

- Advise the woman to review the employment environment in terms of her needs while pregnant and to discuss areas of concern with the health care provider. *The decision to continue employment should be based on several factors. Are there hazards in the workplace that would place additional risk on the pregnancy? Would the woman be under undue physical strain? Would periods of rest be available?*

- Discuss effect of pregnancy on travel. *Travel need not be restricted unless complications develop. Generally, the best time to travel is in the second trimester, when the risks of complications are less. Some airlines may not accept passengers past a certain week of pregnancy without a provider's note. When traveling, the woman should walk for about 10 minutes every 2 hours to prevent venous stasis. The seat belt should be worn snuggly below the abdomen.*

- Encourage the woman to attend childbirth education classes. *Preparation for childbirth usually begins in the third trimester. Many hospitals and birthing centers present childbirth classes. Women should be encouraged to attend these classes so they will be well prepared both mentally and physically. Printed resources are also available to assist in childbirth preparation.*

EVALUATING

Clients should be able to verbalize an understanding of the instructions. A change, or lack of change, in client's behavior is also used to evaluate the instruction provided.

Although the majority of pregnancies are completed with a minimum of discomfort, complications can occur at any time. It is the role of the LPN/LVN to assist in data collection and to report any signs of complications. Chapter 10 describes the most common complications and the related nursing care.

NURSING PROCESS CARE PLAN
Caring for Pregnant Woman Who Wants to Travel

Mrs. Taylor, expecting her first baby, comes to the clinic for a routine visit. She is 22 weeks pregnant and states that she is feeling well and that the baby is becoming very active. She states that she wants to go on a trip with her husband in a few weeks. She also states that she is getting not only excited about labor, but also a little scared.

Assessment
- BP 134/72
- Negative protein in urine
- No edema in ankles
- Weight increase by 1½ pounds in last month

Nursing Diagnosis. The following important nursing diagnosis (among others) is established for this client:

- Deficient Knowledge related to travel during pregnancy and childbirth

Expected Outcomes. The mother will verbalize an understanding of travel guidelines, symptoms of complications, and ways to access health care.

Planning and Implementation

- Discuss travel at this point of the pregnancy, including need for exercise and fluids. Provide information regarding signs of complications and how to access health care if needed.
- Provide information regarding childbirth education classes in the area.
- Schedule a return visit to clinic in 1 month.

Evaluation. Pregnancy progressing in a normal pattern. Mrs. Taylor should verbalize signs of complications and when to contact health care provider. She should be able to begin childbirth education classes.

Critical Thinking in the Nursing Process

1. What are some other topics that should be discussed with Mrs. Taylor at this point of the pregnancy? (*Hint:* Think about changing body shape and safety.)
2. What topics should the nurse plan to discuss at the next appointment in 1 month?
3. What is the role of the LPN/LVN in providing care to the pregnant client in a physician's office?

Note: Discussion of Critical Thinking questions appears in Appendix I.

Note: The references and resources for this and all chapters have been compiled at the back of the book.

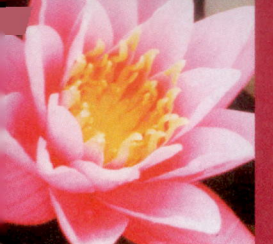

Chapter Review

KEY TERMS by Topic

Use the audio glossary feature of either the CD-ROM or the Companion Website to hear the correct pronunciation of the following key terms.

Preconception
craniofacial, anomalies, teratogens, salpingitis

Fertilization
fertilization, pregnancy, conception, zygote, morula, blastocyst, trophoblast, embryonic disc, implantation, villi, human chorionic gonadotropin (hCG)

Development of Support Structures
chorion, amnion, fetal membranes, "bag of waters," amniotic fluid, lanugo, vernix caseosa, placenta, cotyledons, human placental lactogen (hPL), relaxin, umbilical cord, Wharton's jelly

Stages of Fetal Development
gestation, pre-embryonic stage, embryonic stage, fetal stage

Development of Fetal Body Systems
cephalocaudal, umbilical arteries, umbilical vein, ductus venosus, foramen ovale, ductus arteriosus, yolk sac, surfactant, viability, meconium, ossification

Signs of Pregnancy
presumptive signs, amenorrhea, quickening, pseudopregnancy, ballottement, Hegar's sign, Goodell's sign, Chadwick's sign, fetal heart tones (FHT), uterine soufflé, funic soufflé

Maternal Changes During Pregnancy
trimesters, Braxton Hicks contractions, colostrum, supine hypotensive syndrome, physiologic anemia of pregnancy, hyperemesis gravidarum, linea nigra, chloasma, striae gravidarum, oxytocin, "let-down reflex"

Diagnostic Tests of Fetal Status
ultrasound, amniocentesis, percutaneous umbilical cord sampling, erythroblastosis fetalis, chorionic villus sampling, nonstress test (NST), biophysical profile

Initial Visit
gravida, para, abortion, preterm, term, postterm, miscarriage, Naegele's rule, nulligravida, nullipara, primagravida, primapara, multigravida, multipara, GP/TPAL

Follow-up Visits
abortifacients

Birthing Facilities and Staff
doula

KEY Points

- During fetal development, all body systems are formed in the first 8 weeks.
- Most pregnancies progress as planned. The LPN/LVN is responsible for collecting data and for recognizing and reporting symptoms of complications.
- The key to a healthy pregnancy is regular prenatal care, including client teaching and early detection of complications.
- Nurses have a responsibility to teach good health practices, including nutrition, exercise, and eliminating risky behaviors.

EXPLORE MediaLink

Additional interactive resources for this chapter can be found on the Companion Website at www.prenhall.com/towle.

Click on Chapter 6 and "Begin" to select the activities for this chapter.

For chapter-related NCLEX-style questions and an audio glossary, access the accompanying CD-ROM in this book.

Animations
Pre-eclampsia

Ectopic pregnancy

FOR FURTHER Study

Table 2-1 lists some frequently accessed government programs for women and young children.

Chapter 4 reviews reproductive anatomy; Figure 4-12 shows structures of the uterus; Figure 4-17 illustrates the process of lactation.

See in-depth discussion of reproductive issues and STIs in Chapter 5; Figure 5-18 shows fraternal vs identical twins.

The procedure for performing an external fetal heart monitor reading during labor and delivery is in Chapter 7.

High-risk pregnancies and procedures are discussed in Chapter 8.

Fetal alcohol syndrome is discussed in Chapters 8 and 27.

Chapter 9 discusses newborn care and nutrition.

Chapter 10 includes postpartum complications.

Chapter 12 reviews health promotion and safety issues.

Down syndrome is discussed in Chapter 16.

Fetal and newborn circulation is illustrated in Figure 19-1.

Renal disorders are discussed in detail in Chapter 23.

Caring for an Undernourished Pregnant Woman

NCLEX-PN® Focus Area: Physiologic Integrity

Case Study: Jean, a 17-year-old, comes to the clinic for her first visit. She appears pale and thin. Her weight is 135 lb. Her vital signs are within normal limits. Her urine is negative for protein. It is determined she is 10 weeks pregnant. She states that she is living with her boyfriend in a one-bedroom basement apartment. Both Jean and her boyfriend have had to drop out of high school to get jobs. They are barely able to pay the rent and buy food. Jean begins to cry, stating that she does not know what to do.

Nursing Diagnosis: Imbalanced Nutrition: Less than Body Requirements

COLLECT DATA

Subjective

_____
_____
_____
_____
_____
_____

Objective

_____
_____
_____
_____
_____
_____

Would you report this? Yes/No

If yes, to: _____

Data Collected
(use those that apply)

- Crying
- States she does not know what to do
- Weight: 135 lb
- Vital signs
- Urine negative for protein
- Pale
- Thin
- Money only for rent and food

Nursing Interventions
(use those that apply; list in priority order)

- Teach need for milk products.
- Refer to WIC program.
- Teach need for increased protein, lower carbohydrates in diet.
- Teach need for prenatal vitamins.
- Refer to therapist for depression.

Nursing Care

_____
_____
_____
_____
_____
_____
_____
_____
_____

How would you document this? _____
_____
_____
_____

Compare your documentation to the sample provided in Appendix I.

NCLEX-PN® Exam Preparation

1. After fertilization of the ova, when does the production of hCG begin?
   1. 8–12 hours
   2. 18–36 hours
   3. 4–6 days
   4. 8–10 days

2. Which of the following substances produced by the placenta prevents uterine contractions?
   1. human placental lactogen
   2. human chorionic gonadotropin
   3. progesterone
   4. relaxin

3. Which of the following statements about fetal circulation are true? Choose all that apply.
   1. The fetal respiratory system oxygenates blood.
   2. The ductus arteriosus is located inside the fetal heart.
   3. Osmosis is the means of blood exchange between placenta and fetus.
   4. The umbilical cord contains two arteries and one vein.
   5. The fetal blood and maternal blood do not mix.

4. The nurse, working with a pregnant woman who was eating a well-balanced diet prior to pregnancy, will advise this woman to:
   1. Make no changes in her diet.
   2. Add two milk and one meat servings.
   3. Add two vegetable and one fruit servings.
   4. Decrease the amount of carbohydrates.

5. The nurse, working with a pregnant woman in the last trimester, will advise the woman to sleep on her side mainly to:
   1. relieve pressure on the bladder.
   2. relieve pressure on the fetus.
   3. facilitate sleep.
   4. prevent hypotension.

6. The earliest the nurse will be able to hear the fetal heart tones by using a Doppler is by week number:
   1. 2
   2. 6
   3. 10
   4. 20

7. You are trying to determine the estimated date of delivery for a client whose last menstrual period began on May 6 and ended on May 11. The estimated date of delivery using Naegele's rule is which of the following dates in February?
   1. 6
   2. 11
   3. 13
   4. 18

8. Maria, a 17-year-old single woman, is 12 weeks pregnant. She says to the nurse, "I don't want to be pregnant. How can I take care of a baby and still do all the things I want?" The nurse should reply,
   1. "I can make you an appointment for an abortion."
   2. "You should have thought about that before you had unprotected sex."
   3. "How can I help you problem solve what will be best for you?"
   4. "You should contact a lawyer who handles adoption."

9. Juanita, 32 weeks pregnant, comes to the office stating the baby has not been moving as much as usual. All of the following must be assessed. Place them in priority order.
   1. Report findings to the doctor.
   2. Take Juanita's vital signs.
   3. Measure Juanita's weight.
   4. Listen to the FHT.
   5. Check Juanita's urine for glucose and protein.

10. Nancy, 34 weeks pregnant, calls the clinic at 4:30 P.M. to say that she has had a severe headache all day. She is experiencing some blurred vision and her feet are swollen. She asks the nurse what she should do. The nurse should respond,
    1. "Take two Tylenol every 4 hours and stay in bed until your office appointment next week."
    2. "Go to the hospital to be checked."
    3. "Come to the office at 10:00 tomorrow morning."
    4. "Call back in 30 minutes when the doctor can talk with you."

Answers for Review Questions, as well as discussion of Care Plan and Critical Thinking Care Map questions, appear in Appendix I.

Chapter 7

Health Promotion During Labor and Delivery

BRIEF Outline

Theories About the Beginning of Labor

Signs of Impending Labor

Admission to the Birthing Facility

Variables Affecting Labor

Pain in Labor

Stages of Labor

Delivery Room Care of the Neonate

Nursing Care

LEARNING Outcomes

After completing this chapter, you will be able to:

- Discuss appropriate nursing actions for women who present for admission when in labor.
- Describe variables affecting labor and delivery.
- Identify various methods of pain relief used during labor.
- Differentiate the stages of labor.
- Discuss the mechanisms of labor.
- Identify nursing diagnoses and nursing interventions to assist in the labor process.
- Provide appropriate care for a client during labor and delivery.
- Describe important aspects of nursing care of the neonate immediately after birth.

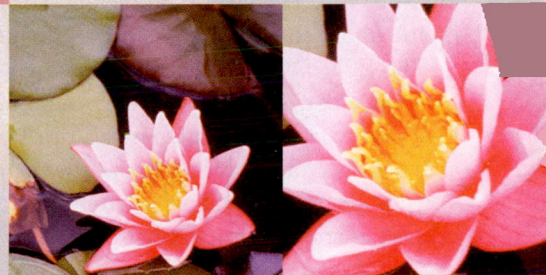

HEALTH PROMOTION ISSUE: Client Wanting Second Labor to Be Better Than First

NURSING PROCESS CARE PLAN: Woman in Active Stage One Labor

CRITICAL THINKING CARE MAP: Caring for a Woman in Transition

Over the past few decades, many changes have been made in birthing practices. At one time, fathers were not allowed in the labor or delivery rooms. They had to stay in a waiting room for hours with little information about the condition of their wives or children. Many women labored in a multiperson ward with curtains separating the clients. Delivery occurred in a cold, white room, with a hard delivery table. Anyone entering the room was dressed in surgical attire with hair and shoe covers and masks. Prior to labor, women received little instruction in the delivery process or in relaxation techniques.

Today, childbirth classes are offered to help the couple prepare for the birth experience. Partners often accompany women through the birthing process. The "traditional" delivery room has given way to modern homelike environments. In birthing centers, labor, delivery, and recovery occur in the same room (Figure 7-1 ■).

This chapter discusses the birthing process and related nursing care. The goal in all instances is to deliver a healthy infant under the safest conditions possible.

The LPN/LVN usually plays the greatest role in postpartum care, not in labor. However, nurses are responsible for knowing what occurs in labor and birth, what complications are possible and how to recognize them, and what care is provided to the mother and infant after birth. The material in this chapter is not only important when studying for licensure. It is preparation for dealing with a birth in emergency conditions or if an RN is not available. It also establishes a baseline of knowledge for further education.

Theories About the Beginning of Labor

Toward the end of pregnancy, the mother and fetus begin preparing for delivery. Although researchers are still unsure of the exact trigger for labor, two theories have been developed to answer the question "Why does labor begin?" Once this question can be answered, preterm labor can be prevented or stopped, and labor can be induced more easily if needed.

OVERDISTENSION THEORY

One theory to explain the onset of labor is based on the principle that hollow organs tend to empty themselves when overdistended. This theory explains the emptying of the bladder and sigmoid colon. This phenomenon may partially explain the beginning of labor. However, it does not fully explain why labor begins early in some women.

HORMONAL THEORY

The hormonal theory relates to the complex relationship of maternal and fetal hormones (Figure 7-2 ■). Fetal cortisol

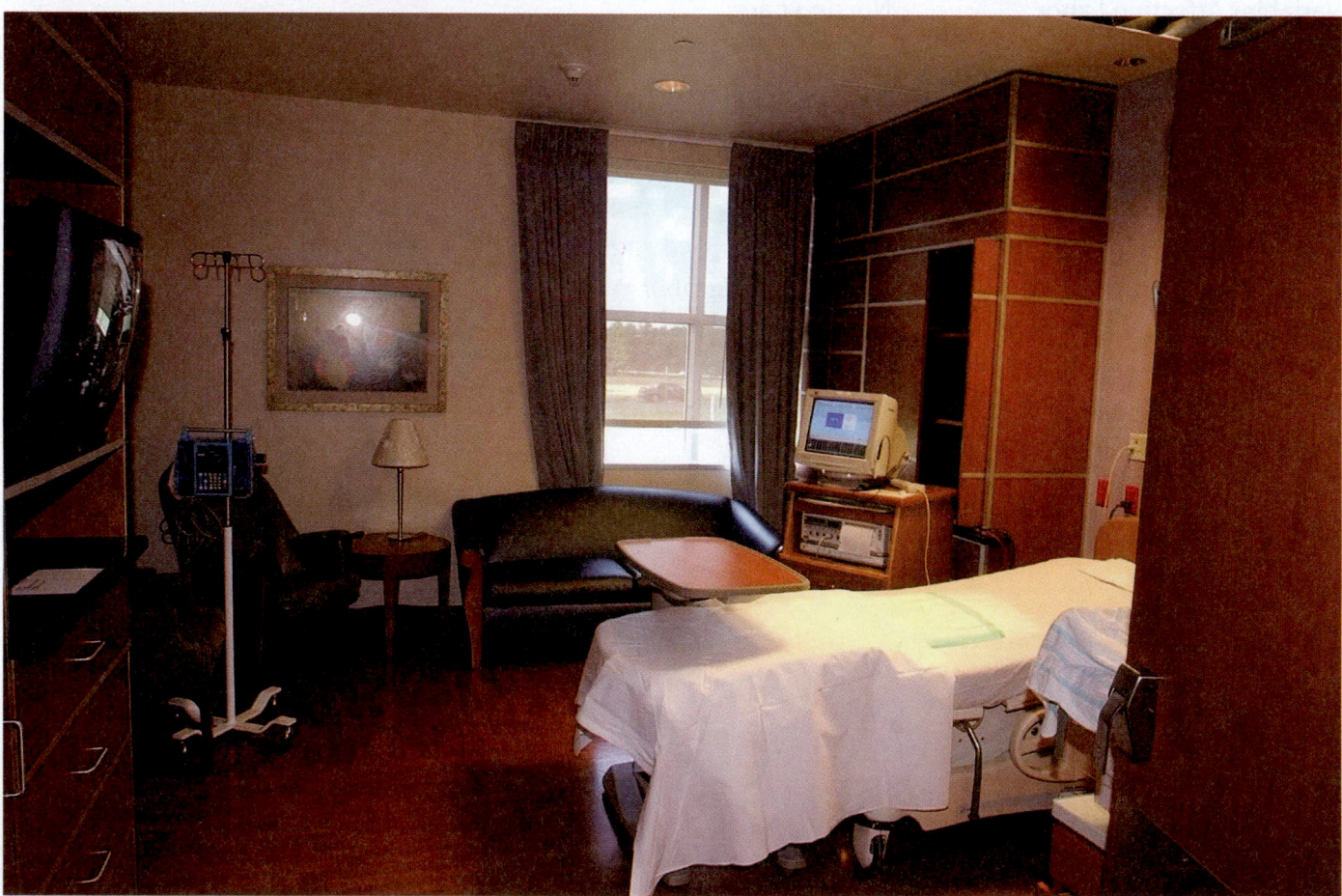

Figure 7-1. ■ Birthing room in a women and babies hospital. (AP Wide World Photos.)

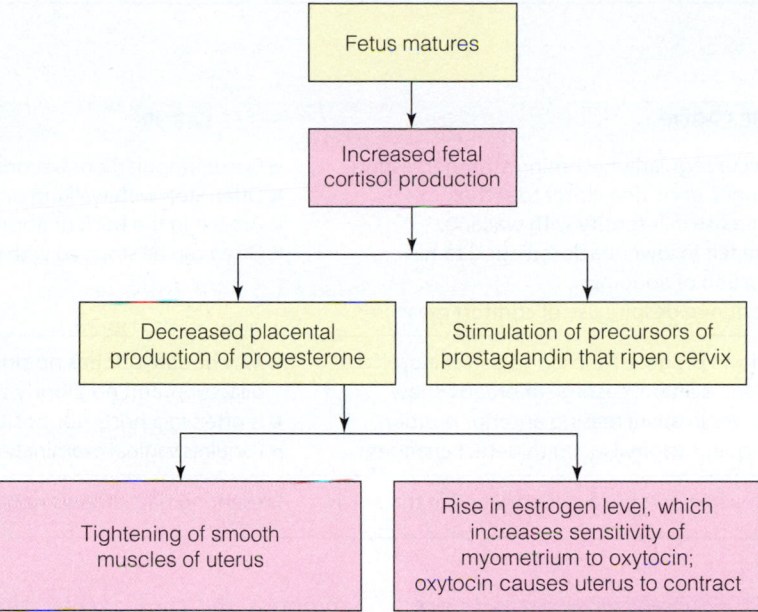

Figure 7-2. ■ Flowsheet showing hormone theory of how labor begins.

production increases as the fetus matures. It is believed that fetal cortisol decreases the placental production of progesterone and stimulates the precursors of prostaglandin that ripen the cervix. Because progesterone causes the smooth muscles of the uterus to relax, a decrease in progesterone allows those muscles to tighten. Also, as the progesterone level declines, the estrogen level rises. Estrogen increases the sensitivity of the myometrium to oxytocin. *Oxytocin,* a hormone produced by the mother's posterior pituitary gland, causes the uterus to contract.

Signs of Impending Labor

Although several signs indicate that onset of labor is close, the exact time cannot be predicted.

LIGHTENING
The descent of the fetus into the pelvis relieves pressure on the diaphragm, allowing the mother to breathe more easily and to "feel lighter" (thus the term **lightening**). The descent of the fetus into the pelvis may occur as long as 2 to 4 weeks prior to the onset of labor. In multipara clients, lightening may not occur until labor contractions begin. Although the ease in breathing may make the mother feel lighter, the fetus's entry into the pelvis puts more pressure on the bladder, resulting in urinary frequency. The descent of the fetus also puts pressure on the femoral veins, increasing venous stasis, and resulting in lower extremity edema. Low back pain and leg cramps result from pressure on pelvic nerves.

BRAXTON HICKS CONTRACTIONS
Irregular painless contractions occur throughout pregnancy. They become more frequent and more noticeable during the last few weeks. At times, they cause the woman to go to the hospital believing that she is in labor. These **Braxton**

Hicks contractions squeeze *around* the uterus instead of from the top down, causing no change in the cervix. Braxton Hicks contractions are termed **false labor**. Table 7-1 ■ compares false labor and true labor.

CERVICAL CHANGES
Due to hormonal changes beginning at about 35 week' gestation, the cervix begins to mature or "ripen" and becomes softer. **Effacement** (the shortening and thinning of the cervix) and **dilatation** (opening of the cervical opening or *os*) may begin (Figure 7-3 ■).

BLOODY SHOW
Bloody show is the release of the mucus plug from the cervix. The plug may contain a small amount of blood. If the client is not already in early labor, it often begins within 48 hours after bloody show. This sign should not be confused with the small amount of blood-tinged drainage that may be produced during a vaginal examination.

RUPTURED MEMBRANES

Spontaneous Rupture of Membranes
Spontaneous rupture of membranes (SROM) is a tearing or perforation of the amniotic sac releasing amniotic fluid. SROM usually occurs after labor begins, but in a small percentage of women the amniotic membranes may rupture before the onset of labor contractions. If SROM occurs outside the medical center, the client should go to the hospital or birthing center for evaluation. If SROM occurs within the medical center, the nurse should obtain FHT and digitally examine the cervix.

When the amniotic fluid drains out of the uterus, the infant moves closer to the mother's pelvic outlet. If the fetal head is tight against the pelvic bones, there is little risk to the baby. If the fetus is **ballotable** (able to be pushed away

TABLE 7-1

False versus True Labor

CHARACTERISTIC	TRUE LABOR	FALSE LABOR
Contractions	■ Occur regularly, becoming stronger, lasting longer, occurring closer together. ■ Increase in intensity with walking. ■ Are felt in lower back, radiating to lower portion of abdomen. ■ Continue despite use of comfort measures.	■ Occur irregularly, or become regular only temporarily. ■ Often stop with walking or position change. ■ Are felt in the back or abdomen above the umbilicus. ■ Often can be stopped with use of comfort measures.
Cervix	■ Shows progressive change, softening, efface-ment, dilation, passage of bloody show. ■ Moves in an increasing anterior position. ■ Requires vaginal exam to detect changes.	■ May be soft, but has no significant change in effacement, dilatation, and no bloody show. ■ Is often in a posterior position. ■ Requires vaginal examination to determine characteristics.
Fetus	Presenting part becomes engaged in the pelvis.	Presenting part often is not engaged in the pelvis.

from the cervix), the mother is asked to remain in bed until the fetus is no longer ballotable.

If the fetus is ballotable, there is a danger that the umbilical cord may be washed out of the cervix with the amniotic fluid. The infant's body (usually the head) may compress the cord against the pelvis, obstructing blood flow through the umbilical cord. This condition, called a **prolapsed umbilical cord**, results in an obstetric emergency in order to save the life of the infant. Umbilical cord prolapse is discussed in Chapter 8 .

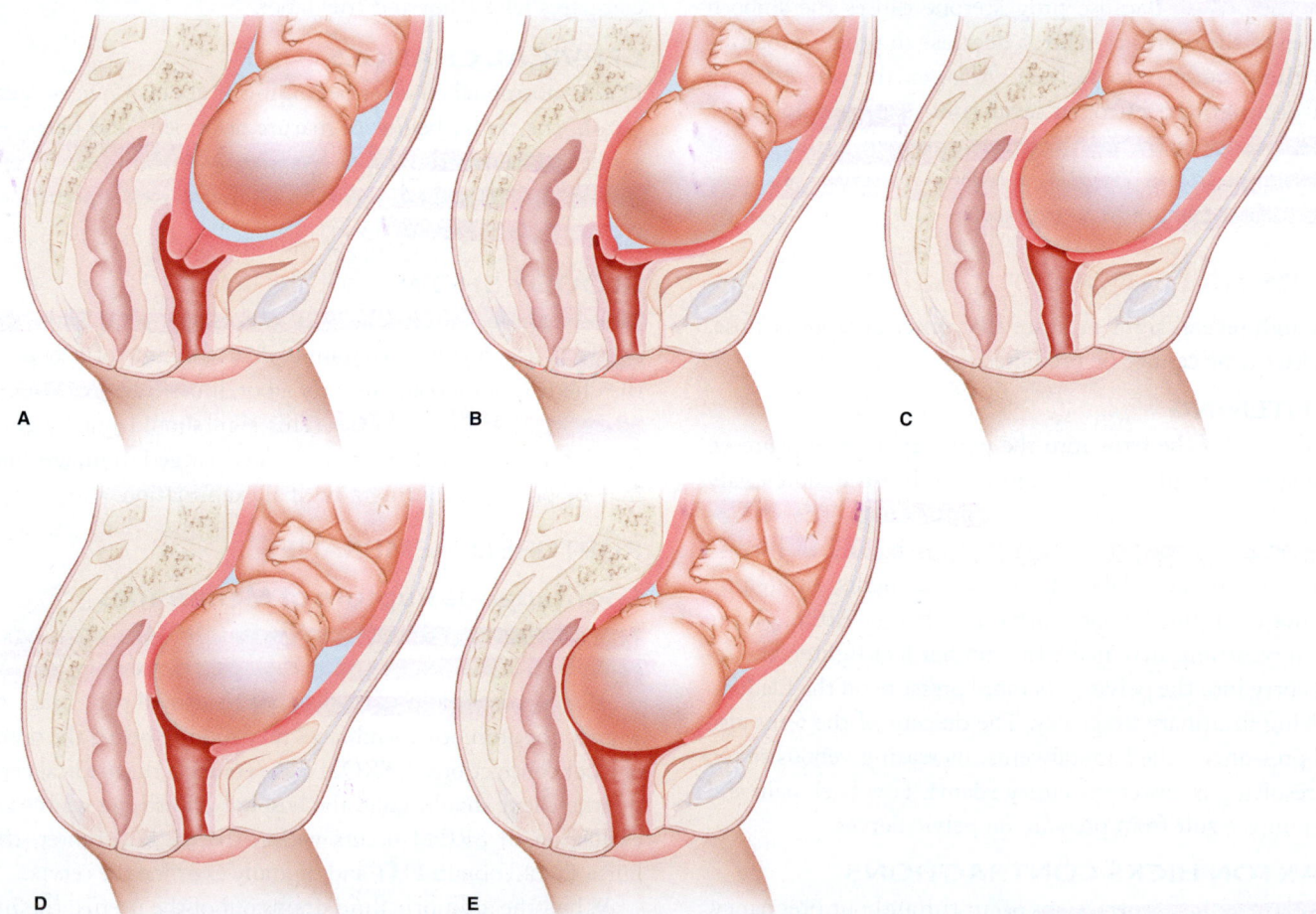

Figure 7-3. ■ Cervical effacement and dilatation of the cervix in a primigravida woman. (**A**) Cervix thick and closed. (**B**) Cervix effaced. (**C**) Cervix effaced and dilated 2–3 centimeters. (**D**) Cervix half open. (**E**) Cervix fully dilated (10 centimeters) and retracted.

In most cases of SROM prior to the onset of labor, contractions begin within 24 hours. Labor may be induced to avoid infection if either of the following applies:

- Labor does not begin within 24 hours after the membranes rupture.
- The pregnancy is near term.

Premature Rupture of Membranes

Premature rupture of membranes (PROM) occurs when the membranes rupture before the 38th week of gestation. This condition (also discussed in Chapter 8) can indicate the onset of premature labor. It requires immediate medical attention.

SUDDEN INCREASE IN ENERGY

Many women experience a sudden burst of energy a few days before labor begins. The woman feels a need to get the "house in order." This urge is sometimes called the "nesting instinct." The reason for the "nesting" is unknown. However, the woman should be careful not to tire herself because she will need energy for labor and for the demands of motherhood after the birth.

Admission to the Birthing Facility

When a client presents at a birthing facility, the staff must carefully assess the woman's condition. The stage of labor, condition of the mother, and condition of the fetus are the most important concerns.

Answers to some initial questions direct how the nurse proceeds with the rest of the admission process. For example, if the nurse determines that the client is in early labor with the first pregnancy, time is available to establish a nurse–client–family relationship, orient the client to the delivery suite, and provide instruction on relaxation techniques. If it is determined that the client is multipara in the second stage of labor, there may only be time to notify the care provider and to prepare for the birth.

Initially, the nurse will want to learn how long ago contractions began, how far apart they are, and how long they last. The nurse will ask whether the membranes have ruptured and whether this is the woman's first pregnancy. If the woman has been in labor before, the nurse will ask how long the previous labor was.

The nurse will review the prenatal record. Any complications during pregnancy will be noted. If the client has had no prenatal care, a more in-depth assessment will be made if time allows.

The assessment of the client should include:

- Maternal vital signs
- Urine dipstick for glucose and protein
- Fetal heart rate

- Contractions (frequency, duration, and intensity)
- Vaginal examination to determine cervical effacement and dilatation, fetal presentation, position, and station (usually done by the RN or physician)

clinical ALERT

If excessive vaginal bleeding is present, the nurse should consult with the care provider prior to the vaginal exam.

- Nitrazine test of vaginal secretions if the client is uncertain whether the membranes have ruptured (To perform a nitrazine test, touch the nitrazine paper to vaginal secretions and compare the paper to the color chart provided. The color will indicate whether amniotic fluid is present, and whether the membranes have ruptured.)
- Signs of pregnancy-induced hypertension (PIH), including edema, altered reflexes, and **clonus** (spasms or seizures).

CLIENT WHO IS NOT IN LABOR

If the client is not in labor, she may be sent home. This can be disappointing to the client and family, and emotional support may be needed. If it is questionable whether the client is in labor, she will be asked to walk for an hour and will then be reassessed.

Variables Affecting Labor

The variables that affect labor are many, but they can be grouped for easier discussion. These variables, known as the **Ps affecting labor,** refer to both maternal and fetal characteristics. The 5 Ps are passage, passenger, powers, position, and psyche.

PASSAGE

The first P, the **passage,** consists of the maternal structures through which the fetus must travel. The size and shape of the maternal pelvis can vary greatly among different women (Figure 7-4 ■). However, the pelvis must be adequate to accommodate the fetus.

Toward the end of pregnancy, the care provider will take measurements of the maternal pelvis to determine the adequacy of the pelvis. (See important landmarks of the maternal pelvis illustrated in Figure 7-4.) In **cephalopelvic disproportion (CPD),** the maternal pelvis is smaller than the fetal head. When this occurs, vaginal delivery will be impossible. Birth must be by cesarean section.

As the due date approaches, the care provider will monitor the station of the fetus. **Station** refers to the relationship between the fetus and the maternal ischial spines. When the fetus reaches 0 station, the head is considered to be fully engaged. Figure 7-5 ■ illustrates stations.

Uterine contractions (discussed under Powers later in this section) push the fetus against the cervix. They cause the cervical mouth (or *os*) to open so the fetus can enter the vagina.

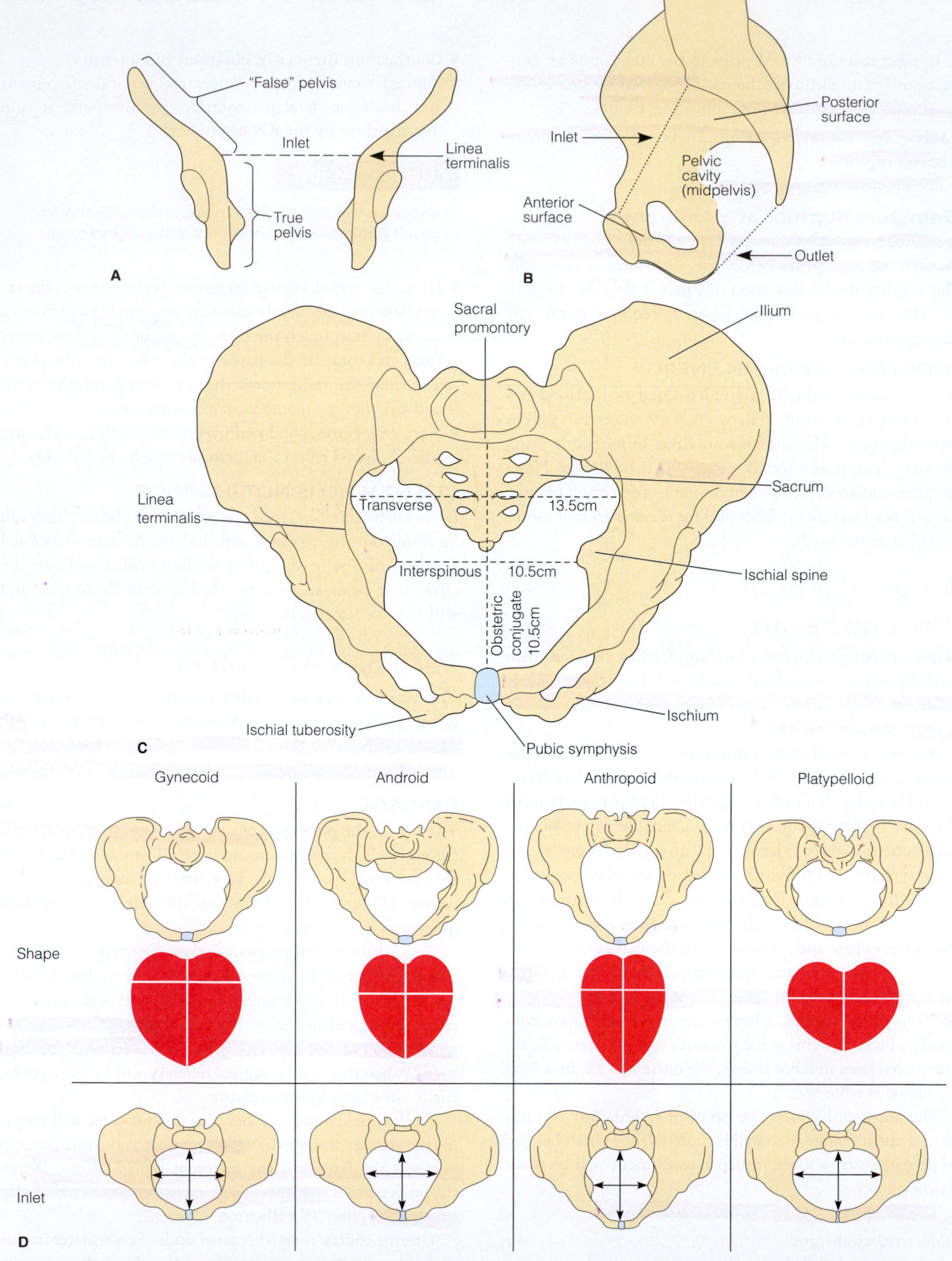

Figure 7-4. ■ Female pelvis. **(A)** False pelvis is a shallow cavity above the inlet. The true pelvis is the deeper portion of the cavity below the inlet. **(B)** The true pelvis consists of inlet, cavity (midpelvis), and outlet. **(C)** Pelvic planes: coronal section and common diameters of the bony pelvis. **(D)** Varying shapes of the female pelvis and inlet can affect the passage of the fetus.

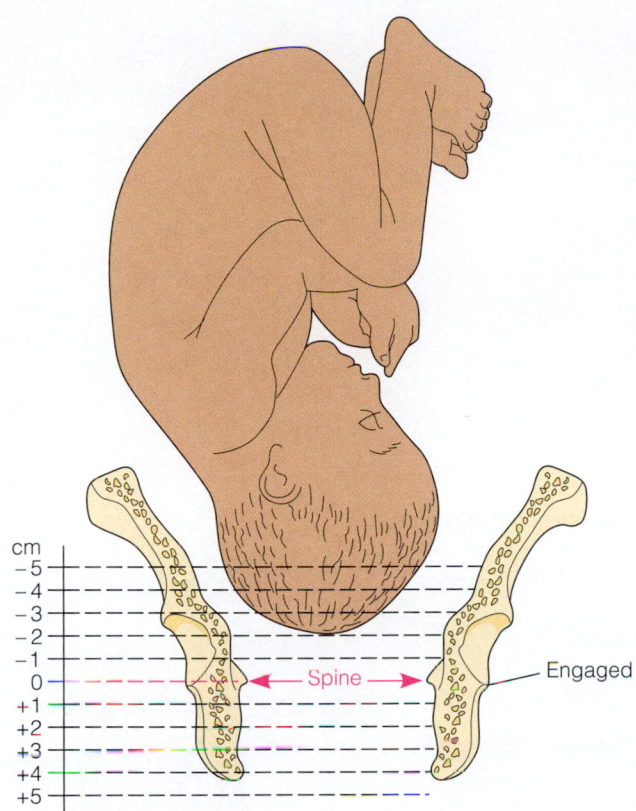

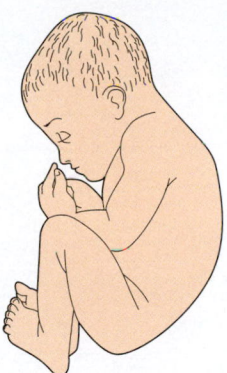

Figure 7-6. ■ Fetal attitude. The relationship of body parts of this fetus is normal. The head is flexed forward, with the chin almost resting on the chest. The arms and legs are flexed.

Figure 7-5. ■ Measuring the station of the fetal head while it is descending. In this view, the station is −2/−3.

the head and arms, labor will be more difficult, and a vaginal birth may not be possible.

FETAL LIE. **Fetal lie** is the relationship of the long axis (head-to-foot or *cephalocaudal* axis) of the fetus to the long axis of the mother. When the long axis of the fetus is parallel to the long axis of the mother, the fetus is in a *longitudinal lie.* If the long axis of the fetus is at a right angle to the long axis of the mother, it is termed a **transverse lie** (Figure 7-7 ■). Obviously, labor with a fetus in transverse lie could be much more

By the end of pregnancy, estrogen has softened the *rugae* (or folds) of the vagina. These changes allow it to stretch enough so the fetus is able to pass through it.

The pressure of the fetus against the muscles of the perineum causes the perineal tissue to thin and stretch. At times the perineum may tear, or it may be surgically cut to lessen trauma to the tissue. In either event, the perineum is sutured after birth to ensure healing.

PASSENGER

The second of the 5 Ps refers to the **passenger,** or fetus. Two things affect how easily the fetus can be delivered:

- The relationship of fetal parts to the maternal uterus and pelvis
- The size of the fetus.

Relationship of Fetal Parts to Maternal Uterus and Pelvis

Three concepts are important in discussing the relationship of fetal parts to maternal structures. These are fetal attitude, fetal lie, and fetal presentation.

FETAL ATTITUDE. **Fetal attitude** is the relationship of fetal body parts to one another. Ideally, the fetus assumes a state of flexion (Figure 7-6 ■), with the head flexed onto the chest, the arms flexed over the chest, and the legs flexed over the abdomen. If any part of the fetus is in extension, especially

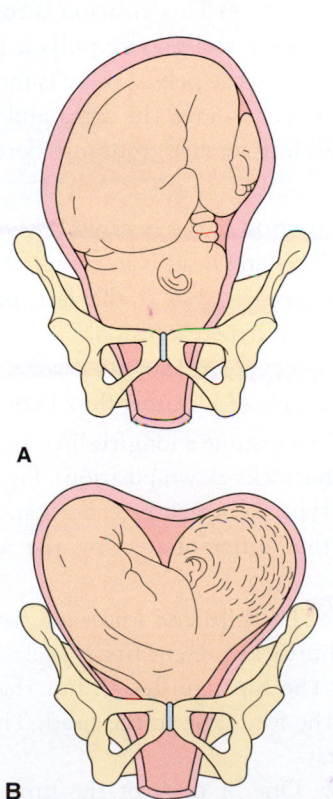

Figure 7-7. ■ Fetal lie. (**A**) Longitudinal. (**B**) Transverse.

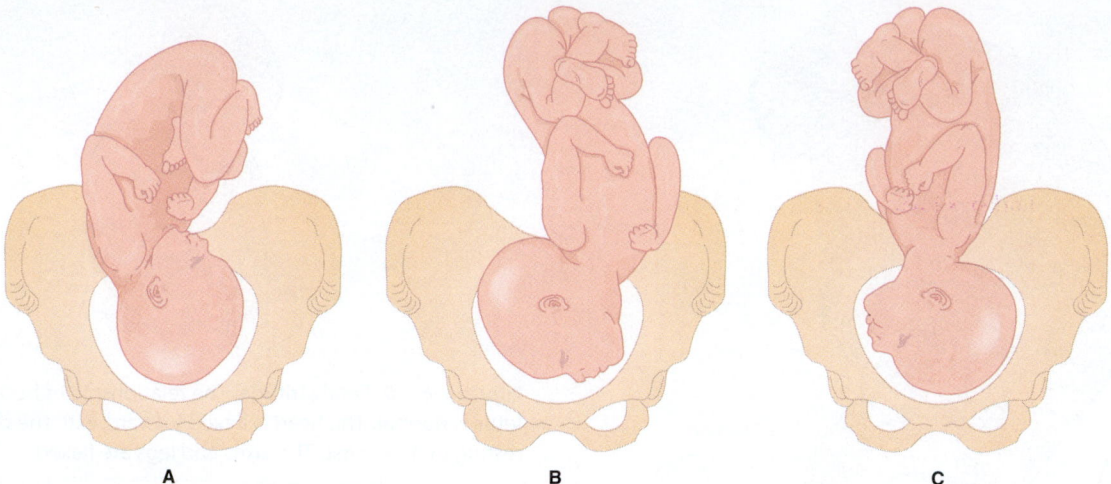

Figure 7-8. ■ Cephalic presentations. (**A**) Vertex/occiput presentation. (**B**) Face (*mentum*) presentation. (**C**) Brow (*sinciput*) presentation.

difficult than one in which the fetus's body is in line with the mother's. If the fetus does not turn to a longitudinal lie, a vaginal delivery will not be possible. Figure 7-7 illustrates fetal lie.

FETAL PRESENTATION. **Fetal presentation,** the body part of the fetus that is closest to the cervix, is determined by the fetal lie. At term, the fetus usually assumes a longitudinal lie with a **cephalic presentation** (head-down position). (See Figure 7-8. ■) This position is common because the fetal head is heavy, and gravity pulls it into the pelvis. With the fetal head in the pelvis, there is more room in the uterus for the fetus to move the arms and legs. Cephalic presentations fall into further groupings determined by the fetal attitude.

- **Vertex presentation** is the **occiput** (crown of head) presenting first. The fetal head is in complete flexion.
- *Face* (**mentum**) *presentation* is the face presenting first. The head is in full hyperextension.
- *Brow presentation* is the **sinciput** (forehead or brow) presenting first. The fetal head is neither flexed nor hyperextended.

The fetus might assume a longitudinal lie with a **breech presentation** (buttocks-down position). Figure 7-9 ■ illustrates different types of breech presentation. Breech presentations are further differentiated by the attitude of the fetus's legs.

- *Complete breech.* The hips and knees are flexed on the abdomen. The buttocks present first.
- *Frank breech.* The hips are flexed, but the knees are extended with the feet close to the head. The buttocks are presenting first.
- *Footling breech.* One or both of the hips and knees are extended, with the foot (feet) being the presenting part.

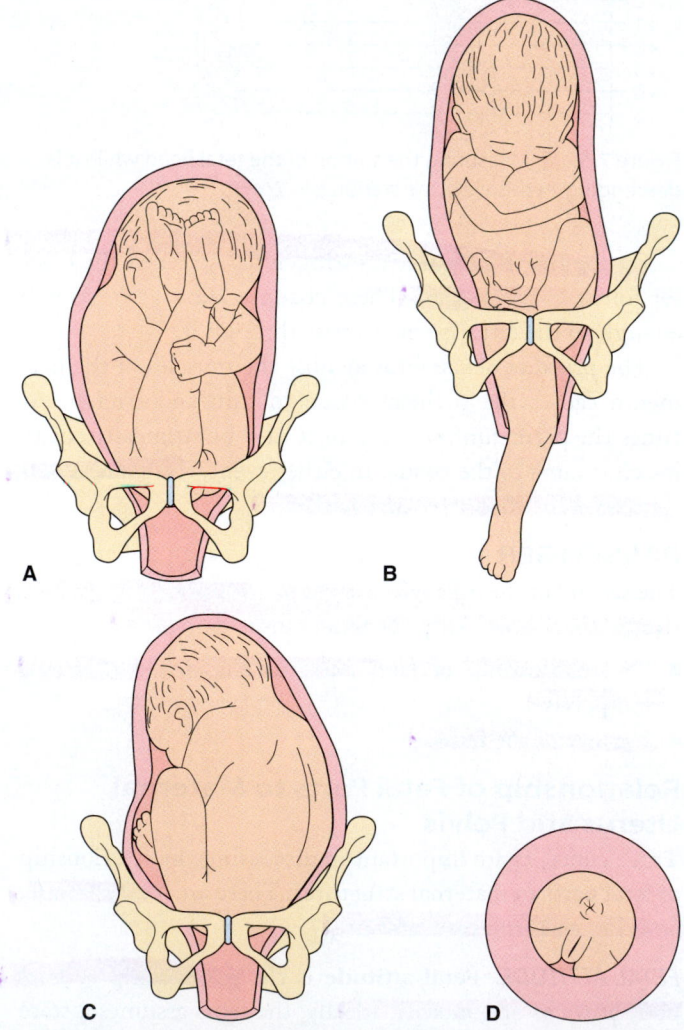

Figure 7-9. ■ Breech presentations. (**A**) Frank breech. (**B**) Incomplete (footling) breech. (**C**) Complete breech. (**D**) Anal sphincter may be felt on examination; buttocks tissue will be soft.

MediaLink Breech birth

If the fetus assumes a transverse lie (see Figure 7-9), the presenting part will be the shoulder, arm, back, abdomen, or side. The fetus in a transverse presentation cannot be delivered vaginally. See discussion of cesarean delivery in Chapter 8 ⚭.

FETAL POSITION. **Fetal position** refers to the relationship of the presenting part to the four quadrants of the maternal pelvis. The fetal landmarks are identified in the right or left, anterior or posterior quadrants of the mother's pelvis. Abbreviations are typically used to indicate fetal position.

- The first letter refers to the mother's right or left side.
- The second letter refers to the fetal landmark.
- The third letter refers to the mother's anterior or posterior quadrant.

The ideal position for a vaginal delivery is either right occiput anterior (ROA) or left occiput anterior (LOA). Table 7-2 ■

(Text continues on p. 178.)

TABLE 7-2

Common Fetal Positions

ABBREVIATION OF PRESENTATION	PRESENTING PART	DESCRIPTION OF FETAL POSITION
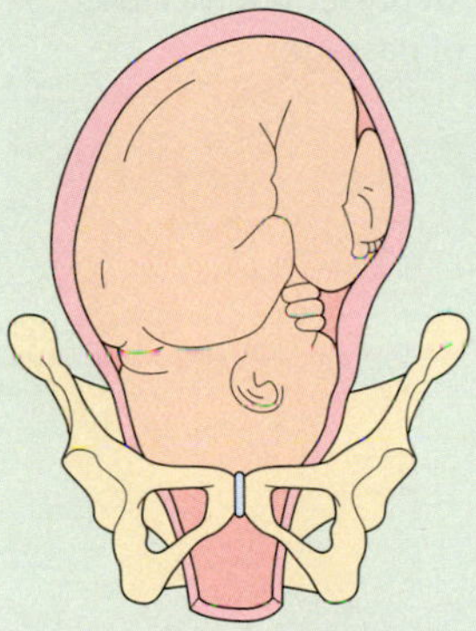 **Figure 7-10.** ■ ROA	Occiput	Right side of maternal pelvis, occiput presenting, occiput directed toward anterior (front) of passage
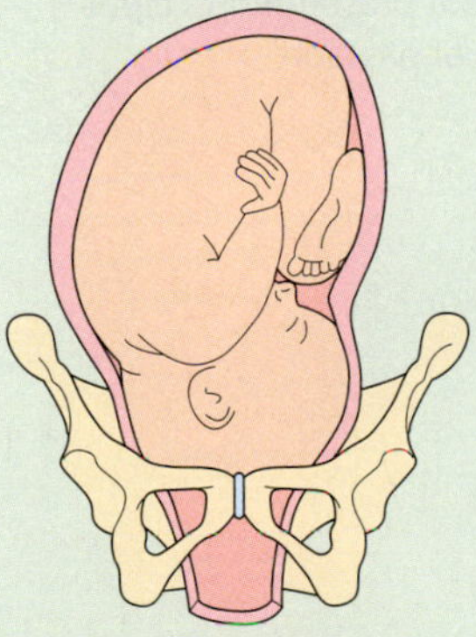 **Figure 7-10.** ■ ROT	Occiput	Right side of maternal pelvis, occiput presenting, occiput transverse (directed toward side of passage)
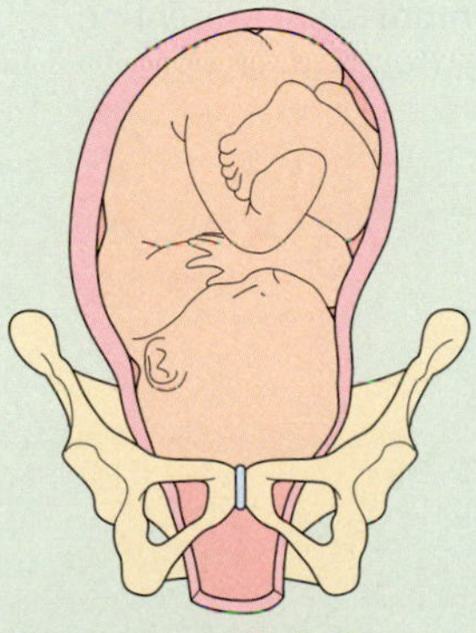 **Figure 7-10.** ■ ROP	Occiput	Right side of maternal pelvis, occiput presenting, occiput directed toward posterior (back) of passage

(continued)

TABLE 7-2

Common Fetal Positions (continued)

ABBREVIATION OF PRESENTATION	PRESENTING PART	DESCRIPTION OF FETAL POSITION
 Figure 7-10. ■ LOA	Occiput	Left side of maternal pelvis, occiput presenting, occiput directed toward anterior (front) of passage
 Figure 7-10. ■ LOT	Occiput	Left side of maternal pelvis, occiput presenting, occiput transverse (directed toward side of passage)
 Figure 7-10. ■ LOP	Occiput	Left side of maternal pelvis, occiput presenting, occiput directed toward posterior (back) of passage
 Figure 7-10. ■ RMA	Mentum (chin)	Right side of maternal pelvis, mentum (chin) presenting, mentum directed toward anterior (front) of passage

TABLE 7-2

Common Fetal Positions (continued)

ABBREVIATION OF PRESENTATION	PRESENTING PART	DESCRIPTION OF FETAL POSITION
Figure 7-10. ■ RMP	Mentum	Right side of maternal pelvis, mentum (chin) presenting, mentum directed toward posterior (back) of passage
Figure 7-10. ■ LMA	Mentum	Left side of maternal pelvis, mentum (chin) presenting, mentum directed toward anterior (front) of passage
Figure 7-10. ■ LSA	Sacrum	Left side of maternal pelvis, sacrum presenting, sacrum directed toward anterior (front) of passage
Figure 7-10. ■ LSP	Sacrum	Left side of maternal pelvis, sacrum presenting, sacrum directed toward posterior (back) of passage

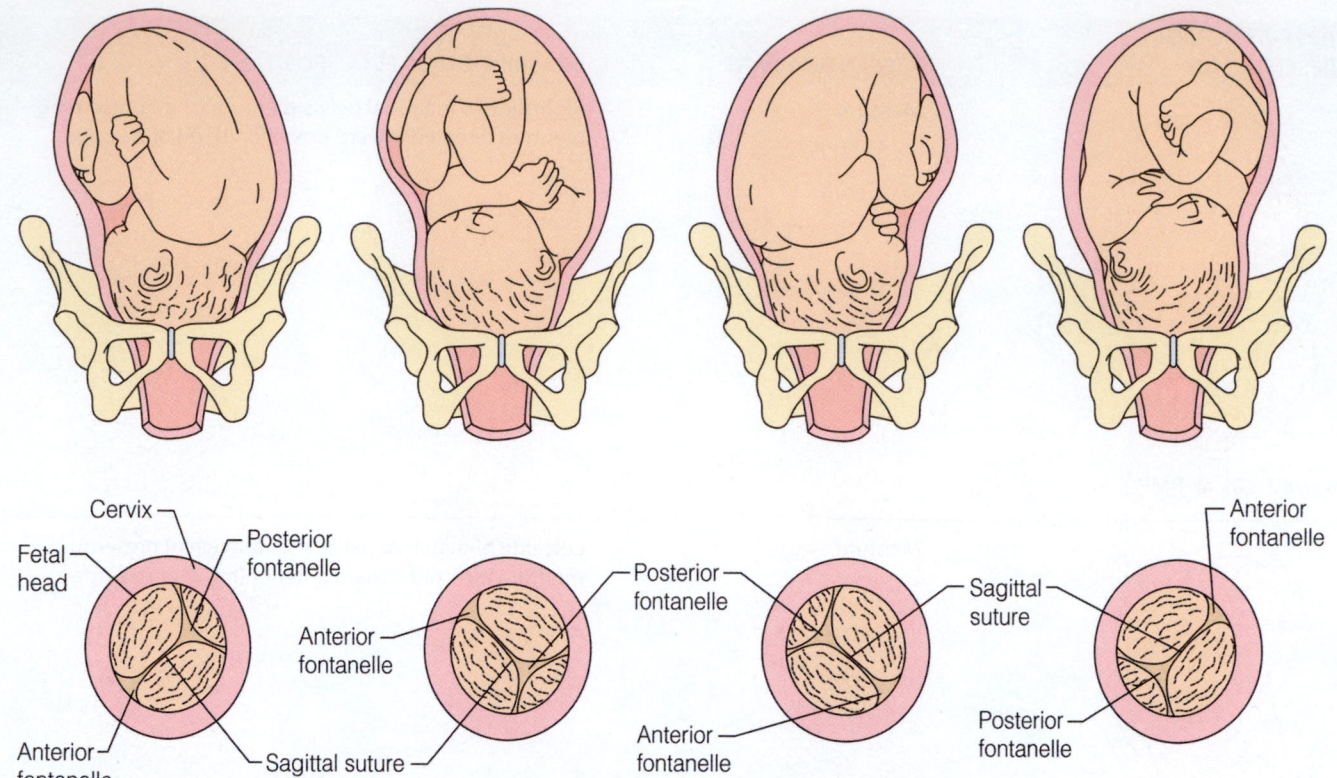

Figure 7-11. ■ Palpating the sutures in the skull to determine position of the fetus. (**A**) Left occiput anterior (LOA). The occiput (area over the occipital bone on the posterior part of the fetal head) is in the left anterior quadrant of the woman's pelvis. When the fetus is LOA, the posterior fontanel (located just above the occipital bone and triangular in shape) is in the upper left quadrant of the maternal pelvis. (**B**) The left occiput posterior (LOP). The posterior fontanel is in the lower left quadrant of the maternal pelvis. (**C**) The right occiput anterior (ROA). The posterior fontanel is in the upper right quadrant of the maternal pelvis. (**D**) The right occiput posterior (ROP). The posterior fontanel is in the lower right quadrant of the maternal pelvis. *Note:* The anterior fontanel is diamond shaped. Because of the roundness of the fetal head, only a portion of the anterior fontanel can be seen in each view, so it appears to be triangular in shape.

(which includes Figure 7-10 ■) describes and illustrates common fetal positions.

Size of the Fetus

The largest part of the fetus is the head. The bones of the fetal skull are not fused but are instead joined by fibrous connective tissue called **sutures**. Large spaces, called **fontanels**, prevent undue pressure on the fetal brain. Figure 7-11 ■ illustrates the bones, suture lines, and fontanels in various presentations. In a cephalic presentation, as the top of the fetal head is pushed through the maternal pelvis, the bones of the skull ride over one another, decreasing the diameter of the head. This shaping of the fetal head to the bones of the maternal pelvis is termed **molding** (Figure 7-12 ■). In a breech presentation, the fetal head moves through the pelvis neck first. This direction of movement prevents pressure on the top of the fetal head, so molding does not occur. The fetal head may be too large to pass through the maternal pelvis, leading to an ominous prognosis.

See Figure 7-11 for the position of fontanels and sutures in relation to the position of the fetus within the birth canal.

POWERS

The third of the 5 Ps affecting labor refers to the powers necessary to push the fetus through the passageway. These powers are (1) the power of uterine contractions and (2) the strength of the mother pushing the baby.

Primary Power

The primary power comes from the involuntary muscle contractions of the myometrium. Uterine contractions begin in response to the posterior pituitary hormone, oxytocin. **Contractions**, which begin in the fundus, are the result of shortening of the muscle fibers.

Muscle fibers of the uterus have several unique properties.

1. Uterine muscle fibers contract and relax in a rhythmic pattern. During relaxation, circulation is restored to the placenta, improving oxygenation of the fetus.

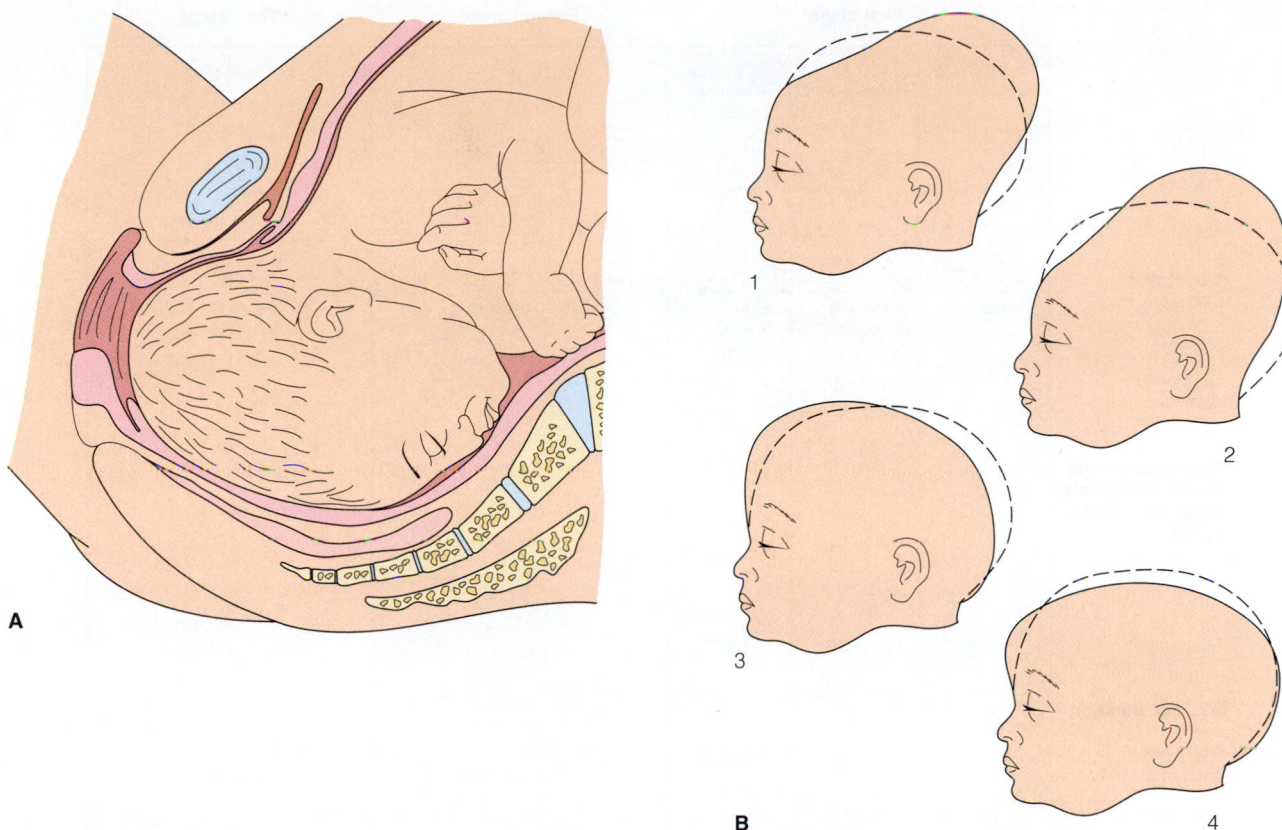

Figure 7-12. ■ Effects of labor on the fetal head. (**A**) The caput succedaneum formation. The presenting portion of the scalp area is encircled by the cervix during labor, causing swelling of the soft tissue. (**B**) Molding of the fetal head in cephalic presentations: (1) occiput anterior, (2) occiput posterior, (3) brow, and (4) face.

2. Contracted uterine muscle fibers remain shortened. This results in a gradual decrease in the size of the uterine cavity. As the uterine muscle fibers shorten, the lower uterine segment is pulled up, and the fetus is pushed down. These actions result in *effacement* (shortening and thinning of the cervix) and *dilatation* (opening of the cervical os). See Figure 7-3 to review effacement and dilatation.

CHARACTERISTICS OF CONTRACTIONS. Contractions are described in terms of frequency, duration, and intensity. Figure 7-13 ■ shows contraction patterns in the first, second, and third stages of labor.

- **Frequency** is the time from the onset of one contraction to the onset of the next contraction.
- **Duration** is the time from the onset of a contraction to the end of that contraction.
- **Intensity** is the strength of the contraction at its peak.

As mentioned, blood supply through the uterus to the placenta is decreased during contractions. Ideally, the fre-

quency of contractions should be every 3 to 5 minutes, with a duration of not more than 90 seconds. This allows time, during uterine relaxation, for circulation to be restored and the fetus to recover. To push the fetus through the cervix, contractions must be of moderate to strong intensity.

Secondary Power

The secondary power comes from the mother actively pushing the fetus through the birth canal. The spontaneous urge to push, known as **Ferguson's reflex**, occurs when the presenting part reaches the pelvic floor. Stretch receptors in the vagina trigger the release of oxytocin, which intensifies contractions. Ferguson's reflex may occur without full cervical effacement. To prevent trauma of the cervix, the woman is discouraged from pushing until the cervix has dilated completely.

POSITION

The fourth P affecting labor is the *position of the mother* during labor. The mother may need frequent changes of

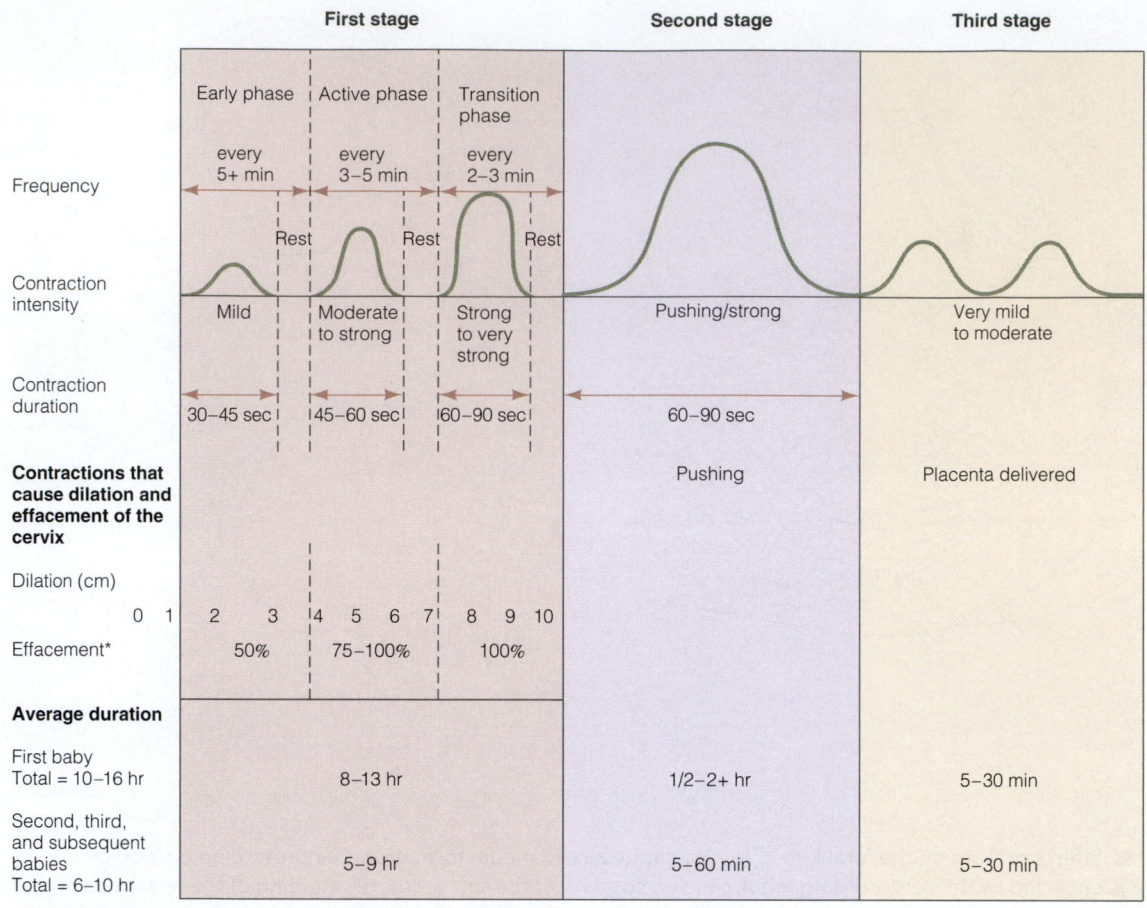

Figure 7-13. ■ Contraction patterns in first, second, and third stages of labor. Primigravidas may be 100% effaced before labor begins.

position as labor progresses. Changes of position relieve muscle tension, support different areas of the body, and provide some distraction. Some options are shown in Figure 7-14 ■. It is important for the nurse to assist the client in finding a comfortable position. There is no single"right" position for labor.

If the mother lies on her back, the contractions are more frequent but of lower intensity. When the mother lies on her side, the contractions are less frequent but of greater intensity. Therefore, it may be helpful to position the mother on her left side, using pillows to support her back and leg. The side-lying position also prevents supine hypotension syndrome.

PSYCHE

Psyche, the fifth P affecting labor, refers to the mother's emotional status during labor. The mother's emotions while delivering a child are determined by past experiences, expectations, culture, and ideas about how to behave during labor.

Cultures vary considerably in their views and expectations of the labor process. Some differences among cultures are highlighted in Box 7-1 ■.

Fear and anxiety can have a profound effect on the labor experience. If the woman is fearful and anxious, a negative cycle can emerge. Fear and anxiety stimulate the mother's adrenal gland to release additional epinephrine and norepinephrine. These "fight-or-flight" hormones have several effects.

■ They constrict blood vessels (restricting placental circulation).
■ They decrease the effectiveness of contractions.
■ They tighten skeletal muscles.

When skeletal muscles of the pelvic floor are tight, they do not stretch easily. To widen them, the uterus needs to contract harder, increasing discomfort. Discomfort increases tension and anxiety. These three factors become a cycle, making the labor a longer and less positive experience. The nurse can provide (or teach a partner to provide)

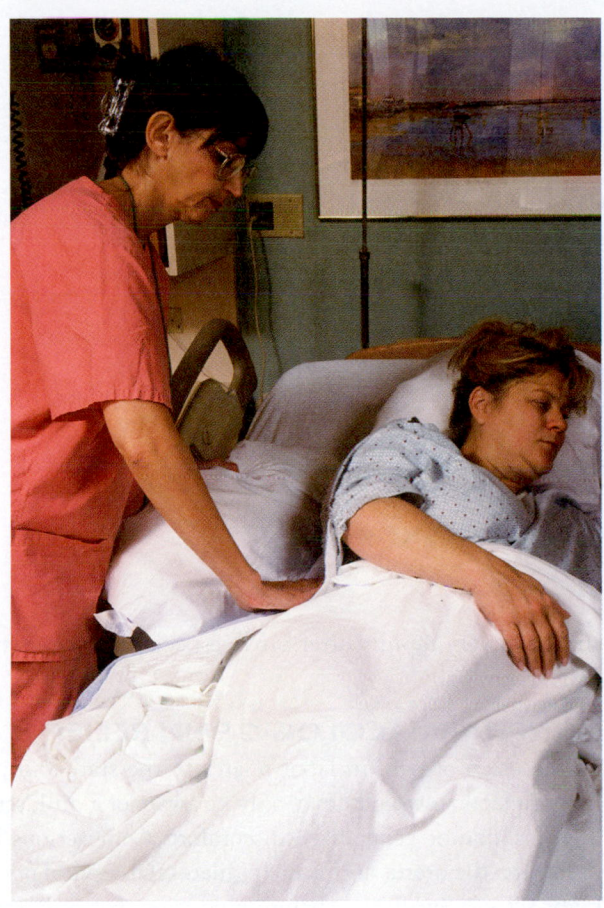

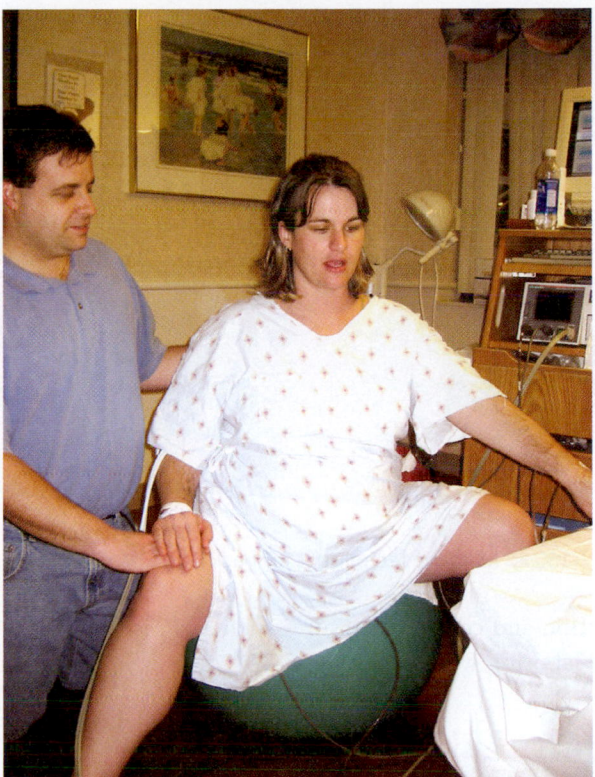

B

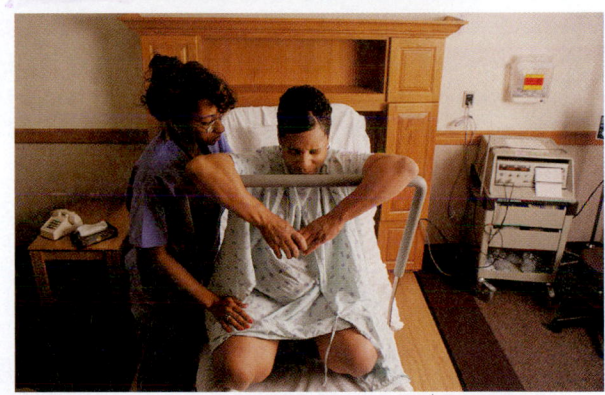

C

A

Figure 7-14. ■ (**A**) The nurse helps the client in labor assume a side-lying position to promote efficiency of contractions and maternal comfort. (**B**) Birthing ball facilitates fetal descent and fetal rotation, and helps increase the diameter of the pelvis. (**C**) Birthing bar.

BOX 7-1	CULTURAL PULSE POINTS

Considerations in Birthing Practices

China
Stoic response to pain. Fathers not present during birth. Prefer side lying during labor and delivery because they believe there is less trauma to fetus.

India
Natural childbirth practices preferred. Fathers usually not present. Female relatives usually present.

Iran
Fathers not present. Prefer female support and female caregivers. (If Muslim, may prefer to retain head covering and have body covered; two long-sleeved gowns may be offered.)

Japan
Natural childbirth methods practiced. May labor silently. Father may be present.

Laos
May want to be active and moving about during labor. May use squatting position for birth. Fathers may or may not be present. May prefer not to have amniotomy until right before birth. Prefer female caregivers. Prefer hot food and warm water during labor (St. Hill et al., 2003).

Mexico
May be stoic about discomfort until second stage, then may request pain relief. Father and female relatives may be present.

South Korea
Stoic during labor. Fathers usually not present.

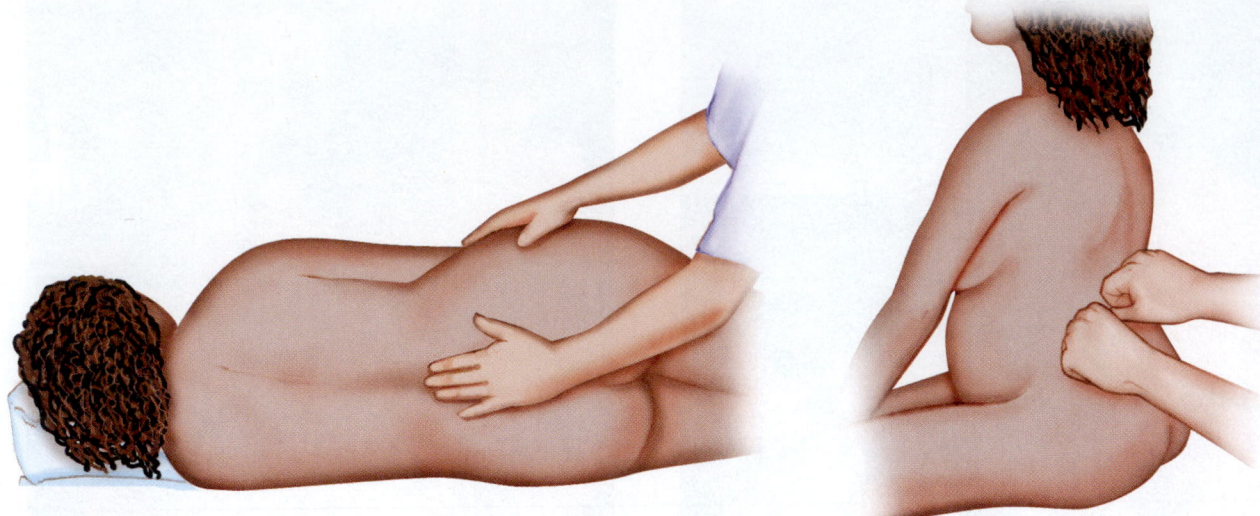

Figure 7-15. ■ Massage techniques for back labor.

distraction and comfort measures such as a sacral massage for the laboring woman (Figure 7-15 ■).

Pain in Labor

The pain of labor has several unique features. Its focus shifts as labor progresses (Figure 7-16A–C ■). It may cause anxiety and some level of fear. However, in most instances it is also associated with excitement and anticipation. Although it may begin as a mild ache, it builds to great intensity within a fairly short period of time. It is relieved abruptly

and often very rapidly after birth, especially in women who deliver vaginally.

NONPHARMACOLOGIC PAIN RELIEF

The location of pain in labor relates to the state and phase. Early in labor, a woman may only be aware of a dull, stretching sensation or generalized discomfort. Contractions begin to shorten the uterus and stretch (dilate) the cervical opening. Light activity (walking, changing position, bathing, rocking on hands and knees) may be acceptable during the latent phase to help distract the mother while labor proceeds. Other

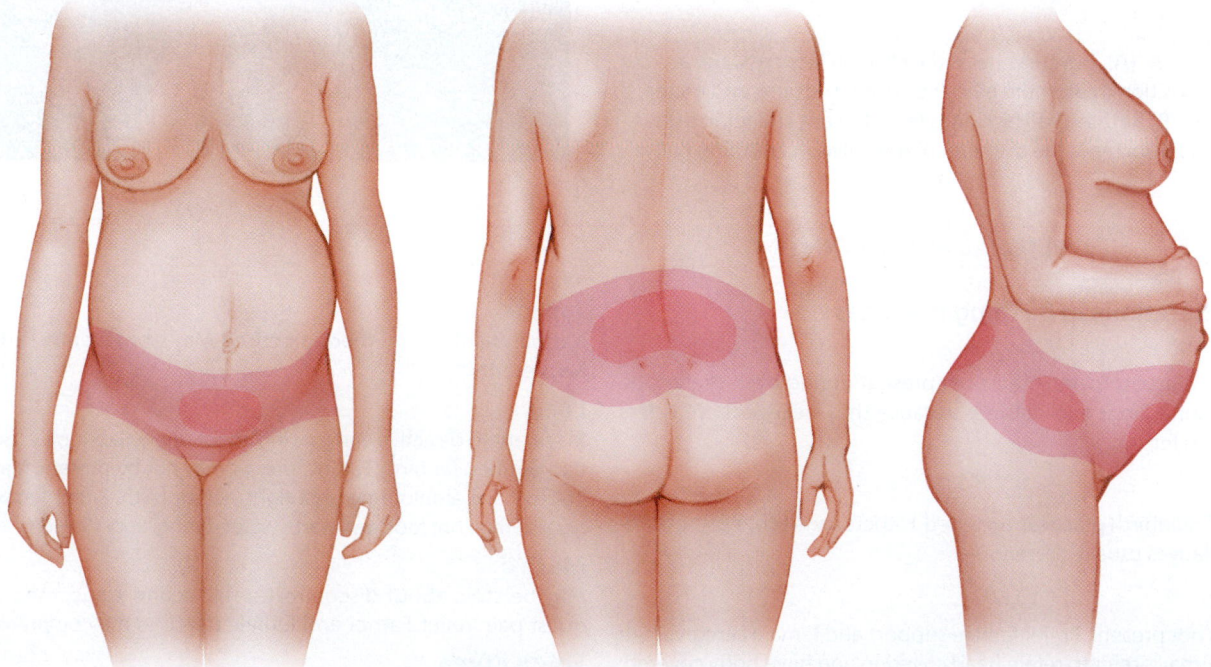

A

Figure 7-16. ■ Distribution of pain in labor. Graduated shades of color indicate intensity of pain. (**A**) Early phase of Stage one labor. (**B**) Latter phase of Stage one and early Stage two labor. (**C**) Latter phase of Stage two and actual delivery. (Adapted, with permission from Bonica, J. J., & McDonald, J. S. [Eds.]. [1995]. *Principles and practice of obstetric analgesia & anesthesia* [2nd ed.]. Baltimore: Lea & Febiger.)

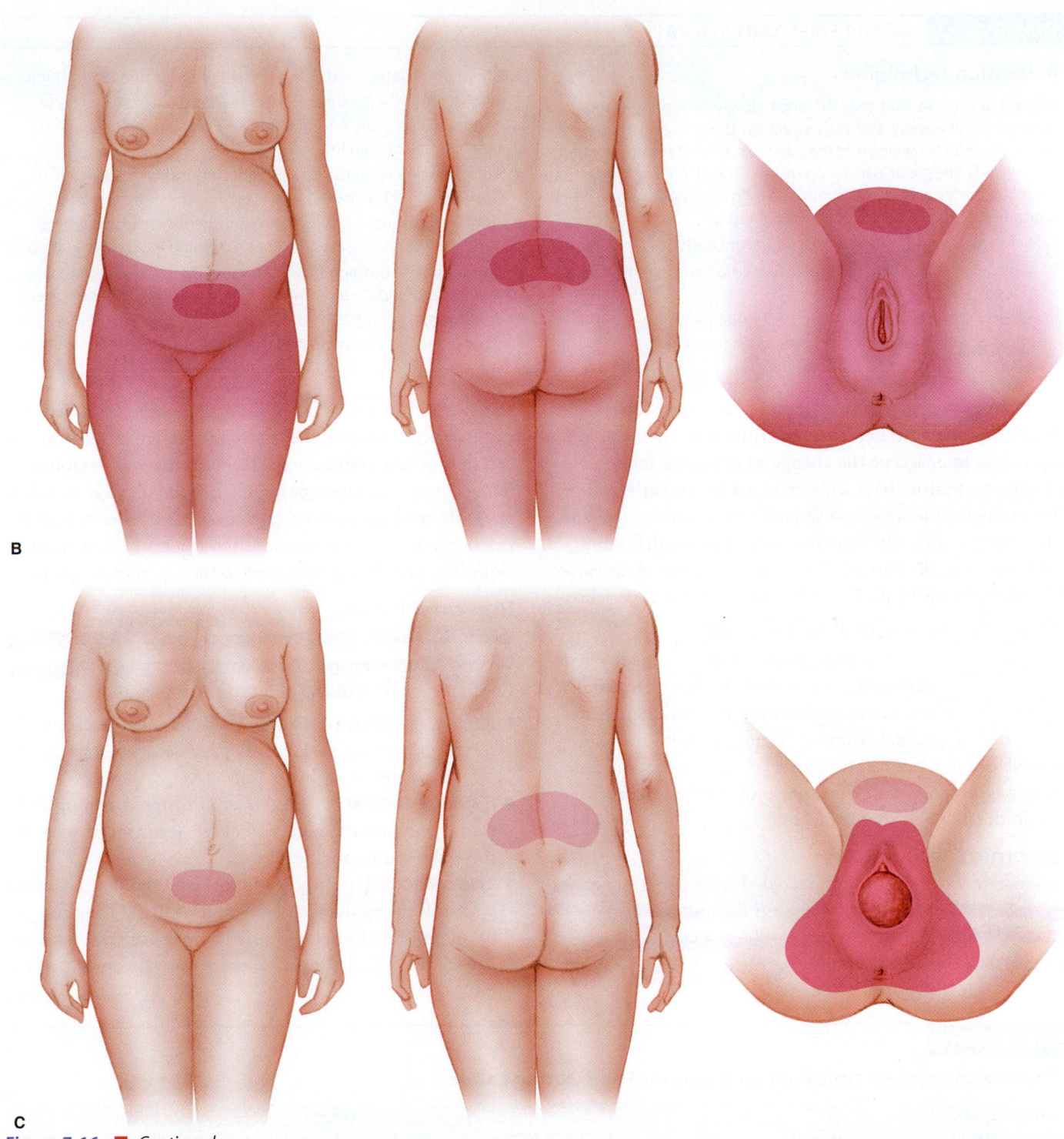

Figure 7-16. ■ *Continued.*

relaxation techniques, such as guided imagery and light massage, can also be useful. Box 7-2 ■ describes several complementary therapies that may be useful to women in labor.

As labor progresses from the latent to the active phase, the pain and pressure shift (see Figure 7-16B). Nurses can teach partners to provide counterpressure to the continuing contractions. For example, a sacral massage (see Figure 7-15) can provide comfort at this phase.

Some women go into labor wanting to experience **natural childbirth** (labor and birth without medical interventions or pain medication). This approach may motivate a woman to "look beyond the pain" and to use breathing and relaxation techniques to work her way through the stages of labor. Natural childbirth may create a tremendous feeling of empowerment. However, if a woman is encountering difficulties or the labor is progressing very slowly, it

BOX 7-2   COMPLEMENTARY THERAPIES

Relaxation Techniques

Labor is a process that may advance slowly or rapidly. It requires great physical energy and puts strain on the musculoskeletal system. It is useful for women as they approach labor to have a variety of methods they can use to provide comfort and/or distraction while the body continues its work. The following options have been found useful and are accessible to all women:

- Hydrotherapy—a warm bath or whirlpool bath
- Application of heat or cold—warm or cold compress directly to an area
- Imagery and visualization—focused, quiet picturing of the uterus opening gently to allow the birth to occur
- Effleurage—(latent and active phases of Stage one labor) rhythmic stroking and massage of the abdomen (see Figure 7-32B)
- Abdominal pressure—(end Stage one labor) deep massage to area of greatest pain intensity
- Biofeedback—response to a painful stimulus with a specific relaxation technique (best if practiced beforehand)
- Comfort measures—rinsing the mouth, gentle cleansing with a warm washcloth, change of clothes if clothing has become damp
- Distractions—soothing or encouraging words, music, watching television, looking out a window, listening to the fetal heartbeat
- Application of childbirth education—using the breathing and other techniques learned in prenatal classes

may be important for her to safeguard her energy by receiving pharmacologic relief. In such situations, the nurse can help the woman accept the change as necessary for her and her infant's health. It is important to be empathetic but firm in these situations, and to remind the woman that she is handling a difficult situation well. The Health Promotion Issue on pages 186 and 187 examines some of the variables that can have a positive effect on the labor experience.

PHARMACOLOGIC PAIN RELIEF

For some women, nonpharmacologic methods of pain relief are not enough, due to the position of the fetus, the length of the labor, the level of discomfort the woman can tolerate, and other individual factors. When nonpharmacologic methods are not sufficient, pharmacologic methods of pain relief may be provided. The choice of method depends in part on the phase or stage of labor.

Systemic Medications

Systemic medications administered during labor are narcotic analgesics. These drugs should be administered only when the client's vital signs are stable, the fetus is at term, the FHR is in a normal pattern between 120 and 160, and

the client is in active labor. Caution is required when administering systemic medications. Systemic medications can slow or stop contractions if labor is not well established. When given in transition or in the second stage of labor, systemic medications can cause respiratory distress in the newborn. Table 7-3 ■ provides information about medications that may be administered to the client during labor.

Regional Blocks

Regional blocks or regional anesthetics are administered by the physician, anesthesiologist, or nurse anesthetist. Common regional blocks (Figure 7-17 ■) include:

- *Paracervical block.* The drug is administered around the cervix during active labor to provide anesthesia to the cervix and upper vagina.
- *Pudendal block.* The drug is administered through the vagina and into the pudendal nerve, resulting in anesthesia of the vagina and perineum.
- *Epidural block.* The drug is administered through a catheter placed in the epidural space (Figure 7-17C). The drug can be administered intermittently or by continuous infusion. Anesthesia usually involves the lower abdomen, pelvis,

(Text continues on p. 188.)

TABLE 7-3

Pharmacology: Systemic Pain Medications Used During Labor

DRUG (COMMON BRAND NAME AND GENERIC)	USUAL ROUTE/DOSE	CLASSIFICATION AND PURPOSE	SELECTED SIDE EFFECTS AND NURSING CONSIDERATIONS	DON'T GIVE IF
Stadol (butorphano tartrate)	1–2 mg IV every 3–4 hours	Opioid analgesic for pain	Respiratory depression, dizziness, euphoria	In second stage of labor
Demerol (meperidine HCL)	2.5–15 mg IV every 3–4 hours	Opioid analgesic for pain	Respiratory depression, sedation	In second stage of labor *or* if allergic to drug
Narcan (naloxone)	0.4–2 mg IV may repeat every 2–3 minutes to total of 10 mg	Narcotic antagonist for relief of respiratory depression in substance abuse	Respiratory depression may recur when Narcan wears off; monitor respiratory status carefully	Total of 10 mg has been given without improvement, *or* if you question narcotic overdose

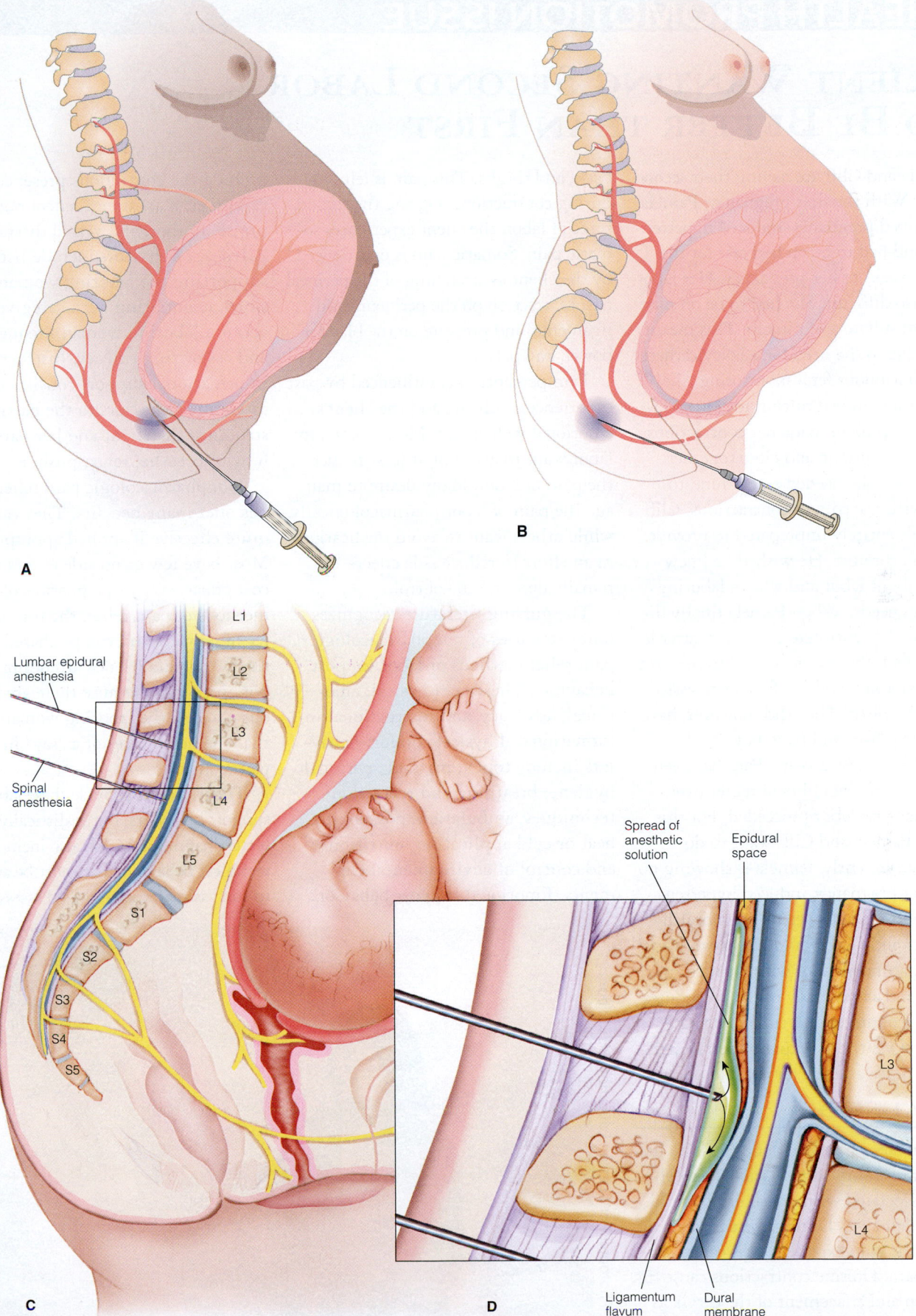

A

B

Lumbar epidural anesthesia

Spinal anesthesia

L1
L2
L3
L4
L5
S1
S2
S3
S4
S5

C

Spread of anesthetic solution

Epidural space

L3

L4

Ligamentum flavum

Dural membrane

D

Figure 7-17. ■ (**A**) Paracervical block (sensory pathways and site of interruption in relation to fetus). (**B**) Pudendal block. (**C**) Placement of epidural and spinal anesthetics. (**D**) Illustrates the epidural space, located between the dura and the vertebra. The slight bulge illustrates the dura being pushed away from the tip of the needle by the force of the injection.

185

CLIENT WANTING SECOND LABOR TO BE BETTER THAN FIRST

Pamela and Cliff are having their second child. With the first pregnancy, Pamela developed pregnancy-induced hypertension and had to be on bed rest for the last 6 weeks of her pregnancy. Her labor was also difficult. She had to be on magnesium sulfate and pitocin. This meant that, due to the need for a Foley catheter and continuous fetal monitoring, she had to stay in bed during the entire labor. The pitocin made her contractions extremely intense and close together. Therefore, she needed an epidural to deal with the pain of contractions. Cliff also felt entirely unprepared to provide her any comfort. He wished he knew more about labor and what a laboring woman needs. When Pamela finally dilated to 10 centimeter, 14 hours after labor began, the physician had to perform an episiotomy and use forceps to assist with the birth. They did, however, have a healthy, 8-pound baby boy.

Over the last 2 years, Pam has been disturbed by thoughts of regret over how her first labor proceeded. For this birth, Pamela and Cliff want to do things differently. Pamela is showing no signs of pregnancy-induced hypertension, and the baby seems to be healthy. Pamela and Cliff would like to go into labor naturally, labor without medications, and avoid many of the procedures they encountered last time. During a prenatal visit, they explain their desires to the nurse and ask for assistance.

DISCUSSION

Pain in labor has been defined as "an unpleasant sensory and emotional experience associated with actual or potential tissue damage." During the first stage of labor, the pain experienced is called visceral pain. Uterine contractions cause dilatation and effacement of the cervix as well as tissue ischemia. Visceral pain is felt by the client in her lower abdomen, back, and thighs. This pain is felt only during contractions. During the second stage of labor, the client experiences somatic pain. Somatic pain is experienced by the client as stretching of the perineal tissues, traction on the perineum and ligaments, and pressure on the bladder, bowel, and pelvis.

Pain perception is influenced by past experiences, culture, and the client's emotional well-being. Most women in labor want to avoid or at least reduce the pain of labor. Many desire to manage the pain of labor pharmacologically, while others want to avoid medications in an effort to reduce side effects and remain alert and in control.

The nursing literature recognizes four categories of nonpharmacologic pain relief methods or labor support behaviors. These are physical, emotional, advocacy, and instructional/informational. Physical comfort behaviors include touch, massage, personal hygiene, breathing and relaxation techniques, ambulation, positioning, heat or cold application, nutrition, and control of environmental elements. Emotional support behaviors include the continuous presence of a caregiver, reassurance, encouragement, praise, humor, and verbal distraction. Advocacy behaviors include listening, supporting the laboring woman's decisions, negotiating with caregivers about a laboring woman's requests, and respecting privacy. Instructional/informational support consists of role modeling behaviors to the partner, instructing the client and her partner how to breathe, relax, push, etc.

Nonpharmacologic pain relief methods offer many benefits. They can be quite effective if applied appropriately. Most have few or no side effects and are cost effective. Unlike pharmacologic methods of pain relief, the responsibility of pain control can be shared with the family and friends attending the labor and birth. Because there are numerous choices, the laboring woman feels that she has choices or a "say" in her pain control.

The nurse can provide these labor support behaviors, but realistically the intrapartum nurses' job also includes technical behaviors that must be attended to such as maternal and fetal assessment,

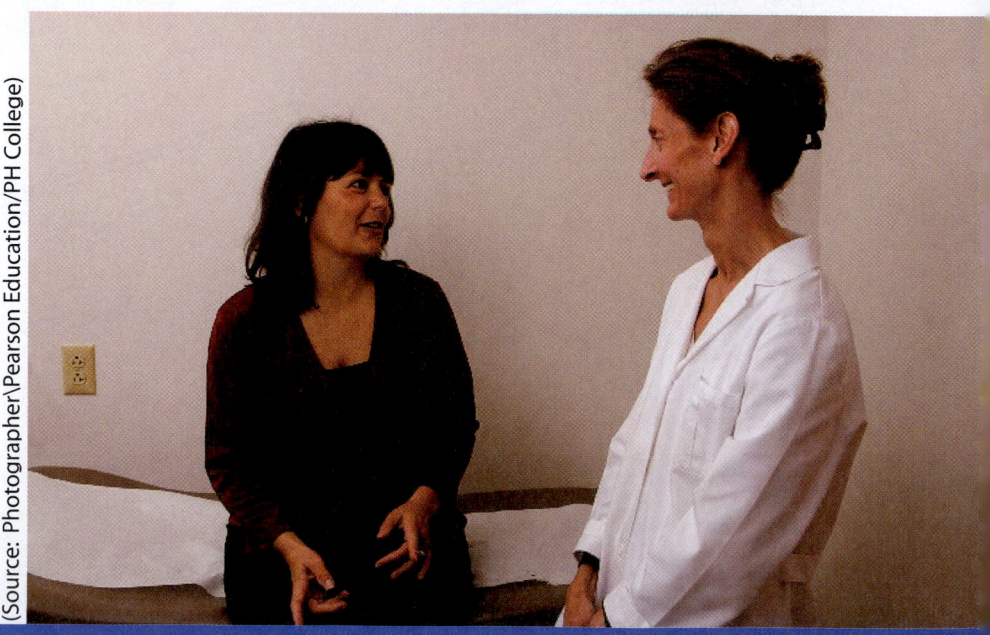

(Source: Photographer\Pearson Education\PH College)

managing equipment, and performing various procedures. Ideally, each laboring woman could have a private support person with her to provide these labor support behaviors. This labor support person may be her significant other, a family member, or a friend, or she could employ the services of a professional labor support person or a doula. The International Childbirth Education Association defines the doula as a trained professional who recognizes birth as a key life experience. The doula attends to the physical, emotional, and social needs of a woman in labor. The doula may be trained formally or informally. Several organizations provide training and certification.

Research studies have demonstrated the numerous positive client outcomes related to supportive care provided by doulas. Labors were shorter, cesareans were reduced, oxytocin use was decreased, and analgesia/anesthesia use was reduced, as was amniotomies, episiotomies, and vacuum extractions.

Some hospitals provide doulas on call for their clients. Other doulas can be hired by the pregnant couple. Some labor and delivery nurse managers are also providing training to their intrapartum nurses in labor support behaviors or doula techniques.

PLANNING AND IMPLEMENTATION

There are many ways that an expectant couple can prepare themselves for labor. The nurse should suggest optimal nutrition, regular exercise, adequate rest, resolution of stress factors, and regular prenatal visits. The couple may also explore issues related to labor in books or on websites.

Childbirth education courses offer couples an opportunity to learn more about pregnancy, labor, birth, and parenting. Many agencies offer a variety of courses such as early pregnancy, childbirth preparation, breastfeeding, and parenting and sibling classes. These courses are offered in many hospitals or by community organizations. The nurse should encourage the expectant couple to explore options thoroughly. Curriculums vary, as do the qualifications and experience of the instructor. Childbirth educators can seek national certification through a number of organizations.

For the couple who wants to attain a more natural birth, the childbirth education course should include a variety of comfort techniques. The course should provide opportunities to practice and perfect these techniques.

The knowledge gained through self-study or childbirth classes can be used by the expectant couple to design a specific plan for their birth. In this plan, the couple can outline their wants, likes, and dislikes related to labor, birth, newborn, and postpartum care. This document should be as detailed as possible. The nurse can be a terrific resource for the expectant couple as they prepare their birth plan. Once this document is drafted, it is important to discuss these issues with both the birth attendant and the staff at the birth facility. The nurse can assist the expectant couple in approaching the birth attendant. The nurse can become an advocate for the client. The nurse can encourage the expectant couple to become familiar with the birth facility where they will give birth. This can reduce stress. They can meet the staff and begin to develop a relationship with the nurses who may assist them during labor and birth. Touring the birth facility offers them an opportunity to review policies and procedures of the unit and negotiate items on their birth plan. If the client expresses an interest in having additional labor support, the nurse can provide information about the benefits and services of a doula. The nurse can provide referrals if necessary.

SELF-REFLECTION

Think about a time when you were in pain. It may have been a physical injury, after a surgical procedure, or simply a trip to the dentist. What non-pharmacologic techniques did you use to provide self-comfort and relieve yourself of pain? What worked? What did not work? Could you teach any of these comfort techniques to a laboring woman? Was there anything you could have done before your encounter with pain that might have assisted you in dealing more effectively with your pain?

SUGGESTED RESOURCES

For the Nurse

Adams, E., & Bianchi, A. (2004). Can a nurse and a doula exist in the same room? *International Journal of Childbirth Education, 19*(4), 12–15.

Bianchi, A., & Adams, E. (2004). Doulas, labor support, and nurses. *International Journal of Childbirth Education, 19*(4), 24–30.

Miltner, R. (2002). More than support: Nursing interventions provided to women in labor. *Journal of Obstetricm, Gynecologic and Neonatal Nursing, 31*(6), 753–761.

Simkin, P., & Bolding, A. (2004). Update on nonpharmacologic approaches to relieve labor pain and prevent suffering. *Journal of Midwifery and Women's Health, 49*(6), 489–504.

For the Client

■ www.birthplan.com or www.childbirth.org These websites offer a blank format that the couple can use to complete a birth plan online. There is also suggestions about how to present this information to the birth attendant.

■ www.dona.org Doulas of North America offers a registry of certified doulas listed by state or province.

■ www.icea.org The International Childbirth Education Association provides listing and contact information for certified childbirth educators.

MediaLink Birthplan

perineum, and lower extremities. Although the client remains fully awake and comfortable, participation in the birth process may be variable. In some clients, a lack of feeling may decrease their ability to push effectively, so the delivery may need to be assisted. The client may experience hypotension, bladder distention, and respiratory depression. For this reason, frequent or constant monitoring by the registered nurse is required. Some clinical facilities also require the physician or nurse midwife to be present.

Local Infiltration

With local infiltration, the drug is injected subcutaneously into the true perineum prior to an episiotomy or repair of a laceration. Figure 7-18 ■ illustrates the technique of local infiltration for episiotomy and repair.

General Anesthesia

General anesthesia is rarely used for vaginal deliveries because it causes the client to lose consciousness. However, it may be used for emergency cesarean section deliveries (see

discussion in Chapter 8 ⚭). Because the drug reaches the fetus in about 2 minutes, there is danger of respiratory depression in the newborn.

Stages of Labor

Labor is a process, or sequence of events, that begins with uterine contractions and ends 1 hour after delivery of the placenta. The labor process is described in four stages.

FIRST STAGE OF LABOR

The **first stage of labor**, also known as the **dilatation stage,** begins with regular contractions and ends with complete effacement and dilatation of the cervix. This is usually the longest stage and is divided into three phases: latent, active, and transition.

Latent Phase

The **latent phase** of the first stage of labor is the period from the onset of contractions until the cervix is dilated 4 centimeters (Figure 7-19 ■). Contractions usually occur

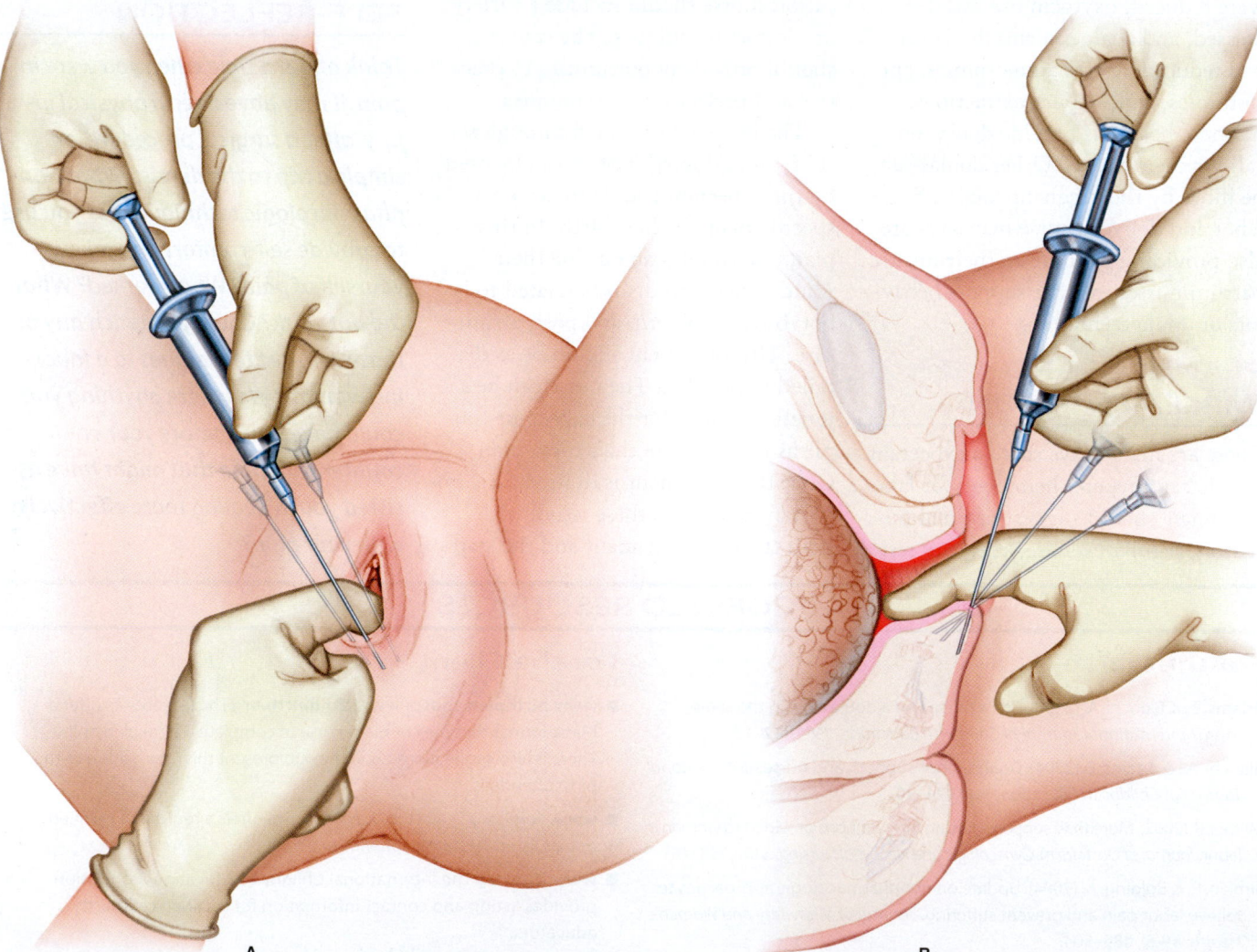

Figure 7-18. ■ Technique of local injection prior to episiotomy. (**A**) Anterior view. (**B**) Sagittal view showing fanwise pattern of injections.

Cervical dilation

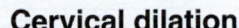

Figure 7-19. ■ Cervical dilatation (actual sizes).

TABLE 7-4	
Breathing Techniques During Labor	
TECHNIQUE	DESCRIPTION
Cleansing breath: Used at beginning and end of each contraction	Relaxed breath in through nose and out through mouth
Slow-paced breathing: Used in early and beginning of active labor	Slower than normal breathing; IN 2-3-4/OUT 2-3-4 (not less than ½ normal rate)
Modified paced breathing: Used in active and transition phases	Faster than normal breathing; IN-OUT/IN-OUT/IN-OUT (not more than twice normal rate)
Patterned paced breathing: Used in active and transition phases. (*Note:* Patterns of 5:1 or higher are tiring.)	<u>3:1 Pattern</u> IN-OUT/IN-OUT/IN-OUT/IN-BLOW <u>4:1 Pattern</u> IN-OUT/IN-OUT/IN-OUT/IN-OUT/IN-BLOW <u>Pattern with Words</u> Client may say phrase such as "Yankee Doodle" or "I think I can" and repeat through contraction <u>Pyramid Pattern of Breaths</u> Client may adapt the IN-OUT-BLOW pattern in a pyramid such as 1:1, 2:1, 3:1, 4:1, 4:1, 3:1, 2:1, 1:1

every 10 to 15 minutes and gradually increase to 5 minutes apart. (To review the pattern of contractions in labor, see Figure 7-13.) Each contraction lasts 30 to 40 seconds and is of mild to moderate intensity.

In the latent phase, the client is aware of the contractions but is relatively comfortable. She is excited that labor has begun and is often anxious about what lies ahead. If the membranes have not ruptured, the woman is encouraged to walk as long as she does not become tired. This is a good time to reinforce teaching to both mother and partner, especially relaxation methods (see Box 7-2) and breathing techniques for different stages of labor (Table 7-4 ■).

The latent phase usually lasts 8 to 10 hours with the first pregnancy. With subsequent pregnancies, it usually lasts about 5 hours.

Active Phase

The **active phase** of the first stage of labor begins when the cervix is dilated 4 centimeters and ends with 8 centimeters of dilatation (see Figure 7-19). Contractions occur every 3 to 5 minutes. They last 60 to 90 seconds and are of moderate to strong intensity. Clients perceive an increased amount of discomfort as the fetus descends through the pelvis, stretching muscles and ligaments. During this phase of Stage one, clients seek a position that reduces discomfort. They may need assistance to change positions. Some devices

that may be useful to women in this phase of labor were shown in Figure 7-14. The client now focuses on relaxation and breathing techniques.

The average length of active labor is 4 to 6 hours for the primagravida client and 3 to 4 hours for the multipara client.

Transition Phase

The **transition phase** of the first stage of labor is the period during which the cervix widens from 8 to 10 centimeters (see Figure 7-19). The contractions are strong, occurring every 2 to 3 minutes and lasting 90 seconds. (To review the pattern of contractions in labor, see Figure 7-13.) As the fetus descends deeper into the pelvis and Ferguson's reflex is triggered, there is a strong urge to push. The client may need to be reminded to focus on relaxation and breathing techniques. As mentioned previously, it is important for the client not to push actively until the cervix is completely dilated. If the client pushes too early, the cervix can tear.

Some behaviors are common during the transition phase of labor. The client frequently becomes restless, irritable, and sometimes angry. Statements such as, "I can't take it anymore" and "Don't touch me!," are common. It is important to help the support person(s) understand that this behavior is a normal part of the labor process.

The average length of the transition phase of Stage one labor is 1 to 2 hours.

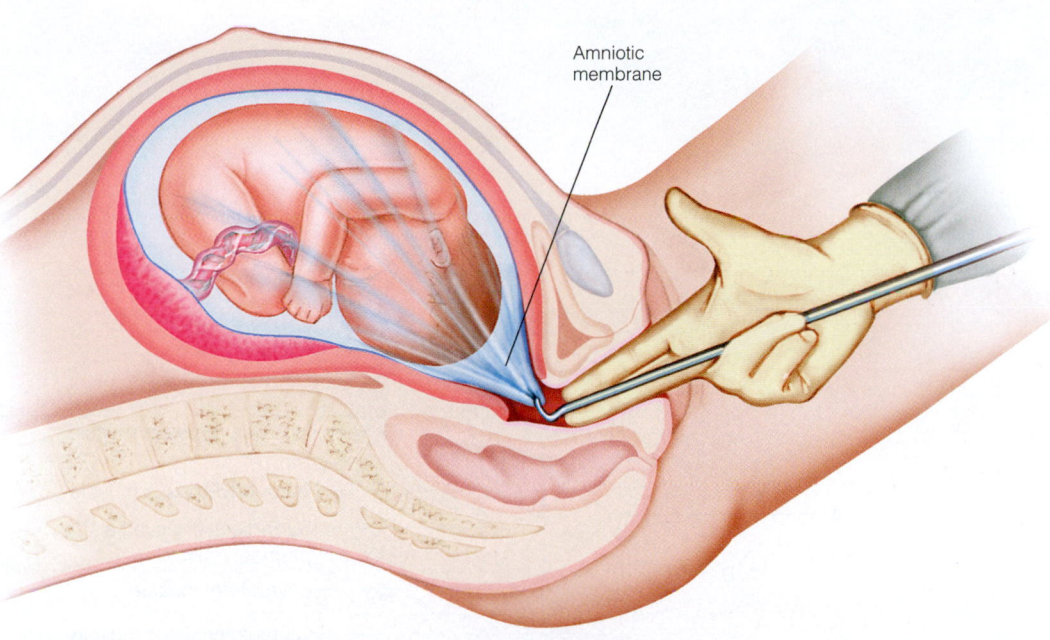

Amniotic
membrane

Figure 7-20. ■ Amniotomy is a very common procedure performed during labor.

AMNIOTOMY. An **amniotomy** is an artificial rupturing of the fetal membranes (Figure 7-20 ■). The procedure may be performed after cervical dilatation has reached at least 2 centimeter. This allows the amnihook to be inserted through the opening in the cervix.

Amniotomy is performed for a variety of reasons.

- It may stimulate the beginning of labor.
- It may shorten the length of labor.
- It allows access to the fetus:
  - To apply an internal fetal heart monitoring electrode (see Chapter 8, Figure 8-18 ⏺⏺)
  - To insert an intrauterine pressure catheter
  - To obtain a fetal scalp blood sample for determining acid–base levels (see Chapter 8, Figure 8-21 ⏺⏺).

There are some disadvantages of amniotomy as well. First, it introduces the possibility of infection because the fetus may be exposed to vaginal and intrauterine micro-organisms. Second, it increases the danger of umbilical cord prolapse. Finally, it may lead to increased molding because the amniotic fluid is not present to cushion the fetal head during contractions.

SECOND STAGE OF LABOR

The **second stage of labor** begins when the cervix is completely dilated (see Figure 7-19) and ends with the birth of the baby. Contractions continue every 2 to 3 minutes, lasting 60 to 90 seconds (see Figure 7-13). The client is encouraged to use her abdominal muscles to bear down actively with each contraction.

The second stage of labor could take 1 to 3 hours for the primagravida client. It often takes 15 to 30 minutes for the multipara client.

As the fetal head pushes on the perineum and the client pushes, the tissues of the perineum thin and bulge. The labia open. The fetal head can be seen with contractions, but it recedes into the vagina between contractions. Gradually, more and more of the fetal head appears with contractions. When the largest part of the fetal head is past the vulva and remains visible between contractions, **crowning** has occurred (Figure 7-21 ■). After a few more pushes, the fetus will be delivered.

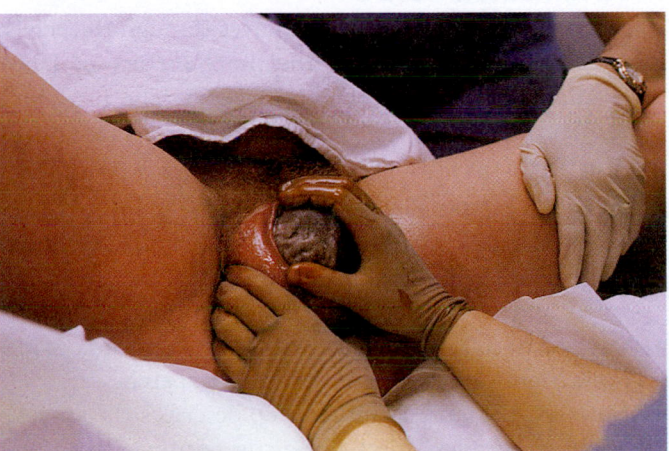

Figure 7-21. ■ Crowning of the fetus.

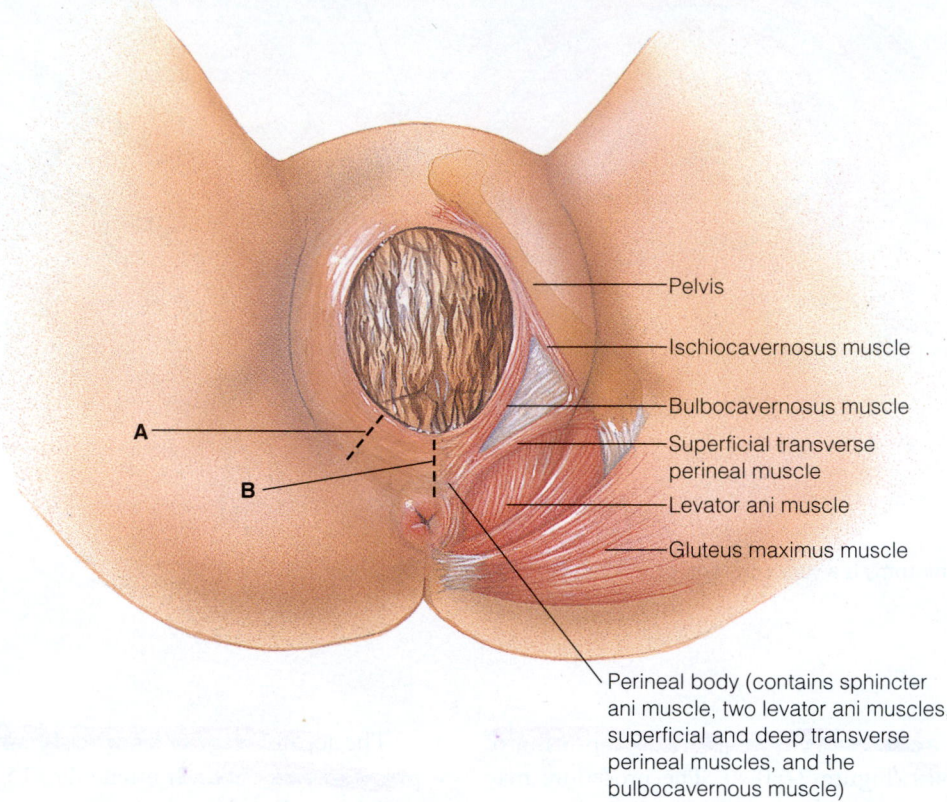

Pelvis

Ischiocavernosus muscle

Bulbocavernosus muscle

Superficial transverse perineal muscle

Levator ani muscle

Gluteus maximus muscle

Perineal body (contains sphincter ani muscle, two levator ani muscles, superficial and deep transverse perineal muscles, and the bulbocavernous muscle)

A

B

Figure 7-22. ■ Two most common episiotomy incisions: (**A**) mediolateral; (**B**) median (midline).

Episiotomy

In many deliveries, an **episiotomy,** or surgical cutting of the perineal tissue, is performed at this time. An episiotomy may aid delivery and prevent tearing of perineal and anal tissue.

Figure 7-22 ■ illustrates the position of midline and lateral episiotomies.

Mechanisms of Labor

The fetus changes positions as it moves through the pelvis. These movements are called the **mechanisms of labor** or **cardinal movements** (Figure 7-23 ■). The first three movements may occur before the first contractions or during the first stage of labor.

- **Engagement** (see Figure 7-23B) is the point at which the presenting part (usually the fetal head) enters the true pelvis. The presenting part is even with or below the ischial spines. The fetus is no longer ballotable.
- **Descent** begins with engagement and continues as the contractions push the fetus through the pelvis.
- **Flexion** (see Figure 7-23C and D) describes the attitude the fetus assumes. Ideal flexion is positive, with head

flexed onto the chest, the arms flexed across the chest, and the legs flexed across the abdomen.

- **Internal rotation** may occur prior to labor, but it most commonly occurs during the first or second stages. The fetus turns to an anterior position (OA). The fetal occiput is next to the maternal symphysis pubis.
- **Extension** (see Figure 7-23E) occurs when the fetus extends its head, pushing its occiput against the maternal symphysis pubis. This movement causes the fetal head to emerge through the vaginal opening. The health care provider may assist with the delivery by applying pressure on the mother's lower perineum, helping the fetus extend its neck by lifting the fetal chin.
- **Restitution** is the turning of the fetal head to be in normal alignment with the shoulders. The fetus then rotates until the shoulders are in an anterior/posterior position (**external rotation**) (see Figure 7-23F).
- **Expulsion** is the delivery of the rest of the fetus after restitution. The assisting health care provider applies gentle, downward pressure on the fetal head, allowing the anterior shoulder to emerge under the maternal symphysis pubis. The head is then raised to allow the posterior

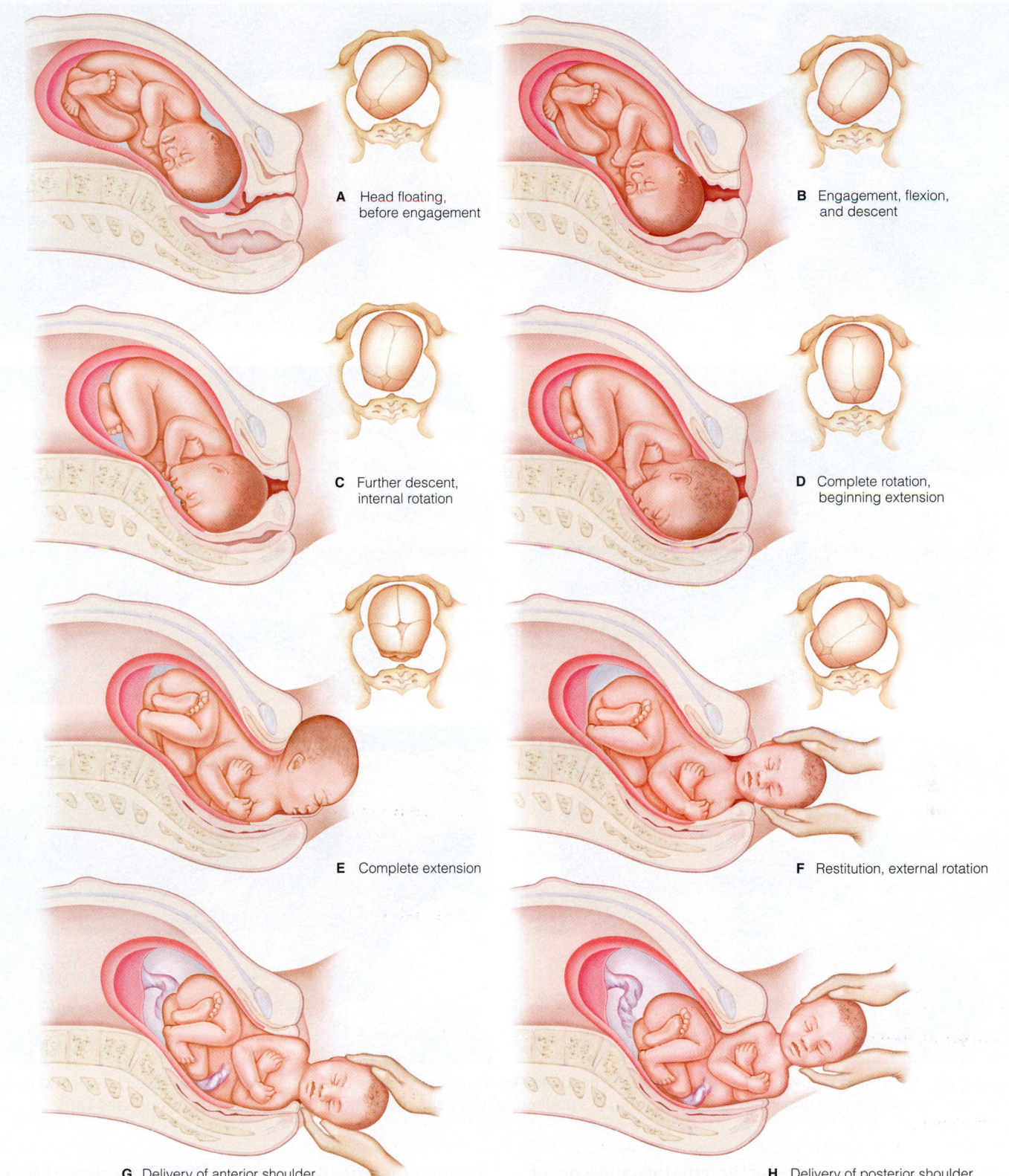

Figure 7-23. ■ Mechanisms of labor: left anterior occiput position. (**A**) Head floating, before engagement. (**B**) Engagement, flexion, and descent. (**C**) Further descent, internal rotation. (**D**) Complete rotation, beginning extension. (**E**) Complete extension. (**F**) Restitution, external rotation. (**G**) Delivery of anterior shoulder. (**H**) Delivery of posterior shoulder. (Adapted, with permission, from McGraw-Hill Companies, Inc. Cunningham, F. G., et al. [Eds.]. [1997]. *Williams obstetrics* [20th ed.]. Stamford, CT: Appleton & Lange, p. 320.)

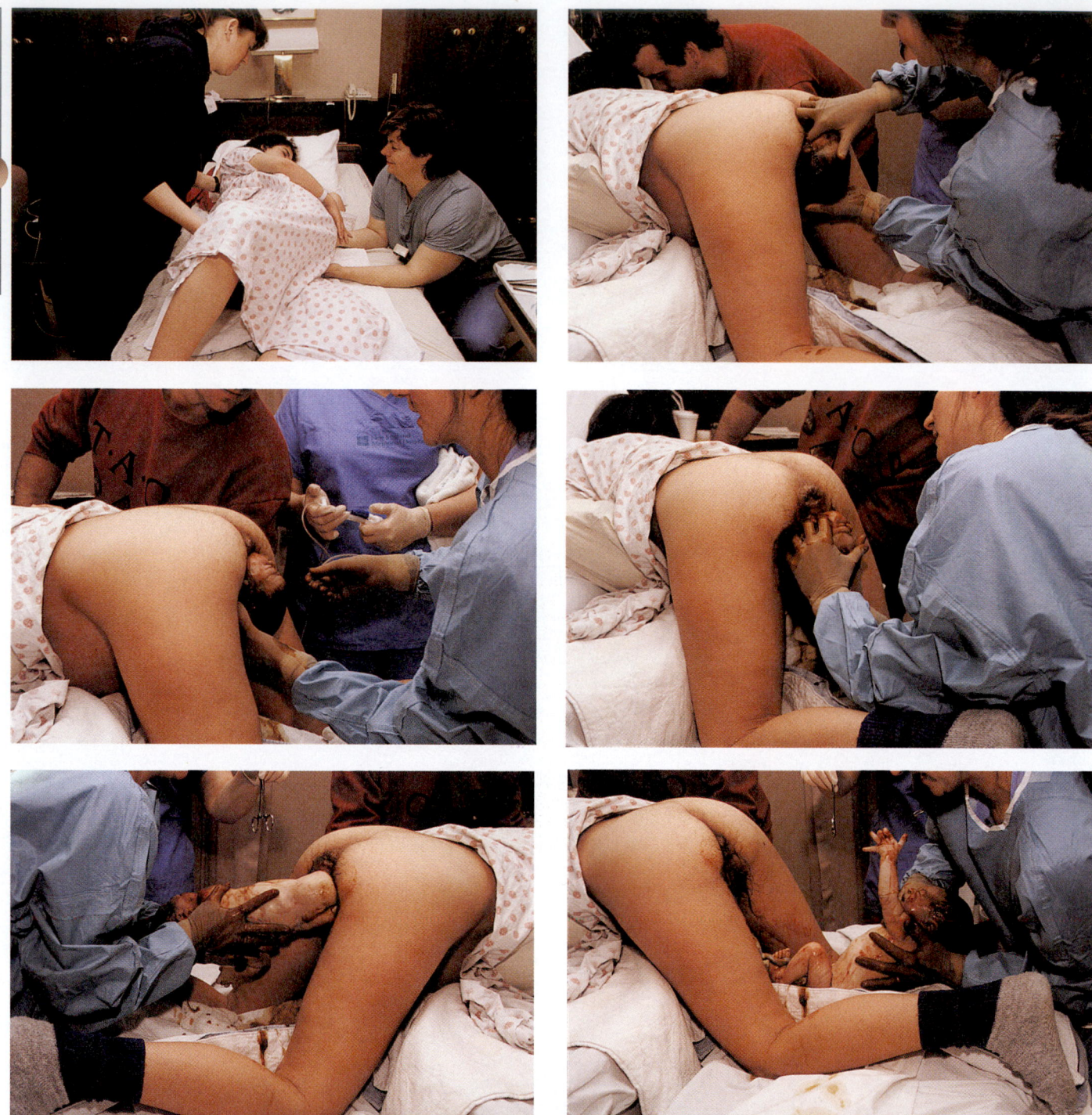

Figure 7-24. ■ Birthing sequence: side-lying position to hands and knees position. Hands-and-knees position (also called knee-chest position) is used when there is a prolapsed umbilical cord. In this position, gravity helps move the fetus away from the compressed cord.

shoulder to emerge. The rest of the fetus then slides out of the vagina.

Figure 7-24 ■ shows one sequence of labor and birth.

Clamping the Umbilical Cord

Clamping of the umbilical cord occurs before delivery of the placenta, although the exact timing is controversial (Olds, London, Ladewig, & Davidson, 2004). Data show that the 50 to 100 mL of blood from the placenta may increase and help stabilize the neonate's temperature. It may also reduce the incidence of iron-deficiency anemia later in infancy. However, it is possible that the added blood may lead to circulatory overload with resulting polycythemia and hyperbilirubinemia.

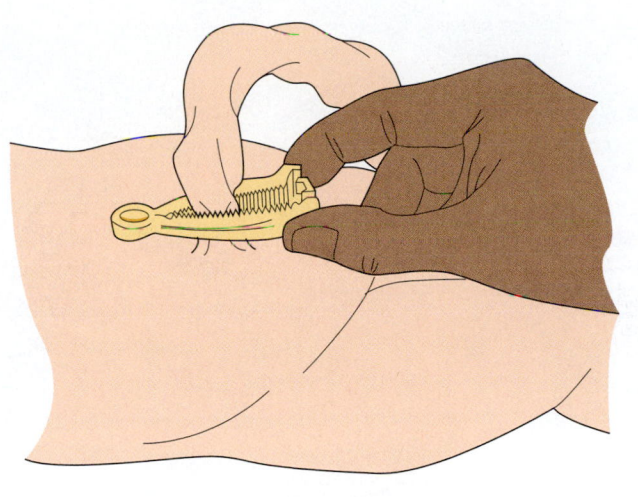
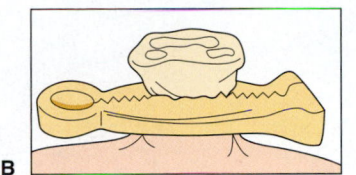
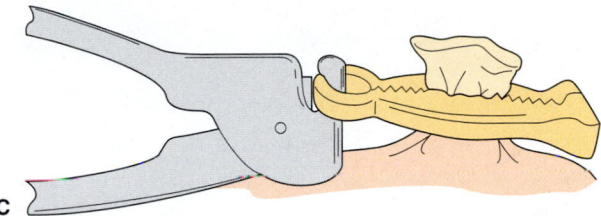

Figure 7-25. ■ Hollister cord clamp. (**A**) Clamp is positioned ½ to 1 inch from the abdomen and then secured. (**B**) Cord is cut. One vein and two arteries can be seen. (**C**) Plastic device for removing clamp after cord has dried. After the cord is cut, the nurse grasps the Hollister clamp on either side of the cut area and gently separates it.

Parents may express specific desires about when the umbilical cord is to be cut. They may also want to assist in cutting the cord. A Hollister cord clamp is illustrated in Figure 7-25 ■.

Once the cord is cut, the end of the cord is observed for the presence of two arteries and one vein. Observations are recorded on the neonatal chart. Presence of only one artery is associated with genitourinary abnormalities (Olds et al., 2004).

Cord Blood

Many parents today arrange for cord blood banking (see Chapter 2 ⦿) and bring a special container from the cord blood registry with them to the birthing facility. Umbilical cord blood is rich in stem cells, which are increasingly being used in fighting disease. The blood may be stored for later use if the child (or perhaps a family member) needs it. The therapeutic possibilities for umbilical cord blood are still being explored.

After the cord is clamped and before the placenta is expelled, the care provider withdraws blood from the umbilical vein using a large-gauge needle. The nurse labels the blood according to directions and arranges for storage and pickup. Even when cord blood banking is not done, a sample of cord blood will be sent to the lab for blood typing.

THIRD STAGE OF LABOR

The **third stage of labor** begins with the delivery of the fetus and ends with the delivery of the placenta. The placenta should be delivered within 30 minutes of birth. Continuous contractions following delivery cause the placenta to separate from the wall of the uterus. As it separates, there is some bleeding. The membranes are peeled from the uterus as the placenta slides into the vagina. Signs that the placenta is ready to be delivered are a gush of blood from the vagina, a lengthening of the umbilical cord, and a globular shape of the uterus. The client pushes one last time to deliver the placenta (Figure 7-26 ■).

The placenta may separate in different ways. Expulsion of the placenta with the fetal side out is termed the **Schultze mechanism** (Figure 7-26A). If the maternal side is out when the placenta is expelled, it is called the **Duncan mechanism** (Figure 7-26B).

FOURTH STAGE OF LABOR

The **fourth stage of labor** is the first hour after delivery. During this period, the mother's body begins to return to a nonpregnant state. Blood pressure has a moderate decline. The pulse increases and then gradually slows. Normal blood loss is between 250 and 500 mL, mostly at the time of placental separation.

The fundus should be located below the umbilicus and in the midline. The uterus should remain firm in order to control bleeding. Saturation of more than one perineal pad with blood during the 1-hour recovery time is considered excessive. (See Figure 10-8 ⦿, which shows how to assess perineal pads visually.) The mother may experience uncontrolled shaking or chills (**postpartal chills**) as a physiologic response to labor and as a result of the rapid weight loss at delivery.

Delivery Room Care of the Neonate

AIRWAY

The newborn has needs that must be met immediately after delivery. Most important, a patent airway must be established. Prior to and during delivery, amniotic fluid, vaginal

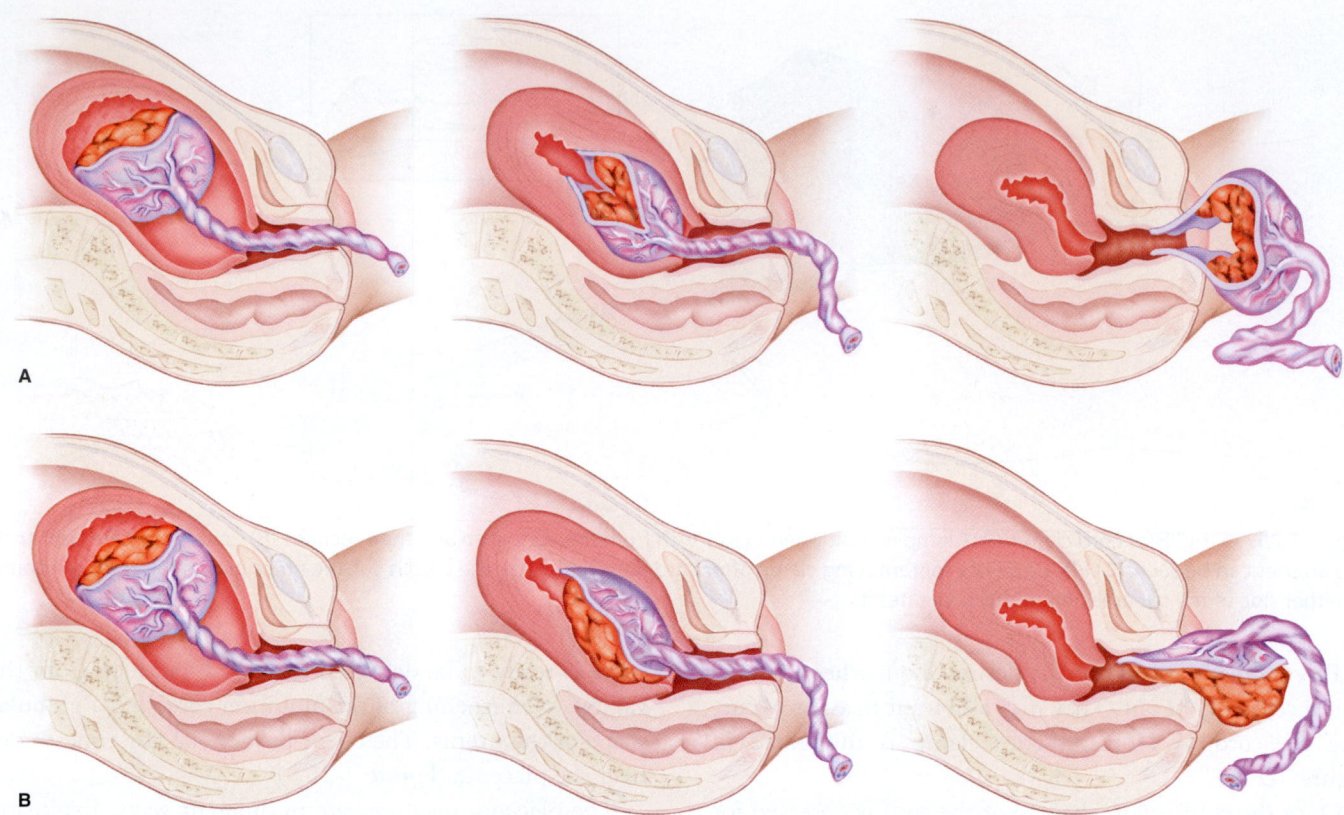

A

B

Figure 7-26. ■ Placental separation. (**A**) Schultze ("Shiny Schultze") mechanism. (**B**) Duncan ("Dirty Duncan") mechanism.

secretions, and pulmonary mucus can get in the infant's airway. These fluids are often removed with a bulb syringe (see Figure 9-23 ⬭) or suction catheter. (The procedure for using a suctioning device is provided later in this chapter under Nursing Care.) The infant's head is placed below its body so that secretions will continue to drain. However, they may need to be removed mechanically.

BREATHING

Breathing is initiated because of several factors.

1. As the infant moves through the birth canal, the chest is compressed, increasing the intrathoracic pressure. *Once the chest has been delivered, the intrathoracic pressure decreases, sucking a small amount of air into the lungs.*

2. When the umbilical cord is clamped, the infant's PCO_2 increases. *This stimulates the respiratory center in the medulla of the infant.*

3. The intrauterine temperature is approximately 20°F higher than the room temperature following delivery. *This change in temperature also stimulates breathing.*

4. The neonate is exposed to sights, sounds, smells, and touch. *Sensory, auditory, visual, and tactile stimulation helps encourage breathing as well.*

CIRCULATION

Circulatory changes occur as a result of change in thoracic pressure inside the heart and large blood vessels. With breathing, more blood flow is needed through the pulmonary arteries. Initially, an increase in pressure inside the aorta causes a reverse blood flow through the ductus arteriosus, increasing the amount of blood that reaches the lungs.

When this increased amount of blood returns to the left atrium, the pressure in the left atrium increases, closing the foramen ovale within minutes. Within 24 to 48 hours, the ductus arteriosus also begins to close. Permanent closure of the foramen ovale and ductus arteriosus may take 1 to 3 months.

TEMPERATURE

Heat loss in a neonate can be life threatening (see discussion in Chapter 9 ⬭), so it is important to dry the infant as soon as possible. Rubbing the infant with warm blankets not only dries the skin but also stimulates breathing. The infant can be placed next to the mother's skin and covered with a blanket or placed under a radiant warmer. The infant's head should be covered with a

TABLE 7-5

Apgar Score

SIGN	SCORE		
	0	1	2
Heart rate	Absent	Slow—<100	Over 100
Respiratory rate	Absent	Slow—irregular	Good crying
Muscle tone	Flaccid	Some flexing of extremities	Active motion
Reflex irritability	None	Grimace	Vigorous cry
Color	Pale blue	Body pink, extremities blue	Completely pink (if light skinned); absence of cyanosis (if dark skinned)

Score: 0–4 requires resuscitation efforts; 4–7 requires administration of oxygen and rubbing the back to stimulate breathing; 8–10 requires no special attention.

cap to prevent heat loss through the scalp. The infant should not be bathed until the temperature has stabilized. When the infant is bathed, care should be taken to prevent heat loss by keeping as much of the body covered as possible.

APGAR SCORE

At 1 minute and 5 minutes after delivery, the newborn will be assessed using the Apgar score (Table 7-5 ■). The **Apgar score** is a rapid evaluation of the infant's adaptation to extrauterine life. The five items are assessed in order of priority. The first is heart rate, followed by respiratory rate, muscle tone, reflex irritability, and color. Each item is assigned a score from 0 to 2. The scores are then totaled.

A score of 8 to 10 requires no special attention. A score between 4 and 7 requires administration of oxygen and rubbing the infant's back to stimulate breathing. If the mother had received a narcotic during labor, Naloxone (Narcan) may need to be administered to the infant to reverse respiratory depression. An Apgar score of 0 to 4 indicates that the infant needs immediate resuscitation (see Chapter 9 ●●). Anytime the infant's condition changes, an Apgar score can be a useful evaluation tool.

MEASUREMENTS OF THE NEONATE

The infant's measurements (height, weight, head circumference, chest circumference) are determined at birth (Figure 7-27A–D ■). Length can be difficult to measure. The infant is placed flat on the back with the legs extended. Usually, a tape measure is stretched from heel to head to determine length. Weight is taken on a balance scale. Head and chest

circumference are taken to obtain a baseline and are part of follow-up care.

IDENTIFICATION

Proper identification must be made in the delivery room before the mother and infant are separated. Identification bands imprinted with the same number, and the mother's name will be placed on the infant and the mother (Figure 7-28 ■). It is important that the infant bands be applied snugly, but not so tightly that they impede circulation.

The identification bands must stay on the infant and mother until both are discharged. Each time the infant is brought to the mother, the identification bands are compared. Some facilities use an identification band equipped with an alarm that would be triggered if the baby were removed from the facility (see Figure 7-28B).

Most hospitals footprint the infant (see Figure 7-28C) and fingerprint the mother. Vernix must be washed from the infant's feet prior to foot printing. The number on the identification bands is also recorded on the footprint sheet. Upon discharge, the mother signs this form as documentation that she has received her infant.

NURSING CARE

PRIORITIES IN NURSING CARE

The first priority in nursing care during labor is to assess maternal and fetal well-being with the progression of labor. Controlling the mother's discomfort can ease the

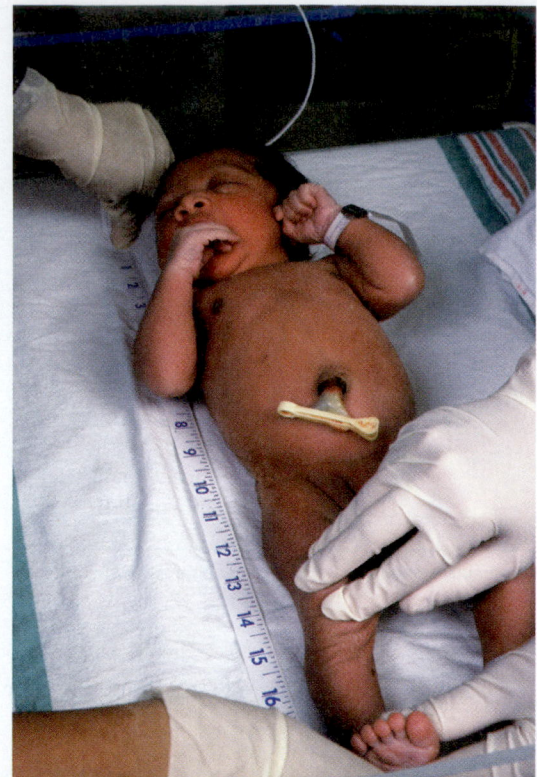

A

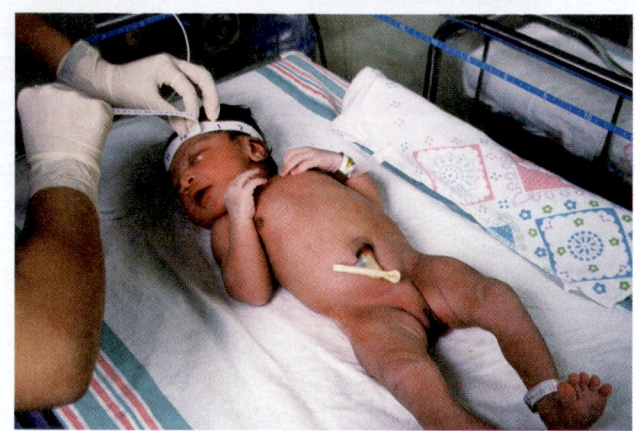

C

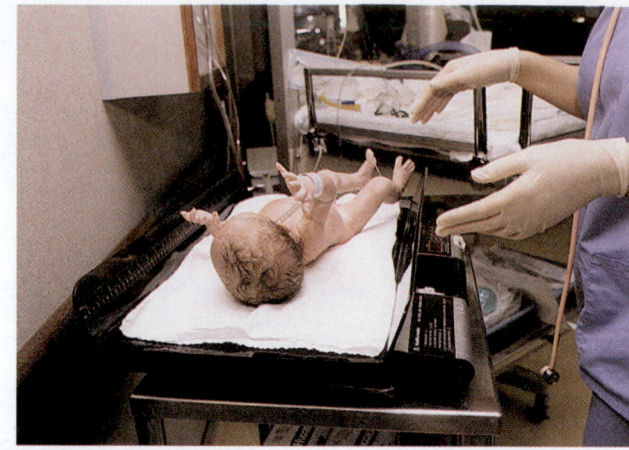

B

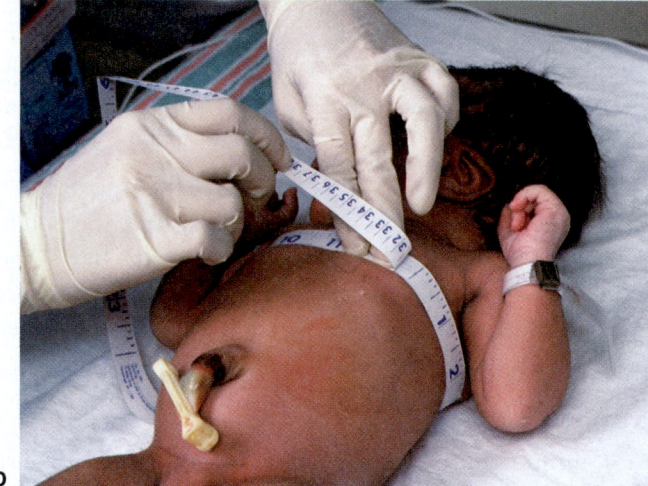

D

Figure 7-27. ■ Neonatal measurements taken immediately after birth. (**A**) Height. It is often helpful to have two staff members work together to ensure the accuracy of the measurement from crown to heel. (**B**) Weight. The caregiver's hands are poised near the newborn as a safety measure. (**C**) Head circumference is usually 33 to 35 centimeter. (**D**) Chest circumference is normally the same as the head circumference but should not exceed it. (**A, C, & D** Pearson Education/PH College) (**B.** © Stella Johnson www.stellajohnson.com)

BOX 7-3	ASSESSMENT

Admission Questions for the Client

The nurse must make a focused assessment of the stage of labor when a woman presents to the birthing facility. The following questions help determine the stage of labor and how quickly labor is likely to progress.

- When did the contractions begin?
- How far apart are the contractions, and how long do they last?
- Have the membranes ruptured? (Has the water broken?)
- Is this your first pregnancy? How long were previous labors?

progression of labor, making the birth experience as pleasant as possible. The nurse also must monitor the progression of labor and report changes to the primary care provider. Last, the nurse must prepare the environment for delivery.

ASSESSING

As described previously under Admission to the Birthing Facility, the nurse first determines the condition of the client, the stage of labor, and the status of the fetus. Initial interview questions the nurse would ask are listed in Box 7-3 ■.

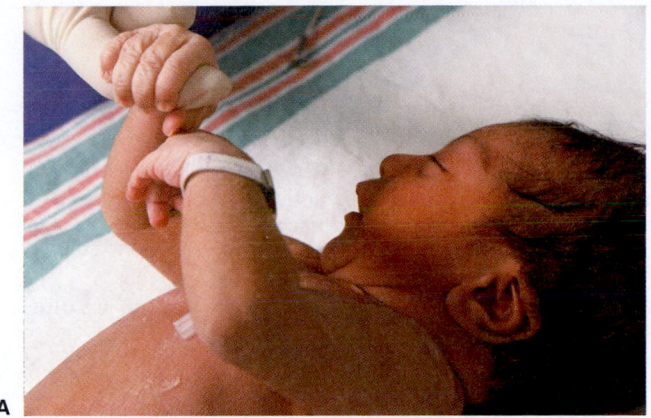

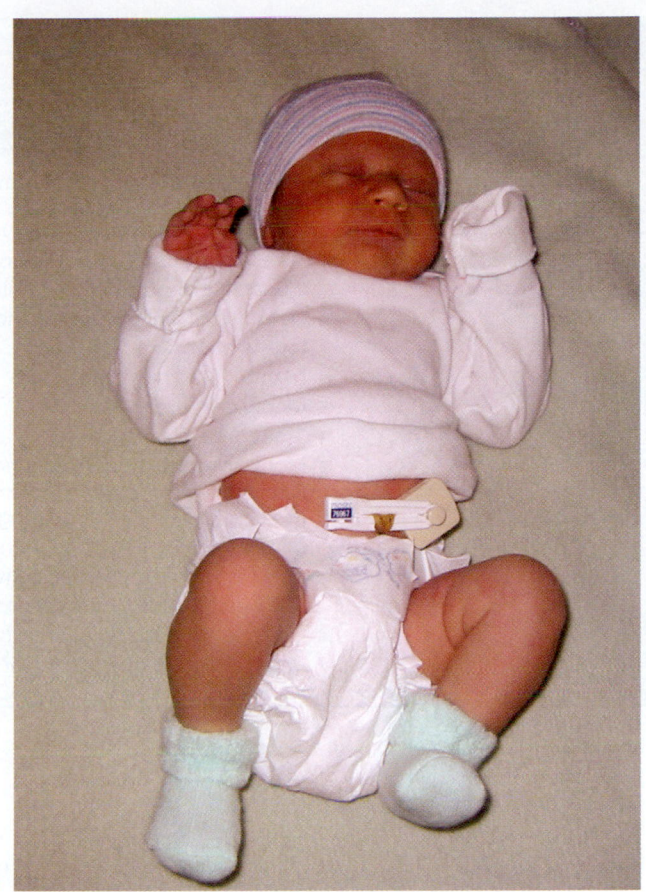

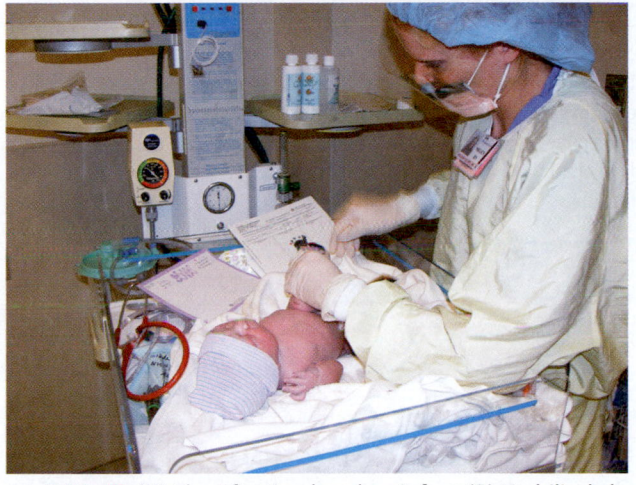

Figure 7-28. ■ **(A)** Identification band on infant. **(B)** Umbilical alarm attached to newborn infant. **(C)** Nurse takes footprint of baby.
(A): Pearson Education/PH College, **(C):** M. C. Schlachter Photography.)

Cultural Aspects of Care

The nurse should be aware of his or her own culture and biases in providing care to a client of another culture during labor. A client's cultural background may affect her assessment and needs during labor. To deliver culturally proficient care, the nurse must be alert to verbal and nonverbal expressions of the client's and family's desires. Box 7-4 ■ identifies some cultural considerations in birth practices.

BOX 7-4   CULTURAL PULSE POINTS

Expression of Pain During Labor

Pain response varies from culture to culture, and pain caused by labor and birth is no different. Some women are very stoic and labor quietly; this is frequently true with African American women. Others are notoriously loud. Many cultures believe that women must experience pain and discomfort during labor (e.g., Mexican, Iranian, Filipino). In fact, very difficult labor usually results in lavish gifts for Iranian women.

Mexican women are frequently heard repeating "aye yie yie" throughout labor. Interestingly, repeating "aye yie yie" in succession requires long, slow deep breaths. This has been described as "Mexican Lamaze." This phrase is more than an expression of pain; it is a culturally accepted method of pain relief.

Initial Data

Assessment data include maternal vital signs and fetal heart rate; the frequency, duration, and intensity of contractions; and the results of a urine dipstick test for glucose and protein. A vaginal exam is performed by the nurse or care provider to determine the amount of cervical effacement and dilatation, as well as fetal presentation, position, and station.

- A nitrazine test is performed if the client is unsure whether the membranes have ruptured. *Status of the membranes is important. Once they have ruptured, the fetus may be exposed to micro-organisms within the uterus.*
- Any signs of pregnancy-induced hypertension (PIH)—edema, altered reflexes, and clonus (spasms or seizures)—are documented and reported. (The procedure for assessing

TABLE 7-6

Standards of Assessment in Labor

ITEM	ASSESSMENT	RATIONALE
Prenatal data	Review prenatal record to determine EDB, gravida/para, history of previous labors, results of laboratory exams.	Identifies risk (i.e., preterm, rapid labor/delivery, and anticipated complications)
Maternal assessment	■ Take vital signs every hour (more frequently if unstable or outside normal limits). ■ Determine level of comfort and effect of intervention. ■ Monitor fluid balance. ■ Monitor reflexes. ■ Monitor cervical changes. ■ Monitor contractions (frequency, duration, intensity).	Determines mother's tolerance and stability during labor Determines if labor is progressing in a usual pattern
Fetal assessment	■ Monitor FHT every hour during early labor, every 30 minutes during active labor, and every 10–15 minutes during transition and delivery. Note change in FHT before, during, and after contractions. ■ Observe amniotic fluid for color (should be clear; green indicates meconium passage by fetus).	Determines fetal tolerance and stability during labor Determines fetal distress during pregnancy and labor

clonus is in Chapter 8, Procedure 8-1 ■.) *The mother with PIH is at greater risk. Care providers must be alerted to the possibility of complications.*

Review of Prenatal Data

■ The nurse reviews the woman's prenatal record to determine the presence of any complications during the pregnancy. If the client has had no prenatal care and labor is not advanced, a more in-depth assessment is performed. *The client who has not had prenatal care may have conditions that could complicate labor or compromise the fetus. Further investigation will help clarify the health status of the woman and fetus.*

Emotional Support for False Labor

Some women present at the birthing facility with false labor or at a very early point in Stage one Phase one labor. If it is not clear whether the woman's labor has begun, she is asked to walk for an hour and is then re-examined. If labor has not begun, the nurse must be sensitive to the disappointment the woman may feel.

■ The nurse provides encouragement and emotional support, as well as reinforcement of the signs of impending labor. *Therapeutic listening can help the woman overcome her disappointment and embarrassment. Encourage her to discuss any concerns she may have about returning home to wait for labor to begin. Review signs of impending labor*

and reassure the woman about her ability to recognize those signs.

Ongoing Data Collection

Once it is determined that the client is in labor, continuous assessment is performed, including frequent vital signs, FHR, and contraction evaluation. Table 7-6 ■ provides guidelines for assessment of the woman in labor.

■ The nurse monitors the client closely. *Most clients will be monitored electronically, either continuously or intermittently. The level of monitoring depends on the stage of labor and the well-being of the client and fetus. In Stage one labor, the nurse's primary roles are to promote comfort, monitor the client's and fetus's status, and report any signs of complications.*

Leopold's Maneuvers

■ If ordered, the LPN/LVN may set up and attach the electronic fetal monitor. Before attaching the monitoring equipment, the nurse will need to assess for fetal position. *Correct placement of the monitor will provide a strong, clear recording of the FHR.*

■ The nurse performs Leopold's maneuvers on the client's abdomen. *Leopold's maneuvers are maneuvers that help caregivers determine the position of the fetus. Procedure 7-1 ■ describes the steps in Leopold's maneuvers.*

External Fetal Heart Monitoring

The external fetal monitor provides continuous data about the heartbeat of the fetus. In some facilities, it may be

(*Text continues on p. 203.*)

PROCEDURE 7-1	# Performing Leopold's Maneuvers

Purpose

■ To determine fetal position and presentation for fetal monitoring or other reasons

Equipment

■ Gloves (optional)

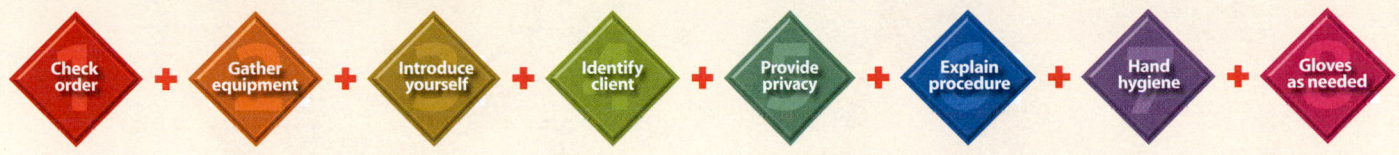

Interventions

1. The first maneuver (Figure 7-29A ■) is to palpate the fundus with two hands, feeling for the fetus' body parts. *The fetal head is firm and round, and it moves independently of the body. The buttocks are softer and round with small bony prominences; they move with the trunk.*

2. The second maneuver (Figure 7-29B) is to find the fetal back and determine if it is to the right or left side of the mother's abdomen. Using the palms, the nurse uses firm but gentle pressure to explore one side of the abdomen and then the other. Supporting the uterus

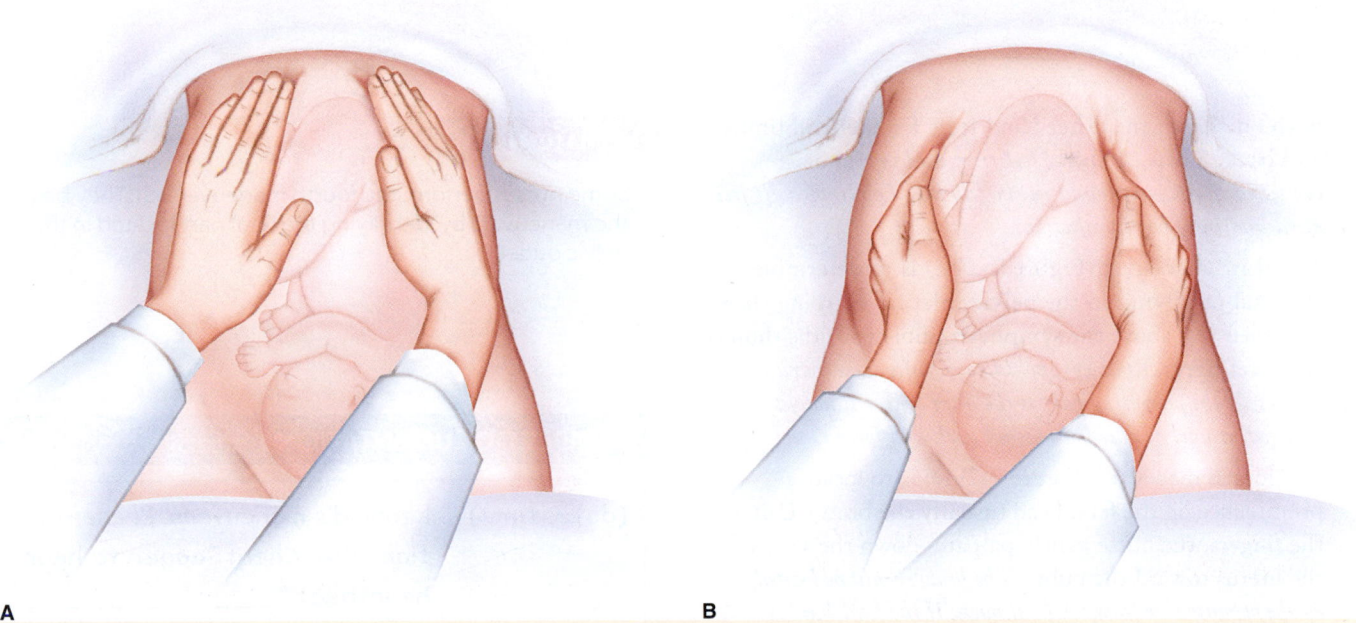

A   B

Figure 7-29. ■ Performing Leopold's maneuvers to determine fetal lie. (**A**) First maneuver. (**B**) Second maneuver. (**C**) Third maneuver. (**D**) Fourth maneuver. (Reproduced, with permission, from McGraw-Hill Companies, Inc. Cunningham, F. G., et al [eds.]. [1997]. *Williams obstetrics* [20th ed.]. Stamford, CT: Appleton & Lange, p. 258.)

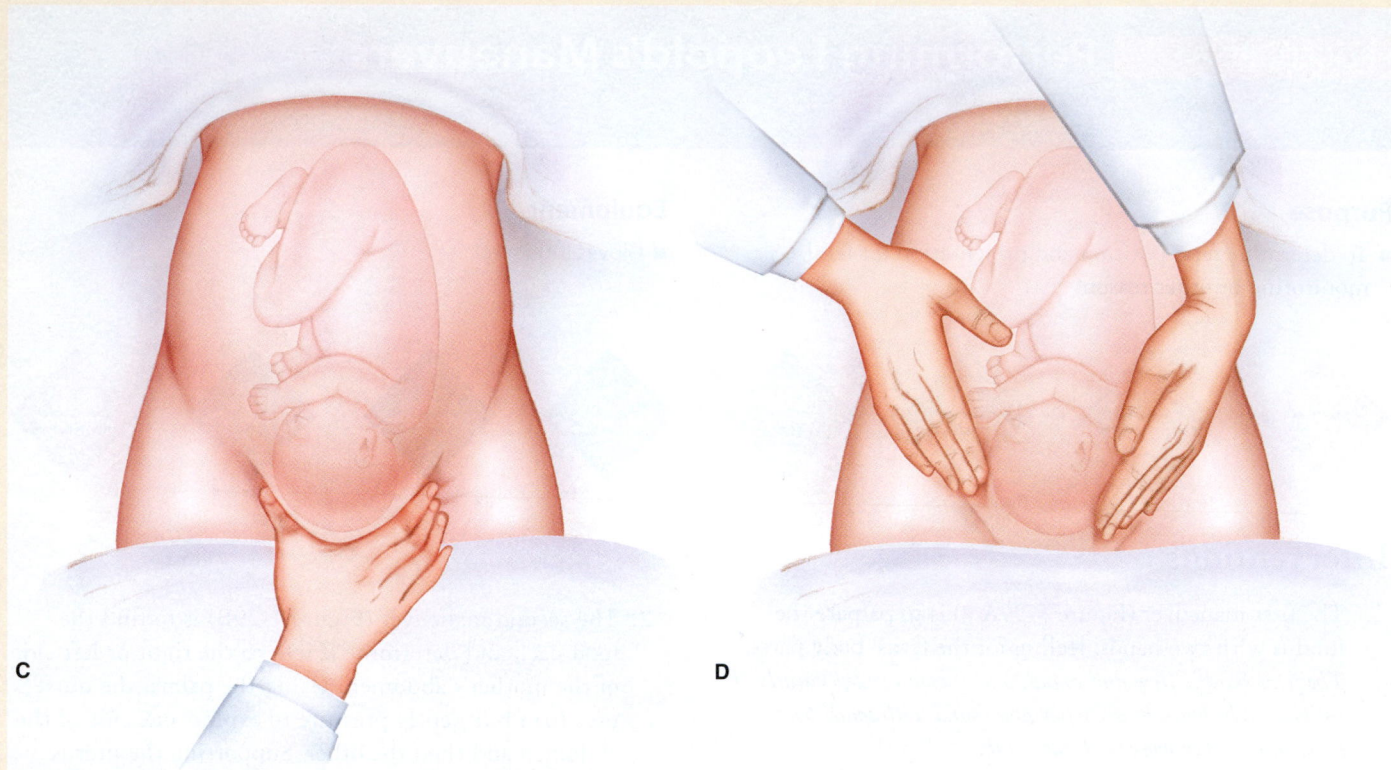

Figure 7-29. ■ *Continued*.

with one hand, the other hand feels for the fetal limbs and back. *The back should feel firm and smooth and connected to the part found in the fundus. The limbs will feel hard and have bony projections.*

3. The third maneuver (Figure 7-29C) is to determine the fetal part lying in the pelvic inlet by grasping the abdomen just above the symphysis pubis with the thumb and forefingers. *Findings should be opposite those found in the fundus. If the presenting part is the head and it is not yet engaged, it will be able to be moved back and forth.*

4. The fourth maneuver (Figure 7-29D) is to locate a prominence on the fetal head (usually the brow). Using the fingers, the nurse gently palpates down the sides of the uterus toward the pubis. *The brow should be located on the opposite side from the fetal back. If the fetal head is extended, the fetal occiput will be felt on the same side as the back* (see Figure 7-11).

clinical ALERT

Some nurses perform the fourth maneuver first. They begin the maneuvers by identifying the fetal part located in the pelvic outlet.

SAMPLE DOCUMENTATION

(date, time)   Leopold's maneuvers. Presentation LOA. Client "eager to hear
heartbeat." _____
J. Roe, LVN

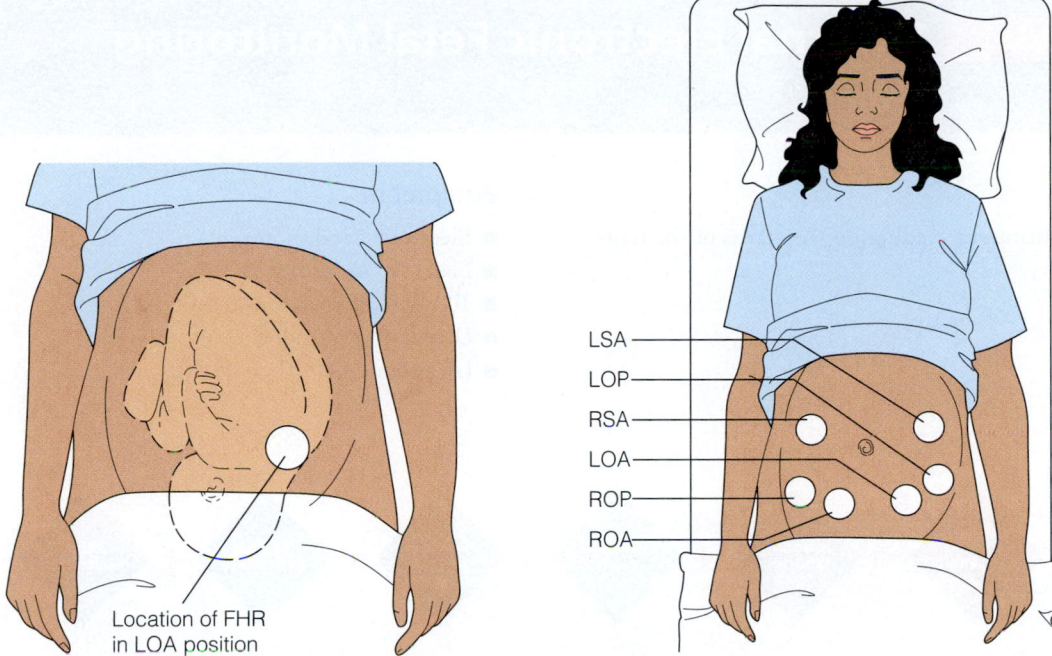

LSA
LOP
RSA
LOA
ROP
ROA

Location of FHR
in LOA position

Figure 7-30. ■ (*Left*) Location of FHR when fetus is in LOA position. (*Right*) Other transducer placements.

used routinely on every client. In others, it is used primarily with high-risk women. The monitor consists of two parts: the *transducer* (which will transmit the fetal heart sounds) and the *tocodynamometer* (which will record uterine contractions).

The FHR is recorded with an ultrasound transducer that is covered with water-soluble conducting gel and then held against the mother's abdomen. If the fetus is in cephalic presentation, the FHR can be located in the right or left lower quadrant of the abdomen. Figure 7-30 ■ shows the location of the FHR when the fetus is in the LOA position (*left*) and where to place the transducer when the fetus is in other positions (*right*). The ultrasound transducer is held in place with a belt or strap around the mother's abdomen. Procedure 7-2 ■ describes steps in performing external electronic fetal monitoring. Refer to Chapter 8 ⌾ for more information on fetal monitoring. See Figure 8-18, and see Figure 8-21 for an illustration of how to obtain a fetal blood sample.

Repeat Vaginal Examination

A vaginal exam is performed at intervals by the care provider (nurse midwife or physician) to assess progression of cervical effacement and dilatation, station, and fetal position. Table 7-6 identifies the standard time frame for assessing the progression of labor. It is not unusual for the FHR to slow to 100 bpm during pushing contractions and then to increase to more than 120 when the uterus relaxes.

clinical ALERT

If the fetal heart rate does not return to 120 bpm or more between contractions, the care provider should be notified immediately. Oxygen may be given to the mother at this time in order to provide adequate oxygen to the fetus.

DIAGNOSING, PLANNING, AND IMPLEMENTING

The following are nursing diagnoses that may be used in planning nursing care for the laboring client:

- Pain related to the labor process
- Anxiety
- Deficient Knowledge
- Risk for Ineffective Individual Coping related to fatigue and the birth process
- Impaired Urinary Elimination
- Deficient Fluid Volume
- Risk for Infection.

Typical outcomes for the laboring woman might include these, as well as others:

- Pain will be controlled within reasonable limits.
- Client will be able to express feelings and listen to instructions during labor.
- Client will understand how, and will have the necessary energy, to participate in labor and birth.

(*Text continues on p. 206.*)

External Electronic Fetal Monitoring

Purpose

■ To obtain a continuous reading on the status of the fetus prior to delivery

Equipment

■ Electronic fetal monitor
■ Elastic monitor belts (2)
■ Tocodynamometer, also called a "toco"
■ Ultrasound transducer
■ Ultrasound gel

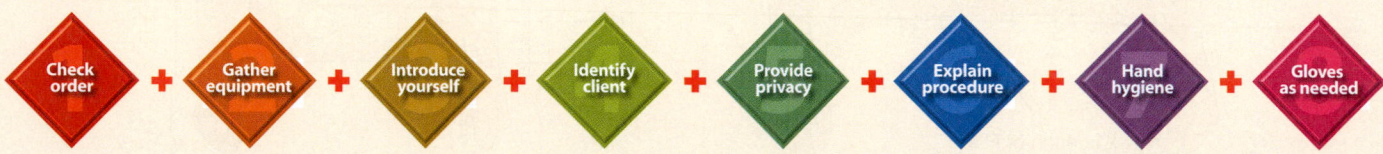

Interventions

1. With the monitor turned on, place the two monitor belts around the woman's abdomen (Figure 7-31 ■).

2. Palpate the area off midline and over the uterine fundus that is most firm during contractions. Place the "toco" in this area, and secure it with one elastic belt. *Because the fundus is the area where contractions are greatest, this placement will provide the best graph of uterine contractions.*

3. Adjust the tracing so it shows 10 or 15 mm Hg between contractions. *Adjustment to this level prevents background static.*

4. Apply gel to the diaphragm of the transducer, and place the diaphragm on the mother's abdomen halfway between the symphysis pubis and the umbilicus. *The gel seals contact between the diaphragm and the maternal abdomen to produce the best quality sound. The midline of the mother's abdomen is most often closest to the fetal heart. When the uterus contracts, pressure is exerted against the "toco" and information is relayed to the electronic fetal monitor and recorded on graph paper.*

5. Move the diaphragm laterally or vertically until the strongest heart sound is heard. (If the fetus is breech, the heart sound will be above the umbilicus.) Attach the second elastic belt snugly to the transducer at this point. *Note:* If a beltless monitor is available (Figure 7-31B), follow specific directions for attaching it. *When the diaphragm directs the ultrasonic beam toward the fetal heart, the whiplike sound of the heartbeat will be heard. Moving the transducer laterally helps determine the position that is most directly over the fetal heart. The belt keeps the transducer in position. A beltless FHR monitor allows the mother to move around the room.*

6. At the beginning of the fetal monitor tape, record the following information: date, time, woman's name, gravida, para, membrane status, and name of the care provider (physician or certified nurse midwife). Follow facility guidelines. *Documentation is a continuous part of quality care. Individual facilities may require additional information to be recorded on the tape.*

7. Follow facility policy about ongoing documentation of information gathered by electronic FHR monitoring, as well as documentation of procedures performed, changes in position, any therapy that might be initiated, etc. The LPN/LVN is not responsible for interpretation of findings but must report unusual

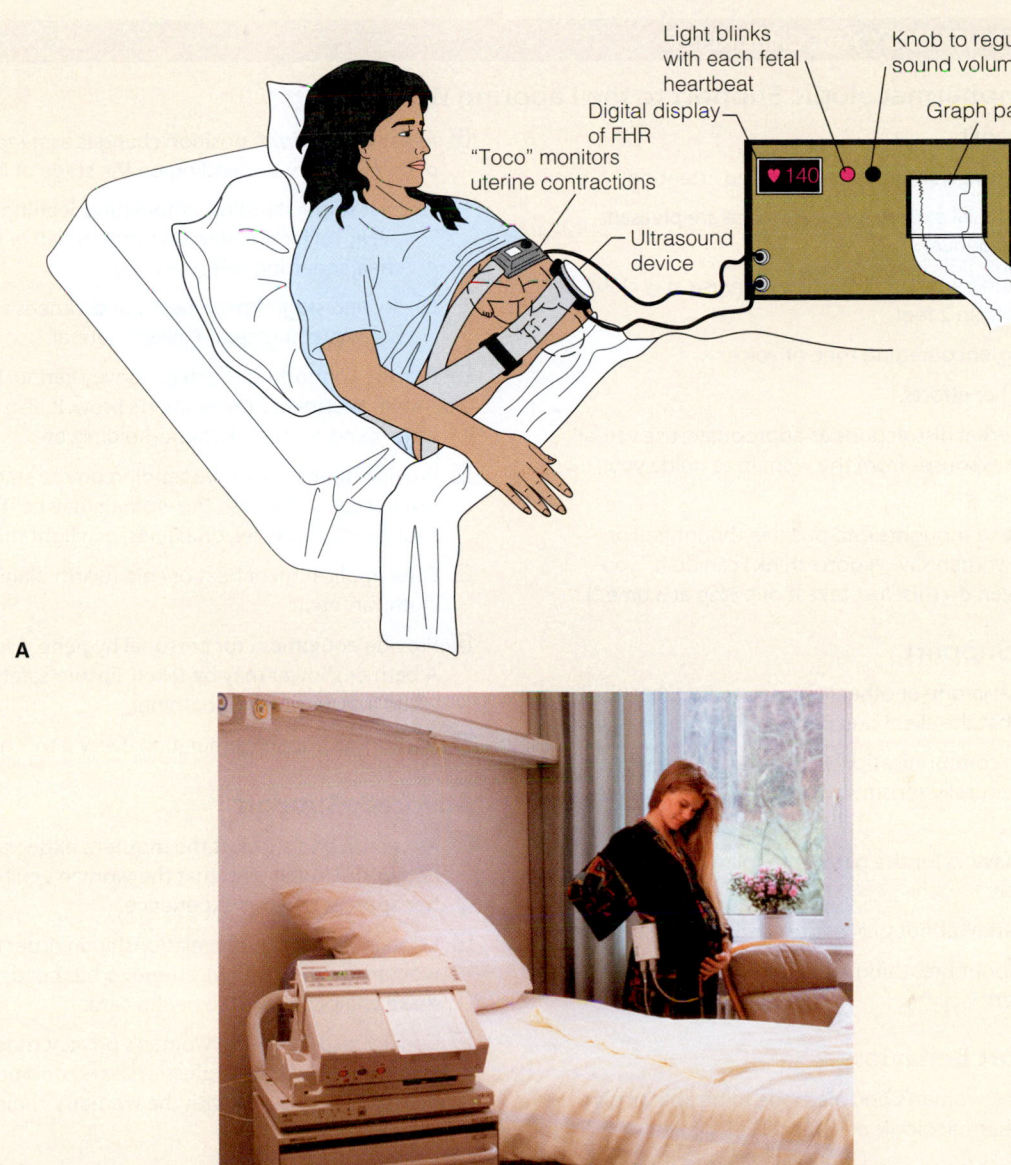

Light blinks
with each fetal
heartbeat

Knob to regulate
sound volume

Digital display
of FHR

Graph paper

"Toco" monitors
uterine contractions

♥ 140

Ultrasound
device

A

B

Figure 7-31. ■ (A) External electronic fetal monitoring device showing graph readout. (B) Beltless tocodynamometer system features remote telemetry that allows the laboring mother more mobility.

findings as directed. *The baseline rate in bpm, plus acceleration and decelerations of FHR in response to maternal contractions, are some of the data that will be recorded. Data either can be reassuring or can provide an early warning of possible complications. Prompt reporting of designated information allows therapeutic intervention. Documentation according to facility policy provides for safe practice and quality care.*

SAMPLE DOCUMENTATION

(date, time)   External fetal monitor applied, FHR 140 bpm, "C" q4m, lasting 45 sec, mod intensity. _____
Margaret Messenger, LPN

BOX 7-5	NURSING CARE CHECKLIST

Providing Nonpharmacologic Support to the Laboring Woman

Emotional Support

☑ Be present. Give the woman your undivided attention.

☑ Make sure your facial expression and stance are pleasant and convey confidence.

☑ Unless the laboring woman requests otherwise, stay close to her, usually within 2 feet.

☑ Use a reassuring, encouraging tone of voice.

☑ Offer praise for her efforts.

☑ Use humor or verbal distractions as appropriate; use verbal and nonverbal responses from the woman to guide your sense of what is useful.

☑ Rephrase negative thoughts into positive thoughts. (For example, if the woman says, "I don't think I can do it," you could say, "You can do this. Just take it one step at a time.")

Informational Support

☑ Interpret medical jargon or other information from health care providers that the client and partner do not understand.

☑ Use therapeutic communication skills (reflecting, rephrasing, choosing culturally sensitive words, using interpreter if needed).

☑ Role model behaviors for the partner to follow, and encourage participation.

☑ Provide information about procedures and progress.

☑ Remind client about breathing, relaxation, or pushing techniques as needed.

Physical Comfort Behaviors

☑ Remember that a woman's body is made to be able to give birth without pharmacologic assistance.

☑ Adjust the environment (including temperature and lighting) as much as possible for the mother's comfort. Mild, familiar scents may be used; avoid candles and strong scents.

☑ Ensure a nonrestrictive environment that allows freedom of movement.

☑ Offer assistive equipment as appropriate (extra pillows, birthing ball, squatting bar, etc.).

☑ Assist woman with position changes as needed. Positions of comfort vary, depending on the stage of labor:

 ☑ First stage: standing, ambulating, leaning, knee/chest, pelvic rocking, sitting on birthing ball or toilet, rocking chair, squatting, left side lying

 ☑ Second stage: knee/chest, hands/knees with birthing ball, squatting, semi-Fowler's, lateral.

☑ Provide comforting touch to convey caring. This can be as simple as stroking the woman's brow. It also includes massage (hand, foot, back), hand-holding, etc.

☑ Provide nourishment. Depending on the stage of labor and level of consciousness, the woman may be offered ice chips, sour candy, Popsicles, oral fluids, or a light meal.

☑ Offer application of heat or cold (warm blanket, cool washcloth, fan, etc.).

☑ Provide equipment for personal hygiene. Assist as needed. A bath or shower may be taken. Ensure safety of the client while transferring and bathing.

☑ Encourage urinary elimination every 2 to 3 hours.

Advocacy Support

☑ Ask about and support the mother's expectations for labor and birth. Understand that the woman's culture may affect her approach to this experience.

☑ Establish a therapeutic relationship in order to protect the woman (provide safety), attend to her needs, and help her make choices related to health care.

☑ Convey respect for the woman's privacy, modesty, relationships, and values. Be professional and nonjudgmental. You do not have to agree with the woman's choices to provide good nursing care.

☑ Provide physical and emotional safety so the woman is able to express both positive and negative emotions.

☑ Encourage problem-solving behavior, and keep the woman at the focus of decision making. Step in if others are trying to interfere.

☑ Support the woman's desires verbally and actively.

Source: Data courtesy of Ellise D. Adams and Ann L. Bianchi (2005). *50 Ways to comfort a laboring woman.* Presented at The AWHONN 2005 Convention, June 14, 2005, Salt Lake City, Utah.

- Client will void every 2 to 3 hours post delivery.
- Client will remain free of infection.

Maintaining Standards of Practice

The goal of nursing interventions is to assist the client and support persons through the labor and delivery process. Nurses provide nonpharmacologic labor support in four ar-

eas: emotions, physical needs, instructions, and advocacy support (Box 7-5 ■). The nurse also assists with pharmacologic interventions as needed.

- Follow the standards of practice for any client. *For example, any client with deficient fluid volume would be given intravenous fluid. Any client with altered urinary elimination would be encouraged to void every 2 hours. If needed, a catheter would be used to drain the bladder. Any client or support person in need would receive emotional support and teaching.*

Preparation for Delivery

As labor progresses to Stage two, the nurse prepares the birthing suite. In some areas, the birth takes place in the same room as labor. In other areas, a special delivery room is used.

- Make sure all necessary equipment is in place. The equipment should include a warmer, suction, oxygen, and emergency drugs for the infant. Check to be sure all equipment is operational prior to delivery. *It is part of quality care to ensure that there is no unnecessary delay in providing for the needs of the client.*
- Cover a table with sterile drapes. Sterile instruments, sterile drapes, gown and gloves, and bulb syringe are arranged for the care provider's convenience. If delivery is imminent, the table can remain uncovered but must remain sterile. If delivery will not occur for some time, the table may be covered with a sterile drape to prevent contamination until it is needed. *Using sterile equipment helps prevent transmission of pathogens to the mother and newborn during the birth process.*

Continuous Monitoring and Support

The role of the nurse during labor is to continue to monitor the client and fetus, assist the physician or nurse midwife, and support the family. Timing of nursing care in the second stage of labor is essential to a smooth delivery.

- A reassuring, professional manner helps the client feel the nurse has the situation under control. The nurse should seek additional assistance if necessary. *The laboring woman, especially the primagravida, is undergoing a challenging and potentially frightening experience. The nurse's calm demeanor and positive approach allow the mother to remain calm and to focus on the demands of labor.*

Pain Control

- Frequently assess the woman's comfort level and her ability to cope. *Although discomfort is unavoidable, empathy can allow the woman to overcome it and stay focused. The woman's ability to understand directions and to cooperate in the laboring process helps guide pain control measures.*
- Evaluate the effectiveness of comfort measures individually, changing methods when needed. *By focusing on individualized care and each woman's responses, the nurse can be sure of providing proficient care.*
- Listen closely to and respect the needs of the client. *Some women prefer to labor and give birth without pharmacologic assistance. Others may prefer to relieve discomfort with medication as soon as possible. There is no "right way" to go through labor. The nurse's role is to provide safety and support to each unique client.*

Nonpharmacologic Comfort Measures

- Teach clients to change position frequently. *Change of position reduces muscle stress.*
- Teach (if there is time) and encourage nonpharmacologic methods of pain control. *Numerous techniques and methods are available to help the woman manage labor discomfort without medication (see Boxes 7-2 and 7-5).*
- Encourage side-lying or upright positions. A supine position should be discouraged. *A side-lying position supports fewer, stronger contractions. In an upright position, gravity can assist labor progression. A supine position puts pressure on the vena cava.*
- Provide ice chips and oral care. Clear liquids may be given in early labor but are prohibited as labor becomes more advanced. *Ice chips and oral care provide some moisture and refresh the mouth. Oral liquids are avoided late in labor because of the possibility of vomiting and aspiration.*
- Encourage muscle relaxation, massage (Figure 7-32A ■), or abdominal **effleurage** (a light stroking with the fingertips in a circular motion). Figure 7-32B ■ illustrates the direction of abdominal effleurage from the symphysis pubis to the iliac crest. *Relaxation techniques and massage promote overall distraction and relaxation. These help relieve the discomfort of labor.*
- Promote use of breathing techniques and monitor the client. Review Table 7-4 for specific breathing techniques that are helpful at different stages of labor. *Proper breathing techniques can smooth labor and decrease pain. It is important, though, to monitor the client closely for signs of hyperventilation.*

clinical ALERT

Numbness and tingling of the tip of the nose, lips, fingers; dizziness; or spots before the eyes are signs of hyperventilation. The nurse should remain with the client and encourage her to take slow shallow breaths. If symptoms become more severe (evidenced by spasms in the hands and feet), have her breathe into a mask or her hands to increase her CO_2 level and alleviate the problem.

Pharmacologic Comfort Measures

- Assist in preparing supplies or equipment for medication administration as ordered. Monitor client closely. *Systemic medications can slow or stop contractions if labor is not well established. Systemic medications given in transition or in the second stage of labor can cause respiratory distress in the newborn.*
- Assist with preparation of equipment for epidural block. Monitor infusion. Be knowledgeable about side effects and complications. *With epidural block, clients may not be able to participate fully in the birth process. Lack of feeling may decrease ability to push effectively, so the delivery may need to be assisted. The client may experience hypotension,*

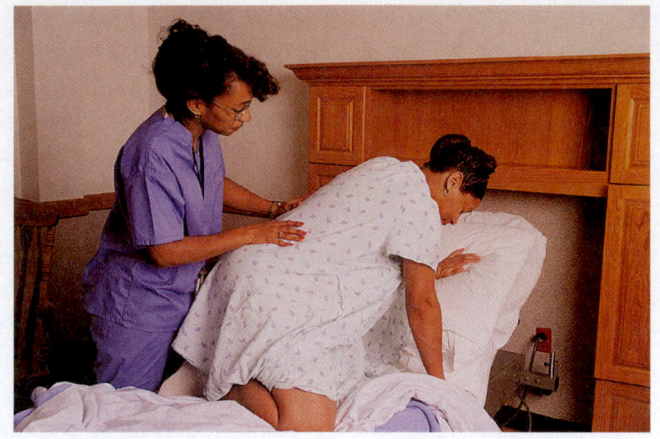

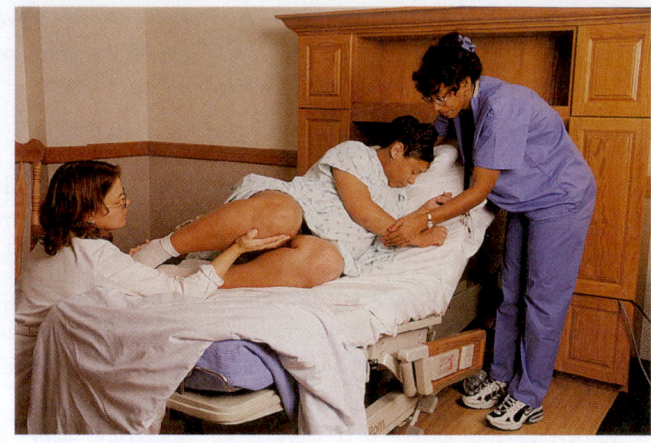

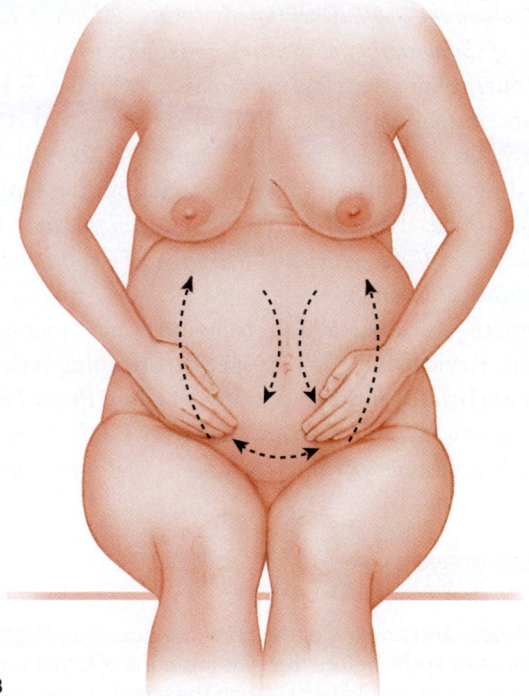

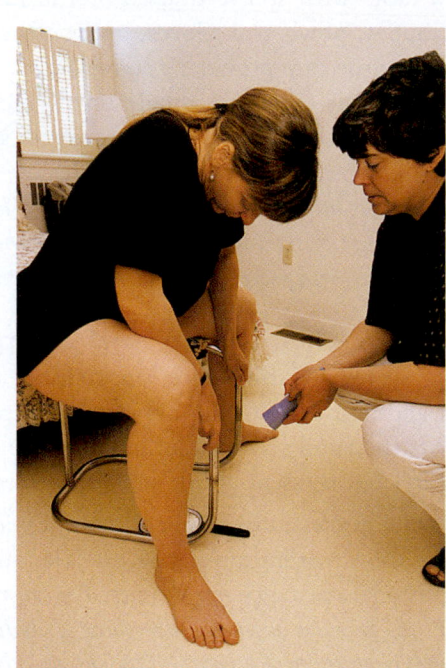

B

B

Figure 7-32. ■ (**A**) Nurse provides massage to sacral area. (**B**) Direction of abdominal effleurage for the latent and active phases of the first stage of labor.

bladder distention, and respiratory depression. For this reason, frequent or constant monitoring by the registered nurse is required. Some clinical facilities require the physician or nurse midwife to be present as well.

- Provide sterile field and sterile equipment as ordered. *The nurse maintains standards of practice and quality care by preventing the spread of infection.*

- Be alert for signs of complications and take immediate action. *Even with the best prenatal care and preparation for childbirth, complications can rapidly change the stability of the laboring mother and the fetus. (Chapter 8 ⦾ discusses the most common complications of labor and the related nursing care.)*

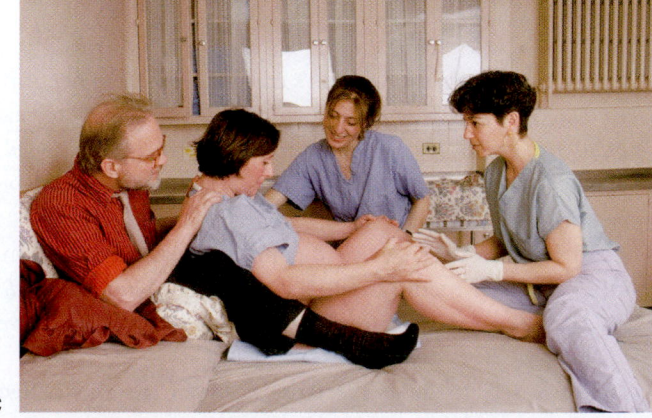

C

Figure 7-33. ■ Some birthing positions. (**A**) Side-lying (left side) with right leg supported. (**B**) Birthing stool. (**C**) Supine with support from partner. (**B**. © Stella Johnson www.stellajohnson.com. **C.** Margaret Miller/Photo Researchers, Inc.)

Maternal Care for Birth

The client is positioned according to the physician/nurse midwife preference. Sometimes the client is placed in lithotomy position with a pillow under the right hip to relieve pressure on the large blood vessels. Legs are abducted with knees bent. Stirrups may be used to support the legs. Other times, the client is placed on her left side with the left leg extended. The right leg is flexed and supported by an assistant. Figure 7-33 ■ demonstrates some common birthing positions.

- The nurse cleanses the perineum with antiseptic soap immediately prior to delivery. *The antiseptic soap prevents the spread of infection.*
- The care provider (physician or nurse midwife) then applies sterile drapes. *This provides a clean environment for the newborn.*

Figure 7-34 ■ provides a visual sequence of the birthing process.

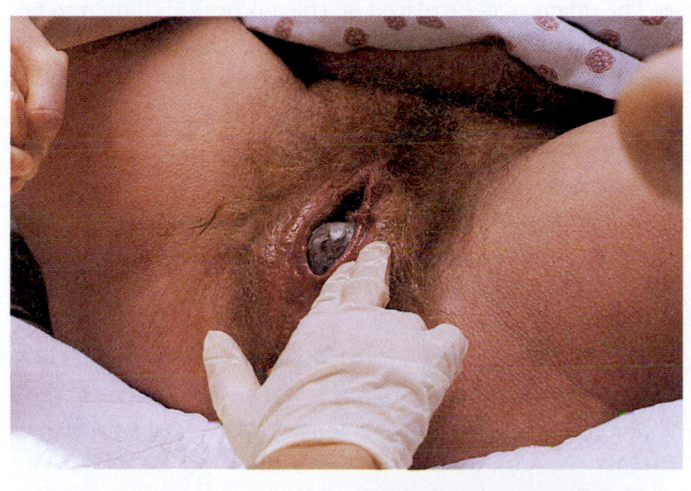
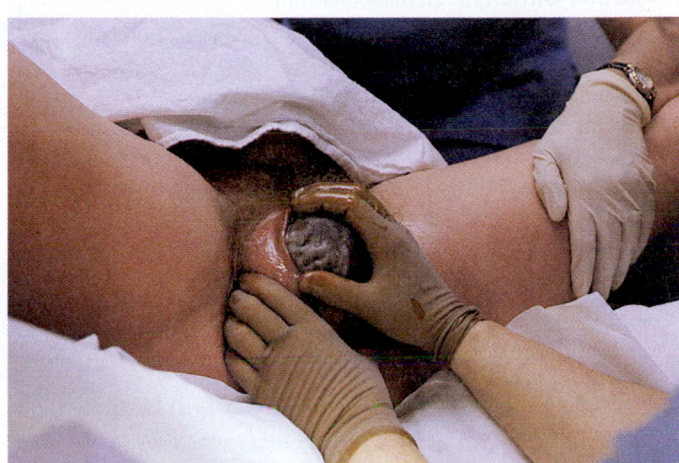
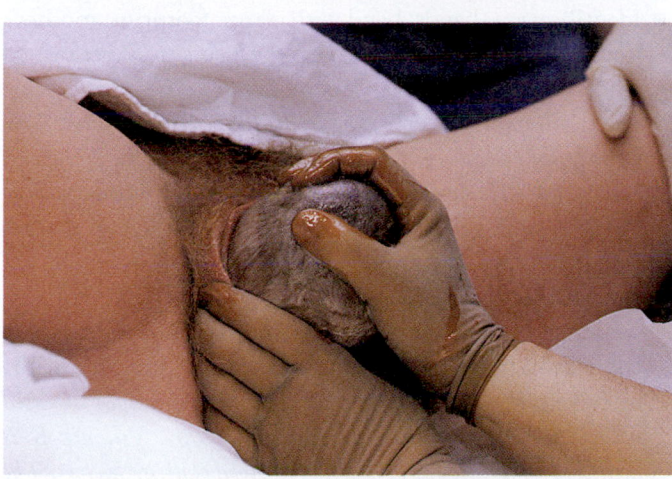
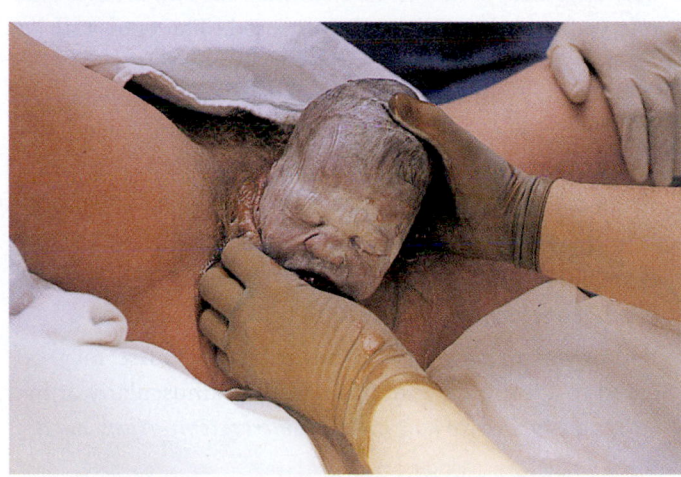
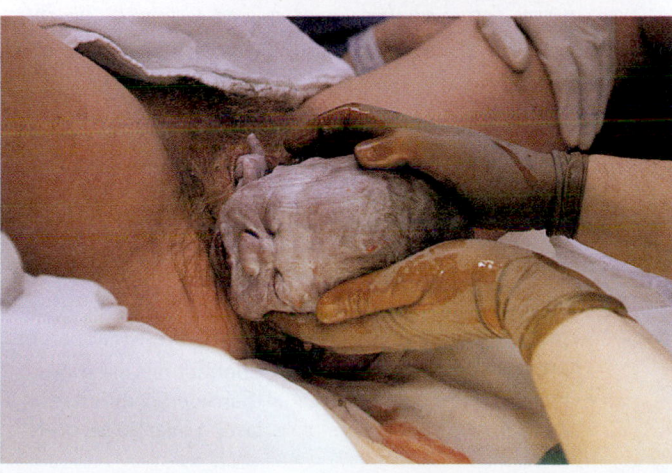
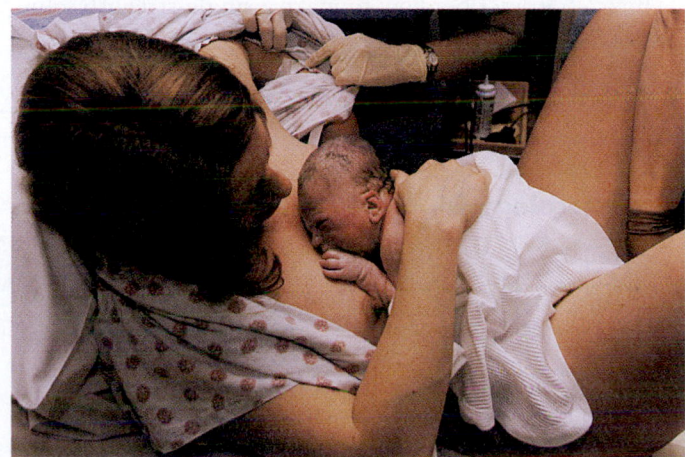

Figure 7-34. ■ Birthing sequence with mother in supine position.

BOX 7-6

Calculations for IV Pitocin Solution

NOTE 1 Unit = 1,000 milliunits

TO MAKE SINGLE-STRENGTH IV SOLUTION: Add 10 Units of Pitocin to 1 liter of compatible IV fluid (lactated Ringer's, or D_5W).

TO INFUSE: Convert prescribed milliunits/min to mL/hr and set infusion pump. *IV infusion pump MUST be used for client safety.*

AMOUNT ORDERED: 20 milliunits/min

CALCULATIONS: 10 Units/1 L = 10,000 milliunits/1,000 mL
OR 10 milliunits/1 mL.
10 milliunits/1 mL = 20 milliunits/X mL
Cross-multiply to get 20 = 10X
X = 2, so 2 mL/min
Multiply by 60 minutes to get amount infused per hour.

THINK: 20 milliunits = 2 mL/min
2 mL/min × 60 min/hr = 120 mL/hr (2 × 60 = 120)
Set the infusion pump for 120 mL/hr.

- Once the infant is delivered, the airway will be suctioned. *Suctioning will help open the airway and promote breathing.*

- The umbilical cord will be examined for two arteries and one vein; results will be documented. The cord will be clamped and cut. A Hollister clamp (see Figure 7-25) or other clamp will be used to clamp the cord. *The presence of two arteries and one vein is normal; the presence of only one artery forecasts genitourinary problems. Cord clamping separates the infant from the placenta and promotes stabilization.*

The vagina and cervix will be inspected for lacerations. Lacerations and an episiotomy will be sutured. The placenta will be delivered and inspected to be sure it is intact.

- Following delivery of the placenta, the nurse may be asked to administer Pitocin, either intramuscularly or intravenously. *Pitocin will stimulate uterine contractions and decrease bleeding.*

Box 7-6 ■ describes how to make a single-strength solution of Pitocin. Table 7-7 ■ provides information about the use of Pitocin.

Initial Neonatal Care

Following delivery, the nurse assumes care of the infant, while the care provider (physician or nurse midwife) focuses on preventing the mother from hemorrhaging following the birth. Several risks exist for the neonate. The most urgent are respiratory distress, circulatory collapse, and hypothermia. These risks require immediate attention. Priorities are for the nurse to maintain the airway, stimulate breathing, and dry the infant.

- The infant may be placed on the mother's abdomen to begin the bonding process, or the infant may be placed under a warmer. *These locations both provide warmth. The infant will lose heat rapidly, so warm, dry blankets should be used. Drying the infant by rubbing its back stimulates crying, which is necessary to expand the lungs.*

- The airway is suctioned as needed. Procedure 7-3 ■ describes nasopharyngeal suctioning with a DeLee mucus trap. *A patent airway is the first priority in neonates, as in adults.*

- The Apgar score is taken at 1 minute and at 5 minutes. *The score creates an objective reading on the neonate's status. It shows that the infant is stabilizing or identifies the need for follow-up care.*

- Identification (bands, band with alarm, footprint, mother's fingerprint) of the mother and the neonate is performed while still in the delivery room. *Identification is done before mother or infant leaves the room in which the birth occurred. This prevents the possibility of misidentification. Follow facility policy closely and make sure the identification bands are neither too loose nor too tight. Loose bands can slip off; tight bands can interfere with circulation.*

- When the infant has stabilized, he or she will be weighed and measured. If ordered, the nurse will give the infant Aqua Mephyton (vitamin K) and an antibiotic eye ointment. *The neonate's height and weight are used as a baseline. The infant's liver is immature. Vitamin K is needed to stimulate the production of blood clotting factors. The eye ointment (often erythromycin) is used to prevent eye infection.* (Chapter 9 ∞ discusses care of the healthy newborn.)

TABLE 7-7

Pharmacology: Drug Used to Stimulate Labor

DRUG	USUAL ROUTE/ DOSE	CLASSIFICATION	SELECTED SIDE EFFECTS	DON'T GIVE IF
Pitocin (oxytocin)	IV To stimulate labor: 0.5–20 milliunits/min To prevent hemorrhage: 20–40 milliunits/min	Oxytocic hormone	Prolonged uterine contractions, which can harm fetus Afterpains	Fetal distress is apparent Contractions are more than every 2 minutes, lasting over 90 seconds

PROCEDURE 7-3

Nasopharyngeal Suctioning of the Neonate

Purpose

- To remove mucus from the neonate's nose and mouth to allow respiration

Equipment

- DeLee mucus trap or other suction device

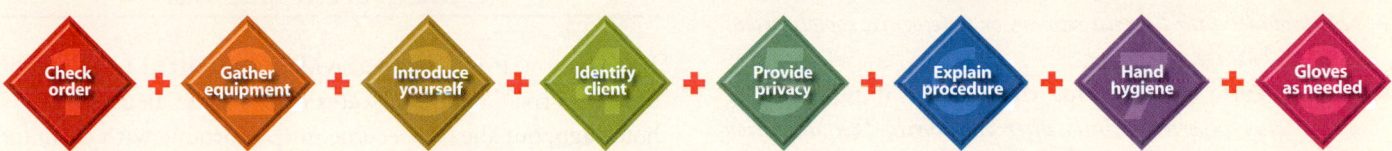

Check order + Gather equipment + Introduce yourself + Identify client + Provide privacy + Explain procedure + Hand hygiene + Gloves as needed

Interventions

1. With gloved hands and without activating suction, insert end of suction device into neonate's nose or mouth (Figure 7-35 ■). *Insertion should be done without suction so the device does not become attached to oral or nasal mucosa.*

2. Place thumb over suction control. Apply suction while removing the tube and rotating it slightly. *The motion of the tube will remove fluids and prevent them from being redeposited in the nasopharynx.*

3. Repeat suctioning as needed. When no fluid is aspirated, stop suctioning. *Excessive suctioning can stimulate the vagus nerve and decrease neonatal heart rate.*

4. If the device is used to suction meconium secretions from the stomach, it should be passed through the newborn's mouth, not the nares. *The neonate's nares are small and delicate. It is quicker and easier to insert the tube through the mouth.*

5. Document completion of the procedure and the type and amount of secretions obtained. *Documentation provides information about the neonate at birth and also provides the record of care.*

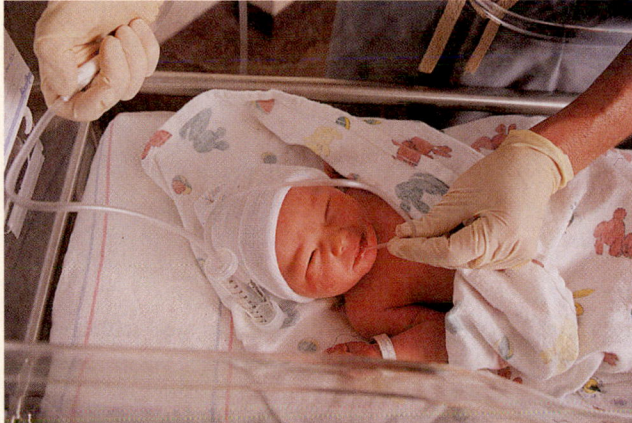

Figure 7-35. ■ A newborn infant being suctioned with a DeLee mucus trap to remove excess secretions from the mouth and nares.

SAMPLE DOCUMENTATION

(date, time)   5 mL meconium-stained fluid suctioned from nares and throat, reported to nurse midwife. ____
P. Bohlen, LPN

- Once the mother and infant are stable, the nurse wraps the infant and allows the mother to hold and, if desired, to breastfeed the infant. The nurse should pick up the delivery room and make the environment presentable for family visitors. *Bonding is important for all members of the family.*

Maternal Care in Stage Four Labor

During the fourth stage of labor and birth, the nurse monitors the mother and newborn.

- Take maternal vital signs every 15 minutes for 1 hour. *This provides data to track recovery or to recognize complications at an early stage.*
- Provide extra blankets for the mother if needed. *The mother may experience chills after childbirth. (See discussion of this topic in Chapter 10 ⚭.)*
- Check the fundus for position and firmness, and assess vaginal flow for amount and character. (See Chapter 10 ⚭.) *The mother's fundus should remain firm, below the umbilicus, and in the midline. Failure of the fundus to remain firm could indicate intrauterine bleeding. If the fundus is not in the proper location, blood clots or a full bladder should be suspected. Vaginal bleeding is assessed by the saturation on the perineal pad.*

clinical ALERT

Total saturation of a perineal pad in the space of one hour is considered heavy bleeding. Report any deviation from normal range to the care provider.

- The fundus may need to be massaged and clots removed. (The procedure for massaging the fundus is provided in Chapter 10 ⚭.) In some facilities and in some states, expelling clots from the uterus is not an LPN/LVN function. *It is important for the LPN/LVN to communicate closely with the RN if the fundus does not remain firm. Always follow facility policy and state nurse practice acts concerning scope of practice.*
- Assess the newborn for signs of respiratory distress. *Notify the charge nurse or care provider if the newborn exhibits these signs of respiratory distress: dusky color, grunting respirations, nasal flaring, and sternal retractions. (See more about respiratory care in Chapter 18 ⚭.)*
- Ensure that the newborn is kept warm, either by warm blankets or by being placed in a warming bed. The newborn may be kept in the room with the mother or placed in the newborn nursery. (Chapter 9 ⚭ details newborn care.)

EVALUATING

The client is evaluated for comfort, stability of vital signs, progression of labor, and response of the fetus. The closer the client progresses toward delivery, the more frequent the evaluation should be. In many cases the nurse remains at the bedside, caring for only one client at a time. After birth, vital signs are taken often to verify that mother and infant are stabilizing.

NURSING PROCESS CARE PLAN
Woman in Active Stage One Labor

Jane, a 20-year-old primagravida, is admitted to the labor unit in active labor. She states contractions began about 5 hours ago, but she has become uncomfortable with them for about 30 minutes. She appears comfortable between contractions but is using controlled breathing techniques during contractions.

Assessment. The following data should be collected as soon as possible after admission:

- Vital signs
- Fetal heart tones
- Urine sample for sugar and protein
- Frequency and duration of contractions
- Dilatation and effacement of the cervix
- Presentation, position, and station of the fetus
- Mother's choice for pain control.

Nursing Diagnosis. The following important nursing diagnosis (among others) is established for this client.

Risk for Ineffective Individual Coping related to birthing process and fatigue of labor

Expected Outcome. Mother will participate actively in the birthing process with no evidence of injury to herself or the fetus.

Planning and Implementation

- Constantly monitor events of second and third stage of labor and birth. *This will ensure maternal and fetal well-being.*
- Provide feedback regarding the progression of labor and delivery. *Feedback helps relieve anxiety and enhance participation.*
- Provide comfort measures such as positioning, dry linen, oral care, and minimal distractions. *Minimizing distractions can decrease discomfort and aid in focusing on the birth process.*
- Remind mother and support person of breathing techniques, positioning, and bearing down during delivery. *These reminders support and encourage participation in the birth process.*

Evaluation

- Labor progresses in a normal pattern.
- Mother verbalizes sufficient comfort.
- Mother remains in control of her behavior.
- Fetal heart rate remains within normal limits.

Critical Thinking in the Nursing Process

1. What are the two top priorities in caring for Jane?
2. Many women in labor are offered a whirlpool bath. Should Jane be offered this method of relaxation? Why or why not?

3. What criteria would the nurse use to determine if Jane should be given a narcotic pain medication that has been ordered PRN?

Note: Discussion of Critical Thinking questions appears in Appendix I.

Note: The references and resources for this and all chapters have been compiled at the back of the book.

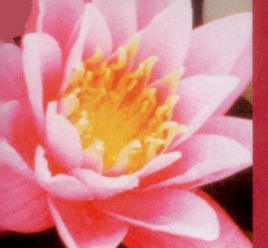

Chapter Review

 **KEY TERMS** by Topics

Use the audio glossary feature of either the CD-ROM or the Companion Website to hear the correct pronunciation of the following key terms.

Signs of Impending Labor
lightening, Braxton Hicks contractions, false labor, effacement, dilatation, bloody show, spontaneous rupture of membranes (SROM), ballotable, prolapsed umbilical cord, premature rupture of membranes (PROM)

Admission to the Birthing Facility
clonus

Variables Affecting Labor
Ps affecting labor, passage, cephalopelvic disproportion (CPD), station, passenger, fetal attitude, fetal lie, transverse lie, fetal presentation, cephalic presentation, vertex presentation, occiput, mentum, sinciput, breech presentation, fetal position, sutures, fontanels, molding, contractions, frequency, duration, intensity, Ferguson's reflex, psyche

Pain in Labor
natural childbirth, regional blocks

Stages of Labor
labor, first stage of labor, dilatation stage, latent phase, active phase, transition phase, amniotomy, second stage of labor, crowning, episiotomy, mechanisms of labor, cardinal movements, engagement, descent, flexion, internal rotation, extension, restitution, external rotation, expulsion, third stage of labor, Schultze mechanism, Duncan mechanism, fourth stage of labor, postpartal chills

Delivery Room Care of the Neonate
Apgar score

Nursing Care
Leopold's maneuver, effleurage

KEY Points

- Labor progresses in an identifiable sequence of events.
- Nursing care during labor involves providing comfort measures for the mother and monitoring the well-being of the infant.
- To determine if labor is progressing in a normal pattern, the nurse must understand the stages of labor and the mechanism by which the infant maneuvers its way through the birth canal.
- The nurse must be constantly on the alert to see whether labor is progressing normally. If it is not, the care provider must be notified at once.

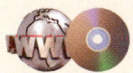 **EXPLORE MediaLink**

Additional interactive resources for this chapter can be found on the Companion Website at www.prenhall.com/towle.

Click on Chapter 7 and "Begin" to select the activities for this chapter.

For chapter-related NCLEX-style questions and an audio glossary, access the accompanying CD-ROM in this book.

Animations

Second stage of labor

Delivery of infant

Breech birth

Applying umbilical cord alarm system

Leopold's maneuvers

Placenta cord blood

FOR FURTHER Study

For additional information on cord blood banking and the cord blood registry, see Chapter 2.

See Chapter 5 for further discussion about dilation and curettage (D&C).

For a complete discussion on complications of pregnancy, see Chapter 8.

Discussion about the care of a healthy newborn appears in Chapter 9.

For a complete discussion on postpartum care, including steps in performing fundal massage, see Chapter 10.

Pediatric respiratory care is discussed further in Chapter 18.

Caring for a Woman in Transition

NCLEX-PN® Focus Area: Physiologic Adaptation

Case Study: 0630 Alyce, a 22-year-old, gravida 2, para 1, is admitted in transition. She states she woke up in labor and her water broke on the way to the hospital. She is obviously uncomfortable and is having difficulty staying relaxed. States previous labor lasted 6 hours.

Nursing Diagnosis: Pain related to contractions

COLLECT DATA

Subjective	Objective
_____	_____
_____	_____
_____	_____
_____	_____
_____	_____
_____	_____

Would you report this? Yes/No

If yes, to: _____

Nursing Care

_____
_____
_____
_____
_____
_____
_____
_____
_____
_____
_____
_____

How would you document this? _____
_____
_____
_____

Compare your documentation to the sample provided in Appendix I.

Data Collected
(use those that apply)

- Cervix 8 cm dilated, 100% effaced
- Station +2
- BP 142/90
- Contractions every 3 minutes, lasting 90 seconds
- Obviously uncomfortable
- Having difficulty maintaining control
- Fetal heart rate 110
- Clear fluid draining from vagina

Nursing Interventions
(use those that apply; list in priority order)

- Prepare sterile field for delivery.
- Oxygen at 10 L per mask.
- Encourage to breathe with each contraction.
- Administer pain medication IV.
- Position on left side.

NCLEX-PN® Exam Preparation

1 The nurse is preparing an expectant mother for a routine prenatal visit. This client asks you to review the hormonal theory of labor with her. When you are finished reviewing, you will evaluate that she understands the hormonal theory of labor if she says fetal production of which of the following hormones increases as the fetus matures and, when sufficient, starts a chain of hormonal events that causes labor?

1. cortisol
2. oxytocin
3. progesterone
4. estrogen

2 When gathering data on a client who has experienced "lightening," the client would most likely claim which of the following?

1. "I can breathe much better."
2. "My ankles are less swollen."
3. "I don't have to urinate as often now."
4. "My lower back pain has been relieved."

3 You are a student nurse assisting in the care of a client who is in labor. If the primary nurse examines this client and finds a prolapsed cord, you realize that the nurse will most likely ask for your assistance in which of the following interventions. Choose all that apply.

1. giving medication to hasten a vaginal birth
2. keeping the client in a back-lying position
3. positioning the client in Trendelenburg
4. arranging for an emergency C-section
5. getting the cord back to its original location
6. monitoring fetal heart rate

4 The student nurse observing a birth hears the obstetrician and the circulating nurse talking about the fetus being "a vertex." The student realizes that the fetal part presenting first is which of the following body parts?

1. forehead
2. face
3. buttocks
4. occiput

5 A client in labor complains of feeling faint, and the nurse turns her on her side. What effect will the side-lying position have on the laboring client's contractions?

1. little or no effect at all
2. increase in frequency
3. increase in intensity
4. will stop the contractions

6 A client is 3 centimeter dilated, excited about labor, and having contractions every 3 to 5 minutes. This phase is best described as:

1. active phase, second stage.
2. latent phase, first stage.
3. transition phase, second stage.
4. active phase, first stage.

7 The nurse explains the phases and stages of labor to first-time expectant parents. The nurse realizes the client understands when she describes the average length of active phase for a primagravida as lasting which of the following lengths of time?

1. 16–18 hours
2. 12–14 hours
3. 8–10 hours
4. 4–6 hours

8 A client in labor has no family or friends to support her during the labor process, so you are supporting her. The physician says the cervix is 8 centimeter dilated. The client's contractions are strong, and she gets irritable with you and tells you not to touch her. Which of the following actions would be appropriate? Choose all that apply.

1. Ask for another nurse to support the client.
2. Tell the client to be cooperative and do as you say.
3. Teach simple relaxation and breathing techniques.
4. Ask the client to push actively with each contraction.
5. Apply warm soaks to her back.
6. Position the client on her left side.

9 You hear the obstetrician, working with a laboring client, say that engagement has occurred. You realize this means which of the following things?

1. The fetus has now become ballotable.
2. Presenting part has entered the true pelvis.
3. Presenting part is just above the ischial spines.
4. There is now observable crowning.

10 You are caring for a client in the fourth stage of labor/birth. At the end of 1 hour, you find the client has saturated two perineal pads. Which of the following actions would be most important?

1. Notify the charge nurse immediately.
2. Assure the client that this is normal.
3. Put the client on the bedpan to void.
4. Start a count of the pads and chart it.

Answers for Review Questions, as well as discussion of Care Plan and Critical Thinking Care Map questions, appear in Appendix I.

Maternal High-Risk Nursing Care

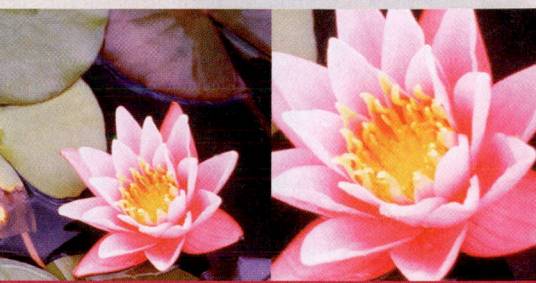

BRIEF Outline

LEARNING Outcomes

After completing this chapter you will be able to:

- Describe factors that put a woman at risk for complications of pregnancy.
- Describe diagnostic tests commonly used during pregnancy.
- Describe common complications of pregnancy, including symptoms, medical treatment, and nursing care.
- Describe common complications during labor and delivery, including symptoms, medical interventions, and nursing care.
- Describe common complications during the postpartum period, including symptoms, medical interventions, and nursing care.

The role of the LPN/LVN is generally one of caring for stable clients, including identifying and reporting signs of complications and teaching clients to prevent them. At times, the RN needs assistance in providing care to clients who are seriously ill. In these cases, the LPN/LVN needs to have a deeper understanding of pathophysiology and treatment. This chapter contains information about care of the woman at risk for life-threatening complications during pregnancy, labor and delivery, and postpartum.

HIGH-RISK PREGNANCY

Risk Factors

Factors associated with high-risk childbearing are grouped according to the threat to health and the outcome of the pregnancy. Box 8-1 ■ identifies these risk factors. Figure 8-1 ■ shows likely referrals for various high-risk issues. Risk factors are interrelated and cumulative. Therefore, a pregnant woman who has multiple risk factors is considered to have a high-risk pregnancy even if each risk factor is not major by itself. Risk factors are identified by verbal interview or written survey. The LPN/LVN may help collect data about risk factors.

Ideally, women prepare for pregnancy by maintaining healthy behaviors, including proper nutrition and the avoidance of risky behavior prior to conception. As stated in Chapter 6 ∞, the woman should obtain prenatal care as soon as she suspects she is pregnant, or within the first 6 to 8 weeks. However, many women do not plan for pregnancy. Some engage in a variety of risk-taking behaviors (large intake of alcohol or other substances, unguarded sexual intercourse with multiple partners, smoking, poor nutritional habits, or fad diets). These behaviors may be part of a woman's lifestyle, and they increase the woman's risk of complications. Once the pregnant woman obtains health care and risk factors are identified, teaching can begin and a plan of care can be implemented to decrease the number and severity of complications.

Even with the best prenatal care, complications can occur. With frequent monitoring and evaluation, though, the severity of complications may be kept to a minimum. If signs of complications are detected, further testing is warranted to evaluate fetal well-being.

BOX 8-1	ASSESSMENT

Risk Factors for High-Risk Pregnancy

Biophysical Factors

Genetic makeup: Abnormalities may interfere with normal fetal development.

Nutritional status: Normal fetal growth and development cannot progress without adequate nutrients.

Medical and/or obstetric history: Mother's health can lead to complications. Examples include history of preterm labor, diabetes, and kidney disease.

Psychosocial Factors

Smoking: Maternal smoking leads to low-birth-weight infants.

Caffeine: Heavy consumption may lead to slight decrease in birth weight.

Alcohol: Consumption of alcohol can lead to fetal disabilities, including fetal alcohol syndrome, learning disabilities, and hyperactivity.

Drugs: Many drugs can affect the fetus, including prescription, over-the-counter, and illicit drugs.

Psychological status: Pregnancy triggers complex psychological responses that affect maternal well-being.

Sociodemographic Factors

Low income: Inadequate financial resources lead to no prenatal care, poor diet, and poor general health.

Lack of prenatal care: Early diagnosis and treatment of complications affect the outcome of the pregnancy.

Age: Adolescents have a higher incidence of complications, including anemia, PIH, and difficult labor. The mature woman is at higher risk for low birth weight, macrosomia, chromosomal abnormalities, congenital malformation, and neonatal mortality.

Parity: First pregnancies and multigravida (especially when pregnancies are close together) carry higher risk.

Marital status: Mortality and morbidity rates are higher for the fetus of nonmarried women.

Residence: Residence is not a risk factor by itself, but health care in some areas is not available or is of poor quality.

Ethnicity: Ethnicity alone is not a risk factor, but it may be impacted by other sociodemographic factors.

Environmental Factors

Many environmental substances can affect the pregnancy, including air quality, chemicals such as pesticides, radiation, and stress. These are found in the workplace, the home, and the community.

Early pregnancy risk identification

Medical history/conditions	Recommended consultation *
Asthma	
Symptomatic on medication	■
Severe (multiple hospitalizations)	△
Cardiac disease	
Cyanotic, prior MI, prosthetic valve, AHA Class ≥ II	△
Other	■
Diabetes mellitus	
Class A–C	■
Class ≥ D	△
Drug/alcohol use	■
Epilepsy (on medication)	■
Family history of genetic problems (Down Syndrome, Tay Sachs)	△
Hemoglobinopathy (SS, SC, S-thal)	△
Hypertension	
Chronic, with renal or heart disease	△
Chronic, on medication or diastolic ≥ 90	■
Prior pulmonary embolus/deep vein thrombosis	■
Psychiatric disease	■
Pulmonary disease	
Severe obstructive or restrictive	△
Moderate	■
Renal disease	
Chronic, creatinine ≥ 3 with/without hypertension	△
Chronic, other	■
Requirement for prolonged anticoagulation	△
Severe systemic disease (examples: SLE, hyperthyroidism)	△

Obstetric history/conditions	
Age > 35 at delivery	■
Cesarean delivery, prior classical or vertical	■
Incompetent cervix	■
Prior fetal structural or chromosomal abnormality	△
Prior neonatal death	■
Prior stillbirth	■
Prior preterm delivery or preterm PROM	■
Prior low birthweight (< 2500 g)	■
Second trimester pregnancy loss	■
Uterine leiomyomata or malformation	■

*At the time of consultation, continued patient care should be determined to be by collaboration with the referring care provider or by transfer of care

Initial laboratory	
HIV	
Symptomatic or low CD4 count	△
Other	■
Rh/other blood group isoimmunizations (excl. ABO, Lewis)	△

Initial examination	
Condylomata (extensive, covering vulva/vaginal opening)	■

Key
■ Specialty
△ Subspecialty

Figure 8-1. ■ Early pregnancy risk identification, showing the likely referral for each condition. Depending on the condition, the client may stay with the original health care provider, who would collaborate with the specialist, or the client might be transferred to the specialist for the duration of the pregnancy. (Data from Committee on Perinatal Health, 1995.)

Tests Used to Assess Fetal Well-Being

A variety of tests can be used to assess fetal well-being.

ULTRASOUND

Ultrasound is a valuable diagnostic test used to visualize both maternal and fetal structures. The test is performed by the doctor, advanced practice nurse (nurse practitioner or nurse midwife), or ultrasonographer. Intermittent ultrasound waves (high-frequency sound waves) are conducted through a transducer applied to the maternal abdomen. The ultrasound waves reflect off the tissue, showing the different tissue densities and creating an image of different organs.

If warranted, a *transvaginal (endovaginal) approach* can be used. A small vaginal transducer, covered with a protective sheath, is inserted into the vagina. Ultrasound waves are conducted through the vaginal transducer. Because the ultrasound waves are emitted closer to the internal structures, a clearer, more defined image may be obtained. With

TABLE 8-1

Benefits of Ultrasound in Diagnosing Complications of Pregnancy

ULTRASOUND USE	WEEK OF PREGNANCY	BENEFIT
Identification of pregnancy	5–6 weeks	Confirmation of pregnancy Calculation of EDC in women with irregular menstrual cycles Early planning of care
Fetal heart rate	6–7 weeks	Determine if fetus is alive
Identification of more that one embryo or fetus	5–6 weeks	Early identification of multifetal pregnancy allows for planning of care
Measure biparietal diameter (between the parietal bones of fetal head) or fetal femur length	Can be made 12–13 weeks; most accurate after 20 weeks	Help determine gestational age; identify intrauterine growth restriction
Estimate fetal weight	8 weeks; more accurate after 30 weeks	Estimation of birth weight is useful in identifying macrosomia (infants greater than 4,000 grams) and risk of birth injury
Identification of fetal anomalies (anencephaly, hydroencephaly, cardiac and renal anomalies, etc.)	18–20 weeks	Identification of fetal anomalies is useful in planning care
Identification of the amniotic fluid index	After 20 weeks	Identification of the amount of amniotic fluid is useful in assessing fetal risk
Location of placenta	5–6 weeks if abnormal, repeat after 30 weeks	Locating the placenta is useful in planning third trimester and delivery care
Placenta grading (maturity of placenta is graded by the amount of calcification present)	30 weeks	Grading the placenta is useful in assessing fetal well-being and predicting fetal risk
Determination of fetal position and presentation	35 weeks (fetus usually assumes cephalic presentation by this time)	Determining fetal position and presentation is useful in planning labor and delivery care

either method, the woman may experience pressure when the transducer is repositioned. Three-dimensional ultrasounds are being developed that will allow for more accurate assessment. Ultrasound has been used for more than 40 years with no clinical studies indicating harmful effects to the mother, fetus, or newborn. Table 8-1 ■ indicates the benefits of ultrasound in diagnosing complications of pregnancy.

AMNIOCENTESIS

Amniocentesis, the withdrawal of amniotic fluid through a needle inserted into the abdomen and the uterus, is used to evaluate the environment surrounding the developing fetus. (See Procedure 6-1 in Chapter 6 ∞ for nursing responsibilities.)

A number of tests can be performed on the amniotic fluid. A *quadruple screen* measures appropriate levels of alpha-fetoprotein, human chorionic gonadotropin (hCG), unconjugated estriol, and Diameric Inhibin-A. Abnormal values in these tests are indicative of Down syndrome (trisomy 21), trisomy 18, and neural tube defect.

At times, it is necessary to evaluate *fetal lung maturity* prior to inducing labor or performing a cesarean delivery. Mature lungs produce *surfactant,* a phospholipid that lines the alveoli and prevents the lungs from collapsing with exhalation. If the infant is born before an adequate amount of surfactant is present, the infant will have difficulty breathing. Lecithin and sphingomyelin are two components of surfactant that can be measured in the amniotic fluid. By 32 weeks, the level of lecithin increases and the level of sphingomyelin decreases. By 35 weeks, the ratio of lecithin to sphingomyelin (L/S ratio) should be at least 2:1 (also reported at 2:0), and the lungs are considered mature. Phosphatidylglycerol (PG) is another phospholipid present in surfactant. PG is present in the amniotic fluid when the lungs are mature at around 35 weeks. When amniotic fluid analysis indicates a mature

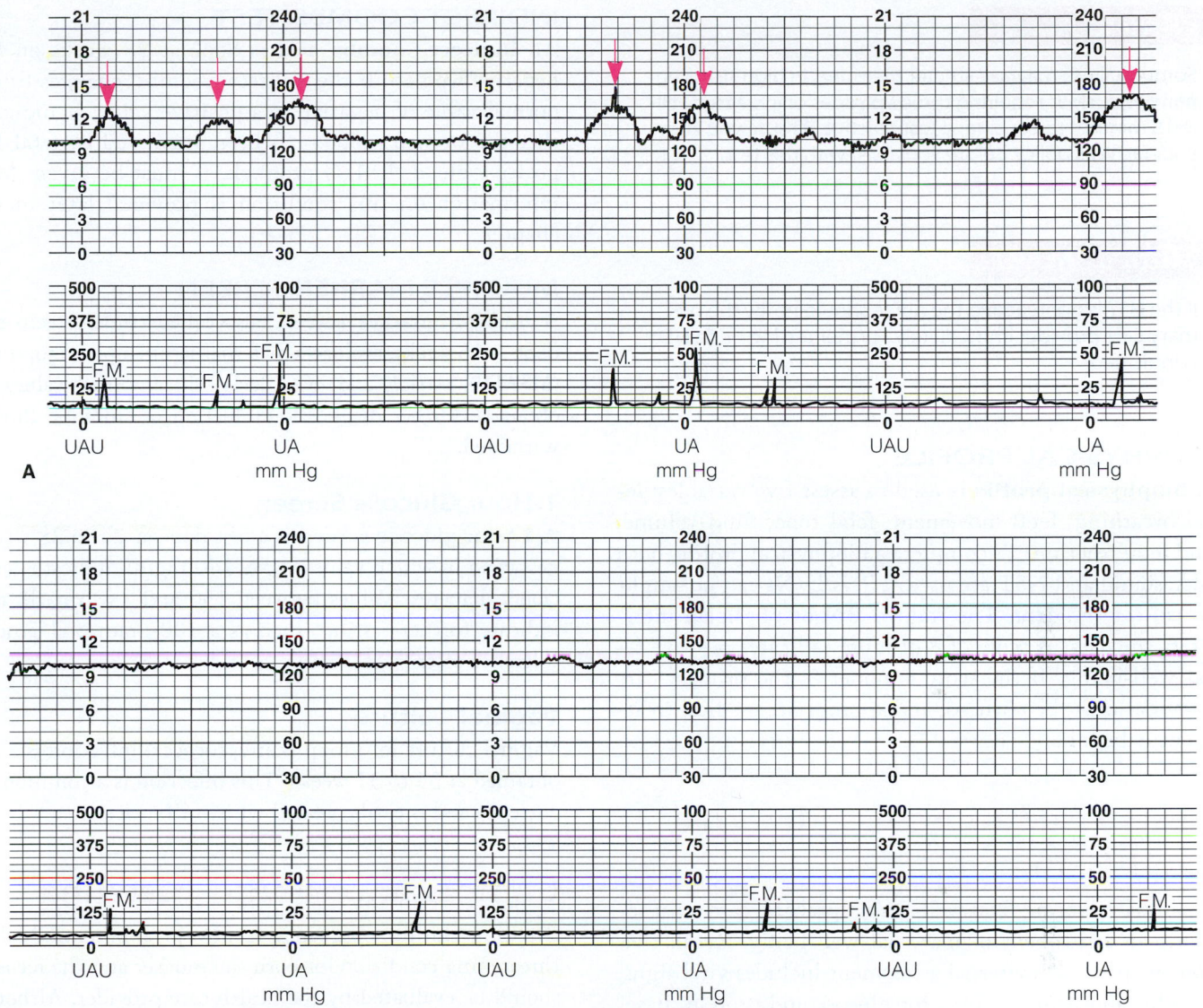

Figure 8-2. ■ **(A)** Normal findings of a reactive nonstress test (NST). **(B)** Examples of a nonreactive NST.

L/S ratio and the presence of PG, the risk of respiratory distress in the infant is low.

Rh factor is another important test. When the mother's blood is Rh negative and the fetus's blood is Rh positive, there is a possibility that the antibodies in the mother's blood will destroy the fetus's blood. This condition, known as **erythroblastosis fetalis** or *hemolytic disease of the newborn,* can be life threatening. During pregnancy, the condition can be monitored by optical density (ΔOD) analysis on the amniotic fluid. The condition is discussed in more depth later in this chapter.

NONSTRESS TEST

A **nonstress test (NST)** is used to assess fetal movement and fetal heart rate (FHR). The test is based on the knowl-

edge that when the fetus has adequate oxygenation and a functioning central nervous system (CNS), there will be accelerations in the FHR with fetal activity (Figure 8-2 ■). The mother is positioned in a semi-Fowler's position, and external fetal monitoring (EFM) equipment is attached to her abdomen. (See Procedure 7-2 in Chapter 7 ⚭) The client identifies fetal movement, and the event is marked on the record. If necessary, fetal movement can be stimulated with a low-frequency vibrator. Usually, the test is considered **reactive** or normal if two episodes of increased FHR occur in a 20-minute period of time.

The heart rate must increase by 15 bpm and last for 15 seconds to be called a reaction. If reactive criteria are not met, the test is considered **nonreactive.** In this case, further testing or immediate birth is recommended.

clinical ALERT

Some facilities may use stricter measures in high-risk pregnancies, such as requiring three episodes of increased FHR in 15 minutes to consider a test reactive. Be sure you know your facility's policy before you assist with this test.

clinical ALERT

If the NST is nonreactive, the nurse should notify the primary care provider immediately. Further testing or delivery is indicated.

BIOPHYSICAL PROFILE

A **biophysical profile** is used to assess five variables: fetal breathing, fetal movement, fetal tone, fluid volume, and fetal reaction. To complete a biophysical profile, both ultrasound and NST are used. LPNs/LVNs can be taught to collect the data. The trained RN or physician interprets the data. A score of 8 or more indicates positive fetal well-being. If the score is under 8, the primary care provider must be notified, and appropriate medical treatment is begun.

Tests Used to Assess Maternal Well-Being

Besides evaluating fetal well-being, prenatal care must include an assessment of maternal well-being. Recall that routine prenatal maternal assessment includes vital signs, weight, and urine analysis for glucose and protein. Baseline blood tests are usually done during the initial prenatal visit and then repeated as indicated. Refer to Table 6-3 in Chapter 6 ∞ for normal values during pregnancy.

MATERNAL HEMOGLOBIN

A **maternal hemoglobin** (measure of the mother's red blood cell [RBC] count) test is repeated at 7 months to assess for anemia. An increased intake of iron or iron supplements may be necessary. There is a tendency for anemia to occur in certain cultural groups (Box 8-2 ■).

BOX 8-2	CULTURAL PULSE POINTS

Erythroblastic Anemia

Women of Mediterranean descent are prone to developing thalassemia, a type of erythroblastic anemia. These women may have a chromosomal defect that results in fragile red blood cells. The stress of pregnancy could cause these fragile cells to be destroyed, resulting in anemia.

INDIRECT COOMBS' TEST

An **indirect Coombs' test** is done at 28 weeks on Rh-negative women. If the indirect Coombs' changes from a normal value of negative to a positive value, it indicates that the woman's blood has been sensitized by fetal Rh-positive blood. RhIgG prophylaxis must be given. More information on this condition is provided later in this chapter.

MULTIPLE MARKER SCREEN

A **multiple marker screen** (also called triple screen) test, done at 16 weeks, evaluates maternal serum alpha-fetoprotein (MSAFP), estriol, and hCG levels. If abnormal values are obtained, further diagnostic evaluation of amniotic fluid is warranted.

1-Hour Glucose Screen

A **1-hour glucose screen** is a test done at 24 to 28 weeks' gestation in which values above 140 mg/dL indicate gestational diabetes. Values between 130 and 140 mg/dL may indicate further testing, such as a 100-gram oral glucose tolerance test.

Vaginal Culture

Vaginal culture for group B streptococcal infection is a test obtained at 35 to 37 weeks. This infection is a common occurrence and is easily treated with antibiotics.

Complications with Bleeding

Bleeding during pregnancy is always a potentially life-threatening condition for both the mother and the fetus. It should be evaluated by the health care provider. Although bleeding could happen at any time, it more commonly occurs in the first and third trimesters.

MENSTRUATION

Menstruation could occur after conception. If the blastocyst implants a few days late, there may not be enough hCG produced to prevent the breakdown of the corpus luteum. A decrease in progesterone would lead to menstrual bleeding. If this occurs, the blastocyst may become detached and the pregnancy could end before the client knew she was pregnant. However, the blastocyst may remain attached to the endometrium and the pregnancy could continue.

SPONTANEOUS ABORTION

Abortion is the term used to identify the loss or termination of any pregnancy, usually before the 20th week of gestation. Although in medical terms abortion is used to describe any pregnancy that ends before the fetus is viable, the public often uses the term to describe a planned event, either a therapeutic or an elective action. In contrast, the public uses the term **miscarriage** to describe the spontaneous event. Some cultures use abortion to describe either occurrence. It is important for the nurse to question the client in a nonjudgmental manner to determine the cause of abortion.

Spontaneous abortion (see Figure 5-20 ⬭) occurs more commonly in the first trimester and can be classified as follows:

- *Threatened.* Bleeding and cramping with the cervix closed and membranes intact.
- *Inevitable.* Bleeding and cramping with the cervix beginning to dilate. The membranes may or may not rupture.
- *Complete.* All products of conception are expelled.
- *Incomplete.* Some of the products of conception are expelled, but the placenta remains attached. Heavy bleeding and severe cramping continue until the placenta is removed.
- *Missed.* The embryo or fetus dies but is not expelled. If the fetus is not expelled within 6 weeks, other complications, including infection and disseminated intravascular coagulation (DIC), can occur. More information regarding DIC is provided later in this chapter.
- *Septic.* An infection of the uterus is present. The infection can be caused by premature rupture of the membranes, an intrauterine device, or an abortion attempted in unsterile conditions.
- *Habitual.* The occurrence of any of the above in 3 consecutive pregnancies. Most commonly, a weak cervix dilates in the second trimester, expelling the fetus. This condition is called **incompetent cervix.**

The treatment of abortion depends on the cause. For a threatened abortion, the client would be placed on bed rest for several days. If the bleeding stops, she should be advised to avoid strenuous activity, fatigue, and sexual intercourse until the pregnancy seems to be progressing normally. If the bleeding does not stop, the pregnancy may be lost and surgical intervention may be necessary. For an inevitable or incomplete abortion, a **D&C (dilation and curettage)** is usually performed under anesthesia. In this procedure, the cervix is dilated, a curette is inserted into the uterus, and the endometrium is scraped, removing all products of conception. For a missed abortion, a D&C may be performed or labor may be induced, depending on the gestational age of the fetus. For habitual abortion caused by an incompetent cervix, a **cerclage (Shirodkar procedure)** is used (Figure 8-3 ⬛). This procedure, done at 16 weeks' gestation, involves surgically placing a suture in the cervix in a purse-string design to hold the cervix closed. The suture can be removed at term, and the fetus can be delivered vaginally. Alternatively, the suture can remain in place for future

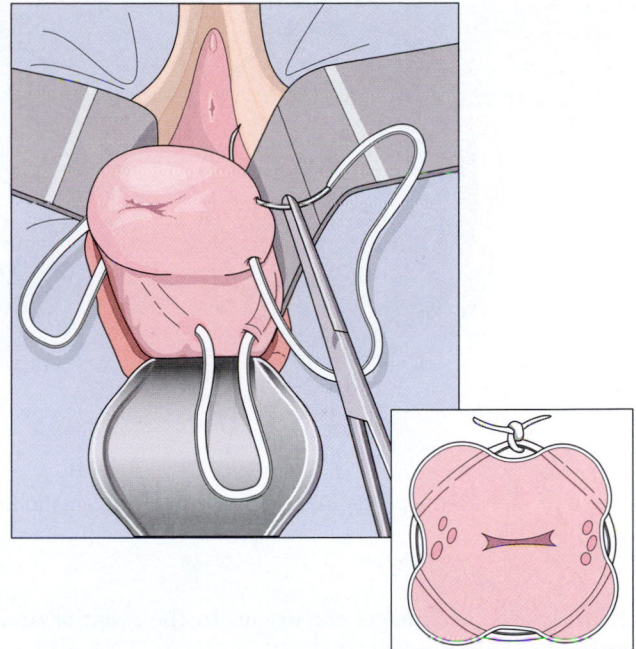

Figure 8-3. ■ A cerclage or purse-string suture is inserted into the cervix to prevent cervical dilation and pregnancy loss. After placement, the string is tightened and secured anteriorly.

pregnancies, and then the fetus will be delivered by cesarean section.

ECTOPIC PREGNANCY

Ectopic pregnancy occurs when the blastocyst implants outside the uterine cavity (Figure 8-4 ■). The most common site for an ectopic pregnancy is the fallopian tube **(tubal pregnancy).** Because the fallopian tubes are not attached to the ovaries, the blastocyst could attach to the ovary or any intra-abdominal structure. The blastocyst could also travel through the uterus and implant in the cervix. As the

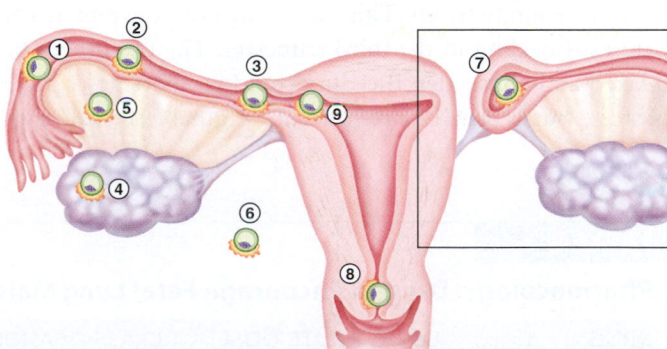

Figure 8-4. ■ Implantation sites of ectopic pregnancy in order of frequency. (1) Ampulla of fallopian tube. (2) Remainder of tube. (3) Interstitial portion of tube. (4) Ovary. (5) Broad ligament (*intraligamentary*). (6) Surface of peritoneum (abdominal). (7) Rudimentary horn. (8) Cervix. (9) Tubouterine junction (angular).

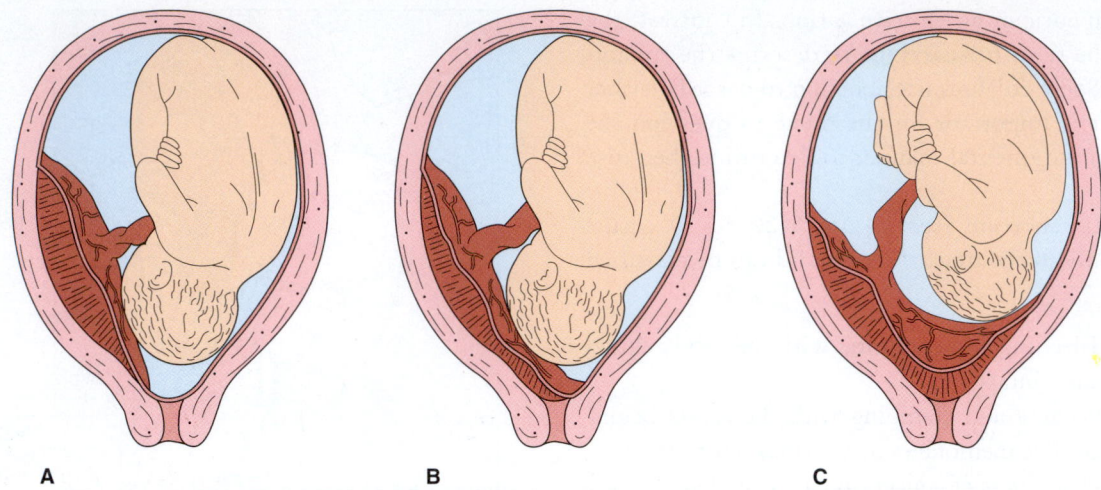

Figure 8-5. ■ Placenta previa. (**A**) Lower placental implantation. (**B**) Partial placenta previa. (**C**) Total placenta previa.

embryo grows, it damages the organ. In the event of tubal pregnancy, the fallopian tube will rupture, causing bleeding into the abdominal cavity, some vaginal bleeding, and shock. Surgery must be performed immediately to stop the bleeding and save the client's life. In most cases, the embryo will not survive an ectopic pregnancy.

PLACENTA PREVIA

Placenta previa results from the blastocyst implanting low in the uterus, allowing the placenta to grow partially or totally across the cervical opening. There are three classifications of placenta previa (Figure 8-5 ■).

- *Marginal or low lying.* The placenta is near the internal cervical opening, but does not cover it.
- *Partial.* The placenta covers part of the cervical opening.
- *Total or complete.* The placenta totally covers the cervical opening.

During the later part of pregnancy, the cervix begins to efface and dilate, resulting in the placenta being torn away from the endometrium. This causes the classic symptoms of painless bleeding in the third trimester. The uterus will be relaxed and nontender. Bleeding could be spotting or more profuse, but is usually intermittent. Vaginal exams are contraindicated until diagnosis can be made by ultrasound. If ultrasound is unavailable, the health care provider may perform a vaginal exam, once preparations for an emergency cesarean section delivery are made.

clinical ALERT

If ultrasound is not available and bleeding is present, preparations for emergency cesarean delivery are made *prior to* any vaginal examination by the health care provider.

The goal of treatment for placenta previa is to stop the bleeding, allowing the fetus time to mature. This may be accomplished by placing the client on bed rest. At times, drugs such as betamethasone (Celestone) may be given to accelerate fetal lung maturity (Table 8-2 ■). If bleeding continues, delivery by cesarean section is begun immediately. The infant and mother should be assessed for anemia.

ABRUPTIO PLACENTAE

Abruptio placentae, or premature separation of the placenta, may occur in late pregnancy or during labor (Figure 8-6 ■).

TABLE 8-2				
Pharmacology: Drug to Encourage Fetal Lung Maturity				
DRUG	**USUAL ROUTE/DOSE**	**CLASSIFICATION**	**SELECTED SIDE EFFECTS**	**DON'T GIVE IF**
Betamethasone (Celestone)	12 mg IM daily for 2–3 days before delivery	Systemic corticosteroid	Low-dose, short-term use has few side effects, fluid retention	Client has active untreated infections (unlabeled use in pregnancy)

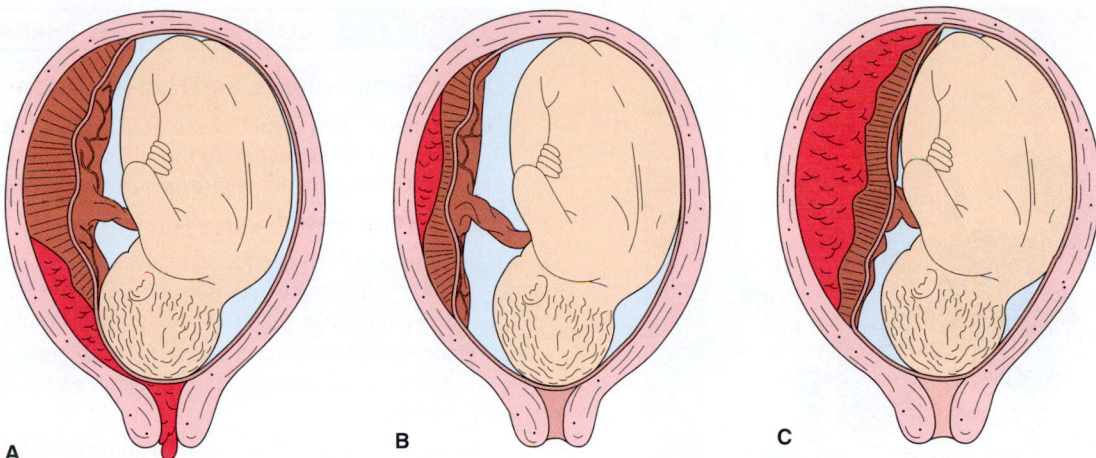

Figure 8-6. ■ Abruptio placentae. **(A)** The marginal abruption with external hemorrhage. **(B)** The central abruption with concealed hemorrhage. **(C)** Complete separation.

The cause is unknown, but contributing factors include maternal hypertension, multiple pregnancy, smoking, use of alcohol and illicit drugs, uterine trauma, and pregnancy continuing past the due date. There are three classifications of abruptio placentae.

- *Marginal.* Edge of the placenta separates and bright red vaginal bleeding occurs.
- *Central.* The center of the placenta separates, trapping blood between the placenta and the uterus. There is no vaginal bleeding, but the uterus becomes painful.
- *Complete.* The entire placenta separates, resulting in profuse bleeding.

If the fetal head is tight against the cervix and maternal pelvis, some blood can be trapped inside the uterus. Bleeding into the myometrium causes a rigid, painful abdomen. After delivery the uterus may contract poorly, resulting in post delivery bleeding.

The goal of treatment for abruptio placentae is delivery as soon as possible. If the separation is small and there are no signs of fetal distress, labor may be induced and allowed to progress. If the separation is moderate or severe, or if the fetus is in distress, an immediate cesarean section is performed. The fetus should be evaluated for anemia and hypoxia. The mother should be evaluated for continued vaginal bleeding and hypovolemia.

Other Complications

HYPEREMESIS GRAVIDARUM

Although "morning sickness" is common in the first 12 weeks of pregnancy, excessive vomiting, or **hyperemesis gravidarum,** leads to dehydration and electrolyte imbalance.

The client vomits everything she tries to eat. She may develop tachycardia, hypovolemia, hypotension, and an increase in blood urea nitrogen. Other signs of dehydration include poor skin turgor, dry mucous membranes, dark concentrated urine, and urinary output less than 30 mL/hr. Lack of nutrition leads to protein and vitamin deficiencies. The embryo or fetus can also suffer from lack of water, lack of nutrients, and a buildup of waste products.

The goals of treatment are to prevent further emesis, regain fluid and electrolyte balance, and maintain adequate nutrition. Antiemetics are prescribed to relieve the vomiting. Oral fluids are withheld until vomiting stops. Oral fluids are then introduced in small quantities at a time. If fluid balance cannot be restored orally, hospitalization may be required to administer intravenous fluids. Once fluid balance is restored and further emesis is prevented, the pregnancy usually progresses normally.

CARDIAC DISORDERS

Pregnancy puts additional work on the woman's heart. Although the cardiovascular system must be routinely assessed, most young women compensate without undue risk. However, not every young woman has a healthy heart prior to pregnancy (Figure 8-7 ■). She may have a heart defect or have sustained cardiac damage from a childhood infection or drug abuse. The added workload on the damaged heart may result in congestive heart failure. The following symptoms are indicative of congestive heart failure and must be reported to the primary care provider:

- Frequent cough with or without hemoptysis (bloody sputum)
- Progressive dyspnea with exertion
- Rales in lung bases

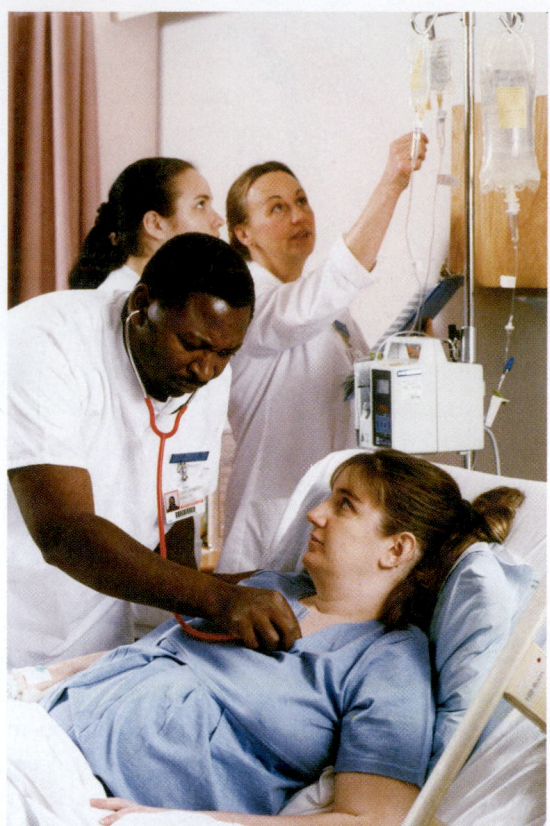

Figure 8-7. ■ When a woman with heart disease begins labor, the caregivers must monitor her closely for signs of congestive heart failure.

■ Progressive generalized edema
■ Heart murmur
■ Fatigue.

The client with cardiac disorders may require constant heart monitoring during labor. Signs of worsening heart failure may necessitate a cesarean section delivery.

HYPERTENSIVE DISORDERS

Several hypertensive disorders can occur during pregnancy. The National High Blood Pressure Education Program (2000) recommends the following classification:

■ Gestational hypertension (formerly pregnancy-induced hypertension or PIH)
■ Pre-eclampsia
■ Eclampsia
■ Chronic hypertension
■ Pre-eclampsia superimposed on chronic hypertension.

Gestational Hypertension

Gestational hypertension is a transient disorder characterized by an increased blood pressure of 140/90 or higher. The hypertensive event occurs for the first time during pregnancy. It is not accompanied by proteinuria.

The blood pressure returns to normal by 12 weeks after the pregnancy.

Clients may be advised about herbs and supplements that affect hypertension (Box 8-3 ■).

Chronic Hypertension

Chronic hypertension occurs when the blood pressure is 140/90 or higher before pregnancy and continues for more than 12 weeks after delivery. It is important for the woman with chronic hypertension to be monitored closely for signs of pre-eclampsia.

Pre-eclampsia and Eclampsia

Pre-eclampsia and **eclampsia,** once called *toxemia,* is a common, complex condition that develops after 20 weeks' gestation. Although the cause is unknown, it is most often seen in primigravidas younger than 20 or older than 35 years of age who have a poor nutritional status. Chronic hypertension, diabetes, and multiple pregnancy (more than one fetus) increase the risk of pre-eclampsia. The only cure is delivery of the baby.

This complication of pregnancy ranges from mild pre-eclampsia to severe pre-eclampsia and eclampsia, depending on the severity of the symptoms. The classic symptoms include progressive hypertension and proteinuria. At one time, edema was included as one of the classic signs, but it is no longer included because it is such a common finding during pregnancy. To be considered sustained hypertension,

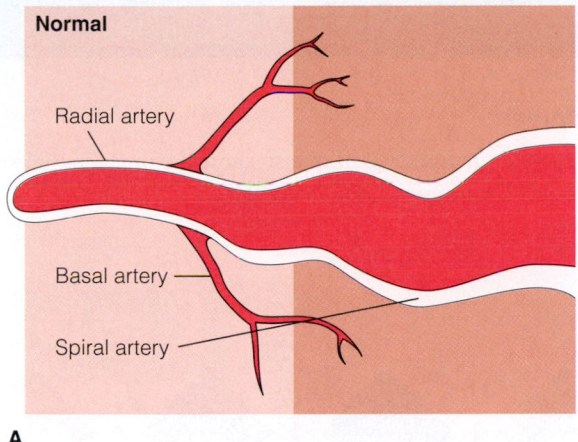

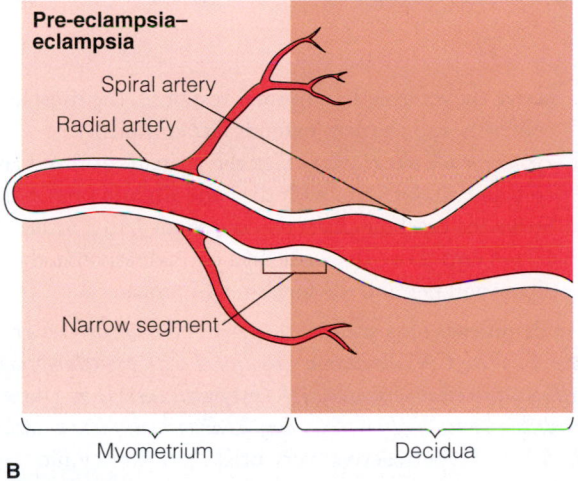

Figure 8-8. ■ **(A)** In a normal pregnancy, the passive quality of the spiral arteries permits increased blood flow to the placenta. **(B)** In pre-eclampsia, vasoconstriction of the myometrial segment of the spiral arteries occurs. This restricts blood flow to the placenta.

the blood pressure elevation is obtained on two occasions 6 hours apart.

Vasoconstriction decreases circulation to the uterus and placenta (Figure 8-8 ■). Blood flow to the kidneys slows, which decreases filtration through the glomerulus, resulting in protein in the urine and edema. Fluid overload leads to cerebral edema, headache, visual disturbances, and hyperactive deep tendon reflexes (Procedure 8-1 ■). The liver enlarges, resulting in epigastric pain and liver damage.

Mild pre-eclampsia is exhibited by a blood pressure of 30 mm Hg systolic or 15 mm Hg diastolic above the client's normal blood pressure reading or a blood pressure reading of 140/90. Edema may be seen in the hands and face, and the client will have a weight gain of more than 1 pound per week (Figure 8-10 ■). The urine may show 1+ protein on a dipstick. Box 8-4 ■ highlights manifes-

tations of mild versus severe pre-eclampsia and eclampsia. In severe pre-eclampsia, the blood pressure increases to 160/110 or higher. Generalized edema is noted in the hands, face, sacrum, lower extremities, and abdomen. Weight gain may be 2 or more pounds in a few days to a week. Protein will be 2+ or more on a dipstick. Urine output may drop to less than 500 mL in 24 hours. The client may exhibit other symptoms, including headache, blurred vision, scotoma (spots before the eyes), irritability, hyperreflexes, and epigastric pain. If left untreated, the condition may progress to eclampsia, as evidenced by grand mal seizures. The client may slip into a coma. The seizures may recur, and the client, the fetus, or both may die. The seizure activity may induce uterine contractions, but the comatose client may be unable to let anyone know.

clinical ALERT

The client with chronic hypertension who develops pre-eclampsia often progresses quickly to eclampsia. The woman with chronic hypertension must be taught to notify the health care provider immediately if any symptoms of pre-eclampsia appear. The nurse must also be alert to and report any manifestations of a seizure. These include:

Partial seizures. Brief change in consciousness with blank stare, blinking of the eyes, fluttering eyelids, or lip smacking

Generalized seizures. Loud cry (called an epileptic cry), loss of consciousness, *tonic* (back-arching) contractions, any cyanosis followed by *clonic* (jerking, contracting and relaxing) contractions, possible frothing, tongue biting, and incontinence

Anticonvulsants (magnesium sulfate or Dilantin) should be available at the bedside for immediate administration.

HELLP Syndrome

Pre-eclampsia with liver damage is characterized by hemolysis, elevated liver enzymes, and low platelet count or **HELLP syndrome.** *Hemolysis* (breakdown of RBCs) occurs when vasospasms cause platelets to aggregate and a fibrin network to form. As RBCs are forced through the fibrin network, they break, resulting in a large decrease in hematocrit. It is believed that the elevation of liver enzymes (AST and ALT) is due to microemboli in vessels in the liver that cause ischemia. A low platelet count of less than $100,000/mm^3$ occurs when platelets aggregate in the arteries. HELLP syndrome results in ischemia and tissue damage. The low platelet count may increase post-delivery bleeding.

Assessing Deep Tendon Reflexes and Clonus

Purpose

- To detect hyperreflexia, which may be a sign of pre-eclampsia
- To determine the presence of clonus, which indicates CNS irritability
- To establish a baseline when beginning medication for pre-eclampsia
- To determine the effectiveness of magnesium sulfate therapy

Equipment

- Percussion hammer (bell of a stethoscope or the radial side of hand if hammer is not available)

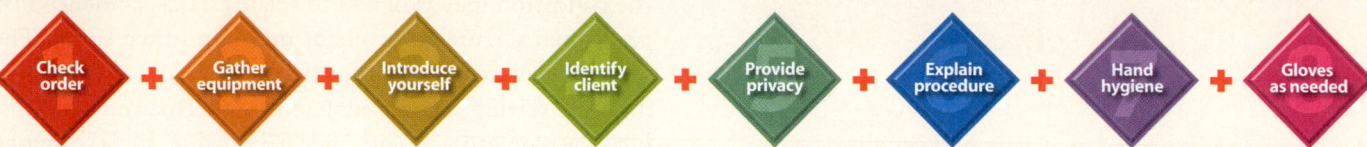

Check order + Gather equipment + Introduce yourself + Identify client + Provide privacy + Explain procedure + Hand hygiene + Gloves as needed

Interventions

1. *Elicit Reflexes.* Usually, the patellar reflex and one other reflex are elicited. *Test of more than one reflex helps ensure that assessment of response is accurate.*
   a. *Patellar Reflex.* Woman in position with legs hanging over the bed or table and not touching the floor. Strike the patellar tendon quickly (just below the patella or "kneecap"). In a normal response, the foot thrusts ("jerks") forward in extension.
   b. *Biceps Reflex.* Support woman's relaxed arm flexed at 45 degrees at the elbow. Place your thumb on the biceps tendon in the antecubital space and your fingers on the posterior elbow. Strike your thumb in a downward motion. In a normal response, the arm flexes.
   c. *Triceps Reflex.* Abduct the woman's upper arm to 90 degrees and have her allow the hand to drop down loosely from the elbow. Strike the triceps tendon (just

   above the elbow). In a normal response, the muscle contracts and the arm extends (straightens).
   d. *Brachioradialis Reflex.* Flex the woman's arm and lay it on your own forearm, with the hand slightly pronated. Strike the brachioradialis tendon, about 1 to 2 inches (2.5–5 cm) above the wrist. In a normal response, the elbow will flex and the forearm will pronate.

2. Grade reflexes on a scale of 0 to 4+. *Normal reflexes are 1+ or 2+. With CNS irritation (associated with pre-eclampsia), reflexes may be abnormally high (hyperreflexia). If magnesium levels become too high, reflexes may be abnormally low or absent.*
   a. 4+ = Hyperreactive; very brisk, jerky, or clonic response
   b. 3+ = Brisker than normal but may not be abnormal
   c. 2+ = Average or normal response
   d. 1+ = Diminished or less than normal response
   e. 0 = No response

3. Assess for clonus. With woman's knee flexed, support the leg and vigorously dorsiflex the foot (Figure 8-9 ■). Hold the foot in dorsiflexion briefly and then release. Note and document normal or abnormal response as one to four beats or sustained. *Normal response is a return to normal position. Abnormal response is a "jerk" or tap of the foot against the examiner's hand before the foot returns to rest in normal plantar flexion. The number of taps or beats must be recorded. This abnormal reaction indicates CNS irritability and a more pronounced hyperreflexia.*

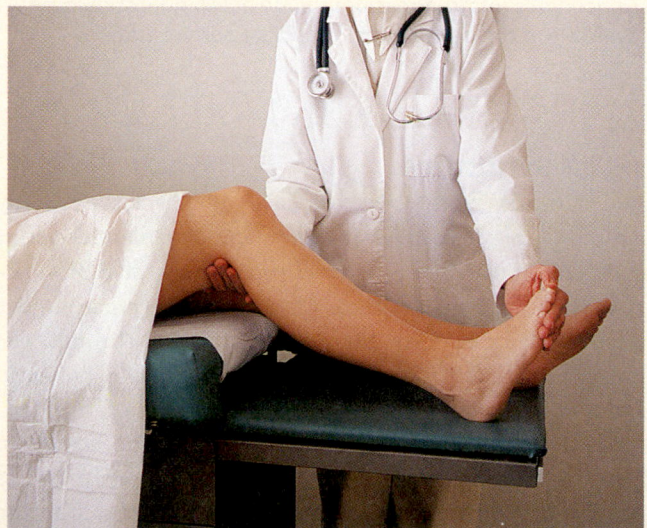

Figure 8-9. ■ To elicit clonus, the nurse sharply dorsiflexes the foot. In an abnormal reaction, the foot performs one or a series of "taps" against the examiner's hand. The nurse records the reaction and the number of taps. (©Elena Dorfman.)

SAMPLE DOCUMENTATION

(date) 1530   T 98.6, P 75, R 20, BP 176/100. Assessed reflexes. Patellar 4+, brachioradialis 4+, clonus sustained; reported reflexes and clonus to care provider. _____

S. Kimini, LVN

Preeclampsia and Eclampsia (Toxemia)

Indications:
Progressive hypertension
Proteinuria

Results:
Vasoconstriction decreases circulation to uterus and placenta. Blood flow to kidneys slows; glomerular filtration decreases; protein in urine increases; edema is marked.
Fluid overload leads to cerebral edema, headache, visual disturbances, hyperactive deep tendon reflexes. Liver enlarges, resulting in epigastric pain and liver damage.

Figure 8-10. ■ Pre-eclampsia edema.

Complications of Pre-eclampsia

Pre-eclampsia may cause a placental infarction. Placental infarction may in turn cause intrauterine growth retardation (IUGR) and acute hypoxia in the fetus, leading to intrauterine death. Abruptio placentae is more common with pre-eclampsia. The fetus may be born preterm due to

BOX 8-4	ASSESSMENT

Pre-eclampsia and Eclampsia

Mild Pre-eclampsia

- Blood pressure (BP) of 30 mm Hg systolic or 15 mm Hg diastolic above the client's normal BP reading *or* BP reading of 140/90
- Possible edema in hands and face
- Weight gain of more than 1 pound per week
- Possible urine output reduction
- Urine may show 1+ protein on a dipstick
- Hyperreflexes
- Complaints of headache, blurred vision, scotoma (spots before eyes), irritability, and epigastric pain

Severe Pre-eclampsia

- BP increases to 160/110 or higher
- Generalized edema in hands, face, sacrum, lower extremities, and abdomen
- Possible weight gain of 2 or more pounds in a few days to a week
- Urine protein 2+ or more on a dipstick
- Urine output reduced, possibly less than 500 miligram in 24 hours

Eclampsia

- Grand mal seizures
- Possible coma
- Initiation of contractions (The seizure activity may induce uterine contractions, but the comatose client may be unable to let anyone know.)
- Death

spontaneous labor or obstetric induction to save the lives of the mother and the infant.

Treatment for Pre-eclampsia

The goals of treatment of pre-eclampsia are to lower the blood pressure, prevent convulsions, and deliver a healthy infant. The client with mild pre-eclampsia may remain at home but is advised to rest in bed. The client is taught not to lie on her back because of the pressure this puts on vena cava and abdominal aorta against the spinal column (see Figure 6-13 ⬭). Blood return will be best with the woman positioned on her left side, but she will need to shift positions for comfort by lying on either side. A well-balanced diet, high in protein and moderate in sodium, should be provided for the client. Excessively salty foods should be avoided, but salt is not restricted. Antihypertensive drugs, diuretics, and sedatives may be prescribed. If severe pre-eclampsia develops, the client is hospitalized and CNS depressants such as magnesium sulfate ($MgSO_4$) are given by intravenous infusion. Magnesium sulfate is usually given for 24 to 48 hours after delivery to ensure that seizures do not develop (Table 8-3 ■).

clinical ALERT

A syringe containing calcium carbonate, the antidote for magnesium sulfate, must be at the bedside in case magnesium toxicity develops.

Nursing Considerations

Nursing assessment involves monitoring blood pressure, urine output, proteinuria, and deep tendon reflexes. In mild pre-eclampsia, the client feels healthy and must be encouraged to follow the plan of care. Teaching regarding diet, activity, and medication must be provided. In severe pre-eclampsia, the client is hospitalized, and fetal and maternal monitoring is more frequent. The nurse should be prepared to assist with induction of labor or cesarean section delivery if the client does not improve. Pre-eclampsia slowly decreases following delivery, but the client remains at risk of seizure for several days. For this reason, clients usually remain hospitalized and frequent blood pressure, urine protein, and deep tendon reflexes are monitored. (See Procedure 8-1.)

GESTATIONAL DIABETES MELLITUS

Appearing only during pregnancy, **gestational diabetes mellitus (GDM)** is an abnormal glucose metabolism caused by the additional requirement for insulin. Many women who develop GDM will develop diabetes mellitus later in life. The client who develops diabetes prior to pregnancy has the same risks to the pregnancy as does the client who develops gestational diabetes, but the blood glucose is more difficult to control.

TABLE 8-3				
Pharmacology: Drug to Reduce CNS Activity and Risk of Seizures				
DRUG	**USUAL ROUTE/DOSE**	**CLASSIFICATION**	**SELECTED SIDE EFFECTS**	**DON'T GIVE IF**
Magnesium sulfate ($MgSO_4$)	4 g/IV infusion, then 1–2 g/hr continuous	Mineral/electrolyte	Arrhythmias, bradycardia, hypotension	Vital signs are not within normal limits (Unlabeled use in pregnancy, but it is routinely given)

In early pregnancy, the mother's pancreas increases insulin production due to an increase in hormones. The tissue's response to the high insulin level is also increased. After the 20th week of pregnancy, an increased resistance to insulin develops as a result of increased placental hormones. Fat is more readily metabolized, resulting in ketonuria. Because the maternal glucose provides energy for the developing fetus, balancing blood glucose levels is more difficult. After delivery of the placenta, there is a rapid decrease in the amount of insulin required. The diabetic client is at greater risk for preeclampsia and ketoacidosis than the nondiabetic client. Refer to a medical-surgical text for information on ketoacidosis.

The client who develops diabetes during pregnancy will need to be taught to monitor her blood sugar (Figure 8-11 ■) and possibly to administer insulin. She will also need instruction in diet and activity. Many areas have diabetes centers where nurses and dietitians who are trained in diabetes management provide this instruction. If a diabetic center is not available, the clinic nurse will need to provide demonstration, written material, and follow-up evaluation.

Maternal hyperglycemia can result in **macrosomia** (excessive growth in the fetus) (Figure 8-11B). Hyperglycemia stimulates fetal insulin production. After birth, the source of glucose is removed, and the infant can develop hypoglycemia within 2 to 4 hours or actually be born in a hypoglycemic state. Gradually, the fetus will produce only the amount of insulin needed. Chapter 9 also discusses hypoglycemia in the newborn.

INFECTIONS

Any infection during pregnancy should be diagnosed and treated. Although many are not harmful to the fetus, some can cause preterm labor, fetal infections, congenital anomalies, or death. Infections that are particularly dangerous during pregnancy and delivery are mentioned in this section.

STIs

Sexually transmitted infections (STIs) are discussed in Chapter 5 ⚭. However, the pregnant woman who has an untreated STI puts her infant at risk (Table 8-4 ■). The intact fetal membranes offer some protection for the fetus, but once they rupture, the fetus will be exposed to the infection. The infecting agent can ascend into the uterus, or the infant can become exposed during the delivery process. Entry sites

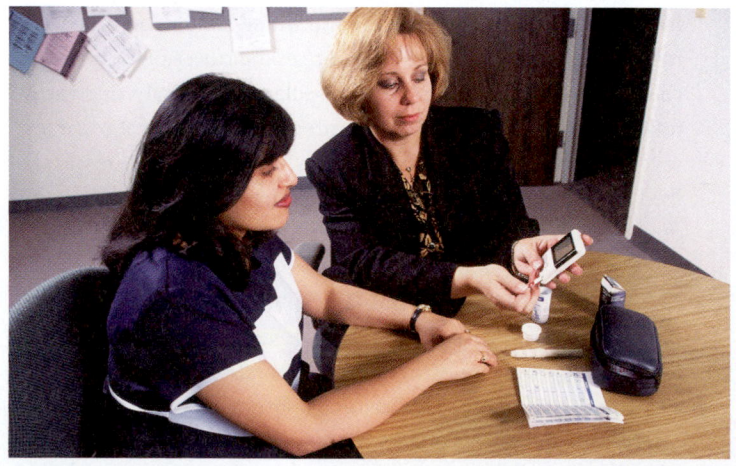

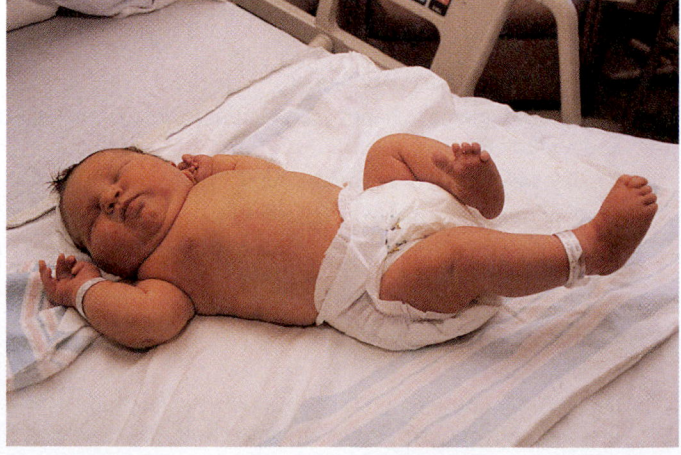

A   **B**

Figure 8-11. ■ (A) Pregnant woman learning to do serum glucose monitoring. (Source: Pearson Education/PH College) (B) Macrosomia. This infant's mother had diabetes during pregnancy.

TABLE 8-4

Maternally Transmitted STIs

INFECTION	FREQUENCY/TIMING	MANIFESTATIONS	TREATMENT
Syphilis	Spirochetes cross placenta after 16–18 weeks	Rhinitis Fissures on upper lip and corners of mouth Red rash around mouth and anus Copper-colored rash on face, palms, soles Irritability Edema, bone lesions, pain in extremities Jaundice, hepatosplenomegaly Congenital cataracts SGA, failure to thrive	Penicillin Isolation until antibiotics have been given for 48 hours
Gonorrhea	About 33% of newborns delivered vaginally to infected mothers acquire infection	Ophthalmia neonatorum, purulent discharge, corneal ulcers Sepsis Unstable temperature, poor feeding response, hypotonia, jaundice	Ophthalmic antibiotic ointment Follow-up referral to check vision
Herpes simplex type 2	1 in 7,500 births usually	Small cluster vesicular skin lesions	Intravenous vidarabine or acyclovir Follow-up referral for possible microcephaly, spasticity, seizures, deafness, or blindness
Oral *Candida* infection (thrush)	Acquired during vaginal birth Appears 5–7 days after birth	White plaques inside mouth Well-demarcated eruptions in diaper area Removal of plaque with cotton-tipped applicator causes raw, bleeding area	Topical gentian violet (1%–2%) on affected mucosa, oral lesions Topical nystatin
Chlamydia trachomatis infection	Acquired during vaginal delivery Appears 3–4 days after birth Pneumonia may appear 4–11 weeks after birth	Pneumonia Conjunctivitis Corneal neovascularization and conjunctival scarring	Ophthalmic erythromycin Follow-up referral for eye complications and late-developing pneumonia
HIV	Acquired through birth process, during pregnancy, or via breast milk Transmission less than 2% in women who have been treated with ZDV, who delivered by cesarean section at 38 weeks and prior to rupture of membranes, and who did not breastfeed	Usually asymptomatic, but possible positive antibody titer, indicating passive immunity from the mother Possible SGA and prematurity Failure to thrive, hepatosplenomegaly, recurrent infections Delayed developmental milestones and loss of acquired skills are common	Zidovudine (ZDV), azidothyamidine (AZT) Prognosis poor

in the infant include the eyes, nose, mouth, and gastrointestinal system. After delivery, antibiotics are routinely administered into the newborn's eyes to prevent bacterial infection (see Figure 9-24 ⬀). However, infections from organisms other than bacteria can still infect the baby, resulting in blindness. If untreated, some of these infections can cause neurologic damage and death.

TORCH Infections

The **TORCH group** includes toxoplasmosis, rubella, cytomegalovirus, and herpes simplex type 2.

TOXOPLASMOSIS. Toxoplasmosis is caused by a protozoan picked up by eating raw or partially cooked meat; it is also transmitted by cat feces. If the mother contracts toxoplasmosis during pregnancy, there is an increased incidence of stillbirth, preterm labor, and neonatal death. If contracted before the 20th week of pregnancy, fetal anomalies involving the central nervous system may occur. The best treatment is to prevent the infection by eating fully cooked meat and avoiding contact with a cat litter box. Infected women may be treated with sulfadiazine (Microsulfon) or pyrimethamine (Daraprim).

RUBELLA. **Rubella,** also known as German or 3-day measles, is a highly contagious airborne virus. The earlier in the pregnancy the mother is infected, the more serious the effects are on the fetus. Congenital rubella syndrome in the fetus is characterized by cataracts (see Figure 16-28), deafness (see Chapter 16), and heart defects. Prevention is the best cure. Rubella immunization prior to pregnancy will allow the client to develop active immunity. Prenatal blood testing for hemagglutination inhibition (HAI) will indicate maternal immunity. A susceptible client should avoid exposure to rubella during pregnancy. The pregnant client who becomes infected may be counseled about having a therapeutic abortion.

CYTOMEGALOVIRUS. **Cytomegalovirus (CMV),** a member of the herpesvirus group, is found in saliva, breast milk, urine, cervical mucus, and semen of infected individuals. Antibodies for CMV are found in half of all adults. The fetus may have no noticeable defects or a variety of CNS anomalies. There is no treatment for mother or fetus.

HERPES SIMPLEX TYPE 2 OR HSV-2 (HERPES GENITALIS)
Herpes simplex type 2 or HSV-2 is an STI that is exhibited by painful vesicles on the genitals. The lesions appear several hours to 20 days after exposure. The first episode is usually the most severe. Although recurrence can happen at any time, stress associated with pregnancy can stimulate a new outbreak. There is no cure for HSV-2, but medications like acyclovir (Zovirax) can reduce the time the lesions contain live virus and shorten healing time. If an acute outbreak occurs during the first trimester, there is a 50% chance the pregnancy will end in spontaneous abortion or stillbirth. If no lesions are noted at the beginning of labor, a vaginal delivery may be performed. If active lesions are present at the beginning of labor, there is a risk the fetus will be exposed during a vaginal delivery. Therefore, a cesarean section delivery is planned.

AIDS

Acquired Immunodeficiency Syndrome (AIDS), caused by the human immunodeficiency virus (HIV), is discussed here as it relates to the mother and fetus. Further discussion appears in Chapter 21 . To understand the transmission, pathophysiology, and treatment of HIV/AIDS, refer to a general medical-surgical textbook.

Although AIDS in the United States remains more prevalent in homosexual and bisexual males, the incidence in women is increasing, and rates among some racial and ethnic groups are significantly higher than others (Box 8-5 ■). The number of pediatric cases is declining, with the majority of reported cases being infants born to HIV-positive mothers. The decline is associated with implementing universal counseling about the risk of transmission from mother to fetus, voluntary testing of pregnant women, and the use of zidovudine (ZDV) therapy for infected women and their infants (Table 8-5 ■).

BOX 8-5	CULTURAL PULSE POINTS

Incidence of HIV and AIDS by Ethnic Group

There continues to be an increase in reported cases of HIV/AIDS among heterosexual women in the United States, especially in the Northeast and the South. A Centers for Disease Control and Prevention report on AIDS cases in 2003 for females age 13 and older also showed that there were strong racial and ethnic correlations among groups. This study, which encompassed the 50 states and Washington, DC, documented the actual number of reported cases of AIDS, the percentage of the total number of cases, and the rate per 100,000 population for five groups of women over age 13: White women, Hispanic women, Black women, Asians/Pacific Islanders, and Native Americans/Alaska Natives.

The study showed White women as having 1,725 cases of AIDS. This is 15% of all reported cases and a rate of 2 infected women per 100,000 population.

Hispanic women had almost an equal number of cases of AIDS (1,744) and a similar percentage (16%). However, this number indicates a rate six times greater than that in White women: 12.4 per 100,000 population.

Black women had the highest number of AIDS cases (7,551) and the highest percentage (68%). These figures translate to a rate of just over 50 infected women per 100,000 population.

Among Asians/Pacific Islanders, the number of cases of AIDS was 86, representing less than 1% of all cases and the lowest rate (1.6 per 100,000 population).

Native Americans/Alaska Natives had the smallest number of reported cases (46) and also less than 1% of all cases of AIDS. However, this number represents a rate three times greater than that of Asians/Pacific Islanders (4.8 per 100,000).

Source: Centers for Disease Control and Prevention. National Center for HIV, STD and TB Prevention. *AIDS cases and rates for female adults and adolescents, by race/ethnicity 2003—50 states and D.C.*

TABLE 8-5

Pharmacology: Drugs for Use in HIV and AIDS

DRUG	USUAL ROUTE/DOSE	CLASSIFICATION	SELECTED SIDE EFFECTS	DON'T GIVE IF
Sulfadiazine (Microsulfon)	PO 2–8 g/d divided dose every 6 hours	Anti-infective	Drug allergy, headache, malaise, anemia	Allergic to sulfa Breastfeeding
Pyrimethamine (Daraprim)	PO 50–75 mg/d with sulfadiazine × 1–3 weeks, then ½ dose for 1 month	Anti-infective	GI upset, anemia, skin rash, CNS stimulation including seizure	Breastfeeding
Acyclovir (Zovirax)	PO 400 mg tid × 7–10 days	Antiviral, anti-infective	Minimal	Breastfeeding
Azidothymidine (AZT) Zidovudine (ZDV)	PO 200 mg every 4 hours	Antiviral, anti-infective	Headache, dizziness, malaise, bone marrow depression	Hematology indicates toxicity Breastfeeding

Many women who are HIV positive actively avoid pregnancy because of the risk to the infant and the probability of their death before the child would be raised. Some women are asymptomatic and may be unaware of HIV exposure until after they become pregnant. Pregnancy is not believed to accelerate the progression of AIDS in the woman who is asymptomatic. However, women with low CD4 counts who are symptomatic have been known to have accelerated progression of AIDS while pregnant. The administration of ZDV (or azidothymidine, AZT) greatly reduces the risk of transmission to the fetus. Most medication used to treat AIDS is safe to administer during pregnancy.

HIV transmission can occur during pregnancy and through breast milk, but most transmission occurs during the birth process. In women who have been treated with ZDV, who delivered by cesarean section at 38 weeks and prior to rupture of membranes, and who did not breast feed, the rate of transmission to the infant is less than 2%. Following delivery, infants are usually asymptomatic. They may have a positive antibody titer, which indicates passive immunity from the mother. Many of these infants are small for gestational age and are likely to be premature. However, this could be due to socioeconomic conditions and not necessarily HIV. The signs of HIV in infants include failure to thrive, hepatosplenomegaly, and recurrent infections, including Epstein-Barr virus and bacterial infections. Delayed developmental milestones and loss of acquired skills are common. The prognosis for the infected child is poor.

HEMOLYTIC DISORDERS

Hemolytic disorders are those conditions that cause fetal red blood cells to break during pregnancy, during labor, or immediately following delivery. There are two types of hemolytic disorders: Rh incompatibility and ABO incompatibility.

Rh Incompatibility

Rh incompatibility can only occur when the mother is Rh negative and the fetus is Rh positive. The placenta normally keeps the maternal and fetal blood from mixing. However, there could be times when tears occur in the placenta. Examples include abruptio placentae, placental infection, abortion, and birth. At that time, fetal blood can enter the maternal circulation (Figure 8-12 ■).

The maternal Rh-negative blood produces antibodies against the Rh-positive fetal blood. This fetus is not harmed because this mixing of blood usually occurs at delivery. However, the mother has been sensitized to the Rh factor. If the next pregnancy is an Rh-positive fetus, the maternal antibodies will attack the fetus, resulting in hemolysis (*erythroblastosis fetalis*). The infant will develop severe anemia, congestive heart failure, and jaundice. The fetus may need blood transfusion upon delivery. In some cases, intrauterine blood transfusion may be indicated.

Blood screening tests done at the first prenatal visit determine the mother's Rh factor, and an indirect Coombs' test (discussed previously) detects Rh antibodies. The indirect Coombs' test may be repeated throughout the pregnancy as necessary. Every Rh-negative mother, following delivery of every Rh-positive fetus, should receive Rh immune globulin (RhoGAM) within 72 hours of delivery. (Some facilities say within 48 hours.) It is also recommended that RhoGAM be given at 28 weeks' gestation to protect the fetus from hemolysis. RhoGAM is administered by IM injection (Table 8-6 ■).

ABO Incompatibility

The second hemolytic disorder affecting the fetus is ABO incompatibility. The most common type of ABO incompatibility occurs when the mother is type O and the fetus is

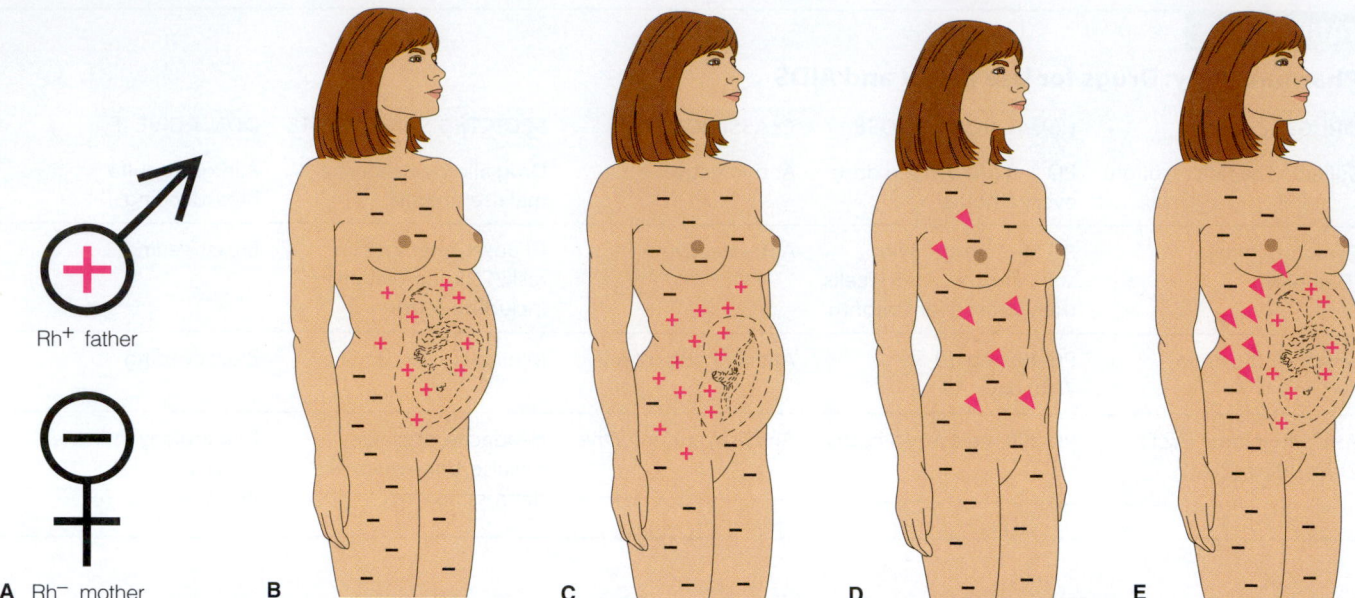

Rh⁺ father

A Rh⁻ mother

Figure 8-12. ■ Rh isoimmunization sequence. (**A**) Rh-positive father and Rh-negative mother. (**B**) Pregnancy with Rh-positive fetus. Some Rh-positive blood enters the mother's bloodstream. (**C**) As the placenta separates, the mother is further exposed to the Rh-positive blood. (**D**) The mother is sensitized to the Rh-positive blood; anti–Rh-positive antibodies (*triangles*) are formed. (**E**) In subsequent pregnancies with an Rh-positive fetus, Rh-positive red blood cells are attacked by the anti–Rh-positive maternal antibodies, causing hemolysis of red blood cells in the fetus.

type A, B, or AB. The mother's blood contains anti-A and anti-B antibodies. If the mother's blood enters the fetal circulation, these antibodies attack the fetal blood. Because only a small amount of maternal blood enters the fetus, the amount of antibodies is limited. The impact on the fetus is not as severe as Rh incompatibility.

MULTIPLE PREGNANCY

Multiple pregnancy is the carrying of more than one fetus. The most common multiple pregnancy is twin pregnancy. Other multiple pregnancies can occur naturally but are more common as a result of infertility treatment. Fraternal twins result from two ova being fertilized by two sperm (see Figure 5-18 ⚭). Fraternal twins could be two boys, two girls, or one boy and one girl. Fraternal twins have two separate placentas, each with an amnion and a chorion layer. Identical twins result from one ovum fertilized by one sperm, dividing into two blastocysts. Because identical

twins come from the same fertilized ovum, they are the same gender. Identical twins frequently share one placenta, with one chorion but separate amnion layers of the fetal membranes. *Conjoined twins* result from incomplete separation of the blastocyst.

Multiple pregnancy is suspected when the fundal height is greater than expected in the first few weeks of pregnancy (see Chapter 6 ⚭). Diagnosis may be confirmed with an ultrasound. As the uterus enlarges, the discomforts of pregnancy are enhanced. Pre-eclampsia, gestational diabetes, and preterm labor are more common with multiple pregnancy. More frequent prenatal monitoring is indicated. Complications affecting one fetus could ultimately affect the other fetus. For example, by the end of the pregnancy, both placentas are close to each other or overlapping. If an abruption develops in one placenta, the other placenta may also detach from the uterus. The umbilical cord from one fetus could become entangled with the other fetus.

TABLE 8-6				
Pharmacology: Drug for Prevention of Hemolysis				
DRUG	**USUAL ROUTE/DOSE**	**CLASSIFICATION**	**SELECTED SIDE EFFECTS**	**DON'T GIVE IF**
Rh immune globulin (RhoGAM)	300 mcg at 28 weeks' gestation 300 mcg within 72 hours of delivery	Immune globulin	Injection site irritation, fever, myalgia	Mother is Rh positive; infant must be Rh positive if postpartum dose is given

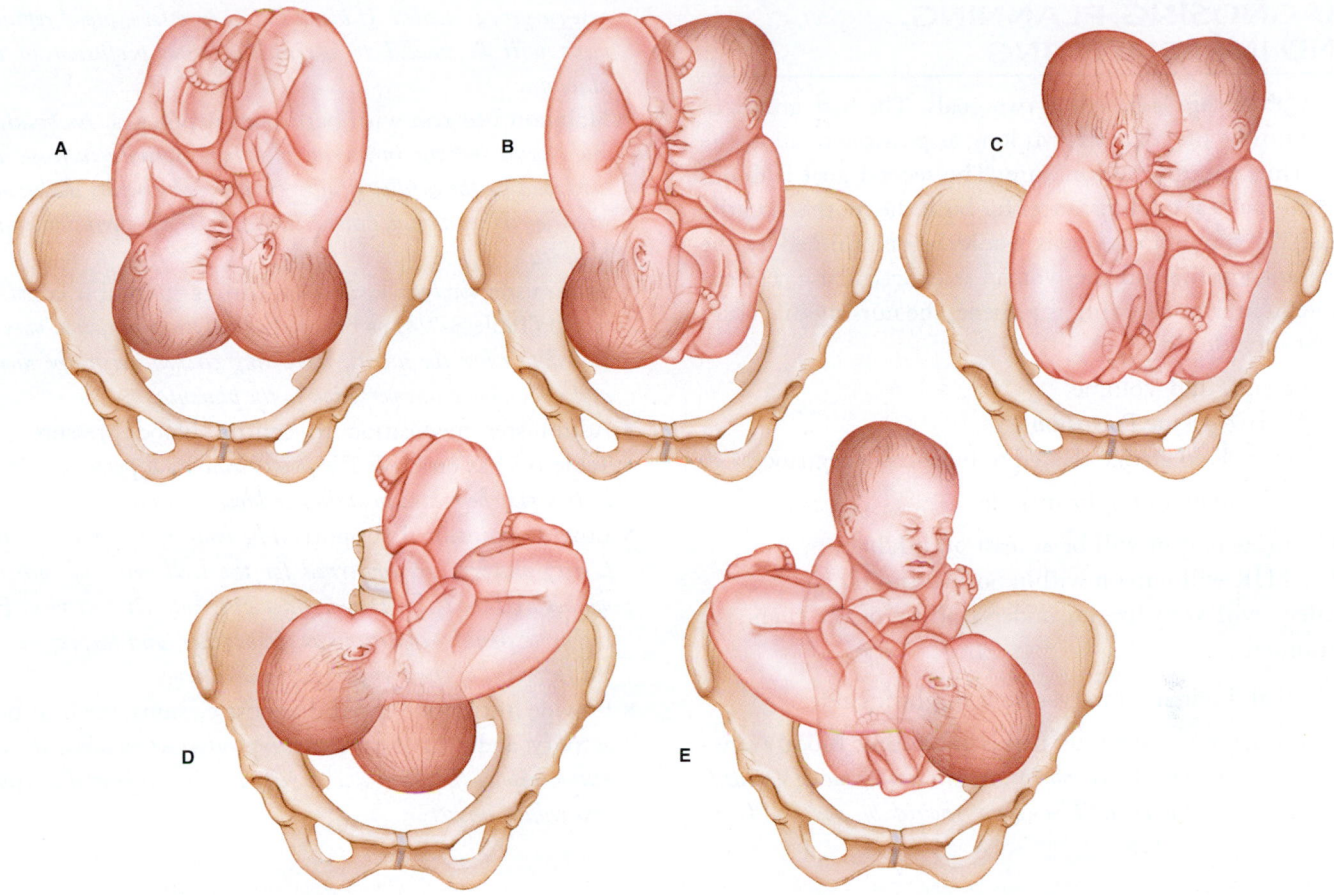

Figure 8-13. ■ Examples of twin presentation. (**A**) Two vertexes. (**B**) One vertex, one breech. (**C**) Two breeches. (**D**) One vertex, one transverse. (**E**) One transverse, one breech.

At the end of the pregnancy, the presentations of the twins will have a great impact on delivery decisions (Figure 8-13 ■). If both twins are in vertex presentation, a vaginal delivery of both infants is possible. However, if one fetus is vertex and the other breech or transverse, a cesarean section delivery is safer for both infants.

NURSING CARE

PRIORITIES IN NURSING CARE

Priorities of care for the at-risk pregnancy focus on the following:

- Detecting complications at an early stage
- Assisting with implementation of medical treatment
- Evaluating the response to treatment as evidenced by stability of the specific condition.

ASSESSING

The assessment of the high-risk mother and fetus consists of frequent monitoring. The time intervals between data col-

lection vary, depending on the severity of the symptoms and the stability of the client. The data that can be collected without a physician's order include:

- Vital signs: mother's temperature, pulse, respiration and blood pressure, and FHR.
- Mother's reflexes and clonus (see Figure 8-9)
- Amount of protein in mother's urine
- Uterine contractions
- Uterine bleeding
- Cervical changes.

clinical ALERT

If there is significant uterine bleeding, an ultrasound to determine placental placement should be done before a vaginal exam for cervical dilatation. With placenta previa, a vaginal examination could dislodge the placenta, resulting in hemorrhage and fetal death.

Data that may be collected with a physician's order include:

- Biophysical profile
- Fetal ultrasound.

DIAGNOSING, PLANNING, AND IMPLEMENTING

The plan of care is based on two goals. The first goal is to maintain the pregnancy for as long as possible to allow the fetus time to grow and mature. The second goal is to deliver in the best circumstances for both the mother and the fetus. The nursing diagnosis would be determined by the specific complication the woman is experiencing. For example, if uterine bleeding is present, the nursing diagnoses might include:

- Deficient Fluid Volume
- Ineffective Tissue Perfusion
- Deficient Knowledge related to high-risk pregnancy.

Expected outcomes might include:

- The urine output will be at least 50 mL/hr.
- The FHR will remain within normal limits.
- Client will verbalize an understanding of the high-risk disorder.

Medical and nursing interventions might include:

- Administer intravenous fluids including blood transfusion as ordered. *To maintain fluid volume, IV fluids must be administered. The client should be kept NPO in case surgery is needed. If blood loss is excessive, blood replacement will be needed to maintain tissue perfusion to the placenta.*
- Maintain bed rest with bathroom privileges. *Ambulation could cause increase in uterine bleeding. Activity increases the workload on the cardiovascular systems, which puts additional stress on the maternal heart, decreasing tissue perfusion to the placenta.*
- Administer *tocolytic medications* (drugs to inhibit contractions) (Table 8-7 ■) as ordered. *Tocolytic medication may be needed to relax the uterus, increasing circulation to the uterus and improving tissue perfusion to the placenta.*
- Administer medication to control blood pressure (see Table 8-7) as ordered. *Fluid loss leads to hypotension. Medication may be needed to maintain blood pressure.*
- Provide emotional support. *The mother, her partner, and family members are concerned for the well-being of both the mother and the baby. Hemorrhage puts both lives at risk. Being professional, remaining at the bedside, and keeping everyone informed of changes provides reassurance.*
- Provide instruction about diagnostic exams, medications, activity, and prognosis. *Providing information about the situation allows the client and family to make informed decisions and reduces anxiety.*

TABLE 8-7

Pharmacology: Medications Used During High-Risk Pregnancies

CLASSIFICATION	DRUG	USE	SIDE EFFECTS
Uterine relaxants (Tocolytic)	Terbutaline (Brethine) Ritodrine (Yutopar)	First-line tocolytic Treatment of preterm labor	Hypotension, cardiac arrhythmia, tachycardia, palpitations, myocardial ischemia, pulmonary edema, maternal hypoglycemia
Macromineral	Magnesium sulfate	Tocolytic, antihypertensive to treat PIH	Warmth, headache, nystagmus, nausea, dry mouth, dizziness
Oxytoxic	Oxytocin (Pitocin)	Induction or augmentation of labor Treat postpartum hemorrhage	Nausea (N), vomiting (V), hypertonicity of uterus, uterine rupture, fetal bradycardia, cardiac arrhythmia
Ergot alkaloids (oxytoxic)	Methylergonovine (Methergine)	Routine management after delivery of placenta, treat uterine atony and hemorrhage	N, V, elevated BP, temporary chest pain, dizziness (D), headache
Prostaglandin	Dinoprostone Prostaglandin E2	Termination of pregnancy, cervical ripening before induction	Before induction: N, V, D, headache, hypotension, chills
Abortifacients	Carboprost tromethamine Hemabate	Termination of pregnancy, evaluation of uterus following missed abortion or fetal demise First-line drug for severe postpartum hemorrhaging	N, V, D, headache, perforated uterus

EVALUATING

Evaluating the effectiveness of the treatment for prenatal complications is essential to determine the well-being of both the mother and the fetus. Evaluation consists of a continual process of collecting data and comparing it to older data to determine if the mother and fetus remain stable. If the complication is controlled with treatment, the pregnancy can usually progress to a normal delivery at 38 to 40 weeks. If the complication cannot be controlled, a premature vaginal delivery or cesarean section delivery may need to be performed.

HIGH-RISK LABOR AND DELIVERY

Although most pregnancies end with a normal labor and delivery, the possibility of anticipated and unanticipated complications exists. The most common complications are discussed in this section.

Factors That Create High Risk

PRETERM LABOR

Preterm labor is the onset of regular contractions, occurring between the 20th and 37th weeks, that cause changes in the cervix. Factors associated with preterm labor include premature rupture of membranes (PROM), multiple pregnancy, vaginal bleeding, cervical abnormalities, and infections. Most women with preterm labor are admitted to the hospital for treatment. Tocolytic agents are frequently ordered. Common tocolytic agents include ritodrine (Yutopar), terbutaline (Brethine), and magnesium sulfate. If labor continues, a corticosteroid, such as betamethasone (Celestone), may be given to accelerate lung maturation in the fetus. If contractions stop and there is no further change in the cervix, the client may be discharged with instructions to limit activity and take prescribed tocolytic medication. If contractions do not stop, labor continues to delivery of a preterm infant. Preterm infants are usually taken to a neonatal intensive care unit (NICU) for specialized care.

INDUCTION OF LABOR

Induction of labor may be necessary if the risk to the mother or infant of continuing the pregnancy is greater than the risk of delivery. Indications for induction of labor include *post dates* (labor does not begin spontaneously by the 41st week), PIH, maternal diabetes, suspected fetal abnormality, history of rapid delivery, and fetal death.

The methods of induction of labor include:

- *Prostaglandins (PGE₁).* At times, the cervix is ripened (softened) by the insertion of prostaglandin gel into and around the cervix. Labor may begin in a few hours or may be induced 12 to 24 hours later by another method.
- *Artificial rupture of membranes (AROM).* The physician or nurse midwife inserts an amnihook through the cervix and perforates the amniotic membranes (see Figure 7-20 ⚭). Labor contractions may begin within a few hours.
- *Pitocin (oxytocin) infusion.* A primary intravenous infusion is begun, and a secondary infusion containing Pitocin is given by piggyback into the primary infusion. If severe side effects of Pitocin occur, the infusion can easily be discontinued and the IV line maintained. The registered nurse increases the dose of Pitocin in small increments until labor is begun. Once labor has begun, it usually progresses like spontaneous labor.

PRECIPITOUS DELIVERY

Precipitous delivery is a birth that occurs rapidly, unexpectedly, and without the attention of a physician or nurse midwife. A precipitous delivery may be accompanied by **precipitous labor,** one that lasts less than 3 hours. Precipitous labor and/or delivery increases the risk of ruptured uterus, cervical and vaginal lacerations, hemorrhage, fetal distress, and fetal cerebral trauma. Steps for assisting a woman with a precipitous delivery are listed in Box 8-6 ■, which contains Figures 8-14 and 8-15.

A physician or nurse midwife should examine the mother and infant as soon as possible after the birth.

PROLAPSED UMBILICAL CORD

Prolapsed cord occurs when the umbilical cord emerges through the cervix before the presenting part. Although the umbilical cord can become trapped between the presenting part and the pelvis at any time, it more commonly occurs when the fetal membranes rupture before the presenting part is engaged. The umbilical cord can be flushed through the cervix. The presenting part then compresses the umbilical cord against the cervix and pelvis (Figure 8-16 ■). If pressure on the umbilical cord is not relieved, the fetus will develop hypoxia and could die. When a prolapsed umbilical cord is identified, the examiner should insert two fingers into the vagina and apply upward pressure against the presenting part to relieve pressure on the cord. While the upward pressure on the presenting part is maintained, the client should be turned to a knee-chest position to allow gravity to help keep the fetus away from the pelvis. If the umbilical cord protrudes from

| BOX 8-6 | NURSING CARE CHECKLIST |

Assisting a Woman in Precipitous Labor

If the client says "the baby is coming," the nurse should check to see if the fetus is crowning. If the baby is crowning, the nurse should:

☑ Stay with the mother.

☑ Call for assistance by putting on the emergency call light. If outside the hospital, have someone call emergency medical services (EMS).

☑ Remain calm and reassure the mother; instruct her to pant.

☑ If time permits, open emergency equipment, wash hands, and put on sterile gloves. If outside the hospital, provide a clean environment and as much privacy as possible.

☑ Provide a sterile or clean area for delivery.

☑ If membranes are intact, tear membranes allowing the amniotic fluid to drain.

☑ Apply gentle pressure to the head with one hand to allow it to be delivered gradually. Do not apply firm pressure or try to stop the head from being delivered.

☑ Check the baby's neck for a wrapped umbilical cord, called a **nuchal cord** (Figure 8-14 ■). If there is a nuchal cord and it is loose enough, slip the cord over the baby's head. If it is too tight, place two clamps on the cord and cut the cord between the clamps. Then, unwind the umbilical cord from the baby's neck.

☑ Suction the baby's nose, mouth, and throat.

☑ Gently apply downward pressure to the baby's head to deliver the anterior shoulder. Then, gently lift the baby's head to deliver the posterior shoulder.

☑ Deliver the rest of the body, being careful not to drop the slippery wet baby.

☑ Suction the airway, and dry the baby.

☑ Clamp the umbilical cord in two places and cut it between the clamps, leaving at least 1 inch (2.5 cm) between the baby and the clamp (Figure 8-15 ■). If outside the hospital, the cord does not need to be clamped and cut until emergency medical personnel arrive. The cord should only be cut using sterile technique.

☑ Deliver the placenta, keeping all tissue for the physician to examine.

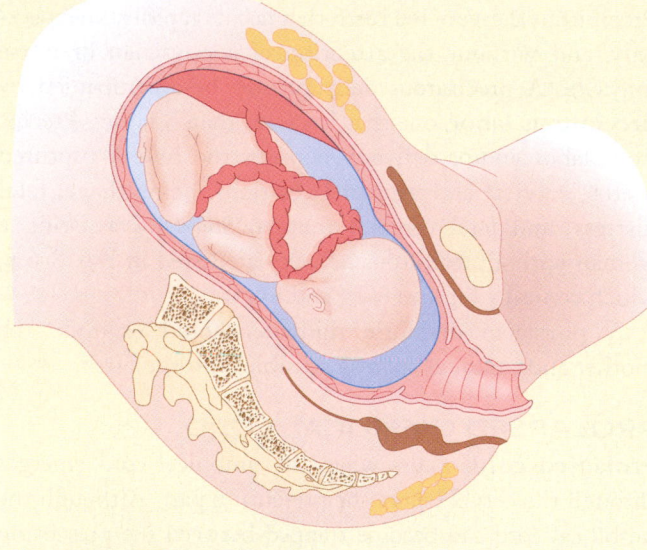

Figure 8-14. ■ Nuchal cord.

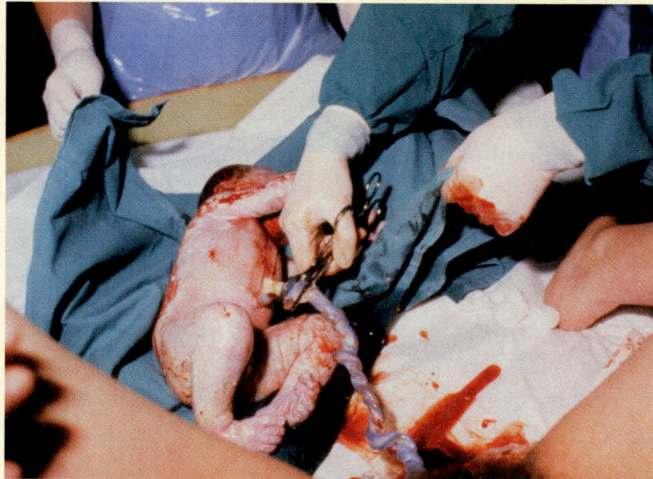

Figure 8-15. ■ Clamp and cut cord, leaving about 1 inch (2.5 cm) between the baby and the first clamp. (John Heseltine/Photo Researchers, Inc.)

the vagina, it should be covered with wet towels to prevent shrinking of the Wharton's jelly and further compression of the umbilical vessels. The physician is notified, and an emergency cesarean section delivery is performed.

DYSTOCIA

Dystocia is defined as a long, difficult, or abnormal labor pattern. It can be caused by a variety of conditions, including ineffective uterine contractions, abnormal fetal presentation or position, a large fetus, or a small maternal pelvic outlet. When labor does not progress in the usual time frame, the nurse should anticipate that further evaluation, tests, and intervention may be necessary.

Electronic fetal monitoring (EFM) involves a continuous tracing of the fetal heart rate (FHR) and uterine contractions. The FHR can be obtained externally by an ultrasound transducer held in place on the abdomen by a belt (see Figure 7-31 ⬭⬭). However, external monitoring of the FHR may not be accurate due to fetal movement or the amount of maternal tissue through which the sound must travel. Contractions

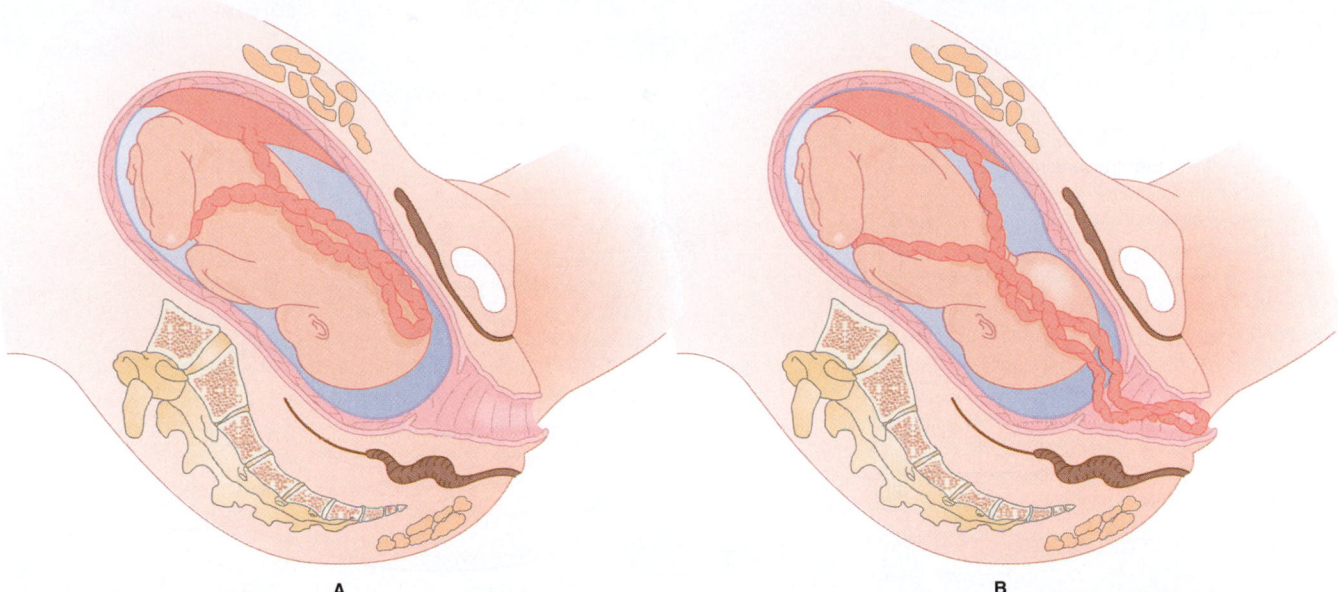

Figure 8-16. ■ Prolapse of the umbilical cord. **(A)** Cord at the inlet. **(B)** Cord prolapsed through the introitus. (Reproduced, with permission, from McGraw-Hill Companies, Inc. Oxorn, H. [Ed.]. [1986] *Oxorn-Foote human labor and birth* [5th ed.]. Norwalk, CT: Appleton & Lange, p. 285.)

are determined by a tocodynamometer attached by a belt to the woman's abdomen at the level of the fundus. This external monitoring of contractions is accurate in determining the frequency and duration of contractions, but may not be accurate in determining the strength of the contractions.

The strength of uterine contractions can be assessed internally. The physician inserts a small plastic catheter through the cervix, past the presenting part (Figure 8-17 ■). The catheter is attached by an adapter to a monitoring system. The strength of contractions is recorded on the labor record. If the contractions are not of an appropriate strength, intravenous Pitocin can be administered to stimulate stronger contractions. If contractions are of sufficient strength, but the

cervix fails to dilate and/or the fetus fails to descend, a cesarean section will be performed.

When labor is not progressing as expected, it is critical to monitor the FHR accurately. Commonly, direct fetal monitoring is used. If fetal membranes have not ruptured, they are artificially ruptured in order for an electrode to be applied to the presenting part (Figure 8-18 ■). A spiral electrode is inserted into the vagina and held firmly against the fetal scalp. The device is rotated until the sharp electrode tip pierces the fetal scalp. The applicator is then removed, and the electrode with attached wires remains. The distal end of the wires is attached to the fetal monitor. The LPN/LVN assists with the procedure, supporting the client and attaching the wires to the monitor.

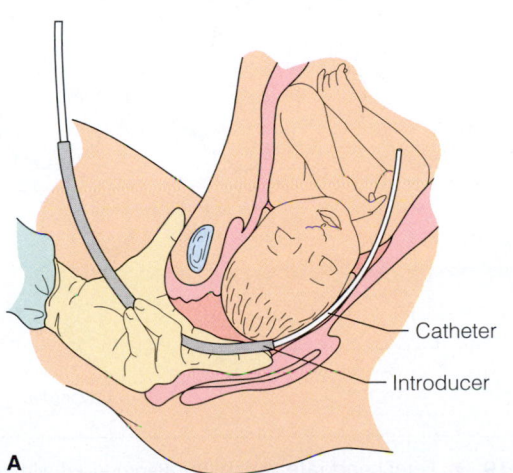

Catheter

Introducer

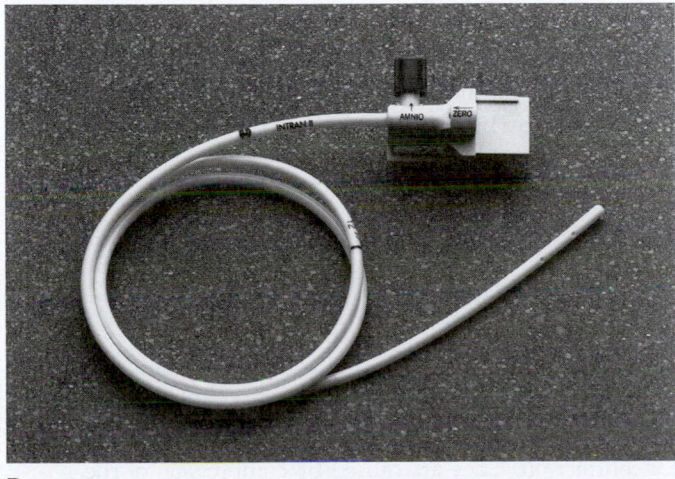

Figure 8-17. ■ **(A)** Technique of inserting a uterine catheter. Note that the introducer (catheter guide) is inserted no farther than beyond the fingertips. **(B)** INTRAN Plus intrauterine pressure catheter. There is a micropressure transducer (electronic sensor) located at the top of the catheter and a port for amnioinfusion at the distal end of the catheter.

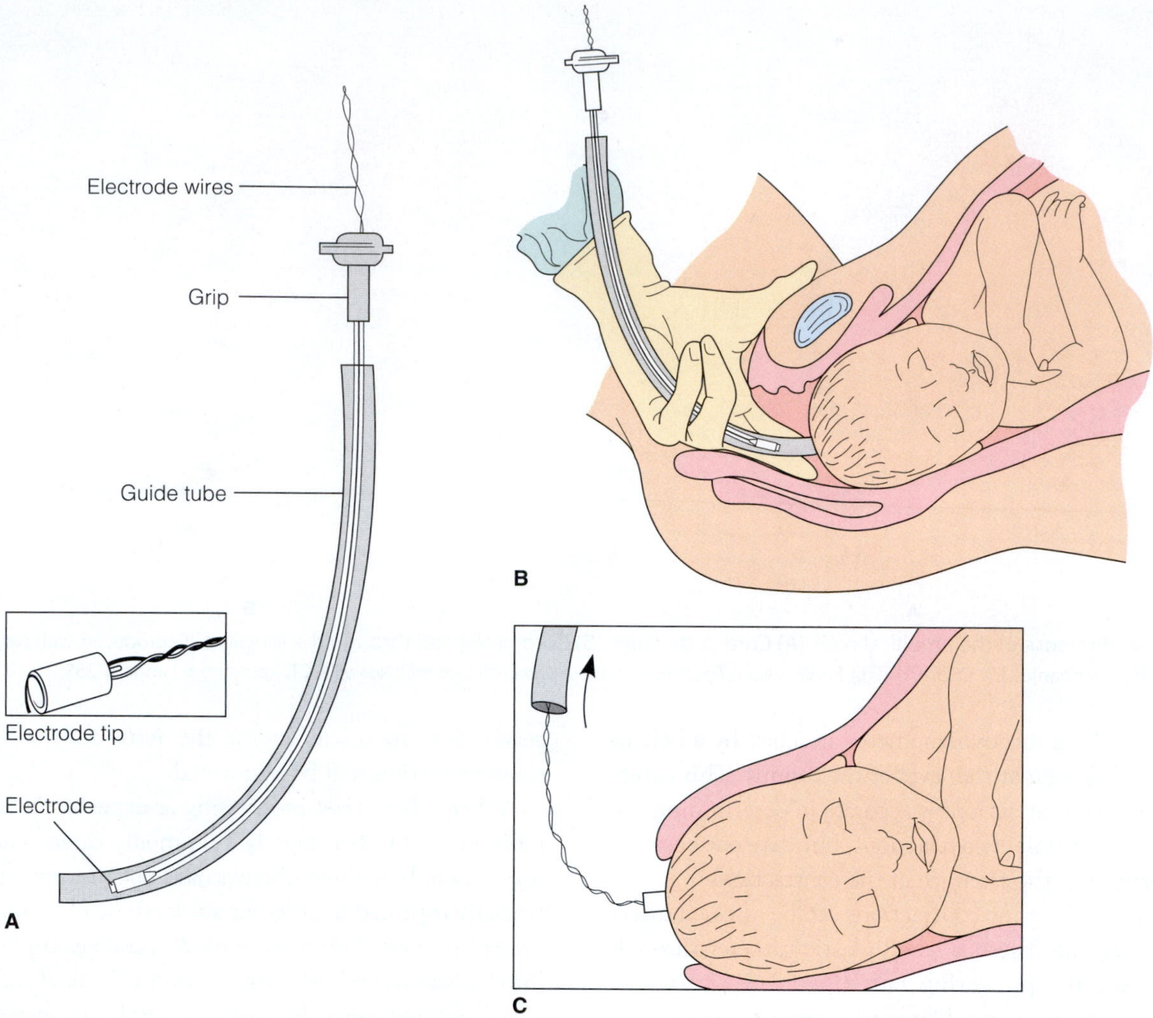

Electrode wires

Grip

Guide tube

Electrode tip

Electrode

A

B

C

Figure 8-18. ■ Technique for internal direct fetal monitoring (**A**) Spiral electrode. (**B**) Attaching the spiral electrode to the scalp. (**C**) Attached spiral electrode with the guide tube removed.

The FHR should change in response to the stress of labor. This change is termed **variability**. Monitoring the FHR with the internal electrode allows for viewing of short-term variability (STV) or the beat-to-beat change. This is noted as short up-and-down waves on the monitor tracing (Figure 8-19 ■). Long-term variability (LTV) is a waviness of the FHR that occurs three to five times a minute. If the variability is normal, the fetus is tolerating the labor process.

Accelerations are an increase in the FHR with fetal activity, just as an adult heart rate increases with exercise. At times, the fetus moves in response to contractions. Accelerations in FHR are a sign of fetal well-being.

Decelerations are a decrease in FHR. They are characterized as early, late, and variable, according to where they occur in the contraction cycle. Early decelerations begin before the start of a contraction. They are caused by compression of the fetal skull, resulting in central vagal stimulation. Late decelerations result from an insufficient blood flow and oxygen transfer from the uterus to the placenta. Late decelerations

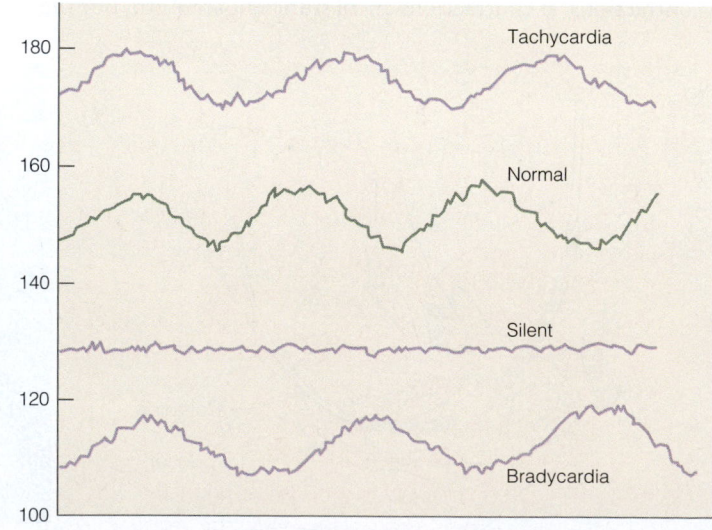

Figure 8-19. ■ Fetal heart rate variability. (Reproduced, with permission, from McGraw-Hill Companies, Inc. Oxorn, H. [Ed.]. [1986] *Oxorn-Foote human labor and birth* [5th ed.]. Norwalk, CT: Appleton & Lange, p. 623.)

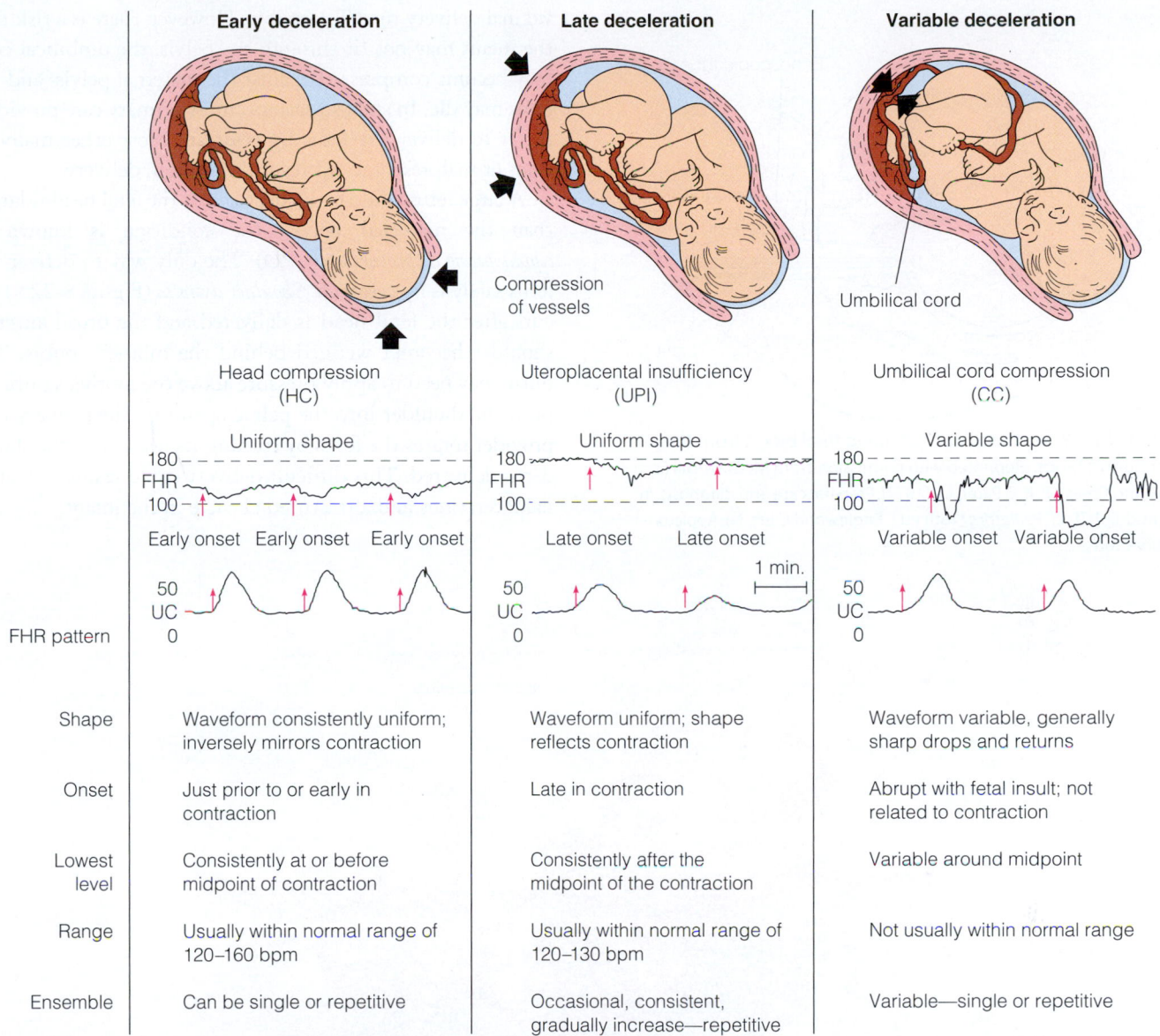

	Early deceleration	Late deceleration	Variable deceleration
	Head compression (HC)	Uteroplacental insufficiency (UPI)	Umbilical cord compression (CC)
FHR pattern			
Shape	Waveform consistently uniform; inversely mirrors contraction	Waveform uniform; shape reflects contraction	Waveform variable, generally sharp drops and returns
Onset	Just prior to or early in contraction	Late in contraction	Abrupt with fetal insult; not related to contraction
Lowest level	Consistently at or before midpoint of contraction	Consistently after the midpoint of the contraction	Variable around midpoint
Range	Usually within normal range of 120–160 bpm	Usually within normal range of 120–130 bpm	Not usually within normal range
Ensemble	Can be single or repetitive	Occasional, consistent, gradually increase—repetitive	Variable—single or repetitive

Figure 8-20. ■ Types and characteristics of early, late, and variable decelerations. (Data from Hon, E. [1976]. *An introduction to fetal heart rate monitoring*, [2nd ed.]. Los Angeles: University of Southern California School of Medicine. p. 29.)

begin after the start of the contraction. The nurse should stop IV Pitocin infusion, reposition the mother, apply oxygen to the mother, and notify the primary care provider. Variable decelerations occur if the umbilical cord becomes compressed. The waveform is variable in shape and occurrence (Figure 8-20 ■). Generally, there is a sharp decrease in FHR and rapid return of the FHR. The nurse should reposition the mother until a more reassuring pattern is found, perform a vaginal exam to determine the presence of a prolapsed cord and cervical dilation, and notify the physician. Immediate assisted delivery or cesarean may be indicated.

If fetal well-being is questionable, the primary care provider may decide to obtain a sample of fetal blood for analysis to determine pH and base deficit. A disposable fetal blood sampling kit is obtained. The woman's vulva and perineum are cleaned and sterile drapes applied. The primary care provider inserts a conical speculum through the vagina and into the cervix to visualize the fetal scalp. The scalp is cleaned. The site is punctured with a 2-maximum microscalpel, and a small amount of blood is collected in two heparinized capillary tubes (Figure 8-21 ■). The sample must be sent STAT to the lab for analysis. Pressure is applied to the site until bleeding stops. Once the results are obtained, a decision regarding the delivery can be made.

Dystocia could occur if the fetus is in a malposition or malpresentation. At times, a fetus in the occiput posterior position may deliver in that position or may be turned to occiput anterior position. The primary care provider can apply lateral pressure to the head by a vaginal exam, causing the fetus to turn in that direction. If the fetus is in a breech presentation,

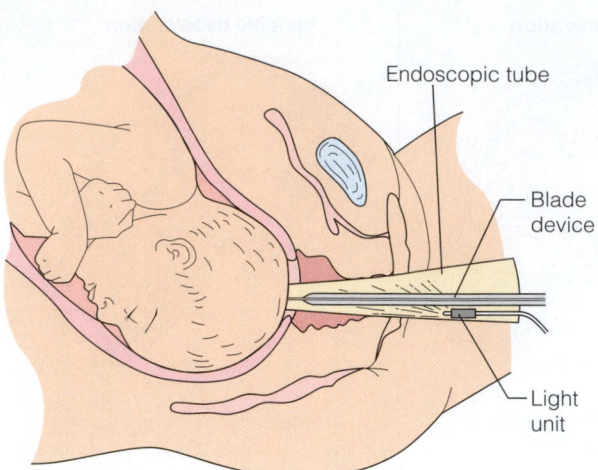

Figure 8-21. ■ Technique of obtaining fetal blood from the scalp during labor. (Reprinted with permission, from McGraw-Hill Companies, Inc. Creasy, R. K. & Parer, J.T. [1977]. Prenatal care and diagnosis. In A. M. Rudolph [Ed.], *Pediatrics* [16th ed.]. Englewood Cliffs, NJ: Appleton-Century-Crofts.)

vaginal delivery may be possible. However, there is a risk that the infant may not fit through the pelvis, the umbilical cord may become compressed against the maternal pelvis, and the fetus may die. In such situations, most primary care providers prefer to deliver the fetus by cesarean. Most other malpositions or malpresentations result in cesarean delivery.

A large fetus could cause dystocia. If the fetal head is larger than the maternal pelvis, the condition is known as *cephalopelvic disproportion* (CPD). The only way to deliver the fetus safely is by cesarean. *Shoulder dystocia* (Figure 8-22 ■) occurs after the fetal head is delivered and the broad anterior shoulder becomes wedged behind the mother's pubis. The nurse may need to apply pressure above the mother's pubis to push the shoulder into the pelvic opening. The primary care provider rotates the fetus by turning its head until the shoulder is delivered. This difficult delivery could result in maternal lacerations and a fractured clavicle in the infant.

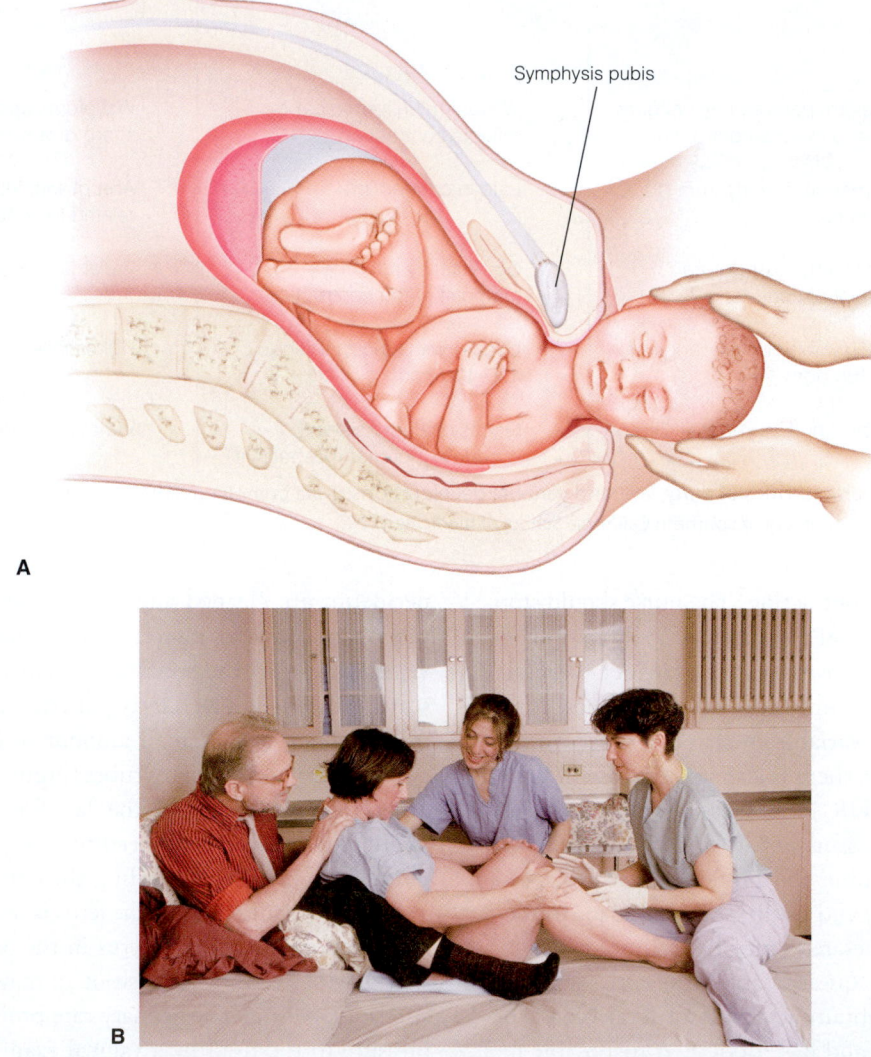

Figure 8-22. ■ (A) Shoulder dystocia. (B) This position with pressure against the mother's knees may be helpful in clients with shoulder dystocia. (B: Margaret Miller/Photo Researchers, Inc.)

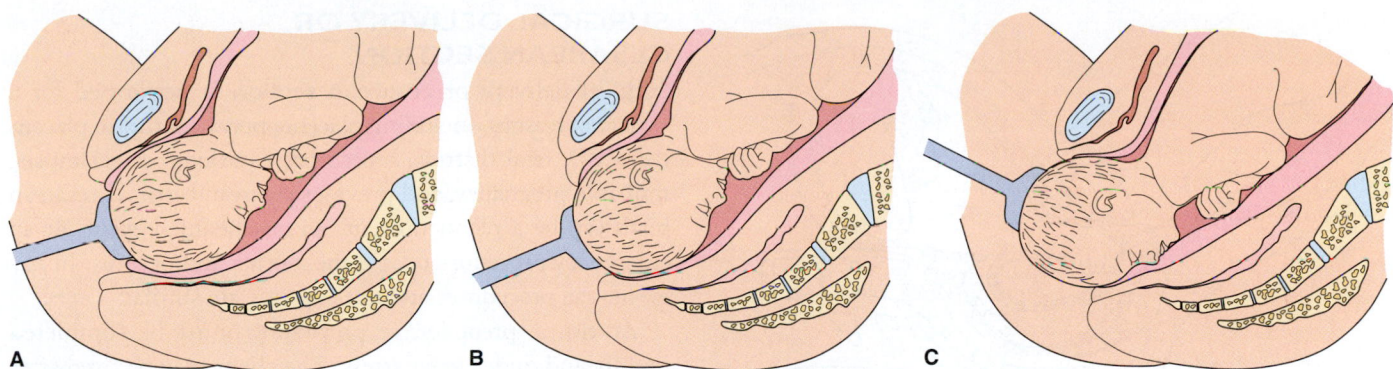

A   B   C

Figure 8-23. ■ Vacuum extractor traction. (**A**) The cup is placed on the fetal occiput, creating suction. Traction is applied in a downward and outward direction. (**B**) Traction continues in a downward direction as the fetal head begins to emerge from the vagina. (**C**) Traction is maintained to lift the fetal head out of the vagina.

ASSISTED DELIVERY

During the second stage of labor, the mother actively uses her abdominal muscles to push the fetus through the birth canal. At times, the fetus is slow to descend through the pelvis. In the absence of documented CPD (cephalopelvic disproportion), the delivery may be assisted with a vacuum or forceps. Because of the risk of fetal and maternal trauma, the use of either appliance should follow strict guidelines and facility policy. CPD is an absolute contraindication to assisted delivery and requires a cesarean delivery.

Vacuum extraction is used when minimal assistance is expected (Figure 8-23 ■). The vacuum extractor is composed of a soft suction cup attached to a suction hand pump. The primary care provider places the suction cup firmly against the occipital area of the fetal scalp. Care must be taken to avoid the area over a fontanel or maternal tissue. The nurse uses the hand pump to apply the amount of suction determined by the primary care provider. During the

next contraction, the primary care provider applies traction. The fetal head should emerge from the vagina with each contraction.

If the suction cup becomes detached from the fetal head, it may be reapplied, and a second attempt at delivery made. If the suction cup becomes detached three times, the procedure should be discontinued and another method of delivery initiated.

Fetal complications include scalp lacerations, bruising, subdural hematoma, cephalhematoma (see Figure 9-17 in Chapter 9 ⬮⬮), intracranial hemorrhage, cranial fractures, neurologic injury, and fetal death. Maternal complications include vaginal, rectal, urethral, and perineal lacerations.

Forceps are indicated when firmer traction is needed. Only a trained obstetrician is certified in the use of forceps. With the development of the vacuum extractor, the use of forceps has decreased.

Forceps consist of two metal spoon-shaped blades attached to handles that lock together (Figure 8-24 ■). The physician

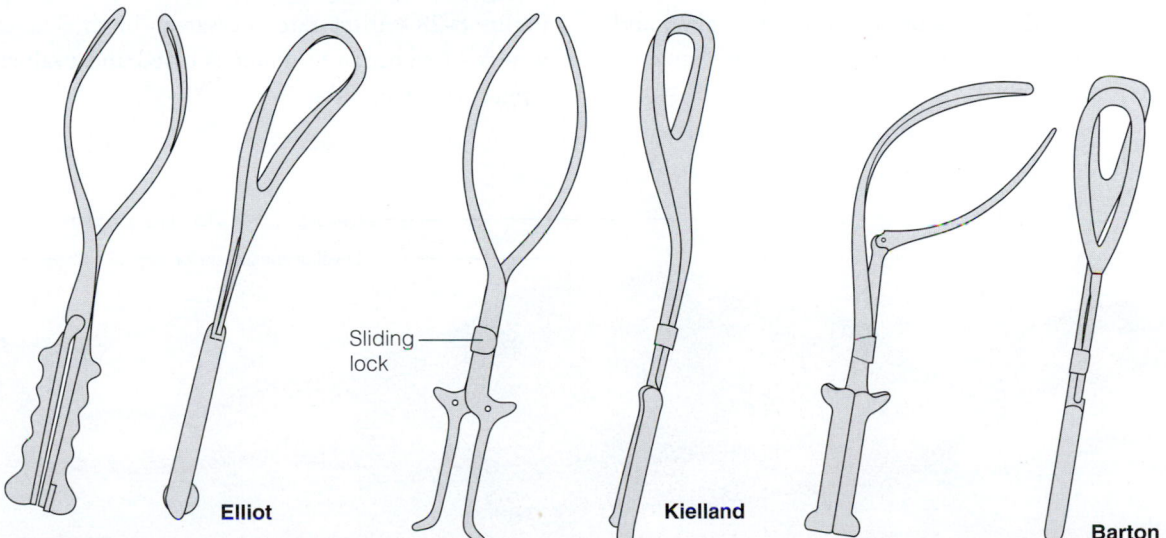

Sliding
lock

Elliot   **Kielland**   **Barton**

Figure 8-24. ■ Forceps are composed of a blade, shank, and handle, and may have a cephalic and pelvic curve. The blades may be *fenestrated* (open) or solid. The front and lateral views of these forceps illustrate differences in blades, open and closed shanks, and cephalic and pelvic curves. Elliot forceps are used as outlet forceps. Kielland and Barton forceps are used for midforceps rotations.

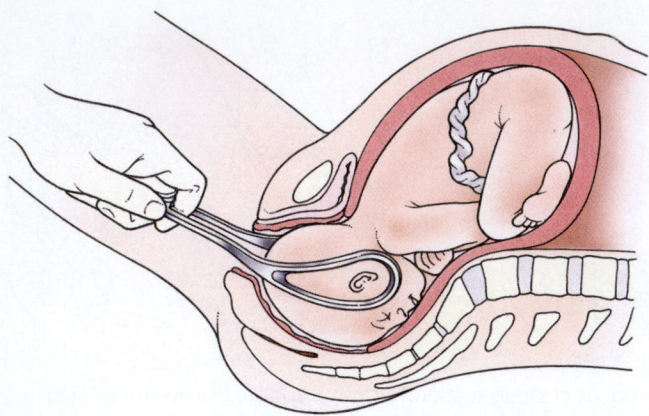

Figure 8-25. ■ Pressure marks from forceps used during delivery may appear on the newborn's cheeks and jaws. They usually disappear within a day (© Dorling Kindersley Media Library.)

slips one blade into the vagina, along one side of the fetal head, past the ear to the level of the jaw. The second blade is then inserted into the vagina past the other side of the fetal head to the level of the jaw. The handles of the forceps are then locked together. If necessary, the fetal head can be rotated to an occiput anterior position. With the next contraction, the physician applies traction. The fetal head should slowly progress through the pelvis until it emerges from the vagina. The forceps are then removed, and the body of the fetus is delivered unassisted.

Complications for the fetus and the mother are the same as for vacuum-assisted delivery. However, due to the position of the forceps, facial trauma (Figure 8-25 ■), including facial paralysis, could also occur. If the forcep blades are not applied correctly, fractures of the fetal skull could occur. Maternal trauma often results in vaginal and perineal lacerations, which may include the rectum and anus.

SURGICAL DELIVERY OR CESAREAN SECTION

Surgical delivery or **cesarean section** is performed for a variety of reasons, including placenta previa, abruptio placentae, CPD, fetal distress, breech presentation, pre-eclampsia, multiple pregnancy, and previous cesarean birth. A cesarean birth can be a planned event, an unscheduled event, or an emergency procedure to save the mother and/or fetus. In any event, the procedures and nursing care are similar.

At times, preoperative procedures must be completed rapidly and under great stress. The client may be tired after hours of labor, worried about the health of her infant, and fearful about her own safety. The nurse must provide teaching and support while performing routine procedures. It will be necessary to have a signed surgical consent. A Foley catheter will be inserted to keep the bladder empty. An intravenous infusion will be started. Hair over the mons pubis is shaved or clipped short. In some areas, the father or a significant other may accompany the client to surgery and will need to change into surgical attire.

Anesthesia is usually administered by the epidural or spinal route (Figure 8-26 ■; see also Figure 7-17C and D ⊙⊙). If an epidural has been used during labor, it will probably be used during surgery. If an epidural has not been used during labor, it will probably be initiated in the surgical suite prior to prepping the abdomen. In the event of an emergency situation, general anesthesia may be used.

Although there are several incisions that can be made to deliver the fetus (Figure 8-27 ■), the most common is a horizontal incision through the skin at the pubic hair border. The bladder is detached from the perimetrium. A horizontal incision is generally made in the lower uterine segment. The infant is then pulled through the opening. If the infant is large, forceps may be needed to extract the infant's head. Figure 8-28 ■ illlustrates a cesarean birth. The infant's airway is suctioned; the infant is dried and evaluated by the Apgar score (see Table 7-5 ⊙⊙).

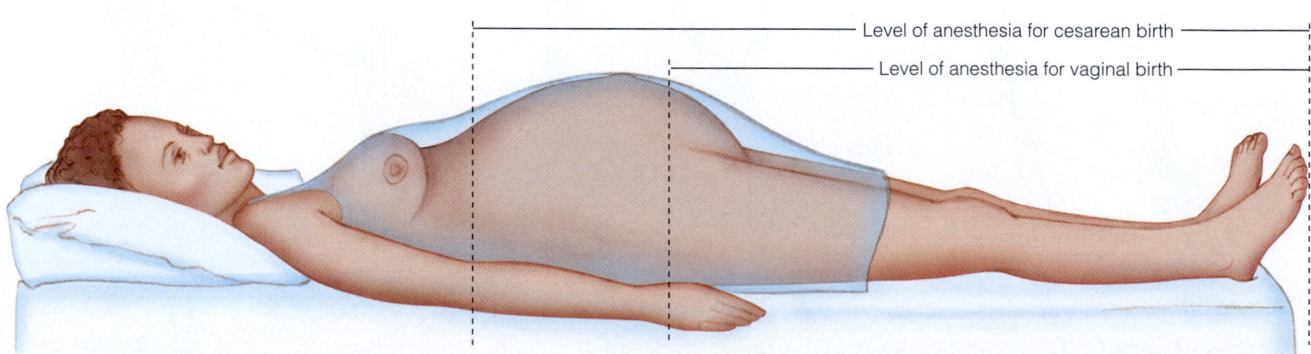

Level of anesthesia for cesarean birth

Level of anesthesia for vaginal birth

Figure 8-26. ■ Anesthesia levels for a vaginal and cesarean birth. (Data from Ross Products Division, Abbott Laboratories, Columbus, OH, from CEA #17, Regional.)

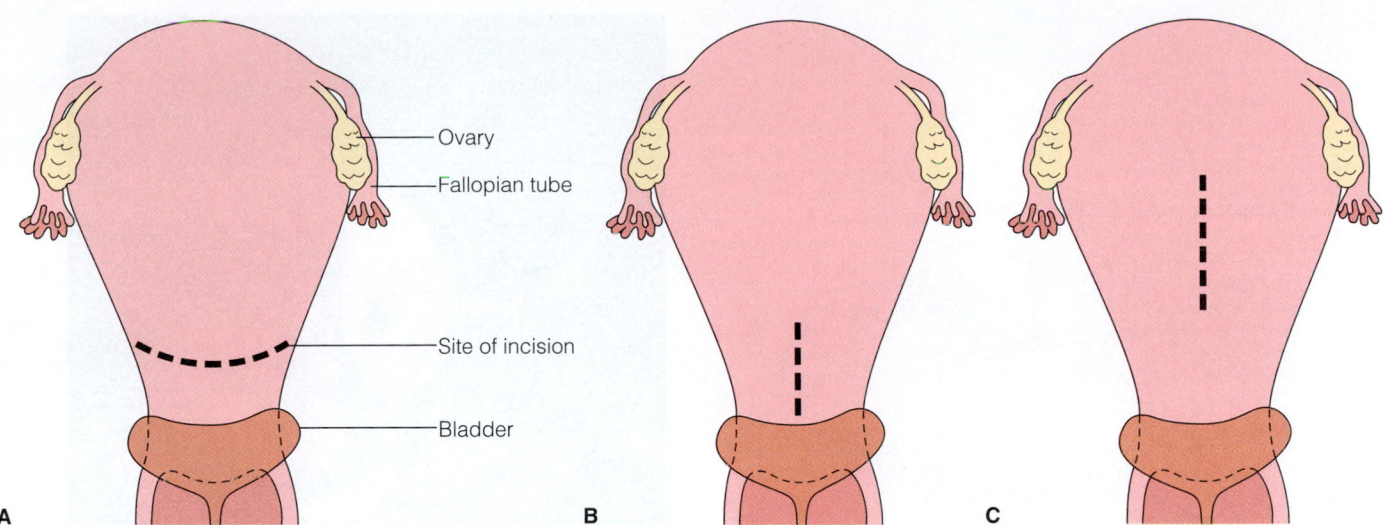

Figure 8-27. ■ The uterine incisions for cesarean birth. (**A**) This transverse incision in the lower uterine segment is called a Kerr incision. (**B**) The Selheim incision is a vertical incision in the lower uterine segment. (**C**) This view illustrates the classic uterine incision done in the body corpus of the uterus. The classic incision was commonly used in the past but is now associated with increased risk of uterine rupture in subsequent pregnancies and labor.

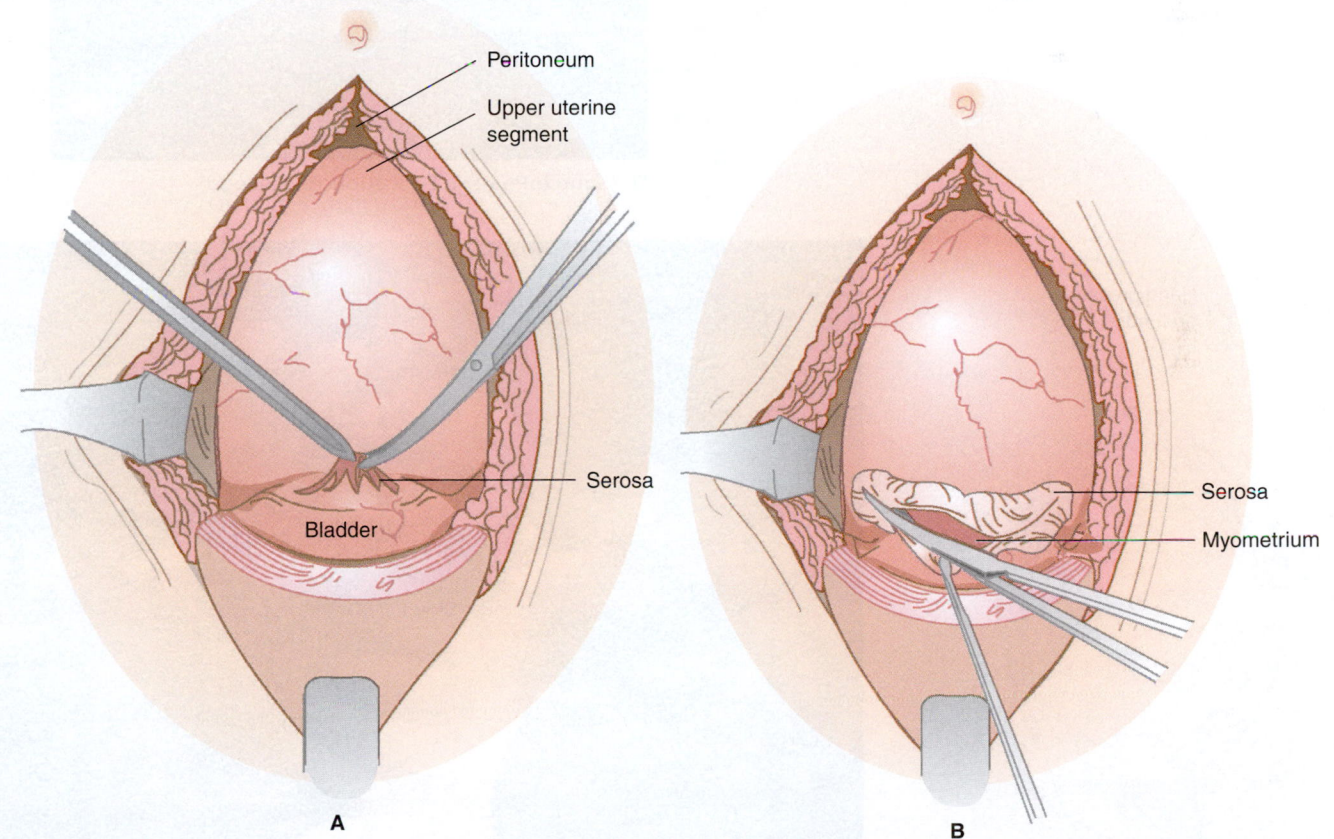

Figure 8-28. ■ Cesarean delivery. (**A**) The loose serosa is held in the forceps. The tip of the hemostat points to the upper margin of the bladder. The retractor is firm against the symphysis. (**B**) Sterile bandage scissors are used to make the incision into the loose serosa. (**C** and **D**) After the incisions are made into the uterus and fetal membranes, the physician reaches into the uterus between the symphysis pubis and the fetal head. The head is carefully lifted to bring it from beneath the symphysis forward through the uterine and abdominal incisions. (**E**) As the fetal head is lifted through the incisions, pressure is usually applied to the uterine fundus through the abdominal wall to help expel the fetus. (**F**) Infant being removed from uterus. (**A, B, C,** and **E**: Adapted, with permission, from McGraw-Hill Companies, Inc. Cunningham, F. G., McDonald, P. C., Gant, N. F., et al. [1997]. *Williams obstetrics* [20th ed.]. Stamford, CT: Appleton & Lange, pp. 516, 519. **D**: Courtesy of Harriette Hartigan/Artemis. **F**: © M.C. Schlachter Photography.)

(Continued)

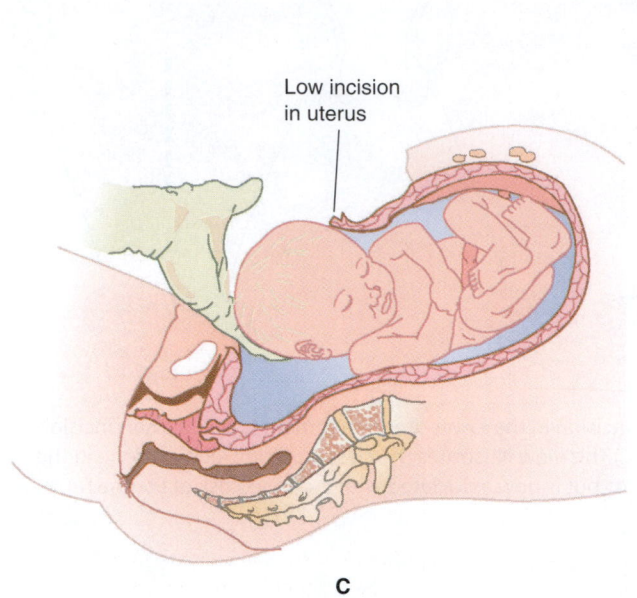

Low incision
in uterus

C

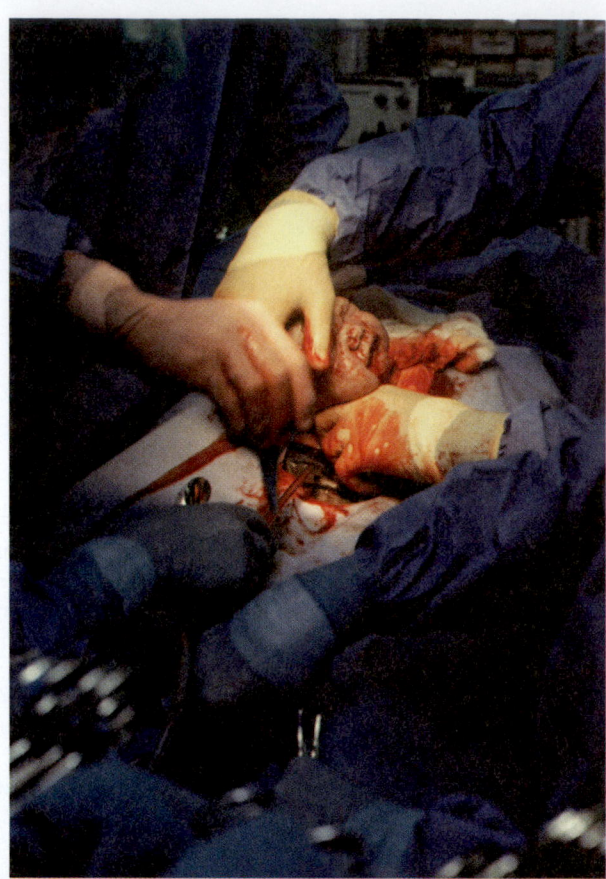

D (Source: Pearson Education/PH College)

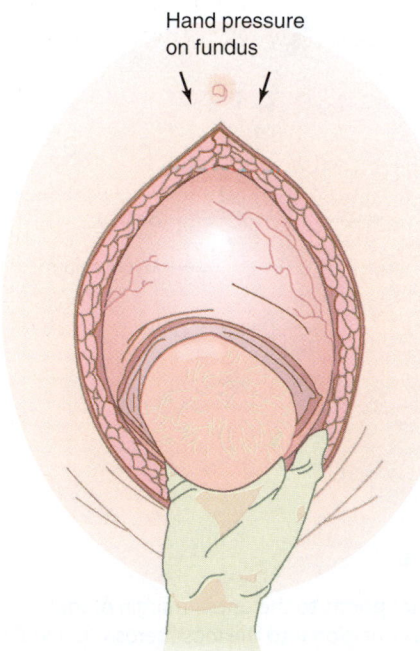

Hand pressure
on fundus

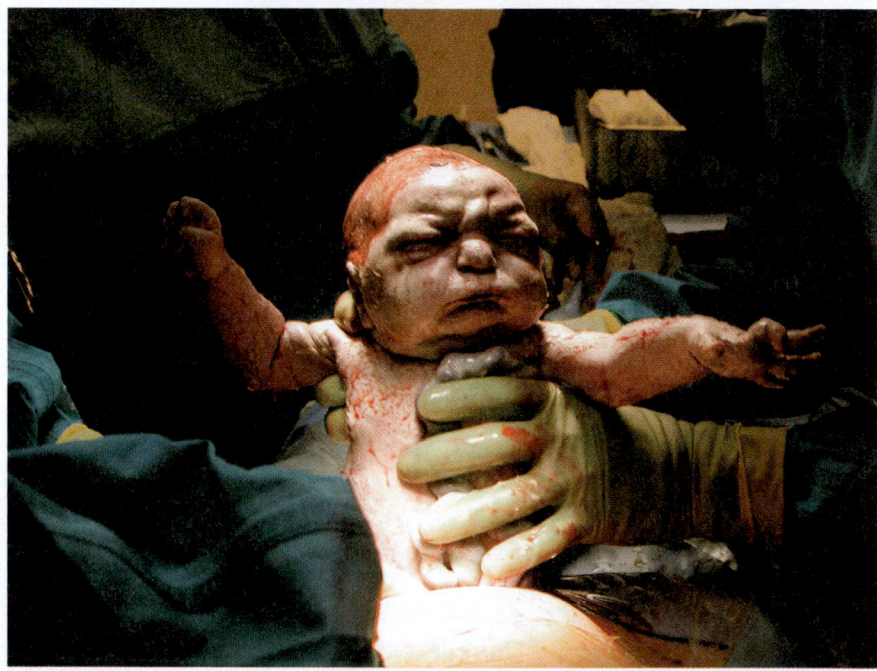

F

Figure 8-28. ■ *Continued.*

After the birth, the uterus, fascia, abdominal muscles, and fat are sutured. Skin staples, clips, or Steri-Strips are used to secure the skin.

The client will be taken to a recovery area for at least 1 hour. Vital signs will be taken. The fundus, surgical dressing, and urinary output are monitored. The airway is maintained until the client is awake and stable. The client is then taken to the postpartum unit.

VAGINAL BIRTH AFTER CESAREAN

Vaginal birth after cesarean (VBAC) may be possible. Success depends on the reason for the cesarean delivery, the condition of the scar tissue, and the size of the fetus. If a vertical uterine incision was made in the cesarean delivery, the risk of rupturing the uterus during labor is great. In this case, a repeat cesarean delivery will be performed. If a VBAC is attempted, a uterine stimulant (Pitocin) is used with caution, and more frequent monitoring may be needed. Anesthesia, a surgical team, and a physician should be available in case emergency cesarean delivery is needed.

Fetal Demise or Fetal Death

Fetal demise (or fetal death) is commonly called **stillbirth.** Although life-preventing fetal anomalies may be identified and discussed with the parents before 20 weeks' gestation, fetal death often occurs without warning. In this case, the mother realizes the fetus has stopped moving and begins to feel "something is wrong." She may or may not be having contractions. The mother may call the primary care provider or the hospital, or she may just arrive at the clinic. If possible, the nurse should recommend that the mother be accompanied by the father or another support person. Ultrasound is used to assess for fetal heart movement. If the diagnosis of fetal death is made, the parents may be allowed a few hours or days to grieve and adjust to the diagnosis. If labor does not begin spontaneously, it will be induced. In either case, the nurse is required to provide emotional support for this grieving family, and monitor the progression of labor and prepare for delivery. The cause of fetal death, such as a knot in the cord, may be obvious at birth, or an autopsy may be required. Figure 8-29 ■ shows a perinatal loss checklist that would assist the nurse in performing interventions.

Although the death of a child is always a traumatic event, when the death occurs prior to or at birth, the parents have not had any time to interact with their child and make positive memories. Following delivery of a stillborn infant, the parents are encouraged to view and hold their infant. Footprints, handprints, and locks of hair are generally collected, and pictures are taken for the parents. They are encouraged to bathe and dress the infant if they desire. Information is provided regarding local support groups and counseling. They may need help in contacting the mortuary. The family should be visited at home by the labor and delivery nurses or health care agency.

NURSING CARE

PRIORITIES IN NURSING CARE

Priorities of care for the pregnancy at risk include:

- Detecting complications at an early stage
- Assisting with implementing the medical treatment and preparing for delivery
- Evaluating the response to treatment as evidenced by stability of the specific condition.

ASSESSING

Assessing the high-risk mother during labor entails frequent monitoring of vital signs and the progression of labor. At times, medication to augment labor will need to be given and must also be monitored closely. When the mother is at risk, the fetus is also at risk and must be evaluated frequently.

The main method of assessing the progression of labor and well-being of the fetus is by EFM. The LPN/LVN can assist with application of the monitoring equipment, should recognize normal and abnormal patterns, and should report abnormal patterns to the supervising nurse immediately.

DIAGNOSING, PLANNING, AND IMPLEMENTING

The plan of care would be designed to alleviate the complication, if possible, and to ensure delivery of a healthy infant. In the case of fetal death, helping the family through this delivery process is coupled with emotional support. Possible nursing diagnoses include:

- Ineffective Tissue Perfusion
- Powerlessness
- Anticipatory (or actual) Grieving.

The medical and nursing plan of care might include:

- Administration of intravenous fluids
- Administration of medications (e.g., tocolytics or uterine stimulants) (see Table 8-7)
- Administration of oxygen
- Application of monitoring devices
- Preparation for a vaginal delivery with suction extractor or forceps, or a cesarean section delivery.

Parents' names _____
Address _____
Phone _____
Description of loss: _____
_____
Description of previous loss(es) _____
_____

L.M.P. _____ E.D.C. _____
Weeks of gestation _____
Sex of baby (if known) _____
Religious affiliation _____

	Office Staff	ER Staff	Labor/Delivery	Postpartum	Neonatal ICU	OR Staff	GYN/Post Op	Community Health	Date(s)
Received pregnancy confirmation									
Lab/amnio results	☐	☐	☐			☐			___
Sonogram photo	☐		☐			☐			
Acknowledgment of loss/impaired fertility	☐	☐	☐	☐	☐	☐	☐	☐	___
Bring up the subject									
Refer to the baby/expected child									
Call the baby by name									
Anticipatory guidance about normal grief									
Mother	☐	☐	☐	☐	☐	☐	☐	☐	___
Father	☐	☐	☐	☐	☐	☐	☐	☐	___
Family members	☐	☐	☐	☐	☐	☐	☐	☐	___
Postloss options given									
To go home/maternity floor/alternate floor	☐	☐	☐	☐		☐			___
Father to remain with mother/private room				☐			☐		
Saw/touched/held baby or products of conception	☐	☐	☐	☐	☐	☐	☐		___
If refused, later offers made									
Family members included in offer	☐	☐	☐		☐	☐			
Received mementos									
Footprints			☐	☐	☐				___
Bracelet			☐	☐	☐				___
Lock of hair			☐	☐	☐				___
Crib card			☐	☐	☐				___
Blanket			☐	☐	☐				___
Tape measure			☐	☐	☐				___
Certificate of life/remembrance	☐	☐	☐	☐	☐	☐	☐	☐	___
Photographs taken									
Given to parents				☐	☐				___
Filed with chart				☐	☐				___
Bathed/dressed baby				☐	☐				___
Postdeath options discussed	☐	☐	☐	☐	☐		☐		___
Need/desire for funeral director									
Type/location/timing of service									
Burial/cremation/hospital disposal									
Parent involvement									
Choosing burial outfit/mementos									
Announcements—public/personal									
Religious options									
Baby baptized	☐	☐	☐		☐	☐	☐		___
Clergy notified	☐	☐	☐	☐	☐	☐	☐	☐	___
Received information about									
Birth/death certificates	☐	☐			☐	☐		☐	___
Autopsy option discussed	☐	☐	☐	☐	☐		☐		___
Marked chart/room with identifying symbol	☐	☐	☐	☐	☐	☐	☐	☐	___
e.g., butterfly, rainbow, rose									
Received literature/suggested readings	☐	☐	☐	☐	☐	☐	☐	☐	___
Hospital admitting office notified	☐	☐							___
SHARE/support group referral made	☐	☐	☐	☐	☐	☐	☐	☐	___

Figure 8-29. ■ Comprehensive checklist for perinatal loss. (Reproduced, with permission, from Ryan, P. F., et al. [1991]. Facilitating care after perinatal loss: A comprehensive checklist. *Journal of Obstetrics, Gynecologic, & Neonatal Nursing, 20,* 385–389. Oxford: Blackwell.)

EVALUATING

Evaluation of the high-risk client in labor is a minute-by-minute comparison of data to normal ranges. Decisions must be made and implemented rapidly in order to maintain the health of the mother and fetus. The role of the LPN/LVN in labor and delivery is one of assisting the RN with delegated tasks.

NURSING PROCESS CARE PLAN
Client with Preterm Labor

A 33-week pregnant client has experienced a 10-day hospitalization for preterm labor. Her husband had to stay home from work all 10 days to care for their 3-year-old child. The physician has ordered complete bed rest with bathroom privileges only. The client states that her husband must return to work and she has no family in town.

Assessment. The following data regarding the client's husband was collected as soon as possible after admission:

- States he must go back to work
- Exhibits anxiety
- States he has not slept in 36 hours
- Unable to continue coaching community soccer team
- States he is afraid his wife will not comply with bed rest if he is not at home.

Nursing Diagnosis. The following important nursing diagnosis (among others) is established for this client's spouse:

Caregiver Role Strain

Expected Outcome. Caregiver is able to identify workable options to care adequately for wife with preterm labor.

Planning and Implementation

- Create an environment in which the caregiver is comfortable relating his fears and concerns. *A trusting environment allows the client to be honest, and this will in turn allow for adequate resolution.*
- Assist the caregiver in identifying his strengths. *Promotes a sense of self-confidence.*
- Assist the caregiver in exploring options for support. *Fears, concerns, and tasks required to manage the care of the pregnant client may be handled by persons other than the husband.*
- If other areas of support are unavailable, refer the husband to community resources. *Community resources can relieve the husband's stress.*
- Encourage the husband to choose one diversional activity weekly. *These activities allow the caregiver to retain a sense of self.*

Evaluation. The client's husband is able to set up a weekly rotation with ladies from his church. He also agreed to referee one soccer game per week.

Critical Thinking in the Nursing Process

1. The client states she is unsure how she will keep from getting bored every day. What suggestions could the nurse give her?
2. The physician orders home tocolytic monitoring weekly for the client. Explain this process to the client.
3. What symptoms does the nurse need to teach the client with preterm labor to report immediately?

Note: Discussion of Critical Thinking questions appears in Appendix I.

HIGH-RISK POSTPARTUM CARE

The postpartum period usually progresses without problems, as described in Chapter 10 ⚭. However, complications that occur during pregnancy or delivery can continue after delivery. For example, the woman who has type I diabetes mellitus will need frequent monitoring of blood sugars and adjustment in insulin dosage until the condition has stabilized. Likewise, the woman who develops gestational diabetes will need frequent blood sugar monitoring until the values remain within normal limits.

Postpartum Assessment

PRE-ECLAMPSIA

Pre-eclampsia, usually beginning during pregnancy, can become worse in the first 24 to 48 hours after delivery. The woman's blood pressure, reflexes, and clonus must be monitored every 2 to 4 hours (see Figure 8-9). The amount of protein in the urine should be measured with each void. The administration of medication to control blood pressure may continue and must be monitored carefully.

In severe cases of pre-eclampsia, there is a risk for seizure, stroke, and kidney or liver damage. Because of the risk to the mother and infant, the woman will probably be delivered by cesarean section. Depending on the prematurity and condition of the infant, the child may be admitted to the NICU (see Figure 9-36). The mother may be admitted to the medical intensive care unit, where constant heart monitoring and observations can be made. Medication to lower the blood pressure and prevent seizures will be given. Once the mother has stabilized (usually in a few days), she may be transferred to the postpartum unit and discharged. Due to the critical nature of this disorder, the role of the LPN/LVN would be to assist the charge nurse.

BLEEDING

Postpartum hemorrhage is most common within the first hour after delivery. There are three main reasons for postpartum hemorrhage: retained placenta, **uterine atony** (lack of muscle tone and firmness), and laceration.

Retained Placenta

Retained placenta occurs when all or part of the placenta or fetal membranes remains attached to the endometrium. When the placenta detaches from the endometrium following delivery, it should detach in one piece (see Figure 6-5). Occasionally, one or more of the cotyledons remain attached to the endometrium and tear away from the rest of the placenta. These torn cotyledons can continue to bleed. The uterus will recognize the intact placenta tissue and fail to contract to stop the bleeding. If the condition is noted during the delivery process, the physician will perform D&C (dilation and curettage), inserting a curette through the cervix and scraping the endometrium. If the retained placenta is not identified at delivery, the uterus will become boggy, and vaginal bleeding will be heavy and uncontrolled. The charge nurse and physician should be notified. The client will probably be taken to surgery for a D&C.

Uterine Atony

Uterine atony is the second most common cause of postpartum hemorrhage. At times, the uterus becomes tired of contracting and no longer responds to hormonal stimulation. This can occur following long labors, a multifetal pregnancy, or a large fetus, or when the mother has had many pregnancies in a short period of time. In such cases, the uterus does not fully contract following delivery of the placenta. The fundus may become firm with massage, but then loses tone within a short time, resulting in free flow of bright red blood. Frequent assessment and fundal massage are necessary. The administration of Pitocin or Methergine may be necessary to cause the uterus to contract.

Laceration

The third cause of postpartum hemorrhage is laceration. Following delivery, the physician examines the cervix, vaginal wall, and perineum for lacerations. If any lacerations are identified, they are sutured. Occasionally, small lacerations are missed and ooze blood. Hemorrhage ensues over time. Bleeding that saturates more than one perineal pad an hour is considered heavy and should be investigated. The physician re-examines the cervix, vagina, and perineum and sutures the tissue as necessary.

The treatment of postpartum hemorrhage begins with identifying the cause. Specific treatment can then be implemented. Intravenous fluids and blood transfusion may be needed. Once the bleeding is controlled and the client is stabilized, routine postpartum care continues.

DISSEMINATED INTRAVASCULAR COAGULATION

Disseminated intravascular coagulation (DIC) is a life-threatening pathologic process of the blood clotting mechanism. The overactivation of the blood clotting mechanism results in a depletion of clotting factors and platelets. Clots form in small blood vessels, blocking circulation to body tissues. Because blood clotting factors are tied up within these small clots, hemorrhage occurs in areas of trauma, such as intravenous puncture sites, the uterus following delivery, and lacerations. Diagnosis is based on laboratory findings and clinical symptoms. In addition to bleeding from wounds, symptoms include bleeding gums, nosebleeds, bruising, and petechiae on the chest and under the blood pressure cuff. Laboratory tests show a decrease in platelets and blood clotting factors, coagulation time shows no clot, and PTT is increased.

There are many causes of DIC, and it is not limited to the events surrounding pregnancy. DIC is seen as a complication of systemic disorders, such as pre-eclampsia or septicemia; lengthy surgery; and pulmonary embolism. Other causes may include fetal demise and abruptio placentae.

Medical treatment involves removing the cause if possible. Intravenous fluids and blood transfusions are used to replace lost fluids. Oxygen is administered to improve tissue perfusion. Anticoagulants such as intravenous heparin may be given to release the blood clotting factors that are tied up in the small vessels.

The nurse must carefully and continuously assess the functioning of all body systems by monitoring vital signs every 15 minutes, and measuring the intake and output, paying close attention to the urinary output and the amount of blood loss. Because DIC could begin prior to delivery, the condition of the fetus must be evaluated frequently. The nursing care focuses on stopping bleeding by pressure and elevation where possible, administering prescribed medical treatment, and providing support to the client and family. Because of the seriousness of this life-threatening condition, the client and family members experience fear, anxiety, and anticipatory or actual grieving. The nurse provides support but may need to contact other resources such as social workers or clergy to assist.

Postpartum Infections

MASTITIS

Mastitis (infection of the breast) occurs primarily in lactating women. The most common causative organisms are *Staphylococcus aureus, Haemophilus parainfluenzae, Haemophilus influenzae,* and *Streptococcus.* Bacteria invade the breast tissue though fissured or cracked nipples. Overdistention of the breast and milk *stasis* (pooling of milk in the mammary glands) are contributing factors. Transmission of bacteria is generally from the mouth and nose of the newborn, but could also be from dirty hands touching the breast or through the mother's blood. Symptoms of mastitis (Figure 8-30 ■) include redness and swelling of one or more lobes of the breast (often in a V-shaped wedge), fever, headache, breast pain, and flulike symptoms.

Mastitis may not occur for several weeks after delivery. It is important for the nurse to teach the mother how to prevent mastitis as well as about its symptoms and treatment. Mastitis can be prevented through good hygiene practices, daily bathing, and hand washing prior to touching the nipple. Wearing a supportive bra, even in bed, will position the

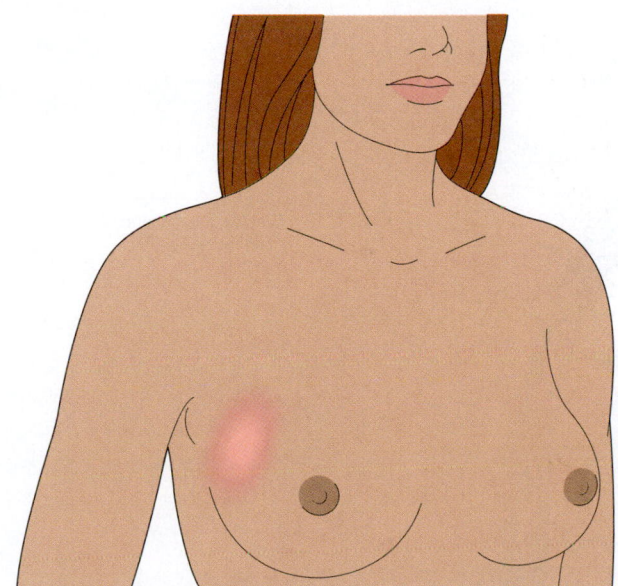

Figure 8-30. ■ Mastitis. Tenderness, swelling, and erythema are present in this example of mastitis in the outer quadrant of the breast. Axillary lymph nodes may be swollen and tender. Mastitis redness often occurs in a V shape because of the shape of breast segments.

breast for proper drainage and prevent pooling of milk. Emptying the breast through nursing or pumping prevents overdistension. Consistently using proper breastfeeding techniques will prevent cracked nipples. If symptoms of mastitis occur, it is important for the client to contact the primary care provider. Medical treatment generally includes antibiotics, moist heat applications, and analgesics. Emptying the breast with frequent breastfeeding or pumping decreases the duration of symptoms and speeds healing. Some mothers are concerned that the baby will become ill from the milk. Generally, this is not the case because of the antibiotic therapy. It is important for the mother to take the antibiotics as ordered.

WOUND INFECTION

A laceration, episiotomy, or cesarean incision could become infected. Redness, swelling, pain, and purulent drainage would indicate a wound infection. An elevated temperature could also indicate an infection. If left untreated, *dehiscence* (opening) of the wound would occur. The client needs to be instructed to report any of these manifestations to the care provider without delay.

Medical treatment includes antibiotics to prevent or treat an infection. When infection is present, healing is delayed. The infected tissue may need to be drained by surgical incision or removal of sutures. If the wound is deep, irrigation and packing may be needed.

Keeping the area clean and dry can prevent wound infection. The client should be taught to shower daily, cover the abdominal incision with a clean dry dressing, rinse the perineum with warm water after each void or stool, and change the perineal pad at least every 2 hours. In most cases, the infection clears without further complication.

POSTPARTUM (PUERPERAL) INFECTION

Postpartum (puerperal) infection is a rare infection of the uterus following childbirth. Strict aseptic technique used in the delivery process prevents this life-threatening complication. Contributing factors are listed in Box 8-7 ■. Often, antibiotics are ordered if any of the contributing factors occurs during the delivery process.

The infection usually begins in the vagina and migrates upward into the uterus **(endometritis),** pelvic lymph nodes, peritoneum **(peritonitis),** and circulation. Once the organisms are growing in the blood, the disease has progressed to **septicemia** (Figure 8-31 ■). If treatment is not started immediately or if treatment is not effective, death can occur.

Although the contamination occurs during the delivery process, it usually takes several days for the symptoms of infection to begin. The client may have been discharged by this time. It is important to teach the client to watch for the

BOX 8-7	ASSESSMENT

Risk Factors for Postpartum (Puerperal) Infection

- Cesarean delivery
- Prolonged rupture of membranes
- Multiple vaginal examinations during labor
- Compromised health status of the mother (due to HIV, anemia, malnutrition, smoking, illicit drug/alcohol use)
- Obstetric trauma (lacerations, episiotomy)
- Intrauterine monitoring equipment
- Instrument-assisted delivery
- Manual removal of placenta
- Pre-existing vaginal infections (STIs)

Antibiotics may be ordered for any of these contributing factors.

classic symptoms, including a fever of 100.4°F (38°C) or higher, chills, pelvic and abdominal pain, and foul-smelling lochia. If these symptoms occur, the client should contact the primary care provider immediately.

Maternal Death

In developed areas of the world, it is rare for the mother to die in childbirth. Prenatal, intrapartum, and postpartum care contributes to the survival of the mother.

If the mother dies, it is usually after her condition has deteriorated over a period of time. She (or family members) may express concern about her condition. They may ask questions that are difficult to answer or for which there is no answer. They may seek information about what is happening physiologically, what treatment is being provided, and why it is not working. The nurse, working alone, may not be able to answer questions thoroughly due to the need to assist the physician and to provide treatments and care. In this situation, the nurse should call for additional assistance from the charge nurse, social worker, or clergy.

When the nurse is able to communicate with the family, care must be taken to listen to their questions and respond appropriately. Generally, the family will ask for reassurance that everything possible is being done. At this time of great emotional stress, a detailed explanation of the pathology and treatment being provided is not the best answer. It is the role and responsibility of the physician or primary care provider to answer these questions. The nurse should respond with statements such as:

- "I know this is extremely difficult. As soon as possible, the doctor will answer your questions."
- "Can you tell me your understanding of what is happening? Maybe I can clarify what is going on."
- "I understand your fear and impatience. It seems to take a long time, doesn't it? Can I call someone to sit with you? A family member or clergy?"

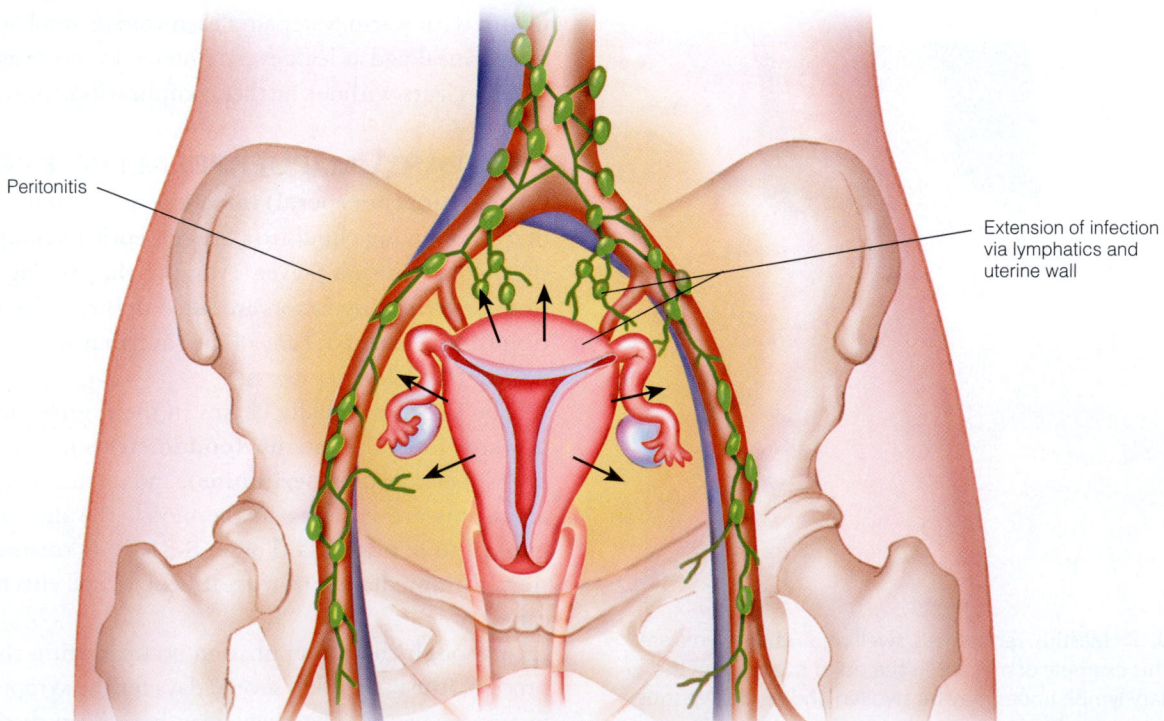

Peritonitis

Extension of infection via lymphatics and uterine wall

Figure 8-31. ■ Peritonitis may develop with the spread of uterine infection via lymphatics.

When death of the mother does occur, the entire family structure is disrupted. The surviving partner is faced with the care of the newborn (and possibly other children) at a time when emotional resources are low. Each family member needs to work through the grief process as with other death events. This process is detailed in Chapter 28 ⬭. Referral to social services can help the family mobilize resources such as counseling before potential problems develop.

The death of the mother also takes an emotional toll on nurses and medical staff. Feeling of guilt, anger, fear, sadness, and depression can impact the care of other clients. The nurses and medical staff need to review the situation surrounding the events, the medical record, and what (if anything) could be done differently in the future. A critical incident debriefing helps cope with feelings and emotions that result from a maternal death.

Postpartum Depression and Postpartum Psychosis

Postpartum depression, a major mood disorder, most frequently appears 4 weeks post delivery and upon weaning the child from the breast (see Health Promotion Issue on pages 254 and 255). The symptoms of postpartum depression are similar to other forms of depression. These include sadness, frequent crying, insomnia, or excessive sleeping, appetite change, difficulty concentrating, feelings of worthlessness, lack of interest in usual activities, and lack of concern for appearance.

Postpartum psychosis, a major psychiatric disorder, usually becomes evident in the first 3 months after delivery. The symptoms of postpartum psychosis include agitation, hyperactivity, insomnia, mood *lability* (changeability), confusion, irrational thoughts and behaviors, difficulty remembering or concentrating, poor judgment, delusions, and hallucinations. Postpartum psychosis is considered an emergency because of the risk of suicide and infanticide. Risk factors for postpartum depression and psychosis are included in Box 8-8 ▪.

Note the symptoms of postpartum blues described in Chapter 10 ⬭. You will see similarities between postpartum blues, depression, and psychosis. Although postpartum blues are common and to some extent expected, the symptoms can progress to postpartum depression and the more serious postpartum psychosis. Several months after delivery, women have limited contact with their health care providers. Therefore, assessment and diagnosis of postpartum depression and psychosis may go undiagnosed. It is critical for the nurse to identify women at risk, teach them

---

BOX 8-8	ASSESSMENT

Risk Factors for Postpartum Depression and Psychosis

Postpartum Depression
- Primipara
- Contradictory feelings about the pregnancy
- History of postpartum depression (most significant)
- History of depression or bipolar illness
- Family history of psychiatric disorders
- Lack of stable relationship with partner or parents
- Lack of social support
- Body image disorders, including eating disorders
- History of drug and/or alcohol abuse

Postpartum Psychosis
- Previous puerperal psychosis
- History of bipolar (manic-depressive) disorder
- Prenatal stressors: lack of social support, lack of a partner, low socioeconomic status
- Obsessive personality
- Family history of mood disorders

---

and their families the signs and symptoms, and encourage them to seek assistance if signs of depression become worse or continue for more than 2 weeks.

The treatment of postpartum depression and psychosis includes a combination of medication, individual and group counseling, and assistance with meeting child care and family needs. The woman needs to be referred to a mental health professional for follow-up treatment. Many of the drugs used to treat depression and psychosis are contraindicated in breastfeeding women.

The role of the LPN/LVN in the care of women with mental health disorders is to:

- Assist the charge nurse and mental health professional in monitoring the symptoms of depression and psychosis
- Monitor for side effects of medication
- Be supportive to the family

The assessment, plan, and evaluation of care of the high-risk postpartum client are similar to the routine care of any postpartum client. The additional treatment of specific complications consists of administering medication and teaching the client and family about this complication.

Note: The references and resources for this and all chapters have been compiled at the back of the book.

RISK FOR POSTPARTUM DEPRESSION AND PSYCHOSIS

The nurse is gathering data at a prenatal appointment from a gravida 3, para 2 at 32 weeks' gestation. The client also has a 4-year-old child and a 2-year-old child. She is a single mother who works as an accountant for an accounting firm and also takes freelance work to supplement her income. The pregnancy thus far has been without any physical complications.

The nurse asks the pregnant woman if she has any concerns about her pregnancy and birth. The woman says she is worried that she will have another episode of postpartum depression (PPD) and not be able to care for her family and keep her job. The nurse asks the client to tell her more about her past experience with PPD. The client relates that during her second pregnancy, she escaped a physically abusive relationship with her now ex-husband. She and her first child had to flee in the night to a community agency for battered women. They lived in the shelter for the remainder of her pregnancy. After the birth of her daughter, they moved to a different state to live with her parents. Although her parents were welcoming, living with them proved difficult. She did not have a job and therefore could not get her own home.

Her emotional condition worsened, and her parents demanded she seek medical help. After several months of treatment, she was able to regain her emotional sense of well-being, find a job, and ultimately get a home of her own.

DISCUSSION

Postpartum Blues

Postpartum blues occur in about 70% of all births. Following birth, from days 1 to 10, the mother may experience sadness and periods of crying. She may also report difficulty sleeping, lack of energy, and anorexia. She may experience anxiety, feelings of being overwhelmed, lack of confidence, and concern over physical changes. These symptoms are believed to result from hormonal shifts following childbirth. It is important for the nurse to communicate to the new mother that this is a normal finding. The nurse should also offer to listen to the mother's concerns, provide her with stress reduction suggestions, and follow-up to determine if the symptoms have resolved or are worsening.

Postpartum Depression

Ten percent of mothers who have recently given birth may experience PPD. Symptoms of PPD may occur 1 to 12 months following birth. Symptoms include those discussed under Postpartum Blues, as well as headaches, hyperventilation, tachycardia and chest pain, dizziness, constipation or diarrhea, and pruritis. The new mother may experience feelings of despair, hopelessness, powerlessness, inadequacy, inability to cope, shame, guilt, and suicidal thoughts. Recognition of the symptoms of PPD is a priority nursing intervention. The nurse is then responsible for notifying the appropriate health care professional so the client can receive the necessary counseling and medication administration. Close follow-up is also necessary to determine if the symptoms have resolved or are worsening.

Postpartum Psychosis

Although rare, occurring in 1% to 2% of all births, postpartum psychosis is serious and must be recognized and addressed promptly. Symptoms develop 1 month after birth and include symptoms of PPD, as well as obsessive behavior, catatonia, amnesia, irrational thoughts, hallucinations, and delusions. Prompt recognition of symptoms and referral to a psychiatric professional can avoid physical harm to both the mother and her infant.

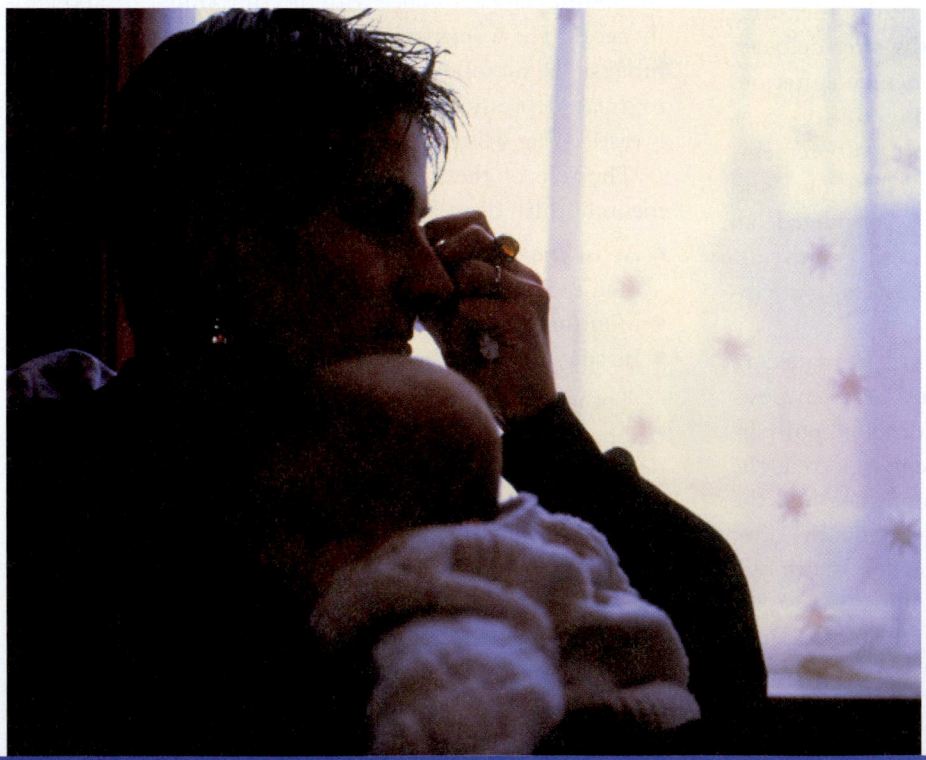

Risk Factors Related to Postpartum Psychological Disorders

Biologic Factors

- Normal and hormonal changes of pregnancy
- Complications of pregnancy and childbirth
- History of
  - Postpartum depression
  - PMS
  - Thyroid disorders
  - Mental/emotional difficulties in the family

Psychological Factors

- Unmet expectations of motherhood
- History of psychological disorders
- Unresolved loss
- Stressful life events such as illness or death of a loved one, job change, financial difficulties, or a move
- History of childhood trauma such as physical or emotional abuse

Relationship Issues

- Expected changes in relationships following childbirth that result from the addition of a new individual in the family and the necessary role changes
- Marriage difficulties
- Social support difficulties or the lack thereof
- Single mothers
- Relationship difficulties with newborn and/or other children. (e.g., a newborn with colic or a child with a disability)

PLANNING AND IMPLEMENTATION

Risk Assessment

It is important for the nurse to perform a thorough risk assessment related to postpartum depression for this client. Several tools are available to assist with this assessment, such as the Edinburgh Postnatal Depression Scale, the Postpartum Depression Checklist, and the Kennerley Blues Questionnaire. (Refer to a psychology text for these assessment tools.)

The client should be taught to recognize symptoms and understand the importance of prompt notification of the health care professional. This client is a single mother, so the nurse should explore what other levels of social support are available to her. If appropriate, the nurse should meet with these individuals to discuss symptom recognition and the importance of prompt reporting.

Prenatal Planning

Much of the stress of motherhood can be avoided with proper prenatal planning and preparation. The nurse can assist the client in taking care of herself physically. She should be encouraged to develop a regular pattern of nutrition, exercise, and rest. The kitchen pantry should be well stocked, and quick meals should be frozen before the birth. Everyone needs rest following birth. The client should seek to avoid interruptions during nap time by taking the phone off the hook and putting a "do not disturb" sign on the door. The nurse can encourage the client to develop a simple wardrobe of comfortable clothes that can be laundered easily.

The client should garner support from trusted individuals to assist with child care, shopping, and household chores. The support system also serves the need for adult socialization and expression of fears and concerns.

The nurse can encourage the mother to adjust her expectations. The client can journal about her fears and concerns. She can stock up on comical movies or books to keep laughter alive in her life. These can provide great stress breaks.

This client is well aware of the added stress of life changes during pregnancy and the postpartum period. The nurse can still encourage her to avoid such changes during this critical timeframe. With these measures, continued assessment, and close follow-up, the effect of postpartum emotional changes can be minimized.

SELF-REFLECTION

There are many high-profile cases related to postpartum emotional reactions. Review the case of Andrea Yates. Do you think Mrs. Yates's caregivers could have implemented any care behaviors that would have prevented this tragedy? What if you had been her nurse? What assessments would you have made? What teaching would you have given? What follow-up care would you have implemented? What are your beliefs concerning the legal charges and convictions related to Mrs. Yates' actions? In your opinion, are there any plausible alternatives to imprisonment?

MediaLink · Mental health in pregnancy

SUGGESTED RESOURCES

For the Nurse

www.ncast.org This site presents materials developed by the University of Washington School of Nursing to promote maternal mental health during pregnancy. The materials include a text, assessment guide, handouts and on-site training for healthcare professionals.

Beck, C. T. (1999) *Postpartum depression: Case studies, research and nursing care.* Washington, DC: Association of Women's Health, Obstetric and Neonatal Nursing.

Johnson & Johnson. (2006). *The compendium of postpartum care.* Washington, DC: Association of Women's Health, Obstetric and Neonatal Nursing.

For the Client

Bennet, S., & Indman, P. (2006). *Beyond the blues: A guide to treating prenatal and postpartum depression.* San Jose, CA: Moodswings Press.

Placksin, S. (2000) *Mothering the new mother: Women's feelings and needs after childbirth: A support and resource guide.* New York, NY: Newmarket Press.

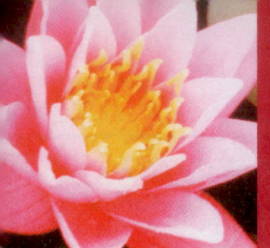

Chapter Review

KEY TERMS by Topics

Use the audio glossary feature of either the CD-ROM or the Companion Website to hear the correct pronunciation of the following key terms.

Tests Used to Assess Fetal Well-Being

ultrasound, amniocentesis, erythroblastosis fetalis, nonstress test (NST), reactive, nonreactive, biophysical profile

Tests Used to Assess Maternal Well-Being

maternal hemoglobin, indirect Coombs' test, multiple marker screen, 1-hour glucose screen

Complications with Bleeding

miscarriage, incompetent cervix, D&C (dilation and curettage), cerclage (Shirodkar procedure), ectopic, tubal pregnancy, placenta previa, abruptio placentae

Other Complications

hyperemesis gravidarum, gestational hypertension, chronic hypertension, pre-eclampsia, eclampsia, HELLP syndrome, gestational diabetes mellitus (GDM), macrosomia, TORCH group, rubella, cytomegalovirus (CMV), herpes simplex type 2, hemolytic disorders

Factors That Create High Risk

preterm labor, precipitous labor, prolapsed cord, dystocia, variability, accelerations, decelerations, cesarean section

Fetal Demise or Fetal Death

fetal demise, stillbirth

Postpartum Assessment

uterine atony, disseminated intravascular coagulation (DIC)

Postpartum Infections

mastitis, postpartum (puerperal) infection, endometritis, peritonitis, septicemia

KEY Points

- Complications can occur at any time during pregnancy, labor, delivery, and postpartum that can put the mother and fetus at risk.

- Through assessment and monitoring, complications can be identified early.

- The nurse must be prepared to assist the physician with diagnostic exams, vaginal and cesarean delivery, and control of postpartum hemorrhage.

- The nurse must be prepared to assist the grieving family when complications result in fetal or maternal death.

- The nurse must be prepared to refer the mother and family for counseling and follow-up home care as appropriate.

EXPLORE Medialink

Additional interactive resources for this chapter can be found on the Companion Website at www.prenhall.com/towle.

Click on Chapter 8 and "Begin" to select the activities for this chapter.

For chapter-related NCLEX-style questions and an audio glossary, access the accompanying CD-ROM in this book.

Animations

Pre-eclampsia

Postpartum assessment

Massage a uterine fundus postpartum

Breech birth

Ectopic pregnancy

Evaluate deep tendon reflexes

FOR FURTHER Study

Sexually transmitted infections (STIs) are discussed in depth in Chapter 5; twins are illustrated in Figure 5-18; spontaneous abortion is shown in Figure 5-20.

Chapter 6 discusses prenatal care, tests for pregnancy, development of the fetus, and nursing care of the healthy pregnant woman; Table 6-3 compares normal lab values during pregnancy and outside pregnancy; Figure 6-5 shows methods of placental separation.

External fetal monitoring is described in Procedure 7-2; Figure 7-17 C and D show epidural and spinal anesthesia; Figure 7-31 illustrates an electronic fetal monitor; Table 7-5 provides the Apgar scoring system.

Chapter 9 discusses hypoglycemia in the newborn; Figure 9-36 shows neonates in the ICU.

The normal postpartum period is described in Chapter 10.

Cataracts and deafness are discussed in Chapter 16.

HIV and AIDS are discussed in Chapter 21.

The grief process is detailed in Chapter 28.

Caring for a Client with Postpartum Depression

NCLEX-PN® Focus Area: Psychological Adaptation

Case Study: Allison, a 23-year-old gravida 3, para 2 mother, delivered a stillborn child 3 weeks ago. She is at the obstetrician's office for a postpartum checkup. She is tearful and states she just does not feel happy anymore. She just cannot get over the death of her baby.

Nursing Diagnosis: Complicated Grieving

COLLECT DATA

Subjective	Objective
_____	_____
_____	_____
_____	_____
_____	_____
_____	_____
_____	_____

Would you report this? Yes/No

If yes, to: _____

Nursing Care

_____
_____
_____
_____
_____
_____
_____
_____
_____
_____
_____
_____

How would you document this? _____
_____
_____
_____

Compare your documentation to the sample provided in Appendix I.

Data Collected
(use those that apply)

- BP 136/82
- Crying
- Breasts expressing small amount of milk
- Wearing maternity clothes
- Fundus at pubis
- States she does not feel happy
- Delivered a stillborn 3 weeks ago
- Negative clonus
- Hair neatly combed
- States she cannot get over baby's death

Nursing Interventions
(use those that apply; list in priority order)

- Ask her if she has family or friends who are helpful.
- Give her a list of support groups.
- Request a urine sample.
- Tell her that if she has not gotten over the baby's death by now, she never will.
- Tell her medication will be needed to clear her thoughts.
- Tell her to stop wearing maternity clothes.
- Ask what she has been doing to overcome her grief.
- Recommend she seek help from a psychiatrist.

NCLEX-PN® Exam Preparation

> **TEST-TAKING TIP** Study the illustrations showing normal pelvic anatomy and normal mechanisms of labor. Try to visualize the high-risk disorders and the physical changes they cause.

1 A client at 34 weeks' gestation is admitted to the delivery unit with preterm labor. An amniocentesis is done to determine fetal lung maturity. Which of the following laboratory tests should the nurse monitor?

1. CBC
2. hCG
3. APTT
4. PG

2 A client is admitted to the emergency department with bright red vaginal bleeding and pelvic cramping. She is 16 weeks pregnant. For which of the following signs should the nurse observe the client?

1. decrease in pulse
2. decrease in FHR
3. decrease in BP
4. increase urinary output

3 A 21-year-old comes to the clinic for her first prenatal appointment. She is at 9 weeks' gestation, and a blood sample is drawn. Which lab result would indicate the fetus is at risk for erythroblastosis fetalis?_____

4 A client who is 30 weeks pregnant was admitted 2 days ago with preterm labor. Oral terbutaline 2.5 mg every 3 hours is ordered. Which of the following nursing measures would have the highest priority in her care?

1. Monitor closely for respiratory depression.
2. Check the pulse before each dose of terbutaline.
3. Monitor the FHR continuously.
4. Place the client on strict bed rest.

5 A client who is 26 weeks pregnant is admitted to the antepartum unit with gestational hypertension. Which of the following symptoms would indicate her condition is getting worse?

1. epigastric pain
2. blood pressure 138/90
3. deep tendon reflexes of 2+
4. dependent edema of 2+

6 A client who is at 32 weeks' gestation is to be admitted with pre-eclampsia. Her blood pressure ranges from 140s/100s to 160s/110s. She has a headache, generalized edema, and 3+ proteinuria. Which environment would be most appropriate for this client?

1. semiprivate room, up ad lib, VS and FHR every shift, 2-gram sodium diet
2. three-bed ward, ambulation four times a day, VS and FHR twice a day, low sodium diet
3. private room, bed rest with bathroom privileges, VS and FHR every 4 hours, regular diet
4. labor room, strict bed rest, VS every 15 minutes, FHR continuous, NPO

7 When admitting a client to the OB unit, the nurse notes the client has a history of IV drug use and is positive for hepatitis B (HBV+). When caring for this client, the nurse would be required to wear personal protective equipment _____. (Select all that apply.)

1. when contacting amniotic fluid
2. when contacting feces
3. when cleaning the bathtub after the client relaxed in the jacuzzi
4. when touching the baby during delivery
5. when providing PO liquids for hydration

8 A gravida 3, para 2 client who is at 39 weeks' gestation is admitted to the OB unit with bright red vaginal bleeding. She states she was just walking around the house when it began. She has not had any pain. The nurse's first priority would be to:

1. determine pulse, blood pressure, and FHR.
2. prepare her for an emergency cesarean delivery.
3. inspect the perineal pad to determine the amount of bleeding.
4. position her in lithotomy position for a vaginal delivery.

9 A client delivered by cesarean 3 days ago and is scheduled for discharge from the OB unit. When the nurse enters the room, she discovers the client crying in the bathroom. There is no evidence of a physical problem. The nurse would:

1. leave her alone in the bathroom to collect her emotions.
2. say, "This is just postpartum blues and they will be over in a few days."
3. say, "Can I call your minister for you?"
4. say, "Tell me what's wrong."

10 A client in the office for a 6-week postpartum checkup states, "I am so sad. I hate taking care of the baby. I'm a terrible mother. I wish it would just go away." The nurse would respond:

1. "I'm sure things will be better in a few weeks."
2. "Do you have some help at home?"
3. "Have you thought about hurting your baby or yourself?"
4. "This is a common feeling of new mothers."

Answers for Review Questions, as well as discussion of Care Plan and Critical Thinking Care Map questions, appear in Appendix I.

Health Promotion of the Newborn

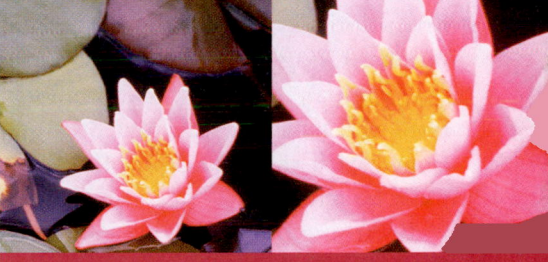

HEALTH PROMOTION ISSUE:
Bioethics of Newborn Male Circumcision

NURSING PROCESS CARE PLAN:
Care of the Preoperative Newborn with a Congenital Heart Defect

CRITICAL THINKING CARE MAP:
Caring for Infant with Depressed CNS

LEARNING Outcomes

After completing this chapter, you will be able to:

- Discuss physiologic adaptation of the newborn.
- Discuss Apgar score.
- Describe physical characteristics of the newborn.
- Describe neonatal reflexes.
- Describe nursery care for the newborn.
- Discuss common procedures and screening tests for the newborn.
- Discuss the newborn's nutritional needs and how they can be met.
- Discuss parent teaching related to care of the newborn.
- Describe signs of respiratory distress in the newborn.
- Discuss conditions and treatment of the high-risk newborn.

The **newborn** is the infant from delivery through the first month of life. Initial care revolves around meeting the basic biologic needs and helping the newborn adjust to life outside the womb.

Physiologic Adaptation

An understanding of the physiologic adaptation to life outside the uterus guides the nurse's actions when setting priorities in the care of the newborn. These adaptations were discussed in Delivery Room Care of the Neonate in Chapter 7 ⚭. They are briefly reviewed here in the order of priority (airway, breathing, circulation, thermoregulation) to set the foundation for newborn care.

RESPIRATORY ADAPTATION

Because the fetus does not breathe inside the uterus, the first priority is to assist the newborn in establishing respirations. Using the bulb syringe or suction catheter, mucus, vaginal secretions, and amniotic fluid are removed from the newborn's airway. Because the infant is positioned with the head down, fluids continue to drain and must be removed.

Breathing usually begins spontaneously (Figure 9-1 ■). However, some newborns need stimulation by rubbing the skin or tapping the feet. If the newborn's respiratory effort is weak or absent, the nurse or respiratory therapist will use an Ambu-bag and mask to breathe for the newborn. Oxygen can be administered by mask to prevent hypoxia (discussed later in this chapter).

CARDIOVASCULAR ADAPTATION

The newborn's cardiovascular system (Figure 9-2 ■) must adapt to life outside the uterus. Recall that fetal circulation contains several structures that must close shortly after delivery. When the umbilical cord is clamped, blood can no longer flow through the umbilical arteries and umbilical vein. The branches of these blood vessels that are inside the newborn's abdomen will eventually become connective tissue.

Other circulatory changes occur as a result of a change in thoracic pressure. The rhythmic increase and decrease in thoracic pressure not only cause respiration but also cause the closure of the foramen ovale and ductus arteriosus. Permanent closure of these structures may take several months.

THERMOREGULATORY ADAPTATION

The body temperature in the fetus is regulated in part by the environment inside the uterus. The mother's body

Figure 9-1. ■ Respiratory adaptation of the newborn. The infant's chest is compressed as it moves through the birth canal. Compression is released as it exits the mother's body, allowing air to be drawn into the expanding lungs to replace the amniotic fluid. As blood levels of oxygen and the infant's pH decrease, and as blood levels of carbon dioxide increase, the respiratory center in the medulla triggers changes that cause the diaphragm to contract. Cold air and light further stimulate the respiratory center, causing the newborn to breathe. (Dorling Kindersley Media Library.)

temperature maintains the amniotic fluid at 98.6°F (37°C). The wet newborn will immediately begin to lose body heat by evaporation (Figure 9-3 ■). The delivery room is generally kept cool for the comfort of the mother and delivery room staff. However, this cool room will cause the newborn to lose heat by convection, conduction, and radiation. To prevent the rapid loss of body heat, the newborn should be dried with warm blankets, placed next to the warm skin of the mother, and covered with warm dry blankets. A warm hat will prevent heat loss through the head. If the newborn is exposed for assessment or nursing interventions, or if close observation is needed, the newborn is placed in a bed under a radiant warmer.

In newborns, **cold stress** occurs when excessive heat is lost. Cold stress is temperature change sufficient to cause the newborn to generate heat by **nonshivering thermogenesis.** Newborns are not able to shiver to produce heat. By moving and crying, the newborn increases metabolism and burns stored brown fat (Figure 9-4 ■). This increase in metabolism results in respiratory distress, hypoxia, and a depletion of glycogen stores. If left untreated, the newborn's life is threatened.

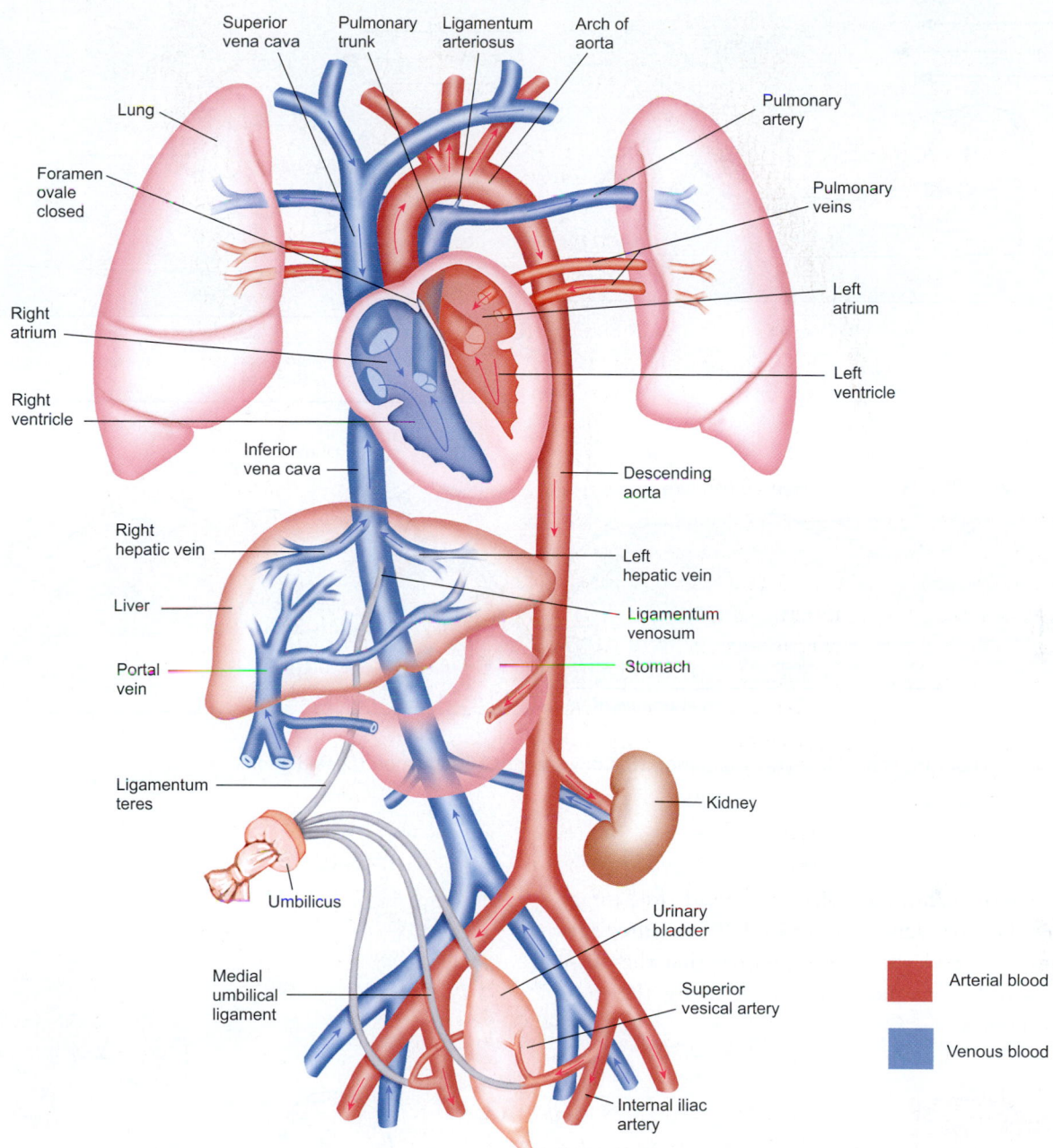

Figure 9-2. ■ The newborn's circulatory system.

Apgar Score

The newborn's adaptation to life outside the uterus will be evaluated using an Apgar score (see Table 7-5 ⚭). This evaluation is typically completed at 1 and 5 minutes, but it can be used anytime the newborn's condition is in question. As you read in Chapter 7 ⚭, each item—heart rate, respiratory rate, muscle tone, reflex irritability, and color—is assigned a score of 0 to 2, and then totaled. A score of 8 to 10 requires no special attention.

A score of 4 to 7 requires the administration of oxygen and stimulation.

If a mother receives a narcotic during labor, it enters the infant through the placenta. Narcotics depress the respiratory center in the infant, leading to hypoventilation and hypoxia. A narcotic antagonist, such as Naloxone (Narcan), may be administered to the infant.

A score of 0 to 3 indicates that the infant needs immediate resuscitation. Figure 9-5 ■ shows some of the

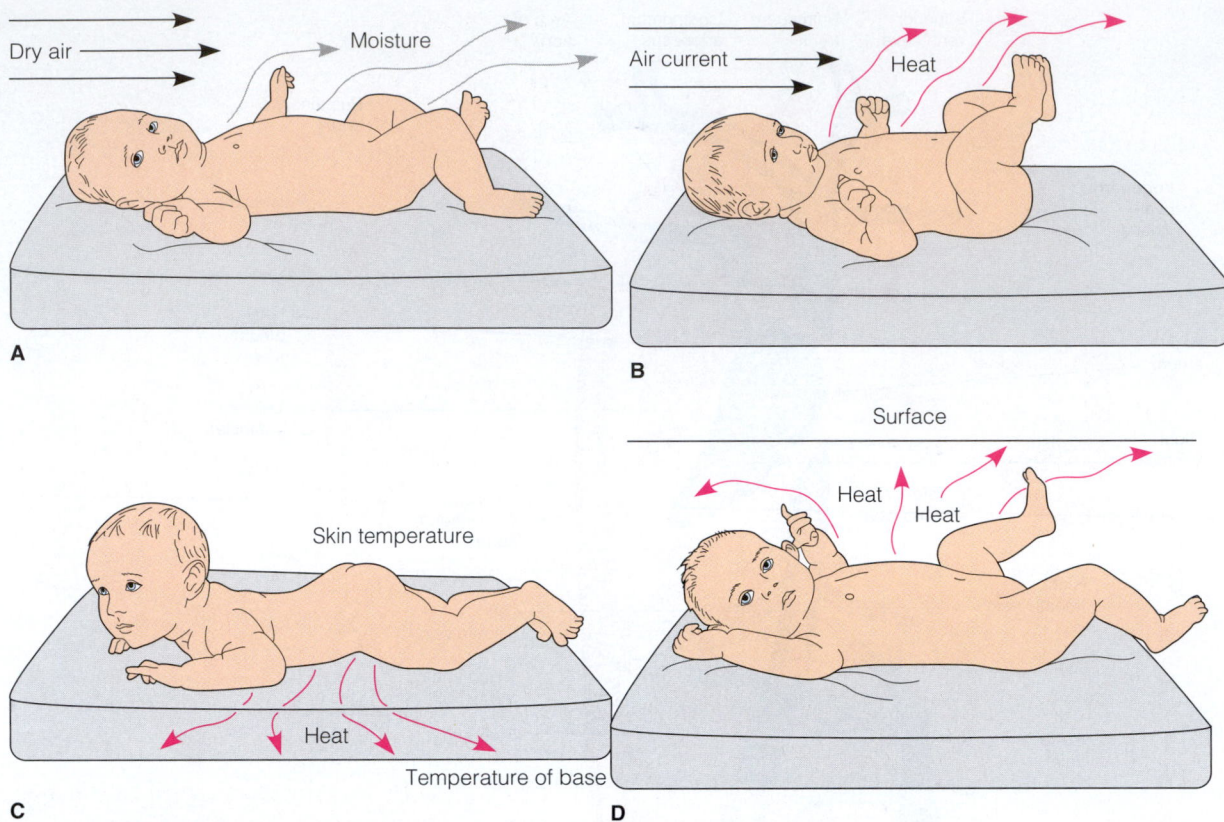

Figure 9-3. ■ Mechanisms of heat loss. (**A**) Evaporation. (**B**) Convection. (**C**) Conduction. (**D**) Radiation.

equipment and techniques that are used for infant cardiopulmonary resuscitation (CPR). CPR requires special training plus review courses to ensure that the nurse is using up-to-date methods and is following the most current guidelines.

clinical ALERT

CPR can be life threatening if performed poorly on an infant. The nurse performing CPR on a neonate or infant must be qualified in pediatric advanced life support (PALS).

Identification

Before the mother and newborn are separated, identification bands are applied (see Figure 7-28A ⚭). Care must be taken not to constrict circulation or scratch the newborn with the clasp. Identification numbers are compared each time the newborn is brought to the mother and at time of discharge. The mother will be asked to sign documents stating that she has received her newborn.

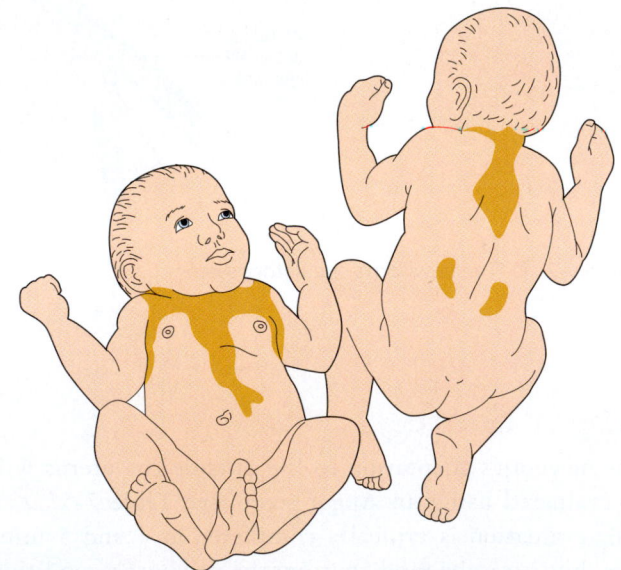

Figure 9-4. ■ The distribution of brown fat (adipose tissue) in the newborn. (Adapted from Davis, V. [1980]. Structure and function of brown adipose tissue in the neonate. *Journal of Obstetrics, Gynecologic and Neonatal Nursing, 9,* 364. Oxford: Blackwell.)

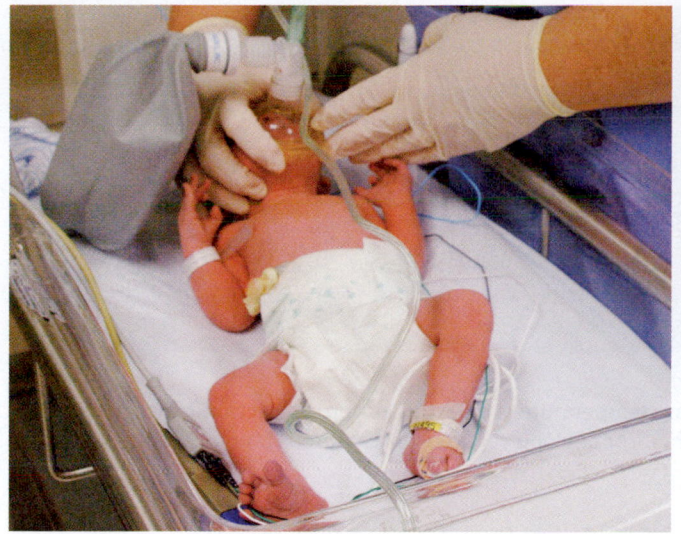

A

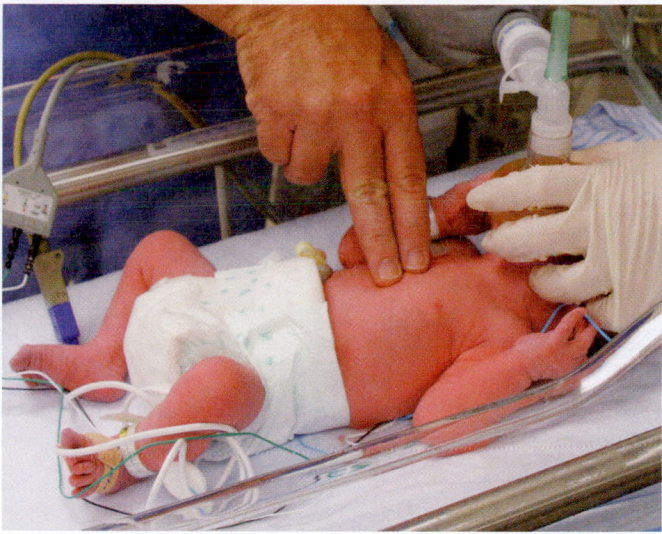

B

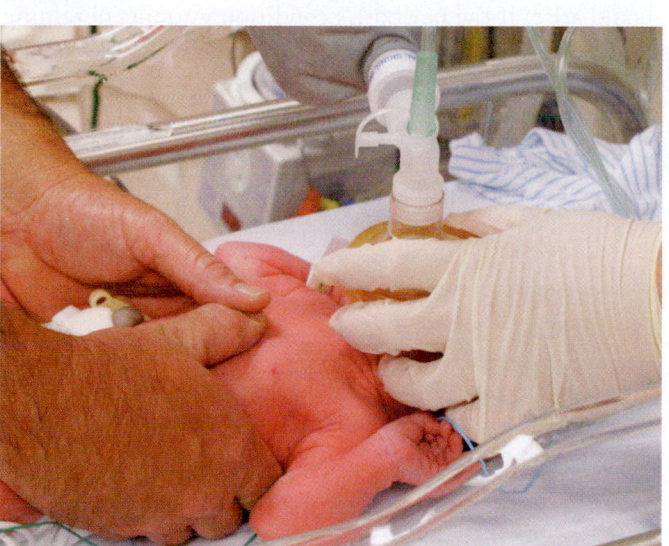

C

Figure 9-5. ■ CPR of an infant. (**A**) Demonstration of resuscitation of a newborn with bag and mask (Ambu-bag). Note that the mask covers the nose and mouth, and the head is in a neutral "sniff" position. The resuscitating bag is placed to the side of the baby so the chest movement can be seen. (**B**) Technique for closed chest cardiac compression (or external cardiac massage) of the neonate. Two fingers of one hand are placed at neonatal nipple line, with the other fingers raised from the surface of the body. In the two-finger method, the tips of two fingers of one hand compress the infant's sternum, and the other hand or a firm surface supports the infant's back. (**C**) Chest compression can also be done using the pads of both thumbs. With either method, the sternum is compressed at a rate of 90 beats per minute.

HEALTHY NEWBORN

The nurse assesses the newborn at the time of delivery to determine the need for resuscitation. The stable newborn can remain with the family. The newborn with complications will be taken to a nursery for further intervention and monitoring. Within the first 1 to 2 hours, the nurse completes a more in-depth assessment to evaluate the newborn's adaptation to life outside the uterus and to identify any complications. The nurse must understand the usual characteristics of the healthy newborn in order to evaluate the newborn's current condition.

Vital Signs

TEMPERATURE
Temperature is assessed frequently in the first hours after delivery. The newborn's temperature ranges are from 97.7–99.4°F (36.5–37.5°C). The axillary temperature is generally taken using an electronic thermometer (Figure 9-6A ■). When the newborn is placed under radiant heat, a skin thermal sensor is placed over soft tissue such as on the abdomen (Figure 9-6B). An alarm will sound if the newborn's temperature rises above the preset value.

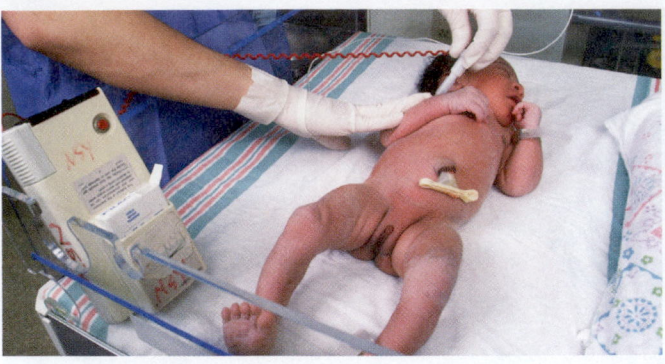 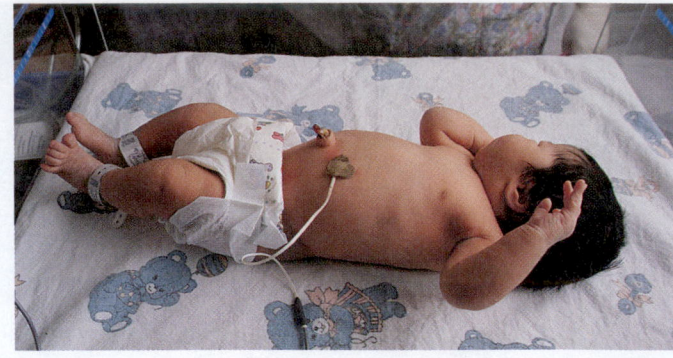

A   **B**

Figure 9-6. ■ Temperature monitoring for the newborn. (**A**) An axillary temperature is measured using an electronic thermometer. (**B**) Skin thermal sensor is placed on the newborn's abdomen, upper thigh, or arm and secured with a porous tape or a foil-covered foam pad.

HEART RATE

Heart rate should be assessed when the newborn is at rest. An apical pulse should be counted for a full minute. The normal pulse rate is 110 to 160 bpm, but it may be as high as 180 bpm if the newborn is crying and as low as 100 bpm if the newborn is sleeping. Brachial and femoral pulses should be palpated (Figure 9-7 ■). However, radial pulses are difficult to feel.

RESPIRATORY RATE

The respiratory rate should be assessed when the newborn is quiet. Respirations should be counted for a full minute. The normal respiratory rate is 30 to 60 breaths per minute.

BLOOD PRESSURE

Measurement of blood pressure (BP) in the newborn varies. Some facilities generally do not take newborn BP. Other facilities routinely take it as a baseline in case cardiac issues should arise. If the newborn's condition warrants obtaining a blood pressure measurement, an electronic Doppler device (Figure 9-8 ■) is used. The cuff can be applied to the upper arm or leg. The size of the cuff must be appropriate for the newborn, usually 1 to 2 inches (2.5–5 cm) wide. Size is determined by measuring the circumference of the upper arm in centimeters.

clinical ALERT

The normal blood pressure for a newborn is 60-80/40-45 mm Hg at birth and 100/50 at day 10. The newborn's extremity must be immobilized during the procedure.

Pain is an unpleasant sensation related to actual or potential tissue damage. Pain exists when the client says it

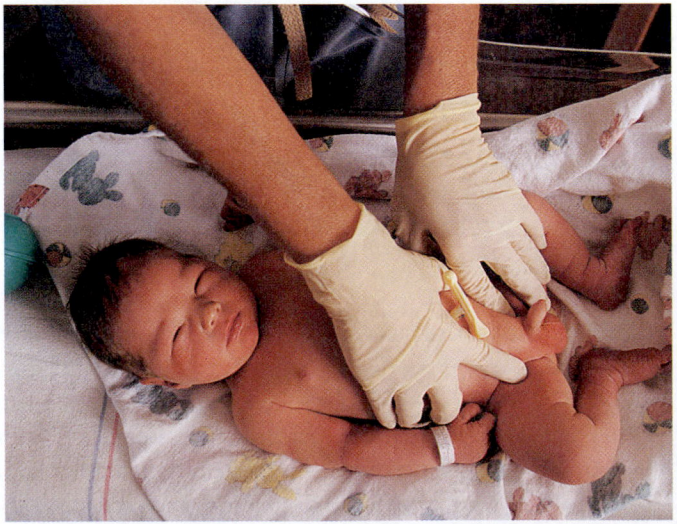 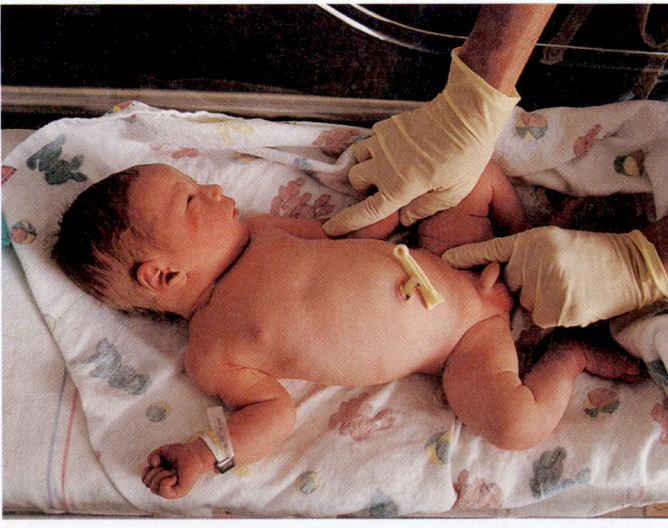

A   **B**

Figure 9-7. ■ (**A**) Bilaterally palpate the femoral arteries for rate and intensity of the pulse. Press fingertip gently at the groin as shown. (**B**) Compare the femoral pulse to the brachial pulse by palpating the pulse simultaneously for comparison of rate and intensity.

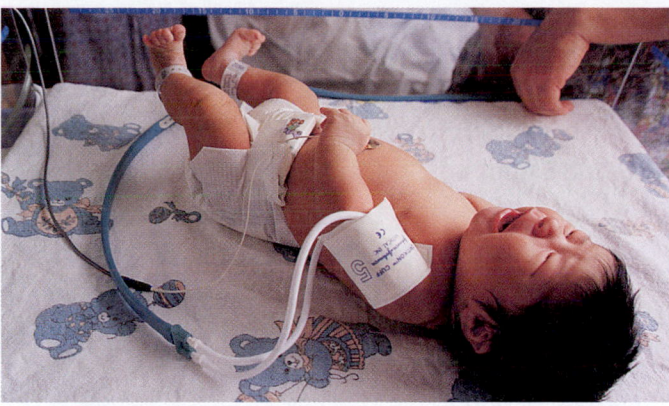

Figure 9-8. ■ Blood pressure measurement using a Doppler device. The cuff can be applied to the upper arm or thigh.

does. The newborn is unable to verbalize the pain experience, but it is widely accepted that the newborn feels pain. Skin sensation is present by 20 weeks' gestation, and the brain centers necessary for pain reception are developed toward the end of pregnancy. The newborn exhibits pain through facial expression and crying. Box 9-1 ■ provides an infant pain rating scale. A facial characteristics pain rating scale is illustrated in Figure 13-12 ⊙⊙.

Gestational Age

An assessment of gestational age is completed within the first 4 hours after birth. Prenatally, the gestational age was determined from the last menstrual period. This estimation is accurate 75% to 85% of the time. A clinical gestational age assessment tool, the Ballard Newborn Rating Scale (Figure 9-9 ■), was developed to determine gestational age more accurately and consistently. In this assessment tool, points from −1 to 5 are assigned to each characteristic. The points are totaled and referenced to the maturity rating scale to determine the gestational age in weeks.

NEUROMUSCULAR MATURITY

The first area of the gestational age assessment is neuromuscular maturity. Some of the assessments taken are illustrated in this section.

BOX 9-1

Infant Pain Scale

S = Sleeping
0 = No pain
1 = Restless
2 = Facial grimacing
3 = Favors body parts (knees at abdomen, pulls at body part)
4 = Crying uncontrollably

Body Position at Rest

At rest, full-term newborns lie in a flexed position, while premature newborns lie extended (Figure 9-10 ■).

Wrist Angle

The square window of the wrist or angle of the hand and fingers when compressed by the examiner (Figure 9-11 ■) is 0 to 30 degrees in the normal newborn and 90 degrees in the premature newborn.

Arm Recoil

Arm recoil (Figure 9-12 ■ on page 268) is exhibited when the arms are held in extension next to the body for 5 seconds and then released. In the healthy newborn, the arms recoil to the flexed position.

Popliteal Angle

The popliteal angle is determined by flexing and holding the thigh to the abdomen while extending the leg at the knee. In the healthy newborn, this angle is less than 90 degrees, while in the premature newborn, the angle is 180 degrees (see Figure 9-9).

Scarf Sign

The **scarf sign** is exhibited by moving the arm in front of the neck (Figure 9-13 ■). In the normal newborn, the elbow will not reach the midline. In the premature newborn, the elbow moves past the midline.

PHYSICAL MATURITY

The second area to be assessed is physical maturity. The skin, lanugo, feet, breasts, ears, and genitals are assigned points based on their degree of development.

Integument

The skin of the premature newborn appears thin and transparent, with numerous blood vessels visible. At term, subcutaneous fat deposits make the skin opaque, with few blood vessels visible. The skin of postmature newborns is dry and peels.

A fine downy hair, *lanugo*, covers the fetus but disappears from the face by 30 weeks and then from the trunk and extremities.

The creases on the bottom of the foot lengthen and deepen with age. This sign of maturity is accurate for up to 12 hours post delivery. After 12 hours, however, the skin on the soles dries and may peel, becoming an invalid reference of age.

At term, the breast tissue, including the areola, measures 0.5 to 1 cm.

Cartilage gives the ear shape. In the premature newborn, this cartilage is not developed, resulting in relatively

NEWBORN MATURITY RATING & CLASSIFICATION

ESTIMATION OF GESTATIONAL AGE BY MATURITY RATING
Symbols: X - 1st Exam O - 2nd Exam

NEUROMUSCULAR MATURITY

	−1	0	1	2	3	4	5
Posture							
Square Window (wrist)	>90°	90°	60°	45°	30°	0°	
Arm Recoil		180°	140°–180°	110°–140°	90°–110°	<90°	
Popliteal Angle	180°	160°	140°	120°	100°	90°	<90°
Scarf Sign							
Heel to Ear							

Gestation by Dates _____ wks

_____

Birth Date _____ Hour _____ am / pm

APGAR _____ 1 min _____ 5 min

MATURITY RATING

score	weeks
−10	20
−5	22
0	24
5	26
10	28
15	30
20	32
25	34
30	36
35	38
40	40
45	42
50	44

PHYSICAL MATURITY

Skin	sticky friable transparent	gelatinous red, translucent	smooth pink, visible veins	superficial peeling &/or rash, few veins	cracking pale areas rare veins	parchment deep cracking no vessels	leathery cracked wrinkled
Lanugo	none	sparse	abundant	thinning	bald areas	mostly bald	
Plantar Surface	heel-toe 40–50 mm:−1 <40 mm:−2	>50 mm no crease	faint red marks	anterior transverse crease only	creases ant. 2/3	creases over entire sole	
Breast	imperceptible	barely perceptible	flat areola no bud	stippled areola 1–2 mm bud	raised areola 3–4 mm bud	full areola 5–10 mm bud	
Eye/Ear	lids fused loosely:−1 tightly:−2	lids open pinna flat stays folded	sl. curved pinna; soft; slow recoil	well curved pinna; soft but ready recoil	formed & firm instant recoil	thick cartilage ear stiff	
Genitals male	scrotum flat, smooth	scrotum empty faint rugae	testes in upper canal rare rugae	testes descending few rugae	testes down good rugae	testes pendulous deep rugae	
Genitals female	clitoris prominent labia flat	prominent clitoris small labia minora	prominent clitoris enlarging minora	majora & minora equally prominent	majora large minora small	majora cover clitoris & minora	

SCORING SECTION

	1st Exam = X	2nd Exam = O
Estimating Gest Age by Maturity Rating	_____Weeks	_____Weeks
Time of Exam	Date _____ Hour_____ am/pm	Date _____ Hour_____ am/pm
Age at Exam	_____ Hours	_____ Hours
Signature of Examiner	_____ M.D.	_____ M.D.

Figure 9-9. ■ Ballard Newborn Rating Scale. (Reprinted from Ballard, J. L., Khoury, J. C., Wedig, K., Wang, L., Eilers-Walsman, B. L., & Lipp, R. [1991]. New Ballard score, expanded to include extremely premature infants. *Journal of Pediatrics, 119*, 417. Used with permission from Elsevier, Inc.)

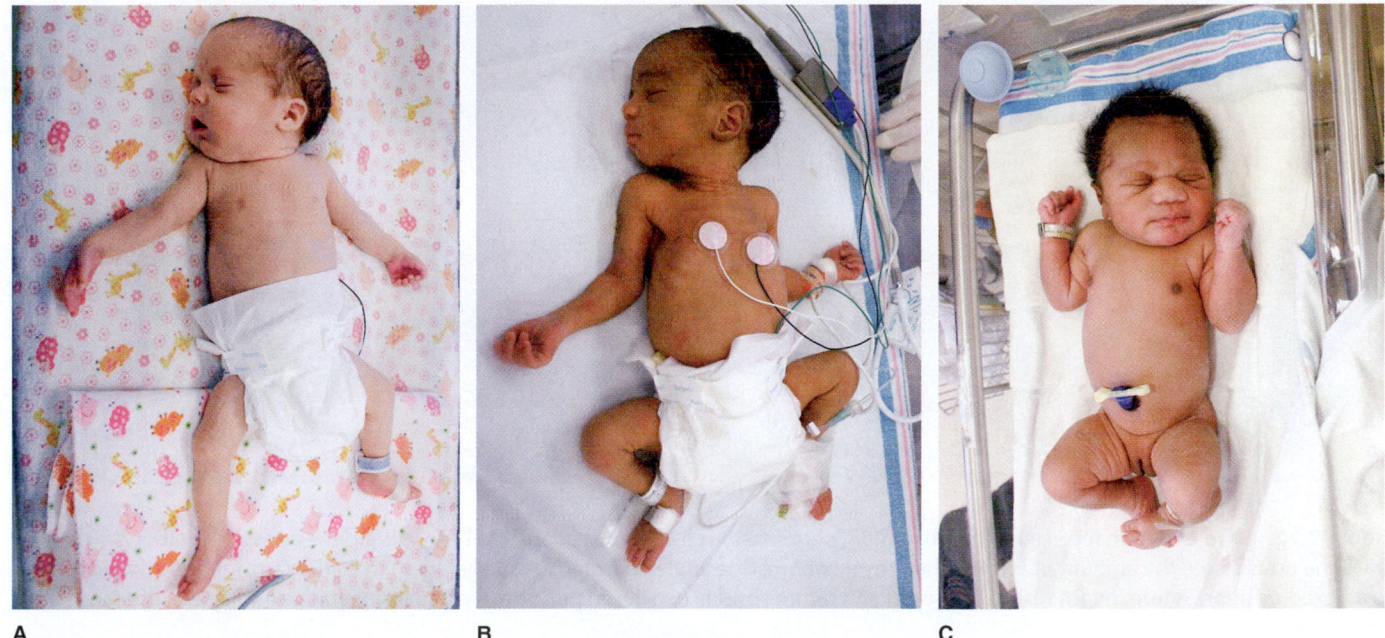

A   B   C

Figure 9-10. ■ Neuromuscular maturity determined by resting posture. (**A**) At a gestational age of approximately 31 weeks, there is extension of the upper extremities and beginning flexion of the thighs. (**B**) At a gestational age of approximately 35 weeks, the newborn shows strong flexion of the arms, hips, and thighs. (**C**) At term, the newborn exhibits hypertonic flexion of all extremities.

shapeless pinna. If the pinna is folded over on itself, it remains folded.

Genitalia

Male genitals are evaluated for the size of the scrotal sac, the presence of rugae, and the descent of the testicles (illustrated later in this chapter). Female genitals are evaluated for size of the labia majora. At term, the labia majora nearly covers the clitoris and labia minora.

Height, Weight, and Head Circumference

The newborn is weighed, and length and head circumference are measured (see Figure 7-27 ⬤⬤). The healthy newborn weighs between 5 lb 8 oz and 8 lb 13 oz (2,500–4,000 g), is 18 to 22 inches (48–52 cm) long, and has a head circumference of 12.5 to 14.5 inches (32–37 cm). These values are recorded on a growth chart for easy reference to national percentile ranges (Figure 9-14 ■). A

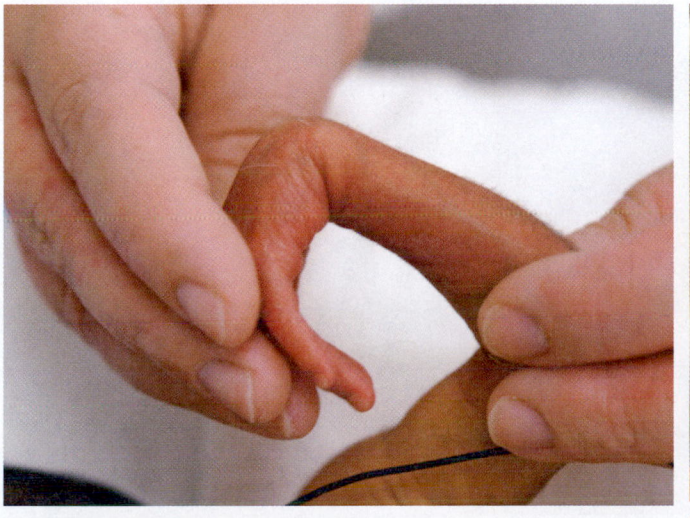
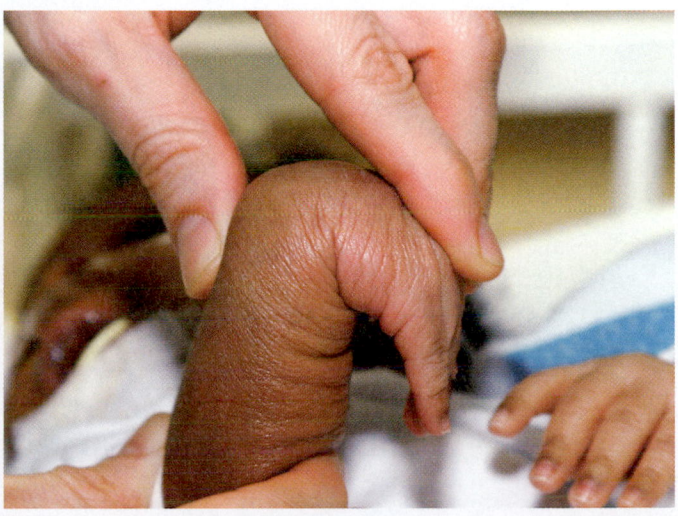

A   B

Figure 9-11. ■ Square window sign. (**A**) At about 28 to 32 weeks' gestation, the angle is 90 degrees. (**B**) At about 39 to 40 weeks, the angle is commonly 30 degrees.

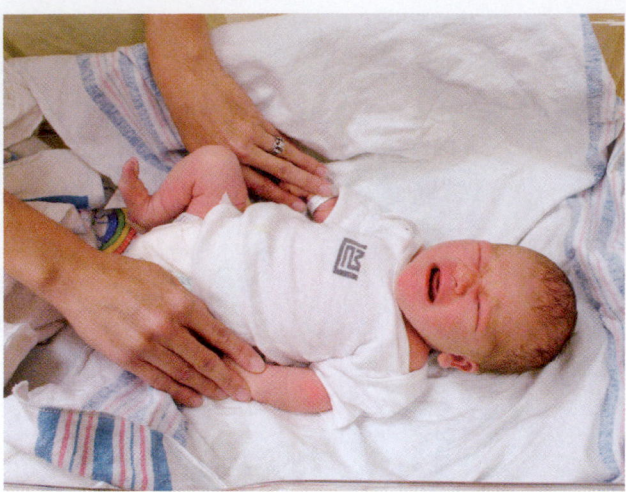
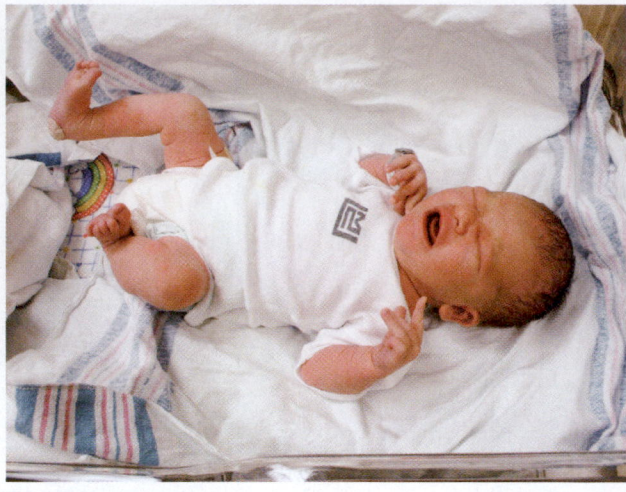

A　　　　　　　　　　　　　　　　　　　　**B**

Figure 9-12. ■ To elicit arm recoil reflex, flex the infant's arms to the chest for 5 seconds. (**A**) Then, extend the arms at the elbows. (**B**) Release the arms to see the amount of recoil. In healthy newborns, the angle of flexion is usually less than 90 degrees, following rapid recoil to a flexed position. A term infant resists extension and returns briskly to a flexed position. A premature infant exhibits less resistance and less recoil.

full set of growth charts is provided in Appendix II ⬭. Infants whose values are in the 10% to 90% range are considered appropriate for gestational age (AGA). Infants less than 10% are small for gestational age (SGA). Those greater than 90% are large for gestational age (LGA).

Characteristics of the Newborn

GENERAL APPEARANCE

The healthy newborn appears plump, pink, and active. The head is disproportionately large for the body. The center of the newborn's body is the umbilicus. The healthy newborn can move all extremities but prefers a flexed position.

SKIN

The skin at birth is red and smooth. **Acrocyanosis** (Figure 9-15A ■), a bluish discoloration of the hands and feet, is common for several hours after delivery. **Ecchymosis** (bruising) and **petechiae** (pinpoint hemorrhages) may be present following a difficult delivery. Some swelling around the eyes is common. The skin may be covered with vernix caseosa, especially in the body folds. The vernix absorbs into the skin, keeping it soft. Lanugo may be present on the face, arms, and back. Within a few days the skin may become dry and peel. A small amount of baby lotion can be used to moisten the skin. Soap should be avoided.

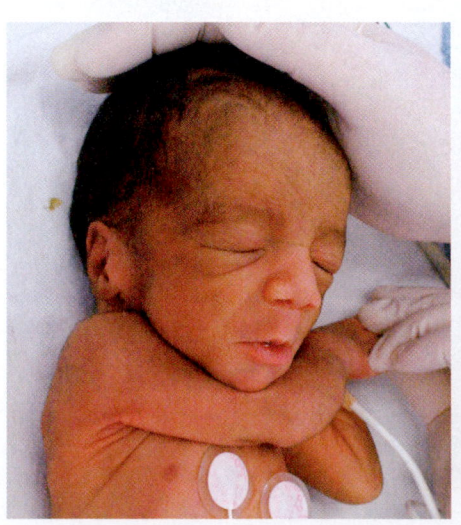
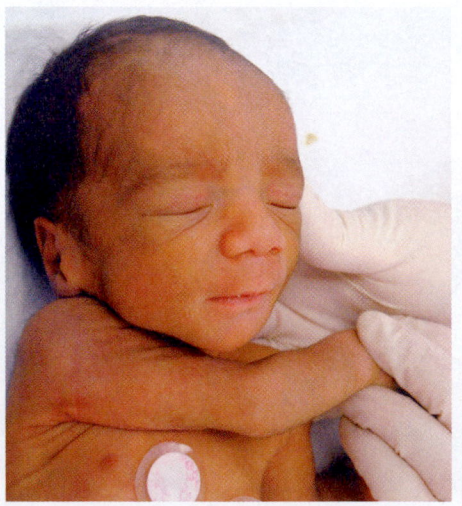
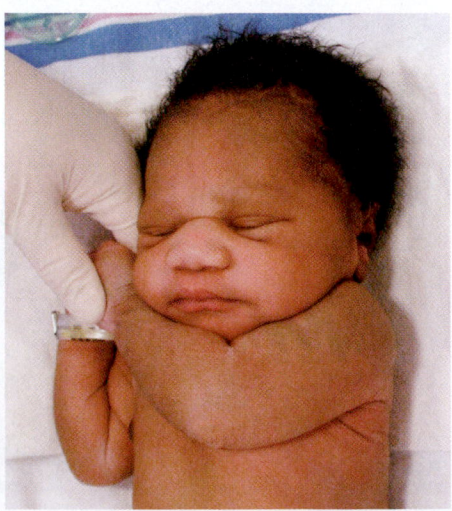

A　　　　　　　　　　　　**B**　　　　　　　　　　　　**C**

Figure 9-13. ■ Scarf sign. (**A**) Until about 30 weeks' gestation, the elbow moves past midline with no resistance. (**B**) At about 36 to 40 weeks' gestation, the elbow is at midline. (**C**) The elbow will not reach midline after 40 weeks' gestation.

CLASSIFICATION OF NEWBORNS—
BASED ON MATURITY AND INTRAUTERINE GROWTH

Symbols: X-1st Exam O-2nd Exam

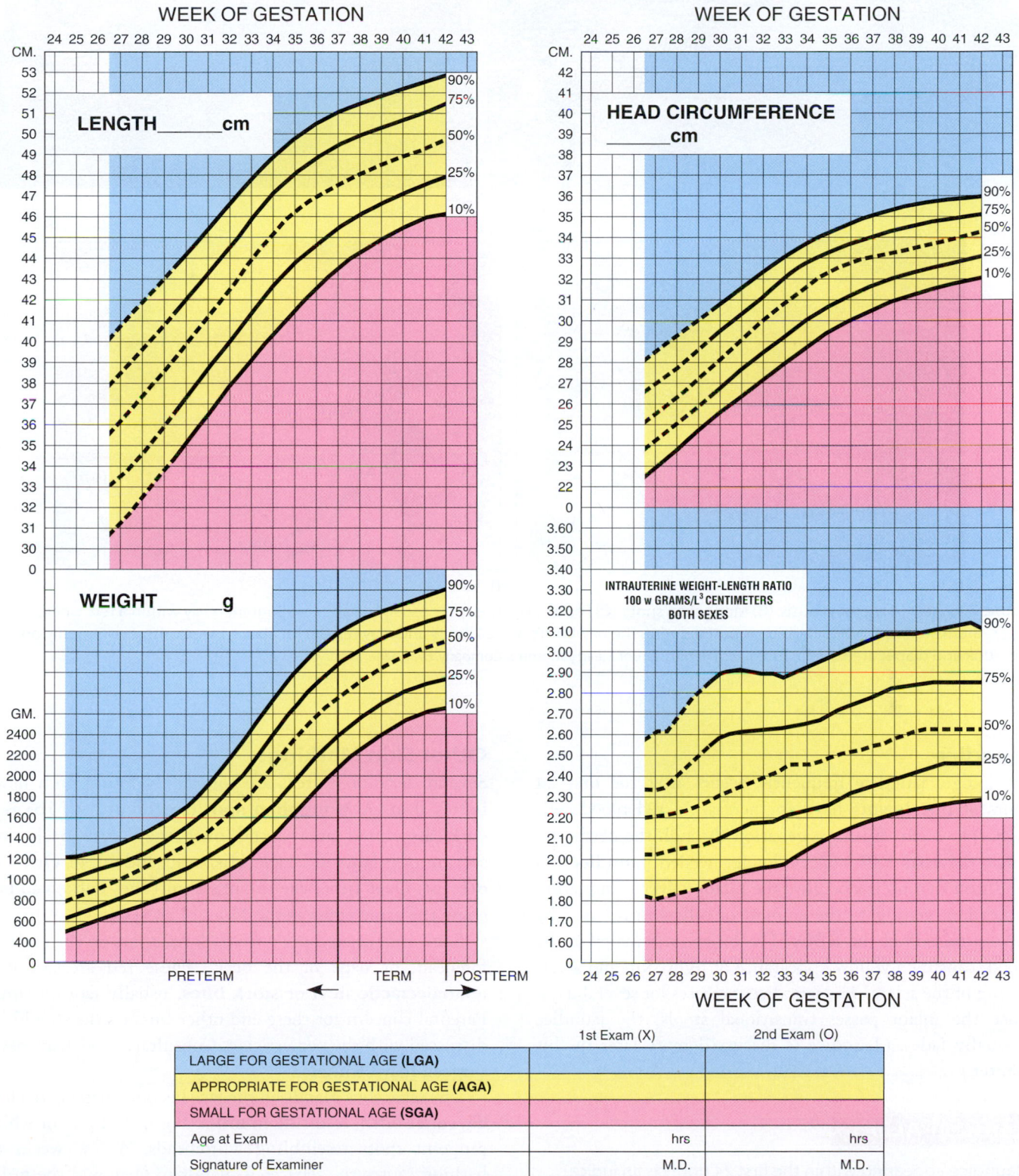

	1st Exam (X)	2nd Exam (O)
LARGE FOR GESTATIONAL AGE **(LGA)**		
APPROPRIATE FOR GESTATIONAL AGE **(AGA)**		
SMALL FOR GESTATIONAL AGE **(SGA)**		
Age at Exam	hrs	hrs
Signature of Examiner	M.D.	M.D.

Figure 9-14. ■ The nurse accurately measures the child and then places height, weight, and head circumference on appropriate growth grids for the child's age and gender. (Adapted from Lubchenco, L. O., Hansman, C., & Boyd, E. [1966]. *Pediatrics, 37,* 404, Figure 1. Reprinted, with permission, from the American Academy of Pediatrics; Battaglia, F. C., & Lubchenco, L. O. [1967]. A practical classification of newborn infants by weight and gestational age. *Journal of Pediatrics, 71,* 161, with permission from Elsevier, Inc.)

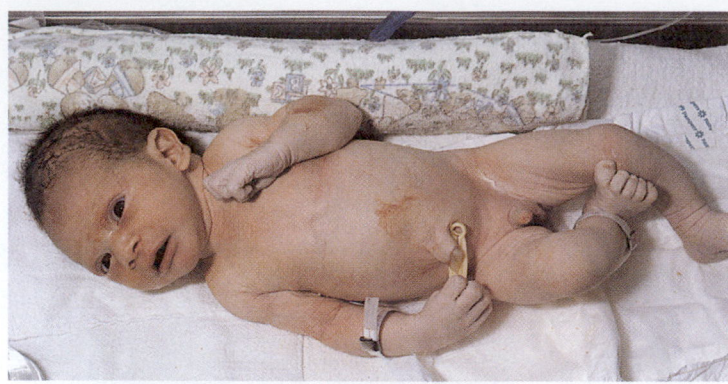

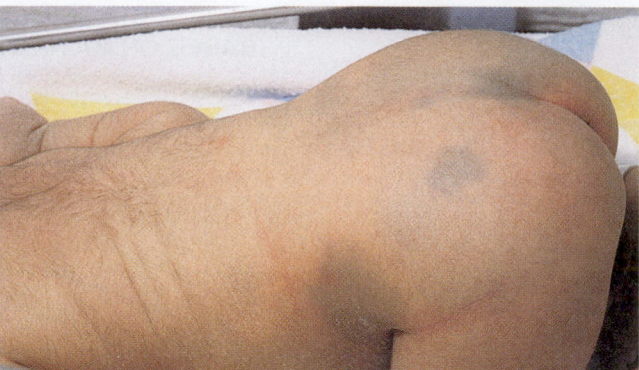

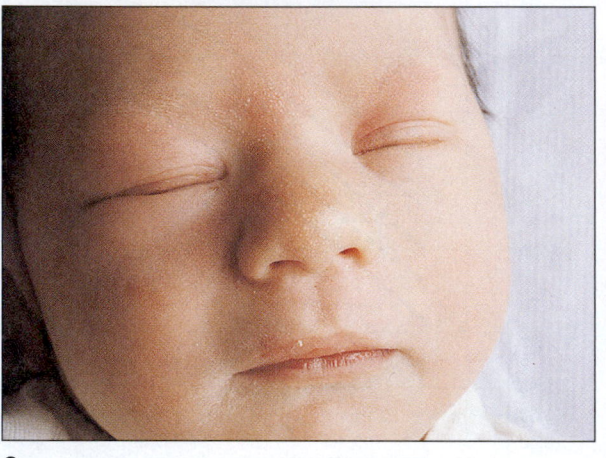

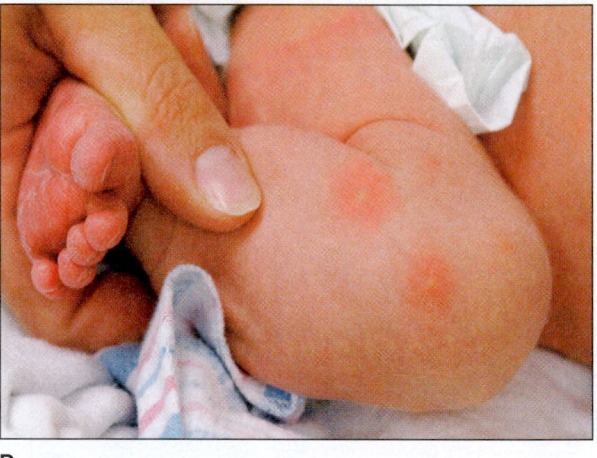

Figure 9-15. ■ **(A)** Acrocyanosis. **(B)** Mongolian spots. **(C)** Facial milia. The spots usually disappear spontaneously within a few weeks. **(D)** Erythema toxicum. The condition is noted during the newborn's first 24 hours and may remain for about 1 week, most commonly on the trunk and diaper area. (Reproduced, with permission, of Mead Johnson & Company, Evansville, IN.)

Jaundice

Physiologic jaundice frequently occurs after the first 24 hours of life. Infants have an increase in red blood cells (RBCs) at birth. With oxygenation through the newborn's lungs, the extra RBCs are no longer needed. **Jaundice** is a condition that occurs because the infant's liver is immature and cannot conjugate the amount of bilirubin released by the destruction of the RBCs. The bilirubin remains in the blood, causing a yellow appearance of light skin and a yellowing of the sclera. The jaundice increases for several days. Once the infant passes transitional stools, the jaundice gradually fades. (Jaundice is discussed more later in this chapter.)

clinical ALERT

Jaundice appearing within the first 24 hours is an indication of a more serious condition, such as hemolytic disease of the newborn or erythroblastosis fetalis (discussed in Chapter 8 ∞), and should be reported to the supervising RN or physician.

Other Skin Markings

Several discolored areas are commonly found on a newborn's skin. A **Mongolian spot** (see Figure 9-15B) is a dark discolored area found over the lower back and sacrum of infants of Black, Hispanic, Indian, or Oriental descent. Over time, the infant's skin tones darken to become the same color as the Mongolian spot.

Some infants are born with dark red spots on the eyelids, forehead, or nape of the neck. These red areas, called **telangiectactic nevi** or **stork bites,** usually fade in time. Parental concern for these and other birthmarks should be discussed with the pediatrician. Consultation with a plastic surgeon may be needed.

The sebaceous glands on the face become distended a few days after birth, resulting in **milia** (Figure 9-15C), or white pinpoint spots resembling whiteheads. A few weeks of bathing causes the sebaceous glands to open and the milia to disappear.

Erythema toxicum neonatorum is a raised pink papule with a light-colored center resembling a mosquito bite (Figure 9-15D). These lesions appear suddenly on the chest, abdomen,

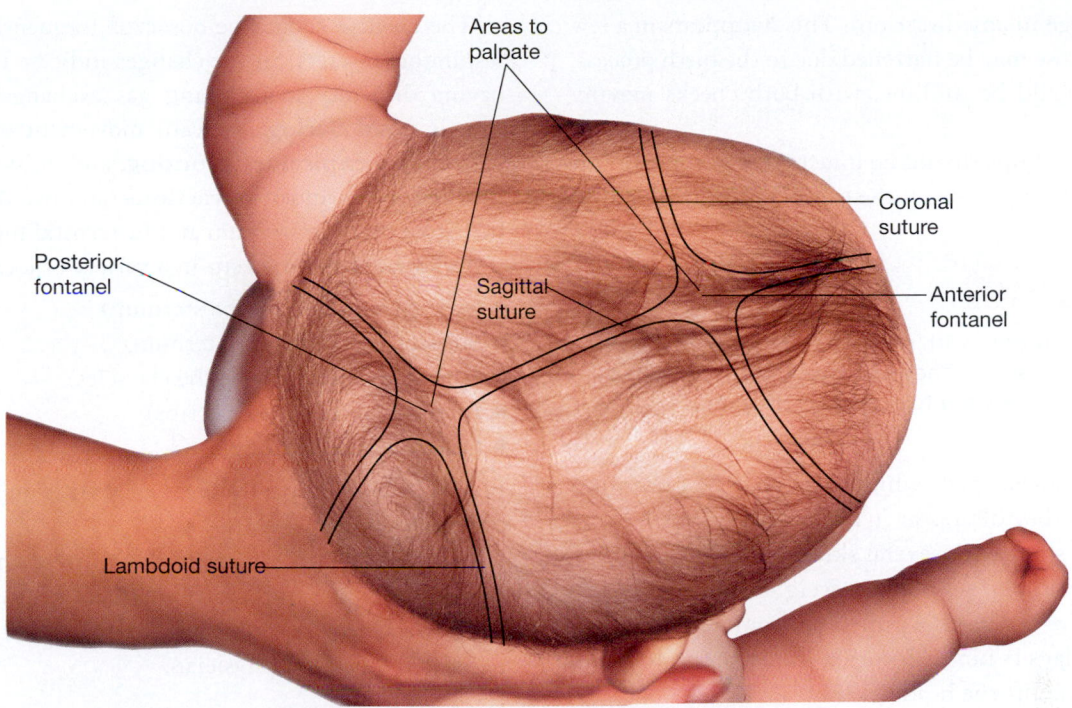

Figure 9-16. ■ Anterior and posterior fontanels. The bones of the skull, showing the fontanel and suture lines.

and back 24 to 48 hours after birth. They are benign and will disappear without treatment. If other birthmarks are found on assessing the newborn's skin, they should be documented.

HEAD

The head of the newborn may be asymmetric at birth. The anterior and posterior fontanels (Figure 9-16 ■) should be firm and flat. The head is 13 to 14 inches (33–34 cm) in circumference. *Molding*, the shaping of the fetal head to the shape of the mother's pelvis, may take several days to resolve (see Figure 7-12 ⬭). Edema of the scalp, called **caput succedaneum**, may cross the suture lines. **Cephalhematoma**, in contrast, is an accumulation of blood between

the periosteum and the skull bone that will not cross the suture lines. Figure 9-17 ■ illustrates caput succedaneum and cephalhematoma. Marks from an internal fetal monitoring electrode, suction (vacuum) extractor, and forceps (see Figure 8-25 ⬭) may be present if they were used in labor and delivery.

The newborn's face should be symmetric. The top of the ears should be in line with the outer canthus of the eye. The pinna may be flat against the head. The eyes of the newborn may show small hemorrhages in the sclera due to the pressure of delivery. The newborn has poor control of the eye muscles resulting in **strabismus** (lack of coordination of the visual axes of the eye; eyes do not stay parallel to each other

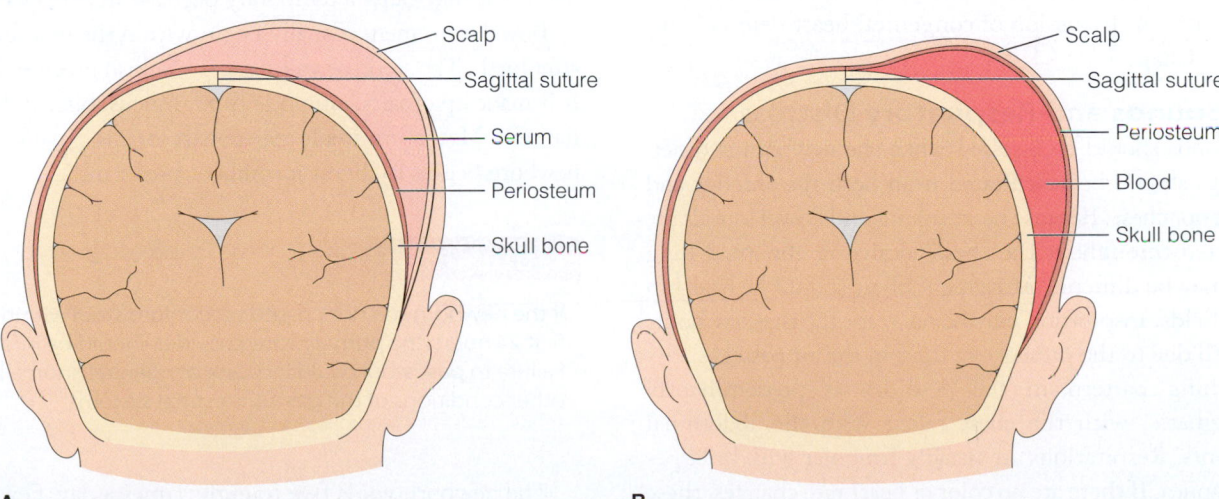

A   B

Figure 9-17. ■ **(A)** Caput succedaneum is a collection of fluid under the scalp. **(B)** Cephalhematoma is a collection of blood between the surface of the cranial bone and the periosteal membrane. This is a cephalhematoma over the left parietal bone.

and may diverge in any direction). This disappears in a few months. The nose may be flattened due to the birth process. The mouth should be midline, with both cheeks moving symmetrically.

The palate and lips should be intact. One or more precocious teeth may be present in the center of the lower gum.

clinical ALERT

If the newborn is born with precocious teeth, they will become loose and fall out. They may need to be removed by the primary care provider to prevent aspiration.

Epstein's pearls, small white cysts, may be present on the palate, but they disappear in a few weeks.

The neck is short with several skin folds. The muscles of the neck are unable to support the weight of the newborn's head. When the newborn is pulled up from a supine position, the head lags behind. However, from a prone position, the newborn can lift the head slightly.

CHEST

The chest should be 12 to 13 inches (30.5–33 cm) in circumference. Two nipples should be identifiable. Some engorgement may be present in both male and female infants due to maternal hormones. The nipple may secrete whitish fluid, called **witches' milk,** for several days.

Heart Sounds

Heart sounds should be assessed when the newborn is in a quiet state. Because of the rapid heart rate, evaluating heart sounds in the newborn takes practice. The normal lub-dub sounds should be heard. A slurring of one sound (usually the lub) may indicate a murmur. Most murmurs are considered normal and disappear within a few months. However, some murmurs indicate an abnormality within the heart. For this reason, the primary care provider should monitor all murmurs. A discussion of congenital heart defects is included in Chapter 19 ⌘.

Lung Sounds and Respiratory Distress

Lung sounds should be assessed when the newborn is quiet. The lungs should be auscultated from both the anterior and the posterior chest. Because heart sounds and bowel sounds are transmitted throughout the chest, localizing abnormal lung sounds may be difficult. Movement of air should be heard in all lung fields. Inspiration may be noisy for the first few hours after birth due to the presence of fluid in the air passages.

Breathing pattern in the newborn is predominantly diaphragmatic, with the chest rising with the abdominal movements. Respirations are usually irregular with brief periods of apnea. If there are no color or heart rate changes, these brief apneic episodes are considered normal.

The neonate should be observed frequently for signs of respiratory distress. Subtle changes indicate the newborn is having difficulty maintaining gas exchange. The earliest sign is **nasal flaring,** outward movement of the nostrils, followed by **expiratory grunting,** and noisy exhalation. If the distress continues, **retractions** (an inward movement of the tissue over the sternum and intercostal muscles) may be seen. Retractions can occur in a variety of locations.

- **Suprasternal** (above the sternum)
- **Substernal** (below the sternum)
- **Supraclavicular** (above the clavicles)
- **Intercostal** (between the ribs)
- **Subcostal** (below the ribs).

Figure 9-18 ■ illustrates areas of retraction in respiratory distress.

Apneic spells (periods without breathing) indicate a worsening of the respiratory distress. Signs of respiratory distress must be reported immediately to the supervising registered nurse and physician.

ABDOMEN

The abdomen should be soft, rounded, and without palpable masses. The umbilical cord should be clamped, and three blood vessels should be identifiable. There should be no distention or bulging. If distention is present, the skin becomes tight and blood vessels appear.

clinical ALERT

Abdominal distention is a sign of many abnormalities of the gastrointestinal tract and should be reported to the primary care provider.

Bowel sounds are present in four quadrants within an hour after birth. These sounds should be assessed before palpation because it may cause a temporary decrease in peristalsis.

Bowel movements usually begin within the first few hours after birth. The stool, or *meconium*, is blackish green and sticky. It is made up of salts, amniotic fluid, mucus, bile, and epithelial cells. Meconium stools may persist for 2 to 3 days until the newborn begins to digest formula or breast milk.

clinical ALERT

If the newborn has not passed meconium stool within the first 24 hours, the primary care provider should be informed. Failure to pass stool could indicate congenital anomalies or other conditions of the gastrointestinal system.

The newborn voids five to eight times a day. Fewer than 5 voids may indicate that the newborn needs more fluids.

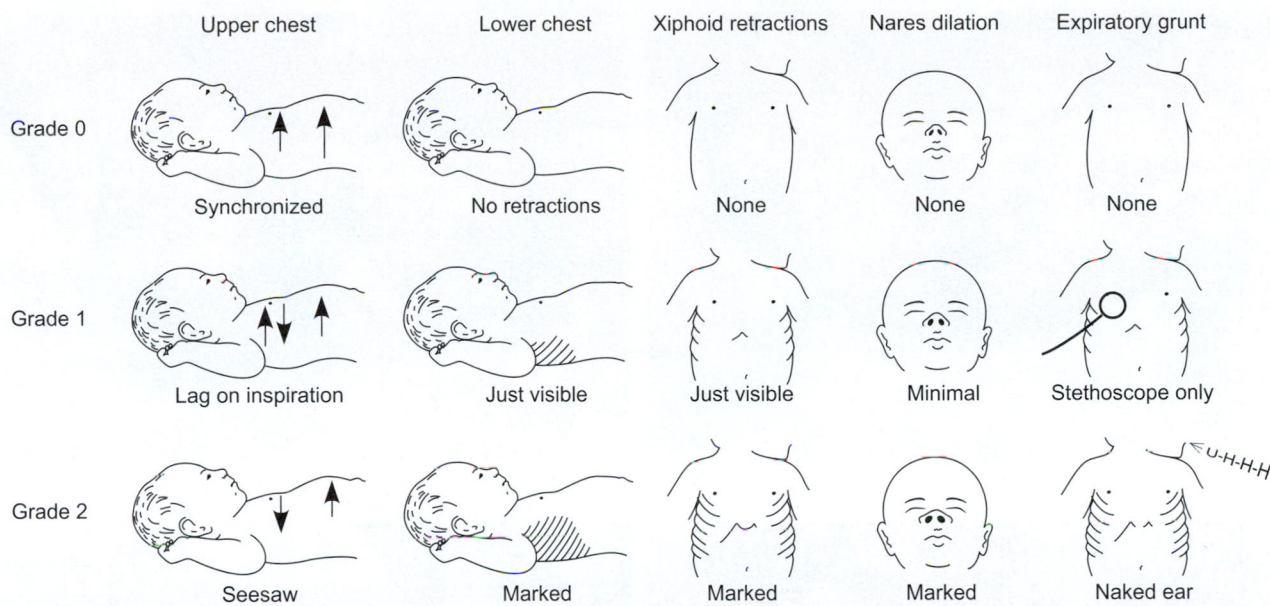

Figure 9-18. ■ Evaluation of respiratory status using the Silverman-Andersen index. The baby's respiratory status is assessed. A grade of 0, 1, or 2 is determined for each area, and a total score is charted in the baby's record or on a copy of this tool and placed in the chart. (From Ross Laboratories, *Nursing inservice aid no. 2,* Columbus, OH; Silverman, W. A., & Andersen, D. H. A controlled clinical trial of effects of water mist on obstructive respiratory signs, death rate and necropsy findings among premature infants. *Pediatrics, 17,* 1: 1956, Figure 2.)

The newborn passes approximately 30 to 50 mL with each voiding. Using disposable diapers may make it difficult to assess the volume of urinary output because the urine is trapped inside the fibers. If an accurate assessment of urinary output is needed, diapers are weighed before and after use. The difference in weight indicates the amount of urine output.

clinical ALERT

If the newborn has not voided within the first 24 hours, the primary care provider should be informed. Failure to void could indicate congenital anomalies or other conditions of the urinary system.

GENITALIA

Genitals should be inspected carefully (Figure 9-19 ■). Some congenital anomalies are discussed in Chapters 22 and 23 ⚭ of this book. In the female newborn, the clitoris varies in size and may be so large that it appears similar to a penis. This is generally due to hormone influence and disappears in a few days. Fat deposited in the labia majora causes them to enlarge and cover the labia minora. This generally occurs before birth, but if the newborn is of low birth weight, there may not be enough subcutaneous fat for the labia majora to cover the labia minora. A mucus or slightly bloody vaginal discharge may be present. This **pseudomenstruation** is related to the influence of maternal hormones and disappears in a few days. **Smegma** (the secretion consisting of epithelial cells found around the external genitalia) may be present in the labial folds. Removing it may traumatize the tissue.

In the male newborn, the penis should be inspected to determine the location of the urinary meatus. The urinary meatus should open onto the tip of the glans. If it opens on the ventral surface, the newborn has *hypospadias.* (Hypospadias is discussed later in this chapter in the Assessment section.) Another condition of the male penis, phimosis, is also discussed later in this chapter and in Chapter 23 ⚭.

The anus is inspected for patency. Abnormalities can usually be identified by visual inspection. If a digital examination is necessary, it should be completed by the primary care provider. The passage of stool verifies the functioning of the gastrointestinal tract. Congenital anomalies of the gastrointestinal tract are discussed in Chapter 22 ⚭.

EXTREMITIES

The extremities should be symmetric bilaterally. Each extremity should end with five digits, without **webbing** (skin between two or more digits), **syndactyly** (the fusion of two or more digits), or **polydactyly** (presence of more than five fingers per hand or toes per foot). Muscle tone should be strong, with full range of motion in each extremity.

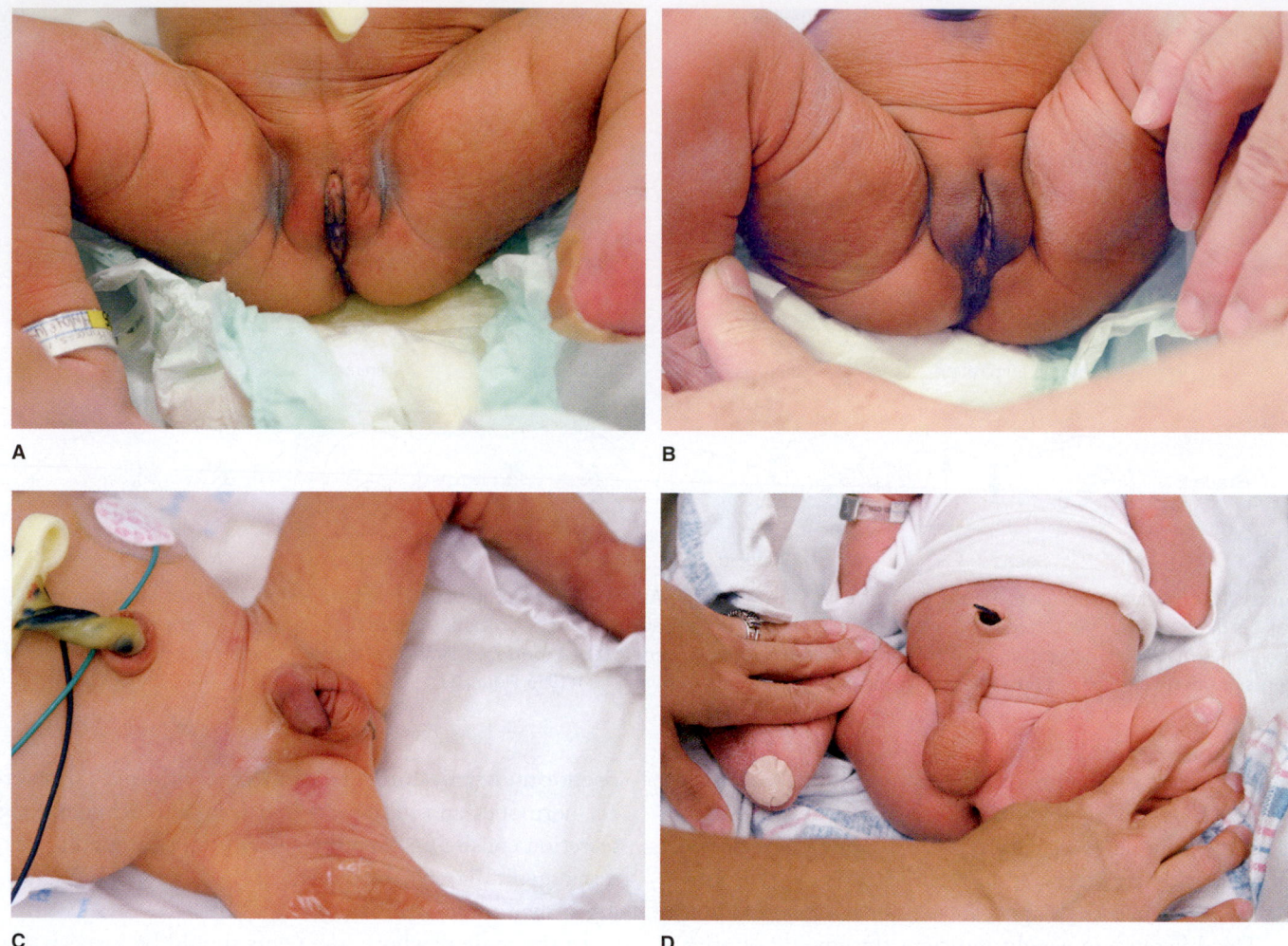

A

B

C

D

Figure 9-19. ■ (**A**) Female genitals. At a gestational age of 30 to 36 weeks, the newborn has a prominent clitoris, widely separated labia majora, and labia minora protruding beyond the labia majora (when viewed laterally). (**B**) At term, the labia majora are well developed and cover both the clitoris and the labia minora. (**C**) Male genitals. Note the absence of the testicles in the scrotum and a scrotum with few rugae in the preterm newborn. (**D**) In the term newborn, the testicles are descended into the scrotum, and the scrotum is covered by rugae.

The femur should be well seated in the acetabulum. The registered nurse or physician should assess the hip for displacement or hip click (Figure 9-20 ■). The ankle of the newborn appears to turn inward due to the position in the uterus. There should not be resistance when the foot is moved to the normal position. If resistance is encountered, evaluation for clubfoot needs to be made by the primary care provider. Musculoskeletal disorders are discussed in Chapter 17 ⬤⬤.

Reflexes

Reflexes in newborns are signs of neurologic integrity (Figure 9-21 ■). Some reflexes, such as blink, cough, and sneeze, remain intact throughout life. Others disappear by 4 to 6 months. Still others will take 2 years to disappear. Absent or slowed reflexes may indicate prematurity

of the infant. They may also result from the CNS depressant medications that were transferred to the infant during labor or in breast milk. Re-examination should be done at a later date. Lingering reflexes (those present after the expected time) may indicate neurologic lesions. The child should be referred for further evaluation by the primary care provider.

The **rooting reflex** occurs when the newborn is searching for food. When the newborn's cheek is stroked, the infant will turn his or her head in that direction. The **sucking reflex** is elicited when the newborn's lips are touched. Together, these two reflexes are important in feeding. Medications, especially pain medications, can be transferred in breast milk and could depress the sucking reflex. (Breastfeeding is discussed later in this chapter.) The rooting reflex disappears between 3 and 4 months; the sucking reflex disappears by 10 months.

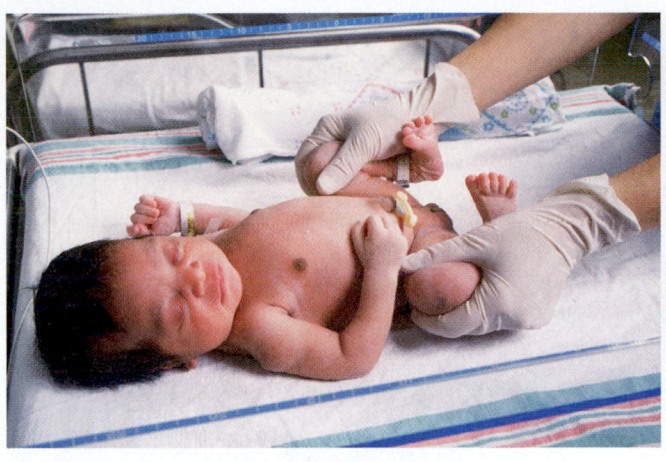
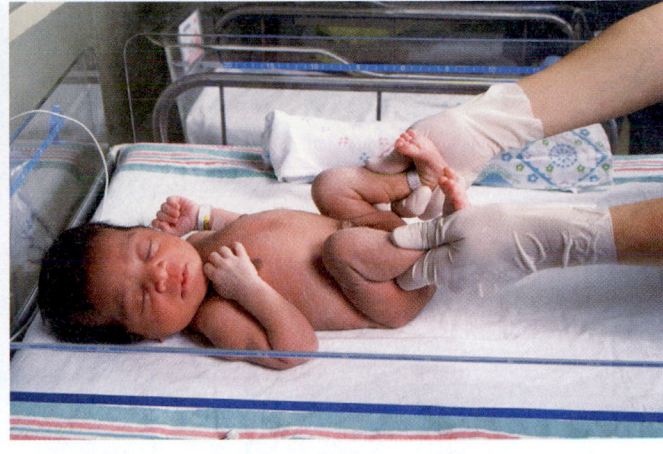

A   **B**

Figure 9-20. ■ Hip integrity is assessed in a newborn by observing and feeling the smoothness of movement in the joint. A "click" is an indication of possible hip dysplasia.

The **palmar grasp reflex** occurs when a finger or small object is placed in the newborn's hand. Newborns grasp the finger tightly enough to be lifted from the bed. This reflex lasts 4 months. The **plantar grasp reflex** (Figure 9-21A), lasting 8 months, occurs when the sole of the foot is touched. The toes curl under as if newborns are trying to "grasp" with their feet. This reflex must disappear before infants are able to walk. The **Babinski reflex** is elicited by stroking the lateral side of the foot from heel to toe. The big toe should dorsiflex and the other toes should flare. This reflex disappears before the infant begins to walk. The **stepping reflex** is obtained by holding newborns with the feet touching the table. Newborns will step as if walking.

The **tonic neck reflex** (Figure 9-21B) is demonstrated by placing newborns supine on a firm surface. When the head is turned to one side, newborns will extend the arm and leg on that side. The opposite arm and leg will flex. The **Moro reflex** or **startle reflex** (Figure 9-21C) occurs when newborns have a sense of falling. This reflex can be elicited by holding the newborn in a sitting position and suddenly lowering the head or by bumping the surface where the newborn is lying. The baby will quickly extend the arms (abduct) with fingers flared and thumb and first finger forming a "C." The arms will then adduct in an embracing motion. The lower extremities may extend and then flex. A slight tremor may be noted.

Behavioral State

Three behavioral states have been identified to describe the normal newborn: sleep state, quiet alert state, and crying state (Figure 9-22 ■).

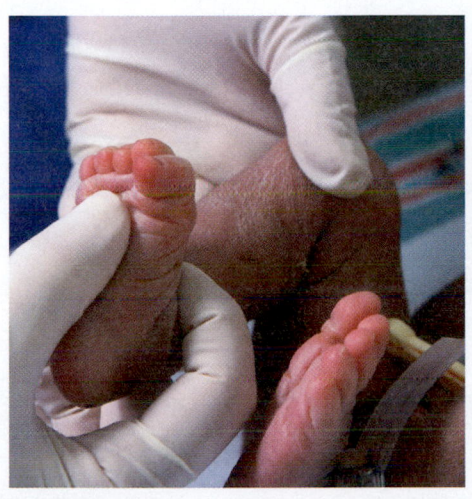
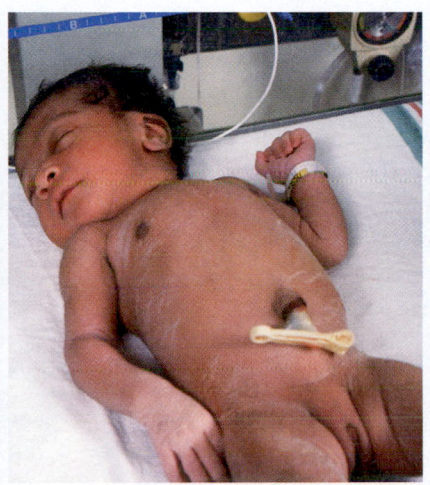
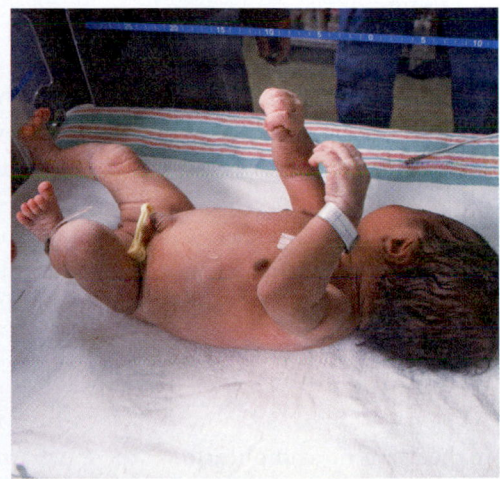

A   **B**   **C**

Figure 9-21. ■ (**A**) Newborn exhibiting plantar grasp reflex. (**B**) Newborn exhibiting the tonic neck reflex. (**C**) Newborn exhibiting Moro reflex.

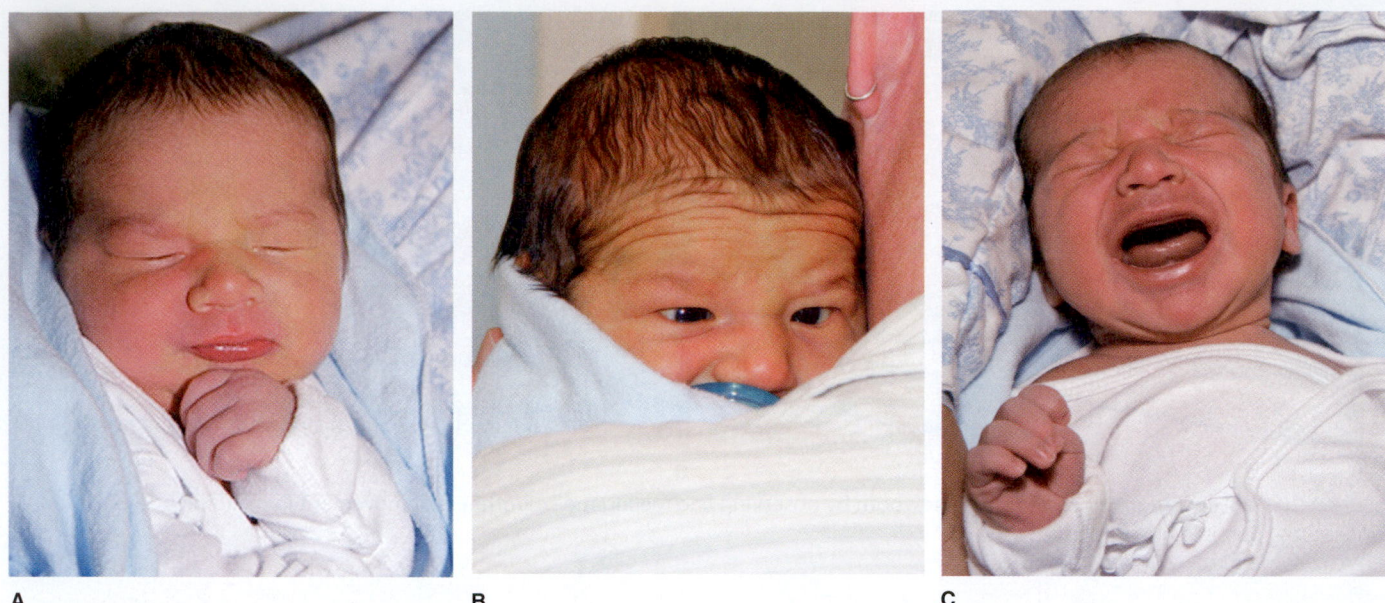

A B C

Figure 9-22. ■ Behavioral states. (**A**) Sleeping state. (**B**) Quiet alert state. The infant may make eye contact or focus on one object. (Note the transient strabismus.) (**C**) Crying state. (M. C. Schlachter Photography.)

SLEEP STATE

Newborns sleep with their eyes closed for 20 to 22 hours a day. There may be periods of rapid eye movement (REM) sleep. Respirations are regular and slow. There may be startle or jerking movements at times. Environmental stimuli may not change the sleep state.

QUIET ALERT STATE

In the quiet alert state (see Figure 9-22B), newborns lie quietly looking around, experiencing their environment. They appear interested in what is happening around them. They may focus on something within their visual field for several minutes. They may remain in the quiet alert state for a period of time before going back to sleep or crying.

CRYING STATE

The cry should be strong, lusty, and of medium pitch. Crying is a method of communicating for newborns. Crying can be used to increase the metabolism when the infant is cold. Crying can indicate that the infant is hungry, wet, or just needing reassurance. Crying may be accompanied by frequent, jerky movements. A high-pitched cry or one that sounds like a "cat cry" requires further evaluation by a primary care provider.

Nursery Care

If there are no complications, the newborn is usually left with the mother in the delivery area throughout the recovery period. The infant may then be either transferred to the newborn nursery or left with the mother. In any case, the following care will be provided. Anytime care is provided in the presence of the mother or significant others, teaching should be provided and documented.

AIRWAY MAINTENANCE

Maintenance of the airway is always the first priority. It is not unusual for the newborn to spit up mucus and fluid. It is critical that the nurse keep the airway clear to prevent aspiration. The bulb syringe is kept at the head of the bassinette for ready access (Figure 9-23 ■). If necessary, the nurse can pick up the newborn, position the newborn with the head down, and use the bulb syringe to suction the airway.

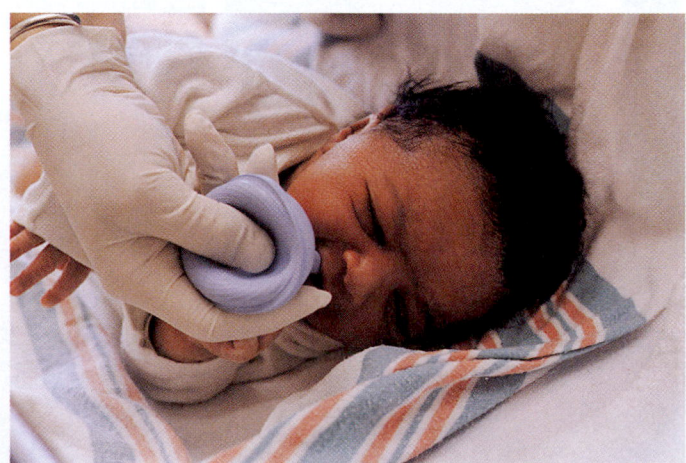

Figure 9-23. ■ Nasal and oral suctioning. The bulb is compressed, the tip is placed in either the mouth or the nose, and the bulb is released. Remember to suction the mouth before the nose.

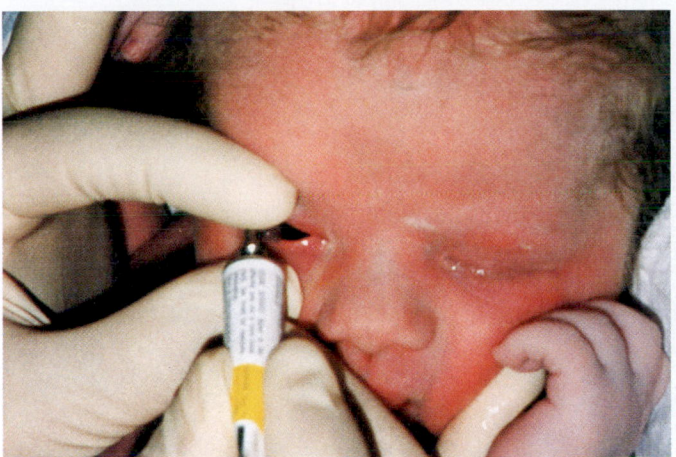

Figure 9-24. ■ Ophthalmic ointment. Retract lower eyelid outward to instill ¼-inch-long strand of ointment from a single-dose tube along the lower conjunctival surface.

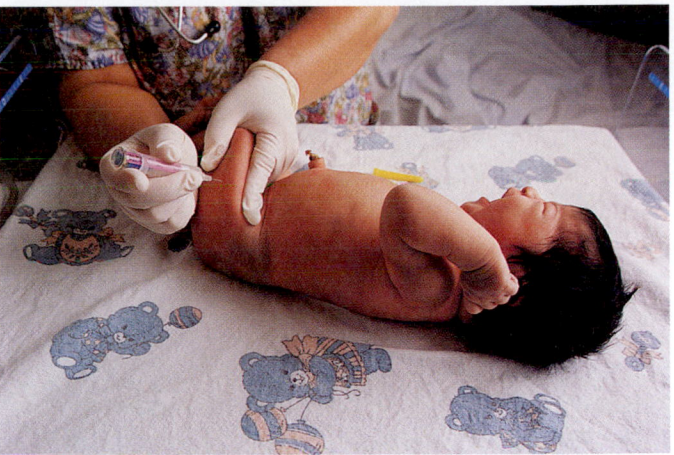

Figure 9-25. ■ Procedure for vitamin K injection. Cleanse area thoroughly with alcohol swab and allow skin to dry. Bunch the tissue of the upper outer thigh (vastus lateralis muscle) and quickly insert a 25-gauge, ⅝-inch needle at a 90-degree angle to the thigh. Aspirate, then slowly inject the solution to distribute the medication evenly and minimize the baby's discomfort. Remove the needle and gently massage the site with an alcohol swab.

EYE CARE

Eye care is necessary to prevent **ophthalmia neonatorum** (inflammation of the eyes of the newborn, resulting from contact with gonorrhea or chlamydia during the birth process). It is mandatory that an antibiotic ointment or solution be placed in the infant's eyes soon after delivery (Figure 9-24 ■).

VITAMIN K ADMINISTRATION

Vitamin K, which is necessary for blood clotting, is normally produced in the intestines from food and intestinal flora. Newborns are unable to produce vitamin K because their intestine is sterile until food is introduced. Within 1 hour after delivery, the newborn is given an IM injection of vitamin K (aquaMEPHYTON) to prevent hemorrhagic disorders (Figure 9-25 ■). Table 9-1 ■ describes the use of this medication.

UMBILICAL CORD CARE

At delivery, a small plastic or metal clamp is generally placed on the umbilical cord approximately 1 inch from the skin, and the cord is cut. The clamp must remain in place until the cord has dried. With each diaper change, the skin at the base of the cord is assessed for redness and drainage. The skin is cleaned with plain water but is not soaked. An aseptic agent such as alcohol, triple blue dye, or betadine is applied to the cord to aid in drying (Figure 9-26 ■). It is important not to get alcohol on the infant's skin surrounding the cord because it would cause drying and irritation. If the cord is completely dry prior to discharge, the cord clamp can be removed. The cord will fall off in approximately 14 days and should not be pulled off, even if it is only partially attached. Until the cord falls off, the newborn should not be submerged in water.

clinical ALERT

Keeping the newborn's cord clean and dry is essential to prevent infection.

TABLE 9-1				
Pharmacology: Drug Used to Prevent Hemorrhagic Disorders				
DRUG	**USUAL ROUTE/DOSE**	**CLASSIFICATION**	**SELECTED SIDE EFFECTS**	**DON'T GIVE IF**
AquaMEPHYTON Phytonadione	Newborn: IM/SC 0.5–1.0 mg immediately after delivery May repeat in 6 hr PRN	Vitamin K	Hypersensitivity, flushing, pain at injection site	None

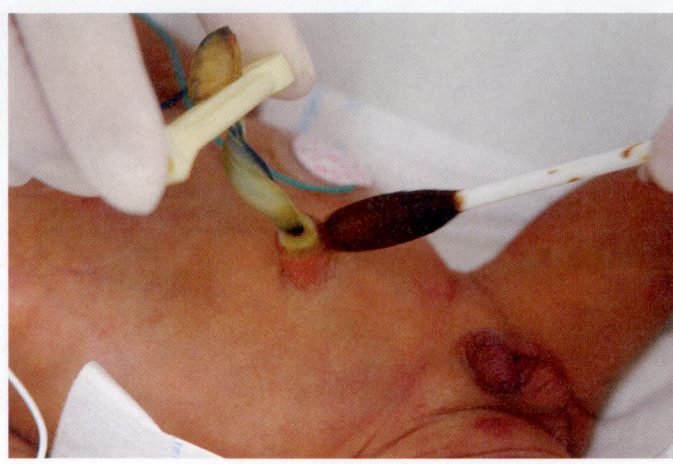
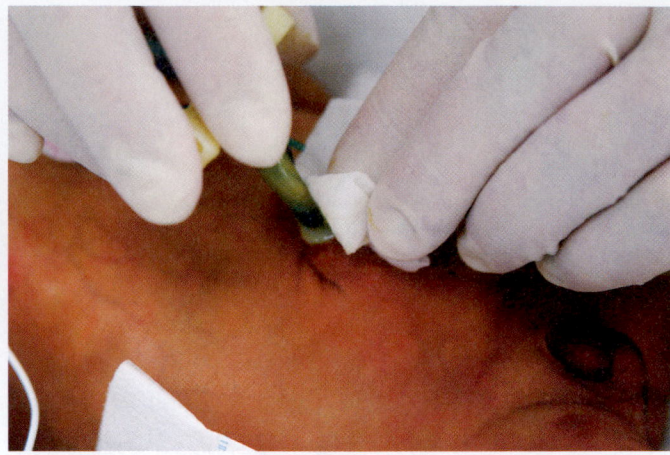

A **B**

Figure 9-26. ■ Two different methods for cord care. (**A**) Betadine cleaning. (**B**) Alcohol cleaning.

BATHING

The newborn has been in contact with maternal body fluids, blood, and amniotic fluid. Following standard precautions, the nurse should not touch the infant without clean exam gloves until the newborn has been bathed. Once the temperature has stabilized, the newborn is bathed with a wet washcloth, exposing only the area being washed. The hair can be washed with warm water and dried with a warm towel. The newborn will be diapered, dressed in a warm t-shirt, and wrapped in two to three warm blankets. Following a bath, the newborn remains under a radiant warmer until his or her temperature stabilizes.

SAFETY

Safety in the newborn nursery involves protecting the newborn from injury and abduction. Safety measures must also be taught to the parents.

Most facilities have procedures that must be followed to protect the newborn from abduction. These might include limiting access to the newborn nursery and the obstetric unit. That is, only personnel or parents with proper identification are allowed to enter. Personnel who transport the newborn from the mother's room to the nursery or other areas of the facility must have proper identification. Parents are taught not to give their baby to anyone who does not have identification.

When the newborn is brought to the mother, the identification band (see Figure 7-28A 🔗) is checked to be sure the infant is given to the correct person. The mother is asked to read the number on the identification bracelet, and the nurse checks it with the identification band on the baby.

When a newborn is carried in someone's arms, there is a possibility of dropping the baby. Therefore, transporting the newborn from room to room in a bassinette is not only the safest method, but it is also often mandatory.

The baby should not be left unattended on a high surface such as the bed. If the mother is tired, the newborn should be placed in the bassinette instead of having the mother sleep with the baby in her arms.

Common Nursery Procedures

NEWBORN SCREENING TESTS

Hypoglycemia

Newborns who are small for gestational age (SGA) or large for gestational age (LGA) are frequently assessed for hypoglycemia by determining the blood glucose level. A small blood sample is obtained from the newborn's heel (Figure 9-27 ■). Because of the possibility of damaging the nerves on the bottom of the newborn's foot, the correct procedure must be followed. The blood is placed on a reagent strip, and the blood glucose level is determined. The nurse must be familiar with the blood glucose monitor used by the facility. If the standards for the equipment are not closely followed, an inaccurate blood glucose level will be obtained.

Phenylketonuria

Another blood test that is done in the newborn period is screening for phenylketonuria (PKU). This screening test, required by law in all 50 states, determines the presence of an autosomal recessive disorder of amino acid metabolism in which the individual is unable to breakdown phenylalanine. This disorder is discussed in Chapter 22 🔗. To meet the legal requirements, facilities obtain the blood sample prior to discharge. For the results of the screening to be most accurate, the test must be done after the baby has received milk (either breast milk or formula). It may take 48 to 72 hours (or more) for the newborn to have an adequate consumption of milk. For this reason, the PKU test may need to be repeated in 1 to 2 weeks. The blood sample

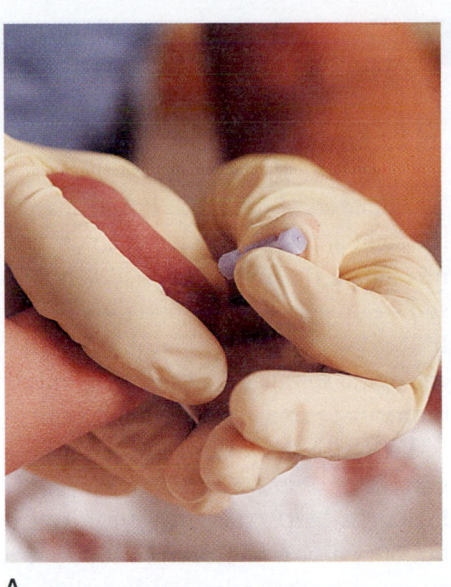
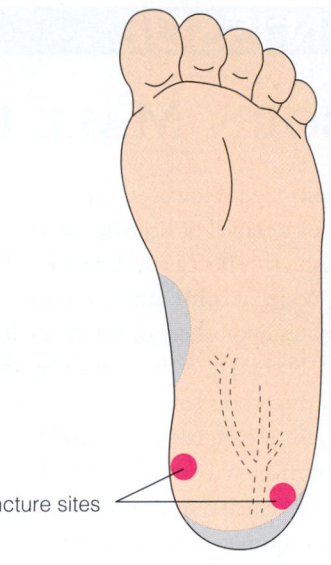
Puncture sites
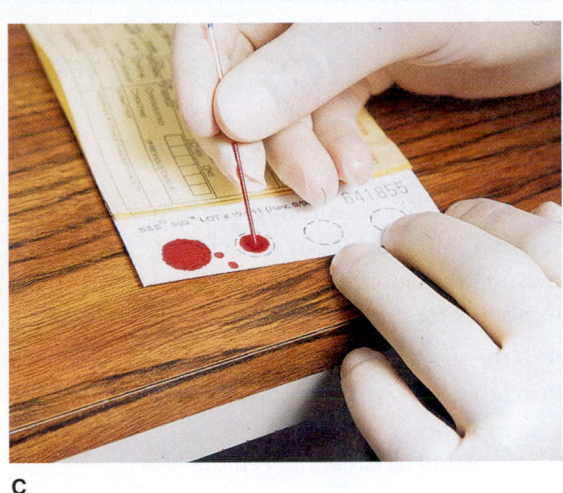

A   B   C

Figure 9-27. ■ (**A**) Heel stick. (**B**) Potential sites for heel sticks. Avoid shaded areas to prevent injury to arteries and nerves in the foot. (**C**) Collecting a blood sample from the newborn for neonatal metabolic screening. The nurse must be sure to saturate the circle on the test sheet thoroughly.

is obtained by heel stick. The blood is placed on a PKU specimen card and sent to the laboratory for analysis.

Bilirubin

The primary care provider frequently orders a bilirubin test to monitor the functioning of the newborn's liver. As stated previously, the newborn needs to break down the excess red blood cells. This is accomplished by the spleen and liver. The excess bilirubin should be broken down by the liver and excreted through the bile. It will take several days for the newborn's liver to be able to complete this process. In the meantime, the bilirubin builds up in the blood, resulting in hyperbilirubinemia. This disorder is discussed later in this chapter. The blood is usually obtained by laboratory personnel. The nurse informs the primary care provider of the results.

NEWBORN PROCEDURES

Circumcision

Circumcision is the surgical removal of the foreskin (*prepuce*) of the penis. Table 9-2 ■ identifies the advantages and disadvantages of circumcision. Parents should make an informed decision prior to signing the consent form. Only full-term infants should be circumcised. Cultural beliefs must be considered when supporting parents' decisions about circumcision. Box 9-2 ■ identifies common cultural considerations. The Health Promotion Issue on pages 280 and 281 discusses the bioethical issue of circumcision.

Before the procedure begins, an informed consent form must be signed. The infant is kept NPO for several hours.

TABLE 9-2

Advantages and Disadvantages of Circumcision

ADVANTAGES	DISADVANTAGES
Religious conviction	No evidence of medical benefit
Culture	Painful procedure
Social norm	Risk of bleeding
Hygiene	Risk of infection

The infant is restrained on a circumcision board, and a blanket should be placed over the infant's chest to prevent heat loss. At this point, the infant frequently begins to cry due to being held in extension. The physician may administer a local anesthetic in the form of an injection or cream. The physician then makes a slit in the prepuce and uses a Yellen

BOX 9-2   CULTURAL PULSE POINTS

Consideration for Circumcision

Male Jewish infants may be circumcised on the eighth day of life during a religious ceremony by the *mohel*, a person trained to do circumcision. Parents should be taught home care before leaving the hospital even though the procedure will occur later.

Muslim parents practice circumcision as a religious rite.

In European countries, circumcision is infrequently performed except for religious reasons.

MediaLink Circumcision

HEALTH PROMOTION ISSUE

BIOETHICS OF NEWBORN MALE CIRCUMCISION

In the United States since the mid-1970s, newborn male circumcision became almost a tradition. Although circumcision is a religious rite in some faiths, most parents circumcised their male newborns for other reasons, including:

- so the son would look like his father
- so other boys would not tease him in gym classes
- so it would be easier to keep the penis clean.

Now more parents are choosing not to circumcise their male infants. Most pediatricians agree that in the absence of a documented medical disorder, there is no medical reason to circumcise the newborn male. The bioethics of removing this healthy tissue is under review by national medical groups and the legal community.

DISCUSSION

Circumcision based on religious beliefs or done for medical reasons (including phimosis, hypospadias, and others) is not being questioned. However, the bioethics of removal of healthy foreskin for the cosmetic effect is under review by medical and legal communities in the United States and other countries around the world. Several questions must be answered in the process of this review.

What are the rights of the child? Under international law, the child has the right to security and freedom from torture or inhumane and degrading treatment. The child has the right to be consulted when decisions are made regarding his welfare. However, most male circumcisions are done within the first few days of life, when the child is unable to be "consulted" about the decision. Because the nontherapeutic procedure is not essential to the current well-being, it may be in the best interest of the child to postpone the procedure until the child can decide for himself.

What are the rights of the parents? The parent has the right and responsibility to the child to make decisions based on accurate information and in the best interests of the child. Parents have the right and responsibility to grant permission for the investigation, diagnosis, and treatment of disease and disorders. In the case of circumcision, it is the psychological well-being of the child in the future that parents are trying to ensure.

What are the benefits of circumcision? The 1999 American Academy of Pediatrics (AAP) statement (reaffirmed in 2006) does not recommend routine circumcision but acknowledges that some medical benefits exist. The AAP recommends that if circumcision is

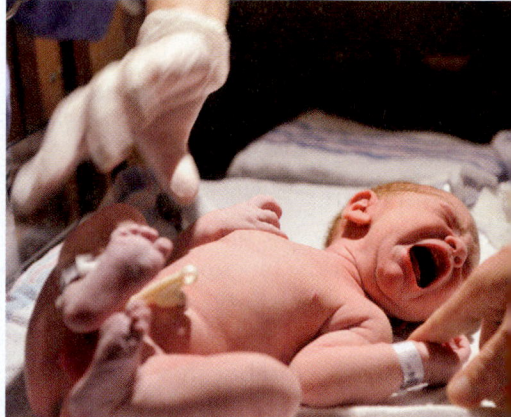

(Carolina K. Smith, M.D./Shutterstock)

(Gomco) clamp or Plastibell (Figure 9-28 ■) to control bleeding. The prepuce is then cut off. The Gomco clamp will be left in place for 5 minutes to ensure bleeding has stopped; it is then removed. When the Gomco clamp is used, vitamins A and D ointment or petroleum jelly may be applied to the penis to prevent the glans from sticking to the diaper. Ointment is not applied when the Plastibell is used. The Plastibell will fall off in 5 to 8 days.

After circumcision, the penis should be checked for bleeding at least every hour for 12 hours. If bleeding occurs, pressure should be applied with sterile 4×4 cotton gauze until bleeding stops. If bleeding cannot be controlled, the charge nurse and physician should be notified. The penis should be washed with warm water with each diaper change. Parents should be instructed to be alert for signs of infection until the circumcision has healed in 7 to 9 days.

Immunizations

Although immunizations can be given at any age, the Centers for Disease Control and Prevention (CDC) and the American Academy of Pediatrics recommend that immunizations be started in infancy. It is recommended that most immunizations begin in the second month of life. However, hepatitis B can be given in the neonatal period and may be given prior to discharge from the hospital after birth. A parental consent must be signed prior to immunization. Immunization schedules are discussed in Chapter 12 ∞.

Nutrition Teaching

Discharge teaching begins as soon as the newborn and mother have stabilized after delivery. Most of the newborn's care is provided with the parents present. The nurse

performed, local analgesic should be administered before the procedure. The circumcised penis is easier to clean. This may prevent urinary tract infections, especially when the boy or man is unable or unwilling to retract the foreskin and clean the glans daily.

Is circumcision harmful? Removal of the foreskin leaves the remaining skin tight and immovable and eliminates the protection of the glans. This allows for drying of the tissue and lessens the gliding action of the tissue during sexual intercourse. Circumcision puts the newborn at risk for infection and bleeding.

Is circumcision lawful? Male circumcision is not unlawful. However, in the absence of a medical indication, some suggestions arise that general laws for the protection of children could be applied to the nontherapeutic

excision of healthy functional tissue. In most developed countries, female circumcision is regarded as genital mutilation. Could or should this same standard be applied to male circumcision?

PLANNING AND IMPLEMENTATION

The nurse and the primary care provider have the responsibility to inform parents of the benefits, the known risks, and the disadvantages of nontherapeutic circumcision. Similar information must be provided regarding noncircumcision as well. Teaching should begin in the prenatal period, with verification of their understanding prior to the procedure. A consent must be signed prior to the procedure. Circumcision care and teaching must be provided before discharge.

SELF-REFLECTION

Circumcision of the newborn male will continue to be discussed in a variety of settings. The nurse must become informed about the bioethical issues as well as the medical benefits and risks on both sides of the issue. Many times, parents will ask the nurse for advice or "what would you do?" Nurses must be able to put their personal bias aside. They should present information in an objective manner, allowing and encouraging the parents to make an informed decision. Parents should understand that nontherapeutic circumcision is an elective procedure that can wait until they have obtained answers to their questions.

MediaLink Circumcision bioethics

SUGGESTED RESOURCES

For the Nurse

■ Committee on Bioethics. (1995). Informed consent, parental permission and assent in pediatric practice. *Pediatrics, 95*(2): 314–317.

For the Client

■ **www.nocirc.org** This is the site for the National Organization of Circumcision Information Resource Centers.

■ American Academy of Pediatrics. (2006). *Pediatrics, 117*(5), 1846–1847.

demonstrates and supervises the parents in providing the necessary care.

A full-term infant needs 50 to 55 kcal/lb (110–120 kcal/kg), which equals 20 ounces (600 mL) of breast milk or formula per day. At birth, the newborn's stomach will hold 20 mL or slightly less than 1 ounce. Because the newborn is initially unable to consume enough nutrition to meet its needs, the infant will lose weight during the first few days. By the end of the first week of life, the newborn can retain 2 to 3 ounces (60–90 mL) with each feeding. The infant will need to be fed every 2 to 4 hours in order to meet nutritional needs.

It is important for parents to receive information about the benefits of both breastfeeding and bottle-feeding. Table 9-3 ■ illustrates benefits for each method of feeding. Some women may choose to breastfeed in the privacy

of their homes and bottle-feed when they are in public or with visitors. Once the parents have decided how to feed the baby, the nurse should support the decision. It is not appropriate to make the parents feel guilty about their decision.

BREASTFEEDING

The American Academy of Pediatrics recommends breast milk for the first year of life. Commercially prepared formula closely approximates breast milk.

Breast milk is produced to meet the newborn's needs and changes as the infant grows. Breast milk contains easily digested nutrients and antibodies. *Colostrum*, the first fluid produced by the breast, is a thin yellow fluid, rich in protein, calories, and immune globulins. Colostrum protects the newborn from intestinal infections. Colostrum also

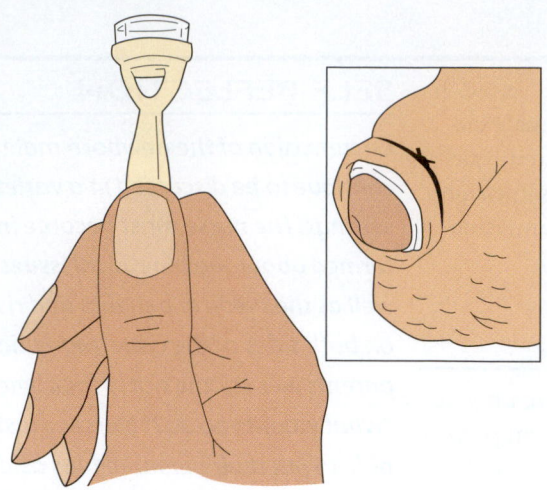

Figure 9-28. ■ Circumcision using the Plastibell. The bell is fitted over the glans. A suture is tied around the bell's rim, and the excess prepuce is cut away. The plastic rim remains in place for 3 to 4 days until healing occurs. The bell may be allowed to fall off. It is removed if it is still in place after 8 days.

contains a laxative that assists in the passage of *meconium,* the first feces of the newborn (Figure 9-29 ■).

Breast stimulation and emptying of the mammary glands stimulates the secretion of prolactin by the mother's anterior pituitary gland (see Figure 4-17 ⬭). Prolactin increases milk production. As the newborn nurses more frequently and for longer periods of time, more milk is produced.

The breastfeeding mother needs a balanced diet in order to provide nutritious breast milk and maintain her own nutritional needs. (The pregnant woman's nutritional needs are discussed in Chapter 6 ⬭.) An extra 500 calories and 1,000 mL of fluid are needed per day to support breastfeeding.

The mother and newborn do not automatically know how to breastfeed. Teaching and support will be needed during the learning process. Several positions (Figure 9-30 ■) can be used for breastfeeding. The *cradle hold*, with the infant's head in the bend of the mother's elbow and the infant's body resting against the mother's abdomen, is the most common. Another position is a *football hold*, with the infant's

TABLE 9-3		
Reasons for Breastfeeding and Bottle-Feeding		
FEEDING METHOD	**BENEFIT TO MOTHER**	**BENEFIT TO INFANT**
Breastfeeding	Decreases incidence of ovarian, uterine, and breast cancer	Breast milk enhances maturation of the GI tract; it is *species specific* (human milk for human babies), so it supplies the exact nutrients needed by the infant; it assists in passage of meconium and stools
	Promotes involution	Breast milk contains antibodies that can protect against some infections
	Return to prepregnant weight sooner	Lower incidence of allergies among breastfed infants
	Unique bonding experience	Breastfed infants have lower incidence of SIDS
	Convenient, no formula and bottles to carry	
	Saves money	
Bottle-feeding	Personal preference	Bonding still can occur
	Provides a good option if mother has breast scarring or HIV infection, or if maternal medication precludes breastfeeding	Others besides mother can feed infant
	Is good choice if mother's place of employment (e.g., hair salon) contains chemicals that could contaminate expressed milk	Provides adequate nutrition
	Provides solution if mother's workplace is intolerant of breastfeeding	Commercial formula comes in three forms for convenience
	Allows several people to share bonding experience while feeding infant	Commercial formula comes in cow's milk and soy milk
	May allow mother to get more rest if others take night feedings	WIC program provides iron-fortified formula

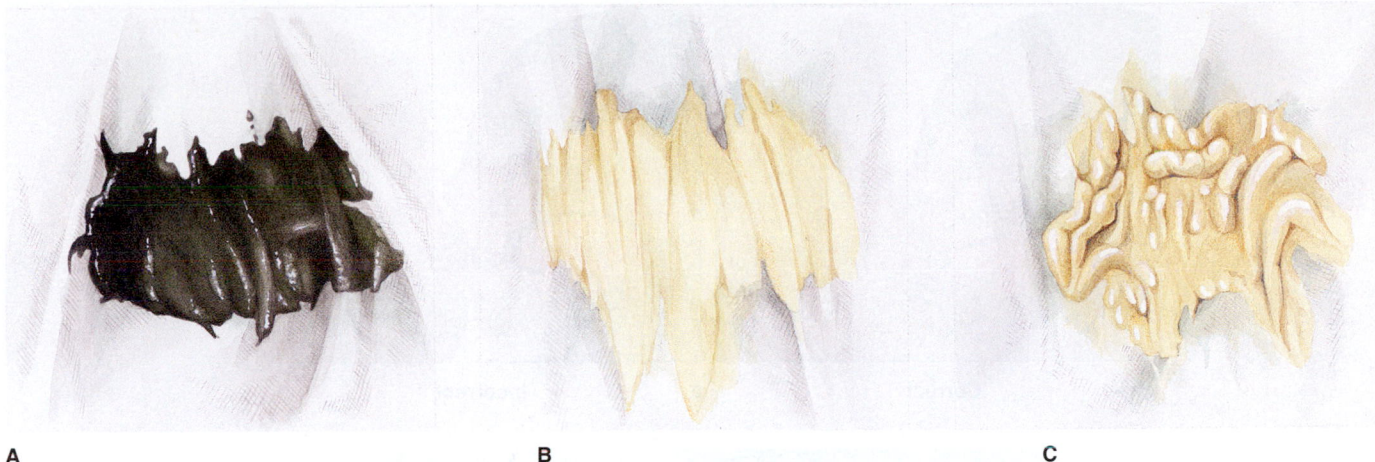

Figure 9-29. ■ Newborn stool samples. (**A**) Meconium stool. (**B**) Breast milk stool. (**C**) Cow's milk stool.

body tucked beneath the mother's axilla and the infant's head positioned against the breast. A *side-lying position* is frequently used in bed. The mother lies on her side with pillows supporting her head and back. The newborn is positioned next to her with the infant's head against the breast and the body parallel to the mother's body. It is important to use a pillow under the mother's forearm to support the weight of the infant.

Once the newborn is positioned against the breast, the infant must open wide enough to take the nipple and areola into the mouth. To help the newborn to latch onto the breast (Figure 9-31 ■), the mother holds the breast in her hand with the thumb and forefinger in the shape of a "C" around the breast and well behind the areola. She tickles the infant's lips with the nipple. The infant will open its mouth (part of the sucking reflex). When the mouth is wide open and the tongue is down, the infant is brought rapidly to the breast. When "latched on" properly, the nipple and areola will be in the mouth, with the tongue under the nipple and the lips flared outward. The suction will be strong, but there will be no discomfort. When the infant latches on properly, milk is sucked easily from the nipple. If the mother experiences discomfort, the infant should be removed from the breast, repositioned, and allowed to latch on again. There are a variety of positions for breastfeeding (see Figure 9-30). In the traditional cradle position, the baby and mother are belly to belly, chest to chest, and the infant's nose and chin should touch the breast. This close position helps the infant to latch on, while also helping prevent nipple soreness.

When removing the newborn from the breast, the mother should gently insert a finger into the corner of the infant's mouth to break the suction. If the nipple becomes sore, cracks, or bleeds, or if blisters form, the nipple needs

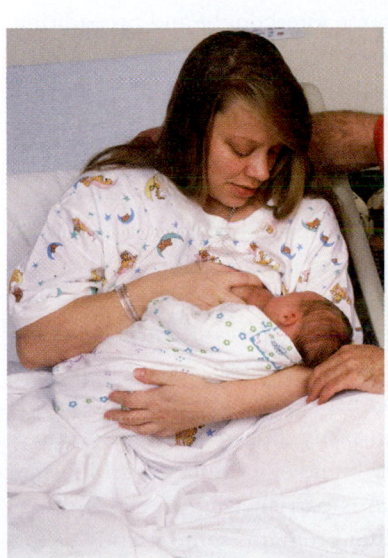
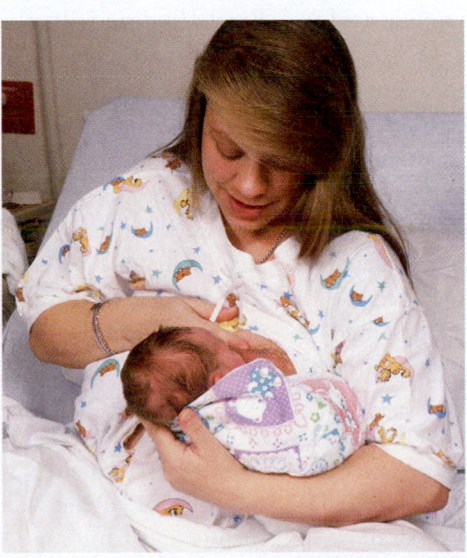
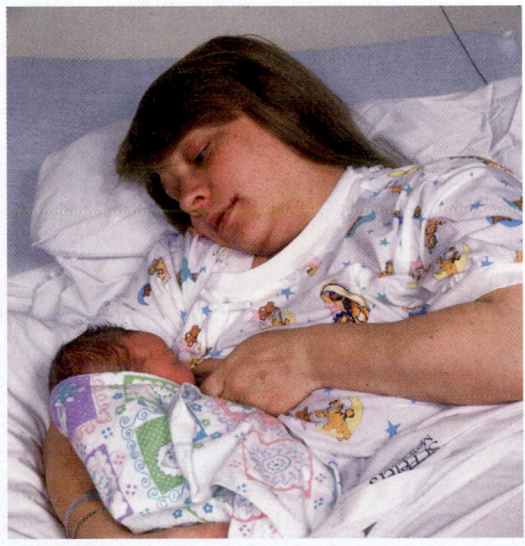

Figure 9-30. ■ Three positions that are often used for breastfeeding. (**A**) Cradle hold. (**B**) Football hold. (**C**) Side-lying position.

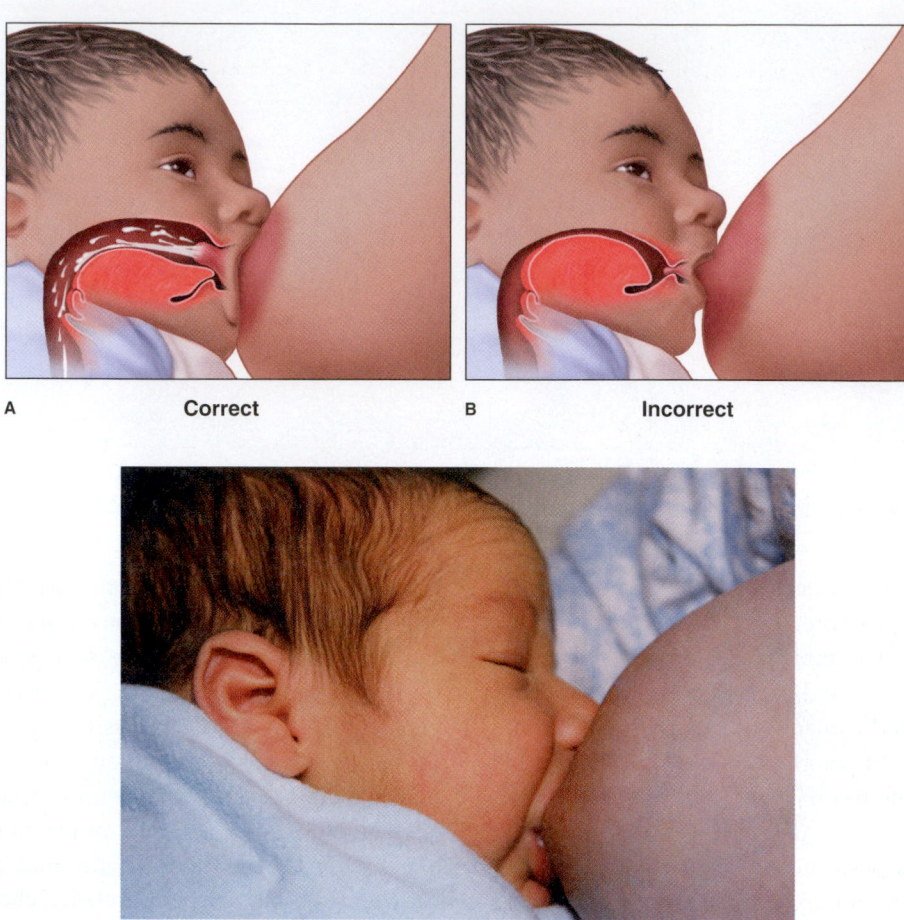

A **Correct**   B **Incorrect**

C

Figure 9-31. ■ Latching on. **(A)** Correct position with tongue over gum ridge. Nipple is down far into mouth and milk flows. **(B)** Incorrect position with tongue behind the lower gum ridge. Only the tip of the nipple is in the mouth. The nipple is pinched and milk cannot flow. **(C)** Newborn properly latched onto mother's breast. **(C:** M. C. Schlachter Photography.)

treatment. Leaving a small amount of milk on the nipple after feeding helps to heal sore nipples. Also the tannic acid obtained by gently rubbing the nipple with a cool wet tea bag can help with healing. A light film of an approved emollient (e.g., Eucerin) may be applied after feedings.

Breastfeeding may range from 10 to 30 minutes a side, depending on the size and health of the infant. Frequency is at least 8 to 12 times a day. However, it is more important to know when the infant is full than to follow the clock. Infants will nurse vigorously at first, and then slow as they become full. The breast will become soft when empty. Infants should be allowed to empty one breast and then be moved to the other breast until they are full. At the next feeding, the infant is started on the breast used last at the previous feeding. This technique allows each breast to be emptied completely every other feeding. As infants grow, both breasts may be emptied with each feeding. Breastfed infants generally do not swallow as much air as bottle-fed infants, but they still should be burped halfway through and again at the end of the feeding.

BOTTLE-FEEDING

Bottle-feeding will take some forethought and preparation. Bottles and nipples should be cleaned regularly with a brush and soapy water and thoroughly rinsed. If there is question about the safety of the water supply, both bottles and nipples should be boiled.

A variety of nipples are available. Generally, babies will feed well from any bottle and nipple, but they may eventually prefer one style. Formulas are available in ready-to-feed, concentrated liquid, or powder forms. There is a great range of prices for formula, and finances should be a factor in choosing what type of formula to use. Accurate mixing is essential to provide the necessary nutrients, the proper number of calories, and an easily digested concentration.

The physician orders the brand of formula. It is important to note that, if the woman is participating in the Women, Infants and Children (WIC) program, some brands of formula may not be funded. Adjustments can usually be made between the physician and the WIC program.

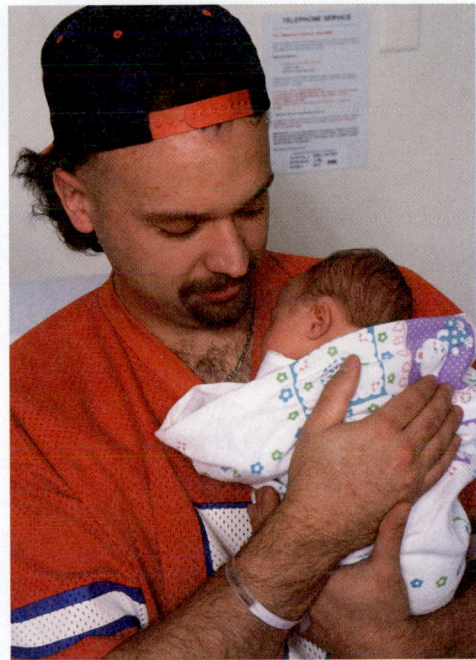

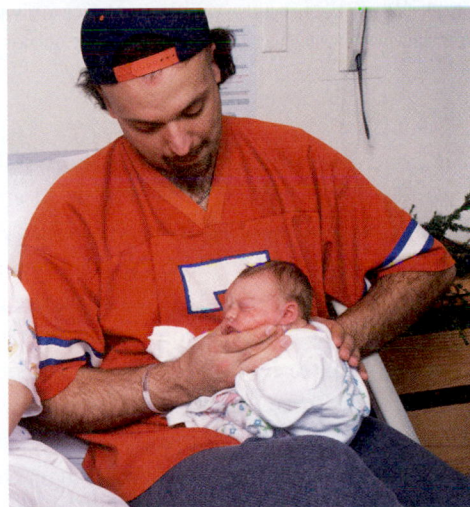

Figure 9-32. ■ Positions in which a neonate may be burped. **(A)** Upright. **(B)** Sitting leaning forward. The infant may also be laid across the lap.

Most newborns will take 15 mL (½ ounce) the first few days but gradually increase the amount of each feeding over time. To avoid wasting formula, only a few ounces should be made until the infant is taking higher volumes.

The infant should be positioned with the head higher than the stomach. The infant should be burped when about half of the feeding is consumed and again at the end of the feeding.

BURPING

To facilitate burping, the infant can be held upright against the feeder's shoulder (Figure 9-32 ■), leaned forward in a sitting position with the head and chest supported, or laid prone across the feeder's lap. Gently rubbing or patting the infant's back can also facilitate burping.

Discharge Teaching

ELIMINATION

The newborn voids 8 to 10 times a day. The perineal area should be washed with warm water or commercially prepared wipes following each void. Diapers should be checked and changed frequently to keep the skin dry.

The newborn should pass meconium stool within the first 24 hours after delivery. Holding the infant's legs across the abdomen for a few minutes may help the newborn pass stool. Meconium is sticky, and the newborn's skin should be cleansed thoroughly. Transitional stools are passed after several feedings. Transitional stools are yellowish- or greenish-brown, thin, and less sticky (see Figure 9-29). Milk curds may be seen. By the fourth day, the stool becomes thicker and pasty. If the infant is breast-fed, stools become yellow to golden and have an odor similar to sour milk. Formula-fed newborns pass pale yellow to light brown stools that are firmer and have a stronger odor. The stool will not be brown and formed until the infant is given solid food.

DIAPERING

Most commonly, disposable diapers are used in the hospital nursery. Disposable diapers are made to draw the urine inside the fibers and away from the newborn's skin. By keeping the urine away from the skin, rashes and skin breakdown are reduced. Although disposable diapers are better for the newborn's skin, there are also some drawbacks. First, disposable diapers are expensive. The young family may not be able to afford them. Second, disposable diapers are not biodegradable. Some argue that disposable diapers are polluting the environment. Parents should not be made to feel guilty for their choice of diapers.

Diapers should be changed at least every 2 hours, or as soon as they become soiled. Figure 9-33 ■ illustrates how to apply a diaper. The diaper area should be washed with each diaper change. If a rash appears, commercially prepared ointments may be beneficial. Laying the newborn on a pad without the diaper fastened exposes the perineum to air and light. This may help prevent or heal skin breakdown.

HYGIENE

Daily hygiene for the newborn includes bathing, umbilical cord care, perineal care, and, if indicated, circumcision care. Until the umbilical cord falls off, the newborn should not be placed in a tub of water. Gentle wiping with a warm, moist

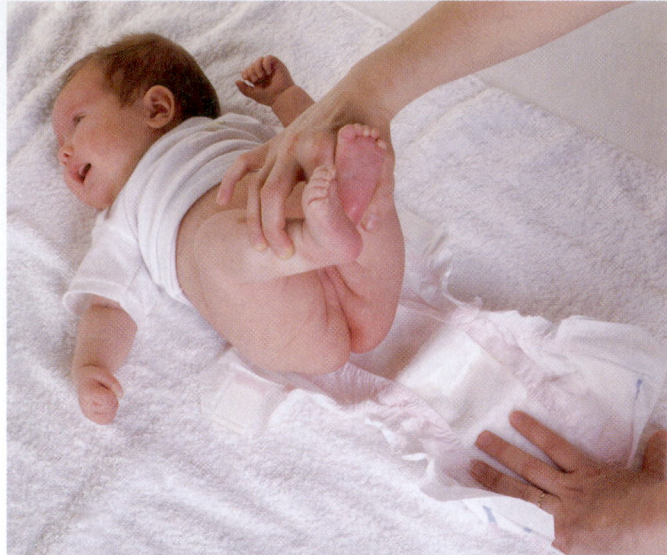

A

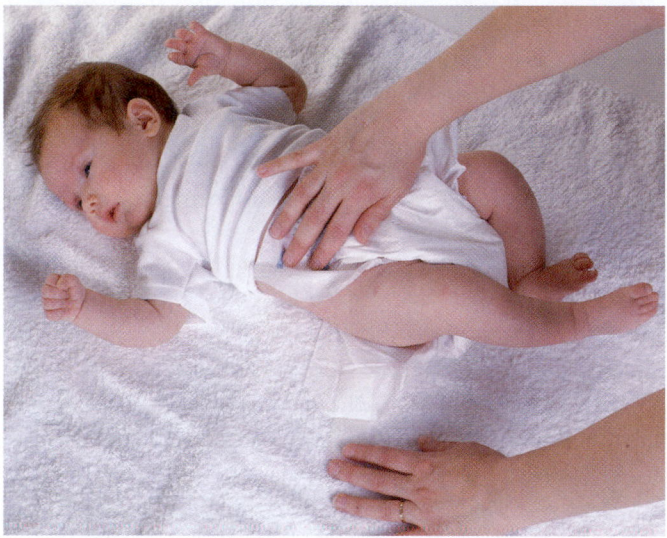

B

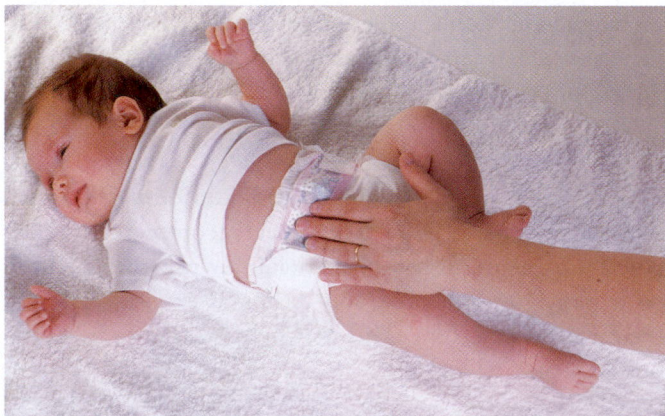

C

Figure 9-33. ■ Diapering. (**A**) Lift the baby by both legs over diaper. (**B**) Make sure the diaper is fully unfolded across the back and buttocks before securing. (**C**) Fasten the diaper snugly but not tightly. (Jules Selmes (c) Dorling Kindersley.)

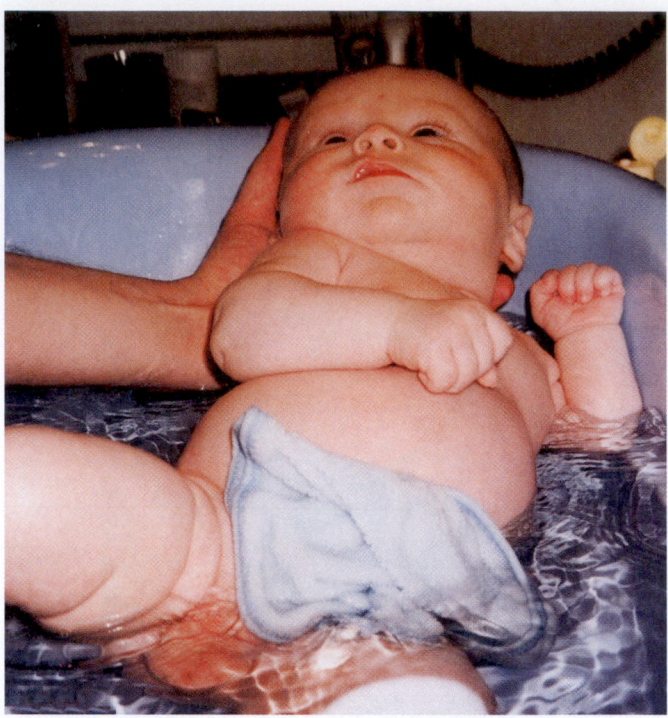

Figure 9-34. ■ When bathing the newborn, the caregiver must support the head and hold the baby carefully. Wet babies are very slippery.

washcloth is generally sufficient. The newborn's skin may become dry and peel within a few days. A small amount of lotion or baby oil may be applied to the dry areas. After the umbilical cord falls off, the newborn can be place in warm water for bathing (Figure 9-34 ■). When wet, the newborn is very slick. Care must be taken to prevent the baby from sliding under the water or hitting its head on the side of the basin. For this reason, many parents bathe the newborn in the sink or a basin of warm water instead of in the bathtub.

Perineal care should be completed with each diaper change. A warm washcloth or commercially prepared diaper wipe may be used. It is important to remove urine and stool from between the labial folds of female infants. If the male infant is not circumcised, the penis should be cleansed with warm water. The foreskin should not be forced back over the penis. The foreskin will retract normally over time, but it might take 3 to 5 years to do so. If the infant is circumcised, squeeze warm soapy water over the penis, rinse, and pat dry. The glans will be sensitive for a few days, so the diaper should be fastened loosely and the baby should not be placed on his abdomen. A small amount of petroleum jelly may be applied (unless a Plastibell is in place). If excessive bleeding, redness, swelling, and purulent drainage occur, the parents should notify the primary care provider.

The umbilical cord should remain clean and dry. Care should be taken to prevent infection of the umbilical cord. The skin around the cord may be pink but should not become red or inflamed. A small amount of dark reddish-brown drainage may be present. The cord should be cleaned with warm water three to four times a day or with each diaper change. Applying a small amount of 70% isopropyl alcohol to the cord (but not to the surrounding skin) will facilitate drying and help prevent infection. The diaper should be folded below the umbilical cord to allow for air-drying. If culture demands binding the abdomen, a clean piece of gauze can be recommended. The umbilical cord should fall off in 7 to 14 days. A small drop of blood may appear when the cord comes off. Parents should be taught never to pull on the cord or attempt to loosen it.

SLEEP

The newborn generally sleeps for approximately 20 to 22 hours a day. The newborn likes the security and warmth offered by swaddling (Figure 9-35 ■). To swaddle the baby, place a blanket on a secure surface in the shape of a diamond. Fold the top corner down slightly. Lay the baby on the blanket with the head at the fold. Wrap the right corner around the baby and secure it under the left side. Do not wrap so tightly that the baby is unable to breathe or move. Pull the bottom corner up to the baby's chest.

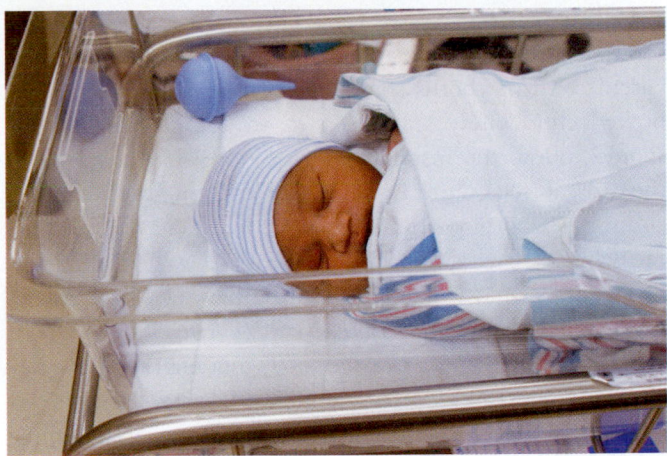

Figure 9-35. ■ It is recommended to position the newborn on the back for sleep. Swaddling maintains warmth and provides security for the infant. (George Dodson/Pearson Education/PH College.)

Wrap the left corner around the newborn's right side. Place the newborn on its back in the crib. A second blanket can be put over the baby, but the head should remain exposed.

A light massage may help the agitated baby to relax before sleep. Box 9-3 ■ provides steps for infant massage.

BOX 9-3	CLIENT TEACHING

Infant Massage

Infant massage has many benefits. It can soothe a tired infant and minimize distress. It promotes bonding and may boost the infant's immune system. It can help relieve colic and promote sleep (Massage, 2006).

General Guidelines

Massage is best done when both parent and child are relaxed and calm. It is best to wait about half an hour after the infant's feeding. The room should be warm (78°F). If the room is cold or humid, a light blanket should be used to cover the body parts that are not being massaged. The infant is placed on a soft surface (like a bed).

Baby lotion may be used for the massage. Put lotion on the hands and rub them together so the hands are warm and soft. Depending on the particular infant, it may not be necessary to keep applying lotion.

The time during massage is an optimum time to bond with the infant. Remember to make eye contact and to speak softly while giving the massage.

Always use gentle pressure (no harder than you would use to rub your own eyes).

Massage Process

■ Start with the infant lying supine (on the back). With light touch, draw fingertips from the center of the nose up and toward the temples, from the mouth out over the ears and down, and up over the top of the head. Bring the fingertips from the center of the chin up to the tops of the ears.

■ Very gently, massage behind the neck and down onto the shoulders. Softly place both hands onto the shoulders. Stroke gently downward from neck to chest.

■ Circle the arm at the armpit with the fingers of one hand. Stroke gently down the arm. Be very careful at the elbow because it is a sensitive area. Gently stroke several times from shoulder to wrist and slide fingers down over the hands.

■ For the abdomen, trace a clockwise circle below the ribs. Do not include the genitalia in the massage. Stroke lightly around the abdomen and down from the abdomen to the thighs.

■ Massage each leg, pressing firmly but gently on the muscles of the thigh and calf. Bend the knees and press the thighs gently against the abdomen.

■ Draw the hands along one foot at a time from ankle to toe. Press each toe lightly. Then stroke the whole foot again. Use a circular motion at the heels.

■ Turn the infant over onto the stomach. Starting at the head, make long stroking motions that include the head, neck, back, and legs. Gently massage the muscles of the back with small, circular motions. Do not massage the spine; instead, place the hands over the spinal cord for a few seconds to warm the area.

■ Massage the backs of the legs from thigh to foot. Then stroke again from head to foot a few times to finish the massage.

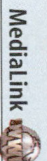

MediaLink   Infant massage

SAFETY

Safety for the newborn cannot be stressed enough with new parents. All newborns should be placed in a federally approved child safety seat when in an automobile. Parents should follow the installation procedure that comes with the car seat (see Figure 12-7 🔗). If carrying both supplies and the newborn, parents should secure the newborn in the car before transferring packages.

Parents should be taught that the newborn is at risk of falling if left unattended on a high surface. Even if the newborn is secured in an infant carrier, the baby's motions can tip the carrier over. For example, if the parent places the newborn in a carrier on the kitchen counter while putting away groceries, the baby's motion can cause the carrier to fall from the countertop.

The need to handle infants gently is stressed. Besides teaching parents to support the baby's head when lifting, teaching is also done about the dangers of shaking infants. Some facilities ask parents to view a video about shaken baby syndrome before being discharged home with the neonate.

NURSING CARE

PRIORITIES IN NURSING CARE

The priorities of nursing care for the normal newborn are:

- Maintaining the airway, breathing, and circulation
- Maintaining body temperature
- Teaching parents to provide care for their newborn
- Providing nutrition
- Ensuring elimination.

ASSESSING

Once the nurse meets the immediate survival needs of the newborn at the time of delivery, the nurse begins the process of preparing the parents to care for their baby. The nurse must assess the learning needs of the parents. If this is the first child, the parents may need more information and support than parents who have had several children. However, the nurse should validate that experienced parents still have the knowledge and skills they require to provide the necessary care.

The assessment of learning needs is accomplished by asking parents what they already know and by watching them handle the baby. Often, a conversational manner not only provides support to the couple, but also makes them feel comfortable about asking questions.

DIAGNOSING, PLANNING, AND IMPLEMENTING

Nursing diagnoses might include:

- Deficient Knowledge related to feeding, diapering, bathing, safety

- Breastfeeding.

Many facilities use prepared teaching plans to provide instruction and documentation of teaching. Nurses often provide and reinforce teaching in the following areas.

- Teach umbilical and circumcision care. *Keeping the umbilical cord and circumcision clean and dry prevents infection and promotes healing.*
- Demonstrate bathing and stress safety concerns. *Keeping the newborn out of water until the umbilical cord falls off promotes drying of the cord. Once the newborn is bathed in water, safety is a high priority because a wet baby is very slippery.*
- Review client decisions about feeding the baby. Support the client's decision about which method to use. Be sensitive to cultural attitudes about feeding. (For example, women of Hispanic culture may want to begin breastfeeding in the privacy of their own home.) Many facilities provide a lactation specialist to discuss breastfeeding methods and concerns. *The newborn needs nutrients every 3 to 4 hours. Mothers need to be taught techniques for breastfeeding. Both parents should be taught how to prepare formula for bottle-fed newborns. They should also be given guidelines for bottle care and for positioning infants for feeding.*
- Provide information about elimination and about what stools should look like. The appearance will depend on whether the child is breastfed or bottle fed. *Parents should be taught to watch for changes in elimination patterns, including changes in stool color and consistency with feeding.*
- Observe the client and others performing routine care such as dressing and diapering. Ensure that caregivers are practicing good hygiene and safety. *The newborn needs to be handled gently. The head needs to be supported. Parents should be taught to provide perineal care with each diaper change.*
- Review safety concerns, including risk for falls and safety car seats. *New parents may not be aware of possible dangers. Experienced parents may need information about how new equipment is used.*
- Encourage the family to take on some daily chores to support the mother. *Family members can participate in the health and care of the mother and infant by providing time for the mother to recover from labor, rest, and care for the baby.*

EVALUATING

Evaluating is best accomplished by watching the parents give care to the newborn. The nurse should document the teaching and list any printed material that was provided to the parents. Follow-up phone calls or home visits may be needed for parents with limited family support.

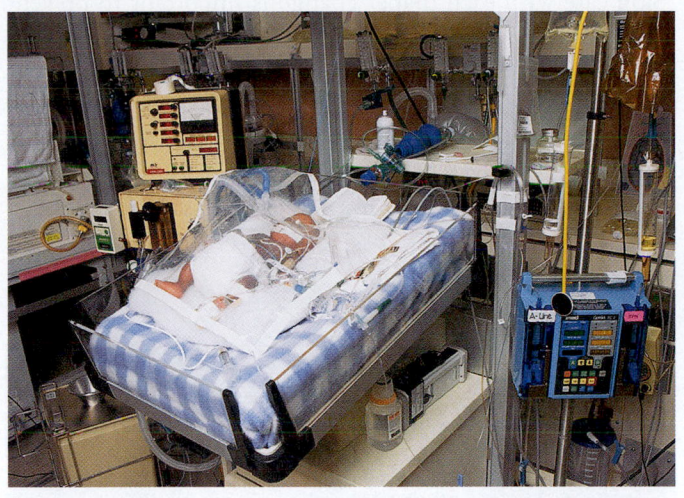

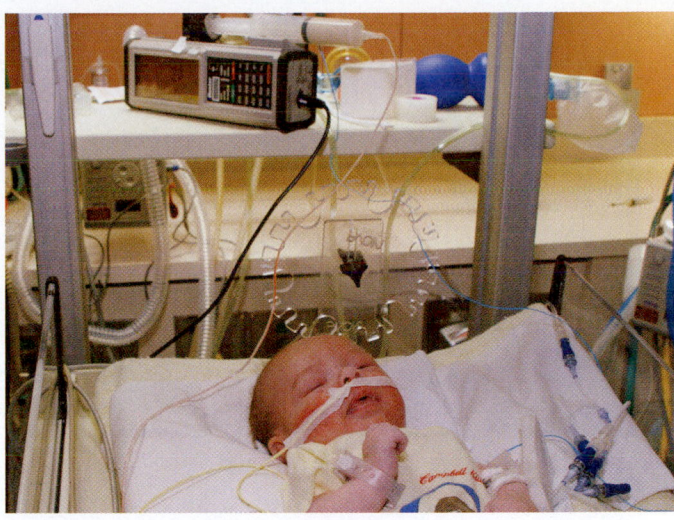

Figure 9-36. ■ **(A)** This premature infant in the NICU is receiving artificial ventilation. **(B)** This premature baby cannot yet coordinate suck and swallow. Gavage feeding is being used until the baby can effectively acquire nutrients.

HIGH-RISK NEWBORN

The high-risk newborn is generally placed in a neonatal intensive care unit (NICU) (Figure 9-36 ■), if available, or in an area of the newborn nursery where the registered nurse can closely observe the baby. The role of the LPN/LVN is one of assisting the RN with data collection, meeting the basic needs of the newborn, and documenting care. If the facility does not have appropriate accommodations, the newborn may be transferred to another hospital that can meet his or her needs.

Many conditions that place the newborn at risk continue past the first month of life. Therefore, the pathology, symptoms, and nursing care of specific conditions are addressed in other chapters of this book. This chapter addresses the basic nursing care of the high-risk newborn and introduces some congenital anomalies, infections, and disorders commonly seen in the high-risk newborn.

General Care of the High-Risk Newborn

MONITORING

The vital signs of the high-risk newborn must be monitored continuously. Electrodes to record the electrical conduction of the heart are placed on the newborn's chest. Respiratory rate and oxygen saturation are also monitored. Blood pressure is monitored electronically. If the newborn's condition warrants, a catheter may be placed through the subclavian or femoral artery to monitor the pressure inside the heart.

Temperature is maintained by radiant heat above the bassinette. A sensor is placed over the soft tissue of the abdomen to ensure that the newborn does not become too warm. The newborn's axillary temperature may also be taken every 2 to 4 hours.

Monitoring intake and output is necessary to ensure adequate fluid balance. Fluids may be given by intravenous infusion, gavage feeding (see Figure 9-36B), or, if the newborn is strong enough, through bottle or cup feeding. Output is monitored by weighing the diaper or, at times, by a suprapubic catheter. Due to the small size of the urethra, a urethral catheter is generally not used.

MEDICAL TREATMENT

Medical treatment is determined by the specific disorder. Common treatments are discussed here. It is important to remember, though, that not every newborn will require all of these treatments.

The premature newborn or newborn in respiratory distress might require mechanical ventilation through an endotracheal tube or, if long-term ventilation is needed, a tracheostomy tube. The nurse or respiratory therapist will maintain an open airway by suctioning mucus from the bronchi. If mechanical ventilation is not needed, oxygen may be administered by an oxyhood (Figure 9-37 ■) or by nasal cannula or catheter.

clinical ALERT

High amounts of oxygen given to the newborn may cause retinopathy. The newborn will need careful monitoring and periodic eye examination.

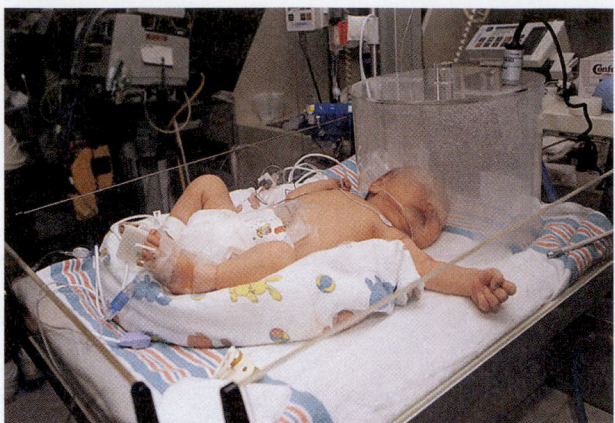

Figure 9-37. ■ An infant under an oxyhood.

Medication is usually administered by intravenous infusion. If the need for IV fluids or medication is determined within the first few hours after birth, the doctor may insert a catheter into an umbilical vein. Another site for a central venous catheter is the subclavian vein. The nurse assists with the insertion of the catheter, maintains the infusion, and administers medication as ordered.

Diagnostic examination, such as MRI scan and ultrasound, may be necessary to determine the specific disorder and provide appropriate treatment. The nurse may need to accompany the newborn to these procedures in order to maintain the necessary care. At times, surgery may be needed to correct life-threatening congenital anomalies. Specially trained operating room personnel provide these services. The newborn returns to the NICU following surgery. Drainage tubes (chest tubes, intraventricular catheter, or wound drainage tubes) may be in place. The nurse must maintain patency of these tubes.

NURSING CONSIDERATIONS

Besides assisting with medical treatment, the nurse must also provide for the newborn's activities of daily living. The newborn needs nutrients in order to grow. The premature newborn may not have the muscle strength or energy to suck from the breast or bottle. Endotracheal tubes may be inserted through the mouth. In these cases, a small amount of formula or breast milk may be given by gavage feeding every few hours. Sometimes the newborn who lacks strength to suck may be taught to drink from a cup. As the newborn gains strength, bottle-feeding may be used. If the gastrointestinal system is not able to function normally, nutrients will be given by total parenteral nutrition (TPN) (see Figure 9-36B).

If the high-risk newborn has adequate fluid intake, he or she should void every few hours. If oral nutrients are administered, the meconium stool should change in a few days to the transitional stools seen in healthy newborns.

Skin care with each diaper change is important to prevent tissue breakdown.

Activity is necessary for muscle development, to prevent skin breakdown, and to prevent hypostatic pneumonia. The high-risk newborn should be turned and repositioned every few hours. The extremities should be free to move as much as possible. If any form of restraint is necessary, it should be removed, and active or passive range of motion should be performed every few hours.

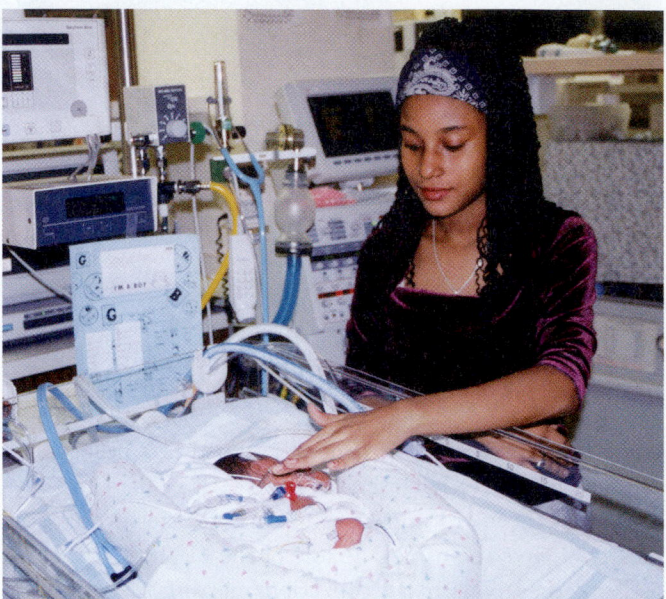

A

B

Figure 9-38. ■ **(A)** Mother of this 26-week gestational age 600-gram baby begins attachment through fingertip touch. **(B)** Kangaroo (skin-to-skin) care facilitates a closeness and attachment between parents and their premature infant. (**A:** Courtesy of Lisa Smith-Pedersen, RNC, MSN, NNP. **B:** Courtesy of Carol Harrigan, RNC, MSN, NNP.)

The skin of the premature or high-risk newborn is thin and fragile. Care must be taken to protect skin and tissue and keep them intact. The skin should be kept clean and dry. The linen should be free of wrinkles. The newborn should not be placed on tubes and monitoring wires.

The skin of the postterm infant is also at risk. Because the vernix caseosa is gradually reabsorbed into the skin, postterm babies may have skin that peels, cracks, or even begins to slough off, making them prone to infection. Very few babies today are postterm. Typically, labor is induced to prevent long delays beyond the EDD.

The newborn needs to be touched and caressed (Figure 9-38 ■). Parents must bond with the newborn. The nurse can promote this bonding process by encouraging the parents to assist with the care of the newborn. It is frightening for parents to see the baby sick, with numerous tubes and monitors attached. They may be frightened to touch or hold their baby. However, parents are encouraged to begin the bonding process by fingertip and palmar touch, followed by stroking, holding, and rocking the newborn as much as possible. Both the parents and the nurses should call the newborn by name. Parents should be encouraged to talk and sing to the baby. They should be allowed to participate as much as possible in daily care—bathing, diapering, and feeding. The nurse must explain all aspects of care and medical treatment, and teach the parents to provide care. The nurse must be alert for parental comments and behavior that indicate their anxiety or comfort with the situation. Support groups may be useful to help parents of high-risk newborns.

Common Conditions Affecting The High-Risk Newborn

Many congenital anomalies are identified at birth or within the first few weeks of life. If the anomaly is life threatening, surgery is usually performed immediately to correct the defect. Less threatening anomalies are not repaired until the child is stronger and better able to withstand the surgical procedure. At times, repair is performed in stages, and complete reconstruction may take months or years.

Infections of the newborn usually result from exposure to the mother before or during delivery. Some infections, such as rubella, syphilis, and HIV/AIDS, are transported across the placenta and infect the developing fetus. Other infections, such as gonorrhea and herpes, can be picked up as the fetus moves through the birth canal (see Table 8-6 ⊙⊙). (In a woman with active herpes, which can be lethal to the baby, delivery is by cesarean section.) The immature immune system of the premature or high-risk newborn makes infection especially dangerous to long-term health.

Some disorders that place the newborn at risk for long-term health concerns are introduced by body system in this section.

CARDIOVASCULAR CONDITIONS

Cardiovascular conditions include congenital anomalies and hemorrhage and hemolytic disorders.

Congenital heart defects are more common when the child has been exposed to rubella, alcohol, or drugs during intrauterine development. Other factors that increase the risk of congenital heart defects include other congenital or genetic defects, advanced maternal age, maternal disorders such as lupus and diabetes, and siblings or parents with congenital defects.

Newborns with congenital heart defects exhibit signs and symptoms of congestive heart failure. These include, but are not limited to, heart murmurs, cyanosis, respiratory distress, fluid retention, and activity intolerance. Some heart murmurs are loud and easily heard. Others are soft and can only be detected by a trained practitioner. Cyanosis can be either constant, generalized cyanosis, or cyanosis around the mouth (**circumoral**), seen only when the newborn is active, nursing, or crying. Signs of respiratory distress include tachypnea, orthopnea, grunting, flaring nostrils, and retractions. Fluid retention may be evidenced by bulging fontanels, fewer than six wet diapers per day, moist lung sounds, and generalized tissue edema. Restlessness, crying, and lethargy can be signs of intracranial edema.

HEMORRHAGE

Although the newborn can hemorrhage from any trauma site, the most common is **intraventricular hemorrhage** (hemorrhage within the cerebral ventricles of the brain), which accompanies premature delivery. Before 35 weeks' gestation, the cerebral ventricles are lined with the germinal matrix; this matrix is susceptible to hypoxia and trauma. If the fetus becomes hypoxic or undergoes labor, hemorrhage from the germinal matrix into the cerebral ventricles is probable. For this reason, premature infants are frequently delivered by cesarean section instead of vaginally.

If intraventricular hemorrhage occurs, the newborn's brain function may be impaired, resulting in mental delay, immobility, or death. The symptoms and condition of the newborn dictate the care required.

HEMOLYTIC DISEASE OF THE NEWBORN (Rh INCOMPATIBILITY, ABO)

Hemolytic disease of the newborn (discussed briefly in Chapter 7 ⊙⊙ and more thoroughly in Chapter 8 ⊙⊙) is a general term for several blood disorders that result in RBC breakdown and an increase in bilirubin (**hyperbilirubinemia**). The most common cause of hyperbilirubinemia is physiologic jaundice, the normal breakdown of RBCs, discussed earlier in this chapter. A secondary cause of hyperbilirubinemia is pathologic jaundice. The most common

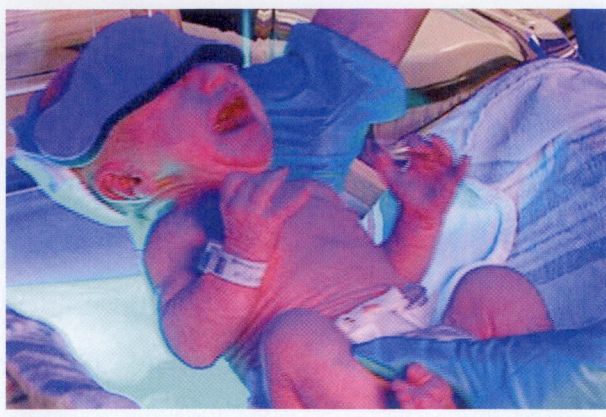

A

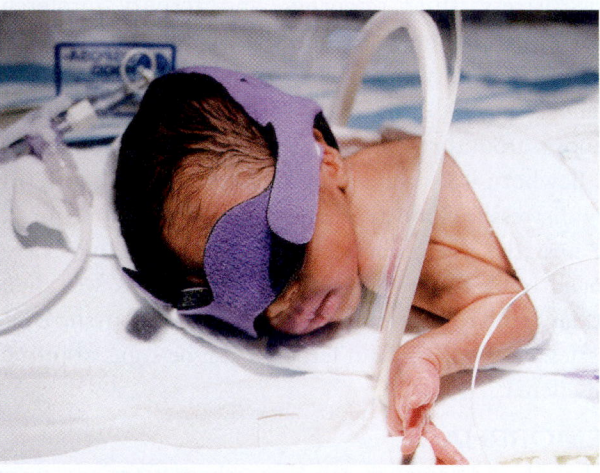

B

Figure 9-39. ■ Phototherapy for hyperbilirubinemia (jaundice). Bilateral eye patches are always used to protect the infant's eyes. (**A**) Newborn on fiberoptic "bili" mattress and under phototherapy lights. A combination of fiberoptic light source mattress and standard phototherapy light source may also be used. (*Note:* The color is distorted because of the reflection of the bililight mattress.) (**B**) Infant receiving phototherapy. The phototherapy light is positioned over the incubator. (**B:** Courtesy of Lisa Smith-Pedersen, RNC, MSN, NNP.)

cause of pathologic jaundice is Rh incompatibility. (You recall that Rh-positive blood contains the Rh protein on the RBC, and Rh-negative blood is missing this protein. If Rh-positive and Rh-negative blood are mixed together in the mother, the Rh-negative blood develops antibodies against the Rh-positive protein. During any future pregnancies with an Rh-positive fetus, the mother's Rh-negative blood will destroy the fetal blood. The destruction of fetal RBCs results in hyperbilirubinemia and pathologic jaundice.) Because the destruction of RBCs occurs before delivery, the newborn exhibits jaundice within the first 24 hours after delivery. The newborn is anemic at birth and has difficulty oxygenating the tissues.

Hyperbilirubinemia may be treated with **phototherapy** (exposure of the newborn to high-intensity light), exchange transfusion, or drug therapy. Figure 9-39 ■ illustrates two

types of phototherapy equipment. If pathologic jaundice is left untreated, the newborn may experience mental delays, congestive heart failure, and death. In the NICU, the newborn may be given blood transfusions of compatible blood until the RBC destruction stops. This condition can be prevented by administering RhoGAM to the Rh-negative mother during pregnancy and again following delivery (see Table 8-6).

RESPIRATORY CONDITIONS

Congenital anomalies that affect the respiratory system commonly involve the esophagus. These anomalies are introduced under gastrointestinal conditions.

The premature newborn's lungs are not fully ready to begin the function of breathing and gas exchange. The premature newborn is unable to produce adequate amounts of *surfactant*, the chemical required to maintain the patency of the alveoli. The collapsed alveoli are unable to exchange oxygen and carbon dioxide. The newborn becomes hypoxic, breathes faster, depletes the energy stores, and develops respiratory distress. To prevent death, the newborn is placed on mechanical ventilation (see Figure 9-36A). However, mechanical ventilation and high oxygen concentration can further damage the alveoli, resulting in permanent lung disease or **bronchopulmonary dysplasia** (BPD).

The passage of meconium by the fetus is a common occurrence in response to hypoxia or stress during the pregnancy. During delivery, the newborn can inhale the amniotic fluid containing meconium **(meconium aspiration)**. Severe meconium aspiration increases the possibility that the newborn will develop persistent pulmonary hypertension, pneumothorax, and pneumonia.

NEUROLOGIC CONDITIONS

Neurologic conditions are very serious and require long-term care. They include congenital anomalies, birth trauma, and acquired deficits.

CONGENITAL DEFECTS

Two congenital defects are introduced here. **Spina bifida** is an incomplete closure of the vertebra and neural tube. Larger defects include **meningocele** (a herniation of the meninges through the vertebral defect) or **meningomyelocele** (a herniation of the spinal nerves and the meninges through the vertebral defect). Although the defect can be found anywhere along the spinal column, the most common area is in the lumbosacral region (see Figure 16-8). The outer covering of the defect may be skin or, at times, the transparent, fragile meninges. It is critical to protect the tissue until surgical correction can be completed. Postoperatively, the infant is observed closely for signs of infection, bowel and bladder function, and movement of extremities. Prognosis is variable, depending on the location and severity of the defect. Chapter 16 ⊂⊃ discusses neurologic defects in more detail.

Hydrocephalus

Hydrocephalus results from increased production, decreased absorption, or blockage of the flow of cerebrospinal fluid. Blockage can be caused by a variety of pathologies, including tumors, cysts, or malformations. At times, hydrocephalus is obvious at birth, but more commonly it develops over time. The classic symptoms include head circumference greater than normal, with the forehead and top of the head being out of proportion to the face. The anterior fontanel bulges as intracranial pressure increases. Surgical placement of a ventriculoperitoneal shunt (see Figure 16-9B ⊂⊃) might be necessary to relieve the increasing intracranial pressure.

Chromosomal Abnormalities

Chromosomal abnormalities can result in congenital anomalies, as well as a decrease in mental and physical functioning. **Down syndrome,** the most common chromosomal abnormality, results from **trisomy 21** (three chromosomes at position 21). (See Figure 4-2C ⊂⊃.) Classic signs of Down syndrome include *microcephaly* (small head), wide short neck, epicanthal folds, and short broad hands with a simian line. There is also an increased incidence of congenital heart defects, diabetes, and hearing loss. The degree of mental retardation is not evident at birth. Down syndrome alone would not necessitate keeping the newborn in the NICU. The newborn with Down syndrome may be hospitalized for some time after birth to allow time for the parents to adjust to the diagnosis and to learn any special care that might be necessary.

Fetal Alcohol Syndrome

Fetal alcohol syndrome (FAS) is a series of malformations found in infants whose mother drank large quantities of alcohol during pregnancy. Facial anomalies, microcephaly, CNS dysfunction, mental retardation, and hyperactivity are common with FAS. (See Chapter 27 ⊂⊃ and Figure 27-5 ⊂⊃.)

GASTROINTESTINAL CONDITIONS

Gastrointestinal conditions are usually the result of congenital defects or immaturity of the organs and surrounding structures.

Congenital Anomalies

Defects of the gastrointestinal system are the most common of the congenital defects. They require surgical correction but are usually not immediately life threatening. However, aspiration, malnutrition, and obstruction could result if detection and correction are not made in a timely manner. For an understanding of these defects, it is important to review the normal structure of the entire gastrointestinal system (see Chapter 22 ⊂⊃).

CLEFT LIP AND PALATE. **Cleft palate** results from failure of the medial nasal and maxillary processes to join, leaving an opening between the roof of the mouth and the floor of the nasal passage. **Cleft lip** results from failure of the upper lip to join medially. Cleft lip can be unilateral or bilateral. Clefts could be complete (through bone and tissue) or partial (involving the bone structure but not the overlying mucous membrane). Cleft lip and cleft palate commonly occur together but can be found separately (see Figure 22-3 ⊂⊃).

The newborn infant will have feeding problems. The infant with a cleft lip will have difficulty making a seal around the nipple. With a cleft palate, the infant will be unable to compress the nipple between the tongue and the palate. The result will be an ineffective suck. With cleft palate, the feeding leaks into the nasal cavity, where it can drain from the nose and not be ingested. Some food can pool in the nasal passage, increasing the risk of sinus and ear infections. Also, some of the feeding may drain down the back of the throat without coordinated swallowing, putting the infant at risk for choking.

The psychological impact on the family is a concern. Families naturally anticipate the arrival of a "pretty" baby. When the infant has a cosmetic defect, the family experiences grief. Even after surgical correction of the cleft lip, the child will still have permanent scarring and some degree of cosmetic defect.

ESOPHAGEAL ATRESIA AND TRACHEOESOPHAGEAL FISTULA. Esophageal atresia and tracheoesophageal fistula are potentially life-threatening defects (see Figure 22-4 ⊂⊃). They may be found separately but are most commonly found together. In **esophageal atresia,** the esophagus ends in a blind pouch before reaching the stomach. **Tracheoesophageal fistula** is a connection between the trachea and esophagus.

The infant with esophageal atresia and tracheoesophageal fistula presents with copious amounts of thin mucus shortly after birth. The secretions clear with suctioning, but they soon reappear. If a tracheoesophageal fistula is present, the stomach may become distended with trapped air. If the defects are not identified prior to feeding, the infant will regurgitate the feeding, or the feeding will be aspirated into the lungs. Severe respiratory distress occurs, and aspiration pneumonia may develop.

In the absence of other anomalies, surgical repair is usually completed in the first few days of life. If other anomalies are present, gastrostomy feedings may be necessary until the infant is stabilized.

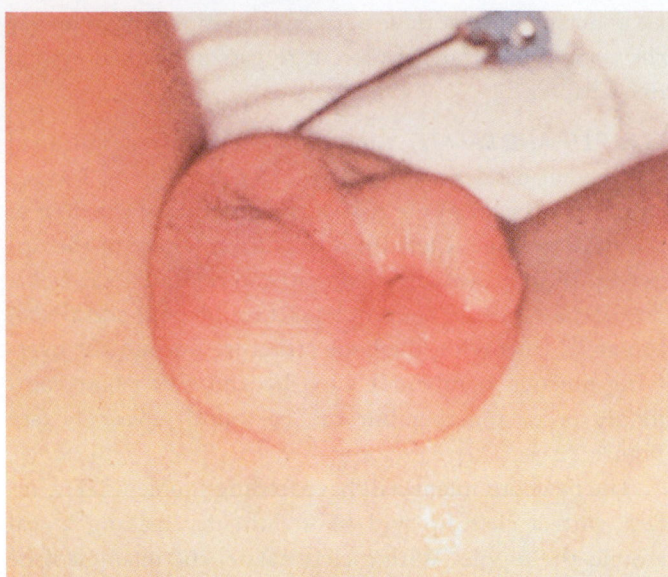

Figure 9-40. ■ Imperforate anus is often obvious at birth. It can range from mild stenosis to a complex syndrome associated with other congenital anomalies.

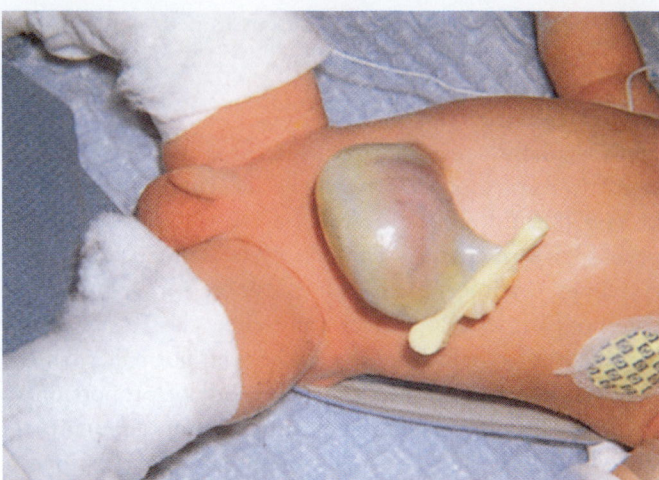

Figure 9-41. ■ In omphalocele, the size of the sac depends on the extent of the protrusion of abdominal contents through the umbilical cord. (Reprinted, with permission, from McGraw-Hill Companies, Inc. Rudolph, A. M., Hoffman, J. L. E., & Rudolph, C. D. [Eds.]. [1991]. *Rudolph's pediatrics* [19th ed.]. Stamford, CT: Appleton & Lange, p. 1040.)

IMPERFORATE ANUS. During fetal development, a pit, forming in the perineum, becomes the outer anal opening. The colon forms and gradually approaches the anal pit, and the connecting tissue breaks down, allowing the colon to open to the outside. **Imperforate anus** results when the connecting tissue fails to break down and the opening of the colon does not develop (Figure 9-40 ■).

Most commonly, there is obvious malformation of the perineum. At times, a thin membrane can be seen covering the anus. At other times, the anus is flat or appears as a deep dimple. Anomalies of the urinary system are commonly present at the same time. If meconium is present in the urine, a fistula has developed.

OMPHALOCELE. **Omphalocele** is a congenital malformation of the abdominal wall allowing the abdominal contents to herniate into the umbilical cord (Figure 9-41 ■). There is generally a thin translucent sac (peritoneum) covering the abdominal organs. The size of the sac varies, depending on the degree of defect. Small defects may be repaired with good prognosis. Large defects may result in long-term gastrointestinal disorders.

PYLORIC STENOSIS. **Pyloric stenosis** is a progressive hypertrophy of the pyloric sphincter resulting in obstruction (see Figure 22-12 ◑). The newborn appears healthy but has increased regurgitation after eating. As the obstruction worsens, projectile vomiting ensues, leading to dehydration, weight loss, and electrolyte imbalance. Surgical correction is the treatment of choice.

HERNIA. **Hernia** is a protrusion of intestines through a weakness in the abdominal or pelvic muscles. The two most common hernias in the newborn are umbilical hernia (Figure 9-42 ■) and inguinal hernia, both of which can be corrected surgically (see Chapter 22 ◑).

GENITOURINARY CONDITIONS

Genitourinary conditions of the newborn are usually caused by congenital defects. Commonly, there is a malformation of the lower urinary system, the gastrointestinal system, and the reproductive system. The first concern is to determine whether the infant is able to urinate. If not, intervention is more immediate.

Urethral Malposition (Hypospadias or Epispadias)

Hypospadias occurs when the urethra opens on the ventral (lower) surface of the penis. **Epispadias** occurs when the urethra opens on the dorsal (upper) surface of the penis

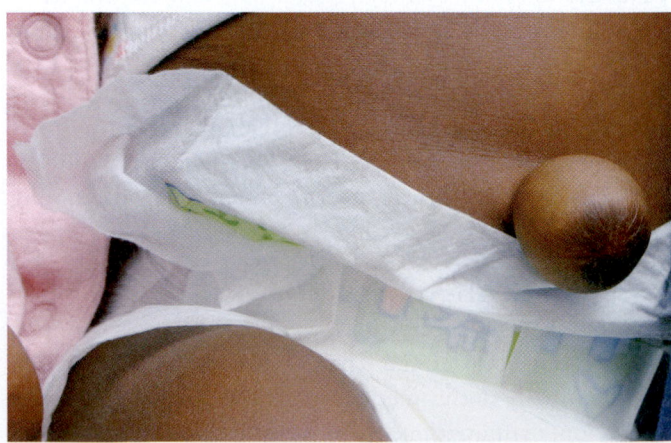

Figure 9-42. ■ Umbilical hernia.

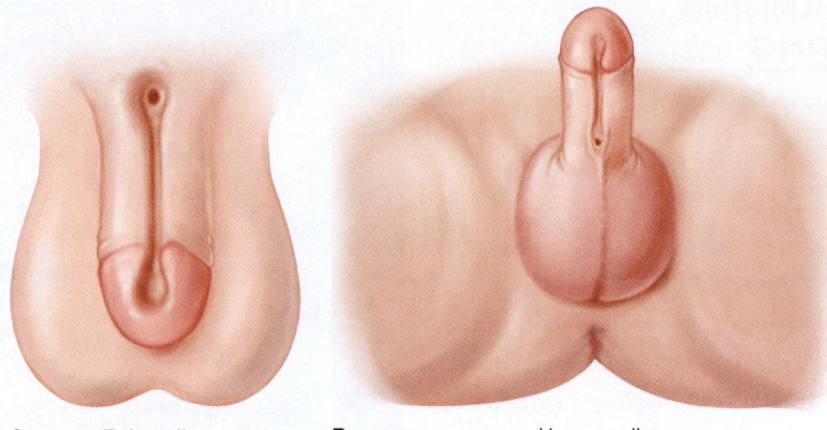

A   Epispadias   **B**   Hypospadias

Figure 9-43. ■ Hypospadias and epispadias. (**A**) In hypospadias, the urethral canal is open on the ventral surface of the penis. (**B**) In epispadias, the canal is open on the dorsal surface.

(Figure 9-43 ■). The opening can be found anywhere along the shaft of the penis. If the urethral opening is on the glans, surgical correction may not be needed. If the urethral opening is well down the shaft of the penis, surgical correction may need to be done in stages.

Phimosis

Phimosis occurs when the opening of the foreskin is small and unable to be retracted over the glans. The primary concern is the adequacy of the urinary stream. In most cases, circumcision is performed to alleviate the problem.

Ambiguous Genitalia

Ambiguous genitalia is a rare condition in which determining the gender of the infant is difficult (Figure 9-44 ■). In this circumstance, chromosomal analysis may be necessary to determine the gender of the infant. Not only is the reproductive system affected, but in many cases, the urinary and in-

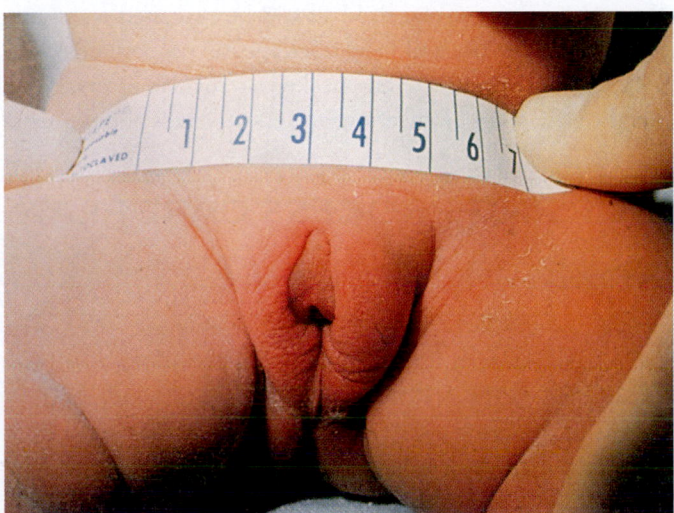

Figure 9-44. ■ Newborn girl with ambiguous genitalia. (Courtesy of Patrick C. Walsh, MD.)

testinal systems are also affected. Surgical reconstruction is usually done in stages, with the primary goal being normal functioning of the urinary and intestinal systems. Depending on the degree of defect, reproductive function may be lost.

Exstrophy of the Bladder

Exstrophy of the bladder (see Figure 23-3 ⚭) is a rare condition in which the abdominal wall fails to fuse, allowing the urinary bladder to protrude to the outside. Other genitourinary abnormalities are associated with exstrophy of the bladder.

NURSING CARE

PRIORITIES IN NURSING CARE

The priorities of nursing care for the high-risk newborn are similar to those for the normal newborn, but the method in which the needs are met may be different. Priorities are:

- Maintaining the airway, breathing, and circulation
- Maintaining body temperature
- Providing nutrition
- Ensuring elimination
- Teaching parents to provide care for their newborn.

ASSESSING

The high-risk newborn requires a more frequent and in-depth assessment than the normal newborn. The high-risk newborn may have equipment such as a heart monitor, a mechanical ventilator, or a feeding tube. The nurse must ensure that the equipment is functioning properly. The high-risk newborn may have had surgery to correct a congenital anomaly, or he or she may have infections or other conditions that require assessment and monitoring. Parents and family members require assessment information and support in the care of their high-risk newborn.

DIAGNOSING, PLANNING, AND IMPLEMENTING

Nursing diagnoses might include:

- Ineffective Airway Clearance
- Risk for Infection
- Risk for Impaired Skin Integrity
- Deficient Knowledge related to specific disorder, medical equipment, or care of the high-risk newborn.

Nursing care might include these and other interventions:

- Suction the airway as needed. *The premature or high-risk newborn may be unable to clear the airway, resulting in hypoxia.*
- Monitor for respiratory distress (Box 9-4 ■). *The high-risk newborn's condition is less stable and can change quickly.*
- Prevent and/or treat infection. *The high-risk newborn may undergo invasive procedures and may have puncture sites or open areas that can become infected. If an infection exists, treatment must be provided to prevent worsening of the condition.*
- Provide skin care, including bathing, turning, and protecting the skin under tape/monitor electrodes, etc. *The skin of the high-risk newborn is thin and fragile. Monitor elec-*

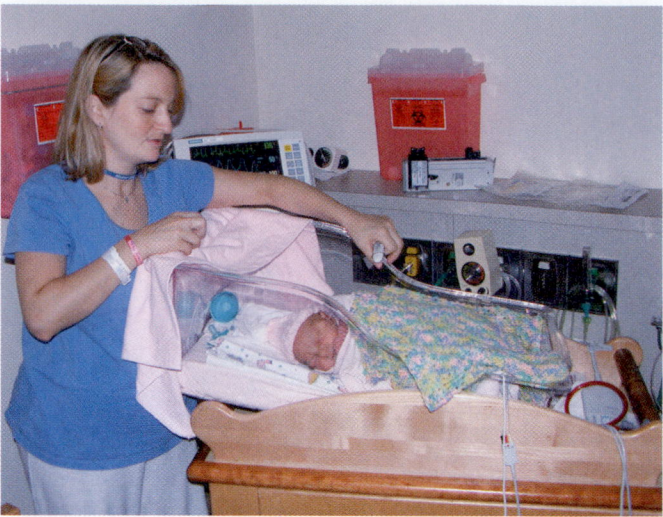

Figure 9-45. ■ It is important to allow new mothers to assist in the care of infants in the NICU as much as possible. This reduces parental anxiety and helps establish bonding. (M. C. Schlacter Photography.)

trodes, IV lines, and dressings are taped to the skin. Care must be taken to prevent skin breakdown.

- Give parents knowledge and support to make the best decisions about the care of their newborn. *By understanding the specific disorder, the parents can make informed decisions. Parents can provide some of the necessary care in the NICU with instruction and support from the nurse* (Figure 9-45 ■).
- Model acceptance and loving response of the newborn who appears different. *Parents may be uneasy about touching and caring for a baby who is not cosmetically normal or who is premature. The nurse's modeling of loving behaviors and good caring skills will help the parents adjust and begin to cope.*

EVALUATING

Parents' reactions to the child should be evaluated on an ongoing basis. Parents will need teaching and support along the way. The infant should be checked at regular intervals for weight gain, signs of infection, and effectiveness of treatment.

NURSING PROCESS CARE PLAN
Care of the Preoperative Newborn with a Congenital Heart Defect

Jeremy, 24 hours old, has been transferred from a small rural hospital to the NICU of a major medical center with a diagnosis of aortic stenosis. Jeremy is breathing room air with minimal respiratory distress. His condition is stable, and he is scheduled for surgery within the next few days. His parents are asking questions regarding his care and prognosis.

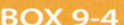

BOX 9-4	ASSESSMENT

Newborn Distress

In assessing the infant, the nurse would monitor for these manifestations of newborn distress:

- Increased respiratory rate (more than 60/minute) or difficult respirations
- Sternal retractions
- Nasal flaring
- Grunting
- Excessive mucus
- Facial grimacing
- Cyanosis (central: skin, lips, tongue)
- Abdominal distension or mass
- Vomiting of bile-stained material
- Absence of meconium elimination within 24 hours of birth
- Absence of urine elimination within 24 hours of birth
- Jaundice of the skin within 24 hours of birth or due to hemolytic process
- Temperature instability (hypothermia or hyperthermia)
- Jitteriness or blood glucose less than 40 mg%

(Data from Olds, S. B., London, M. L., Ladewig, P. A. W., Davidson, M. R. [2004]. *Maternal-newborn nursing & women's health care.* [7th ed.]. Upper Saddle River, NJ: Prentice Hall; Sherwen, L. N., Scoloveno, M. A., Weingarten, C. T. *Maternity nursing care of the childbearing family.* [3rd ed.]. Stamford, CT: Appleton & Lange; Tappero, E. P., & Honeyfield, M. E. [1996]. *Physical assessment of the newborn* [2nd ed.]. Petaluma, CA: NICU Ink.)

Assessment
- Jeremy is breathing on his own.
- There are no signs of respiratory distress.
- Parents are asking questions regarding pre- and postoperative care.

Nursing Diagnosis. The following important nursing diagnosis (among others) is established for this client:

> Deficient Knowledge related to preoperative and postoperative care of the newborn following heart surgery

Expected Outcomes. The parents will have an adequate knowledge base concerning aortic stenosis, as well as the upcoming surgical procedure and care, as evidenced by their ability to state information correctly.

Planning and Implementation
- Reinforce information on aortic stenosis presented by physician. Obtain pictures to increase parents' understanding of the condition and possible complications.
- Provide information regarding the expected medical equipment to be used in the postoperative period, including mechanical ventilator, heart monitoring equipment, and chest tubes.
- Correct any misinformation.
- Repeat teaching as needed.

Evaluation
- Parents verbalize understanding of aortic stenosis and related complications.
- Parents verbalize understanding of medical equipment that may be used postoperatively.

Critical Thinking in the Nursing Process

1. What are some other topics that should be discussed with Jeremy's parents before surgery?
2. What topics should the nurse plan to discuss with Jeremy's parents before discharge?
3. What is the role of the LPN/LVN in providing care to the NICU client and family?

Note: Discussion of Critical Thinking questions appears in Appendix I.

Note: The references and resources for this and all chapters have been compiled at the back of the book.

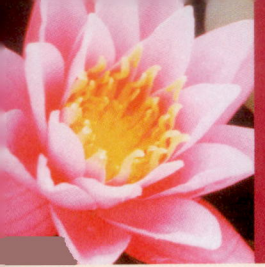

KEY TERMS by Topic

Use the audio glossary feature of either the CD-ROM or the Companion Website to hear the correct pronunciation of the following key terms.

Introduction
newborn

Physiologic Adaptation
cold stress, nonshivering thermogenesis

Gestational Age
scarf sign

Characteristics of the Newborn
acrocyanosis, ecchymosis, petechiae, jaundice, Mongolian spot, telangiectactic nevi, stork bites, milia, erythema toxicum neonatorum, caput succedaneum, cephalhematoma, strabismus, Epstein's pearls, witches' milk, nasal flaring, expiratory grunting, retractions, suprasternal, substernal, supraclavicular, intercostal, subcostal, apneic spells, pseudomenstruation, smegma, webbing, syndactyly, polydactyly

Reflexes
rooting reflex, sucking reflex, palmar grasp reflex, plantar grasp reflex, Babinski reflex, stepping reflex, tonic neck reflex, Moro reflex, startle reflex

Nursery Care
ophthalmia neonatorum

Common Nursery Procedures
circumcision

Common Conditions Affecting the High-Risk Newborn
circumoral, intraventricular hemorrhage, hyperbilirubinemia, phototherapy, bronchopulmonary dysplasia, meconium aspiration, spina bifida, meningocele, meningomyelocele, Down syndrome, trisomy 21, fetal alcohol syndrome (FAS), cleft palate, cleft lip, esophageal atresia, tracheoesophageal fistula, imperforate anus, omphalocele, pyloric stenosis, hernia, hypospadias, epispadias, phimosis, ambiguous genitalia, exstrophy of the bladder

KEY Points

- Most infants are born without complications and require routine care.
- The LPN/LVN must know the normal appearance and reflexes of the newborn, and report deviations to the supervising nurse or physician.
- Common neonatal conditions, including SGA or LGA and drug addiction, require additional data collection and treatment.

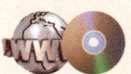

EXPLORE MediaLink

Additional interactive resources for this chapter can be found on the Companion Website at www.prenhall.com/towle.

Click on Chapter 9 and "Begin" to select the activities for this chapter.

For chapter-related NCLEX-style questions and an audio glossary, access the accompanying CD-ROM in this book.

Animations

Cord care to a newborn's cord stump

Breastfeeding and first foods

Circumcision

Applying umbilical cord alarm system

Congenital heart defects

FOR FURTHER Study

Figure 4-2C illustrates changes seen in Down syndrome; Figure 4-17 shows the influence of hormones on milk production.

The pregnant woman's nutritional needs are discussed in Chapter 6.

Hemolytic disease of the newborn is discussed briefly in Chapter 7 and more thoroughly in Chapter 8.

Physiologic adaptation to life outside the uterus is discussed in Chapter 7; the Apgar test is shown in Table 7-5; molding is illustrated in Figure 7-12; Figure 7-27 shows newborn measurements; Figure 7-28A shows a neonatal identification band.

Table 8-6 details infections that can be transmitted at birth.

Figure 13-12 provides a pain rating scale for infants.

Immunization schedules and safety issues are provided in Chapter 12.

Chapter 16 discusses neurologic defects in more detail; Figure 16-8 shows some spinal defects; Figure 16-9B shows a shunt used to treat hydrocephalus.

Musculoskeletal disorders are discussed in Chapter 17.

A discussion of the normal heart and heart defects or disorders is found in Chapter 19.

Phenylketonuria (PKU) is also discussed in Chapter 20.

Normal anatomy, congenital anomalies, and disorders of the gastrointestinal tract are discussed in Chapter 22.

Phimosis is also discussed in Chapter 23; bladder exstrophy is shown in Figure 23-3.

Fetal alcohol syndrome (FAS) is discussed in Chapter 27; effects are shown in Figure 27-5.

Appendix II provides a full set of growth charts for infants and children.

Caring for Infant with Depressed CNS

NCLEX® Focus Area: Physiologic Adaptation

Case Study: Timothy was born 1½ hours ago following a long difficult labor and delivery. His mother received a total of five doses of morphine sulfate during labor, with the most recent dose 30 minutes before delivery. He has been admitted to the newborn nursery for continued care.

Nursing Diagnosis: Ineffective Breathing Pattern related to mother receiving morphine sulfate

COLLECT DATA

Subjective	Objective
_____	_____
_____	_____
_____	_____
_____	_____
_____	_____
_____	_____
_____	_____

Would you report this? Yes/No

If yes, to: _____

Nursing Care

_____
_____
_____
_____
_____
_____
_____
_____
_____
_____
_____

How would you document this? _____
_____
_____
_____

Compare your documentation to the sample provided in Appendix I.

Data Collected
(use those that apply)

- Respiration 64/minute
- Mother received morphine sulfate 2 hours ago
- Apgar score 10
- Flaring nostrils
- Color pink
- Temperature 97.2°F (36.2°C)
- Crying
- Grunting respirations
- Passed large meconium stool

Nursing Interventions
(use those that apply; list in priority order)

- Bathe with antimicrobial soap.
- Start oxygen per nasal catheter.
- Place under radiant warmer.
- Administer Narcan (naloxone hydrochloride).
- Take to mother for feeding.
- Suction airway.
- Apply pulse oximeter.
- Monitor vital signs every hour.
- Place under bilirubin light.

NCLEX-PN® Exam Preparation

1 The mother of 1-month-old Jason tells the nurse that she props the baby's bottle on pillows because he wiggles so much. The best response from the nurse would be:

1. "It is probably a good idea to prop the bottle until you feel more comfortable holding him."
2. "It is not a good idea because he could choke on the formula."
3. "You need to hold the baby when you are feeding him."
4. "Are you afraid of dropping him?"

2 Routine newborn care includes the administering of antibiotic ointment or drops into the infant's eyes to prevent _____ and _____ infection.

3 The respirations of the normal newborn will be in a _____ pattern at the rate of _____ to _____ breaths per minute.

4 Two days after birth, a newborn in the nursery appears jaundiced. The LPN should:

1. report this to the nurse in charge because it indicates a liver malfunction.
2. document the finding but not report this normal condition.
3. report this to the nurse in charge because it indicates ABO and Rh incompatability.
4. document the finding but wait another 24 hours before reporting it.

5 A new mother examines her infant and says, "Look, her hands and feet are blue. I know there must be something wrong with her." The best response should be:

1. "Blue hands and feet are normal in newborns. It could last a few days."
2. "You are correct, there must be something wrong. I'll call the doctor right away."
3. "Your baby is cold. We need to wrap her in warm blankets."
4. "This must be birth trauma. I will let the charge nurse know."

6 Seeing his son, who was born with spina bifida, for the first time, a father exclaims, "What is that on his back!" An appropriate response would be:

1. a complete description of the condition, including long-term complications.
2. "That is spina bifida. Your son's spinal column did not fuse completely before birth."
3. conversation that would direct his attention away from the defect.
4. "I don't know. I'll have the doctor call you."

7 Shortly after delivery, the mother asks how she will know if the baby is having problems breathing. The best response would be:

1. "He will not cry and will begin to turn blue."
2. "His nostrils will flare out, he will grunt, and the skin over his ribs will sink in."
3. "You won't; he will just stop breathing."
4. "His respirations will become irregular and be more than 30 per minute."

8 Kathy, a new mother, is learning to breastfeed before she leaves the hospital. Kathy demonstrates correct breastfeeding technique when she:

1. has the baby take only the nipple in his mouth.
2. nurses on one side at each feeding.
3. has the baby take as much of the areola as possible into his mouth.
4. nurses for 20 minutes on each side.

9 A new mother needs further teaching in regard to circumcision care when she states:

1. "I will clean the penis with alcohol three times a day."
2. "If the penis becomes red and swollen, I will call the doctor."
3. "The Plastibell will fall off by itself, so I don't need to do anything with it."
4. "If I see bleeding, I will apply pressure until it stops."

10 Peter was born with developmental dysplasia of the hip. His father states, "I am glad we will only have to triple diaper Peter for a few days. They look so uncomfortable." The nurse should reply:

1. "What did the doctor tell you about Peter's hip problem?"
2. "You are wrong. Peter will have to have triple diapers for 3 to 4 months."
3. "You are right. Peter will only need triple diapers for a few days."
4. "Triple diapers are uncomfortable, so you will need to medicate Peter every 4 hours."

Answers for Review Questions, as well as discussion of Care Plan and Critical Thinking Care Map questions, appear in Appendix I.

Chapter 10

Health Promotion in the Postpartum Period

BRIEF Outline

Physical Changes
Psychological Changes
Fathers, Siblings, and Others

Cultural Influences in the Postpartum Period
Nursing Care

LEARNING Outcomes

After completing this chapter, you will be able to:

- Describe physical changes in the mother during the postpartum period.
- Discuss psychological changes in the mother during the postpartum period.
- Discuss important aspects of postpartum assessment and nursing care.
- Describe the complications commonly seen during the postpartum period.
- Discuss topics for client teaching about self-care in the postpartum period.
- Discuss client teaching about warning signs in infants in the postpartum period.

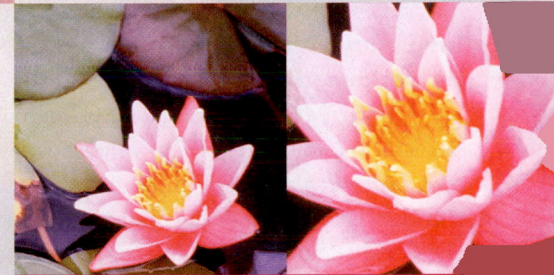

HEALTH PROMOTION ISSUE:
Pregnant 15-Year-Old Giving Child Up for Adoption

NURSING PROCESS CARE PLAN: Client at Risk for Deep Vein Thrombosis

CRITICAL THINKING CARE MAP: Caring for a Client at Risk

The **puerperium** or **postpartum** period begins immediately after the birth of the baby and continues for 6 weeks, or until the woman's body has nearly returned to a prepregnant state. This chapter describes the physiologic and psychological changes that occur during the postpartum period and the nursing care of the new mother.

Physical Changes

Every body system undergoes changes during pregnancy. Following delivery, the body systems must change again and return to the nonpregnant state. Some of these changes are noticeable, whereas others are subtle.

REPRODUCTIVE SYSTEM

Uterus

The return of the uterus to the nonpregnant state is called **involution.** When the placenta separates from the uterus, the **decidua** (tissue that lines the uterine wall during pregnancy) is irregular in thickness. Over the next 3 weeks, the decidua separates from the innermost layer of the uterus (the *endometrium;* see Figure 4-12 ⬭⬭) and is expelled through the vagina. This discarded blood, mucus, and tissue is called **lochia.** The placenta attachment site contains large blood vessels. Bleeding from these vessels is controlled by contraction of the *myometrium* (muscle fibers of the uterus). The placenta attachment site heals by **exfoliation** (a shedding of the outer layer) instead of by scar formation, which would prevent uterine attachment of future pregnancies. During exfoliation, the endometrium grows from the margins and from the basal layer under the site. The superficial tissue becomes necrotic and is sloughed off. This sloughing of tissue continues for approximately 4 weeks.

To control bleeding from the large vessels at the placenta site, the uterus must remain contracted, as evidenced by the fundus remaining very firm. If blood pools in the body of the uterus, it will clot, causing the uterus to enlarge, stopping contractions, and causing more bleeding. When the uterus stops contracting, the fundus becomes soft and spongy, which is termed **boggy.** If the fundus is boggy and located above the umbilicus, bleeding is suspected. If the fundus is boggy, the nurse should massage it in a circular manner to stimulate contractions. Clots can be expelled by pushing on the fundus (discussed later in this chapter). In many facilities, expelling clots from the uterus is an RN function. It is important for the LPN/LVN to know facility policy and to communicate closely with the charge nurse if the fundus does not remain firm or if excess bleeding is noted.

The ligaments supporting the uterus in the pelvic cavity stretch during pregnancy. A full bladder can easily push the

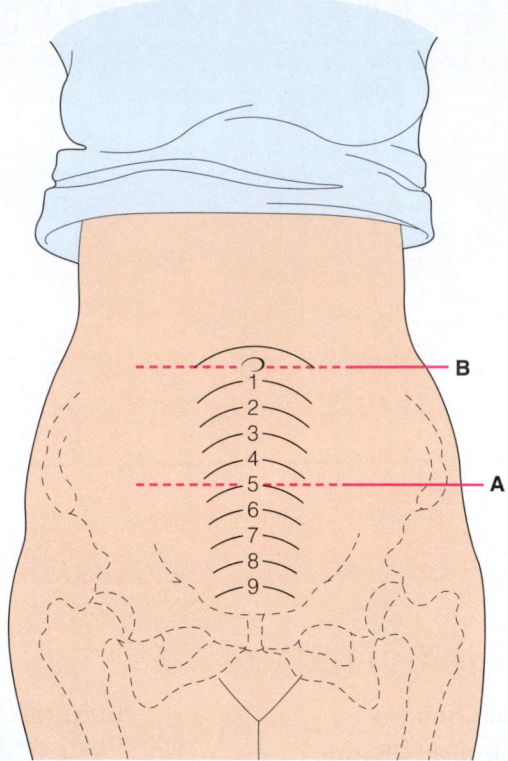

Figure 10-1. ■ Involution of the uterus. (**A**) Immediately after delivery of the placenta, the top of the fundus is in the midline and about halfway between the symphysis pubis and the umbilicus. (**B**) About 6 to 12 hours after birth, the fundus is at the level of the umbilicus. The height of the fundus then decreases about 1 fingerbreadth (about 1 cm) each day.

uterus up and to one side. When the fundus is higher than expected and deviated to the side, a full bladder is suspected. The displaced uterus stops contracting, leading to bleeding. To prevent excess bleeding, the nurse should teach the mother to keep the bladder empty.

The height of the fundus decreases approximately 1 centimeter per day until it is located below the symphysis pubis (Figure 10-1 ■). Factors that enhance involution of the uterus include an uncomplicated labor, complete expulsion of the placenta and membranes, breastfeeding, and early ambulation. Factors that slow involution include a full bladder, difficult birth, grand multipara, and retained placenta or membrane fragments.

As previously stated, lochia is the tissue and fluid expelled vaginally after delivery. The total amount of lochia shed from the uterus after birth is 240 to 270 mL.

Lochia is classified by its appearance.

■ **Lochia rubra** is dark red and contains epithelial cells, red blood cells, pieces of decidua, and sometimes meconium, lanugo, and vernix caseosa. It may contain small blood clots (quarter size or less), but large clots suggest the possibility of excessive bleeding and should be investigated. Approximately 3 days after delivery, the drainage changes.

- **Lochia serosa** is pinkish in color. Present from days 4 to 10, it contains serous exudate, red blood cells, mucus, and many bacteria. Gradually, the number of red blood cells decreases, again changing the color of the lochia.
- **Lochia alba** is a creamy white or pale yellow. It consists of the last pieces of decidua, white blood cells, mucus, and bacteria. Discharge of lochia alba continues for approximately 2 weeks. Once it stops, the cervix is considered to be closed, and the risk of an infection ascending from the vagina to the uterus is minimal.

It is common for an increase in lochia to be noted during or shortly after breastfeeding. Breast stimulation causes endogenous oxytocin to be released by the pituitary gland, stimulating uterine contractions and causing more lochia to be discharged.

Vagina

The vagina, cervix, and perineum appear swollen and bruised for approximately 1 week after delivery. The muscles of the vagina and perineum are flabby for several days but gradually regain tone. Kegel exercises, described in Chapter 6 ⬤⬤, help strengthen these muscles. The edges of an episiotomy or lacerations, sutured under the skin, should be well approximated. Occasionally, a **hematoma,** an accumulation of blood under the skin, is present. A hematoma may look like a bruise, feel like a solid mass in the tissues, and can be extremely painful when touched. The physician should be notified of changes in a hematoma or of any signs of infection. By 3 weeks, the tissue returns to a nonpregnant state, and lacerations heal.

Breasts

In preparation for lactation, the breasts begin secreting **colostrum** (a thin, yellowish fluid that is high in protein) a few weeks before or shortly after delivery. Even if the mother is not breastfeeding, the mammary glands begin to fill and the breasts become enlarged. After several days without the stimulation of nursing, the milk production stops and the breast tissue becomes soft. If the mother is breastfeeding, the breasts will become

engorged within 2 to 3 days. The breasts will cycle between empty and full but will remain firm until breastfeeding stops. (See Breastfeeding section of Chapter 9 ⬤⬤ for more details.)

Ovaries

The return of ovulation and menstruation varies with each individual. For most women, ovulation and menstruation resume in 2 to 3 months, but it may take as long as 6 months. For nursing mothers, this process is usually delayed.

MUSCULOSKELETAL SYSTEM

Abdominal Muscles

After delivery, the abdominal muscles appear flabby. It takes several months of exercise for them to regain tone. In the woman who had poor abdominal muscle tone before pregnancy or who had overdistention of the uterus, return of muscle tone may be delayed. The abdomen may remain flabby. Occasionally the abdominal muscle separates during pregnancy, resulting in **diastasis recti abdominis** (Figure 10-2 ■). If diastasis occurs, only skin, fat, and peritoneum support the abdominal contents. Inadequate support results

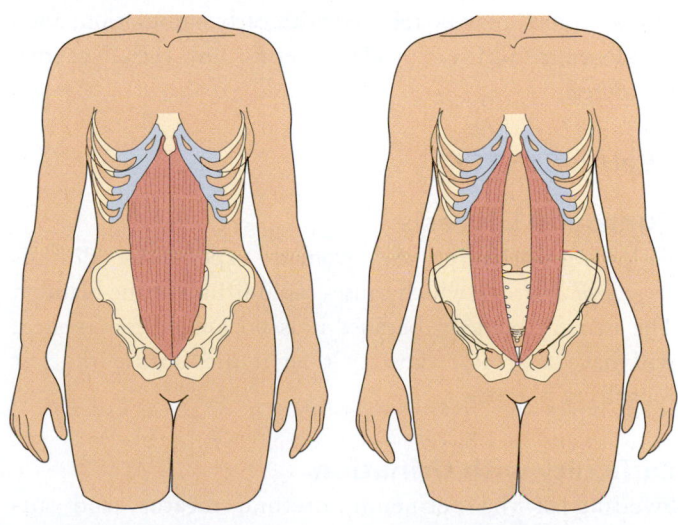

Normal location of rectus muscles of the abdomen

Diastasis recti: separation of the rectus muscles

Figure 10-2. ■ Diastasis recti abdominis, a separation of the abdominal musculature, commonly occurs after pregnancy.

in a pendulous abdomen and backache. Fortunately, diastasis responds well to abdominal exercise.

Pelvis

The cartilage supporting the joints of the pelvis stretches in the last months of pregnancy to allow more flexibility during delivery. The cartilage regains its firmness, but the diameter of the pelvis will never return to the nullipara state. The result is a widening of the hips.

GASTROINTESTINAL SYSTEM

Need to Replenish Energy

Following delivery, the woman may be hungry. She has expended a lot of energy during the delivery process, and a light meal can help replace the spent calories. She usually drinks a large amount of fluid to replace what was lost in labor.

Return of Peristalsis

Peristalsis has been sluggish during pregnancy due to the effects of progesterone and the pressure of the enlarged uterus. It will take several days for peristalsis to return to normal. The woman may be reluctant to strain to defecate due to fear of perineal pain or rupturing sutures. The nurse can teach that delaying a bowel movement may increase constipation. Therefore, stool softeners and a diet high in fiber plus adequate fluid may be advised to relieve or to prevent constipation.

Postcesarean Diet

Following a cesarean section delivery, the woman may be placed on a liquid diet until bowel sounds are present. Her diet will then be advanced quickly. Flatulence, which adds to discomfort, may be relieved with early ambulation, antiflatulence medication, or Harris return flow (HRF) enema, if ordered.

RENAL SYSTEM

Puerperal Diuresis

Following delivery, the woman experiences diuresis (*puerperal diuresis*), which causes rapid filling of the bladder. The urinary bladder, because it is no longer compressed, will have a greater capacity than it did during the last months of pregnancy.

Difficulty with Urination

Swelling of the perineum, urethral meatus, and surrounding structures may make urination difficult, especially if the woman has had an epidural. Also, there may be a decreased sensation of bladder filling due to tissue trauma and swelling. Together, these aspects put the woman at risk for overfilling, incomplete emptying, and urinary retention. As mentioned, a full bladder can increase uterine bleeding as well. Catheterization may be ordered to relieve discomfort and prevent increased uterine bleeding.

CARDIOVASCULAR SYSTEM

Temperature

Changes in the cardiovascular system following delivery can be seen in alterations in vital signs and blood values (see Table 6-3 ⊙⊙). During labor, the mother's temperature may have risen to 100.4°F (38°C) due to dehydration and physical exertion. Commonly, the mother begins to chill shortly after delivery. The *postpartal chill* is the result of body temperature being higher than the surrounding environment. It also results from neurologic and vasomotor changes during labor. Covering the woman with warm blankets may alleviate the chill and provide comfort. The temperature should return to normal after birth.

clinical ALERT

The postpartal woman should be afebrile 24 hours after delivery. If fever continues, infection should be suspected and the fever should be reported to the primary care provider.

Blood Pressure

The mother's blood pressure should remain stable following delivery. Commonly, the blood pressure rises slightly during labor and returns to the mother's baseline within 1 hour post delivery. Hypotension could indicate a reaction to medication or excessive bleeding. Hypertension, especially accompanied by headache, could indicate pregnancy-induced hypertension (PIH). If hypertension was a problem prior to labor, the blood pressure must be monitored frequently during the postpartum period.

Blood Values

Blood values should return to normal range during the postpartum period. During pregnancy, coagulation factors have been activated. Delivery trauma or decreased mobility may predispose the mother to **thrombosis** (formation of clots in blood vessels). The white blood cell count may temporarily rise to 25,000/mm^3, with granulocytes as the predominant cell type. The hemoglobin and hematocrit may be difficult to interpret in the first few days after delivery because of rapid changes in blood volume. Excessive blood loss is not suspected until the hematocrit decreases more than two percentage points from the level on admission to the labor unit.

Many women gain 25 to 30 pounds during the pregnancy. Figure 6-22 ⚭ shows how this weight gain is distributed. A woman who has gained this amount of weight during pregnancy may be able to return to prepregnancy weight during the postpartum period. She will lose 10 to 12 pounds during the birthing process. Another 5 pounds may be lost in the first few days due to puerperal diuresis. A woman who is physically active will have less difficulty with weight loss than a woman who is sedentary.

ENDOCRINE SYSTEM

Estrogen and Progesterone

Recall that one function of the placenta is to produce estrogen and progesterone to maintain the endometrium and to prevent ovulation during pregnancy. Following delivery of the placenta, the blood levels of estrogen and progesterone decline rapidly (see Table 6-3 ⚭). The decline of these hormones contributes to the sloughing of the decidua. The return of the menstrual cycle usually occurs 2 to 3 months after delivery. However, because ovulation precedes menstruation, the woman can become pregnant again before the first menses.

Prolactin

Stimulation of the breast increases the production of prolactin by the anterior pituitary gland (see Figure 4-17 ⚭). Prolactin is responsible for milk production by the lactiferous glands in the breast. Once lactation is well established, prolactin decreases.

Oxytocin

Oxytocin was discussed under changes in the reproductive system earlier in this chapter.

Psychological Changes

The woman needs time to adjust to the role of mother. This adjustment occurs in stages.

TAKING-IN STAGE

During the first day or two, the mother is said to be in the **taking-in stage.** She is "taking in" information about her baby, recalling the experience of delivery, and storing this information in her memory. The mother is tired and may depend on others to help meet her needs. She allows others to care for the baby, participating mainly in feeding the infant. She has a need to talk about her perception of the labor and delivery, and readily shares the experience with visitors.

TAKING-HOLD STAGE

By the third day after birth, the mother is usually ready to resume control. She is moving into the **taking-hold stage.**

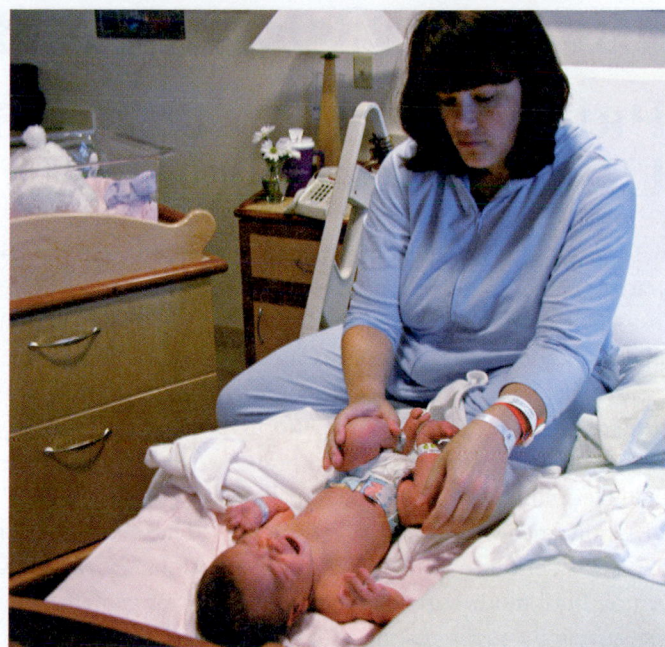

Figure 10-3. ■ As the woman takes hold of her new role, she will begin to perform care activities on the newborn. (M. C. Schlachter Photography.)

She is "taking hold" or control of the activities of caring for herself and her newborn (Figure 10-3 ■). She may become preoccupied with her bodily functions, such as elimination. If she is breastfeeding, she begins to be concerned about the quality and quantity of the milk. Although she is ready to meet her physical needs and the infant's needs, she may not be ready to resume responsibility for household activities. It may take several weeks for her to have the physical and mental energy to return to her full activities. In most cases, it takes 3 to 10 months for a woman to be comfortable with the role of mother.

Women and their partners discover that social interactions become increasingly important. The support of family and friends is important at this time. Mothers and fathers must learn to care for the infant and to make decisions about meeting the infant's needs. Obtaining information from others who have experienced parenthood is a valuable part of the normal adjustment process. Mothers who have little social interaction and support find the adjustment to motherhood more difficult.

ADOPTION

Emotional care of the mother is important for mothers who are giving their babies up for adoption. Even if a woman has decided that she does not want to keep her baby, she may still experience feelings of grief. The Health Promotion Issue on pages 306 and 307 explores this topic further.

(Text continues on p. 308.)

HEALTH PROMOTION ISSUE

PREGNANT 15-YEAR-OLD GIVING CHILD UP FOR ADOPTION

A 15-year-old female in your pediatric practice comes to the office with nausea (usually occurring in the morning), amenorrhea for the last 2 months, and breast tenderness. The nurse asks for a clean catch urine specimen and performs a rapid pregnancy test. The test is positive. Her mother asks if they can make an appointment for the following week to discuss her care and her plans for the future. Both mother and daughter are too distraught to discuss the issues today.

When they return the following week, both mother and daughter seem resigned to the pregnancy. They have discussed how they will handle the situation with the client's father, their minister, the father of the baby, and several family members. They want to pursue adoption but have some questions. Do they need to contact anyone during the pregnancy? Can they have some say in who adopts the baby? Will they ever be able to see the baby again or at least find out how the baby is doing? What does it cost to put your baby up for adoption?

DISCUSSION

Types of Adoptions

There are confidential and open adoptions. A *confidential adoption* is a legal arrangement whereby a child is placed with a family who has been screened by an agency. The adoptive family has background information on the birth mother, but the birth mother does not know the details of the adoptive couple. In an *open adoption,* both the birth mother and the adoptive family will have some degree of exposure to one another. The birth mother can review prospective adoptive families, without knowing their names. She makes a choice from these families and never has a face-to-face meeting. Another degree of exposure between the adoptive parties would be a telephone interview, in which first names are exchanged but, again, no face-to-face meeting occurs. The parties could also meet in the prenatal period or during the selection process. Continuing contact after birth can be arranged for in the open adoption agreement. Some birth mothers desire to see the child on special occasions or just to be allowed to send cards and letters to the child. For the birth mother to have a confidential adoption, an adoption agency must be selected. These agencies can be for profit, nonprofit, or sponsored by certain religions. Some agencies provide counseling to both the birth mother and other family members of her choosing. They may also provide medical and legal assistance.

Open adoptions are more typically handled by an attorney. Open adoptions are not legal in every state. Some states allow the adoptive parents to cover the legal fees for the birth mother. In the states where this is not allowable or if the adoptive parents are not willing to cover these expenses, the birth mother may need to apply for legal aid in her community.

There are several ways a birth mother can find families who want to adopt a child. Some families run advertisements in the newspaper. Local physicians may be able to refer families in their practice who want to adopt. Some communities have prospective adoptive parent support groups who would be able to provide a list of families desiring to adopt. Also the National Adoption Information Clearinghouse provides a matching service for parties interested in adoption.

PLANNING AND IMPLEMENTATION

The nurse should help the birth mother explore her desires for the child's life. The following questions would be appropriate: Is it important to you to have a say in who adopts your child? Will it matter what type of family the child lives with—a single parent, a

Source: Evan Johnson

nuclear family? It is okay with you if a homosexual couple adopts your child? Does the race of the family matter? Does the religion of the family matter? Do you think that the family should have substantial amounts of money? Do you desire for the child to have siblings? Would you rather the child live in the city or in the country? Do you have any medical history that it would be important to share with an adoptive family?

It is important for the nurse to determine the birth mother's motivation for deciding to put her child up for adoption. The following questions could assist in this process: Is anyone trying to coerce you, shame you, embarrass you, or provide you with a bribe to adopt your child? Is your decision solely based on your desires? The nurse should ask the birth mother who she has consulted with regarding her decision.

The nurse can assist the birth mother to understand the permanence of adoption. The long-term stability of the adoptive child is partly determined by the birth mother's decision to totally relinquish any control over the child's life. This is not to say that the birth mother may never contact her child later in life. Following a confidential adoption, records are not available to either party. There are, however, several agencies that provide a registry for birth parents and

the adoptee to gain contact information. The registries include Concerned United Birth Parents, American Adoption Congress, and the International Soundex Reunion Registry. For private adoptions, a letter containing contact information for the birth mother can be held by the attorney who handled the adoption. If the adoptee decides that he or she wants to contact the birth mother, the attorney can forward the letter to him or her.

When the birth mother makes a firm decision to put her baby up for adoption, the nurse can be instrumental in providing her with the necessary resources. Contact information for community adoption agencies and/or legal services can be provided. Referrals to support groups for birth mothers would provide emotional support for the teenage girl. If there are no support groups available, a counselor could provide this emotional support. The birth mother will experience a wide range of emotions. She may feel guilt, shame, sorrow, and grief. She may also feel relief. It is important for the nurse to include in the plan of care a mechanism for follow-up visits to monitor her emotional health. The nurse should assess the level of support available to the birth mother. Birth mothers should have someone they can rely on to give them support and encouragement when they experience doubt. The nurse can

encourage activities to assist the birth mother in dealing with her emotions. These activities could include journaling her thoughts, or creating a scrapbook of the pregnancy and birth experience. In 1990, Mary Jean Wolsh-Marsh created Birth Mother's Day to be celebrated on the Saturday before Mother's Day in May. Ms. Wolsh-Marsh wanted a day to commemorate the sacrifice of birth mothers who had lost a child to adoption. Birth mothers may find solace in this type of celebration.

The nurse can also assist the birth mother in making future plans for herself. The birth mother should be encouraged to express her hopes and dreams for the future. The nurse could be instrumental in helping the birth mother take action to make these dreams a reality.

SELF-REFLECTION

What are your feelings about teenage pregnancy? If your teenage daughter were pregnant, what would you counsel her to do? Why? Do you know anyone who grew up in an adoptive home? How would you characterize their life? What are the benefits of adoption to the pregnant woman? To the infant? What do you see as the negative aspects of adoption to the pregnant woman? To the infant?

SUGGESTED RESOURCES

For the Nurse

Narad, C. & Mason, P. (2004). International Adoption: Myths and realities. *Pediatric Nursing, 30*(6) 6. 483–487.

Salladay, S. (2004). Ethical Problems: Adoption dilemmas. *Nursing, 34*(12), 29.

For the Client

www.crisispregnancy.com This site includes a pregnancy workbook meant to aid the prospective birth mother in making an adoption decision.

Russell, M. (2004). *Adoption wisdom: A guide to the issues and feelings of adoption.* Santa Monica, CA: Broken Branch Productions.

POSTPARTUM BLUES

Postpartum blues are a transient period of mild depression that often occurs in the early postpartum period. This state may be manifested by tearfulness, feeling let down, and being unable to sleep. Postpartum blues usually begin on the third or fourth day post delivery and last for a week or two. They may be associated with changing hormone levels and psychological adjustment to motherhood. Fatigue, discomfort, and overstimulation may make postpartum blues worse. If postpartum blues persist or worsen, the woman must be evaluated for postpartum depression and postpartum psychosis. (See Chapter 8 🔗 for these high-risk complications.)

Attachment

During pregnancy, the woman begins to develop an emotional attachment to the infant. Personal characteristics of the mother affect the extent of attachment. For example, the woman with a high level of self-esteem enters motherhood with a more positive outlook than the mother who is depressed, angry about her situation, or overly anxious. The mother who has developed a level of trust in her own abilities will be confident in her ability to care for the infant. At the time of birth, each mother has developed an emotional attachment of some kind with the infant.

New mothers generally follow a regular pattern of behavior when meeting their infants for the first time. Touch usually begins with fingertip exploration of the infant's limbs, followed by palmar touch of the torso, and finally enfolding the infant with the entire hand and arms. As the mother spends more time with her infant, she positions the newborn so she can look into its eyes (Figure 10-4 ■). She uses her sense of sight, hearing, and touch to get to know her infant. She responds verbally to the sounds the newborn makes. She may make comments or have questions about the normality of the infant's features, especially if the delivery was difficult or if a previously delivered infant was not healthy. The mother's interest in and loving behaviors toward the newborn are part of the bonding process. **Bonding** is the establishment of a strong emotional attachment between two unique individuals.

Negative Feelings

The mother may have negative feelings about the baby. She may be disappointed about the baby's gender or angry that her lifestyle will need to change. Because mothers are "supposed to love their children," the mother may not express these negative feelings. If she does express them, the reaction of friends or family may be, "You don't mean that." The nurse must identify these blocks to therapeutic

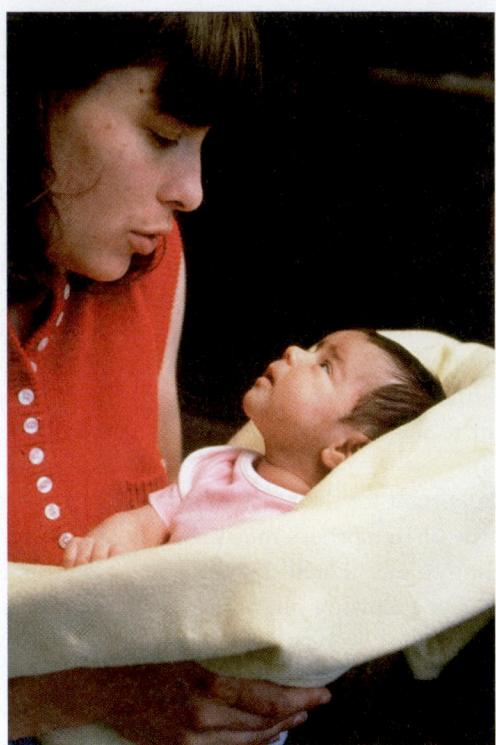

Figure 10-4. ■ Mother-child bonding is strengthened as infant and parent look into each other's eyes. (Elizabeth Crews/The Image Works.)

communication and help the mother and family explore the basis of the negative feelings. (Prolonged negative feelings and depression in the postpartum period are discussed in Chapter 8 🔗.)

Fathers, Siblings, and Others

Fathers, siblings, grandparents, and others also need time to bond with the infant. The father will express a strong attachment to the infant, similar to that of the mother (Figure 10-5 ■). He will demonstrate **engrossment** (a sense of

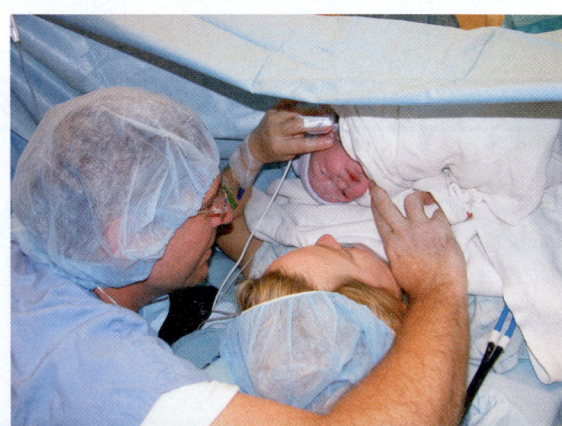

Figure 10-5. ■ The father's intense concentration shows engrossment in his new child. (M. C. Schlachter Photography.)

interest and preoccupation) by holding, maintaining eye contact with, and talking to the infant.

Siblings and grandparents are important members of the family who also need time to develop a bond with the infant. Each family member who has the opportunity to view, hold, and interact with the infant will begin to establish a relationship. With open visiting hours and rooming-in practices, family bonding can begin early.

Cultural Influences in the Postpartum Period

The mother's beliefs about hygiene, food choices, and activity during the postpartum period are influenced by her culture. Western culture places a great deal of emphasis on the birth process itself. Other cultures place more emphasis on postpartum practices. Many women of European heritage want to eat a full meal and drink plenty of cold fluids in the belief that they will replace the nutrients lost during the delivery process. They will want to shower right away, wash their hair, and put on a clean gown.

The women of Mexican, Asian, and African descent often avoid cold, including cold air, food, and drink. They may put off showering to prevent a chill.

Certain cultures teach choices that are meant to help the woman regain harmony or a balance between "hot and cold" within the body. They may avoid heat, including some foods that are considered "hot."

In most Native American cultures, family plays an important role during the postpartum period. The baby's grandmother is the primary helper and teacher for the new mother. She brings experience and knowledge, and allows the new mother time to rest and regain her strength. Some other areas of cultural beliefs and practices related to the postpartum period are provided in Box 10-1 ■.

BOX 10-1   CULTURAL PULSE POINTS

Beliefs and Practices Related to the Postpartum Period

Cultures may have taboos concerning reactions during labor, presence of men, position for delivery, preferred types of health practitioners, and location of the birth. A new mother may need to follow practices of her culture in the postpartum period related to bathing, cord care, exercise, foods, and roles of men. Some cultures even have specific practices related to care and disposal of the placenta.

Source: Ramont, R. P., Niedringhaus, D. M., & Towle, M. A. (2006). *Comprehensive nursing care.* Upper Saddle River, NJ: Prentice Hall, p. 1117.

If the mother's beliefs are different from those of the nurse, the physician, or hospital practices, adjustments may need to be made. It is the nurse's responsibility to advocate for the rights of the mother, father, and family.

NURSING CARE

PRIORITIES IN NURSING CARE

The nurse may use the mnemonic of BUBBLE to help remember important areas of assessment: **B**—breasts, **U**—uterus, **B**—bowel, **B**—bladder, **L**—lochia, **E**—episiotomy/incision.

The first priority for nursing care in the postpartum period is to assess for complications that may slow or prevent the mother from returning to the prepregnant state of health. Some complications may threaten the mother's life if they are not treated promptly.

The second priority is to teach the mother how to care for herself and her infant.

ASSESSING

The postpartum assessment begins by obtaining information about the pregnancy and delivery. This information is used to identify the risk of postpartum complications. Table 10-1 ■ identifies common risk factors and areas that must be included in the assessment. The greater the degree of risk, the more frequently the assessment must be made.

Many parts of the assessment are the same as for any other client. For example, monitoring vital signs and observing for an increase in bloody drainage is the same for the postpartum woman as it is for the postsurgical client. Listening to heart sounds, lung sounds, and bowel sounds is the same as for any other client. The LPN/LVN must know the normal findings in order to report abnormal readings to the charge nurse or physician. Only those parts of the assessment that are particular to the postpartum client will be included here. While performing the assessment, the nurse has an opportunity to teach the new mother about normal body changes and signs of complications.

Vital Signs

The vital signs should be assessed first. Vital signs were assessed every 15 minutes during the first hour after delivery. When the vital signs are stable and within normal range, the time interval between measurements is lengthened. Vital signs should be recorded every 30 minutes for an hour, every hour for 2 hours, every 2 hours for 4 hours, and then

MediaLink Postpartum assessment

TABLE 10-1

Postpartum Risk Factors and Areas of Assessment

RISK FACTOR	IMPLICATIONS	AREA TO ASSESS
Cesarean section birth	Risk for impaired healing Risk for paralytic ileus Risk for urinary retention	Incision pain every 2–4 hours Incision for infection and healing Bowel sounds, flatus every 2–4 hours Voiding after catheter removed
Prolonged labor	Risk for exhaustion Risk for nutrition and fluid depletion Risk for uterine atony and hemorrhage	Verbalizes adequate rest Intake, output, % of diet consumed Fundus firmness every 1–2 hours Amount of lochia every 1–2 hours Vital signs every 1–2 hours
Precipitous delivery	Risk for uterine atony, hemorrhage Risk for lacerations of birth canal	Fundus firmness every 1–2 hours Amount of lochia every 1–2 hours Vital signs every 1–2 hours
Delivery complications (retained placenta, lacerations)	Risk for lacerations of birth canal Risk for hemorrhage	Fundus firmness every 1–2 hours Amount of lochia every 1–2 hours Vital signs every 1–2 hours
Diabetes	Risk for insulin regulation Risk for periods of hyperglycemia and hypoglycemia Risk for poor wound healing	Obtain blood glucose readings every 2–4 hours Signs of hyper- and hypoglycemia Episiotomy or incision for healing
Pregnancy-induced hypertension (PIH)	Risk for neurologic and cardiovascular damage	Vital signs every 1–2 hours Reflexes and clonus every 1–2 hours Headache and blurred vision
Overdistended uterus (large fetus or multiple gestation)	Risk for uterine atony and hemorrhage	Fundus firmness every 1–2 hours Amount of lochia every 1–2 hours Vital signs every 1–2 hours

every 4 hours. By the second to third postpartum day, the vital signs can be taken once every 8 hours, as long as they have remained stable.

Abnormal findings direct the nurse to pay closer attention to other areas of the assessment. For example, if the temperature is elevated, the nurse should assess for other signs of infection. An elevated temperature coupled with premature or prolonged rupture of membranes prior to delivery may indicate a genital infection. Further assessment of the uterus and lochia may be indicated. A slight elevation in pulse is expected in the early postpartum period, but the pulse should return to a normal range within the first 24 hours. Tachycardia after 24 hours can indicate hemorrhage, so further assessment is needed. Tachypnea is also an indication of respiratory stress to the body and should be investigated.

The blood pressure should remain consistent with the baseline blood pressure during pregnancy. As excess body fluids are eliminated during the first few weeks postpartum, the blood pressure should return to the prepregnant state.

clinical ALERT

A marked elevation in blood pressure in the first 24 to 36 hours postpartum could be an indication of PIH and should be reported. If PIH occurred prior to delivery, the blood pressure should begin to decrease in the first few days postpartum.

Pain

Pain should decrease during the postpartum period. Any increases in pain or swelling of incisions should be reported promptly. There will be some discomfort as breasts fill. The nurse can teach the mother to know whether discomfort is within a normal range. Breastfeeding mothers, especially multiparas, should be taught that afterpains may be strong during feedings.

New mothers experience pain from engorged breast tissue, the traumatized perineum or abdominal surgical site, and uterine contractions. **Afterpains,** or discomfort from uterine contractions after delivery, occur in most women but are generally more noticeable in multipara mothers. They are stronger during breastfeeding because breast stimulation causes release of oxytocin (see Figure 4-17), which stimulates contractions. Oral analgesics may be prescribed for discomfort.

Nursing mothers may express concern about the effect of pain medication on the infant. The nurse should explain to the mother that pain can make her tense and anxious, which may decrease milk production. The nurse should also explain that some analgesics may be excreted in breast milk. This medication will not harm the infant but would make the infant sleepy. It is important, therefore, for the mother to feed the infant before she takes the analgesic.

Breasts

The breast assessment begins with checking the bra for design and fit. The postpartum mother should wear a well-fitting bra at all times. The bra should provide support to prevent the weight of the breast from stretching the supporting ligaments and connective tissue. A nursing bra with proper fit provides the needed support and should be used even by nonnursing mothers. The straps should be made of cloth instead of elastic. The back should be wide, with at least three rows of hooks to adjust the fit. The cups of a nursing bra have a supportive inner cup and a partial outer cup that can be unhooked for breastfeeding. Cotton is often recommended instead of synthetic material because it "breathes" and does not hold perspiration inside against the woman's skin.

The bra should be removed so the breast can be inspected and palpated. The breast should be inspected for redness and cracked or inverted nipples. The breast should be palpated for softness, slight firmness associated with filling, or firmness associated with full or engorged glands. Warmth and tenderness should also be noted. Colostrum or milk may drain from the nipple. The mother should be taught to report signs of complications, such as redness, heat, and pain. These may signify mastitis (discussed in Chapter 8). She should also report cracked, sore nipples.

Abdomen

To assess the abdomen accurately, the urinary bladder must be empty and the mother should be supine. Placing one hand on the symphysis pubis to support the uterus, the nurse places the middle finger of the other hand on the umbilicus and pushes down on the abdomen to palpate the location of the fundus.

clinical ALERT

Support of the uterus is crucial when palpating the abdomen. Pressure on the fundus without the hand supporting the uterus at the symphysis could lead to uterine prolapse.

The fundus should be firm, in the midline, and between the umbilicus and symphysis. The distance from the umbilicus is measured in finger widths (also called fingerbreadths) and recorded as a number above or below the umbilicus. The following are two methods of documenting the information:

1. For finger widths above the umbilicus, write the number before a capital U (1 finger width above the umbilicus = 1 U). For finger widths below the umbilicus, write the number after a capital U (e.g., 2 finger widths below the umbilicus = U 2). *OR*
2. You may write the number, followed by FB for fingerbreadth(s) and an arrow up, followed by U (for 1 fingerbreadth above the umbilicus, write: 1 FB ↑ U). For fingerbreadths below the umbilicus, write the number, followed by FB, an arrow down, and a capital U (e.g., 2 fingerbreadths below the umbilicus = 2 FB ↓ U).

If the fundus is not firm or in the proper location (Figure 10-6 ■), complications should be suspected. Procedure 10-1 ■ illustrates the proper technique for assessing the fundus.

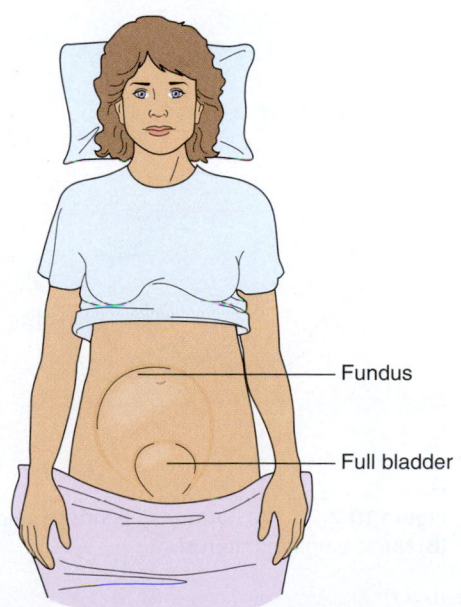

Fundus

Full bladder

Figure 10-6. ■ The uterine fundus becomes displaced and deviated to the right when the bladder is full.

PROCEDURE 10-1	**Fundal Assessment**

Purpose

■ To assess the fundus for complications following delivery

Equipment

■ Clean exam gloves
■ Clean perineal pad
■ Impervious (leak-proof) bag

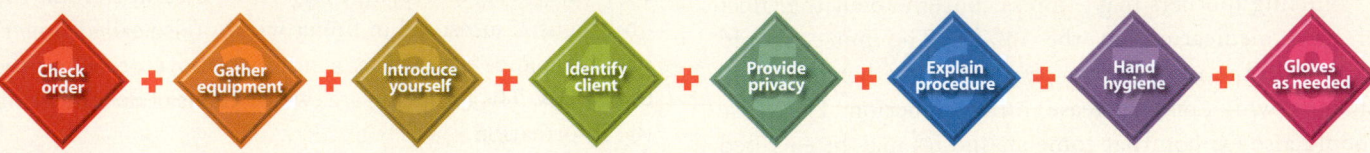

Interventions

1. Ask the woman to void. *A full bladder can cause the uterus to deviate from midline and produce uterine atony and hemorrhage.*

2. Position the woman supine with the knees slightly flexed and her head on a pillow. *Flexing the knees relaxes abdominal muscles. The supine position prevents falsely high measurement of the fundal height.*

3. Gently place one hand on the lower uterine segment just above the pubic symphysis. With the other hand, gently palpate the abdomen until the fundus is located (Figure 10-7 ■). The fundus should feel like a hard mass about the size of a large grapefruit. *One hand supports and stabilizes the uterus to prevent prolapse, while the other determines the location and condition of the fundus.*

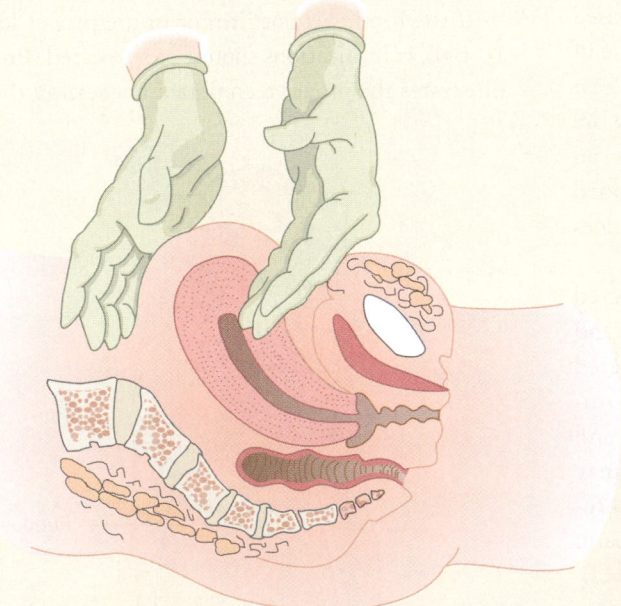

A

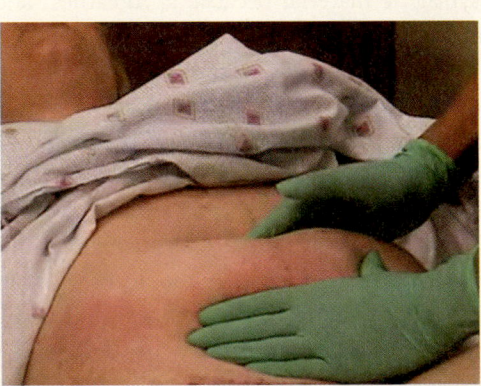

B

Figure 10-7. ■ (**A**) Position of hands to palpate the uterus, assess its firmness, and promote contraction. (**B**) Nurse palpating uterus.

4. If the fundus is boggy, gently massage the fundus in a circular motion while continuing to support the lower uterine segment. If the fundus does not become firm within a few minutes, summon assistance by using the call light. *A boggy uterus indicates uterine bleeding that could lead to hemorrhage. Gentle massage stimulates uterine contractions. Do not leave the client when there is risk of hemorrhage.*

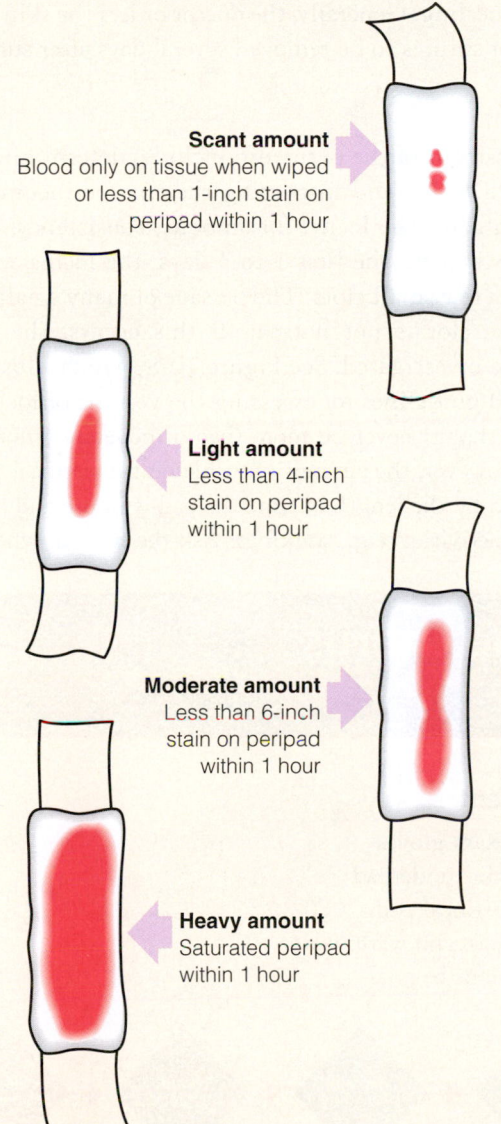

Scant amount
Blood only on tissue when wiped or less than 1-inch stain on peripad within 1 hour

Light amount
Less than 4-inch stain on peripad within 1 hour

Moderate amount
Less than 6-inch stain on peripad within 1 hour

Heavy amount
Saturated peripad within 1 hour

Figure 10-8. ■ Suggested guidelines for assessing lochia volume. (Data from Jacobsen, H. [1985]. A standard for assessing lochia volume. *Maternal–Child Nursing,* May/June.)

5. Measure the height of the fundus in fingerbreadths above, below, or at the umbilicus. *The fundal height is useful in determining the degree of involution.*

6. Determine the location of the fundus in relation to the midline of the body. If the fundus is not in the midline, evaluate for a full bladder. *A full bladder can push the uterus up and to one side, and may result in uterine atony.*

   a. If the woman did not empty her bladder before the procedure and the fundus is not in the midline, the bladder may be full. The client should be asked how long it has been since she has voided. If it has been longer than an hour, the woman should be assisted to the bathroom to void. The mother should then return to bed, and the fundus should be reassessed. *The bladder will fill rapidly in the postpartum period. Assessment of a full bladder does not provide accurate data.*

   b. If the bladder is empty and the fundus remains off center, ask the mother about the position of the baby in the last few weeks of pregnancy. *If an infant lies mostly on one side of the uterus during the last few weeks of pregnancy, the uterus may be tipped in that direction.*

7. Look at the perineal pad to determine the volume, color, and consistency of lochia (Figure 10-8 ■). *The lochia should be red, of moderate amount, and without clots.*

8. Provide the woman with a clean perineal pad. Dispose of all contaminated articles in the impervious bag following standard precautions. *A clean pad decreases the risk of infection and provides a point from which to assess future blood loss. Standard precautions prevent the spread of infection.*

9. Document the completion and findings of the procedure. *This provides a record of the intervention and data for ongoing assessment of the mother's progress.*

SAMPLE DOCUMENTATION

(date and time)   Fundus in midline, 2 FB ↓ U. Moderate amt lochia rubra without clots. Peripad changed. _____
M. Rodriguez LVN

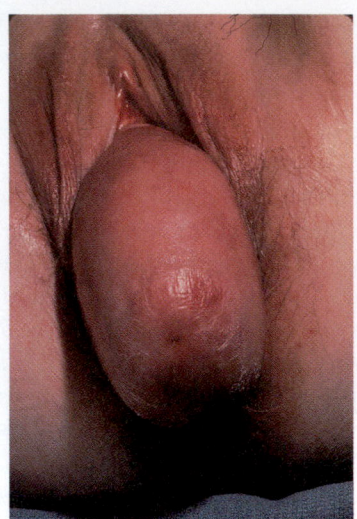

Figure 10-9. ■ Complete uterine prolapse with inversion of the vagina.

If the fundus is boggy, the LPN should begin to massage the fundus gently in a circular manner. Procedure 10-2 ■ reviews the proper procedure for fundal massage. If the fundus does not regain or maintain firmness within a few minutes, the LPN/LVN should summon assistance. The RN or physician may apply strong pressure on the fundus to remove

clots. As mentioned, this is generally not an LPN/LVN function, due to the risk of uterine prolapse (Figure 10-9 ■).

The abdomen of the woman who has had a cesarean section delivery should be assessed as for any other abdominal surgical client. The abdomen may be tender, so palpation must be done gently. Bowel sounds should be assessed, and the mother should be asked about the passage of flatus. The abdominal dressing should be assessed for abnormal drainage. The incision should be assessed for signs of infection and healing. Generally, the doctor orders the skin clips, staples, or sutures to be removed several days after surgery.

Perineum

The assessment of the perineum includes determining the amount of lochia and inspecting the true perineum. The nurse evaluates the lochia for amount, consistency, color, and odor. During the first 1 to 3 days, the lochia will be red with a few small clots. The passage of many small clots or a large clot is not normal. If this occurs, the cause should be investigated. See Figure 10-8, which illustrates suggested guidelines for assessing the volume of lochia.

There should never be more than a moderate amount of lochia. However, the amount of lochia on the perineal pad is influenced by the length of time the pad is in use and by the woman's activities (e.g., walking). Ask the woman when she

---

PROCEDURE 10-2 | # Removing Clots from the Uterus

Purpose

■ To remove clots from the uterus in order to evaluate the amount of uterine bleeding and prevent hemorrhage

Equipment

■ Clean exam gloves
■ Clean blue underpad
■ Clean perineal pad
■ Washcloth and warm water
■ Impervious bag

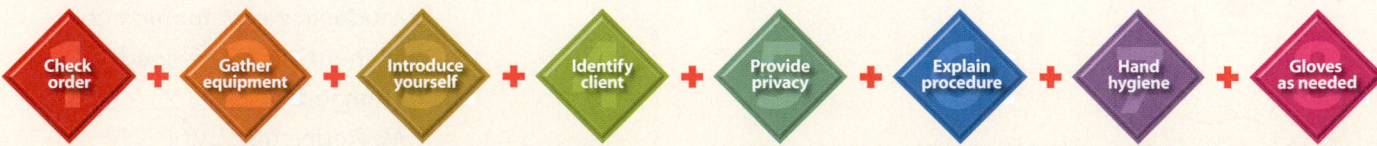

Check order + Gather equipment + Introduce yourself + Identify client + Provide privacy + Explain procedure + Hand hygiene + Gloves as needed

Interventions

1. Assess the fundus as outlined in Procedure 10-1. *Assessment of the fundus determines the need for blood clot removal. If the fundus is boggy and above the umbilicus, blood clots are suspected.*

2. Gently massage the fundus to stimulate contractions. *The fundus must be firm in order to remove clots safely.*

3. Explain to the woman the need to remove clots. The procedure will be uncomfortable but should only last a few minutes. *Explanation should help the woman to relax.*

4. Supporting the lower uterine segment, apply firm pressure from the fundus toward the vagina (Figure 10-10 ■).

changed the pad last, the amount of lochia on the pad, and the presence of any clots. If heavy bleeding is reported or suspected, change the pad, have the woman remain in bed, and reassess in 1 hour. Do not discard the saturated pads, but save them in the bathroom until the bleeding is controlled and the physician has determined the estimated blood loss. In some cases, the physician will ask that the saturated pads, blue underpads, and bloody linen be weighed to determine blood loss.

Assess the odor of lochia. It should be similar to the odor of menstruation and should never be strong or foul. The cause of foul or offensive odor should always be investigated. A specimen may need to be obtained for culture and sensitivity.

To assess the perineum, position the mother in left Sims' position and lift the buttocks to expose the true perineum (Figure 10-11 ■). Observe for discoloration, bruising, and generalized swelling. If an episiotomy or lacerations were repaired, the tissue should be well approximated. Generally, stitches are not visible. Report signs of infection or wound dehiscence to the physician. If hemorrhoids are present, assess for bleeding and tenderness. Generally, the swelling of hemorrhoid tissue resolves in a few weeks. Procedure 10-3 ■ details steps in perineal assessment.

Swelling of the perineum can make voiding difficult. Urinary output should be measured for at least the first two voidings after delivery. The woman should be encouraged

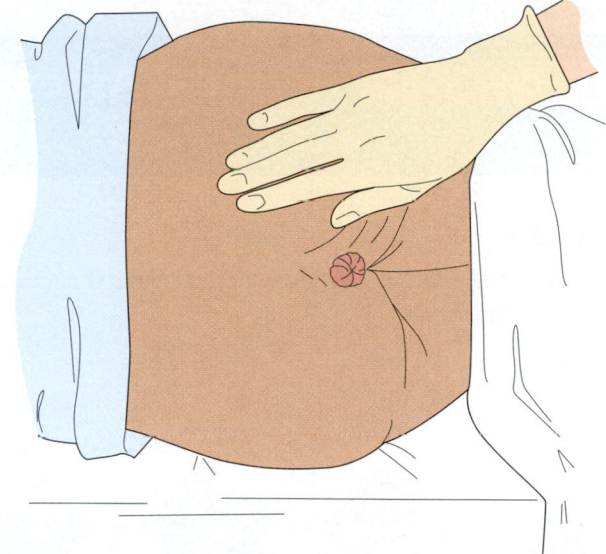

Figure 10-11. ■ Intact perineum with hemorrhoids. Note how the nurse's hand raises the upper buttocks.

to void every 2 to 4 hours. If the bladder can be palpated or urinary retention is suspected, further assessment with a bladder scan may be necessary, and the woman may require urinary catheterization.

It may be several days before bowel elimination occurs due to slowing of peristalsis during pregnancy. If the woman has

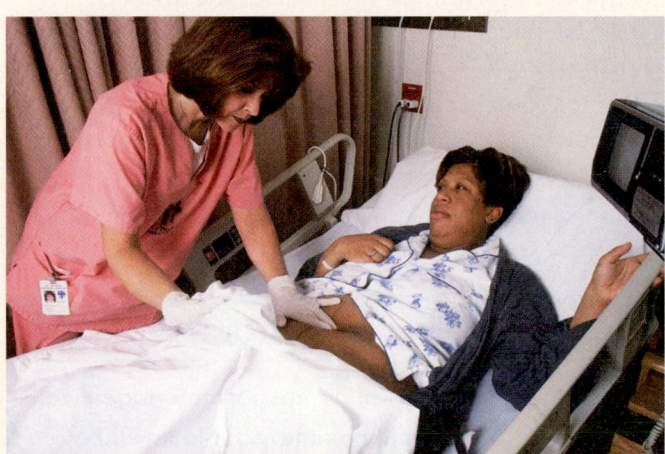

Figure 10-10. ■ Nurse removing clots from uterus. Note that lower hand supports the uterus.

Observe the perineum for expulsion of blood clots. *Uterine support is necessary to prevent prolapse of the uterus.*

5. Reassess the fundus for firmness and location. *The fundus should regain tone once clots are removed.*

6. Remove all bloody pads, provide a wash to the perineum, and apply a clean blue underpad and perineal pad. Follow standard precautions for disposal of contaminated articles. *Cleanliness promotes comfort. All bloody supplies may need to be*

saved until the amount of blood loss is determined. Following standard precautions prevents the spread of infection.

7. Assess the fundus every 15 minutes until it remains firm for a minimum of 1 hour. *If the fundus becomes boggy, further bleeding could occur.*

SAMPLE DOCUMENTATION

(date and time)	Fundus boggy and 2 FB ↑ U. Fundus massaged until firm. Manual fundal pressure applied resulting in approximately 10-cm blood clot. Fundus regained tone at U. Dr. Williams notified. _____ K. Chi, RN
(date and time)	Fundus assessed every 15 minutes. Fundus firm at U. Moderate amount red lochia noted on peripad. _____ A. Adams, LPN

Perineal Assessment

Purpose

- To assess the perineum for signs of healing and complications following delivery

Equipment

- Clean exam gloves
- Clean perineal pad
- Small light such as a pen light may be necessary
- Impervious bag

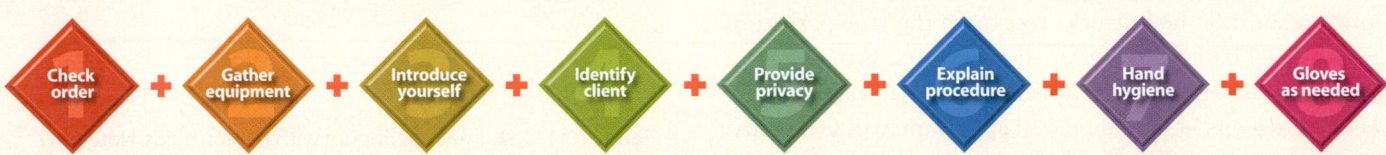

Check order + Gather equipment + Introduce yourself + Identify client + Provide privacy + Explain procedure + Hand hygiene + Gloves as needed

Interventions

1. Ask the woman about perineal discomfort. "Is it getting better or worse? Is it greater than expected?" *Pain greater than would be expected or that is becoming worse is an indication of complications and must be investigated.*

2. Position the woman in the left Sims' position. *When the woman is supine, the posterior perineum may be difficult to see. Sims' position allows for adequate exposure of the perineum.*

3. Lift the buttocks to expose the perineum (see Figure 10-11). Use a small light to visualize the perineal tissues. *Adequate visualization is necessary for complete assessment.*

4. Assess the perineum in a systematic order. The mnemonic REEDA (redness, edema, ecchymosis, discharge, approximation) may be a helpful reminder.
   - **R** = redness. *Redness is a sign of infection.*
   - **E** = edema. Palpate for softness of tissue. *Some edema is usual following a vaginal delivery. Edematous tissue is soft. A firm mass is a sign of a hematoma and must be reported to the charge nurse.*
   - **E** = ecchymosis. *The tissue may be somewhat bruised, but an increase in bruising or excessive bruising is a sign of a hematoma.*
   - **D** = discharge. Look for drainage from episiotomy or lacerations. *There should be no drainage from repaired episiotomy or lacerations. Purulent or foul-smelling drainage is a sign of infection.*

   - **A** = approximation. The edges of repaired episiotomy or lacerations should be touching. *Within 24 hours, the wound edges should be "glued" together. Sutures are placed under the skin and therefore will not be visible.*

5. Assess the anus for hemorrhoids (Figure 10-11). If hemorrhoids are present, the size, number, and degree of tenderness should be noted. *Hemorrhoids often develop during pregnancy and labor and delivery. Comfort measures may be needed.*

6. Apply a clean perineal pad. Replenish ice pack, if necessary. *Ice packs prevent swelling and may relieve some discomfort.*

7. Dispose of contaminated pads using standard precautions. *Standard precautions prevent the spread of infection.*

SAMPLE DOCUMENTATION

(date and time)   Midline episiotomy edges well approximated. No swelling, ecchymosis, or drainage noted. States comfort measure effective in relieving tenderness. _____

J. Jones, LVN

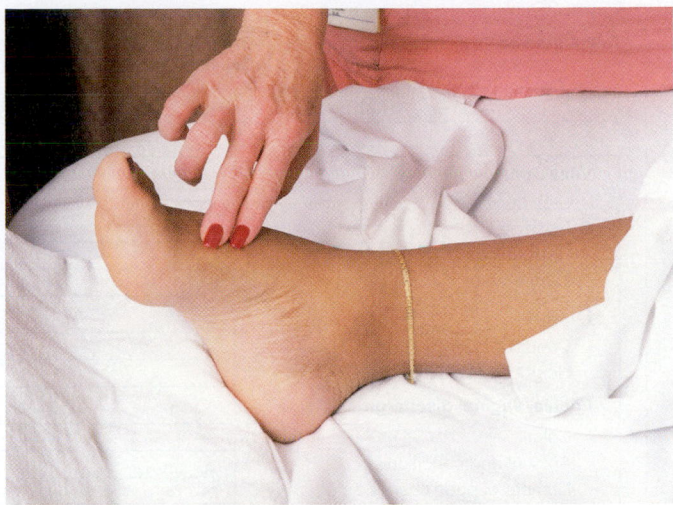

A

had a large episiotomy or laceration, the resulting swelling, pain, and fear of tearing the tissue may make defecation difficult. The woman can prevent constipation by increasing her intake of oral fluids, eating a diet high in fiber, and ensuring early ambulation. At times, a stool softener is ordered. Complementary therapy may also be useful (Box 10-2 ■).

Lower Extremities

The legs should also be assessed for abnormalities caused by pregnancy, including varicose veins and edema (Figure 10-12 ■). If varicose veins are present, care should be taken to protect them from injury. Reassure the woman that edema from pressure on the pelvic veins or PIH should resolve in a few days.

Assess the legs for signs of *thrombophlebitis* (positive Homan's sign: see Figure 10-12B). Note any areas of redness, swelling, or tenderness. With the legs straight and knees slightly flexed, the woman's foot should be sharply dorsiflexed. No discomfort should be present. Pain with dorsiflexion is an indication of an inflamed vessel in the leg. The charge nurse or physician should be notified at once because of the risk of deep vein thrombosis and **thromboembolism** (a blood clot moving within the blood vessels).

Psychological Assessment

Psychological assessment is an important part of postpartum care. Figure 10-13 ■ illustrates a postpartum assessment sheet. The mother's attitude and feelings affect her ability to care for herself and the infant. Fatigue from a long labor makes everything seem more difficult to manage. A tired mother may seem disinterested in the infant and be labeled as a "potential attachment problem." After a nap, the mother is often more receptive to her baby.

Some mothers have little experience caring for a newborn and feel overwhelmed. They may show these feelings by asking frequent questions and reading all the information that is available. Feeling inadequate may cause others to become passive and quiet. The nurse must help the mother explore these feelings in order to assess the need for further outside support.

To assess for early attachment or bonding with the infant, the nurse needs to observe the mother handling the

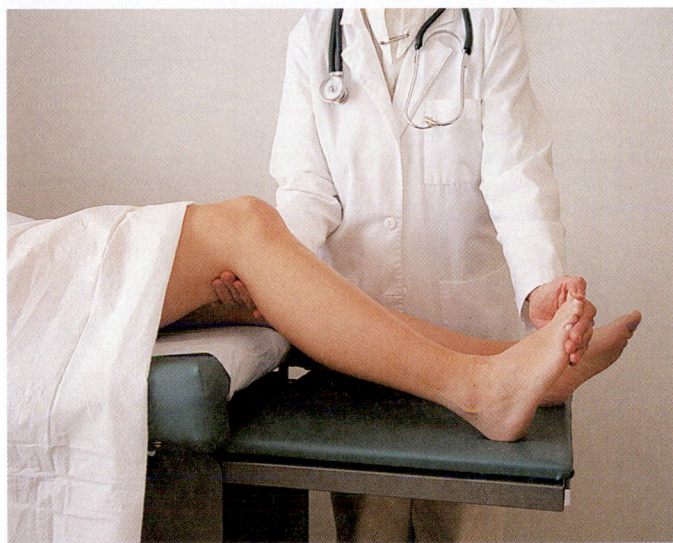

B

Figure 10-12. ■ (A) Nurse assessing client's foot for edema. (B) Assessing for thrombosis. (B: Elena Dorfman.)

baby. Through observation, the nurse can answer the following questions:

- To what extent does the mother seek face-to-face interaction with the infant?
- Has she progressed from fingertip touch to enfolding the infant in her arms?
- Is interaction increasing or decreasing?
- Is she sensitive to the newborn's needs?
- Does she seem pleased with her infant? Is she upset by baby's appearance or gender?
- Does she call the baby by name?

Once the nurse has observed the mother-baby interaction, three more questions must be answered: Is there a problem with attachment? What is the problem? What is the source of the problem? The LPN/LVN refers any concerns about attachment to the charge nurse.

Client's name _____   Gravida _____ Para _____
                                   Delivery date _____

Physical assessment			
	Remarks		
Vital signs			
Blood pressure			
Pulse			
Respirations			
Temperature			
Fundus			
Condition			
Height and location			
Lochia/vaginal discharge			
Color			
Amount and condition			
Number of pads changed			
Breast			
Breast or bottle feeding			
Breast assessment			
Nipple assessment			
Incision/lacerations (REEDA)			

Perineum
  Episiotomy site
  Lacerations			

Abdominal incision
  Appearance
  Dressing change
  Wound irrigation			

Nutrition Diet Intake			

Fluids
  Type and amount
  IV solution, rate, site			

Elimination
Voided
  Amount
  Any discomforts			

Bowel movement
  Number and type
  Constipation
  Treatments			

Comfort measures Rest Pain (type, location, intensity)			

Interventions
  Sitz bath
  Witch hazel pads
  Surgigator
  Pericare
  Analgesic perineal spray
  Analgesic (name, route, time)
  Other			

Figure 10-13. ■ Postpartum flow sheet of physical and psychological assessment and possible educational needs of the client.

DIAGNOSING, PLANNING, AND IMPLEMENTING

Once an assessment is completed, problems must be identified. Generally, new mothers can provide for their own physical needs but may have deficient knowledge about the specifics of postpartum care. Common nursing diagnoses include:

- Pain
- Deficient Knowledge regarding breast care
- Deficient Knowledge regarding perineal care
- Imbalanced Nutrition: Less than Body Requirements
- Constipation
- Impaired Urinary Elimination.

Some possible outcomes include the following:

- Client expresses that pain is reduced with medication.
- Client asks for information she can read about breastfeeding and self-care.
- Client states understanding the importance of nutrients to self and infant, and states "maybe I don't have to lose all my pregnancy weight in 2 weeks; maybe I can take a little more time."
- Client asks for dried fruit and extra liquids with meal to assist bowel elimination.
- Client states that pain on urination has lessened from 5 to 2 on scale of 1 to 10.

The plan of care centers on teaching the new mother to meet her needs and the needs of the infant. Teaching care of the infant is addressed in Chapter 9 ⬀.

Pain Management

- Assess the client's level of pain. Pain may be described by various pain rating scales, by location (incision, leg, back, head), and by type (dull, aching, throbbing, radiating, etc.). Box 10-3 ■ provides guidelines for the nurse in assisting the client in pain. *The nurse uses information from the client, plus objective data gained by observing the client, to report the level of pain.*
- Advise the breastfeeding mother with discomfort from engorged breast tissue to take a warm shower or nurse her baby. *These actions will stimulate the let-down reflex and relieve the pressure in the breast.*
- Evaluate breastfeeding technique if the nipples become sore or cracked. *A lanoline ointment may be applied with an order from the primary care provider. This type of ointment is safe for use with breastfeeding infants.*
- A nonnursing mother may express breast discomfort due to beginning lactation. Assist by applying ice and a breast binder to the chest. Administer analgesics as ordered. Teach that it may take several days to suppress lactation and alleviate the problem. *Ice and breast binders*

| BOX 10-3 | NURSING CARE CHECKLIST |

Helping a Client in Pain

☑ Ask the client when the pain started. If it is a recurring pain, ask what starts the pain and what causes it to stop.

☑ Ask the client to describe how bad the pain is on a scale of 0 to 10, with 0 being no pain and 10 being the worst imaginable pain.

☑ Ask where the pain is, or have the client show the nurse by pointing to the area of pain. Also, determine if the pain begins in one area and moves to another.

☑ Ask the client to identify what kind of pain exists.
  - ☑ Throbbing
  - ☑ Shooting
  - ☑ Stabbing
  - ☑ Sharp
  - ☑ Gnawing
  - ☑ Burning
  - ☑ Dull
  - ☑ Tender
  - ☑ Radiating
  - ☑ Other _____

☑ Provide medication as ordered. Review standing orders for administering pain medications. Consult with charge nurse as needed.

☑ Return to client 20 to 30 minutes after administering pain medication to determine effectiveness of medication.

---

can prevent engorgement. Analgesics may be given for discomfort. Knowing that discomfort will subside in several days will usually help the person tolerate it better.

- Administer analgesics as needed to control perineal discomfort. Provide ice packs and anesthetic spray to the perineum, as ordered by the primary care provider. Recommend other interventions to alleviate perineal discomfort, such as sitting in a reclined position. A sitz bath (discussed in Procedure 10-4 ■) may also be helpful. *The woman will be better able to provide for the needs of herself and her infant if she is comfortable.*
- The woman who has had a cesarean section birth may have epidural analgesia or patient-controlled analgesia (PCA). Follow facility guidelines on the use of these methods of pain relief. Provide information about the prescribed medication, its uses, and side effects. Oral pain medication will be ordered as soon as bowel tones are present and oral intake is tolerated. *As in any situation, medication administration must be carefully carried out. Once peristalsis has ended, oral medications can be tolerated.*

PROCEDURE 10-4 Sitz Bath

Purpose

- To relieve discomfort and promote healing of the perineum

Equipment

- Disposable sitz tub kit, containing disposable basin and plastic bag with tubing
- Clean perineal pad
- Impervious bag
- Towel

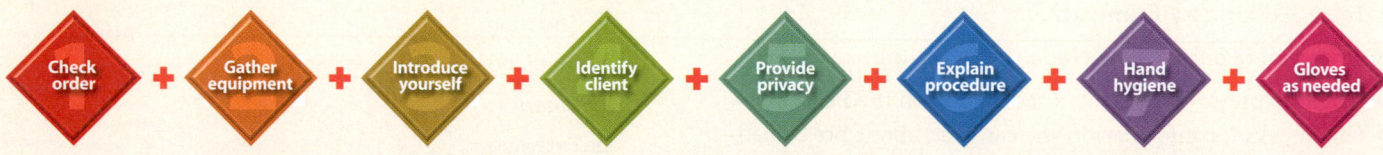

Check order + Gather equipment + Introduce yourself + Identify client + Provide privacy + Explain procedure + Hand hygiene + Gloves as needed

Interventions

1. Provide client teaching about sitz baths, including the benefits and use of the equipment. *Instructing the client in the use of equipment and the benefits of the sitz bath helps ensure compliance.*

2. Raise the toilet seat, and place the disposable basin on the toilet. *The toilet seat should be raised and basin placed directly on the toilet for maximum support.*

3. Close clamp on tubing. Fill plastic bag with very warm water. Attach tubing to inside bottom of basin in groove provided. *The water in the bag will drain into the basin to keep the water comfortably warm. If the water in the bag is too cool, the water in the basin will cool and not be as effective.*

4. Fill the basin with comfortably warm water. *Warm water will increase circulation to the perineum and promote healing of tissues.*

5. Have the woman remove the perineal pad, dispose of it in the impervious bag, and sit directly on the basin. *Sitting directly on the basin will allow the perineum to be covered by the warm water. If the woman sits on the toilet seat, the perineum would not reach the water.*

6. Instruct the woman to open the tubing clamp periodically to drain the very warm water into the basin, keeping the basin water comfortably warm. As the basin fills, the water will drain into the toilet. *The very warm water should keep the basin water at a comfortable temperature.*

7. Instruct the woman to sit in the warm water for 10 minutes, three to four times a day as ordered. *Sitting in warm water for 10 minutes stimulates circulation without traumatizing the tissues.*

8. Instruct the woman to pat the perineum dry and to apply a clean perineal pad. *Patting the perineum dry prevents further perineal trauma and discomfort.*

9. Assess the perineum following treatment. *The perineum should show signs of healing over time.*

10. Clean the disposable sitz basin, bag, and tubing and store for future use by this client. Equipment should be sent home with client at time of discharge. When healing is complete and treatment is discontinued, dispose of the equipment. *The disposable sitz basin is intended for individual use to prevent cross-contamination between users.*

SAMPLE DOCUMENTATION

(date and time)	Up to bathroom. Sat in sitz bath for 10 minutes. Perineum dried, clean peripad applied. Perineal swelling decreased. Laceration edges well approximated. _____ B. Abbs, LVN

MediaLink Sitz bath

TABLE 10-2

Pharmacology: Oral Pain Medications

DRUG	USUAL ROUTE/DOSE	CLASSIFICATION	SELECTED SIDE EFFECTS	DON'T GIVE IF
Motrin (ibuprofen)	400–800 mg 3–4 times/day	NSAID (nonsteroidal anti-inflammatory drug)	Nausea, dyspepsia, blurred vision, dizziness	Allergic to drug
Tylenol (acetaminophen)	325–650 mg every 4–6 hours	Nonopioid analgesic	Few in usual dose; liver toxicity if dosage guidelines are ignored	Pain not controlled by usual dose
Percocet (oxycodone with acetaminophen)	5 mg oxycodone with 325 mg acetaminophen	Opioid agonist/ nonopioid analgesic	Confusion, sedation, respiratory depression	Respiratory rate is less than 10/min
Morphine (morphine sulfate)	4–10 mg IV every 3–4 hours Patient-controlled analgesia (PCA); dose varies	Opioid agonist	Respiratory depression, confusion, sedation, vomiting, constipation	Respiratory rate is less than 10/min Allergic to drug
Demerol (meperidine HCl)	50–100 mg IM every 3–4 hours; PCA; dose varies	Opioid agonist	Respiratory depression, confusion, sedation, vomiting, constipation	Respiratory rate is less than 10/min Allergic to drug

■ Provide nonpharmacologic methods of pain relief. *Many women prefer to "forget about" the pain by using alternate methods of pain relief, such as baths, backrubs, distraction, etc.*

Table 10-2 ■ provides information about oral pain medications.

Client Teaching

Client teaching is an important part of the LPN/LVN role. Because many new mothers remain in the hospital for only 24 to 48 hours, the nurse must take every opportunity to teach health-promoting activities.

Hygiene

■ Instruct the new mother to bathe daily. Teach that showers are preferable to tub bathing because they can help prevent contamination carried from the feet to the perineum or breast. If a shower is not available, the mother should be taught to clean the tub and rinse the residue away before sitting in the tub. The new mother should be taught to wash the breast without soap and to allow the nipples to air-dry. *Cleanliness is the main technique used to prevent infection. Washing the nipple with soap might cause it to become dry and to crack.*

If delivery was by cesarean section, instruct the woman to keep the incision clean until healing is complete. Once the dressing is removed, the woman may shower without any special precautions. Instruct her to allow the incision to dry completely after washing and to apply a small dressing if desired. *A small dressing will absorb any drainage from the incision site. If Steri-Strips have been applied to the incision, they will not be harmed by the shower and will come off in about 1 week.*

■ Teach the client to rinse the perineum with clear water after each voiding and bowel movement and to pat it dry. Instruct the new mother to wipe the perineum always from front to back. *Cleansing removes micro-organisms. Wiping the perineum from front to back prevents contamination from the anus to the vagina and urethra.*

Sitz Baths

The doctor may order a sitz bath to relieve perineal swelling and discomfort. Some hospitals have porcelain sitz tubs, which must be cleaned between clients. Other facilities use portable individual sitz basins (Figure 10-14 ■) that are sent home with the client.

■ Teach the mother to shower before using the sitz bath. *This will wash away contaminants that could infect the perineum or vagina.*

Postpartum Nutrition

The new mother needs a balanced diet in order to regain her strength. Most facilities provide written information about proper nutrition after delivery. The hospital dietitian is also a valuable resource.

■ Teach the client that her diet should be high in fiber and fluids. *This diet will prevent constipation.*

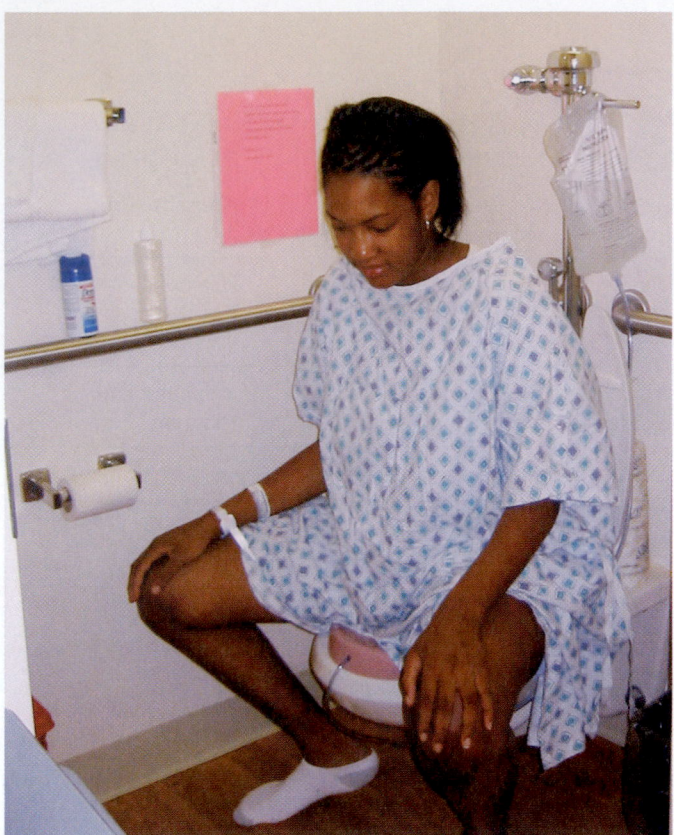

Figure 10-14. ■ A sitz bath promotes healing and provides relief from perineal discomfort during the initial weeks following birth.

- If the woman has a good understanding of basic nutrition, it may be sufficient to advise her to decrease her daily caloric intake by 300 calories and resume her prepregnancy level of other nutrients. *The 300 calories a day that provided for the needs of the fetus are no longer necessary. The woman will return to her prepregnancy weight more quickly if she reduces the daily intake of calories.*
- Teach the breastfeeding mother to consume an additional 500 kcal per day, to drink at least 8 glasses of fluid a day (1,000 mL), and to consume 65 g of protein and 1,000 mg of calcium. Most physicians request that the new mother continue to take prenatal vitamins with iron for 3 months (see Breastfeeding section of Chapter 9 ⬮). *These will balance the nutrients used up by milk production and breastfeeding. The prenatal vitamins help ensure that the woman's system is balanced.*

Exercise

- After delivery, assist the woman to begin activity with ambulation. *Early ambulation promotes healing and prevents complications such as thrombophlebitis.*
- Encourage the woman to begin with simple postpartal exercises (Figure 10-15 ■). *The new mother may want to engage in abdominal exercises to tighten stretched muscles.*

Inform the woman that an increase in lochia or pain means she may be overdoing exercise and should decrease her activity. Most agencies provide a booklet describing suggested postpartum exercises.

Postpartum Immunizations

Two different immunizations are commonly given following delivery, if needed. A **RhoGAM blood stick** (a test to identify incompatibility of mother's and infant's Rh factor) is done within the first hour after birth if Rh status is not known. (Discussion of Rh incompatibility is found in Chapter 8 ⬮.) For the mother who has Rh-negative blood and delivers an infant with Rh-positive blood (see Figure 8-12 ⬮), the doctor usually prescribed an injection of RhoGAM (Rh$_o$ [D] immune globulin) (see Table 8-6 ⬮). This immune globulin can be given as soon as there are test results, but it must be given within 72 hours of delivery (some facilities say within 48 hours). RhoGAM prevents the production of Rh antibodies that could harm a future pregnancy. The purpose of the injection and the usual side effects should be explained to the mother prior to the immunization. Table 10-3 ■ provides information about postpartum immunization.

Exposure to rubella virus can cause congenital malformation in the fetus, so immunization is avoided when pregnancy is possible. If the mother has a negative rubella titer, most physicians recommend an MMR (measles, mumps, rubella) immunization in the postpartum period. If the immunization is given shortly after delivery, there is no chance of exposure to the next fetus. (*Note:* In some facilities, the MMR immunization is given immediately prior to discharge to prevent accidental exposure of other pregnant women to this virus.)

All other adult immunizations can be given in the postpartum period, if necessary.

Building a Support Network and Healthy Patterns

- Inquire about family and friends who might be available to assist the mother when she returns home. *The mother may need encouragement to realize that people want to help her during this time. It is good to explore specific ways that people can help. Some people do best with a written list.*
- Discuss and encourage a pattern of good eating, exercise, and rest. *Good nutrition, regular exercise, and periods of rest will help the mother return to her prepregnant state most efficiently.*
- Respect the mother's rest periods as much as possible, and teach that it is important to listen to her body when a rest is needed. *Many women ignore their own need for rest. Teach the mother that getting rest will benefit not only herself, but also the infant and the family.*

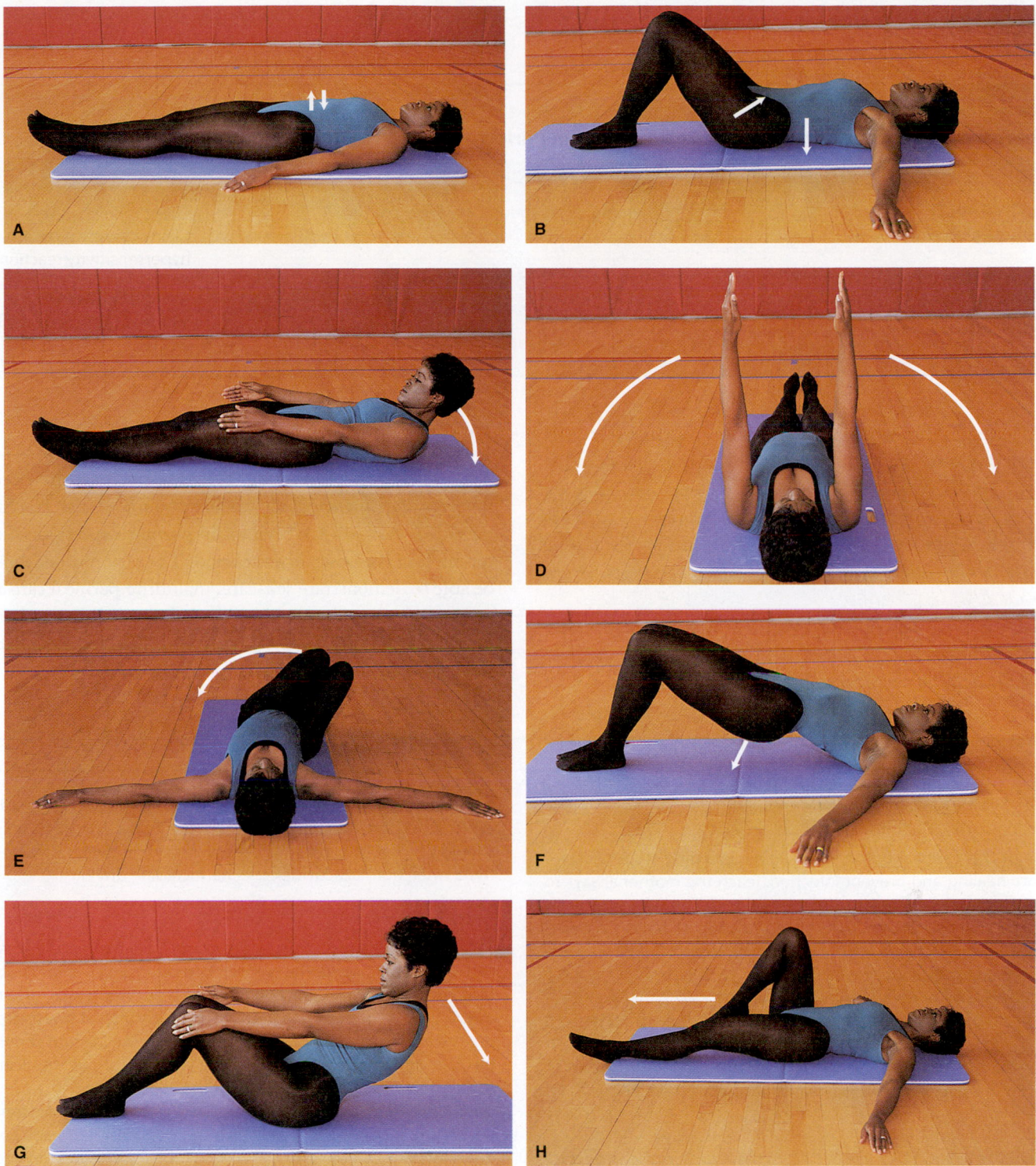

Figure 10-15. ■ Postpartal exercises. Begin with 5 repetitions two or three times daily, and gradually increase to 10 repetitions. First day: (**A**) Abdominal breathing. Lying supine, inhale deeply, using the abdominal muscles. The abdomen should expand. Then exhale slowly through pursed lips, tightening the abdominal muscle. (**B**) Pelvic rocking. Lying supine with arms at sides, knees bent, and feet flat, tighten abdomen and buttocks, and attempt to flatten back on the floor. Hold for a count of 10; then arch the back, causing the pelvis to "rock." On the second day, add (**C**). Chin to chest. Lying supine with legs straight, raise head and attempt to touch chin to chest. Slowly lower head. (**D**) Arm raises. Lying supine, arms extended at a 90-degree angle from body, raise arms so they are perpendicular and hands touch. Lower slowly. On fourth day, add (**E**). Knee rolls. Lying supine with knees bent, feet flat, arms extended to the side, roll knees to one side, keeping shoulders flat. Return to the original position, and roll to opposite side. (**F**) Buttocks lift. Lying supine, arms at side, knees bent, feet flat, slowly raise the buttocks and arch the back. Return slowly to starting position. On sixth day, add (**G**). Abdominal tighteners. Lying supine, knees bent, feet flat, slowly raise head toward knees. Arms should extend along either side of legs. Return slowly to original position. (**H**). Knee to abdomen. Lying supine, arms at sides, bend one knee and thigh until foot touches buttocks. Straighten leg and lower it slowly. Repeat with other leg. After 2 to 3 weeks, more strenuous exercises, such as push-ups and side leg raises, may be added as tolerated. Kegel exercises, begun before birth, should be done many times daily during postpartum to restore vaginal and perineal tone.

TABLE 10-3

Pharmacology: Immunizations in the Postpartum Period

DRUG	USUAL ROUTE/DOSE	CLASSIFICATION	SELECTED SIDE EFFECTS	DON'T GIVE IF
RhoGAM (Rh$_o$D immune globulin)	300 mcg IM	Immunizing agent	Local pain, fever	Client is Rh positive Client has history of hypersensitivity reaction
MMR (measles, mumps, rubella)	1 vial IM	Vaccines	Local pain, fever	Allergic to eggs History of hypersensitivity reaction

■ Encourage the woman to simplify routines for this period of time and not to make any major changes. *The nurse can reinforce that changes are natural and necessary when an infant is brought home. It will take time to adjust to the new person and new roles. Encourage the mother to keep maintenance tasks simple and to expect energy to return gradually.*

■ Ask the client how she is feeling. *The woman may have anxieties or concerns about parenting. Asking open-ended questions can allow her to raise these issues.*

EVALUATING

The evaluation of nursing care for postpartum clients involves documenting an understanding of the teaching provided. Box 10-4 ■ reviews important aspects of client teaching in the postpartum period. The new mother should be able to demonstrate self-care, including perineal care and suture line care. She should select a balanced diet and consume adequate fluids. She should verbalize an understanding of the use and side effects of medications.

BOX 10-4 **CLIENT TEACHING**

Self-Care After Discharge

Episiotomy/Perineal Laceration Care

Use of the perineal bottle until vaginal bleeding stops can promote healing and prevent infection. Teach the mother always to rinse the perineal area, to cleanse and wipe from front to back, and to change perineal pads after urinating or having a bowel movement. Tell the mother to wait to use tampons until after the follow-up exam.

The doctor or midwife may recommend a sitz bath (see Procedure 10-4) to decrease perineal discomfort. Sitting in a sitz bath 10 to 15 minutes, three times a day, can soothe the perineal tissue. It may be more comfortable to place a bath towel in the tub to sit on. Some hospitals provide a plastic sitz bath to take home.

Vaginal Discharge

Teach the woman that it is normal to have vaginal discharge after delivery. Vaginal discharge may last as long as 5 to 6 weeks, although it should decrease in amount every day. The color will also change from bright red to dark red or brown. After 4 to 5 days, the discharge will become pinkish-red and then change to yellowish or white in color. Excessive activity may cause discharge to become red again with some small clots. If this occurs, the mother should lie down and rest with her feet elevated. If she fills a perineal pad in 1 hour or less, bleeding is excessive. Instruct her to call the doctor or midwife immediately.

Cesarean Section

Teach the woman who has had a cesarean section that it is important not to overdo activity for 4 to 6 weeks. Activity should be limited to taking care of oneself and the baby. The women should avoid lifting anything heavier than the baby. Climbing stairs should be kept to a minimum. The doctor or midwife will determine when normal activities resume, including driving.

Incision Care

Teach that an incision from a C-section does not need special care. Showering should be sufficient to cleanse the area. Scrubbing the incision is not necessary. Paper tape (Steri-Strips) on the incision can be gotten wet. Pat the incision dry after showering, or dry the area with a hairdryer on cool setting. The incision should be inspected in a mirror or by another person. It should be clean, dry, and intact; it should heal without redness, swelling, or foul odor. It is normal to have a small amount of clear fluid ooze from part of the incision. However, teach that bleeding or pearly colored discharge is not normal and should be reported to the doctor or midwife. Instruct the woman to call the doctor or midwife if the incision appears red and feels hot to the touch. Sutures underneath the incision will dissolve. If the staples were not removed in the hospital, it will be necessary to see the doctor or midwife to have them removed.

Hemorrhoids

Hemorrhoids often appear outside the rectum due to the pressure of pushing the baby out during delivery. Often, they will shrink with time. The doctor or midwife may prescribe ointment or suppositories. Teach the woman that ice packs can help decrease pain and swelling, and that some women find that a sitz bath is soothing after the first 24 hours post delivery.

Bowels

Teach the woman to avoid constipation. The mother should drink 6–8 glasses of water a day, and more if breastfeeding. The woman should be instructed to eat a balanced diet, which includes fruits, vegetables, and whole grains. The doctor or midwife may prescribe a stool softener or a laxative.

Menstruation

Instruct the woman that the time before periods begin again varies from woman to woman. Most women start their period within 2 to 3 months after delivery, unless they are breastfeeding. The woman who is breastfeeding may not have a period until after she stops breastfeeding.

Family Planning

Reinforce that the woman should not have sexual intercourse for 4 to 6 weeks after birth. It is recommended to wait until after the follow-up exam to resume intercourse. Birth control methods should be discussed with the doctor or midwife at this appointment. A woman can still become pregnant, even if she does not have a period.

Adjustment to Parenthood

Remind the woman that—although she may feel normal once she goes home—she is still recovering from the delivery of the baby. She needs time to adjust to having a new baby in the home. She should gradually resume activities, but allow time for rest. She should sleep when the baby sleeps. Allow family members and friends to help around the house and to prepare meals. The baby needs the woman to take care of herself.

Remind the woman that many women experience "baby blues." Teach that if weepiness, exhaustion, and anxiety last longer than a couple of weeks, she should see a physician to rule out postpartum depression. Emphasize that symptoms of "baby blues" or postpartum depression do not mean she is a "bad" mother. The period after the birth of the baby is a time of many changes and a whole new type of pressure. It is important not to try to deal with these feelings alone. Teach the mother these ways to ease "baby blues":

- Nap at every opportunity.
- Have small, nutritious, and easy-to-prepare meals throughout the day.
- Express her feelings to nonjudgmental family and friends. Ask for help with cooking and cleaning.
- Make time for herself!

Source: Ramont, R. P., Niedringhaus, D. M., & Towle, M. A. (2006). *Comprehensive nursing care.* Upper Saddle River, NJ: Prentice Hall, p. 1123.

Discharge Considerations

It is the nurse's responsibility to ensure that client teaching has occurred and that the woman has been given written information about care after discharge. Many parents will be concerned about going home with their new baby. They will worry about what to do if something is wrong. Box 10-5 ■ provides a list of criteria to help parents know when to call care providers for help.

The nurse can also assist by helping the client identify support people for the postpartum period. It may be helpful

---

BOX 10-5	CLIENT TEACHING

Postpartum Emergencies

Teach the woman/parents to look for these signs in her infant and to call the pediatrician in the following situations:

- An axillary temperature above 100.4°F (38°C) or an axillary temperature below 97.8°F (36.6°C)
- Projectile vomiting or frequent vomiting
- Refusal to feed for 2 feedings or 6 hours
- Listlessness or difficulty in waking baby
- Excessive fussiness during which comfort measures are not effective
- Jaundice increasing and working its way down the baby's trunk
- Two or more loose black or green watery stools
- Fewer than 6 wet diapers in a 24-hour period (after the mother's milk has come in)
- If baby is blue or is not breathing, call 911 or your local emergency number.

Teach the woman to call the obstetrician or midwife if any of the following occurs in herself:

- A temperature above 100.4°F (38°C)
- Sudden bright red bleeding or blood clots that are lemon-size or larger
- Foul-smelling lochia
- Painful urination
- Unexplained, sudden pain
- Hot or reddened area on breast
- If experiencing sudden shortness of breath or chest pain, call 911 immediately.

Provide these special discharge instructions about reasons to call the care provider after a cesarean section:

- Incision not changing for the better; pearly colored, white, or bloody drainage
- Reddened or hot area on incision
- Gaps between edges of incision or opening of incision.

Source: Ramont, R. P., Niedringhaus, D. M., & Towle, M. A. (2006). *Comprehensive nursing care.* Upper Saddle River, NJ: Prentice Hall, p. 1124.

for the client to list a set of tasks with which she could use help. Only trusted family and friends should be asked to help with child care.

NURSING PROCESS CARE PLAN
Client at Risk for Deep Vein Thrombosis

C. S., a 35-year-old gravida 3, para 2, is transferred from labor and delivery following a primary cesarean section for severe pre-eclampsia (see Chapter 8 ⚭). She is on a PCA pump for postoperative pain. Her husband is at the bedside.

Assessment. The following data should be collected as soon as possible after admission:

- Vital signs and pain
- Lung sounds
- Bowel sounds
- Fundus firmness and bleeding
- Deep tendon reflexes
- Response to test for Homan's sign
- Skin on legs—color, moisture, temperature
- Urine output
- Edema
- Capillary refill
- Incision (if woman had cesarean or episiotomy).

Nursing Diagnosis. The following important nursing diagnoses (among others) are established for this client:

Risk for Ineffective Peripheral Tissue Perfusion related to surgical procedure and immobility

Acute Pain related to surgical procedure

Risk for Respiratory and Incisional Infection related to surgical procedure

Expected Outcomes. Client will have adequate tissue perfusion in lower extremities as evidenced by lack of symptoms of deep vein thrombosis.

Client will have adequate pain control as evidenced by verbalizing pain relief.

Client will have no infection as evidenced by lack of respiratory or incisional symptoms.

Planning and Implementation

- Discuss with client the importance of increasing mobility following surgery. *Compliance may be increased when the client understands the risks of immobility.*

- Increase mobility as tolerated. *Mobility causes calf muscle contraction, which enhances venous return and thus decreases the risk for thrombus formation.*
- As ordered, implement thromboembolic stockings, intermittent pneumatic compression devices, or venous foot pump compression devices. *These devices work in the same manner as ambulation to prevent thrombus formation.*
- Continue to assess for signs and symptoms of thrombus formation. *Symptom recognition will facilitate prompt treatment.*
- Administer pain medication as ordered. *Pain medication will allow client to rest and will facilitate healing.*
- Encourage use of relaxation techniques such as imagery and massage. *Relaxation decreases muscle spasms and relieves discomfort.*
- Encourage client to do turn, cough, and deep breathe (TCDB) exercises every 2 hours. *Pooling of lung secretions increases risk for respiratory infection. TCDB will help client remove secretions from airways. Repositioning the client also facilitates comfort.*
- Provide dressing changes as ordered. *Changing wet dressings eliminates a reservoir for micro-organisms and decreases the risk of incisional infection.*

Evaluation. The client verbalizes an understanding of the risks of thrombus formation and implements preventive measures. There will be no development of symptoms of deep vein thrombosis or infection. Client verbalizes comfort.

Critical Thinking in the Nursing Process

1. How can the nurse encourage movement when the client is in pain and states that movement greatly increases her pain?

2. What is the nurse's responsibility when he or she assesses that the client's husband is not allowing his wife to get out of bed in an effort to conserve her energy?

3. Discuss hygiene issues related to *TED* (support) hose.

Note: Discussion of Critical Thinking Questions appears in Appendix I.

Note: The references and resources for this and all chapters have been compiled at the back of the book.

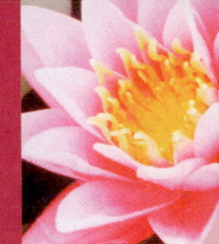

Chapter Review

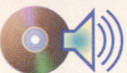 ## KEY TERMS by Topic

Use the audio glossary feature of either the CD-ROM or the Companion Website to hear the correct pronunciation of the following key terms.

Introduction
puerperium, postpartum

Physical Changes
involution, decidua, lochia, exfoliation, boggy, lochia rubra, lochia serosa, lochia alba, hematoma, colostrum, diastasis recti abdominis, thrombosis

Psychological Changes
taking-in stage, taking-hold stage, postpartum blues, bonding

Fathers, Siblings, and Others
engrossment

Nursing Care
afterpains, thromboembolism, RhoGAM blood stick

KEY Points

- Physical changes in the mother during the postpartum period progress in an expected pattern as the body returns to a nonpregnant state.

- The woman experiences psychological changes while adjusting to the role of mother.

- The nurse assesses the postpartum client for signs of healing and adaptation.

- Puerperal complications must be identified early in the postpartum period to prevent serious life-threatening conditions.

- Client teaching about self-care in the postpartum period is a continuous process that occurs with each interaction.

- New mothers must be taught to care for both themselves and their infant.

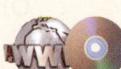 ## EXPLORE MediaLink

Additional interactive resources for this chapter can be found on the Companion Website at www.prenhall.com/towle. Click on Chapter 10 and "Begin" to select the activities for this chapter.

For chapter-related NCLEX-style questions and an audio glossary, access the accompanying CD-ROM in this book.

Animations

Postpartum assessment

Sitz bath

Massage a uterine fundus postpartum

Breast, uterus, bladder, bowel, lochia, episiotomy, Homan's sign, emotional status

FOR FURTHER Study

High-risk complications, including pre-eclampsia and postpartum depression, are discussed in Chapter 8.

Chapter 9 addresses teaching of infant care.

Critical Thinking Care Map

Caring for a Client at Risk

NCLEX® Focus Area: Coping and Adaptation

Case Study: Mandy, a 19-year-old, G1, P1 is transferred from labor and delivery to the postpartum unit following vaginal birth of a 5-pound, 2-ounce, male. Mandy labored for 15 hours and had a second-degree, midline episiotomy. Her history reveals she had no prenatal care, her drug screen was positive for cocaine, and she is unemployed.

Nursing Diagnosis: Risk for Impaired Parent-Infant Attachment

COLLECT DATA

Subjective	Objective
_____	_____
_____	_____
_____	_____
_____	_____
_____	_____
_____	_____
_____	_____

Would you report this? Yes/No

If yes, to: _____

Nursing Care

_____
_____
_____
_____
_____
_____
_____
_____
_____
_____
_____
_____
_____

How would you document this? _____
_____
_____
_____

Compare your documentation to the sample provided in Appendix I.

Data Collected
(use those that apply)

- Positive drug screen
- No prenatal care
- No employment
- States "Leave the child in the nursery."
- "Where can my boyfriend sleep tonight?"
- VS: T 99.0, P 58, R 12, BP 120/70
- Fundus firm, 1 FB above umbilicus
- Scant amount of lochia
- No eye contact made with baby
- Asks "Will the nurses change the baby's diapers? I don't ever want to do that."

Nursing Interventions
(use those that apply; list in priority order)

- Take the newborn into the client's room, even if she has not requested him.
- Inquire about the child's name.
- Reassess fundal height every 4 hours.
- Report to the charge nurse behaviors that indicate impaired bonding.
- Encourage the client to put the baby up for adoption.
- Teach the client about birth control methods.
- Teach the client about caring for a newborn.
- Continue to assess mother-child interaction.

1 Which of the following assessment findings are related to uterine atony in the postpartum client? Choose all that apply.

1. a boggy uterus
2. increased vaginal bleeding
3. large amounts of clots expressed
4. fundus midline
5. fundus displaced to left or right
6. scant amount of lochia rubra

2 On the second day postpartum, the nurse palpates the fundus one fingerbreadth below the umbilicus. The fundus was found to be firm. What nursing action is appropriate?

1. Document the finding.
2. Call the physician.
3. Catheterize the client.
4. Administer Lortab PO.

3 Which client would the nurse expect to be at risk for decreased rate of involution?

1. primiparous client
2. precipitous birth
3. client with indwelling catheter
4. client nonimmune for rubella

4 The nurse observes a creamy white vaginal discharge at the client's 2-week postpartum clinic visit. Which of the following terms would she use in documenting this finding?

1. lochia rubra
2. lochia serosa
3. lochia alba
4. lochia nigra

5 The postpartum client plans to breastfeed her newborn. She is concerned about birth control. Which of the following methods would the nurse recommend?

1. no method necessary; breastfeeding prohibits ovulation
2. combined oral contraceptives
3. barrier methods such as a diaphragm
4. intrauterine device

6 The postpartum client calls the office nurse and states that she is constipated. Which of the following suggestions would the nurse offer? Choose all that apply.

1. Restrict fluid intake.
2. Walk 30 minutes per day.
3. Eat a diet consisting of soft foods.
4. Increase fluid intake.
5. Eat a diet consisting of high fiber.

7 Following birth, the nurse encourages the Asian client to place an ice pack on her episiotomy. What is the expected response from the client?

1. placing the ice pack on her perineum
2. requesting to take a shower instead
3. refusing the ice pack
4. asking for a chemical cold pack instead

8 On the second day postpartum, the nurse assesses the client's temperature to be 100.6°F. What nursing action is most appropriate?

1. Assess for further signs of infection.
2. No action is necessary; this is a normal finding.
3. Administer Lortab PO.
4. Encourage the mother to breastfeed.

9 The LPN/LVN understands that which of the following breast assessment findings is considered to be normal for the client who gave birth less than 24 hours ago?

1. firm, hard to palpation
2. red streaks surrounding the areola
3. cracks noted on the nipple
4. thin yellow drainage noted from the nipple

10 The nurse is to give Colace (docusate sodium) 250 mg PO. On hand is Colace 100 mg/tablet. The nurse will give _____ tablets.

Answers for Review Questions, as well as discussion of Care Plan and Critical Thinking Care Map questions, appear in Appendix I.

Thinking Strategically About...

You are a new graduate LPN, employed in a small hospital obstetric unit. The unit is staffed with one RN and one LPN per 8-hour shift. In report, you learn that a gravida 4, para 3 woman is laboring rapidly and is currently 8 cm dilated. The RN will need to remain with this client and assist in the delivery. You will be assigned to the other clients. There is an RN in another part of the hospital who can assist you if necessary.

At 0700, you receive the following report:

Mrs. Jessie Owens, a 22-year-old gravida 2, para 2, had a 7-lb 2-oz boy at 1300 yesterday by spontaneous vaginal delivery. She had no episiotomy or lacerations. She has had no postpartum complications. She is breastfeeding and plans to go home late this afternoon. Her baby, Philip, is nursing 8 minutes per breast. He has voided and stooled. Jessie has blood type B−, rubella positive. Philip has blood type A+. He is to be circumcised before discharge.

Miss Monica McQuire, a 19-year-old, gravida 1, para 1, delivered an 8-lb 10-oz girl at 0130 this morning by primary cesarean section for failure to progress in labor. Prior to delivery, Monica had pregnancy-induced hypertension with a blood pressure of 154/92. She had 2+ pitting edema in her ankles. Her reflexes were brisk without clonus. She has an IV of lactated Ringer's solution with magnesium sulfate and a Foley catheter that can be discontinued this morning. Her baby, Amanda, has voided but not stooled. Monica has only tried to breastfeed once since delivery, with poor results.

Mrs. Chung, a 24-year-old, gravida 7, para 6, is scheduled for admission and Pitocin induction of labor because she is overdue. She has just arrived at the hospital with her husband. They have only been in the United States for 4 months. They need to return to China as soon as possible after the baby is born because Mr. Chung's mother is extremely ill.

CRITICAL THINKING

- At what point do you become concerned that baby Amanda has not stooled?

- Is baby Philip nursing enough? What would indicate he is not obtaining enough nutrition?

COLLABORATIVE CARE

- Which of your assigned clients may need referral to an outside agency for follow-up care? Why?

PRIORITIES IN NURSING CARE

- Identify the order in which you will assess these assigned clients.
- What is your rationale for your prioritization of care?

MANAGEMENT OF CARE

- How frequently should you monitor Miss McQuire?
- What part of Mrs. Chung's induction can you begin before the RN returns from the delivery room?

DELEGATING

- If a CNA is available to assist with your assignment, what care would you delegate?

COMMUNICATION AND CLIENT TEACHING

- Due to your responsibilities with postpartum clients, what communication should be given to Mrs. Chung?
- What teaching should be provided to Mrs. Owens before she is discharged?

DOCUMENTING AND REPORTING

- What changes in Miss McQuire would indicate a decline in her condition? How and to whom would you report them?
- Document the teaching provided to Mrs. Owens regarding circumcision care.

CULTURAL CARE STRATEGIES

- What cultural strategies should be incorporated into the care of Mrs. Chung?

Pediatric Care

UNIT III

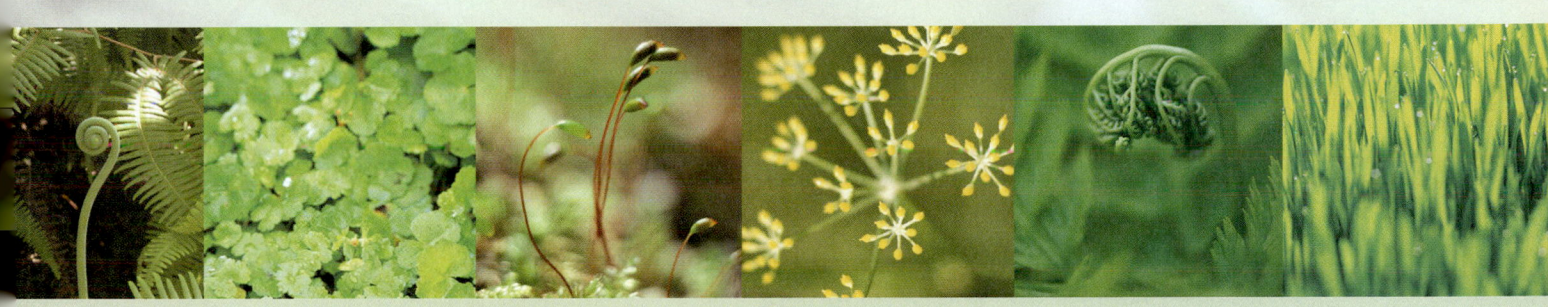

Chapter 11

Life Span Growth and Development

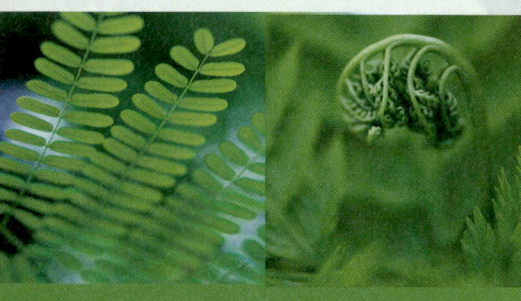

HEALTH PROMOTION ISSUE:
Internet Safety for Children

NURSING PROCESS CARE PLAN:
Infant with Delayed Growth and Development

CRITICAL THINKING CARE MAP:
Caring for Client with Risk for Injury

BRIEF Outline

Principles of Growth and Development

Theories of Development

Standards of Physical Growth and Development

Stages of Physical Growth and Development

Nursing Care

LEARNING Outcomes

After completing this chapter, you will be able to:

- Differentiate growth from development.
- List factors that influence growth and development.
- Describe Piaget's stages of cognitive development.
- Describe Erikson's levels of psychosocial development.
- Describe Freud's stages of psychosexual development.
- Describe Kohlberg's levels of moral development.
- Describe the usual physical development for each age group.
- Describe characteristic milestones and deviations from the norm for each age group.
- Provide some guidelines for age-appropriate teaching to each age group.

Growth and development are continual processes of change. They begin at the moment of conception and continue until the moment of death. **Growth** is the process of increasing in physical size. **Development** is the process of maturation, including the refinement of body systems, thought processes, and judgment.

Principles of Growth and Development

Growth and development occur individually but follow a general pattern of progression from simple to complex. Although orderly, they are usually uneven, with growth spurts followed by periods of little or no growth. Changes are often gradual and blur or blend together, instead of having a definite starting point. Box 11-1 ■ identifies the principles of growth and development. (*Note:* This chapter includes all stages of the life span, just as we included all phases of the family in Chapter 3 ⚭. Mother and child exist within this larger web.)

DIRECTION OF DEVELOPMENT

The directional patterns of development are fundamental to all humans and are equal bilaterally. Development is **cephalocaudal,** proceeding from head to toe (Figure 11-1 ■). For example, the infant must be able to raise its head before it can sit up. It must gain control of its trunk before it can walk (Figure 11-2 ■). Development is also **proximodistal,** meaning from the center of the body to

BOX 11-1
Principles of Growth and Development
■ Growth and development are continuous, bilateral processes.
■ Not all parts of the body mature at the same time.
■ Growth and development are individualized.
■ Growth and development are orderly and proceed from simple to complex.
■ Growth and development are uneven at times, with growth spurts followed by plateaus.
■ Growth and development changes are insidious, blurring and blending together.
■ Growth and development proceed from head to toe (cephalocaudal).
■ Growth and development proceed from center to periphery (proximodistal).
■ Growth and development proceed from general to specific.

the periphery and proceeding from general to specific. For example, the infant can close its hand and grasp before it has finger pinch. The child has gross motor control before fine motor control.

FACTORS THAT INFLUENCE GROWTH AND DEVELOPMENT

Heredity

There are many factors that influence normal growth and development (Box 11-2 ■). Heredity plays an important

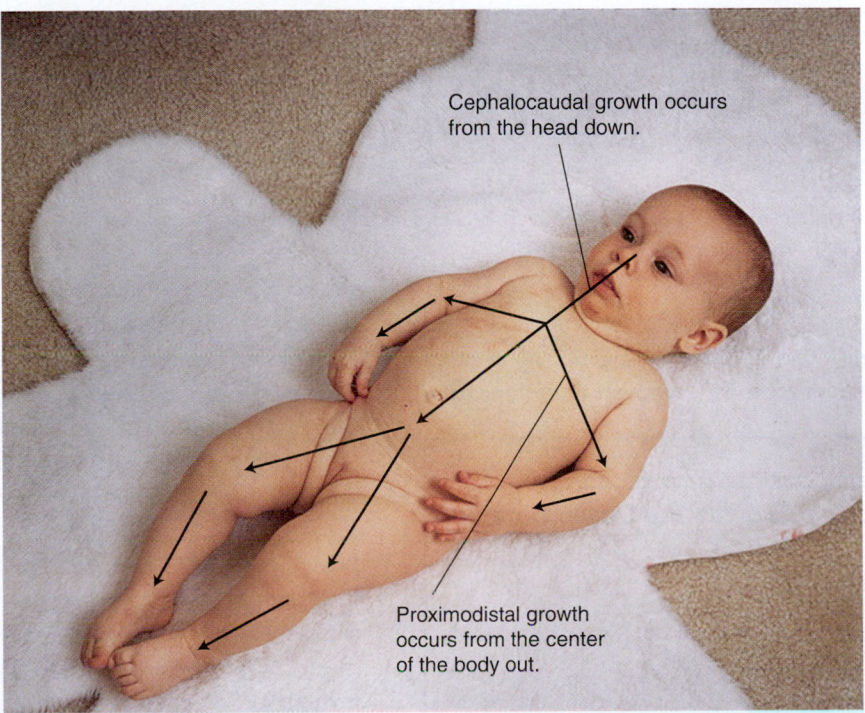

Cephalocaudal growth occurs from the head down.

Proximodistal growth occurs from the center of the body out.

Figure 11-1. ■ Illustration showing growth and development direction in a small child.

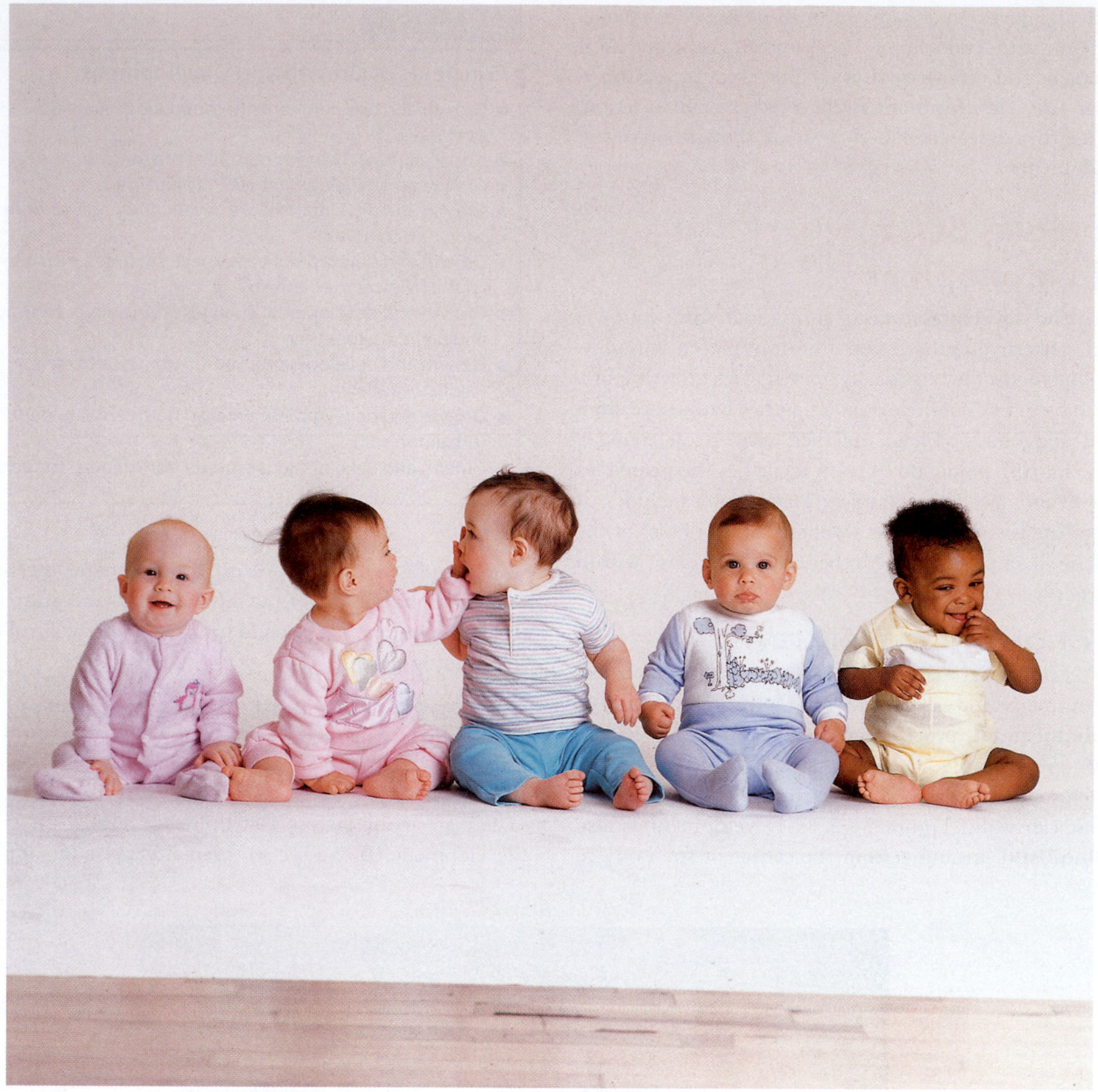

Figure 11-2. ■ Infants learn to sit by about 6 months. They communicate with body language long before they speak. (Barbara Campbell/Getty Images, Inc.)

role. Characteristics from ancestors are determined at conception through countless combinations of genes. Some characteristics from one parent are more dominant than those from

BOX 11-2

Influences on Normal Growth and Development
- Heredity
- Nationality, race, and culture
- Ordinal position in family
- Gender
- Family function or dysfunction
- Physical environment

the other parent. Eye and hair color and physical stature are examples of hereditary characteristics. If both parents are tall with blond hair and blue eyes, the children will probably be the same. If one parent is tall and blond with blue eyes and the other parent is short with brown hair and brown eyes, the children will probably show a mixture of these characteristics.

Nationality, Race, and Culture
One's nationality, race, and cultural customs can influence the rates of growth and development. To some extent this might appear to be genetic, but we are finding that growth and development are more complex. At one time, both parents came from the same town, were of the same

Thinking Clearly About Clients of Other Cultures

When culture is an issue in the delivery of client care, the nurse must make use of his or her critical thinking ability. Cultural awareness does not take the process far enough. Cultural awareness can be used to categorize, rather than individualize, care. It may cause too great a focus on race, culture, and ethnicity.

Nurses must not label people by culture and race. We must not assume that the characteristics of a certain cultural group are true for every client who belongs to that racial, ethnic, or cultural group. Assumptions close our minds to the real information we can obtain through our senses and through insightful questions addressed to the client.

The information we learn about cultural groups is no more than an overview. Nurses must always be aware of what people may be thinking that may differ from our own thoughts. We must recognize that other sources outside the traditional medical community exist to help clients.

Source: Adapted from Ramont, R. R., Niedringhaus, D. M., & Towle, M. A. (2006). *Comprehensive nursing care.* Upper Saddle River, NJ: Prentice Hall.

race and nationality, and had the same cultural customs. Children from these towns grew and developed at similar rates. As our world has become more mobile, and race and cultural customs have blended, growth and development patterns have changed. As these changes are studied, we are learning that cultural customs affecting diet, activity, and family dynamics influence childhood development. For example, it was once believed that people of Asian descent were short in stature. Today, a person of Asian descent who is born in the United States grows to a height comparable to other U.S. children. Box 11-3 ■ discusses the importance of viewing a client's culture as only one aspect of the whole person.

Order of Birth

The order of birth (**ordinal position**) in the family can influence development. People who are just learning to be parents influence the development of the oldest child. The development of the middle child is influenced not only by parents who have some experience, but also by learning from the older child. The youngest child may develop differently in some areas because he or she learns from the older children. At other times, the youngest child is slower in development because of the tendency to do things for "the baby." An only child might mature faster intellectually because of the amount of time spent with adults instead of other children. Parents of an only child might "spoil" the child or slow the development in an attempt to "hold on to their baby."

Gender

The gender of the person influences growth and development. Males are usually longer and heavier at birth. This growth difference continues into adulthood. Development and **maturation** (the process of becoming fully developed) also occur at different rates. They are influenced by different expectations of the genders. For example, the girl who is expected to play in the house with dolls may not gain physical strength as rapidly as the boy who plays soccer. In this example, the children might assume girls are weaker or boys are less nurturing. Culture also has a big influence on gender roles. For example, a culture may dictate that men must be dominant and that women must be submissive. Children of these cultures develop these beliefs and may have difficulty interacting with people of different cultures.

Family Stucture

The family structure influences the development of the child. The traditional roles of the mother and father have changed. In many families, parents are employed outside the home, so children spend a lot of time interacting with other children and adults in child care facilities. Families may consist of one parent, homosexual parents, or grandparents assuming the role of parents. Children may live in poverty, lack proper nutrition, and have limited access to health care. The function or dysfunction of the family affects the development of the child. Family systems are discussed later in this chapter. See also Chapter 3 ⚭.

Physical and Emotional Environment

The physical environment in which the child lives will influence the development of the child. A clean, secure, and stable environment with adequate nutrition and health care allows a child to focus energy on healthy growth and development. A tense environment, in which the child feels unloved, or an insecure environment, where there is limited nutrition and health care, interferes with the development process.

Theories of Development

Theories provide a framework for studying the world around us. Many individuals have devoted their life's work to understanding the process of human growth and development. They have developed theories to organize their findings. Some have used a "systems approach," believing that everyone in the system or family is influenced by everyone else in the family. Others have studied various aspects of the individual such as physical growth, cognitive ability, or moral development. The LPN/LVN must have a basic understanding of these theories in order to assist in the assessment of the growth and development of the child and individual members of the family. These theories will be applied to each stage of development.

COGNITIVE DEVELOPMENT

The intellectual ability of an individual is called cognition or **cognitive development.** Children are born with an innate cognitive ability that must be developed. Jean Piaget, a Swiss psychologist, was a pioneer and an outstanding authority on cognitive development. Piaget believed intelligence consists of interaction and coping with one's environment. He proposed four interrelated levels of cognitive development. These are shown in Table 11-1 ■.

The first level, the **sensorimotor,** is from birth to 2 years of age. During this stage, the baby and young child begin interaction with the environment by reflex response. (More information about typical infant reflexes is provided in Chapter 9 ⚭.)

As children learn to interact with members of the environment, they move into the **preoperational** level at ages 2 to 7. The child at age 2 begins to use symbolism (mainly in the form of language) and progresses to the use of other symbols, such as numbers and letters, by age 7.

From ages 7 to 11, the child is oriented in the here and now. In this stage, called **concrete operational,** the child interacts with the local environment. The development of technology has expanded that environment, but the child's main focus remains relatively narrow. Everything in the environment is "black and white," "right or wrong." The child has difficulty with "gray" areas or abstraction.

From ages 11 to 16, the child's interaction with the environment rapidly expands to include abstract comprehension. This includes being able to predict future outcomes of today's behavior. In this final stage, called **formal operations,** the child gradually completes the intellectual development that is necessary to function as an adult.

PSYCHOSOCIAL DEVELOPMENT

Psychosocial development is a much more complex process, and, likewise, more theorists have contributed to our understanding. Although there are differences in the theories, there are also many similarities. Erikson's theory is widely used and is described here. It is important to note that this is not the only theory on psychosocial development. (Psychosocial issues are also discussed in Chapter 27 ⚭.)

Erikson described eight stages of development in which the individual moves between two opposing themes. These stages are listed in Table 11-2 ■. The first stage is infancy. In this stage, the infant (from newborn to 1 year) is developing trust. For example, when the infant is hungry, it cries in an attempt to make its needs known. There is a brief period of mistrust as the infant waits for satisfaction. As the mother holds and feeds the infant, the infant learns to trust her to meet needs that he or she cannot meet. Over time, the infant learns to trust and is less stressed in time of need. This basic stage of trust versus mistrust is very important. Children who do not have these first needs met often have a lot of difficulty trusting anyone as adults.

The second stage is early childhood, from ages 1 to 3 years. In this stage, the toddler learns autonomy versus shame and doubt. As the child becomes more mobile, he wants to do increasingly more on his own. When he is unsuccessful, he feels shame and doubts his abilities. Through repeated tries and successes, the child gradually develops confidence. For example, the toddler shows autonomy by learning to use the toilet. If parents focus on "accidents" and put him down for soiling himself, he learns shame and doubt, and he may not

TABLE 11-1

Piaget's Levels of Cognitive Development

LEVEL	AGE (YEARS)	TASK
Sensorimotor	Birth–2	Interacts with the environment by reflex response
Preoperational	2–7	Begins to use language and progresses to use of numbers and letters
Concrete operational	7–11	Sees everything in "black and white," "right or wrong" terms
Formal operations	11–16	Interactions include abstract thought; able to predict future outcomes of today's behavior

TABLE 11-2

Erikson's Eight Stages of Development

STAGE	AGE (YEARS)	OPPOSING THEMES
Infancy	0–1	Trust vs. mistrust
Early childhood	1–3	Autonomy vs. shame and doubt
Late childhood	3–6	Initiative vs. guilt
School age	6–12	Industry vs. inferiority
Adolescence	12–18	Identity vs. role confusion
Young adult	20–40	Intimacy vs. isolation
Middle adult	40–65	Generativity vs. self-absorption/stagnation
Elder adult	Older than 65	Ego integrity vs. despair

try as hard. If parents praise his efforts and calmly accept the times when he is not successful, his feelings of trust (from Stage one) help him feel positive about his developing autonomy. His bowel and bladder control will develop over time, and eventually he will become successful. However, his feelings about himself can be either positive or negative.

The third stage, late childhood, is one of initiative versus guilt. In this stage, ages 3 to 6 years, the child learns to take initiative to meet her own needs. She may become quite creative in an effort to accomplish what she sets out to do. If she does not receive praise for her efforts, she will feel guilt about being a failure or about not giving pleasure to those she loves. For example, if the child's hair is hanging in her face, she might get the scissors and cut it instead of combing it. If the parent reacts by yelling or punishing, the child will feel guilty. If the parent quietly explains to the child reasons for not cutting her hair, she will not experience guilt. Through positive reinforcement of her initiative, she will continue to develop a positive attitude.

The fourth stage, school age, from 6 to 12 years, is a time of developing industry versus inferiority. As a child progresses through school and applies what he learns to a variety of life experiences, he becomes more industrious. He seeks praise from both teachers and peers. If the child is unsuccessful or does not receive praise, he feels inferior and may become withdrawn. He might become quiet, have few friends, and not participate in any outside activities. Other children may use different behaviors to get attention. They might act out in groups, become bullies, or become physically or verbally abusive in an attempt to feel better about themselves. The child who receives praise for something he does well will be able to work for improvement in difficult areas, while excelling in others. The child will learn that everyone has areas of strength and areas that need improvement.

The fifth stage is adolescence. This stage, ages 12 to 20 years, is the time of identity versus role confusion. The teenager is developing a sexual identity, is becoming more independent, and is beginning the process of separation from the parents. The teenager has a strong desire to make her own decisions and "live her own life" but at the same time has a real need to know the boundaries or rules. The teenager is examining the world and trying to decide where she fits, what her life's work will be, and how she can accomplish her goals. She is beginning to use peers for support instead of relying on parents for help in making decisions. With positive reinforcement of her progress, she can develop a strong identity. However, with continual negative feedback, coupled with feelings of inferiority and guilt, she can become confused, ambivalent, and withdrawn. If the parents do not allow her to separate from their influence, to develop peer relationships, and make her own decisions, she will remain dependent.

The sixth stage, young adult, ages 20 to 40 years, is a time of intimacy versus isolation. The young adult has made decisions regarding his life's work and is now interested in finding a companion, someone with whom to share his life. This is a time when many people marry and begin a family. The relationships developed are usually deep, long-lasting bonds. If the young adult has difficulty finding a companion, he fears a life of loneliness and isolation. This fear can either be a motivating force or be immobilizing. If motivated, the young adult settles into a life of companionship, special friends, and raising children. If immobile, the young adult settles for a life of few or no close friends, where leisure time is spent by oneself.

The middle years, ages 40 to 65, constitute the seventh stage. This is a time of generativity versus self-absorption and stagnation. Generativity comes from the same root word as generation, generator, and generous. This is the time in life when the adult becomes a great generator of ideas and beliefs. He thinks of what he has contributed to society and the next generation. He is generous in sharing what he has learned from his life experiences. This is a time when most adults become grandparents and are proud to see their life's work carried on by their offspring. Sometimes, though, adults becomes absorbed in their own lives. People who do not complete this stage successfully become stagnant and lack creativity. They have difficulty seeing any value and meaning in their lives.

The final state is the older adult, older than 65 years. This time is devoted to ego integrity versus despair. Most adults have learned to trust as infants, have developed a sense of identity during adolescence, and have enjoyed an adult life full of rich relationships. If older adults have had these positive life experiences, they will probably enter old age with a strong identity. They can look at their life and know the world was a better place because of them. They can truly say, "I've had a good life." However, if the older adult has had a life of mistrust, guilt, and feelings of inferiority, if they have been isolated and stagnant, they will enter old age in self-despair. They find no joy in life. They become angry and bitter in their old age and can drive others away, leading to more isolation.

PSYCHOSEXUAL DEVELOPMENT

Freud, an Austrian physician, worked with adults who were experiencing nervous disorders. By studying the results of psychoanalysis, he developed the belief that early childhood experiences led to unconscious motivation for actions in later life. He believed that sexual instincts were important to the development of the personality. He termed the need for sensual pleasure **psychosexual.**

Freud viewed the personality in three parts. The **id** is the basic energy that drives the individual to seek pleasure. The **ego** is the realistic part of the personality that searches for acceptable methods of meeting pleasure needs. The **superego**

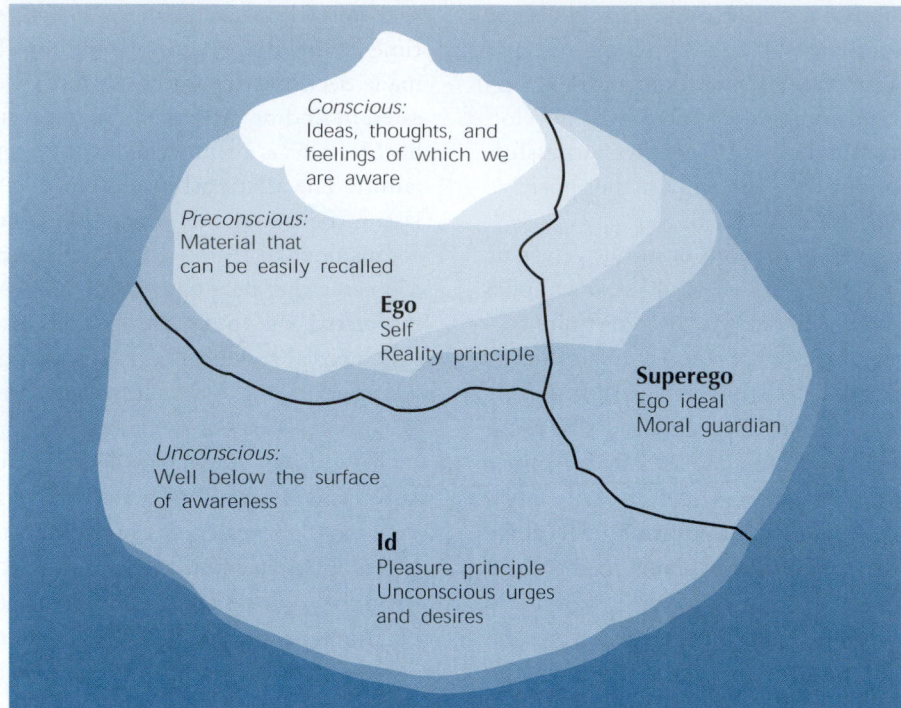

Figure 11-3. ■ Freud saw the vast importance of the unconscious in people's lives. He said that most actions are motivated by subconscious thought. He viewed the personality in three parts: the id (the basic energy that drives the individual to seek pleasure), the ego (the realistic part of the personality that searches for acceptable ways of obtaining pleasure), and the superego (the moral system that contains learned values and conscience). People are aware of their conscious thoughts, but it is often the subconscious that drives us. (Reprinted from Morris, C. G., & Maisto, A. A. [2001]. *Understanding psychology* [5th ed.]. Upper Saddle River, NJ: Prentice Hall.)

is the moral system that contains learned values and conscience (Figure 11-3 ■). Freud described five stages of psychosexual development. Table 11-3 ■ identifies these stages. Freud also emphasized that much of what people experience is governed by the subconscious parts of the mind. In other words, we are often not aware of the feelings and buried thoughts that

motivate us and cause us to respond the way we do. He first introduced the idea that a client could uncover problems by talking, remembering dreams, and associating thoughts freely. Although many of Freud's theories have been refuted by later theorists, two aspects of his thinking still prevail:

1. Behavior is motivated (not accidental) and is often unconscious.
2. People have ways of "protecting the ego from threatening impulses or painful realities of life experiences" (Eby, 2005). These ways of protecting oneself are called **defense mechanisms.** Common defense mechanisms are described in Chapter 27 ⬭). Four defense mechanisms are commonly used by children. These are shown in Table 11-4 ■.

KOHLBERG'S THEORY OF MORAL DEVELOPMENT

Kohlberg focused his theoretical study on the moral development of people. He worked with children in his native Germany and in other countries. He presented stories involving a moral dilemma and asked children and adults to solve the problem. He then analyzed their expressed motives for the decisions they made. In this way, Kohlberg established three levels of moral development. He noted that the age guidelines he presented are approximate and that many people never reach the highest level. Table 11-5 ■ describes these levels of moral development.

TABLE 11-3

Freud's Stages of Psychosexual Development

STAGE	AGE (YEARS)	DESCRIPTION
Oral	Birth–1	Baby obtains comfort and pleasure through the mouth
Anal	1–3	Child achieves pleasure through control of waste elimination from the body
Phallic	3–6	Child works out relationships with parents and relatives of the same and opposite genders
Latency	6–12	Sexual energy is at rest
Genital	12 to Adulthood	Development of mature sexuality and the establishment of relationships with others

TABLE 11-4

Defense Mechanisms Commonly Used by Children

DEFENSE MECHANISM	DEFINITION	EXAMPLE
Regression	Returning to an earlier stage of behavior	A 7-year-old who does not suck his thumb, suddenly begins to suck his thumb when hospitalized
Repression	Involuntary forgetting of hurtful situations	A child witnessed the brutal death of her parent, cannot consciously recall the incident
Rationalization	Attempting to make unacceptable feelings acceptable	A child explains pulling another child's hair because "she won't give me my doll"
Fantasy	Creating a story in the mind to help deal with unacceptable fears	A child with a history of abuse pretends to be Cinderella

Standards of Physical Growth and Development

Physical growth is usually measured by height, weight, and head circumference. Before the child can stand, horizontal length is measured instead of vertical height. The standard measurements for height and head circumference are inches or centimeters. Weight is measured in pounds

TABLE 11-5

Kohlberg's Levels of Moral Development

STAGE	APPROXIMATE AGE (YEARS)	DESCRIPTION
Preconventional	4–7	Decisions are based on desire to please others and avoid punishment
Conventional	7–11	Rules are important and must be followed Conscience begins to develop
Postconventional	12 and older	Individual has internalized ethical standards and recognizes social responsibility

and ounces or in grams. These measurements are recorded on a growth chart (see Appendix II ⚭). The growth chart has lines to correspond to 5th, 10th, 25th, 50th, 75th, 90th, and 95th percentile. **Percentile** is a measure of the portion of the overall population that is the same. For example, if a child is at the 75th percentile for height, he or she is taller than 75% of the population and shorter than 25% of the population. The use of growth charts is valuable for the following reasons:

- The child's growth can be compared to the average for his age. A difference of 2 or more percentile between height and weight may indicate an overweight or underweight condition that should be further investigated.
- The current measurements can be compared to the child's previous measurements. If the child's growth pattern falls outside the normal pattern, further investigation may be suggested (see Appendix IV ⚭).

Stages of Physical Growth and Development

INFANT (BIRTH TO 1 YEAR)

At no time is rapid change as notable as during the first year of life. The infant enters the world totally dependent and by year's end can walk and communicate. Over years of study into growth and development, researchers have developed tables showing standard milestones for each age group. It is important to compare the progress of the growing child with these standards. With them, problems can be identified early and intervention begun. Table 11-6 ■ illustrates the milestones the infant should reach during the first year of development. (*Note:* The nurse's adaptations to different stages of growth and development are discussed in Chapter 13 ⚭.)

Physical Growth

With good nutrition, the infant gains weight rapidly, doubling its birth weight by 5 months and tripling the birth weight by 12 months. It grows about 12 inches during this time. With this growth comes a change in body proportion (see Figure 12-10 ⚭). The head, growing rapidly during fetal development, now slows its growth, while the torso and limbs become longer and stronger.

Organs and body systems are completely formed early in the fetal development process, but are not fully mature for several years. The liver and kidneys begin to mature and are able to detoxify and excrete drugs and other chemicals. The nervous system is able to coordinate muscle movements. The senses are able to discriminate visual images, sound, and taste. As teeth erupt, beginning at about 6 months, the stomach and intestines are also able to digest more complex foods.

TABLE 11-6

Growth and Development Milestones During Infancy

AGE (MONTHS)	PHYSICAL GROWTH	FINE MOTOR SKILLS	GROSS MOTOR SKILLS	SENSORY ABILITY
Birth–1	Gains 5–7 oz (140–200 g)/wk Grows ½ in. (1.5 cm) in first month Head circumference increases ½ in. (1.5 cm)/month	Holds hand in fist (1) Draws arms and legs to body when crying Tight grasp	Inborn reflexes such as startle and rooting are predominant activity May lift head briefly if prone (2) Alerts to high-pitched voices Comforts with touch (3) Arm/leg movement jerky	Prefers to look at faces and black and white geometric designs Follows objects in line of vision (4)

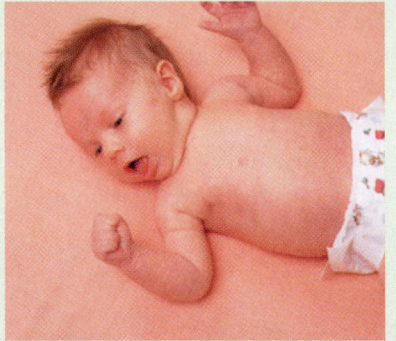

(1) Picks up small objects

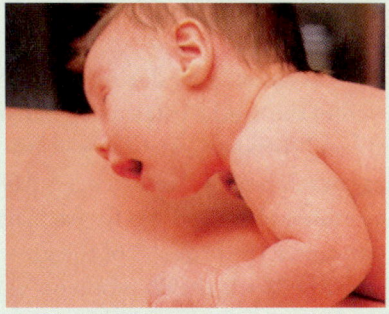

(2) May lift head

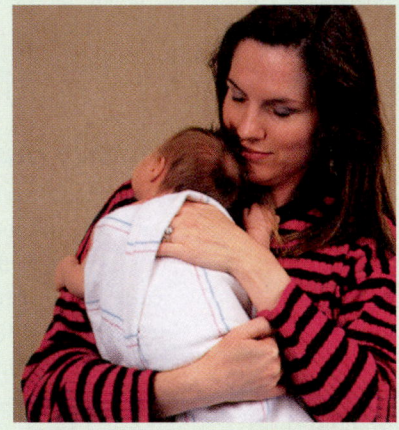

(3) Comforts with touch

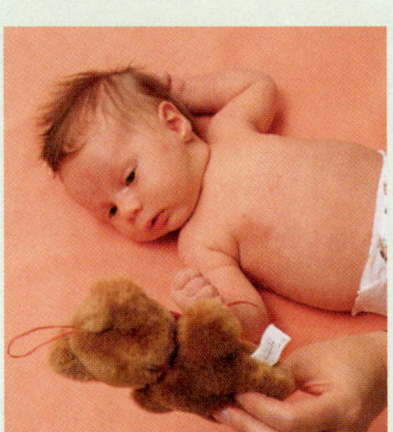

(4) Follows objects

| 2–4 | Gains 5–7 oz (140–200 g)/wk
Grows ½ in. (1.5 cm)/month
Head circumference increases ½ in. (1.5 cm)/month
Posterior fontanel closes
Eats 120 mL/kg/24 hr (2 oz/lb/24 hr) | Holds rattle when placed in hand (5)
Looks at and plays with own fingers
Readily brings objects from hand to mouth | Moro reflex fading in strength
Can turn from side to back and then return (6)
Decrease in head lag when pulled to sitting; sits with head held in midline with some bobbing
When prone, holds head and supports weight on forearms (7) | Follows objects 180 degrees
Turns head to look for voices, sounds |

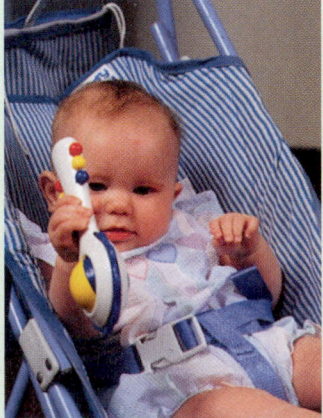

(5) Holds rattle

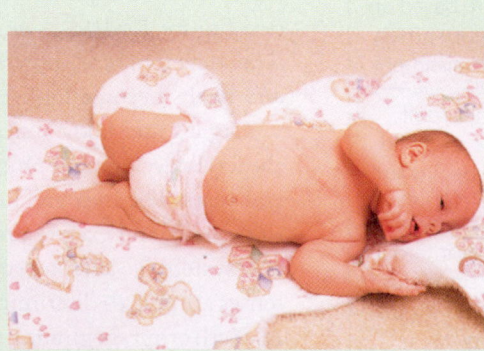

(6) Can turn from side to back

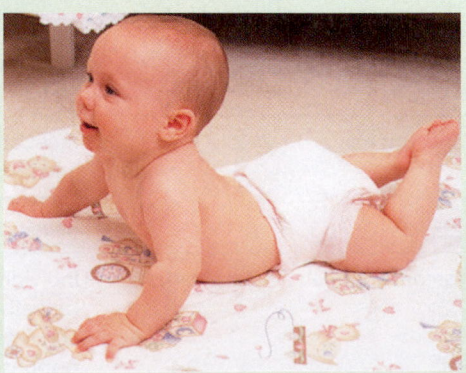

(7) Holds head up and supports weights with arms

AGE (MONTHS)	PHYSICAL GROWTH	FINE MOTOR SKILLS	GROSS MOTOR SKILLS	SENSORY ABILITY
4–6	Gains 5–7 oz (140–200 g)/week Doubles birth weight by 5–6 months Grows ½ in. (1.5 cm)/month Head circumference increases ½ in. (1.5 cm)/month Teeth begin to erupt by 6 months Eats 100 mL/kg 24 hr (2 oz/lb/24 hr)	Grasps rattle and other objects at will; drops them to pick up another offered object (8) Mouths objects Mouths feet and pulls to mouth Holds bottle Grasps with whole hand (palmar grasp) Manipulates objects (9)	Head held steady when sitting Turns from abdomen to back by 4 months and then back to abdomen by 6 months When held standing, supports much of own weight (10)	Examines complex visual images Watches the course of a falling object Responds readily to sounds

(8) Grasps objects at will   **(9)** Manipulates objects   **(10)** Supports most of weight

| 6–8 | Gains 3–5 oz (85–140 g)/week
Grows 3/8 in. (1 cm)/month
Growth rate slower than first 6 months | Bangs objects held in hand
Transfers objects from one hand to other
Beginning pincer grasp at times | Most newborn reflexes extinguished
Sits alone without support by 8 months (11)
Likes to bounce on legs when held in standing position | Recognizes own name and responds by looking and smiling
Enjoys small and complex objects at play |

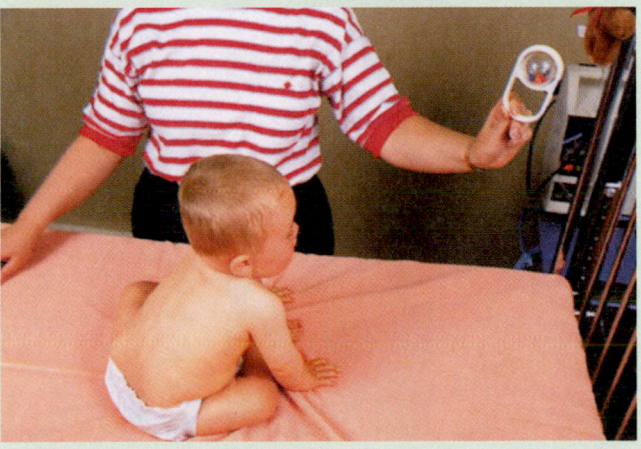

(11) Sits alone without support

(continued)

TABLE 11-6

Growth and Development Milestones During Infancy (continued)

AGE (MONTHS)	PHYSICAL GROWTH	FINE MOTOR SKILLS	GROSS MOTOR SKILLS	SENSORY ABILITY
8–10	Gains 3–5 oz (85–140 g)/week Grows 3/8 in. (1 cm)/month	Picks up small objects (12) Uses pincer grasp well (14)	Crawls or pulls body along floor by arms (13) Creeps by using hands and knees to keep trunk off the floor Pulls self to standing and sitting by 10 months Recovers balance when sitting	Understands words such as "no" and "cracker" May say one word in addition to "mama" and "dada" Recognizes sound without difficulty

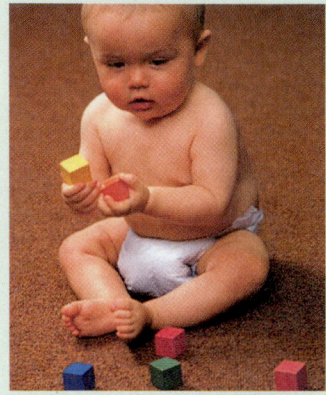

(12)   Picks up small objects

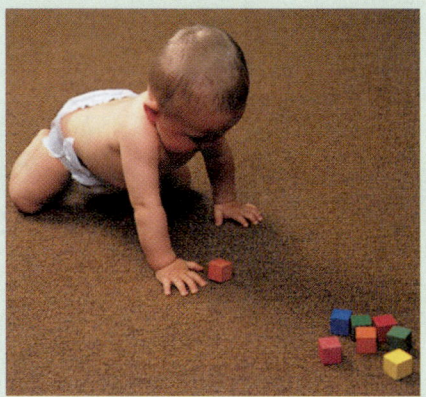

(13)   Crawls or pulls body by arms

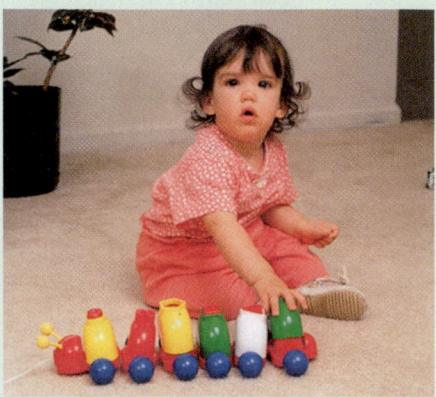

(14)   Uses pincer grasp well

AGE (MONTHS)	PHYSICAL GROWTH	FINE MOTOR SKILLS	GROSS MOTOR SKILLS	SENSORY ABILITY
10–12	Gains 3–5 oz (85–140 g)/week Grown 3/8 in. (1 cm)/month Head circumference equals chest circumference Triples birth weight by 1 year	May hold crayon or pencil and make mark on paper Places objects into container through holes (15)	Stands alone (16) Walks holding on to furniture Sits from standing (17) May walk alone for short distance	Plays peek-a-boo and patty cake

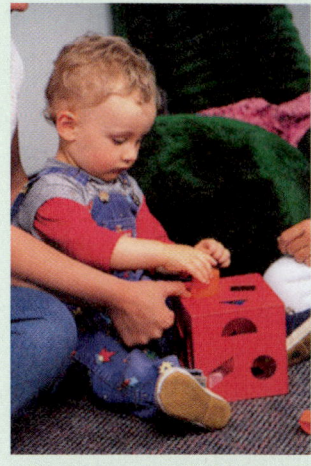

(15)   Places objects in container

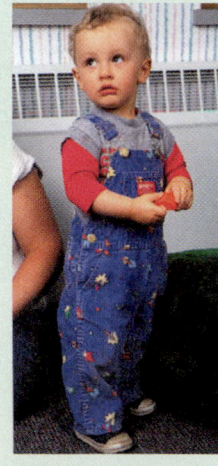

(16)   Stands alone

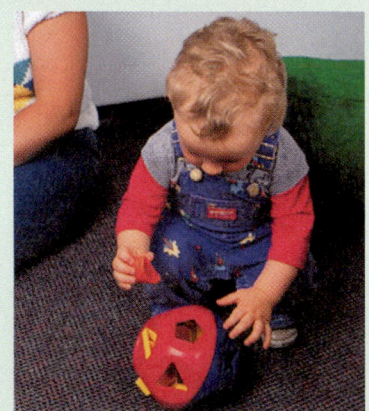

(17)   Sits down from standing

Source: Ball, J., & Bindler, R. Pediatric nursing care for children. 3rd ed. [2003]. pp. 41–43. Upper Saddle River, NJ: Prentice Hall.

Cognitive Development

The infant's behavior provides clues to brain function. There is a great change between a newborn, which interacts with its environment on a reflex level, and a 1-year-old, who interacts with the environment and interprets sights and sounds. During the course of a child's first year, the brain has learned to input and store impulses for future reference. The 2-month-old learns to make noise in response to voices, and by the end of the year can understand many words and say a few of them.

The newborn sleeps for 20 to 22 hours a day. Over the next few months, the infant gradually stays awake for longer periods of time. By 4 months, the infant will be

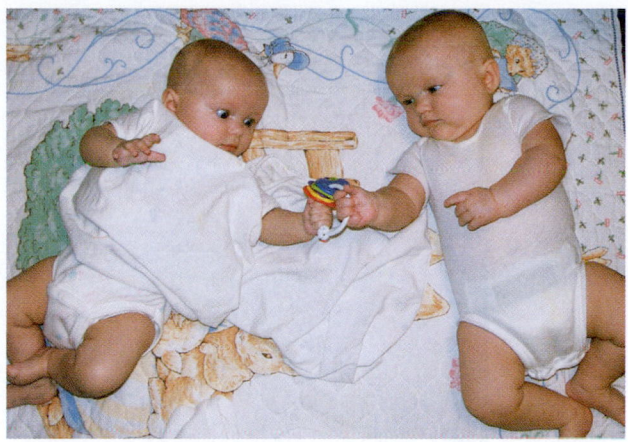

Figure 11-4. ■ In the first year, reflex actions gradually evolve into deliberate actions. Until the infant becomes mobile, the "world" of the infant consists of things within his or her reach. (Courtesy of J. Tobias)

awake for 2 to 3 hours at a time during the day and sleep through the night. During these hours of wakefulness, it is important for the infant to begin to explore the environment. With little mobility, the infant's "world" is the area within reach (Figure 11-4 ■). As he moves and stretches to explore, he learns to turn over and roll. He learns to explore by touch and taste. He learns he can manipulate things in

his grasp and produce pleasure. He is developing the foundation of play. As the infant's strength grows, he learns to sit alone, to crawl, and finally to stand. With movement comes a wider and wider environment to explore.

TODDLER (1 TO 3 YEARS)

The word *toddle* means to walk with short unsteady steps. The child in this age group fits this definition well. As he learns to walk, he is unsteady, falling frequently. His steps are short, with the feet far apart to broaden his base of support. Once he gains security and practice in walking, he begins to walk faster and finally to run. At the same time, he is learning to climb and wants to stand on everything. By age 3, he can stand briefly on one foot and can ride a tricycle.

Physical Growth

During the second year of life, the toddler's growth slows, but his body proportions continue to change. His legs become longer and his head smaller in relation to body size. At first, he appears pot bellied because his abdominal muscles lack strength. Over time, the child's activity strengthens the muscles, and the abdomen becomes flatter (see Figure 17-3).

The toddler continues to cut teeth, with complete eruption of 20 deciduous teeth by 34 months (Figure 11-5 ■).

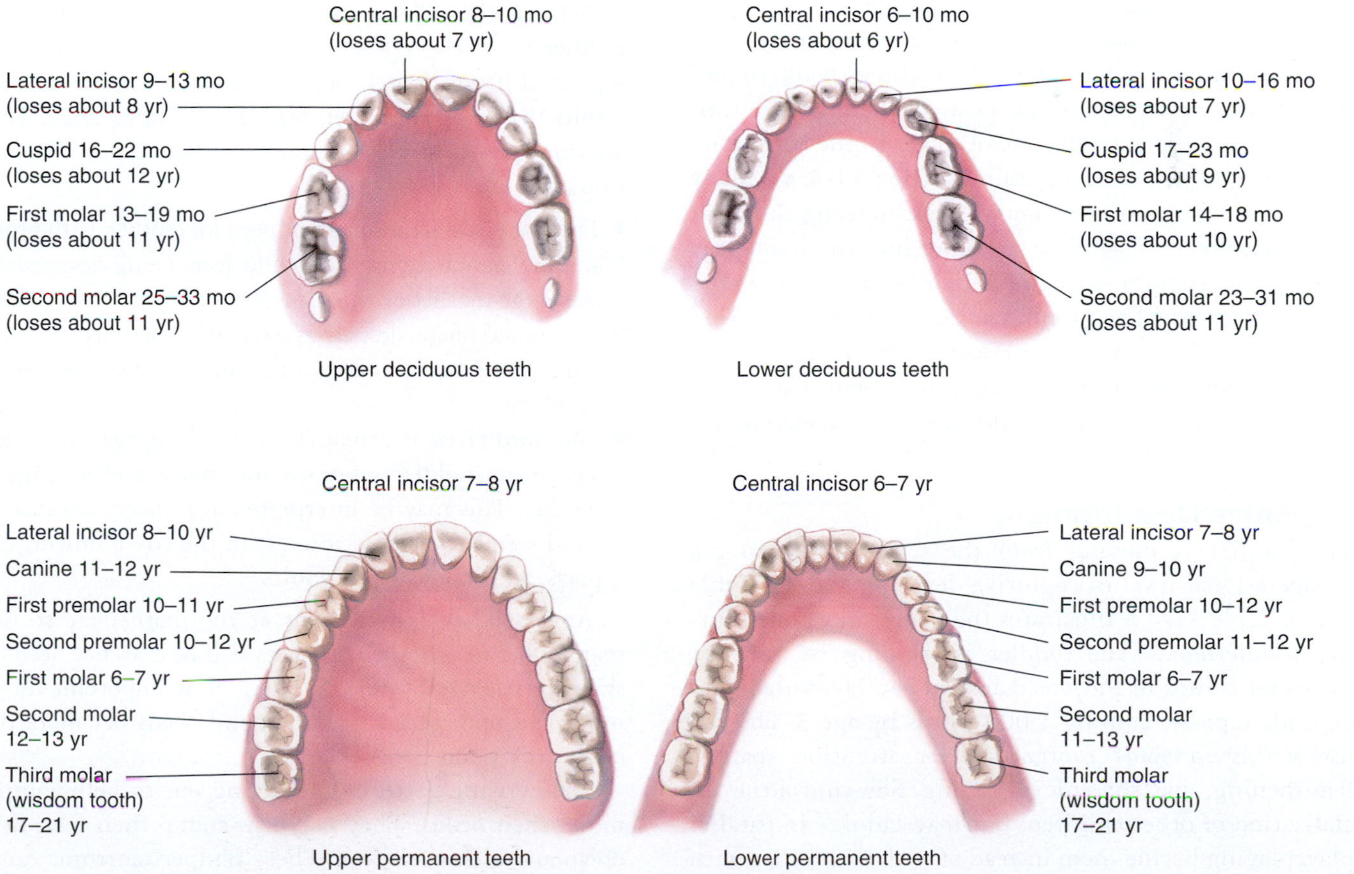

Central incisor 8–10 mo (loses about 7 yr)

Lateral incisor 9–13 mo (loses about 8 yr)

Cuspid 16–22 mo (loses about 12 yr)

First molar 13–19 mo (loses about 11 yr)

Second molar 25–33 mo (loses about 11 yr)

Upper deciduous teeth

Central incisor 6–10 mo (loses about 6 yr)

Lateral incisor 10–16 mo (loses about 7 yr)

Cuspid 17–23 mo (loses about 9 yr)

First molar 14–18 mo (loses about 10 yr)

Second molar 23–31 mo (loses about 11 yr)

Lower deciduous teeth

Central incisor 7–8 yr

Lateral incisor 8–10 yr
Canine 11–12 yr
First premolar 10–11 yr
Second premolar 10–12 yr
First molar 6–7 yr
Second molar 12–13 yr
Third molar (wisdom tooth) 17–21 yr

Upper permanent teeth

Central incisor 6–7 yr

Lateral incisor 7–8 yr
Canine 9–10 yr
First premolar 10–12 yr
Second premolar 11–12 yr
First molar 6–7 yr
Second molar 11–13 yr
Third molar (wisdom tooth) 17–21 yr

Lower permanent teeth

Figure 11-5. ■ (*Top*) Typical eruption of deciduous ("baby") teeth. (*Bottom*) The school-age child loses teeth at a rate of 4 a year and, by age 12, has 26 of the 30 permanent teeth. The remaining molars appear during adolescence.

BOX 11-4   CLIENT TEACHING

Toilet Training

Determining Readiness

Although readiness is individualized, the child must have achieved the following developmental skills:

- Stand and walk
- Pull pants up and down
- Recognize need to "go"
- Can wait to reach bathroom

Helpful Hints

- If child is afraid of toilet, use small chair or small toilet seat insert.
- If using toilet, place sturdy stool in front of toilet for child to stand on to reach the seat.
- Place child on seat upon rising in the morning, before and after naps, before bath, before bed, and at regular intervals through the day.
- Teach hand washing after toileting.
- Praise success. Do not punish accidents.
- If child does not cooperate, wait a few weeks and try again.

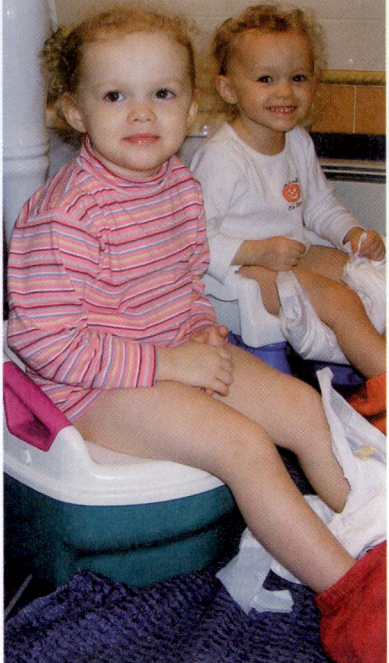

Figure 11-6. ■ Toilet training requires consistency and commitment on the part of the caregiver to schedule regular trips to bathroom.
(Courtesy of J. Tobias)

This helps the child eat a bigger variety of foods. Wanting to be independent, the toddler wants to feed himself and should be encouraged to do so.

During the second year, the toddler begins to gain control of his elimination. Once he is able to walk, to pull his pants up and down, to be aware of the urge to eliminate, and to have enough control to get to the bathroom, it is time to begin toilet training (Box 11-4 ■). Many children prefer their own "potty" chair to using the adult toilet (Figure 11-6 ■). Fear of falling into the water may prevent successful toileting. The toddler should be placed on the toilet for a few minutes at regular intervals during the day. Toddlers should be rewarded for success. If the toddler seems uninterested or confused about what is expected of him, the parent should wait a few weeks and try again.

Cognitive Development

The toddler is moving from the sensorimotor to the preoperational level of cognitive development (see Table 11-1). Table 11-7 ■ illustrates the major milestones during toddlerhood. The toddler is learning to associate words for things in the world around her. Her vocabulary expands rapidly, gaining 1,000 words by age 3. She can use words in short sentences. Her attention span is lengthening, and she enjoys playing. She enjoys the socialization of other children, but may indulge in parallel play, playing beside them instead of with them. Play with a variety of toys encourages both gross motor and fine motor development.

Being close to parents, especially the mother, is important in helping the toddler feel safe and secure. An infant or toddler experiences a state of extreme discomfort when separated from loved ones. This **separation anxiety** results in feelings of anger, fear, grief, and revenge. There are three phases of grief or mourning as a result of separation anxiety.

- The first phase is the apparent need for mother, with protest and prolonged crying. The child fears being deserted and needs the mother at this time.
- The second phase, despair, is seen by less activity. The child is not crying but is in deep mourning. He does not respond to others.
- The third phase is denial. This is defense against anxiety. The infant/toddler represses the image and feelings for mother. This may be interpreted as recovery because the child seems to take an interest in the environment, eats, plays, and accepts other adults.

Anger and disappointment at the mother are so deep that, on her return, the child acts as if he does not need her, showing revenge by rejecting her. It is important for the mother to understand that the child needs her more than ever at this point.

Toddlers use gestures and acting out to help communicate their needs. They may cry, stamp their feet, or lie down and kick their feet. These temper tantrums can be frustrating to parents. It is best to acknowledge the toddler's feelings and then to set limits for the toddler. For

TABLE 11-7				
Growth and Development Milestones During Toddlerhood				
AGE (YEARS)	**PHYSICAL GROWTH**	**FINE MOTOR SKILLS**	**GROSS MOTOR SKILLS**	**SENSORY ABILITY**
1–2	Gains $1/2$ lb (227 g) per month Grows 3.5–5 in. (9–12 cm) during this year Anterior fontanel closes All deciduous teeth present by 33 months	By end of second year, builds tower of four blocks (1) Scribbles on paper (2) Can undress self (3) Throws a ball	Runs Walks up and down stairs (5) Likes to push toys	Visual acuity 20/50 Increasing vocabulary of 200 words by 2 years
2–3	Gains 3–5 lb (1.4–2.3 kg)/year Grows 2–2.5 in. (5–6.5 cm)/year	Draws a circle and other rudimentary forms Learns to pour Learning to dress self (4)	Jumps Kicks ball (6) Throws ball overhand Rides tricycle	Communication improves Uses short 3- to 5-word sentences Vocabulary 1,000 words Displays frustration by temper tantrums

(1) Tower of four blocks

(2) Scribbles on paper

(3) Can undress self

(4) Learning to dress self

(5) Walks up and down stairs

(6) Jumps and kicks ball

Source: Ball, J., & Bindler, R. Pediatric nursing care for children. 3rd ed. [2003]. p. 48. Upper Saddle River, NJ: Prentice Hall.

example, "I know you are upset because you cannot have a cookie now. When you stop crying, you can come out of your room." When the child stops crying and comes out of his or her room, the parent should not bring up the bad behavior, but could say, "I am glad you are ready to help me set the table for dinner."

PRESCHOOL CHILD (3 TO 6 YEARS)

The preschool child is becoming more independent. He is learning to obey rules and is becoming self-disciplined. He is very curious and is developing an imagination. Table 11-8 ■ illustrates growth and development milestones during the preschool stage of development.

TABLE 11-8

Growth and Development Milestones During Preschool Years

AGE (YEARS)	PHYSICAL GROWTH	FINE MOTOR SKILLS	GROSS MOTOR SKILLS	SENSORY ABILITY
3–6	Gains 3–5 lb (1.5–5 kg)/year Grows 1½–2½ in. (4–6 cm)/year	Uses scissors **(1)** Draws circle, square, cross Draws at least a six-part person Enjoys art projects such as pasting, stringing beads, using clay Learns to tie shoes at the end of preschool years **(3)** Buttons clothes **(4)** Brushes teeth **(5)** Eats three meals with snacks Uses spoon, fork, and knife	Throws a ball overhand Climbs well **(6)** Rides tricycle **(7)** May learn to ride bicycle with/without training wheels	Visual acuity continues to improve Can focus on and learn letters and numbers **(8)** Begins to write letters, numbers

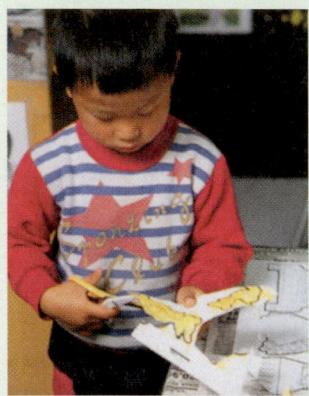

(1) Uses scissors

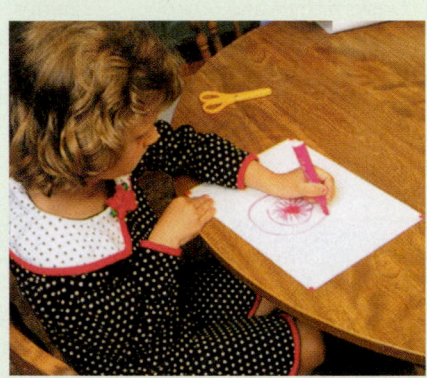

(2) Draws circle, square, cross

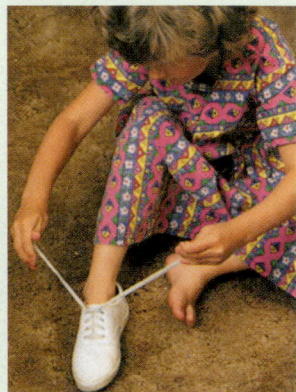

(3) Ties shoes

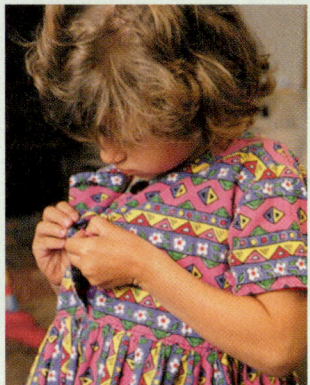

(4) Buttons clothes

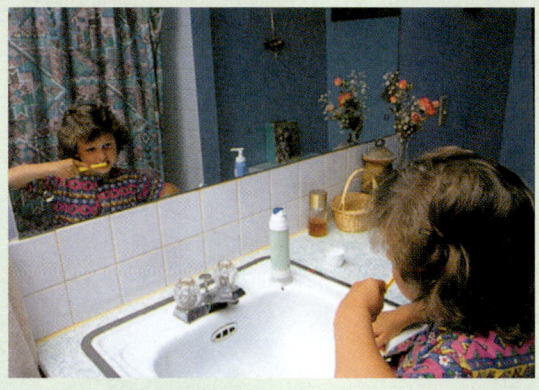

(5) Brushes teeth

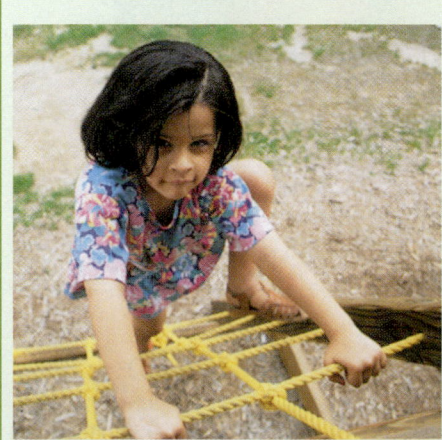

(6) Climbs well

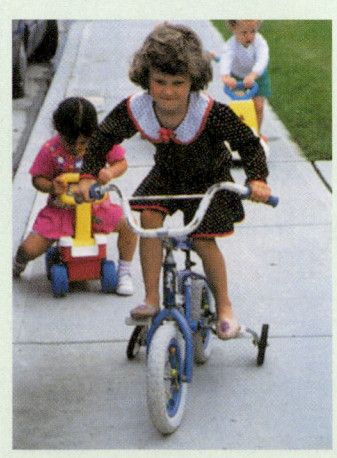

(7) Rides bicycle or bicycle with

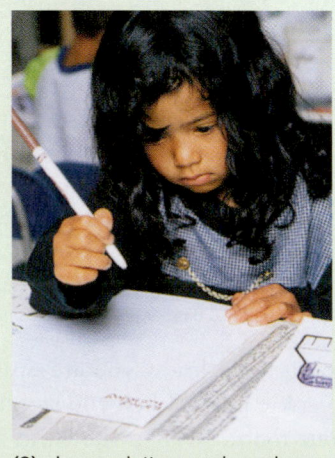

(8) Learns letters and numbers

Source: Ball, J., & Bindler, R. *Pediatric nursing care for children.* 3rd ed. [2003]. p. 53. Upper Saddle River, NJ: Prentice Hall.

TABLE 11-9

Growth and Development Milestones During School-Age Years

AGE (YEARS)	PHYSICAL GROWTH	FINE MOTOR SKILLS	GROSS MOTOR SKILLS	SENSORY ABILITY
6-12	Gains 3–5 lb (1.5–5 kg)/year Grows 1½–2½ in. (4–6 cm)/ year Loses teeth	Enjoys crafts projects Plays cards, board games, and computer games	Rides two-wheeler **(1)** Jumps rope **(2)** Roller skates/blades or ice skates Balance and muscle strength increase Group sports (i.e., football, soccer, basketball, gymnastics, dance)	Can read Able to concentrate for longer periods on activities by filtering out surrounding sounds **(3)** Knowledge increases through school subjects Concentrates for longer periods

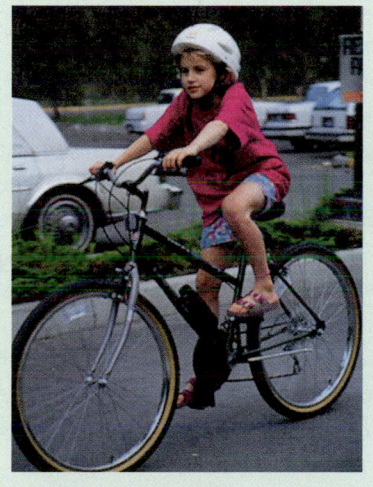

(1) Rides two–wheeler

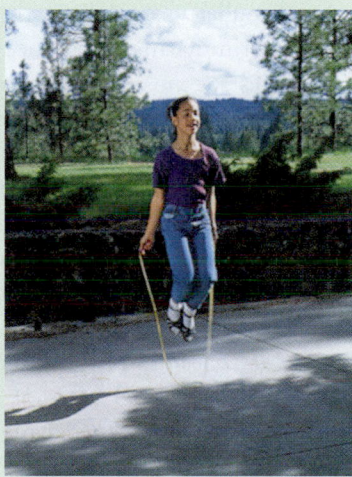

(2) Jumps rope

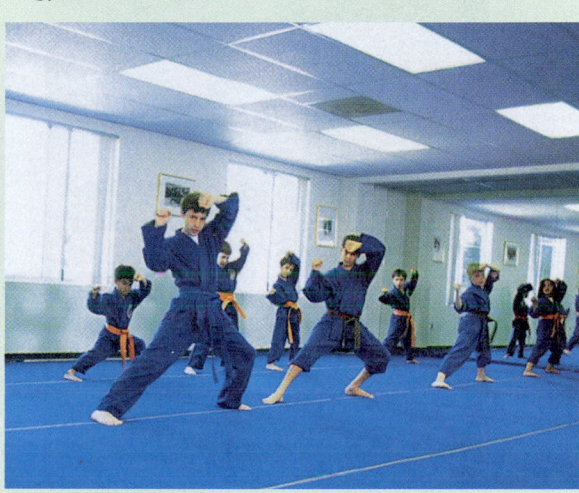

(3) Concentrates on activities for longer periods

Source: Ball, J., & Bindler, R. *Pediatric nursing care for children.* 3rd ed. [2003]. p. 58. Upper Saddle River, NJ: Prentice Hall.

Physical Growth

The preschool child continues to grow steadily, averaging an increase of 2 to 2½ inches (5–6 cm) and 4 to 5 pounds (about 2 kg) a year. The growth is mainly in the long bones of the arms and legs. Muscles are gaining strength and coordination.

Cognitive Development

The preschool child continues to progress in the preoperational level of cognitive development. He knows his name and age. He is developing an understanding of relationships and gender identification. By age 5, he has a better concept of time, day, week, month, and year. He knows the main colors and can count to 10. His attention span is getting longer, and he can spend 30 minutes with an activity.

The preschooler's vocabulary continues to increase, with more than 2,000 words by age 5. His sentence structure is also increasing to 7 to 8 words. The preschooler can describe drawings in detail. He can follow three simple commands given at the same time. He talks a lot, often asking "why" and "what."

SCHOOL-AGE CHILD (6 TO 12 YEARS)

The school-age years are a time of exciting growth and development. The child has reached many milestones that allow him to explore his ever-expanding world. Table 11-9 ■ illustrates the milestones during the school-age years.

Physical Growth

The school age child continues to grow about 2 inches and 2 pounds a year. Although the rate of growth is generally even, there may be a prepuberty growth spurt. The "childlike" appearance is replaced by a more adult appearance as the body proportions continue to change. Curvature of the spine (scoliosis) can be detected (see Chapter 17 ⚭).

The school-age child loses teeth at a rate of 4 a year and, by age 12, has 26 of the 30 permanent teeth. The remaining molars appear during adolescence (see Figure 11-5).

Cognitive Development

The school-age child is moving into the concrete operational stage of cognitive development. She can be expected to complete tasks, working both independently and in groups. She is learning to compromise and cooperate with others. She is

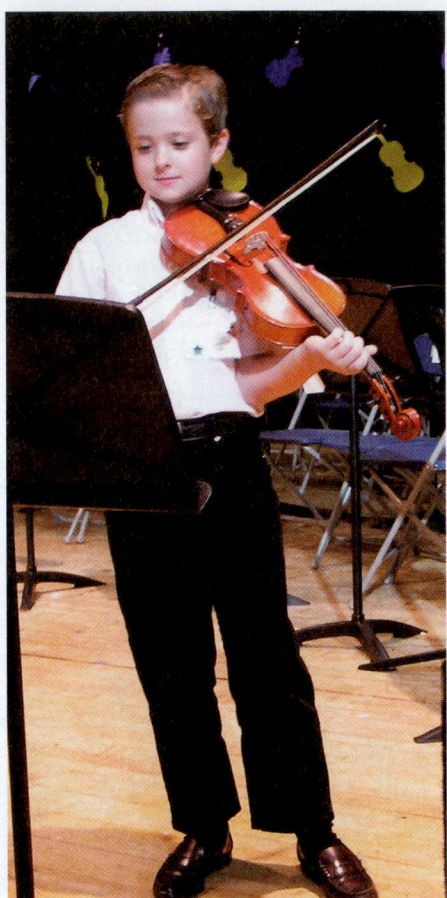

Figure 11-7. ■ School-age children have fine motor coordination and higher cognitive ability. This allows them to develop skills such as playing an instrument.

developing confidence in herself but can be disappointed with her own skills at times. If she feels left out, or behind her peers, she may develop "attention-getting" behaviors.

As the child moves through the school-age years, she learns to be more logical and coherent. Through school subjects, she learns to reason and to understand cause-and-effect and reversibility. For example, $2 + 2 = 4$ and $4 - 2 = 2$ teaches not only a mathematical computation, but also concepts of reason. Her vocabulary increases to more than 2,500 words, and she uses increasingly complex grammar in sentences. She is able to understand the multiple meaning of words. She can also learn complex physical-mental skills (Figure 11-7 ■).

During these years, the school-age child begins to question family rules and traditions. She moves away from fantasy, giving up Santa Claus and the Easter Bunny. As she looks to adults other than parents as role models, she may begin to question family values, religious beliefs, and culture.

Group play becomes important, and the school-age child joins clubs and teams. Through group play and team effort, the child learns "fairness." At about age 10, gender differences become more apparent in play activities.

ADOLESCENT (12 TO 20 YEARS)

The term "adolescence" means to grow up. Indeed this is a time of maturation, where the individual moves from childhood to adulthood. Table 11-10 ■ illustrates the growth and development milestones for this stage.

Physical Growth

Adolescence is the second fastest growth period. This is the first time growth patterns differ by gender. Both height and weight begin to increase in females earlier than in males. Table 11-11 ■ sketches height and weight information for normal adolescent physical growth.

Females usually start to mature sooner than males. At puberty, increases in the four primary sex hormones (follicle-stimulating hormone [FSH], luteinizing hormone [LH], estrogen, and progesterone) cause the physical changes. There is a change in the rate of skeletal growth, a widening of the pelvis, and a change in fat distribution. The breast tissue begins to develop, and course hair forms under the arms and over the mons pubis. At about 13 years old, the female experiences menarche, the beginning of menstruation, and, a few months later, ovulation begins. These changes take several years to complete. The female usually reaches full physical maturation by age 16, but it might be as late as 18 years of age. Sexual maturity can be documented in stages (called *Tanner's stages*), as shown in Table 11-12 ■.

Male development usually begins 2 years after female development. Changes in hormones guide the physical changes. FSH and LH trigger the increase of testosterone. There is rapid growth with an increase in height, lengthening of the jaw, and a doubling of muscle mass. The penis and testicles develop, and course hair forms on the face, axilla, and pubis. The voice deepens. Ejaculation signals the beginning of spermatogenesis. Although these changes are apparent by age 16, the male may not reach his adult height until 19 to 21 years of age.

Cognitive Development

Although emotional maturity is usually reached sooner in females, cognitive development progresses equally. The adolescent is moving from the concrete operational level to the abstract comprehension level of cognitive development. Cognitive milestones include the following:

- Ability to examine hypothetic situations and apply the concepts to current issues
- Ability to examine philosophic ideas and compare real-world situations to the ideal
- Ability to plan for the "what if"
- Development of adult proficiency with language (although adolescents frequently use slang to "fit in" with the group).

TABLE 11-10

Growth and Development Milestones During Adolescence

AGE (YEARS)	PHYSICAL GROWTH	FINE MOTOR SKILLS	GROSS MOTOR SKILLS	SENSORY ABILITY
12–18	Variation in age of growth spurt, girls gain 15–55 lb (7–25 kg) and grow 2–8 in. (2.5–20 cm); boys gain approximately 15–65 lb (7–29.5 kg) and grow $4^1/_2$–12 in. (11–30 cm) Puberty results in body changes	Skills are well developed (1)	New sport activities attempted and muscle development continues (2) Some lack of coordination common during growth spurts	Fully developed

(1) Motor skills are well developed

(2) New sports activities attempted

Source: Ball, J., & Bindler, R. *Pediatric nursing care for children.* 3rd ed. [2003]. p. 63. Upper Saddle River, NJ: Prentice Hall.

In the early years (13–14 years) adolescents may be self-centered, but they gradually mature and develop a strong identity. This is a difficult transition, however. A changing body and an increase in hormones bring about confusion and doubt. Adolescents want to feel attractive, but skin changes, awkwardness of a rapidly changing body, and mood changes can make them feel ugly. Hormonal changes and a physiologic drive to reproduce put many pressures on sexuality development. Peers are most important at this time and can have a positive or negative influence on behavior. Strong peer pressure and feelings of immortality ("it won't happen to me") can lead to unwise choices and risk-taking behaviors (Figure 11-8 ■).

TABLE 11-11

Normal Adolescent Physical Growth Patterns

AGE	HEIGHT—FEMALES (in.)	HEIGHT—MALES (in.)	WEIGHT—FEMALES (lb)	WEIGHT—MALES (lb)
12	55–64	54–63.5	68–136	66–130
14	59–67.5	59–69.5	84–160	84–160
16	60–68	63–73	94–172	104–186
18	60–68.5	65–74	100–178	116–202

Source: Ramont, R. R., Niedringhaus, D. M., & Towle, M. A. (2006). *Comprehensive nursing care.* Upper Saddle River, NJ: Prentice Hall.

MediaLink Internet safety

TABLE 11-12	
Tanner's Stages of Sexual Maturity	
STAGE OF SEXUAL MATURITY	**DESCRIPTION**
1	The preadolescent has no pubic hair except for a fine "peach fuzz" body hair.
2	There is a sparse growth of long, slightly darkened, downy hair, mostly along the labia in females or at the base of the penis and sometimes on the scrotum in males. This hair is usually straight or only slightly curled.
3	The pubic hair becomes darker, coarse, and curlier. It now grows sparsely over the mons veneris area in females; it remains in the Stage 2 area in males.
4	The hair grows in more densely. It becomes as coarse and curly as in the adult, but there is not as much of it.
5	Pubic hair is the classic coarse and curly hair that extends onto the inner thighs.
6	The final amount, color, and distribution of pubic hair are quite variable.

Source: Data from Tanner, J. M. *Growth at adolescence.* [1966]. New York: Appleton; Tanner, J. M. *Growth of adolescents.* [1962]. Oxford: Blackwell; Marshall, W. A., and Tanner, J. M. Variations in the pattern of pubertal changes in boys. *Arch Dis Child 45*(239): 13–23, 1970; Marshall, W. A., and Tanner, J. M. Variations in the pattern of pubertal changes in girls. *Arch Dis Child 445*(235): 291–303, 1969.

Parents often look for guidance at this period in their children's lives. The simple rules of the family are giving way to larger influences. Educational, religious, and health care professionals can provide valuable information to help parents provide guidelines for their teens. (See Health Promotion Issue box on pages 352 and 353.)

ADULT (18 TO 65 YEARS)

The adult years are subdivided into young adult, middle adult, and older adult. Young adults are adjusting to the "loss" of their place in the family. They move out of the home to attend school, begin a career, or start a family. This causes a change in the organization of the family (see Table 3-1). They seek intimacy and a long-term relationship. Without them, they face isolation.

As members of the family become young adults, the parents reach middle age. This is not only a time for them to "let go," but also to take pride in their children becoming independent adults.

Physical Growth

Young adults (20–40 years) are resilient, and their bodies function at peak efficiency. The posture is erect, with optimal muscle tone and coordination. The skin is taut and smooth. There is a high reproductive capability, and sexuality is a powerful response. Sexual performance peaks for males at age 18 and for females at age 30. (See also Reproductive Issues, Chapter 5 ⚭.)

As the years pass and people become middle age (40–65 years), the body gradually decreases in its abilities. With a slowing of metabolism, there can be an increase in weight and a change in fat distribution, and people generally need to pay more attention to diet and exercise to maintain strength and mobility (Figure 11-9 ■). **Presbyopia** (farsightedness) and **presbycusis** (loss of hearing) are common with age. At about age 50, women enter menopause, the ovaries stop releasing ova and estrogen, and progesterone levels fall. Men also experience a change in hormone levels that causes a decrease in sperm production. As middle-age adults struggle to cope with these changes in body function, they may become depressed or have affairs with younger partners. The emotional struggles of this period are rightly called a *midlife crisis.*

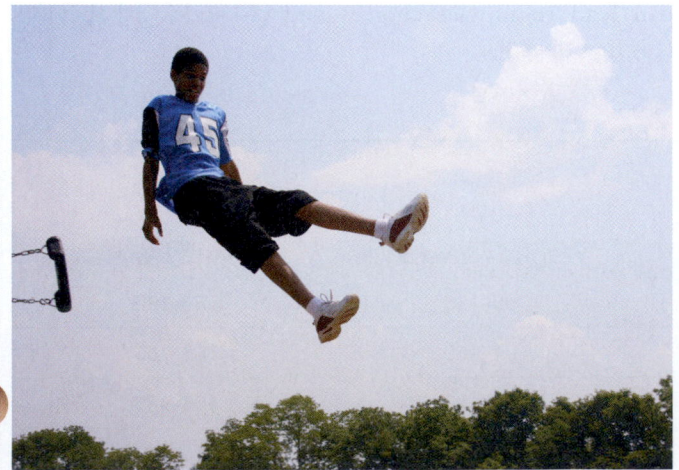

Figure 11-8. ■ Teens typically engage in high-risk behaviors and exhibit an attitude of "it can't happen to me." (M. C. Schlachter Photography.)

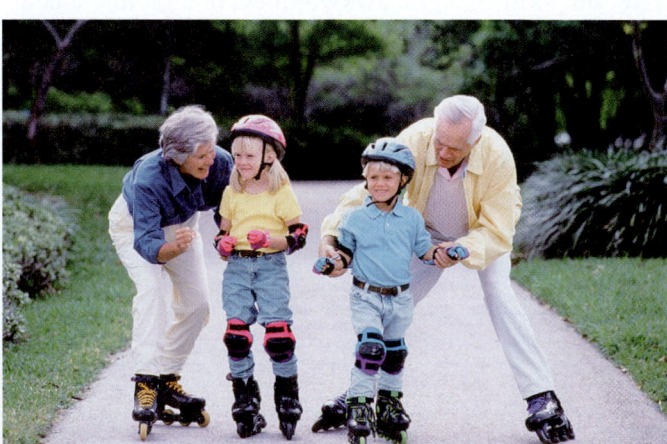

Figure 11-9. ■ Today's more health-conscious middle and older adults may be more than just observers of their grandchildren's activities. (Paul Barton/CORBIS.)

Cognitive Development

Young and middle-age adults have all the cognitive skills necessary for a productive life. Their main challenges are adjusting to life's crises (career, marriage, purchasing a home, raising a family, coping with an empty nest, and participating in the lives of grandchildren or great grandchildren). Perceptions of time, productivity, and self change as the middle-age adult plans for retirement.

SANDWICH GENERATION.   Middle-age adults have often been called the "sandwich generation." This term describes their simultaneous responsibilities to children who are not quite established outside the home and aging parents who begin to rely on them for physical, emotional, or cognitive support.

OLDER ADULT (OLDER THAN 65 YEARS)

The average life expectancy in the United States is 75 years. With the technologic advances in health care, improved nutrition, and health promotion activities at all ages, the quality of health in the elderly is much improved. Chronic disorders may not affect everyone, but are often seen in this age group.

Physical Growth

When the body ages, there is a slowing or decreased function of all organ systems. As the skin ages, it becomes dry, thin, and pigmented. A loss of elasticity causes wrinkles. The hair becomes thin, dry, brittle, and gray. Male pattern baldness, a hereditary condition evident in younger men, usually has stopped progressing. The skeletal system undergoes changes in degree of calcification. Some bones become porous and more subject to fracture. Other bones degenerate, forming an uneven edge and spurs. This results in decreased mobility of joints. The spine (especially the low cervical and thoracic vertebrae) may develop compression fractures that result in curvature of the spine and shorter stature. The costal cartilage attaching the ribs to the sternum becomes hard and fixed. The result is a decreased expansion of the chest cavity and decreased respiratory ability. Years of smoking and inhaling air pollutants damage the bronchi, alveoli, and capillary bed and result in progressive lung disease.

One of the most significant changes associated with aging is a decrease in function of the heart and blood vessels. If fat deposits build up inside the blood vessels, the lumen narrows, blood pressure increases, and blood supply to distal tissues decreases. These changes can lead to heart attack, stroke, hypertension, and other vascular disease.

The number of functioning nephrons decreases by about 50% by age 75, so the kidney is less able to produce urine. As tissues lose their elasticity, there might be a decrease in capacity of the bladder, a prolapse of the bladder, and incontinence. Changes in the prostate can result in difficulty urinating.

The sense organs show a slow decline with age. Vision is affected by a clouding of the lens called *cataracts*. A hardening of the lens affects accommodation, resulting in farsightedness. In the ear, a decrease in the number of hair cells in the organ of Corti causes a significant decline in hearing. There is also a decrease in taste and smell that may affect appetite and food preferences.

Although both men and women remain sexually active, a decrease in hormones affects the ability to reproduce. In men erection may be more difficult to obtain and sustain, and sperm count decreases. In women, symptoms commonly seen with menopause include hot flashes, cessation of menstruation, and a thinning and drying of the vaginal wall.

Cognitive Development

Cognition shows some decline with age. This is due in part to decreased circulation, decreased oxygenation, and disease processes. Most seniors can process mentally as they did in younger years. However, there is a slow loss of memory, with recent memory affected more than distant memory. Seniors experience more extreme cognitive deficits. Although parents need to exercise judgment in leaving small children with seniors who have cognitive deficits, most families value interaction among generations.

The main task in this stage of development is to "age gracefully." Seniors look at their life as one of meaning, where they can see that they have made a contribution to the world. Without meaning, they can easily sink into despair and depression.

NURSING CARE

PRIORITIES IN NURSING CARE

Nursing priorities for clients throughout the life span include:

- Establish a therapeutic relationship with the client.
- Communicate appropriately for age level, stage of development, and cognitive level.
- Verify teaching through appropriate means to ensure client understanding.

ASSESSING

The role of the LPN/LVN is to assist in the assessment of the pediatric client and the family. Several tools are available to guide the data collection and assessment. Instruction in the detailed use of these tools is covered in the orientation to each facility. Although there are differences in the tools, the kinds of information collected are the same. Measurements of height, weight, and head circumference (for a small child or neonate) are taken and recorded on a growth chart. Other observations, such as activity, gross and fine

(*Text continues on p. 354.*)

HEALTH PROMOTION ISSUE

INTERNET SAFETY FOR CHILDREN

The school nurse conducts a parents' meeting with the eighth-grade parents each year as school is beginning for these junior high students. She discusses the issues that she will present during health class throughout the year. These issues include personal health, disease prevention, sexual behavior, and peer pressure. She describes for the parents some of the things they may expect from a child this age. She ends the parents' meeting with time for questions and answers. This fall, a father of a 13-year-old daughter asks her what she thinks about the dangers of the Internet. The father also asked for the nurse's help in setting guidelines for his daughter related to the Internet. The nurse decided that this topic required more than a quick response and planned another parents' meeting to adequately address the issue.

DISCUSSION

A survey of 19,000 students, conducted by i-SAFE America (a government-funded Internet safety program), reviewed their online behavior. The survey found that 80% of students spend at least 1 hour per week on the Internet. Thirty percent say e-mail, chat rooms, or instant messaging is the main way they stay in contact with their friends. Fifty-five percent of the students admit giving out personal information such as name, gender, and age over the Internet. Almost half of the students say they have visited inappropriate sites on the Internet. It's frightening, but 10% of students have met someone face-to-face following an encounter on the Internet.

One in five children in the United States has been solicited sexually online, according to the Justice Department. This includes teenagers such as a 16-year-old girl lured into a face-to-face meeting by a 24-year-old parolee for sexual assault. This young woman's parents claim they were vigilant in monitoring her online behavior. However, they are now searching for their daughter after she met this parolee online.

How are teens accessing the Internet? They can e-mail, get into discussions in chat rooms, enter newsgroups, or engage in instant messaging. Web sites cannot only be accessed by computer, but also by cell phones, pagers, personal digital assistants (PDAs), and video game systems. Cell phones allow teens to exchange digital photographs or videos, instant messages, or text messages; to contact websites; or even to watch TV. They can engage in file sharing of music, videos, pictures, and other data over the Internet. These services may contain spyware that tracks Internet activity and that can possibly share this information with others. Interactive gaming sites allow participants to play a game with an unknown individual on a computer at another location.

Many aspects of an adolescent's growth and development make them susceptible to engaging in risky behaviors online. Adolescents are attempting to separate from their family and are seeking independence. This makes them seek privacy and rebel when their privacy is invaded. The Internet provides teens with a way to figuratively venture away from their family. Fear of rejection and developing confidence can cause them to conform to the risky actions of their peers. A teen who wants to become independent, but who also wants to be loved and accepted, may not be able to discern the difference between the luring of a sexual predator and the true adoration of someone who loves her.

The unsupervised, unchecked use of the Internet can lead to many dangers. Unhealthy relationships can develop. These relationships can lead to physical, emotional, and sexual abuse. There are also many instances when these relationships lead to the fatal demise of teenagers.

Many predators online seek important information so they can steal another person's identity. Predators may

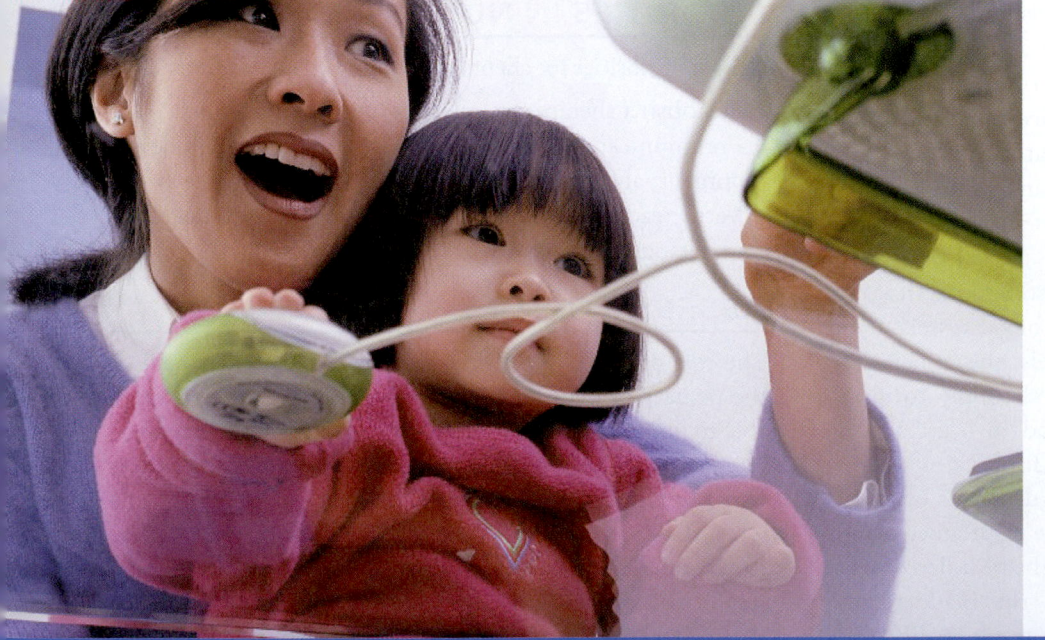

(© Larry Williams/CORBIS)

tap directly into financial information that can be used to delete bank accounts and ruin credit. Teens need to learn the dangers of identity theft as soon as they open a bank account.

The nurse can be effective in assisting families to safeguard against the dangers of the Internet. Parents need to be able to assess the online behaviors of their teens, set guidelines, and take swift action if risks are identified. The nurse can provide teaching and suggest resources to assist the family.

PLANNING AND IMPLEMENTING

The nurse discusses with parents how to manage Internet use in their home. These are the teaching points the nurse uses:

- Learn to use your computer as efficiently as your child. Regularly review your web browser's history to see exactly where your child has gone while surfing the web. Be sure your child knows that you are going to do this.
- Learn the lingo (shortcuts and acronyms) for instant messaging and text messaging. Comprehensive lists of chat abbreviations are available on some Internet sites.
- Screen names should be gender neutral and never contain sexual innuendos or personal descriptive information.
- Chat sites, instant messaging, and e-mail profiles should never contain personal information that a predator could use to make a connection. Personal information would include gender, age, address, phone number, likes, dislikes, hobbies, and interests. (Some parents have discovered that their child's "away"

message for instant messaging contained their cell phone number.)
- Free e-mail accounts are simple to obtain. Children could have numerous ones without the parents' knowledge. The computer's web browser history would give a clue if the child has been to these sites.
- Create some clear house rules with clearly defined parameters for time spent on the computer, what is allowed, and what is not allowed. Remember also that it is not just the home computer that a teen uses. They can also access the Internet at grandma's house or at a friend's house. Discuss how the rules apply to these sites as well.
- Use a filtering program to block the computer from a predetermined set of websites, block e-mail except from a preset list, or block individual web pages with offensive words.
- Install a "firewall" and antivirus software that is updated regularly to protect your computer from unwanted intrusions.
- Software can be added to the computer to ensure that teens cannot share pictures online, set certain profiles, or use a webcam (camera).
- The teen's privacy can be respected when trust is earned. However, computer access should be in a common area of the home.
- Use a search engine to search weekly for their name, screen names, address, and telephone numbers. This assists in discovering postings that predators or even personal enemies may have posted.
- The computer should be password protected. If the teen has a password, it should be known to the parents. Change passwords frequently.

- Search recently downloaded file folders for more information about where the teen is surfing. Regularly review their other files and folders, not secretively but with their knowledge and perhaps in their presence.
- Sharing music, digital, and video files increases the risk of viruses that can infect the computer. It could also be illegal. Parents should learn about and discuss recent cases in which teens have been charged with theft when sharing digital files.
- Regularly review your child's cell phone bill to monitor calls received and sent.

Many services allow records to be reviewed online for more frequent monitoring. The nurse also decides to include a class on Internet safety in her health class. She invites law enforcement officials to discuss the hazards of the Internet, a student who was solicited online to discuss personal dangers, and an Internet/computer expert to discuss technical issues.

SELF-REFLECTION

How often do you access the Internet? What methods do you use for access? Carefully review your Internet practices. Do you participate in any risky behaviors that might compromise your safety or personal information? Do you know about the Internet practices of other family members in your home? Do you have any cause for concern? List three ways you could improve your Internet practices or those of family members within your home.

SUGGESTED RESOURCES

Gralla, P. (2002). *The complete idiot's guide to internet privacy and security.* Indianapolis, IN: Alpha.

- **www.missingkids.com** This site provides parents with information about this organization's NetSmartz program and offers suggestions on reporting information that might assist in apprehending child predators.

- **www.wiredkids.org** The purpose of this site is to protect children using the Internet from cybercrime and abuse.

- **www.isafe.org** i-SAFE is a nonprofit foundation dedicated to protecting the online experiences of youth. It has been endorsed by the U.S. Senate.

MediaLink Apprehending child predators

motor control, and language development, are compared to the normal milestones for the age group. Parents and grandparents may supply information about development and maturation of family members. The LPN/LVN documents these observations and reports any deviations from normal.

DIAGNOSING, PLANNING, AND IMPLEMENTING

Nursing diagnoses for clients with growth and development delays might include, among others:

- Altered Parenting
- Altered Growth and Development
- Situational Low Self-Esteem.

Outcomes for these clients might include the following:

- Client expresses understanding of need for support and joins spina bifida parents group.

- Parent schedules follow-up physical therapy for 20-month-old child who does not walk.
- Teenage client agrees to talk with counselor about abuse by father of her newborn.

When planning and implementing care, the nurse may use the following interventions:

- Consider the client's age and stage of development. *An understanding of what is normal is crucial when providing nursing care.*
- Be sensitive to developmental issues. *Parents of children with growth or developmental delays may be very anxious about what these delays might mean for the child. Establish a therapeutic relationship by asking open-ended questions and allowing space for the client to express feelings.*
- Use age-appropriate communication (Box 11-5 ■). *Like other factors, the child's communication level develops over time. The nurse can improve communication and learning by*

BOX 11-5	NURSING CARE CHECKLIST

Providing Age-Appropriate Communication

The way the nurse communicates with children and parents will have a great effect on their understanding, learning, and cooperation. The following guidelines will help the nurse understand how to communicate with children at different stages of development. The nurse can also teach parents these guidelines.

Infant (Birth to 1 Year)

☑ Speak softly.

☑ Communicate through touch.

☑ Avoid overstimulation.

☑ Comfort by holding or rocking.

☑ Encourage parents to participate.

☑ Be aware that older infants may be fearful of strangers.

Toddler (1 to 3 Years)

☑ Allow the child to complete a thought without interruption.

☑ Avoid frightening discussions.

☑ Say specifically what you want the child to do.

☑ Do not offer a choice if there really is none.

☑ Speak at the child's eye level.

☑ Have as few teachers as possible (one nurse).

☑ Use parallel play or toys to teach.

☑ Encourage parents to participate.

☑ Expect that the child will not understand time or "why."

Preschooler (3 to 6 Years)

☑ Keep instruction brief for short attention span.

☑ Use simple, direct language.

☑ Speak with a simple vocabulary.

☑ Make learning fun.

☑ Allow the child to act out or express thoughts or feelings.

☑ Reinforce learning immediately.

☑ Use body outlines or drawings to explain illness.

☑ Separate fantasy from reality.

School-Age Child (6 to 12 Years)

☑ Determine the child's understanding about illness, treatment, and prognosis.

☑ Dispel myths and fears.

☑ Give child the opportunity to speak for him- or herself.

☑ Allow and encourage children to communicate their needs.

☑ Provide information in clear terms; they are able to learn more about body parts.

☑ Be aware that children may respond to third-person prompts: "I know a boy who is afraid of the x-ray machine."

Adolescent (12 to 20 Years)

☑ Show respect by listening and explaining clearly.

☑ Allow for more independence.

☑ Give adolescent privacy and opportunity for confidentiality.

☑ Help adolescents trust adults by being honest about their treatment.

☑ Use peer support when possible.

☑ Never use a "baby" voice; speak as to another adult, but be sure language is clear.

☑ Provide space for questions.

gearing body language and verbal communication to the appropriate age.

EVALUATING

The LPN/LVN assists in the collection of evaluation data. If goals are not achieved, interventions may be changed or adapted.

NURSING PROCESS CARE PLAN
Infant with Delayed Growth and Development

Jim, a 9-month-old infant, is brought to the clinic by his single, 19-year-old mother for his first well-baby checkup. His mother states that he weighed 7 pounds at birth. She states that he takes 6 to 8 ounces of formula three times a day, but does not take solid food. She states that Jim spends most of the day in his crib, so she can work from her home.

Assessment

- Weight 15 pounds
- Height 26½ inches
- Skin pale
- Makes limited verbal response
- Smiles only occasionally.

Nursing Diagnosis. The following important nursing diagnoses (among others) are established for this client:

- Delayed Growth and Development (as evidenced by height and weight under 5th percentile, limited verbal sounds, and infrequent smiles)
- Impaired Parenting (as evidenced by putting infant in crib for most of the day, limited social interaction with infant, and not providing adequate nutrition for stage of development).

Expected Outcomes. The expected outcomes for Jim are that:

- Height and weight will be at 5th percentile by 1 year of age.
- Social interaction will be appropriate for 1-year-old.

Expected outcomes are that the mother will:
- Provide meals appropriate for age daily.
- Provide toys appropriate for age daily.
- Verbalize appropriate parenting skills.

Planning and Implementation

- Teach mother about nutrition and the need for social interaction. *Mother cannot be expected to provide needed care without instruction.*
- Monitor infant's height, weight, and social skills monthly. *Generally, single assessments are not as revealing of problems. This infant is obviously delayed, and progress must be monitored frequently.*
- Encourage mother to attend parenting classes. *This mother will need parenting skills and in-depth instruction in child care in order for infant to progress and maintain normal pattern of growth and development.*

Evaluation. It is critical to evaluate this child's progress. If further slowing of growth and development occurs, the child's life could be in danger. Evaluation by social services may be necessary to ensure the child is not being neglected. Because the child is 9 months old and has not had well-baby checkups prior to this visit, other health care issues may be present. For example, immunizations may be off schedule. It may be important for the nurse to maintain contact with the mother to help ensure compliance and return visits to the health care practitioner.

Critical Thinking in the Nursing Process

1. What questions should the nurse ask Jim's mother to determine if other health issues are present?
2. What other information would have been helpful in this situation?
3. What data would indicate a need to call social services to protect Jim?

Note: Discussion of Critical Thinking Questions appears in Appendix I.

Note: The references and resources for this and all chapters have been compiled at the back of the book.

Chapter Review

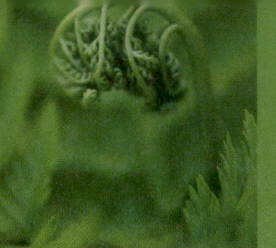

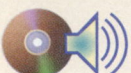 **KEY TERMS** by Topics

Use the audio glossary feature of either the CD-ROM or the Companion Website to hear the correct pronunciation of the following key terms.

Introduction
growth, development

Principles of Growth and Development
cephalocaudal, proximodistal, ordinal position, maturation

Theories of Development
cognitive development, sensorimotor, preoperational, concrete operational, formal operations, psychosexual, id, ego, superego, defense mechanisms

Standards of Physical Growth and Development
percentile

Stages of Physical Growth and Development
separation anxiety, presbyopia, presbycusis

KEY Points

- Growth and development are influenced by genetics and environment. Development begins at conception and continues until death.

- Growth and development have five major components: physiologic, psychosocial, cognitive, moral, and spiritual.

- Health assessment and promotion activities assist the client in meeting developmental milestones.

- As the population grows older, growth and development needs of the elderly will impact health care to a greater extent.

- Parenting styles affect family dynamics.

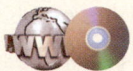 **EXPLORE Media**Link

Additional interactive resources for this chapter can be found on the Companion Website at www.prenhall.com/towle.

Click on Chapter 11 and "Begin" to select the activities for this chapter.

For chapter-related NCLEX-style questions and an audio glossary, access the accompanying CD-ROM in this book.

Animations

Infancy: A major life transition

Communicating with toddlers

Handling temper tantrums

Health maintenance for school-age children

Teens: Mental & spiritual health

Health promotion & health maintenance

The importance of physical activity

FOR FURTHER Study

See Table 3-1 and Chapter 3 for discussion of family development.

Reproductive issues are discussed further in Chapter 5.

Information about typical infant reflexes appears in Chapter 9.

For additional information on the care of the neonate, see Chapter 10.

Figure 12-10 shows some body proportion changes.

Nursing adaptations for children of different ages are discussed in depth in Chapter 13.

Defense mechanisms and other psychosocial information is provided in Chapter 27.

Appendix II shows growth charts for ages birth to 20 years.

Caring for Client with Risk for Injury

NCLEX-PN® Focus Area: Safety

Case Study: Jane, a 4-month-old, has been brought by her 17-year-old mother to the well-child clinic. When you enter the room, Jane is lying on the exam table with her mother at her side. Jane's vital signs are T 98, P 120, R 30, Wt 15 lb, Ht 22½ in. Head circumference is 16 in. Her history indicates she weighed 7 lb 3 oz at birth and was 20 in. long with a 13½-in. head circumference. Jane's mother tells you Jane rolls from front to back and enjoys putting her toys in her mouth. Jane drops her rattle on the floor. Her mother walks away from the exam table to pick it up.

Nursing Diagnosis: Risk for Injury/Trauma

COLLECT DATA

Subjective	Objective
_____	_____
_____	_____
_____	_____
_____	_____
_____	_____
_____	_____

Would you report this? Yes/No

If yes, to: _____

Nursing Care

_____
_____
_____
_____
_____
_____
_____
_____
_____
_____
_____
_____

How would you document this? _____
_____
_____
_____

Compare your documentation to the sample provided in Appendix I.

Data Collected
(use those that apply)

- 4-month-old child
- VS: 98-120-30
- Weight: 15 lb
- Height: 22½ in.
- Head: 16 in.
- Activity: turns front to back, puts toys in mouth

Nursing Interventions
(use those that apply; list in priority order)

- Instruct mother to keep syrup of ipecac in first aid kit.
- Teach parent to avoid foods that could cause choking (raisins, peanuts, whole grapes).
- Instruct mother to begin adding soft pureed food to child's diet.
- Teach mother need for close supervision because the child is becoming mobile.
- Instruct mother on toys for age.

NCLEX-PN® Exam Preparation

1 A woman has brought her 2-year-old to the well-child clinic. Which of the following would be recommended to encourage autonomy in a toddler?

1. Help the toddler complete tasks.
2. Provide the toddler opportunities to play with other children.
3. Help the toddler learn the difference between right and wrong.
4. Encourage the toddler to do things for herself when she is capable.

2 Five-year-old Sally is in the hospital and is becoming bored. The best activity for her would be:

1. books.
2. TV.
3. puppets.
4. oil paint by number.

3 In terms of cognitive development, which of the following would a 5-year-old be expected to do?

1. Use magical thinking.
2. Think abstractly.
3. Understand conversation about matter.
4. Comprehend another person's perspective.

4 Which of the following would the nurse reasonably expect a 2-year-old to be able to do?

1. Jump rope.
2. Ride a bicycle.
3. Skip on alternate feet.
4. Balance on one foot for a few seconds.

5 The parents of an 8-year-old tell you that their daughter wants to join a soccer team. Which suggestions about participation in sports at this age should be made?

1. Organized sports such as soccer are not appropriate at this age.
2. Competition is harmful in establishing a positive self-image.
3. Sports participation is a good idea if the sport is appropriate for the child's abilities.
4. Girls should compete only against girls because at this age boys are larger and have more muscle mass.

6 The mother of a 13-year-old tells you that her daughter is a good girl, but does not seem to do what she is told anymore. Your response would be guided by the knowledge that the adolescent is most influenced at this stage by _____.

7 A disruptive 10-year-old is having difficulty with other children at school. Which nursing action would be best for the school nurse to use first?

1. Have a meeting with the teachers and discuss strategies to solve the problem.
2. Talk with the child about the behavior that is causing the problem and identify possible solutions.
3. Tell the other children to stop teasing the client and observe the changes in behavior.
4. Tell the child's parents that they need to take care of the problem.

8 A 52-year-old woman talks about her changing family. She is upset that "her baby" recently married and moved to New Jersey, and her son lives far away with his wife and three children. This woman is experiencing _____.

9 Exploratory abdominal surgery is planned for tomorrow on a 3-year-old girl. How would the nurse best prepare this child for the procedure?

1. The evening before the procedure, demonstrate by pointing on the child's body where the incision will be made.
2. Ask the child's parents to leave the room while the preoperative medication is given.
3. Ask the parents to hold the child down while sedation is given.
4. Explain the procedure to the child in simple terms just before giving preoperative medication.

10 An 18-year-old is upset about his 83-year-old grandfather, who is dying of lung cancer. The boy says, "I don't understand how he can be so calm and accepting about death." Which of the following is the best response, based on an understanding of development?

1. Your grandfather is just trying to be brave for your sake.
2. When we are young, it is hard to understand that we can be content with our life's accomplishments and be ready to die.
3. It is the pain medication that is keeping your grandfather calm.
4. We will keep him comfortable, and this will be over soon.

Answers for Review Questions, as well as discussion of Care Plan and Critical Thinking Care Map questions, appear in Appendix I.

Chapter 12

Illness Prevention, Health Promotion, and Nutrition in Children

BRIEF Outline

Role of the Nurse in Illness Prevention and Health Promotion

Client and Family Teaching

Illness Prevention

Health Promotion

Nursing Care

Infant

Toddler

Preschooler

School-Age Child

Adolescent

Nursing Care

LEARNING Outcomes

After completing this chapter, you will be able to:

- Describe techniques for client and family teaching.
- Describe illness prevention activities.
- Describe health promotion activities for children in each age group.
- Discuss important aspects of nutrition for each age group.

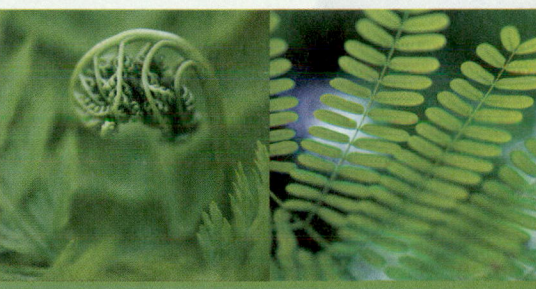

HEALTH PROMOTION ISSUE:
Types of Learning

NURSING PROCESS CARE PLAN:
Pediatric Client with Unintentional Poisoning

CRITICAL THINKING CARE MAP:
Caring for a Client with Inadequate Nutrition

Health promotion and health maintenance

MediaLink

In community-based nursing practice, nursing care is provided wherever the client and the family are found. Nursing care is not just the treatment of illness. It also includes teaching of good health practices in order to prevent illness and injury. Publications such as *Healthy People* (U.S. Public Health Service 1979), *Promoting Health/Preventing Illness: Objectives for the Nation* (U.S. Public Health Service, 1980), *Healthy People 2000* (U.S. Department of Health and Human Services, 1991) and *Healthy People 2010* (U.S. Department of Health and Human Services, 2000) have documented the need for activities to help Americans become healthier. See more on this program in Chapter 1 ⚭.

Role of the Nurse in Illness Prevention and Health Promotion

As described in previous chapters, the role of the LPN/LVN is diverse. The nurse collects data from the client and family, reports to the charge nurse, assists in establishing the plan of care, and helps implement quality care. The nurse follows good health practices and acts as a role model for the client and family. Once a formal teaching plan has been established, the nurse implements the teaching plan and reports back to the charge nurse. Informal teaching occurs with each family interaction (Figure 12-1 ■). Client teaching techniques can be reviewed in a fundamentals of nursing textbook. This chapter reviews client teaching principles as they apply to illness prevention and health promotion in the care of children.

Client and Family Teaching

Every interaction between the nurse and client and/or family needs to be one of assessment and teaching. Through the assessment process, the nurse determines specific areas of needed

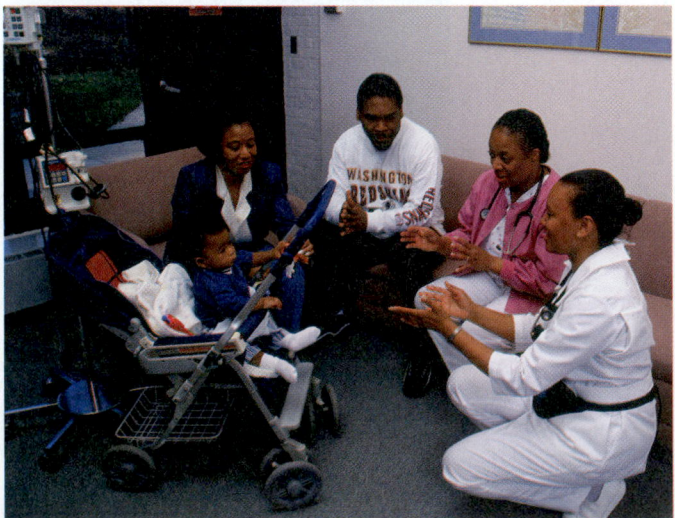

Figure 12-1. ■ The nurse begins assessment of the infant's family when they are seen in the waiting room and called in for care.

Guidelines for Teaching

The following guidelines should be used for client and family teaching:

- ☑ Be a role model.
- ☑ Maintain a distraction-free environment.
- ☑ Use age-specific communication techniques.
- ☑ Have accurate and complete information.
- ☑ Be familiar with printed material.

instruction and the effectiveness of prior teaching. Some teaching needs to be a planned, formal event that might take several hours or days to complete. Other teaching is a spontaneous informal event, with one-to-one dialogue. Box 12-1 ■ outlines teaching guidelines the nurse should use in order to be efficient and effective with client and family teaching.

The nurse is a role model for good health practices. It is difficult to convince a client or family to be compliant with good health practices and instruction if the nurse does not practice them. For example, if the nurse is providing instruction on insulin administration and does not keep the needle sterile, the client or family will not see the need to use sterile techniques either. If the nurse teaches about the effects of smoking on health and then is seen having a cigarette, the family will not view the nurse as credible.

For the client and family to get the most out of the instruction, the environment must be free from distraction. For example, if cast care instruction needs to be given to a mother who has her four other children with her at the pediatrician's office, one of the office staff members can take the other children to the playroom, providing the mother with a distraction-free environment. If the instruction is to be given in the home primarily to older children and adults, the nurse should ask someone to turn off the television, request no telephone calls, and ask family members to leave the room so privacy can be provided.

The nurse must use age-specific communication techniques, audiovisual aids, and vocabulary (see Box 11-5). If instruction is too simplistic, an older child might feel "put down" and not pay attention to or follow it. If the instruction is too advanced, the client might be confused and will either do nothing or be poorly equipped to perform the needed care. If the client and/or family speak a language different from the nurse, an interpreter may be needed to ensure accurate communication.

The instruction provided must be accurate and complete. The nurse must keep up to date with the latest research, techniques, and technology. The nurse might use an outline or other notes so important points are not forgotten, resulting in incomplete instruction.

If questions arise that the nurse cannot accurately answer, she should say she does not know but will find out the answer. Then the nurse should be diligent in getting the information to the client. It is better to give no instruction than inaccurate instruction.

The nurse needs to be familiar with the printed material provided to the client and family. By reviewing the printed material in its entirety prior to the client interaction, the nurse can discuss the content, using eye contact and a relaxed approach. Printed material should be individualized so the client and family will have complete written instructions at home. The nurse never assumes that the parents or the clients know, understand, and will practice good health promotion activities. The nurse must validate whether the pediatric client and his or her caregiver understand the teaching before ending the interaction.

Illness prevention and health promotion activities are designed to help the client regain and maintain the highest level of health possible for as long as possible. The health of the mother and father have an impact on the health of the developing infant. Therefore, both parents should practice a healthy lifestyle prior to pregnancy.

Parents are responsible for helping maintain their children's health. Parents do this by providing a healthy environment and nutritious food, and by teaching their children healthful behaviors. The nurse encourages the parents by providing information and by being a positive role model. (See the Health Promotion Issue on pages 362 and 363 for different types of learning among pediatric clients.)

Illness Prevention

Illness prevention is encouragement of specific behaviors that can prevent illness and injury. Illness prevention can be divided into three categories: primary, secondary, and tertiary prevention.

LEVELS OF PREVENTION

Primary Prevention

Primary prevention includes activities to keep the individual from developing health problems. This includes activities such as immunizations to prevent communicable disease, wearing a seat belt to protect from injury during a motor vehicle crash, and learning about proper preparation of infant formula to avoid disease.

Secondary Prevention

Secondary prevention involves activities directed at early detection and treatment of health problems. The following are examples of secondary prevention:

- Voluntary drug screening in the school system
- Checking each child in a classroom for lice if one child is found to have lice
- Screening for developmental delays using the Denver Developmental Screening Test (DDST) (see Appendix IV ⚭).

Tertiary Prevention

Tertiary prevention includes treating existing diseases to prevent the disease from developing complications. Tertiary prevention activities include antibiotics to prevent the spread of an infection, range of motion to prevent the effects of immobility, and rehabilitation after a car crash.

Many health disorders can be prevented by a healthy lifestyle. Children learn from their parents, and when the parents practice healthy behaviors, the children are more likely to practice good health as well. Health-promoting behaviors include exercising regularly, eating a balanced diet, obtaining adequate rest, limiting caffeine and alcohol consumption, and omitting the use of illicit drugs.

Cigarette smoking is not only harmful to the smoker's lungs and blood vessels, but the exhaled smoke can also stimulate respiratory disorders in children who live with the smoker. Children are more likely to begin smoking when one or both parents smoke. When a pregnant woman smokes, there is a greater risk that the baby will have a low birth weight. For these reasons, every family member should be encouraged to stop smoking. For those smokers who need assistance to quit, help is available through prescription medication and support groups. Nurses should become familiar with the groups in their community.

Alcohol use during pregnancy can damage the infant's growing brain, resulting in mental and physical deficiencies (see Figure 27-5 ⚭). When parents drink alcohol, they are teaching their children that drinking is accepted. Although an occasional drink may not be harmful, frequent consumption can lead to liver, heart, and behavior issues. The amount of alcohol needed to intoxicate varies from individual to individual. Intoxication leads to poor judgment, unpredictable behavior, and sometimes criminal actions. Adults need to consider the effects of alcohol on their children and families before choosing to drink.

WELL-CHILD VISITS

The child should be assessed by a pediatrician or family practice physician or family nurse practitioner at regular intervals. An accepted schedule is 2 weeks, 2 months, 4 months, 6 months, 9 months, 12 months, 15 months, 24 months, and yearly thereafter. Well-child visits gather data about physical health, including growth and development, nutritional health, emotional health, and neurologic status. These visits would also include immunizations, health promotion teaching, and assessment of parent–child

HEALTH PROMOTION ISSUE

TYPES OF LEARNING

The LPN/LVN works for a family practice office. Job responsibilities include health promotion teaching for all age clients. She teaches the importance of immunizations, health screening, contraception control, sexually transmitted infection prevention, cardiac health, etc. The content for the teaching plan has been carefully researched and written in collaboration with the entire health care staff, including the physician and the supervising registered nurse. Although she is knowledgeable about the content, the LPN/LVN has noticed that some clients respond enthusiastically while others seem only to tolerate the teaching. She has become increasingly concerned that the teaching may be ineffective for some clients. She discusses her concerns with the supervising nurse.

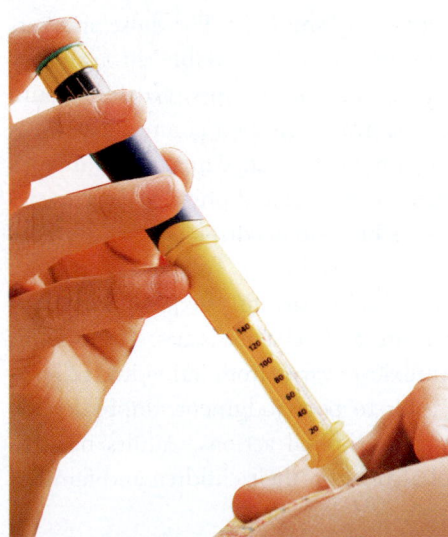

(Ben Edwards\Getty Images Inc.- Stone Allstock)

DISCUSSION

People learn in different ways. Many theorists have developed ideas of how learning occurs. Dr. David Kolb developed the following categories of learning styles:

■ *The Accomodator.* This learner is flexible and needs an overview of the content prior to having the details. In fact, this learner will get lost if the teacher begins with the details. The accommodator also learns by trial and error. He or she needs activities such as games, written exercises, or role play.

■ *The Assimilator.* This learner is a logical, structured, and task-oriented individual. The content should be presented in a practical manner with clear application of the principles. The teacher should provide concrete methods so the learner can put the principles into practice. This learner learns best through lectures, questioning, watching, and through reasoning-type exercises such as thought questions. This learner desires an organization to the teaching, including expected time frame and an outline of goals or objectives. The teacher must be diligent or the learner will become frustrated.

■ *The Diverger.* This learner looks for multiple solutions to the topic being taught. He or she needs to own the content, to feel it, and to attach emotion to the subject. The teacher can assist this learner by relating personal

stories. Using audiovisual aids will assist this learner. The teacher should also allow the diverger to participate in the learning experience by expressing his or her opinion.

■ *The Converger.* This learner is task-oriented and loves to handle the content him- or herself. He or she enjoys researching the content, and will take notes and learn better when the teacher has prepared a handout. Much of this learner's learning occurs on his or her own time as he or she continues to dig into the content. Homework assignments work well for this learner. The teacher must be available outside the teaching session for this learner to discuss the content further.

Other theorists have defined learning styles as *visual, auditory,* and *kinesthetic*:

■ The visual learner needs to see the content. The teacher will assist this learner best by providing visual material.

■ The auditory learner needs to hear the content, and he or she also needs to verbalize the content. The teacher can lecture to this learner, but also needs to allow this learner to discuss the content.

■ The kinesthetic learner needs to touch the content. The teacher should provide a physical activity for this learner, such as handing him or her a syringe or an anatomic model.

The teacher must also keep in mind that a typical learner needs a variety of

relationships. During a visit with the toddler, information about toileting should be gathered. Health screenings such as vision, hearing, urinalysis, hematocrit, and tuberculosis are usually initiated in the preschool years. Screening for scoliosis is done during the school years. The adolescent should be screened for involvement in sexual activity, and appropriate health care should begin when the teen is sexually active.

HYGIENE

Children are at high risk for contracting communicable diseases. This risk can be lowered through careful attention to matters of hygiene. Hand washing (Figure 12-2A ■) is an important measure for the nurse to teach parents. Children need to understand the importance of washing their hands vigorously before and after meals and after toileting. Germs are also spread among children by sharing toys and snacks

teaching methods to grasp the content. Learners will retain 10% of what they read, 20% of what they hear, 30% of what they see, 50% of what they hear and see, 70% of what they say, and 90% of what they say and do.

PLANNING AND IMPLEMENTATION

The supervising nurse and the LPN/LVN spent time reviewing different learning styles. They then reviewed their teaching plans and discovered that they were basically designed for an auditory learner. They decided that it was necessary to re-work the health promotion teaching plans. They first wanted to assess the learning styles of their clients. They obtained a learning style inventory tool and asked clients to complete it while waiting for their appointments. The results of this inventory were then attached to each client's chart so the nurse providing health promotion teaching could adapt his or her content appropriately.

Second, they redesigned the health promotion teaching plans to accommodate each type of learner. They developed teaching and learning activities that would best meet the needs of each learning style. For example, when teaching cardiac health, the nurse will:

- For the accommodator, present an overview of cardiac risks and prevention methods, followed by written activities about diet, exercise, and risk factors.
- For the assimilator, present a written agenda of the teaching, followed by a short lecture on cardiac risk and prevention methods. Then, together with the client, the nurse will help him or her outline a specific plan that fits his or her lifestyle.
- For the diverger, present the content in a visual format using pictures of people and objects rather than graphic drawings. The nurse will also incorporate personal stories of success and failure with cardiac health prevention.
- For the converger, present the content in a logical, straightforward manner, with a handout to give to the client. The nurse will also suggest several websites and other resources where the client can learn more about the content.

Last, the supervising nurse and the LPN realized the need to add an evaluation tool to their teaching plan. It became apparent that they needed to know whether learning had occurred. They incorporated a variety of methods such as verbal reviews of the content, written reviews of the content, quizzes, and crossword puzzles and matching games for younger clients.

SELF-REFLECTION

What is your particular learning style? When you encounter teaching that is not presented in your learning style, how do you adapt so you can learn? When you teach, do you accept responsibility for the learning that occurs? What expectations do you have for those you teach? Are they realistic? Why or why not? What teaching methods do you use most often when presenting health content to clients? Are these methods always effective? Do you vary your teaching methods according to your client's needs? List 5 things you could do to improve your teaching style.

MediaLink   Learning styles

SUGGESTED RESOURCES

For the Nurse

Wilkinson, B. (1983). *The 7 laws of the learner: How to teach almost anything to practically anyone.* Sisters, OR: Multnomah Press.

- **http://pss.uvm.edu** This website offers an inventory for assessing learning styles.
- **www.clat.psu.edu** This learning style inventory differentiates visual, auditory, or kinesthetic learners.

- **www.haygroup.co.uk** This website offers information on obtaining the learning style inventory to assess David Kolb's learning styles.
- **www.reviewing.co.uk** This website offers information on the learning styles developed by David Kolb.

(see Figure 12-2B). Children in church nurseries, day care centers, and schools should be monitored for hand-to-mouth activities and encouraged to wash their hands frequently.

The child who is ill can spread germs to other children by coughing, sneezing, and indiscriminately disposing of used tissues. The nurse can teach parents and children the importance of covering their mouth and nose when coughing or sneezing (see Figure 12-2C). School officials are now encouraging children to sneeze and cough into their elbow rather than into their hands. This will prevent germs from getting onto the child's hands, where they can be more easily passed to others. Children should be taught to dispose of used tissues in trash receptacles and avoid leaving them where others may come in contact with them.

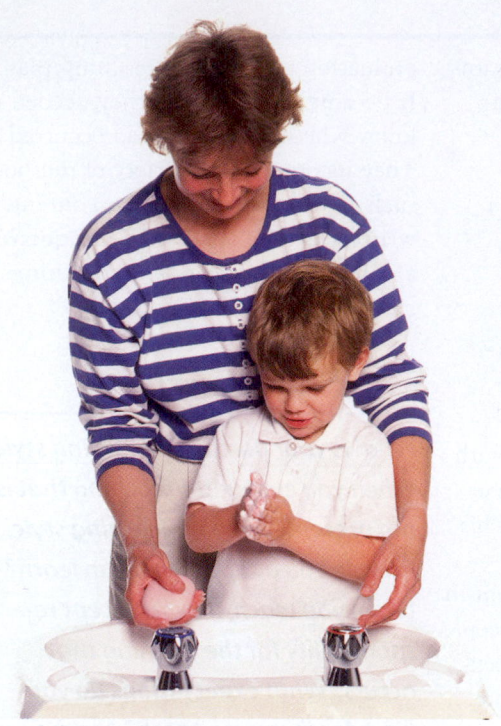

A

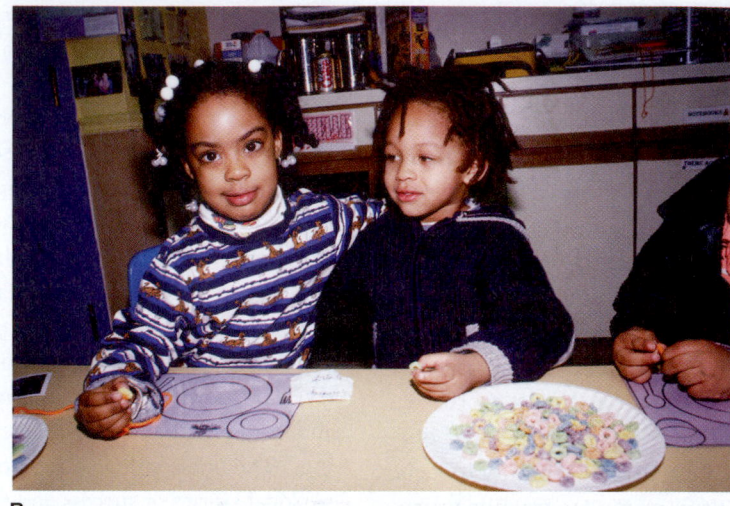

B

C

Figure 12-2. ■ **(A)** Adults teach children the proper technique for washing and drying hands. They can also teach children that this action is the single, most effective way to prevent transmission of infection. (Dorling Kindersley Media Library.) **(B)** When preschoolers and kindergarten children share snacks or supplies, there is always the potential for transmitting infection. For this reason, children with highly transmissible infections (e.g., conjunctivitis) are asked to stay at home until the infection has cleared. (Nancy Sheehan Photography.) **(C)** Many respiratory infections are transmitted by droplets from person to person. Children need to learn to cover the nose and mouth completely when coughing or sneezing. Some now recommend coughing into the sleeve at the elbow so hands are not contaminated. (Photo Researchers Inc.)

IMMUNIZATIONS

To prevent dangerous illnesses, vaccines have been developed. By injecting dead or weakened organisms, inactivated toxins, or toxoids, active immunity is produced. To be effective, repeat injections (immunizations) must be given on a schedule. The American Committee on Immunization Practices, the American Academy of Pediatrics (AAP), and the American Academy of Family Practitioners annually update the immunization schedule. A copy of the current schedule can be obtained from the client's local health

DEPARTMENT OF HEALTH AND HUMAN SERVICES • CENTERS FOR DISEASE CONTROL AND PREVENTION

Recommended Childhood and Adolescent Immunization Schedule   UNITED STATES • 2006

Vaccine ▼ Age ▶	Birth	1 month	2 months	4 months	6 months	12 months	15 months	18 months	24 months	4–6 years	11–12 years	13–14 years	15 years	16–18 years
Hepatitis B[1]	HepB	HepB		HepB[1]	HepB	HepB					HepB Series			
Diphtheria, Tetanus, Pertussis[2]			DTaP	DTaP	DTaP		DTaP			DTaP	Tdap	Tdap		
Haemophilus influenzae type b[3]			Hib	Hib	Hib[3]	Hib								
Inactivated Poliovirus			IPV	IPV	IPV					IPV				
Measles, Mumps, Rubella[4]						MMR				MMR	MMR			
Varicella[5]						Varicella				Varicella				
Meningococcal[6]									MPSV4		MCV4	MCV4 / MCV4	MCV4	
Pneumococcal[7]			PCV	PCV	PCV	PCV			PCV	PPV				
Influenza[8]					Influenza (Yearly)				Influenza (Yearly)					
Hepatitis A[9]						HepA Series								

Vaccines within broken line are for selected populations

This schedule indicates the recommended ages for routine administration of currently licensed childhood vaccines, as of December 1, 2005, for children through age 18 years. Any dose not administered at the recommended age should be administered at any subsequent visit when indicated and feasible. ▨ Indicates age groups that warrant special effort to administer those vaccines not previously administered. Additional vaccines may be licensed and recommended during the year. Licensed combination vaccines may be used whenever any components of the combination are indicated and other components of the vaccine are not contraindicated and if approved by the Food and Drug Administration for that dose of the series. Providers should consult the respective ACIP statement for detailed recommendations. Clinically significant adverse events that follow immunization should be reported to the Vaccine Adverse Event Reporting System (VAERS). Guidance about how to obtain and complete a VAERS form is available at **www.vaers.hhs.gov** or by telephone, **800-822-7967**.

▨ Range of recommended ages   ▨ Catch-up immunization   ▨ 11–12 year old assessment

Figure 12-3. ■ Immunization schedule.

department. Figure 12-3 ■ illustrates an immunization schedule. Table 12-1 ■ lists routine pediatric immunizations. See Chapter 26 ◉◉ for more information on childhood diseases and prevention methods.

The nurse is responsible for reviewing the medical record and determining the need for immunization. Federal legislation requires written informed consent from the parent or guardian prior to administering a vaccine. The nurse must provide literature about the vaccine and its possible adverse effects. Parents should be given a copy of the child's immunization record because schools may require proof that immunizations are up to date before admitting a child.

TABLE 12-1

Pharmacology: Routine Pediatric Immunizations

DRUG (COMMON BRAND NAME AND GENERIC)	USUAL ROUTE/DOSE	SELECTED SIDE EFFECTS	DO NOT GIVE IF
Diphtheria, tetanus toxoid and acellular pertussis vaccine (Acel-Immune, Tripedia)	IM 0.5 mL*	Erythema and induration at site; fever; malaise	Children have symptoms of infection; seizure activity
Measles, mumps, rubella vaccine (M-M-R II)	SQ 0.5 mL*	Arthralgia; pain at injection site	Children have allergy to eggs
Hepatitis B vaccine (Engerix-B, Recombivax HB)	IM 10 mcg Engerix-B; IM 2.5 mcg Recombivax HB*	Soreness at site	Children have hypersensitivity to yeast

* See immunization schedule.

There are many reasons why a child's immunization schedule may be interrupted. Well-meaning parents can forget to schedule appointments. Parents may not see the need for immunization. The following guidelines can be used to prevent missing immunization opportunities:

- Several immunizations can be given at the same visit.
- Immunizations can be given when the child has a minor illness with or without low-grade fever.
- Immunizations can be given when the child is receiving antibiotics.
- Immunizations can be given even if the child has been exposed to an infectious disease.
- Premature infants have the same requirement for immunization as full-term infants.
- Immunization can be given when there has been a local reaction to previous immunizations.

For parents who refuse immunization of their children, it is important to teach about the development of immunity. Box 12-2 ■ provides information about alternative ways to strengthen the immune system.

Contraindications to immunization are anaphylactic reactions to the vaccine, moderate to severe acute illness, or pregnancy. Nonimmunized women of childbearing age are not only at risk for becoming infected, but also of exposing an unborn child to infection. Because immunization is contraindicated during pregnancy, it is important for women of childbearing age to remain current with the recommended immunization schedule.

When preparing and giving immunizations, the nurse should check the expiration date on the vaccine. Outdated vaccines may be weak and ineffective. Vaccines must be stored properly in the refrigerator. Some vaccines must be mixed with the solution provided. These vaccines usually have a short shelf-life, so it is important to put the date the solution was mixed on the bottle. Once the vaccines have been prepared, they should be given quickly and efficiently. Allow the child to select the site where the injection will be given. The site needs to be gently restrained to prevent injury from the needle. This is best done by obtaining help from a colleague and allowing parents to give emotional support only. Give the child honest answers, and do not say that the needle will not hurt. Children become anxious, so do not hesitate in giving the injection even if the child begins to cry or scream. After the injection, allow the parent to comfort the child. Compliment the child for being brave, for holding as still as possible, or for other positive behavior.

Health Promotion

Health promotion is the encouragement of lifestyle changes that result in a healthier state for the individual. **Health,** a sense of physical, psychological, emotional, and

---

BOX 12-2 **COMPLEMENTARY THERAPIES**

Boosting the Immune System

Some parents may choose not to immunize their children. They may be fearful of the negative effects of childhood immunizations. When parents make an informed decision, the nurse can assist parents in keeping their children healthy. The following are suggestions for boosting a child's immunity:

- Teach children to be diligent about washing their hands before and after meals, after handling pets, after blowing their nose, and after using the bathroom.
- Quarantine children from other children who have known illnesses.
- Give the child a diet containing plenty of foods with vitamin C and carotenoids, such as carrots, green beans, oranges, and strawberries.
- Ensure that the child gets adequate sleep each night. The newborn should sleep 18 hours/day. The toddler should sleep 12 to 13 hours/day, and the preschooler should sleep at least 10 hours/night.

- Encourage regular exercise to boost immunity.
- Decrease exposure to secondhand smoke, which lowers immunity.
- Consider acupuncture during the cold and flu season. (Improved immunity is linked to use of acupuncture.)
- After consultation with the physician, give vitamin and mineral supplementation to boost immunity.
  - Vitamin C can be given to children under 6 at a dose of 250 mg/day and for children older than 6 at 500 mg/day.
  - Zinc supplements can be given to children under 6 at 10 to 20 mg/day and for children older than 6 at 20 to 40 mg/day.
- Provide the herbal product *Echinacea* to improve immunity. During the cold and flu season, children under 6 can be given 450 to 500 mg/day and children older than 6, a dose of 225 to 250 mg/day.

spiritual well-being, is not just the absence of disease. Activities that promote health include eating a proper diet, getting adequate rest, and exercising. Activities such as chiropractic care, massage, taking herbs or nutritional supplements, meditation, and religious services can also promote a healthier individual. (*Note:* Encourage parents to discuss any alternative health care practices with their care provider, especially herbal and nutritional supplements.) Health promotion encourages the individual to take charge of personal health by making lifestyle changes.

Because of their broad knowledge base and experience in assisting in medical treatment of illness, nurses are the obvious choice for directing health promotion activities. (See also Chapters 5, 6, and 10 ∞ for health promotion in women and Chapter 11 ∞ for health promotion in children.) This chapter introduces illness prevention and health promotion concepts through the stages of growth and development. Additional topics related to health promotion are addressed by body system in the remaining chapters of Unit III.

ENVIRONMENTAL SAFETY

Injuries resulting from accidents are a leading cause of death in children ages 1 to 19 (Anderson, 2005). Although accidents occur and not all injuries can be prevented, striving to keep the family as safe as possible is an important nursing intervention. As the child grows and becomes more mobile, keeping the environment safe becomes a greater challenge. Key safety issues are discussed for each age group.

PSYCHOSOCIAL HEALTH

Promoting Self-Esteem

The child growing up in today's American culture will have challenges never faced by previous generations. To face those challenges in a healthy manner, the child will need to have a strong sense of self. Promotion of self-esteem begins early in child development. By praising accomplishments, the parent gives positive feedback for hard work. This teaches the child that hard work will result in positive outcomes. For example, as the infant tries and tries to turn over, and finally accomplishes the task, parents can smile, clap, and praise the infant. Infants will learn that certain behaviors cause parents to smile. They will continue to try to elicit this response. The toddler learns to use the toilet through praise for his or her efforts and success. (Toilet training is discussed later in this chapter.) When parents emphasize the positive work the preschooler does in trying to make the bed and compliment that behavior, they build the child's self-esteem and pride in the task. If they add ways to improve, the child will be more willing to try to make it nicer. But if the parents repeatedly criticize the child because the bed is not made perfectly, the child will become discouraged and may stop trying to do the task at all.

Soon-to-be parents and new parents also need encouragement. If adults enter parenthood with a high level of self-esteem, they will generally have skills to help them be supportive parents. However, if parents have low self-esteem, they will need teaching and support to strengthen their self-esteem in order to be better parents. The nurse provides information about illness prevention and health promotion activities, and then praises the parent for their effort in making changes. By being a role model, the nurse helps the parents understand the effect of praise for good behavior and success.

Providing Discipline

To function in society, the child needs to learn rules and the consequences for breaking rules. The key to effective discipline is consistency. Both parents need to agree ahead of time on the family rules and the consequences of breaking the rules. The AAP (2004) defines **spanking** as one or two flat-handed swats on a child's wrist or buttocks, and states that corporal punishment is of limited effectiveness and has potentially dangerous side effects. The AAP recommends that parents develop methods other than spanking for managing undesired behavior. Striking the child, other than spanking as defined here, is considered to be child abuse. For ideas about the best way to discipline a child, see Box 12-3 ■.

More acceptable forms of discipline for the young child include "time-out" in the child's room or a corner

---

BOX 12-3

Child Development Experts' Views on Discipline

T. Berry Brazelton, MD, a well-known expert in pediatric care, clinical professor of pediatrics at Harvard Medical School, and professor of psychiatry and human development at Brown University, views spanking as an unnecessary and potentially harmful method of discipline.

William Sears, MD, associate clinical professor of pediatrics at the University of California, Irvine School of Medicine, pediatrician in practice, and author of more than 30 books on parenting, does not advocate spanking. He sees this form of punishment as a method of teaching children that it is okay to hit and strike out at one another when a wrong has been done.

John Rosemond, a family psychologist who writes for 225 newspapers nationwide on parenting issues, believes children should be spanked only as an immediate response to an unacceptable behavior. He teaches that the spanking should be followed by a short explanation and an additional consequence if the unacceptable behavior is repeated.

James Dobson, a clinical psychologist with a PhD in child development, former clinical professor of pediatrics at the University of Southern California School of Medicine, and current chairman of Focus on the Family, believes that if spanking is delivered in anger and with intimidation, negative outcomes may occur. However, he teaches that spanking can be used effectively for willful disobedience.

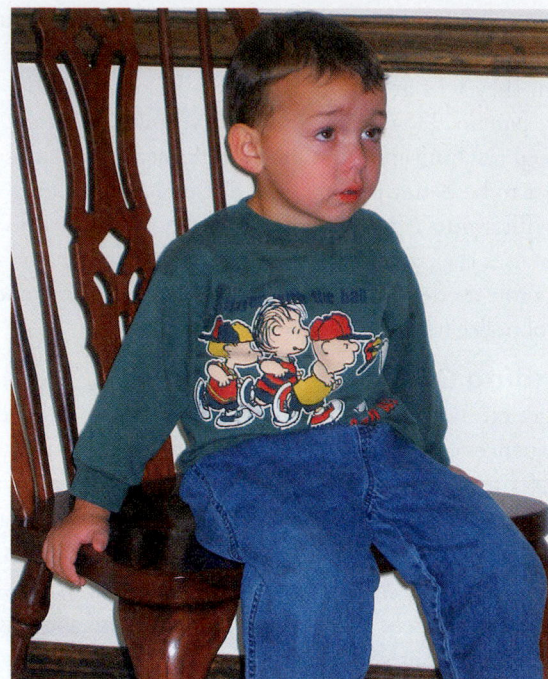

Figure 12-4. ■ One effective discipline method is to move the child to an isolated area where no interaction with children or adults can occur and no toys are present. This is used to demonstrate that there is a consequence to misbehavior. For older children, consider the loss of phone, computer, or other privileges for a set period of time.

(Figure 12-4 ■). For the older child, restricting the use of the computer, telephone, or outside activities may be effective. Discipline becomes ineffective when the parent does not allow the child to experience the consequences of his or her actions. The nurse needs to help parents explore their method of discipline and work toward setting effective consequences for bad behavior. The nurse must continually be alert for signs of child abuse. Child abuse is discussed in Chapter 27 ◯◯ of this text.

Promoting Play

Children play together wherever they gather. Play occurs in the home with siblings or friends, in the neighborhood at parks or backyards, at day care or other formal programs such as mother's morning out, and in the nursery at church. Play can be spontaneous, encouraged, or organized.

"To play" has many meanings, but in general it means to take part in an activity for entertainment and recreation. For the young child, play also has a valuable purpose. Through play, the young child learns and practices many skills that will be necessary in adulthood. For example, when preschoolers play with chalk and a chalkboard, they develop eye–hand coordination (Figure 12-5 ■). For 6-year-olds, playing a board game is practice in "taking turns" and "cooperating." Adolescents also need time to play. Engaging in sports activities such as golf, tennis, fishing, and

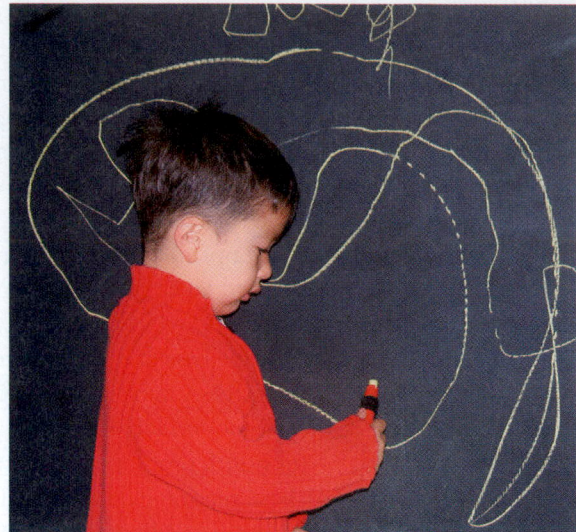

Figure 12-5. ■ Preschoolers develop eye–hand coordination in a variety of settings. (M. C. Schlachter Photography.)

swimming can help both adolescents and adults stay fit, gain confidence, receive positive feelings through competition, and interact socially.

NUTRITION

Malnutrition is often associated with emaciated-looking children with protuberant abdomens from underdeveloped countries. However, malnutrition in the United States presents more often as obesity. According to Carmona (2004), 15.3% of American children are considered to be clinically obese. For the most part, improper nutrition is not due to a lack of finances but to a lack of knowledge coupled with readily accessible convenience food.

The goal of *Healthy People 2010* is to reduce the prevalence of obesity in children and adolescents to 5% (US Department of Health and Human Services, 2000). Proper nutrition is the first line of defense against obesity. The standard American diet is high in fat, carbohydrates, and sodium, and deficient in fruits, vegetables, fiber, and water. Oversized portions are a cause of obesity, providing excessive calories. A typical fast-food meal is a double patty hamburger with cheese, super-sized french fries, and an extra large soft drink. This meal contains approximately 1,480 calories. The nurse can assist clients in making more appropriate choices. For example, the following is a healthier lunch: 2 cups green salad with low-fat dressing, 3 oz grilled chicken breast with the skin removed, and unsweetened iced tea or diet soda. This meal contains approximately 250 calories.

The foundation fat cells are established in childhood. When parents choose high-fat diets for their children, the lifelong struggle to maintain normal weight begins. The nurse can teach parents the importance of serving healthy foods. The U.S. Department of Agriculture's Center for Nutrition Policy and Promotion has improved the food pyramid (Figure 12-6 ■). My Pyramid is a helpful tool that

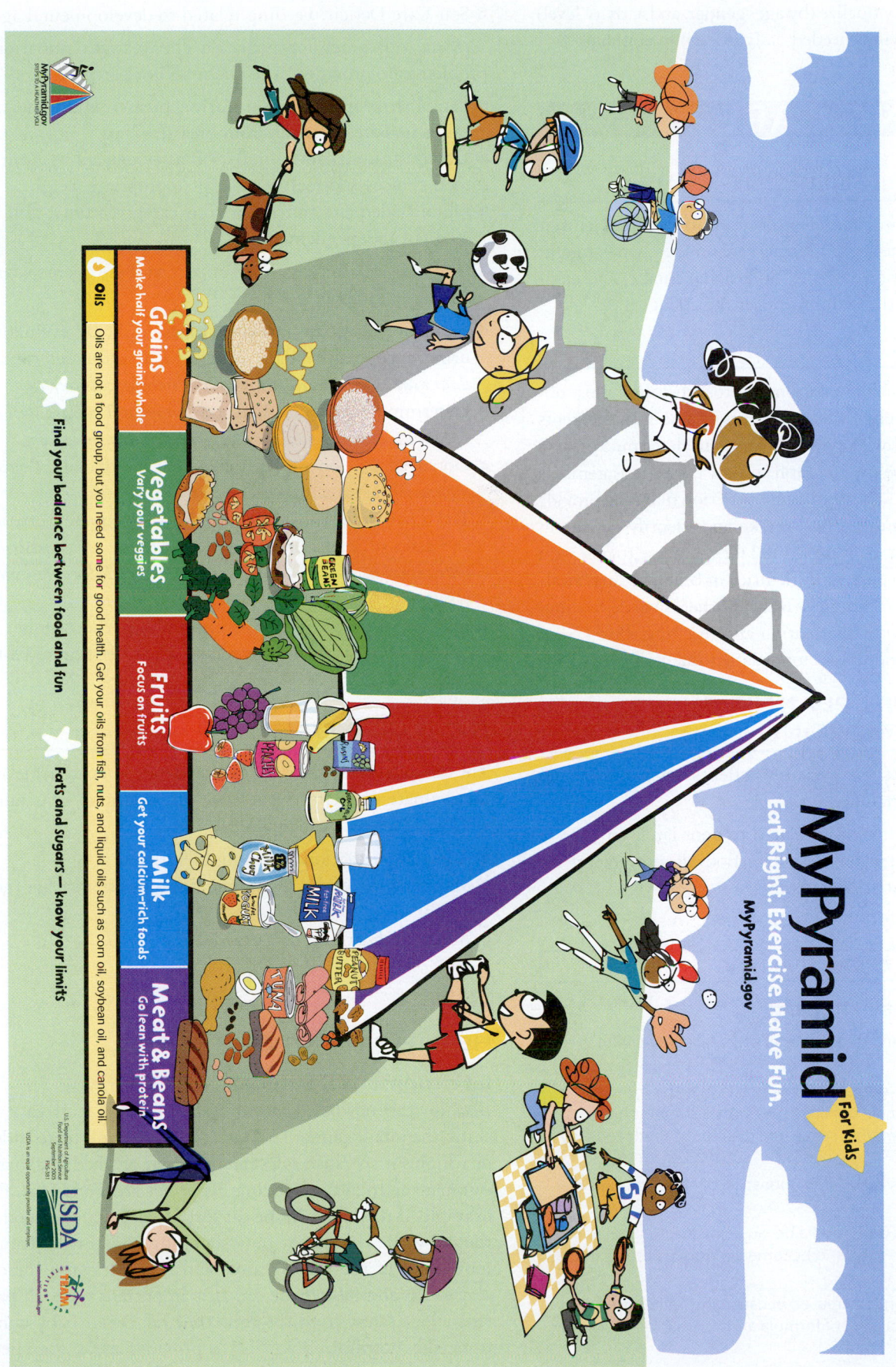

Figure 12-6. ■ Food pyramid. (Reprinted from the U.S. Department of Agriculture and U.S. Department of Health and Human Services.)

can be used to individualize (by age, gender, and activity level) the number of servings needed daily in each food group.

NURSING CARE

PRIORITIES IN NURSING CARE

When caring for pediatric clients with nutrition problems, it is important for the nurse to focus care on the client's weight and height, nutritional status, nutritional intake, and environmental factors that might impact the client's diet.

ASSESSING

To determine adequate nutritional status, the nurse must obtain height and weight measurements. These measurements are then compared with previous values to determine growth patterns. The nurse uses a graph to plot these measurements (see Appendix II ⚭). A 24-hour nutrition diary can provide information about the child's intake and identify deficits in the diet. With infants, it is optimal for the nurse to observe a feeding in order to observe difficulties in breastfeeding, swallowing, or feeding techniques. If the mother is bottle-feeding, the nurse can provide information and teaching. Box 12-4 ■ discusses bottle-propping in formula-fed infants.

DIAGNOSING, PLANNING, AND IMPLEMENTING

Nursing diagnoses for pediatric clients with nutritional problems might include:

- Ineffective Breastfeeding related to poor latch-on
- Imbalanced Nutrition: Less than Body Requirements related to poor nutritional choices

BOX 12-4	CLIENT TEACHING

Dangers of Bottle-Propping

- Decreases bonding due to lack of physical contact with caregiver.
- Increases risk for dental caries or bottle mouth syndrome because the formula or juice in the bottle contains high amounts of sugar, which coats the deciduous teeth and may erode enamel.
- Overfeeding may result from ingestion of large amounts of formula.
- Increases risk for otitis media because the formula can pool in the Eustachian tube and become a medium for bacterial growth.
- Risk for aspiration is increased because the infant may fall asleep with a mouthful of formula and be unable to swallow appropriately.

- Self-Care Deficit: Feeding related to developmental age.

Some outcomes for pediatric clients with nutritional problems are provided. The client and/or parent will:

- Establish proper latch-on during breastfeeding and obtain adequate nutrition from breastfeeding.
- Demonstrate balanced nutrition as evidenced by healthy food choices and maintenance of appropriate weight.
- Obtain adequate nutrition from caregiver until able to feed self independently.

The nurse's role in providing support to these clients would include the following:

- Assess for adequate intake of breast milk by evaluating urine output and infant weight. *This assessment provides data used to prevent dehydration and imbalanced nutrition.*
- Determine child's adequate body weight. *The data will assist the caregiver in planning for appropriate interventions.*
- Obtain a nutrition history from parent and/or child. *Provides information about nutritional elements that are deficient.*
- Teach parent and child the benefits of adequate nutrition and risks of inadequate nutrition. *Compliance to prescribed nutritional regime may be improved with knowledge of risks and benefits.*
- Instruct the parent and/or child about the number of calories needed and healthy food options (see Figure 12-6), etc.

EVALUATING

The care plan is revised until expected outcomes are achieved. To evaluate the effectiveness of interventions, the nurse would gather data concerning:

- Adequate urination following breastfeeding
- Maintenance of body weight appropriate for age and height
- Adequate nutrients consumed daily.

Infant

HEALTH PROMOTION

Environmental Safety

Because the newborn has limited mobility, it is easy to think the infant cannot fall. However, when left unattended on a high surface, such as a changing table or a bed, the infant can manage to fall by moving his or her arms and legs. For example, if the infant in the car seat is placed on the hood of the car while the parent puts shopping bags in the trunk, movement of the infant's arms and legs can cause the car seat to tip and fall off the car. It is important to teach parents about safety from the time they take their baby home from the hospital. Box 12-5 ■ provides areas for client teaching about physical injury and safety.

BOX 12-5   **CLIENT TEACHING**

Guidelines About Physical Injury and Safety

- Support the infant's head carefully when carrying the infant or picking him or her up.
- Never leave the infant unattended on any surface other than the floor. He or she may fall.
- Never leave the child unattended in the bathtub or near any other source of water such as swimming pools or spas. Swimming pools and spas should have locked gates surrounding them. Children may also drown in water left in buckets.
- Raise the siderails on the crib and lock them into place.
- Position safety gates at the top and bottom of staircases, no matter how few steps. Gates are also appropriate in entrances to areas such as the kitchen or laundry room, where dangerous products are stored.

Burns

- Carefully test the temperature of heated formula or bottled breast milk before giving it to the infant.
- Carefully test the temperature of bathwater before immersing the child.
- Never place the child close to fireplaces, space heaters, or stoves.
- Do not smoke or carry hot beverages when holding an infant.
- Cover electrical outlets.
- Adjust the temperature of hot water heater to 120° F (48.8° C).

Car Safety

- Never leave a child unattended in a motor vehicle. Temperatures inside of cars can quickly become dangerous.
- Only use age-appropriate, approved car safety seats.
- Place an infant in the back seat to avoid injury from airbags.

Choking

- Never place the infant's crib near drapes or blinds because the child could choke on the cords.
- Secure electrical cords out of reach.
- Remove pillows and plastic from an infant's reach. Do not place an infant on a bean bag, feather bed, or sheepskin rug.
- Be diligent about keeping small objects out of the infant's reach.
- Do not give infants small foods such as hard candy, grapes, hot dogs, or popcorn.
- Do not prop bottles.

Poisoning

- Keep toxic products in locked areas.
- Keep houseplants out of reach.
- Keep prescribed and over-the-counter medicines in locked cabinets.
- Ensure that the child is not exposed to paint containing lead.
- Keep the local Poison Control Center phone number by the phone.

The baby begins to roll from side to back and can crawl as early as 6 months. It is important to begin the habit of protecting the child from falls at birth. Parents should be taught to use safety gates to prevent the infant from falling down stairs. Particularly when the infant becomes mobile, it is important to secure the gate to the wall following manufacturer's guidelines. Safety in bed may also be a consideration (Box 12-6 ■). Also, in older cribs, the child's head may become trapped between slats because these cribs were not designed to prevent this.

CHOKING. **Choking** (asphyxiation by a foreign object lodged in the respiratory tract) and suffocation are a particular concern during infancy. Because the baby becomes mobile within a few months and frequently brings hand to mouth, parents

BOX 12-6   **CULTURAL PULSE POINTS**

Sleeping with Infants in the Same Bed

Consider the family's cultural norms when discussing the risks of parents and children sleeping in the same bed. For example, it is common for Bosnian families to allow children up to age 2 to sleep in the same bed with the parents. Safety teaching about the dangers of the practice must occur, but be sensitive to the client's cultural beliefs.

must be constantly aware of small objects within the infant's reach and be vigilant to remove them from the baby's environment. The parent should be encouraged to get down on the floor and look for small objects from the infant's perspective. Toys should be inspected to be sure there are no small parts that could come loose and be swallowed by the infant. Any toy labeled "not intended for use by those under 3 years" should be kept out of the infant's reach. Other choking or suffocation hazards include stuffed toys, pacifiers, pillows, and plastic-type materials, including plastic bags and balloons.

The crib should not be close to the drawstring on the curtains or blinds because the infant can get the cord around his or her neck and strangle. Parents should also be aware that hanging mobiles can cause a choking hazard. An infant's crib slats must be close together so he or she cannot get his or her head caught between the slats. Any crib with slats spaced more than $2\frac{3}{8}$ inches (6 cm) should be discarded. The mattress should fit tightly against the crib rails to prevent body parts from becoming lodged in the crib frame.

CAR SAFETY. The most common injuries to a newborn are caused by car crashes, falls, and choking. All infants must be transported in a rear-facing infant car seat. The car seat should be secured according to directions provided by the manufacturer. The safest place for the infant is in the back seat. With the infant in the rear-facing position in the back seat, the

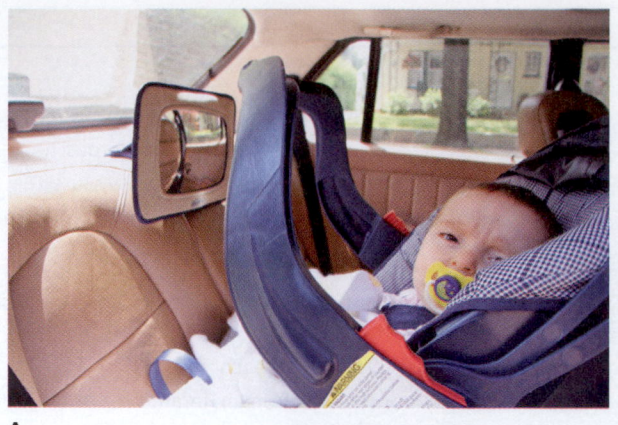

A

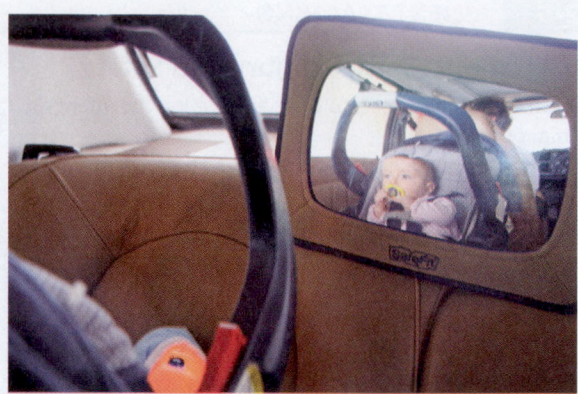

B

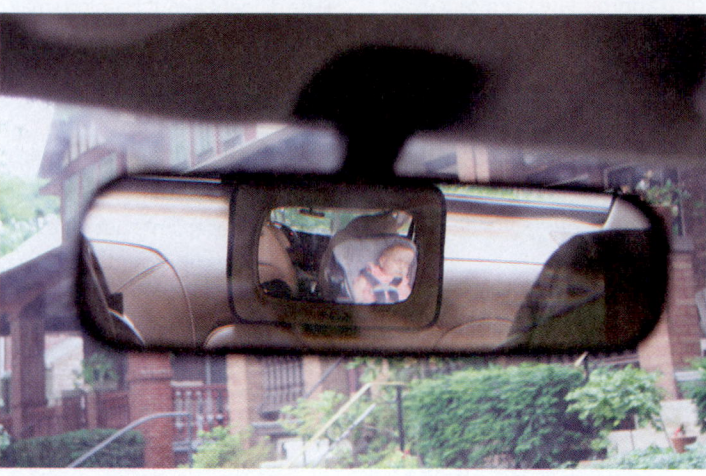

C

Figure 12-7. ■ Adjustable mirrors are available to allow the driver to see the infant via the car's rearview mirror. (**A**) The mirror is positioned next to the infant's car seat. (**B**) *(Facing rear of car)* There is no obstruction between the front seat and the mirror next to the car seat. (**C**) The driver attaches a small mirror to the rearview mirror in front and slants it so the infant can be seen from the driver's seat. (M. C. Schlachter Photography.)

parent may have difficulty seeing the infant. Adjustable mirrors are available to allow the driver to see the infant through the car's rearview mirror (Figure 12-7 ■). The driver should not allow a crying infant to distract from safe driving practices; he or she should pull off the road and stop before attending to the infant. Information can be obtained from the National Safety Council. *Federal Motor Vehicle Safety Standards* (AAP, 2006) should be followed regarding use of infant car seats and booster seats. Table 12-2 ■ identifies the recommended use of infant and child car seats. Small or premature infants may not be able to breathe in a sitting position in the car seat. In these cases, they need to use an approved infant car bed until their weight increases. The infant car bed will need to be secured to the automobile's rear seat, and the infant secured into the bed following manufacturer instructions. Infants should never be left alone in a car. In the summer, temperatures inside the car can reach more than 130°F in just a few minutes, subjecting the infant to hyperthermia, brain damage, and even death.

PSYCHOSOCIAL HEALTH

Promoting Self-Esteem
Many child development experts agree that one of the best ways to promote self-esteem in children is to give them a sense of security and to assist them in developing trust. In infancy, trust is developed as needs are met promptly. Nurses can help parents recognize the infant's cues for hunger, sleep, and nurture. The nurse should also encourage parents to respond promptly to these cues. This allows the infant to learn to trust the parent and will facilitate the process of bonding or attachment.

Promoting Play
Each age group has patterns of play that indicate its level of social development. Many changes occur in the first year of life. Infants rapidly learn about the world around them. Play for the 2- to 3-month-old infant involves learning to

TABLE 12-2

Use of Infant and Child Car Seats

CHILD SIZE OR WEIGHT	INSTRUCTIONS
Weight below 20 lb (9 kg)	■ Place infant or convertible seat in back seat of car facing backward. ■ Never place the infant in the front passenger seat. ■ Recline infant at 45 degrees or less (some small infants must be flat in a car bed). ■ Following manufacturer's instructions, fasten seat securely to car using car seat belt. ■ Adjust harnesses to fit snugly at shoulders and legs. ■ Move to a larger seat before the infant's head reaches top of the shell. ■ When using a convertible seat from birth, use one with a five-point harness.
Birth to 40 lb (18 kg)	■ Use reclined for rear-facing and upright for forward-facing position. ■ Follow manufacturer's instructions for proper position at specified child weights for that product. ■ Move to a high-back child seat or booster when child's ears are above the seat. ■ Always place the seat in the back seat of the vehicle.
Above 40 lb (18 kg)	■ Use booster seat for children who have outgrown convertible toddler seat. ■ Follow manufacturer's instruction for instillation and for specified child weights for the product. ■ Use booster seat until the vehicle lap and shoulder belts fit correctly. ■ Have all children 12 years and younger ride in the back-seat regardless of whether in a car seat.

Note: Airbags can cause serious injury and death when a child is in a car seat in the front passenger seat. Even when not in a car seat and when the vehicle is not equipped with a passenger side air bag, the back seat is the safest location for all children.

Source: From National Safety Council. (2004). *Child Passenger Safety Fact Sheet.* Washington, DC: Author.

grasp and move small, lightweight toys. The infant enjoys seeing bright colors and hearing rattling noises coming from the toy. As the infant grows in strength and learns to sit and crawl, play becomes exploring the world. This exploration involves seeing, touching, and tasting the environment.

APPROPRIATE TOYS. Toys for infants should be age appropriate and safe. They should not have small, removable parts or long cords that could be a choking hazard. Rattles are interesting to infants because they make noise and can be easily grasped. Mobiles and baby gyms should be brightly colored or black and white to attract the infant visually. Blocks should have smooth, rounded corners. The older infant is able to stack these successfully. Books with pictures and few words will interest the infant. Many books are soft sided and easy to grasp.

NUTRITION

Breastfeeding provides optimal, complete nutrition for infants and is recommended for "all infants in whom breastfeeding is not specifically contraindicated" by the AAP (2005). Some mothers, however, have difficulty breastfeeding due to low milk production or latch-on issues. Some mothers choose not to adjust their lifestyle to manage breastfeeding. Many hospitals have lactation consultants to assist new mothers in learning to breastfeed their infants and manage difficulties as they arise. Breastfeeding is discussed in detail in Chapter 9 .

Commercially produced formulas are available in powder, concentrate, and ready-to-use forms for mothers who choose to bottle-feed or to breastfeed and bottle-feed their infants. The powder form may be more convenient when traveling or when the infant goes to a day care center. Warm water is added to make individual servings. If the water is contaminated, it must be boiled to remove harmful bacteria. Leftover formula needs to be refrigerated or discarded because it is a rich medium for bacteria growth. Formula is given throughout the first year. Due to the possibility of milk allergy, the use of cow's milk is generally not recommended until after 1 year of age. Bottles and nipples need to be washed and rinsed thoroughly. Unless there is concern over contaminated water, the bottles and nipples do not need to be sterilized.

clinical ALERT

The microwave oven is not appropriate for heating infant formula. Burns could occur due to uneven heating. Also, the rubber used in bottle nipples can deteriorate with frequent microwave use (Pediatric Nutrition Practice Group of the American Dietetic Association, 2003).

Formula intake is adjusted according to infant weight. Keep in mind that the infant has both caloric needs and fluid needs. Infants need 100 to 120 kcal/kg/day and 1 to 1.5 mL/kcal/day. Table 12-3 ■ provides information about nutrition needs at different ages. In an effort to prevent childhood obesity, parents should limit infant intake of fruit juices and avoid beverages with high sugar content such as powdered and carbonated drinks. The AAP (2001)

TABLE 12-3

Recommended Caloric Intake by Age Group

AGE GROUP	RECOMMENDED CALORIC INTAKE
Infant	100–200 kcal/kg/day
Toddler	1,100–1,300 kcal/day
Preschooler	1,300–1,600 kcal/day
School age	1,600–2,200 kcal/day
Adolescent	2,200–2,800 kcal/day

suggests that fruit juices never be given to an infant in a bottle but only in a covered cup. This will avoid dental caries and decrease the intake amount.

Solid food is gradually introduced beginning around 6 months. Usually, a thin rice cereal is given once or twice a day. As the infant learns to control his or her tongue and swallow, a thicker consistency of the cereal can be given. Generally, pureed vegetables and fruits are then added to the diet, with meats added last. Once teeth erupt, the infant can be given soft finger foods such as crackers, bananas, and cheese. By 12 months, the infant should be encouraged to use a covered cup exclusively for fluid intake.

Infants generally thrive with three set meals and several snacks a day. Placing the infant in a high chair or seat at the table and letting him or her eat only in the kitchen or dining room helps the infant learn social skills associated with meals.

Food allergies or sensitivities (e.g., lactose intolerance) are growing concerns. Parents should be taught to pay attention to any unusual reactions to foods their infants are eating. Some pediatricians recommend avoiding certain foods prior to the age of 2 years, when the child's immune system is more developed. Such foods include eggs, peanut butter, and shellfish. See more about gastrointestinal issues in Chapter 22 ⚭.

Oral Health

Infants may show signs of teething at 4 months of age. These signs include increased drooling, increased hand-to-mouth activity, attempting to clench hard on objects, disturbed sleep patterns, difficulty in being consoled, and loss of appetite. Teething does not cause gastrointestinal disturbances or fever. Parents should be taught that these symptoms indicate a disease process and that they should consult a health care professional if symptoms do not resolve.

Parents can be taught to apply cold to the infant's gums for relief. Freezing the teething ring or wrapping a piece of ice in a thin towel and applying it to the gums are appropriate methods. The nurse should warn parents not to place a piece of ice in the infant's mouth because this could cause

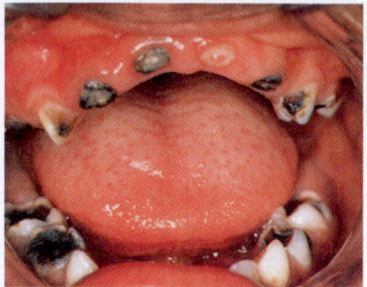

Figure 12-8. ■ Bottle mouth. This child has major tooth decay related to sleeping as an infant and toddler while sucking bottles of juice and milk. (Courtesy of Dr. Lezley McIlveen, Department of Dentistry, Children's National Medical Center, Washington, DC.)

aspiration. Topical anesthetics are available over the counter and can provide temporary relief from the discomfort of teething. If these relief measures are ineffective, systemic analgesics can be used on a short-term basis. Dosing should be discussed with the pediatrician or family practitioner.

Parents should be encouraged to model dental health as soon as teeth begin to erupt. A soft brush or cloth without toothpaste can be used to clean the teeth and gums. The American Academy of Pediatric Dentistry (2003) suggests that children receive fluoride supplementation if the drinking water in the home contains fluoride levels of less than 0.6 ppm.

Infants engage in nonnutritive or recreational sucking. They may suck a pacifier or their thumb, or spend extra time at the breast. There appear to be benefits to this type of sucking, both physically and emotionally. Some parents may be concerned about tooth alignment and forming unwanted habits. The nurse can encourage parents to view this type of sucking during infancy as harmless. However, nurses should teach parents not to allow an infant to suck on a bottle after feeding. This can result in "bottle mouth" (Figure 12-8 ■).

Toddler

HEALTH PROMOTION

Environmental Safety

The toddler is becoming more mobile and inquisitive, so safety becomes more of a challenge. Parents often claim the toddler is "into everything" when he or she is learning to walk and climb. The most common injuries of this age group include automobile injury, falls, burns, poisonings, and drowning. The toddler is not big enough to use car seat belts, but still needs to use a safety seat at all times. The shoulder strap on adult seat belts should not be used because it could cause strangulation. Figure 12-9 ■ illustrates proper use of toddler safety car seats. Again, the

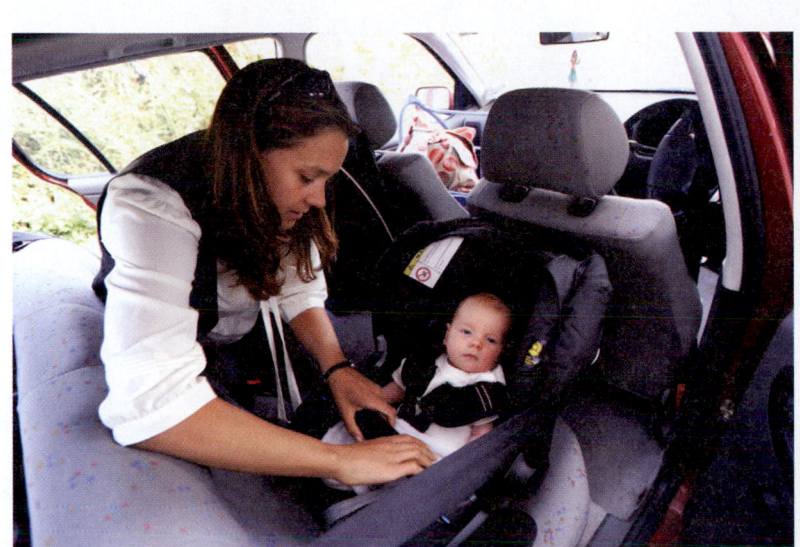

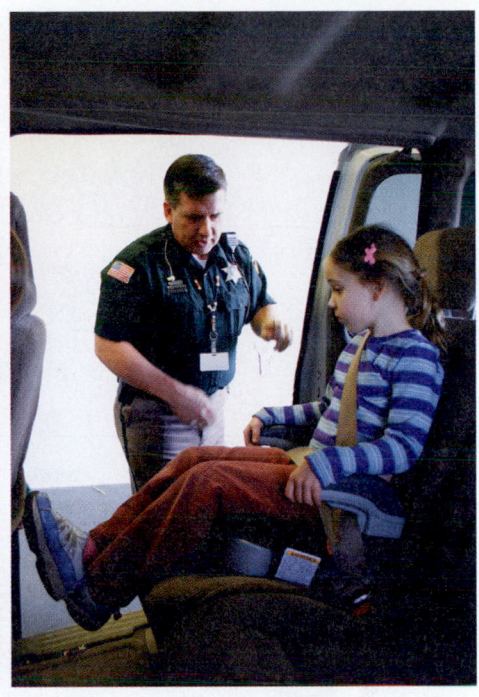

A   **B**

Figure 12-9. ■ It is important to be consistent in use of safety-approved car seats for infants and children. (**A**) Infants should be in the back seat facing the rear. (David Bagnall/Alamy) (**B**) Toddlers and older children can face forward but should still have the protection of being in the back seat. Front seat air bags can suffocate a child if they inflate, so the general guideline is that children younger than age 12 should not ride in the front seat of a car. (Pearson Education/PH College)

safest place for the toddler is in the back seat. The toddler may be able to unfasten the seat belt and may resist being restrained in the seat. However, the parent must insist on safety for all trips, regardless of the distance. Once the car has come to a complete stop with the engine off, the seat belt can be removed.

The toddler must not be left alone in an automobile. Not only can he or she suffer from extreme temperature inside the vehicle, but also the toddler might disengage the brake, put the car in neutral, or start the engine, allowing the car to move and causing a crash.

Inquisitive toddlers often want to explore their environment. As a result, parking lots can be dangerous places. Toddlers are not capable of sensing the hazards of cars as they pull in and out of parking spaces. Parents must devise a plan for toddler safety when entering or exiting the car. This plan can be complicated by younger children who must be held and by loading groceries or shopping bags. For the overly adventurous toddler, parents may limit outings to times when another trusted adult can accompany them.

Toddlers learn to ride tricycles and other wheeled vehicles. This mobility carries a risk for injury. As toddlers learn to ride these vehicles, they must be taught to wear properly fitting helmets and both knee and elbow pads. Riding in a park where the sidewalks are surrounded by grass is safer

than riding on a sidewalk along the street. When riding on a sidewalk, toddlers could ride into the street without being aware of the risk for injury. Therefore, it is important for parents to supervise toddlers who are riding a tricycle outside a fenced area.

Falls continue to be a concern for toddler safety. Body shape changes continually throughout childhood (Figure 12-10 ■). The body shape of a toddler compromises stability. A protuberant abdomen and short legs increase the risk of falls. Toddlers are also learning to climb stairs. At first they go up and down stairs on their knees, but as soon as they are more steady on their feet, they want to walk up and down. They should be taught to use the handrail. Toddlers may be able to move chairs and climb onto the counter. Close supervision is needed at all times. The toddler should be provided with safe climbing toys and be taught acceptable places to climb. Most playgrounds have climbing toys. Parents should be taught to inspect them for damage. The ground in and around the toys should be covered with a soft material such as loose bark to decrease injury in the event of a fall.

As toddlers climb onto chairs and counters, medicines, cosmetics, and cleaning supplies become easy to reach. Therefore, all poisonous substances must be kept out of reach and/or locked away. Childproof lids, electrical outlet covers, and cupboard closures are helpful but not perfect (Figure 12-11 ■).

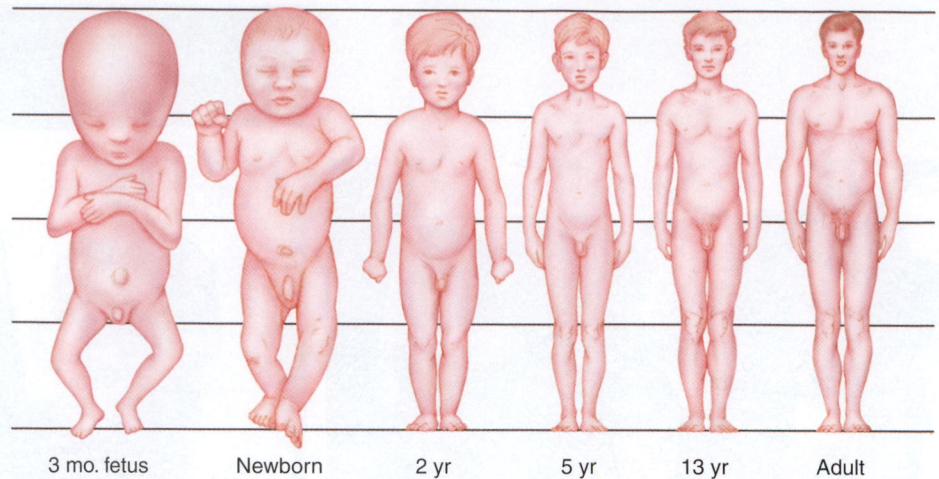

Figure 12-10. ■ Body proportions at various ages.

3 mo. fetus   Newborn   2 yr   5 yr   13 yr   Adult

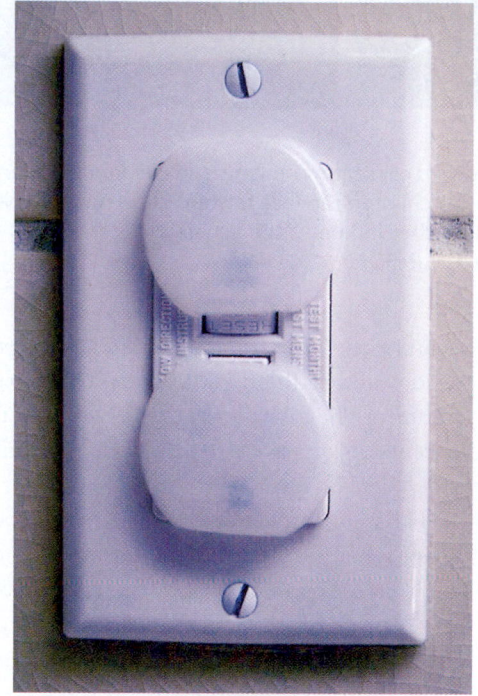

A

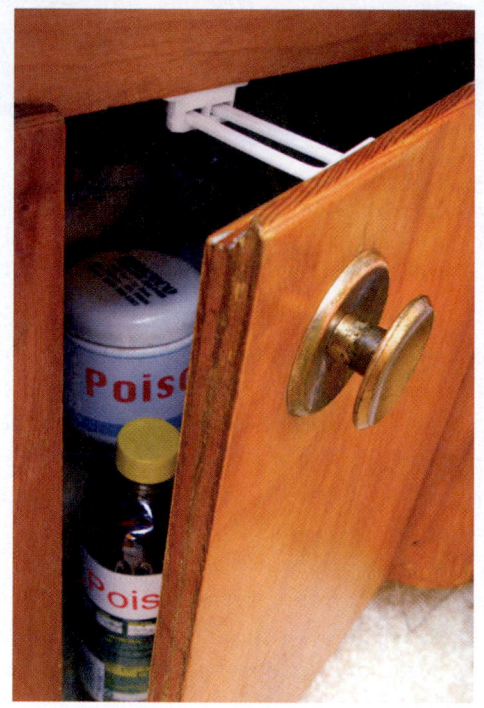

B

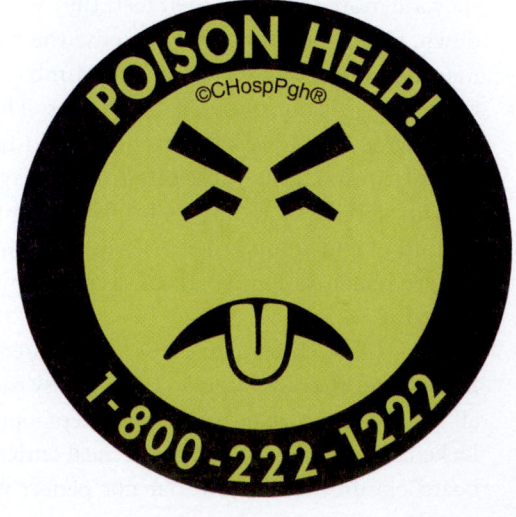

C

Figure 12-11. ■ The home needs to be childproofed for safety. (**A**) Safety covers for electrical outlets. (**B**) Childproof locks on drawers and cabinets. (**C**) Mr. Yuk stickers on toxic substances. (**A**: Jerry Marshell. **B**: Michael Newman/Photo Edit. **C**: Children's Hospital of Pittsburgh.)

Teaching toddlers to play with toys is an important step in reducing the risk for poisoning. Parents should be aware that many houseplants are poisonous if the child chews the leaves and stems. Poison Control Center phone numbers and syrup of ipecac should be readily available. Plant reference books are also available with handy guides on plant safety.

Choking remains a hazard for toddlers, even though they do not explore their environment by putting objects in their mouth like infants do. They are eating a greater variety of whole foods, which increases the risk for aspiration. Nuts and meat can be particularly risky for toddlers to swallow. Children should not be given peanuts until they have enough teeth to chew the nut well before swallowing. Meat should be cut into small pieces for the toddler. Other foods that could be dangerous are hot dogs, grapes, and hard candy. Parents should insist that children eat in a controlled environment, such as at the dining table, where adult supervision is available. To prevent choking, children should not be allowed to talk with their mouths full or to play while eating.

Injury to the mouth can occur if children are allowed to run or play with things in their mouths. For instance, running or rough play with a popsicle stick, lollipop stick, or toothbrush in the mouth could cause injury to the palate, tongue, gums, or teeth. These objects should be placed out of the toddler's reach.

As toddlers watch routine activities in the kitchen, their curiosity is aroused. They are tall enough to reach the stove and can pull hot pans, spilling contents onto their head, arms, or entire bodies. They can touch the hot burner or open an oven door and turn on stoves with front controls. They can even turn on the burners. Toddlers are fascinated with fire and might reach into a lit fireplace or touch burning candles. They want to mimic adults who are lighting matches and using cigarette lighters. Toddlers should be taught that all heat-producing objects are dangerous and off limits. Parents must not forget that electric cords pose a strangulation hazard to toddlers and also pose a risk for electrical burns or electrocution if they are chewed.

Most toddlers enjoy playing in water. Constant supervision is critical when the toddler is in the bathtub (Figure 12-12A ■). The toddler should be taught to sit and never to stand while in the tub. Nonskid surfaces should be used to prevent falls in the tub. Children might try to play in the toilet water, fish tanks, and mop buckets. The child can fall into these seemingly safe, shallow water sources. Children who fall head first into these tanks do not have the upper body strength to right themselves. Therefore, parents need to protect children from water hazards. Buckets should be emptied when not in use. Fish tanks should have childproof lids. Toilet seat lids should be down and the bathroom door closed at all times. Swimming pools, hot tubs, ponds, ditches, canals, and rivers are other places in which the toddler might try to play. When possible, fences with locking gates should be used to prevent young children from accessing water hazards. The use of child life jackets near water and on boats is essential. However, flotation devices such as arm or doughnut inflatables are not certified life preservers (Figure 12-12B).

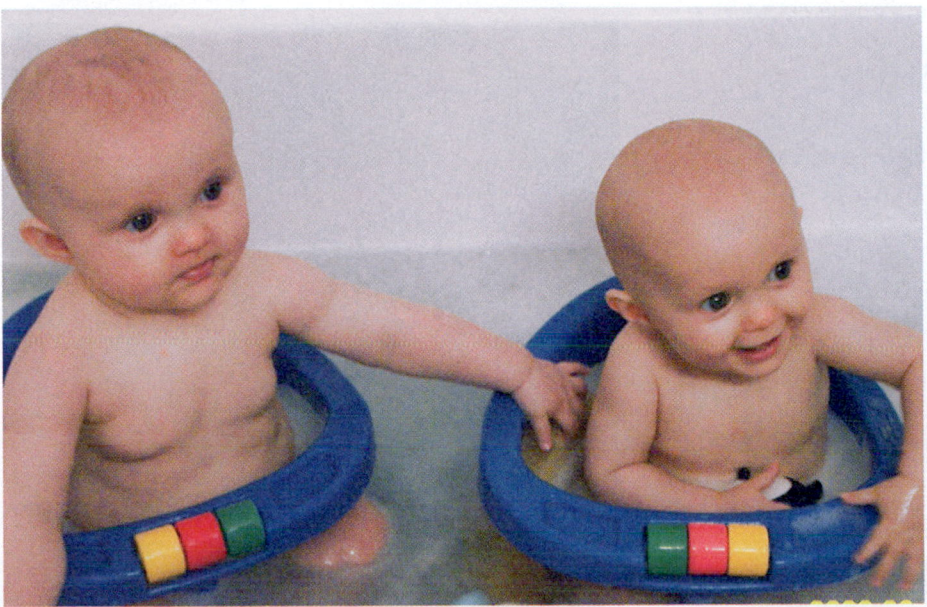
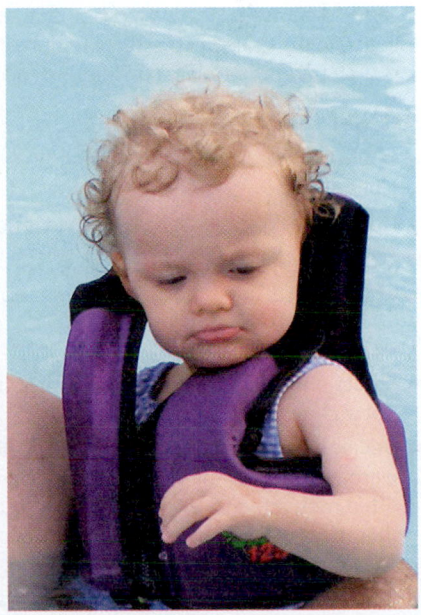

A   B

Figure 12-12. ■ **(A)** Infants and toddlers can easily lose their balance in a bathtub, and they do not have the muscle strength and coordination to pull themselves back up. These bathing devices allow the parent to bathe both twins at once in the bathtub. **(B)** Toddlers should not be allowed to play in swimming pools or other deep water without a flotation device. Teach parents to look for life vests that help support the head above water. (Courtesy of J. Tobias)

Swimming lessons at an early age might be valuable but cannot guarantee that a child will not drown. Adult supervision is always necessary.

PSYCHOSOCIAL HEALTH

Toilet Training

Children are expected to learn to use the toilet and abandon wearing diapers. This often presents a struggle for both the child and the parent. Parents need to understand how to determine whether the toddler is ready to be toilet trained. They also need assistance in accomplishing this task without bringing shame to the toddler. The nurse can provide this information and teaching to parents. Box 12-7 ■ provides some tips for helping a toddler succeed at toilet training.

Providing Discipline

Toddlers are beginning to develop a measure of independence, even though they are still dependent on the mother or caregiver. Consistency in limit setting is important at this age. Children can begin to learn social expectations (to sit at the table when eating, not to eat food that has fallen on the ground, etc.). The more consistent the parent is in establishing norms, the easier it will be for the child to accept them.

This is the time when children learn to say "NO." When the child performs a negative behavior or refuses to partici-

pate in a desired behavior, it is important for the parent to respond in clear and consistent ways. The following steps are generally recommended for toddler discipline:

1. Give the child a warning that the behavior is unacceptable and name the consequence if the child continues.
2. If the toddler continues the behavior, provide the consequence. Usually, "time-out" is a good method for disciplining a toddler (1 minute of time-out per year). The toddler should be removed from the physical situation and placed where there are no toys or other diversions so the time-out is focused on thinking about the behavior.
3. After time-out, direct the child's attention to an activity that is not associated with the previous behavior.

Temper tantrums are also common in this age group. Teach parents that tantrums are normal for toddlers, and that it is most important for them to remain calm and not to give in to the behavior. Time-out may be useful. If tantrums occur in public, it may be necessary to remove the child from the situation or to hold the child firmly until the tantrum has subsided. Remind parents to reinforce good behavior by praising the child when he or she regains control.

Promoting Play

Toddlers enjoy the company of others, even though they may not play together. This side-by-side play is known as **parallel play** (Figure 12-13 ■). Toddlers imitate the behavior of others, such as talking on the telephone, hammering, or sweeping. The toddler also likes to climb, ride big-wheeled toys, and swing. Fine motor skills are continuing to develop by scribbling with a pen and turning pages in a book.

BOX 12-7	CLIENT TEACHING

Teaching Toileting

Bladder and bowel control is possible physiologically between 18 and 24 months. However, other factors must be in place for toilet training to be successful. The nurse can review these factors with parents who are considering toilet training.

Assessing for Readiness

- Interest in mimicking the toileting behavior of parents and siblings
- Noticeable indications that the child is defecating or urinating
- Genital awareness
- Child reports that defecation or urination has occurred

Tips for Toilet Training

- Create enthusiasm by purchasing the child a proper-sized potty chair.
- Develop a reward system, possibly giving the child a small reward when he or she uses the potty chair. Some children are often motivated by "big girl or big boy underwear." Establish that there will be no punishment for accidents.
- Use transitional diapers. They are easier for the child to manipulate, and give a better sense of bladder and bowel awareness.
- Establish a routine. Take the child to the potty following meals and snacks and before bedtime.
- Create an environment of patience and praise.

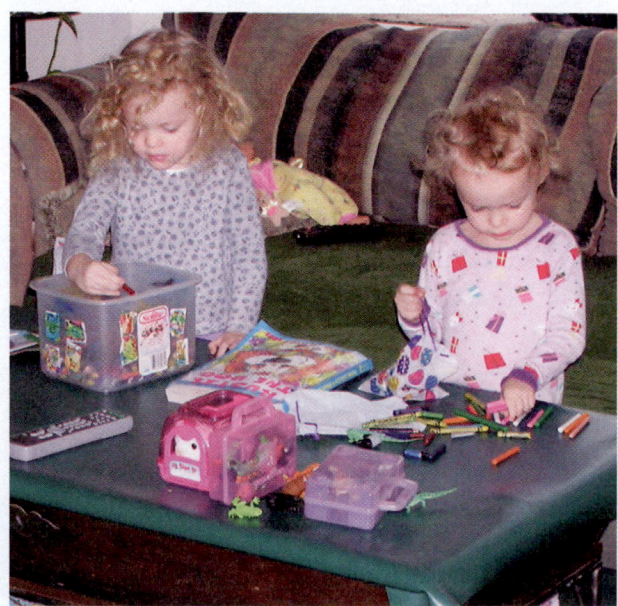

Figure 12-13. ■ In toddler and preschool years, children often participate in parallel play, enjoying each other's presence while having separate playthings.
(Courtesy of J. Tobias)

| BOX 12-8 | CLIENT TEACHING |

Toy Safety

Younger Than Age 3

Children younger than age 3 tend to put everything in their mouths.

- Avoid buying toys intended for older children that may have small parts that pose a choking danger.
- Never let children of any age play with uninflated or broken balloons because of the choking danger.
- Avoid marbles, balls, and games with balls that have a diameter of 1.75 inches or less.

These products also pose a choking hazard to young children. Children at this age pull, prod, and twist toys.

- Look for toys that are well made, with tightly secured eyes, noses, and other parts.
- Avoid toys that have sharp edges and points.

Ages 3 to 6

- Avoid toys constructed with thin, brittle plastic that might easily break into small pieces or leave jagged edges.
- Look for household art materials, including crayons and paint sets, marked with the designation "ASTM D-4236." This means the product has been reviewed by a toxicologist and, if necessary, labeled with cautionary information.
- Teach older children to keep their toys away from their younger brothers and sisters.

Ages 6 to 12

- For all children, adults should check toys periodically for breakage and potential hazards. Damaged or dangerous toys should be repaired or thrown away.
- If buying a toy gun, be sure the barrel, or the entire gun, is brightly colored so it is not mistaken for a real gun.
- If you buy a bicycle for any age child, also buy a helmet and make sure the child wears it.
- Teach all children to put toys away when they are finished playing so they do not trip over or fall on them.

Read the Label . . .

The U.S. Consumer Product Safety Commission (2003) requires toy manufacturers to meet stringent safety standards and to label certain toys that could be a hazard for younger children. Look for labels that give age recommendations and use that information as a guide. Labels on toys that state "not recommended for children under 3 . . . contains small parts" are labeled that way because they may pose a choking hazard to children younger than age 3. Toys should be developmentally appropriate to suit the skills, abilities, and interests of the child.

Shopping for toys during the holidays can be exciting and fun, but it can also be frustrating. There can be thousands of toys to choose from in one store, and it is important to choose the right toy for the right age child. Toys that are meant for older children can be dangerous for younger children.

APPROPRIATE TOYS. Toddlers need toys that provide action. Examples of these types of toys are pull toys, puzzles, shape sorters, dolls, and sports equipment. Toddlers also need toys to improve their creativity. Crayons, washable markers, and musical instruments will spark the toddler's creativity. Toys that challenge a toddler, such as books and blocks, are also good choices. Box 12-8 ■ provides information for teaching parents and caregivers about toy safety.

NUTRITION

Parents are often concerned that the toddler is not eating enough food. As the rate of growth slows, a toddler's body needs decrease. The amount of food consumed over several days is more indicative of adequate intake than the intake meal by meal. The general rule is 1 tablespoon of each food offered per year of age. For the toddler to consume the needed nutrients, a variety of foods from all food groups should be offered. The pediatrician or family practitioner may recommend a daily multivitamin for the picky eater. Allowing the toddler to choose between healthy options, such as the kind of juice or a choice between two kinds of cereal, will encourage positive eating habits and satisfy the toddler's search for independence.

After 12 months of age, parents may introduce cow's milk into the diet of their child. Prior to 1 year of age, cow's milk is an insufficient source of iron and exclusive use of cow's milk would put the infant at risk for anemia. There is also considerable evidence that many children have an allergy to cow's milk. Parents should observe closely for adverse reactions when they introduce cow's milk into the diet of their toddler.

It is also time to help the toddler learn to use a spoon and fork. At first, toddlers may pick the food up in one hand and put the food onto the spoon before putting it into the mouth, or they may hold the utensil backwards (Figure 12-14 ■). With practice, they learn to scoop the food into the spoon with one hand. Using a bowl instead of a plate may help the toddler practice this fine motor skill. It is important to cut the food into small, bite-size pieces. The toddler has not yet learned how much food to put into his or her mouth at a time. Close supervision will avoid a choking hazard.

Oral Health

As the toddler gains more teeth, caring for the teeth becomes a higher parental priority. This is a good time to take the child to the dentist for the first time. This will help the child get used to going to the dentist at regular intervals. Pediatric dentists are available in many communities, providing a child-friendly environment.

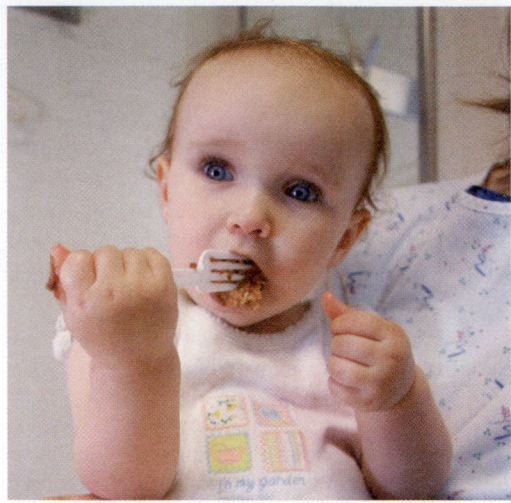

Figure 12-14. ■ Bit by bit, toddlers learn the complicated task of eating with utensils. (M. C. Schlachter Photography.)

Preschooler

HEALTH PROMOTION

Environmental Safety

The preschooler is becoming more independent. The parent may begin to feel comfortable with leaving the preschooler to play by him- or herself for a brief period of time. As the preschooler learns numbers and letters, he or she can be taught to call 9-1-1 to reach emergency help. However, the preschooler does not completely understand cause and effect and needs to be provided with a safe place to play. For example, the preschooler may not understand that climbing on a stool to reach the cookie jar could lead to a fall. Motor vehicle crashes, burns, and drowning remain the leading causes of injury.

The older preschooler can independently get into the car and fasten the seat belt. However, he or she may forget to fasten the seat belt correctly. It is important for the driver to verify that the seat belt is fastened before the car is started. Because the child is growing physically, eventually the booster seat will no longer be needed and the regular car seat belt will be best. The back seat continues to be the best location for the child. It may be tempting to have an older preschooler sit in the front seat, but front and side air bags still pose a danger to the smaller child.

clinical ALERT

Teach parents always to place infants in rear-facing, safety-approved car seats until the infant is at least 1 year old *and* weighs at least 20 pounds. Car seats should be used until the child reaches the maximum weight for the car seat or until straps do not fit over the shoulders. Children should then use booster seats until a seat belt fits properly over the shoulder and across the hips. This is usually when the child is 4 feet 9 inches tall and between 8 and 12 years of age (AAP, 2006).

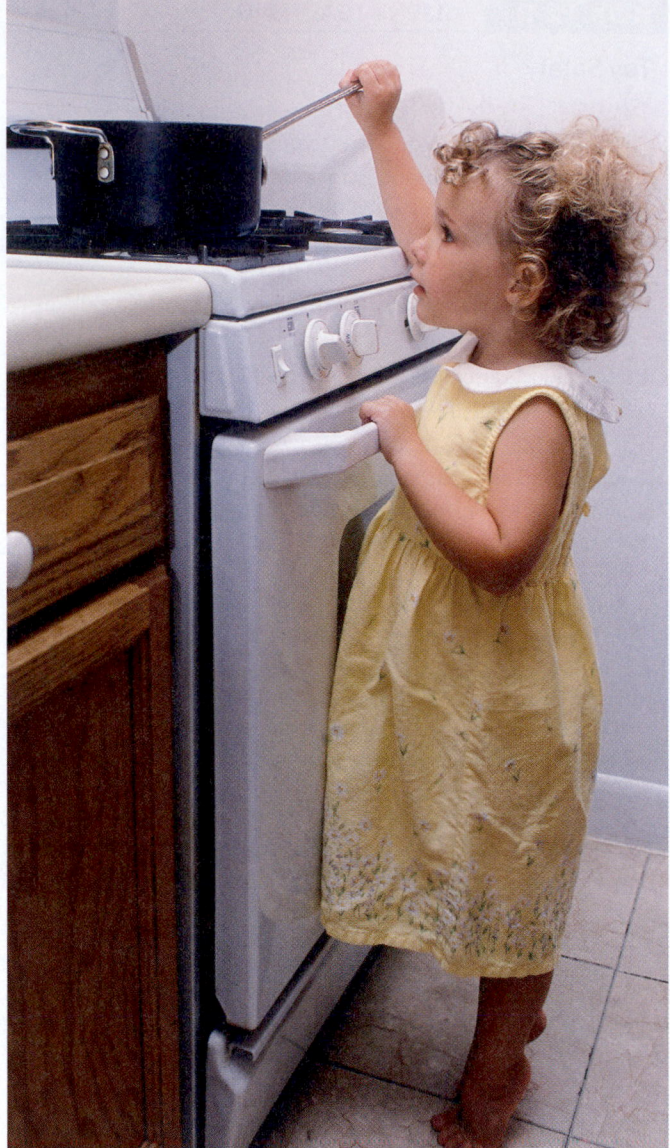

Figure 12-15. ■ Placing hot pots on back burners with handles turned inward is one way to prevent injury to children.

Striving for independence, the preschooler may choose to go into a lake or pool unsupervised. He or she is not cognizant of the dangers of swimming alone. Running water in ditches and canals also poses a danger. The preschooler likes to watch toy boats, sticks, or other items float in moving water; he or she might try to reach them and fall into the current. It continues to be important to provide constant supervision in and around water.

The preschooler has an understanding of "hot" and the hazard of fire but still needs to be watched near stoves and fires (Figure 12-15 ■). With reminding, he or she can blow on hot food before eating. The preschooler should be taught not to play with matches, and to stop, drop, and roll if his or her clothes are on fire. He or she can learn escape routes in case of fire and should practice them on a monthly basis. If the preschooler is in a day care facility, basic fire safety

BOX 12-9	CLIENT TEACHING

Fire Safety for the Home

- Place a fire detector on every floor of the home. Check the batteries regularly.
- Maintain at least two working fire detectors in the home.
- Discuss an exit strategy with children in case of fire. Have rehearsals regularly.
- Store flammable liquids such as gasoline and paint away from heat sources, and do not smoke around these substances.
- Regularly inspect electrical cords and discard any that are frayed.
- Never leave candles unattended.
- Store matches and lighters in locked cabinets.
- Post emergency numbers where the child can easily read them.

may also be taught there. Box 12-9 ■ lists fire safety rules for the home.

"TEACHING ABOUT STRANGERS." It is never too early to talk to children about trusting people they do not know. They should also be taught about appropriate and inappropriate touch. Although parents do not want to scare children unnecessarily, they have to be taught not to get into a car or go anywhere with someone they do not know. A family "password" could be used to identify those individuals whom the child could trust. Children should be taught to close the bathroom door when using the toilet, to dress and undress in private, and to keep their "private parts" covered. The preschooler is old enough to wash themselves with parent supervision, and should be taught to do so, instead of having others wash or touch their breasts or perineum.

Preschoolers should also be taught to tell parents if they believe they have been or are being touched in bad ways. Abusers are most often people children already know, so they may not think of them as "strangers."

Health Education

During the preschool years, a child's brain is rapidly developing. This is an optimal time to promote learning that will influence a lifetime of healthy behaviors. Organized learning often begins during this period when the child attends day care, mother's morning out programs, or preschool programs. These settings provide an excellent opportunity to learn about healthy behaviors.

Learning in the school setting can be quite appealing to the child, and it promotes retention of the information. Games and skits that incorporate peers and friends entice the child to listen attentively. Craft activities provide the child with an ongoing reminder of the lessons learned. Many health topics are appropriate for the school environment. These include seat belt use, personal hygiene, disease prevention, importance of daily exercise, and proper nutritional habits.

PSYCHOSOCIAL HEALTH

Providing Discipline

During the preschool years, the goal of discipline is for the child to develop a sense of responsibility for his or her actions. The child is able to understand the cause and effect of most of his or her actions and can choose behavior accordingly. The preschooler also desires to please the adults in his or her life. He or she wants to be obedient and often feels guilty if he or she is not.

One form of discipline found to be effective during the preschool years is the use of isolation or "time-out" for disobedient behavior. After the expected behavior is clearly defined and the child chooses an alternative action, the child can be placed in a safe setting for a defined period of time. This safe setting could be a certain chair in a specific room or an area of a room that is devoid of toys and other forms of entertainment. After the child has been isolated for the defined period of time, he or she should be asked by the caregiver what he or she learned as a result of this discipline. The parent may need to help the child understand the lesson by supplying hints and further teaching.

It is important for all caregivers in the child's life to provide the same type of discipline and expect the same behaviors. This will enhance the child's expected behavior. These caregivers must be careful to communicate to the child that the unwanted behavior is why the discipline is implemented, not because the child is "bad."

Play and Appropriate Toys

Preschoolers begin to socialize and indulge in **associative play** by learning to share and by working together on a project. Associative play occurs when children are engaging in the same activity but without formal organization. The preschooler develops fine motor skills by using scissors, crayons, and glue. They enjoy making art projects with adult supervision. They are learning colors, shapes, numbers, and letters. The preschooler uses dramatic play in acting out the events of daily life. By using dolls, furniture, and clothing, the preschooler not only portrays the events of the world, but can also learn new things. The nurse should use playtime to assess the child's social skills and get clues into the family interaction from the child's point of view. The nurse should also use this time to teach the preschooler about health care issues and upcoming procedures. For more information, see Chapter 13 ⌾.

NUTRITION

The preschooler generally eats three meals and two snacks a day. Mealtime is a social event because the preschooler enjoys participating in conversation. The preschooler also wants to be involved in food preparation. This is a good time to teach about nutritious foods, food preparation, refrigeration, cleanliness, and safety around stoves and other kitchen utensils and appliances. The preschooler can be given routine tasks such as setting the table, clearing away dirty dishes, and putting away left-over food.

A balanced diet, with adequate amounts of fruit, vegetables, protein, grains, and dairy, is desirable for the preschooler. Some fat is necessary to absorb fat-soluble vitamins and to ensure proper metabolism; however, saturated fat must be limited. Unfortunately, foods high in saturated fats, such as hamburgers, french fries, and chicken nuggets, satisfy the preschooler's taste. Parents can be encouraged to serve these foods only on special occasions instead of routinely.

Oral Health

By age 7, children begin to lose their baby teeth. It is not uncommon to have several missing teeth at a time. Soft, easy-to-chew foods may be needed until the permanent teeth come in. Dental care is important to be sure permanent teeth are well cared for and in proper alignment.

School-Age Child

HEALTH PROMOTION

Environmental Safety

School-age children are learning to take responsibility for their own safety. Automobile safety continues to be of concern. Pedestrian and bicycle safety also poses a risk. School-age children may travel to and from school by themselves or in small groups. If they ride a school bus, they must be taught to cross well in front of the bus so the driver can see them. They also need to follow the safety rules of pedestrian travel consistently (Box 12-10 ■). They need to be told to watch for cars because the driver may not see them. School-age children should be taught to cross the street at crosswalks or intersections, being alert for cars making turns at the corner. When sidewalks are not available, they should walk on the side of the road facing traffic. This would allow them to move completely off the roadway if a car is approaching them too closely.

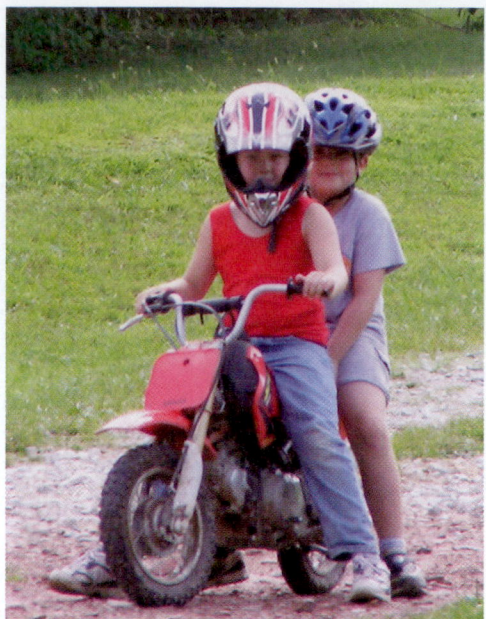

Figure 12-16. ■ Children on motorized bikes are at risk for injury. Helmets are essential. Knee pads and elbow pads can help reduce the risk. (Courtesy of J. Tobias)

They might ride a bicycle and need to learn safety rules, including how to ride in traffic. School-age children should be taught to ride their bicycles on the side of the road, in the same direction as traffic flows. Wearing a properly fitted helmet is essential, and both elbow and knee pads are recommended (Figure 12-16 ■). In-line skates and skateboards must never be used in traffic. Protective equipment, including a helmet and elbow and knee pads, should be worn at all times.

School-age children can be depended on more often to follow directions. They are learning cause and effect but may become careless as they "show off" for friends. Injury from fire, drowning, and poison usually occurs as a result of carelessness and experimentation rather than from unknown dangers. It is important for parents to talk frequently with their children about safety and family rules. Parents should know where and with whom their children are at all times. School-age children still need general supervision in order to prevent careless behavior.

School-age children may come home from school to an empty house and may remain unsupervised until parents return from work. The term **latch-key children** has been used to describe these children who may be as young as 5 years. As a result of spending a large amount of time alone, these children are at greater risk for dangers related to drugs, smoking, crime, behavior problems, and peer pressure. They may become lonely or bored and feel more stress than children who are supervised after school. The National Crime Prevention Council (O'Neil, Kelly, and Kirby, 1995) recommends that communities offer afterschool programs to prevent children's involvement in dangerous activities and to encourage academic excellence.

BOX 12-10   CLIENT TEACHING

Pedestrian Travel

- Walk on sidewalks.
- Walk along the side of the road when sidewalks are not available.
- Walk facing traffic when sidewalks are not available.
- Cross the street at corners or cross-walk.
- Cross the street when the signal indicates it is okay.
- Check traffic in all directions when crossing without a light.
- Ride bicycle along the side of the road or in the bike lane.
- Ride bicycle in the same direction as traffic flow.

As school-age children become more independent and mobile, they must also be aware of injury from assault. Many children have been taught "not to talk to strangers" and presume a "stranger" to be an evil-looking individual. However, most child molesters seem nice, friendly, and gentle. They use ploys such as "help me find my dog" to lure children into unsafe areas.

Children who arrive home from school before their parents should be taught not to open the door to strangers and should demonstrate that they are responsible before being left alone. Older children should not be expected to care for younger siblings until they are mature enough to handle the responsibility. Community resources, available through the local public health department and local police department, help parents talk with their children about the danger of assault.

School-age children may begin to experiment with fire, including matches, lighters, and fireworks. Fire dangers include setting themselves on fire, starting a fire resulting in property damage, and causing injury to others trapped in the burning building. Fire safety must be reviewed frequently.

School-age children may have witnessed adults using, caring for, and storing firearms. They may find firearms in their house and want to show them to friends. Even when children have received instruction not to touch a firearm, research shows that most children are fascinated with a gun when they find it. They pick it up (Figure 12-17 ■) and

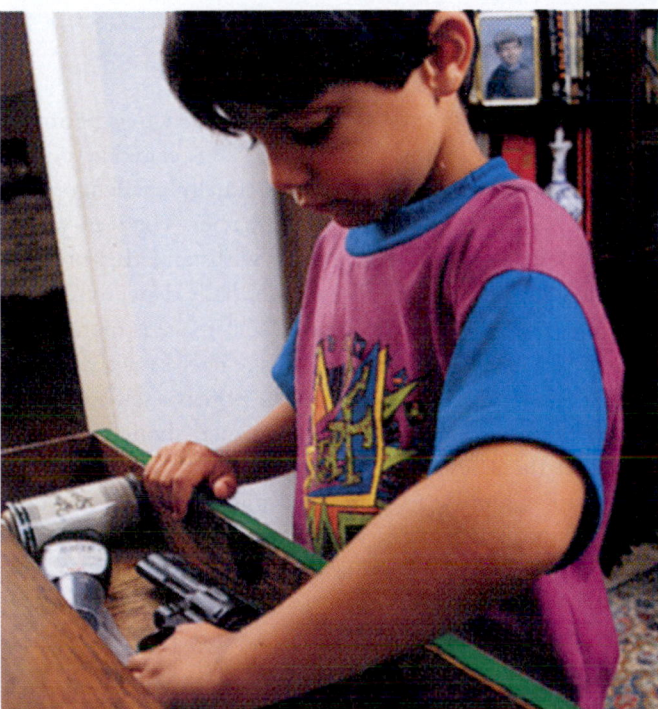

Figure 12-17. ■ Teach children never to touch guns without a parent present. Be sure to teach parents that all ammunition must be removed from guns and kept safely locked away from all weapons. Safety locks should always be in place on weapons.

even point it at friends. Firearms must be unloaded, locked with a trigger lock, and stored in a locked cabinet. Some states provide trigger locks free of charge. Ammunition should be kept in a separate locked storage area.

PSYCHOSOCIAL HEALTH

Promoting Self-Esteem

The school-age child is developing his or her sense of self-concept. The ability to make appropriate decisions, to problem solve, and to be successful contributes to his or her self-esteem. The school-age child also begins to address issues of body image and sexuality. The nurse can help parents promote the school-age child's self-esteem by encouraging them to praise the child for successes. When a child experiences a failure, the parents should be encouraged to assist the child in problem solving and should promote a sense of accomplishment in seeking alternative solutions to the problem.

Promoting Play

The school-age child has learned that everyone has a role and can take part in **cooperative play.** Cooperative play is organized play such as games at school or sports. School-age children understand that games have rules and are eager to follow them. They become frustrated when others do not follow the rules and may act out their frustration. School-age children learn competition and the concepts of winning, losing, teamwork, and doing your best. Children in this age group have an increasing desire to spend time with friends and begin to develop long-term relationships.

Providing Discipline

School-age children like to know the rules, and they generally want to play by the rules. They are gaining an understanding of "fair play" and may complain "it's not fair" when they see peers getting special favors.

School-age children are learning how to solve problems and regulate their own activities. They can be invited to participate in finding solutions to problems among family or friends. Parents should be encouraged to ask for their children's input while still realizing that their children need their guidance and discipline.

This is often the stage at which hyperactivity, attention deficit, and anxiety disorders are identified. The nurse can provide information and referrals to help the parents set up the care they may need. (See also Chapter 27 ⬤⬤.)

Bullying is also identified in the school-age child. Nurses can teach parents to interrupt bullying behaviors in their own children and to follow up if they hear of bullying in their child's school or play group.

NUTRITION

As children enter school, they begin to eat at least one meal a day away from home. Many school-age children have not been exposed to food outside their home. They may not like or eat the food found at school. Parents should thoroughly assess the child's likes and dislikes when deciding whether to purchase cafeteria food or to pack the child a lunch. Eating in a busy cafeteria may be distracting to 6-year-olds, and they may not have enough time to finish their meal. For this reason, nutritious afterschool snacks and a balanced evening meal are essential. Eating at school makes mealtime more of a social occasion for school-age children. Table manners should be encouraged and reinforced in the home and at school. School-age children are capable of using utensils properly, contributing to conversation, listening when others speak, and assisting in serving food to others. Proper hygiene should also be encouraged.

Toward the end of the school-age period, there might be a period of rapid growth as the child prepares for adolescence. With this period of rapid growth comes an increase in appetite and the need for adequate nutrition.

Oral Health

Loss of primary teeth and the eruption of permanent teeth occur during the school-age period. The nurse can teach parents and the child proper ways of pulling these primary teeth. The nurse can also discourage improper ways of pulling teeth, such as tying a string to the tooth and attaching the other end of the string to a doorknob while the door is closed quickly. This method may cause further injury to the child's mouth, jaw, and head.

As the permanent teeth appear and the jaw line grows, the school-age child may have crooked teeth or a misaligned bite. Parents often consult an orthodontist during this period. If the orthodontist determines that the child will need braces, preliminary measures may be implemented in the school-age period.

Adolescent

HEALTH PROMOTION

Environmental Safety

Adolescents are at increased risk for injury related to their tendency toward risk-taking behavior and their belief that no harm can come to them (see Figure 11-8). In fact, motor vehicle crashes and suicide are the leading causes of adolescent death. For more information about suicide, see Chapter 27 . The ability to drive a car gives the adolescent freedom from parental supervision. Although teenagers may have developed the skills to maneuver a car though traffic, they may not be mature enough to handle the responsibility. Conversation, use of cell phones, joking, and loud music are common when teens get together, and they cause distraction for the driver. The use of alcohol clouds judgment, resulting in great risk for accident and injury. The risk is not limited to the automobile. These same dangers and concerns relate to the operation of off-road vehicles, snowmobiles, jet skis, and motorcycles. The use of safety devices such as seat belts and helmets is important. Adult supervision can help only when the adult teaches and enforces safety rules.

Many teens participate in physically challenging sports such as soccer, football, baseball, basketball, track, and swimming. They may overestimate their endurance, competence, and athletic ability, causing them to take more risks. Proper training, supervision, and correct use of protective equipment may prevent unnecessary injuries.

Health Education

Many schools provide a health course for the adolescent. This course provides an opportunity for the educator to present topics related to the health care needs of the adolescent, while also assessing the health behaviors of the class. The nurse is an ideal educator for this type of program.

Topics covered in this class include decision making, peer pressure, dating, sexuality and sexual intimacy, sexually transmitted diseases, substance abuse, mental health concerns such as depression and anorexia nervosa, and accident prevention. Because some of this content may be uncomfortable to present in a mixed gender setting, students are often divided into male and female groups.

PSYCHOSOCIAL HEALTH

Promoting Self-Esteem

Teens are faced with pressure from their peers to experiment with tobacco, alcohol, illegal drugs, gang-related activities, and premarital sex. These activities usually challenge what the teen has learned as acceptable behavior. The teen with a positive self-image may be able to withstand this pressure and make a choice to avoid these potentially dangerous activities. The teen with a compromised self-image is more likely to conform to peer pressure and engage in risky activities.

The nurse can help to promote a positive self-image by first assessing whether the teen feels good about himself or herself. If the assessment reveals a lowered self-image, the nurse can explore the teen's feelings and refer the teen and parents to community resources aimed at promoting positive self-image. For more information on issues of teen sexuality, see Chapters 5 and 23 . For information on substance abuse and psychosocial disorders of the adolescent, see Chapter 27 .

TYPES OF PLAY. The adolescent is rapidly making the transition from childhood play to adult play. As a result, team sports, extracurricular activities, and attending movies and concerts often occupy the adolescent's free time.

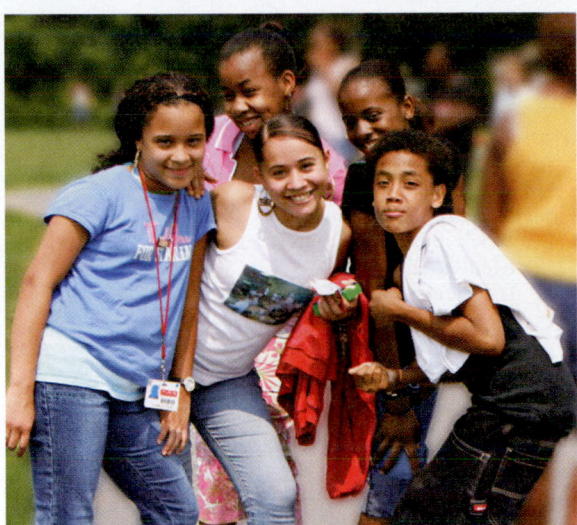

Figure 12-18. ■ Peers are the most important group among teens. (M. C. Schlachter Photography)

The adolescent begins to try out more risky adult activities, including car racing, motorcycle riding, and jet boating. Being with friends and peer groups soon becomes more important than spending time with parents. Teens look to each other for approval (Figure 12-18 ■). By late adolescence, male-female relationships are developing, and sexual encounters might be part of the "play." Unfortunately, other activities such as use of alcohol and illegal drugs might become part of the adolescent's recreational time. Nurses should help parents and teens prepare for the responsibilities and consequences of adult play.

Providing Discipline

Although teenagers are learning the important task of setting their own rules and boundaries, they still need guidance and discipline during this developmental stage. Remind parents of the value of positive feedback at this time. Praise can reinforce desired behaviors, such as keeping up with their studies, helping with tasks at home, and maintaining good hygiene.

This is a time to emphasize a few basic and crucial rules. Emphasize respect, and show respect for the teenager by never belittling the teen in front of peers. Discuss the teen's unacceptable behavior, rather than labeling him or her as a "bad person." Keep rules simple and fair (e.g., "Avoid risky behaviors that could hurt you and others."). Gradually increase the teen's independence as he or she exhibits more responsibility. Irresponsible behavior can be tied to a restriction in freedom. For example, if a teen deliberately stays out past curfew, the parent may restrict the teen from going out the following weekend. Try to discuss rules in terms of how they apply in the adult world. Teens are more likely to cooperate with behaviors that all adults should follow than with limits that seem like power plays by figures in authority.

NUTRITION

Meeting the nutritional needs of the adolescent is a challenge. The rapid growth spurt and increased muscle mass result in the need for 2,000 to 3,000 calories daily. Teens active in sports require an even higher caloric intake. Requirements for iron, calcium, zinc, and vitamins all increase. To meet these requirements, three meals per day, with nutritious snacks between meals, are needed (Abrams, 2001). Figure 12-19 ■ shows an example of a dietary screening survey for adolescents.

Calcium intake has been found to be particularly important during adolescence, and adequate intake has been linked with the prevention of osteoporosis. The deposition of calcium is five times greater prior to menarche than that of adult women. Adequate calcium and vitamin D during early adolescence is effective in enhancing bone mineral composition.

Adolescents can prepare much of their own food and frequently eat with friends. Their diet should contain protein, milk, and fresh fruits and vegetables daily; however, many adolescents choose high-calorie, high-fat, convenience foods. The adolescent should be taught to make healthy food choices. Nutritional teaching and counseling are most effective when conducted in a group setting with the teenager's peers.

Oral Health

During adolescence, individuals are at increased risk for caries. This risk is due to immature enamel, a diet high in refined carbohydrates and acid-containing beverages, and poorly established oral habits. The nurse should assess for and encourage regular dental checkups, brushing, and flossing.

The adolescent may pierce his or her tongue, lip, cheek, or uvula. These piercings have been found to compromise oral and overall health. If they are done in nonaseptic conditions, disease transmission may occur. Such diseases include hepatitis, tuberculosis, tetanus, and other bacterial or viral infections. Other hazards of oral piercings include hemorrhage, airway obstruction, pain, scarring, tooth damage, speech impediment, and nerve damage. The nurse should assess a client's oral cavity for the presence of these piercings and include the risks and hazards in health promotion teaching.

NURSING CARE

PRIORITIES IN NURSING CARE

When assisting clients and their families with issues related to illness prevention and health promotion, the nurse should focus on recognizing environmental hazards that would place a child's health or safety at risk. The nurse should also teach parents and other caregivers to develop strategies to prevent injury or illness.

1. Which of these meals or snacks did you eat yesterday?
   _____ Breakfast
   _____ Morning snack
   _____ Lunch
   _____ Afternoon snack
   _____ Dinner/supper
   _____ Evening snack

2. Do you skip breakfast three or more times a week?
   _____ Yes   _____ No

3. Do you skip lunch three or more times a week?
   _____ Yes   _____ No

4. Do you skip dinner/supper three or more times a week?
   _____ Yes   _____ No

5. Do you eat dinner/supper with your family four or more times a week?
   _____ Yes   _____ No

6. Do you fix or buy the food for any of your family's meals?
   _____ Yes   _____ No

7. Do you eat or take out a meal from a fast-food restaurant two or more times a week?
   _____ Yes   _____ No

8. Are you on a special diet for medical reasons?
   _____ Yes   _____ No

9. Are you a vegetarian?
   _____ Yes   _____ No

10. Do you have any problems with your appetite, like not feeling hungry, or feeling hungry all the time?
    _____ Yes   _____ No

11. Which of the following did you drink last week?
    _____ Regular soft drinks
    _____ Diet soft drinks
    _____ Fruit-flavored drinks
    _____ Whole milk
    _____ Reduced fat (2%) milk
    _____ Low-fat (1%) milk
    _____ Fat-free (skim) milk
    _____ Flavored milk (for example, chocolate, strawberry)
    _____ Coffee/tea
    _____ Tap/bottled water
    _____ Juice
    _____ Sports drinks
    _____ Beer/wine, hard liquor

12. Which of these foods did you eat last week?

Grains
   _____ Bread   _____ Cereal/grits
   _____ Rolls   _____ Popcorn
   _____ Bagels   _____ Noodles/pasta/rice
   _____ Crackers   _____ Tortillas
   _____ Other:_____

Vegetables
   _____ Corn   _____ Greens (collard, spinach)
   _____ Peas   _____ Green salad
   _____ Potatoes   _____ Broccoli
   _____ French fries   _____ Green beans
   _____ Tomatoes   _____ Carrots
   _____ Other:_____

Fruits
   _____ Apples/juice   _____ Peaches
   _____ Oranges   _____ Pears
   _____ Grapefruit/juice   _____ Berries
   _____ Grapes/juice   _____ Melon
   _____ Bananas
   _____ Other: _____

Milk and Other Dairy Products
   _____ Whole milk   _____ Yogurt
   _____ Reduced-fat (2%) milk   _____ Cheese
   _____ Low-fat (1%) milk   _____ Ice cream
   _____ Fat-free (skim) milk   _____ Flavored milk
   _____ Other:

Meat and Meat Alternatives
   _____ Beef/hamburger   _____ Sausage/bacon
   _____ Pork   _____ Peanut butter/nuts
   _____ Chicken   _____ Eggs
   _____ Turkey   _____ Dried beans
   _____ Fish   _____ Tofu
   _____ Cold cuts
   _____ Other: _____

Fats and Sweets
   _____ Cake/cupcake   _____ Chips
   _____ Pie   _____ Doughnuts
   _____ Cookies   _____ Candy
   _____ Other: _____

13. Do you have a working stove, oven, and refrigerator where you live?
    _____ Yes   _____ No

14. Were there any days last month when your family didn't have enough food to eat or enough money to buy food?
    _____ Yes   _____ No

15. Are you concerned about your weight?
    _____ Yes   _____ No

16. Are you on a diet now to lose weight or to maintain your weight?
    _____ Yes   _____ No

17. In the past year, have you tried to lose weight or control your weight by vomiting, taking diet pills or laxatives, or not eating?
    _____ Yes   _____ No

18. Did you participate in physical activity (for example, walking or riding a bike) in the past week? If yes, on how many days and for how long?
    _____ Yes   _____ No

19. Do you spend more than 2 hours per day watching television and videotapes or playing computer games? If yes, how man hours per day?
    _____ Yes   _____ No

20. Do you take vitamin, mineral, herbal, or other dietary supplements (for example, protein powders)?
    _____ Yes   _____ No

21. Do you smoke cigarettes or chew tobacco?
    _____ Yes   _____ No

22. Do you ever use any of the following?
    _____ Alcohol/beer/wine
    _____ Steroids (without a doctor's prescription)
    _____ Street drugs (marijuana/speed/crack/heroin)

Figure 12-19. ■ Dietary screening for adolescents. (Reprinted from Story, M., Holt, K., & Sofka, D. [Eds.]. [2002]. *Bright futures in practice: Nutrition* [2nd ed.]. Arlington, VA: National Center Education in Maternal and Child Health and Georgetown University, Nutrition Tools Appendix. Used with permission.)

ASSESSING

The nurse plays an important role in assisting parents to learn and teach health-promoting behaviors. As children gain cognitive abilities and become increasingly more responsible for their own wellness, the nurse can be involved in assessing the degree of ability the child has developed.

DIAGNOSING, PLANNING, AND IMPLEMENTING

Nursing diagnoses for health promotion and illness prevention might include:

- Deficient Knowledge related to unidentified or unmanaged environmental safety hazard
- Disturbed Thought Process related to deficits in reality orientation and problem-solving abilities due to immature cognitive abilities
- Imbalanced Nutrition: More than Body Requirements, related to familial pattern of eating dinners and snacks at fast-food restaurants
- Compromised Family Coping related to lack of information about successful methods of providing discipline.

Some outcomes for these diagnoses are as follows. The client and/or parent will:

- Identify current hazards in or around the home and develop a plan to protect the child and avoid injury.
- Demonstrate the ability to make reasonable choices between two or more alternatives.
- Exhibit an understanding of good nutrition by identifying the most healthful choices from a fast-food menu.
- Explain why discipline helps the child, and describe the steps the parent will take in upholding discipline.

The nurse's role in providing support to these clients would include the following:

- Assess the child's gag reflex. *A present gag reflex gives an indication of a child's ability to swallow properly, although aspiration may still occur.*
- Teach parent to feed an infant in an upright position and maintain this position for 30 minutes after feeding. *Aspiration can be avoided when the child is in an upright position.*
- Teach parent to remove small objects from the infant's or toddler's environment. *Small objects may become lodged in the child's airway.*
- Teach parents to observe for symptoms of aspiration: coughing, choking, or excessive drooling. *Response time to aspiration is decreased with prompt symptom recognition.*
- Teach parents to assess the home environment for safety hazards and to prevent the child's access to hazardous areas. *Children are at increased risk for injury in the presence of environmental hazards. Parents should be proactive in avoiding*

injuries. *This includes a range of items: safety catches on medicine cabinets, locks on gun cabinets, and separate cupboards for alcoholic beverages.*

- Encourage the use of personal protective equipment. *Seat belts, bike helmets, knee and elbow pads, etc., can protect the child from injury. Teens who drive should be asked if they routinely use seat belts.*
- Encourage parents to attend a course that teaches lifesaving techniques such as the Heimlich maneuver. *All parents and caregivers should know the Heimlich maneuver. The ability to perform the maneuver immediately may mean the difference between life and death.*
- Ask about the child's activities outside school. *The child's activities outside school give a clearer picture of behaviors that are health promoting (e.g., an outside sport) or risk creating (e.g., hours of video games each day).*
- Ask how the child likes school, or what is his or her favorite activity at school. *This question can help create discussion about behavior issues or learning difficulties. It may also raise other psychosocial problems, such as low self-esteem.*
- Assess the child's ability to reason and make appropriate safety decisions. Observe the parent's ability to provide adequate care. *Assessment identifies level of ability to provide self-care. If the nurse observes a parent who is endangering the child by poor decisions, the nurse must report the behavior.*
- Teach parent and child the associated risks of behaviors that compromise personal health. Provide information in a nonjudgmental manner. *Knowledge of risks may lead to changed behaviors. A nonjudgmental approach is more easily accepted and leads to greater cooperation.*

EVALUATING

The care plan is revised until expected outcomes are achieved. To evaluate the effectiveness of interventions, the nurse would gather data concerning:

- The parent/client's injury prevention plan
- Identification of environmental hazards
- Avoidance of aspiration
- The client's decisions regarding self-care behaviors.

NURSING PROCESS CARE PLAN
Pediatric Client with Unintentional Poisoning

The parent of a 3-year-old male child calls the poison control center and states that her child had been playing in the neighbor's yard. The child and his friend went into the neighbor's garage, and the child came running out suddenly, crying. The parent noticed a white powdery substance around the child's mouth and a foamy substance in the child's mouth. The parent brings the child to the neighborhood clinic for assistance.

Assessment. The following data should be collected as soon as possible.

- Condition of pupils
- Moderate irritation of the mucous membranes with edema and erythema
- VS: T 98.6°F tympanic, P 96, R 24, BP 90/60.
- Parent and child deny nausea, vomiting, or diarrhea
- Pain: child is experiencing mouth and throat pain
- Description of possible toxic substances

Nursing Diagnosis. The following important nursing diagnosis (among others) is established for this client:

- Risk for Injury related to possible poisoning and the presence of toxic substances and physical manifestations.

Expected Outcome. Client will not have complications related to ingestion of toxic substances.

Planning and Implementation

- Obtain a specimen of the substance found on the child's face and in his mouth. *Identifying the substance assists in the treatment process.*
- If the poisonous substance is suspected to be corrosive or a hydrocarbon, rinse the mouth with water. *Vomiting should not be induced if there is evidence of mucosal irritation because it would cause further damage.*
- If the poisonous substance is suspected to be medication, induce vomiting. *Vomiting removes the poison from the child's system.*
- Observe for signs of respiratory obstruction and signs of shock. *Various substances may cause respiratory obstruction or shock.*

Evaluation. The client does not experience complications related to poisoning.

Critical Thinking in the Nursing Process

1. What substances, commonly found in a garage, could the child have ingested?
2. What prevention methods would be appropriate for the nurse to discuss with the parent?
3. What is the expected emotional response from the parent following this event?

Note: Discussion of Critical Thinking questions appears in Appendix I.

Note: The references and resources for this and all chapters have been compiled at the back of the book.

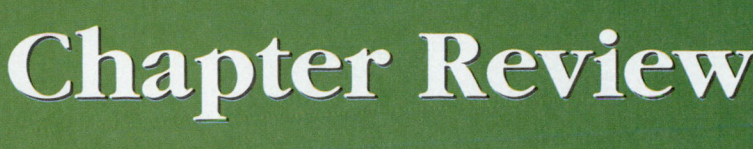

Chapter Review

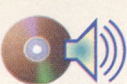 **KEY TERMS** by Topic

Use the audio glossary feature of either the CD-ROM or the Companion Website to hear the correct pronunciation of the following key terms.

Illness Prevention
illness prevention, primary prevention, secondary prevention, tertiary prevention

Health Promotion
health promotion, health, spanking

Infant
choking

Toddler
parallel play

Preschooler
associative play

School-Age Child
latch-key children, cooperative play

KEY Points

- It is important for the nurse to use each contact with the client and family as a time to assess and promote health behaviors and illness prevention.

- The nurse promotes healthy individuals, families, and communities by role modeling appropriate healthy behavior, providing encouragement to family members, reinforcing the need for change, and recognizing positive efforts.

- The nurse is involved in three levels of illness prevention: primary, secondary, and tertiary. Primary prevention helps the child avoid illness. Secondary prevention allows for early detection and treatment of illness. Tertiary prevention involves treating illnesses to prevent complications.

- An essential nursing intervention is health promotion, which includes promoting environmental safety and psychosocial health.

- Nutritional assessment, teaching, and monitoring of the child's nutritional status are important nursing tasks.

- Nursing measures to protect the infant include preventing injury from falls and aspiration, promoting the development of trust, and implementing appropriate feeding measures whether formula feeding, breastfeeding, or introducing solid foods.

- The nurse can be instrumental in protecting the toddler from injuries during play, promoting appropriate toilet training, and discussing methods of discipline with parents.

- Preschoolers begin to be independent, and the nurse can assist in health promotion by discussing protecting the child from strangers, promoting the use of seat belts, and helping both parent and child make nutritious food choices.

- The nurse can help the school-age child take responsibility for his or her own safety by discussing with the child how to stay safe at school, during sporting activities, and after school, especially when home alone.

- Adolescents frequently compromise their safety by participating in risk-taking activities. The nurse can provide teaching to the adolescent regarding risks associated with certain behaviors such as sexual contact and substance abuse.

EXPLORE MediaLink

Additional interactive resources for this chapter can be found on the Companion Website at www.prenhall.com/towle.

Click on Chapter 12 and "Begin" to select the activities for this chapter.

For chapter-related NCLEX-style questions and an audio glossary, access the accompanying CD-ROM in this book.

Animations

Children and overweight

Health promotion and health maintenance

FOR FURTHER Study

For more information on *Healthy People 2000* and *Healthy People 2010*, see Chapter 1.

For more information on issues of teen sexuality, see Chapters 5 and 23.

For nutrition for the pregnant woman, see Chapter 6.

Breastfeeding is discussed in detail in Chapter 9.

For nutrition for the breastfeeding woman, see Chapter 10.

See Chapter 11 for additional information on safety and life span issues; see Box 11-5 for some age-specific communication techniques.

See Chapter 26 for more information on childhood diseases and prevention methods.

For more information on psychosocial issues and disorders, see Chapter 27

See Appendix II for growth charts and an immunization schedule.

See Appendix IV for a Denver Developmental Screening test.

Critical Thinking Care Map

Caring for a Client with Inadequate Nutrition

NCLEX-PN® Focus Area: Physiological Integrity: Basic Care and Comfort

Case Study: An adolescent is being interviewed by the school nurse. She is asked to complete a 24-hour nutrition diary. For breakfast, the teen writes "none." For lunch, the teen writes "chips and cola." For dinner, the teen writes "chicken fingers, fries, and sweet tea." She also states that this is fairly typical for her daily diet.

Nursing Diagnosis: Imbalanced Nutrition: Less than Body Requirements

COLLECT DATA

Subjective	Objective
_____	_____
_____	_____
_____	_____
_____	_____
_____	_____
_____	_____

Would you report this? Yes/No

If yes, to: _____

Nursing Care

_____
_____
_____
_____
_____
_____
_____
_____
_____
_____
_____
_____

How would you document this? _____
_____
_____
_____

Compare your documentation to the sample provided in Appendix I.

Data Collected
(use those that apply)

- Current weight 100 lb
- T 98.8, P 66, R 12, BP 110/60
- Lungs sound clear bilaterally
- Previous weight 110 lb
- States typical diet is low in calories
- Skips breakfast
- Deep tendon reflexes (DTRs) 2+
- All peripheral pulses present
- Chips and cola for lunch
- Chicken fingers, fries, and sweet tea for dinner

Nursing Interventions
(use those that apply; list in priority order)

- Present a sample daily meal plan.
- Discuss the hazards of obesity.
- Refer to a dietitian prn.
- Use the food pyramid to discuss essential nutrients.
- Discuss exercise as a method of weight reduction.
- Discuss ways to overcome difficulties related to food preparation and food acquisition.
- Explain importance of nutrition during adolescence.
- Consider hospitalization and feeding tube for nutrition.

NCLEX-PN® Exam Preparation

1 The nurse is preparing to give a hepatitis B vaccine to a newborn. The order reads hepatitis B vaccine 10 mcg IM. The vaccine is supplied in 20 mcg/mL. How many milliliters will the nurse give? _____ (Fill in the blank.)

2 The registered nurse discusses a teaching plan for primary prevention for a newborn with the LPN/LVN. Which of the following interventions would be appropriate?

1. immunizations
2. bimonthly visits with the pediatrician
3. treating diaper rash
4. changing the formula to a soy product

3 The adolescent admits to being sexually active. Which of the following secondary prevention methods is appropriate for the client?

1. monthly pregnancy tests
2. yearly Pap smears
3. attending an abstinence support group
4. increasing iron in the diet

4 The toddler has been diagnosed with otitis media. The nurse assists in providing tertiary prevention. Which of the following interventions is a method of tertiary prevention?

1. hearing screening
2. administering cephalosporins
3. keeping the child from interacting with other children for a period of 48 hours
4. reading books to the child

5 A new mother asks the nurse to suggest appropriate toys for her newborn son. Which of the following are appropriate choices?

1. balloons on ribbons
2. stuffed animals of any variety
3. plastic keys on a plastic ring
4. bright music box attached to the outside of the crib

6 The nurse is assisting the mother of a 6-month-old infant to make appropriate solid food choices. Which of the following could be suggested? Choose all that apply.

1. rice cereal mixed with breast milk
2. cheerios
3. thinly sliced hot dogs
4. pureed bananas
5. commercially prepared vegetable puree

7 The nurse has an order to administer *Haemophilus b* conjugate vaccine. He or she should document all of the following, except:

1. lot number of the vial used.
2. expiration date of the vial.
3. site of the injection.
4. temperature and blood pressure at time of injection.

8 A 17-year-old client states that she smokes and is unwilling to attend smoking cessation classes. Choose the most appropriate nursing intervention.

1. Contact social services to report parental neglect.
2. Discuss reducing the number of cigarettes daily.
3. Obtain a prescription for the nicotine patch.
4. Inform the client that she will have to deal with lung cancer later in life.

9 A 16-year-old female visits the family physician. Height is 5 ft 1 in. Current weight is 159 lb. The nurse is concerned about the risk for obesity when the client reveals which of the following?

1. Her single mother works two jobs and is rarely home.
2. Client enjoys smoothies at breakfast and rarely snacks.
3. Client states she is doing well academically.
4. Client has two siblings and lives with her mother and grandmother.

10 The school nurse recognizes pinpoint pupils and drowsiness for several days in a student. Which of the following drugs might the nurse suspect the teen is abusing?

1. narcotics
2. amphetamines
3. depressants
4. hallucinogens

Answers for Review Questions, as well as discussion of Care Plan and Critical Thinking Care Map questions, appear in Appendix I.

Chapter 13

Adapting Procedures in the Care of Children

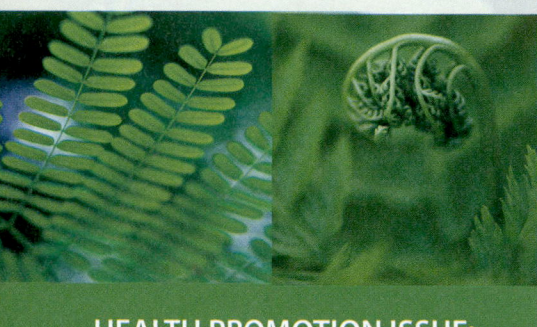

HEALTH PROMOTION ISSUE:
Developing a Therapeutic Relationship with a Pediatric Client

NURSING PROCESS CARE PLAN:
Client with Fractured Arm

CRITICAL THINKING CARE MAP:
Caring for a Child Requiring Restraints

BRIEF Outline

Assessment of the Child
Discussing Procedures with Children
Common Procedure Steps
OBTAINING VITAL SIGNS
Temperature
Pulse
Respiration
Blood Pressure
Pain, the Fifth Vital Sign
GROWTH MEASUREMENTS
Height
Weight
Body Mass Index
Head Circumference
Chest Circumference
CARE OF THE CHILD DURING DIAGNOSTIC PROCEDURES
Restraining the Child

SPECIMEN COLLECTION
ASSISTING WITH NUTRITION
Feeding a Child
ASSISTING WITH ELIMINATION
Enema
Urinary Elimination
RESPIRATORY PROCEDURES
Airway Clearance
Oxygen Administration
PHARMACOLOGY AND MEDICATION ADMINISTRATION TO CHILDREN
Oral Administration
Rectal Suppository
Medications by Injection
Intravenous (IV) Administration
Storage of Medication
Nursing Care

LEARNING Outcomes

After completing this chapter, you will be able to:

- Describe why procedures need to be adapted in the care of children.
- Identify specific adaptations for selected procedures in the care of children.
- Discuss the role of the LPN/LVN in adapting procedures in the care of children.

Many of the same nursing and medical procedures used in the care of adults are used in the care of children. However, some procedures must be adapted to the size and age of the child. This chapter describes the common adaptations that should be made to provide safe nursing care to children.

Assessment of the Child

Assessment involves the collection of data and interpretation of the findings in order to make a decision about care of the individual. The assessment of the child is organized like the assessment of an adult, but the approach is quite different (Table 13-1 ■). The reason for assessment, the environment in which the assessment is done, and the condition of the child all influence the extent of data collected. For example, if the child is brought to the clinic for a well-child checkup, an in-depth assessment of the child's physical and cognitive growth and development and emotional well-being is completed. If the child is brought to the office because of a minor injury, the physical assessment is focused on that cause. The cognitive assessment might be directed at the cause of the injury so the child can be taught about safety issues. If the child is acutely ill in the hospital, the physical assessment is more in depth. In-depth cognitive assessment is not done because the child could regress during the illness, and the cognitive and emotional assessment would, therefore, not be accurate.

Although an assessment of an adult is generally conducted from head to toe, it may be better to assess the child in a different order. For example, it is easier to hear heart and lung sounds when a child is quiet. Because touching a child's ears might cause the child to cry, it would be better to take a tympanic temperature after listening to heart and lung sounds.

To begin, the nurse assesses the general condition of the child by answering questions such as the following:

1. What is the child's general appearance? Does the child appear sick or well? Is he or she clean or dirty?
2. What is the child doing? Playing, laughing, crying? (*Note:* The child may be crying because of the illness.) Is the child being held by a parent or sitting alone?

Answers to these questions will help guide the nurse in determining the subsequent order of the assessment.

It is important to obtain the cooperation of both the child and the parent (Figure 13-1 ■). At times, much of the assessment can be done while the child is sitting on the parent's lap. This parental contact provides needed security for the small child. Any part of the assessment that might be painful, embarrassing, or frightening should be done last. A more detailed assessment of each body system is outlined in Chapters 15 to 28 ⊙⊙.

TABLE 13-1	
Gathering Data from the Pediatric Client	
SUBJECTIVE DATA	
Demographic data	Full name, contact information, birth date, gender, race, religion
Reason for visit	Statement of the problem in the child's or the parent's words; onset, symptoms, and relieving factors of the problem
Past medical history	Illnesses, hospitalizations, surgeries, accidents (including dates and treatments); current medications (including over-the-counter medications and vitamins); immunization record; known drug, food, and environmental allergies; hazardous substances—alcohol intake, tobacco intake (including smokeless tobacco products), illegal drugs
Family history	Diseases, congenital anomalies, deaths, genogram, review level of support, type of dwelling, source of family income
Review of systems	*Note:* Begin with the system of the presenting problem. Integumentary, head-ears-eyes-nose-throat (HEENT), respiratory, cardiovascular, gastrointestinal including nutritional history, genitourinary, musculoskeletal, neurologic, and endocrine; include psychosocial concerns
OBJECTIVE DATA	
Baseline data	Height, weight, head and chest circumference, vital signs
Physical examination	General appearance, level of consciousness (LOC) *Note:* Begin with the system of the presenting problem. Integumentary, HEENT, respiratory, cardiovascular, gastrointestinal including nutritional history, genitourinary, musculoskeletal, neurologic, and endocrine

MediaLink   Child physical assessment

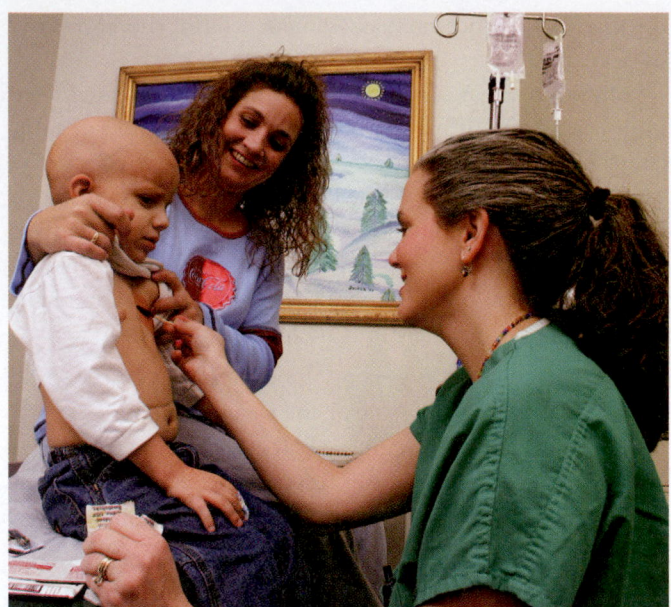

Figure 13-1. ■ A family-centered care policy permits parents to be present during a procedure performed on their child. The parent plays an important role in providing security and comfort to this child who is having his port accessed for an IV infusion treatment.

Discussing Procedures with Children

With the infant and very young child, parents need to be informed about the procedure. The nurse should provide a simple explanation that defines the rationale for the procedure, outlining the steps of the procedure, and describing how the parent can assist with the procedure. Allowing the child to touch or play with the equipment may increase the child's sense of security. Parents need an opportunity to ask questions about the procedure. It is best to give them time to ask questions before the procedure begins.

Older children, with greater cognitive ability, need a simple explanation of the procedure. It is often better to time the explanation for immediately before the procedure. This prevents the child from focusing on a painful or invasive procedure and becoming more afraid. The nurse should also allow children ample opportunity to ask questions and discuss fears. Older children and adolescents are curious about their bodies and about the planned procedures. They may even be asked to sign informed consent forms, along with their parents, allowing procedures to be done (see more in Chapter 2 ∞).

Common Procedure Steps

When performing procedures with children, certain basic steps are taken, just as they are with adults. Adaptations of the basic interventions may be made based on age or developmental level. These steps are represented by an icon bar in each procedure in this book as shown below:

1. Check the client chart for an appropriate physician's order.
2. Gather all necessary equipment so the procedure can be completed more efficiently, without interruption.
3. Make introductions to increase the child's comfort level. When the child is young, fear can be decreased when introductions are made to the parent first. The child can then view the nurse as safe because the parent was comfortable with the nurse.
4. Identify the client by checking the identification band or bracelet.
5. Provide privacy. Age and developmental level are important. A young child will want the parent's presence. An adolescent might not.
6. Explain the procedure. Obtain consent if necessary.
7. Wash hands. Follow standard precautions and facility policy. Often, rinse-free hand sanitizers can be used.
8. Don gloves if necessary. Again, follow standard precautions and facility policy.

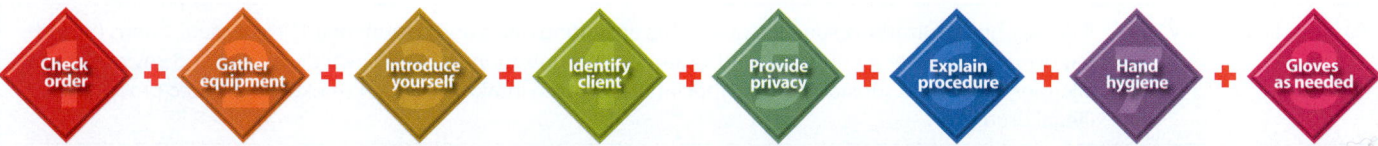

OBTAINING VITAL SIGNS

Temperature

The safety of the child must be taken into consideration in choosing a thermometer and route of measurement. Mercury thermometers have mostly been eliminated from health care facilities due to possible mercury exposure from a broken glass shaft (Box 13-1 ■). Temperatures can be recorded in both Fahrenheit and Celsius. Box 13-2 ■ provides conversion formulas.

Electronic thermometers are commonly used. There are a variety of routes for obtaining a temperature with an electronic thermometer. A young child may not be able to follow the directions to keep the mouth closed and not bite the thermometer, so an oral route may not be safe and may not provide an accurate measure. An axillary temperature is safe, but it often takes longer to obtain.

BOX 13-1

Glass Thermometers

The use of glass thermometers in public health care facilities is rare. Glass thermometer have several disadvantages and hazards, including difficulty reading the temperature, increased time required to obtain the temperature, risk of mercury exposure, and risk for injury related to broken glass. Many parents may still have glass thermometers in their homes. Therefore, the nurse needs to discuss these disadvantages and hazards with the family.

The hazards of mercury exposure are affected by the method of exposure. The amount of mercury contained within most thermometers is very small. If the mercury is swallowed, it is rarely absorbed in the stomach and usually passes through the digestive system. If the mercury is touched, it may cause a skin rash. The greatest risk from mercury occurs with inhalation.

The LPN/LVN can discuss with families the proper methods for handling a mercury spill in the home. Caution the family not to sweep the mercury because this causes it to break into many pieces. Recommend wearing heavy rubber gloves to avoid skin exposure. The mercury may be picked up with an eyedropper, scoop and heavy cardboard, or duct tape. The mercury, and all utensils and clothing exposed to the mercury, must be triple bagged and then sealed in a plastic container. Instruct the client to call the local health department for proper disposal locations. Caution them not to wash material exposed to the mercury in the washing machine because this could contaminate the whole washing machine. The client should ventilate the area for 48 hours.

Note: Sphygmomanometers may also contain mercury.

clinical ALERT

The axillary temperature is one degree *lower* than the oral temperature. Chart the axillary temperature as the numeric value read from the thermometer. Include in your documentation the route of the temperature as "AX."

BOX 13-2

Temperature Conversion Formulas

Celsius to Fahrenheit

From °C **up** to °F:

$$°F = 1.8 \times °C + 32$$

First **multiply** ° by 1.8, then **add** 32.

Fahrenheit to Celsius

From °F **down** to °C:

$$°C = °F - 32 \text{ divided by } 1.8$$

First **subtract** 32 from °F, then **divide** by 1.8.

A rectal temperature is accurate, but it is not a common procedure because taking a rectal thermometer runs the risk of perforating the anus if the child moves.

clinical ALERT

The rectal temperature is one degree *higher* than the oral temperature. Chart the rectal temperature as the numeric value read from the thermometer. Include in your documentation the route of the temperature as "R."

A tympanic thermometer, which bounces infrared light off the tympanic membrane to measure body temperature, is generally less traumatic for the child and obtains a reading quickly. Measurement of tympanic temperature is described in this section.

Chemically treated tapes that are placed on the child's forehead may also be used to determine temperature. Normal temperature ranges for children are the same as for adults. Table 13-2 ■ shows the normal ranges in vital signs for different ages. Methods for obtaining temperature readings are provided in Procedure 13-1 ■.

TABLE 13-2

Normal Vital Sign Ranges by Age

AGE	TEMPERATURE IN DEGREES FAHRENHEIT/CELSIUS	PULSE (AVERAGE AND RANGE)	RESPIRATIONS (AVERAGE AND RANGE)	BLOOD PRESSURE (mm HG)
Newborns	98.2/36.8 (axillary)	130 (80–180)	35 (30–80)	73/55
1–3 years	99.9/37.7 (rectal)	120 (80–140)	30 (20–40)	90/55
6–8 years	98.6/37 (oral)	100 (75–120)	20 (15–25)	95/57
10 years	98.6/37 (oral)	70 (50–90)	19 (15–25)	102/62
Teen years	98.6/37 (oral)	70 (50–90)	18 (15–20)	120/80
Adult	98.6/37 (oral)	80 (60–100)	16 (12–20)	120/80
Older adult (older than 70 years)	96.8/36 (oral)	80 (60–100)	16 (15–20)	Possible increased diastolic

Measuring Temperature

Purpose

- To determine a child's body temperature and compare to normal ranges
- To identify variances in normal temperature ranges
- To report abnormal temperatures, in a timely fashion, in an effort to facilitate treatment

Equipment

- Electronic or tympanic thermometer, or thermometer tape
- Disposable probe covers
- Water-soluble lubricant
- Disposable gloves

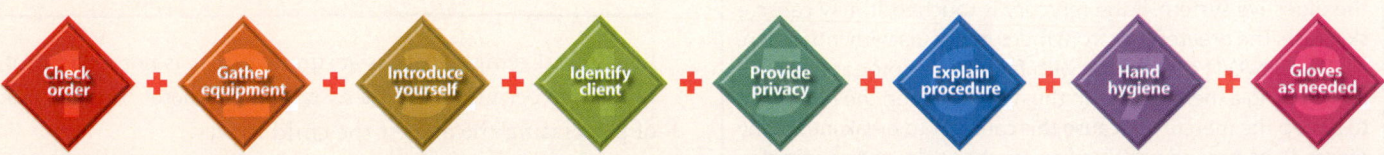

Check order + Gather equipment + Introduce yourself + Identify client + Provide privacy + Explain procedure + Hand hygiene + Gloves as needed

Interventions

1. Perform preparatory steps (see icon bar).

2. Determine client's normal range of temperature by reviewing the chart.

3. If applicable, apply a disposable probe cover to the thermometer shaft. *This prevents transmission of infection. Devices such as thermometer tapes do not have covers.*

4. Position the child in a supine, side-lying, or seated position. *It will be easier for the nurse to manage the child's movements in these positions.*

5. For all methods, take the temperature, safely dispose of any probe cover, document the temperature reading and route, and report abnormalities. *Quality care includes safe practice to prevent spread of micro-organisms. It also requires timely documentation and reporting.*

TAKING A TYMPANIC TEMPERATURE

6. Position the pinna.
   - For the child younger than 3 years, pull the pinna down and back (Figure 13-2A ■).

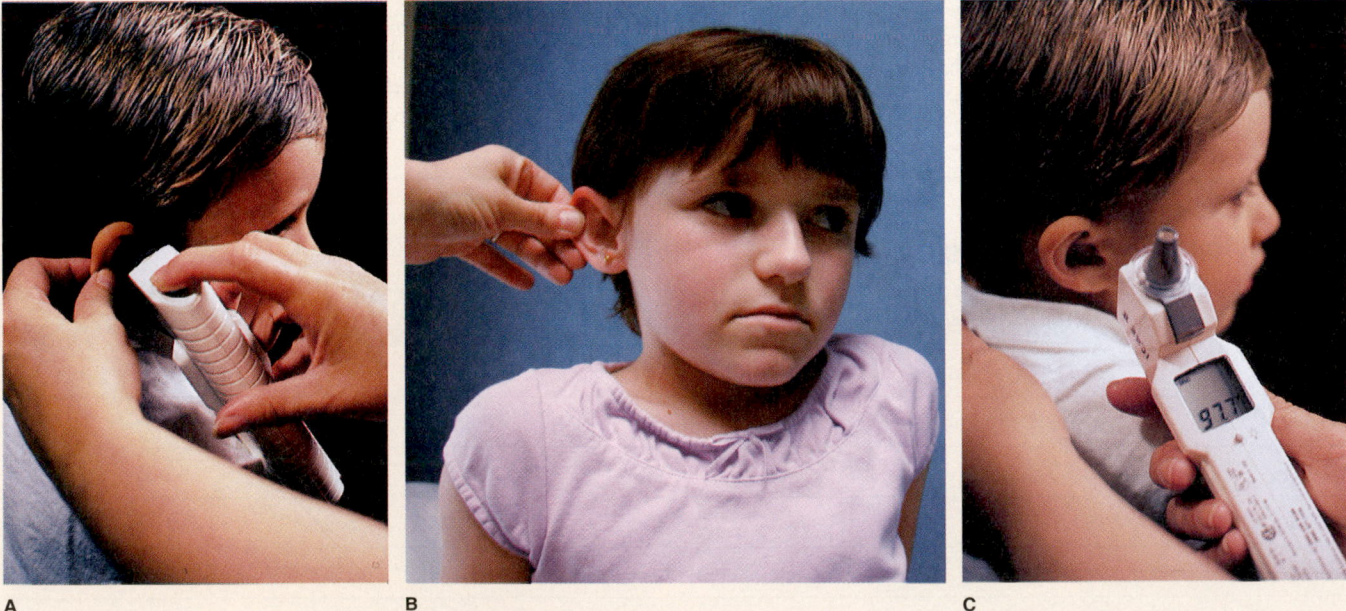

A   B   C

Figure 13-2. ■ Position for inserting thermometer when tympanic route is used. (**A**) Younger than 3 years of age. (**B**) Older than 3 years of age. (M. C. Schlachter Photography) (**C**) Digital readout of temperature appears within 1 minute.

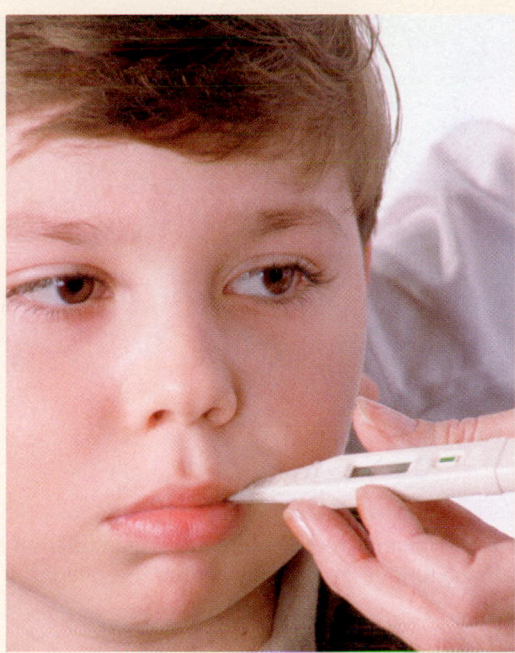

Figure 13-3. ■ Measuring oral temperature. It is important to position the tip of the thermometer under the child's tongue and to make sure the child's lips are closed around the base. (Carolyn A. McKeone/Photo Researchers, Inc.)

- For the child older than 3 years, pull the pinna up and back (Figure 13-2B). *These positions straighten the ear canal*

7. Place the probe in an anterior position, occluding the outer canal. *The temperature will be more accurate if the probe is positioned toward the tympanic membrane. Occluding the canal will provide core body temperature.*

8. Take the temperature according to manufacturer's recommendations. *In most models, a reading appears on a screen (Figure 13-2C).*

9. Return thermometer to the base. *This restores the battery charge.*

10. Review steps 1 to 4 above.

TAKING AN ORAL TEMPERATURE

6. See step 2 above. *This protects the child from micro-organisms on the equipment.*

7. Place the probe under the child's tongue and ask the child to close the mouth but not clamp down with the teeth (Figure 13-3 ■). *Accurate body temperature is detected when the probe is placed near the large blood vessels in the posterior sublingual pocket.*

8. Leave the thermometer in place according to manufacturer's recommendations. *Most digital and electronic thermometers will signal completion with a beep.*

9. See step 4 above. *Following safe practices will help prevent the spread of infection.*

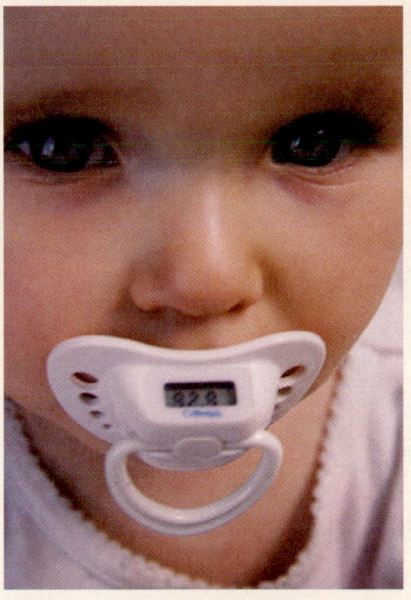

A

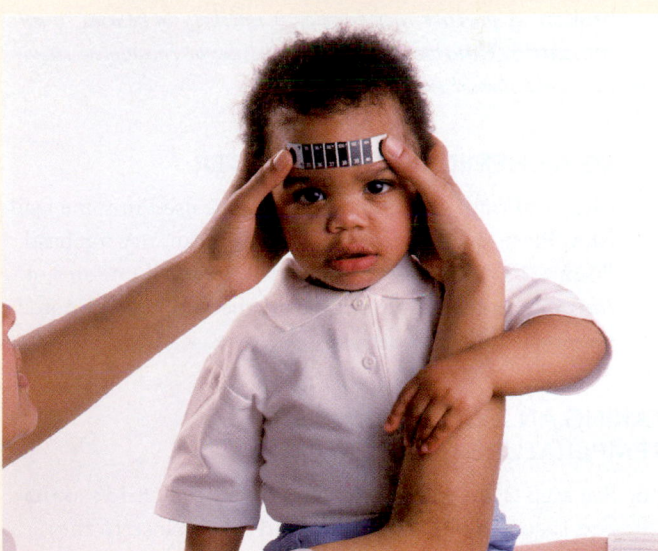

B

Figure 13-4. ■ **(A)** Thermometers within pacifiers may be used by some parents. (M. C. Schlachter Photography) **(B)** A chemically treated tape can provide temperature readings when pressed firmly against a clean, dry forehead. Usually these temperature-measuring devices are only accurate within 1 or 2 degrees. (© Dorling Kindersley Media Library)

TAKING ORAL TEMPERATURE WITH PACIFIER THERMOMETERS

6. Although they are not common in health care facilities, the nurse should be aware of thermometers within pacifiers (Figure 13-4A ■). Teach parents to follow manufacturer's directions and to cleanse the thermometer carefully after each use. Teach that the instrument should not be used as a regular pacifier and that

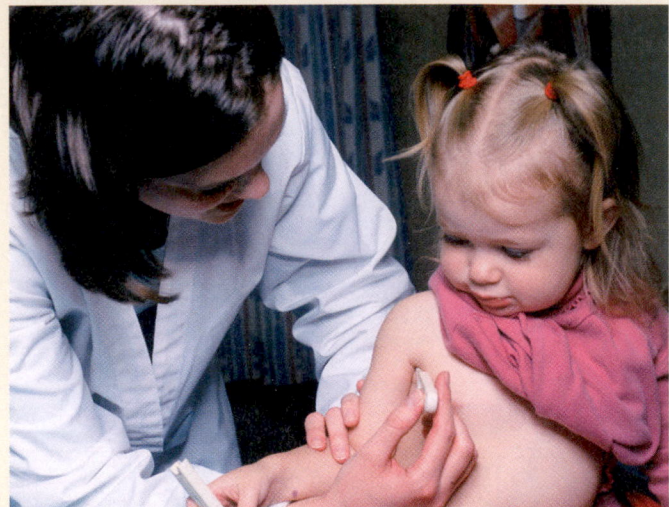

Figure 13-5. ■ Measuring the axillary temperature.

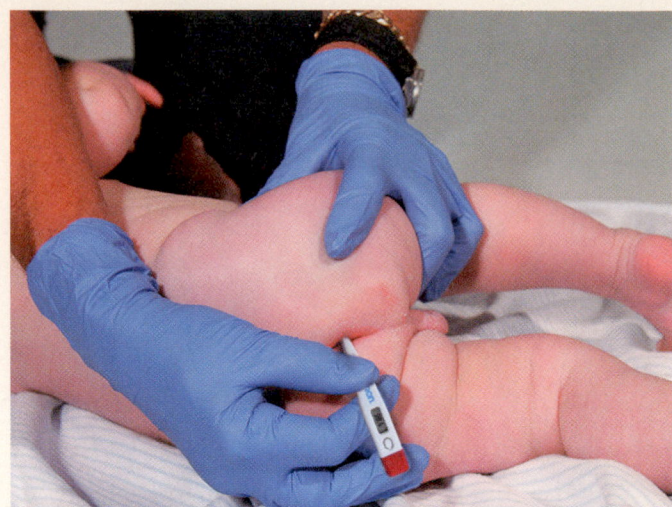

Figure 13-6. ■ Taking a rectal temperature reading from an infant. (Nathan Eldridge\Pearson Education/PH College)

it should be discarded if any part becomes cracked or broken. *A pacifier thermometer is unlikely to be used in an institution. Caution parents that misuse or incomplete cleaning could spread infection.*

USING A CHEMICAL THERMOMETER

6. Chemical (tape) thermometers may be used in some facilities. Place the tape firmly against a clean, dry forehead (Figure 13-4B) and hold it at the ends until one area of the tape becomes lighter. Record the temperature noted under the lightest portion of the tape.

TAKING AN AXILLARY TEMPERATURE

6. See step 2 above. Place the probe in the child's axilla and secure by holding the child's arm close to the side (Figure 13-5 ■). *Accurate body temperature is detected when the probe is placed near the large blood vessels in the axilla.*

7. Leave the thermometer in place according to manufacturer's recommendations. *Most digital and electronic thermometers will signal completion with a beep.*

8. Follow step 4 above.

TAKING A RECTAL TEMPERATURE (FIGURE 13-6 ■)

6. Follow step 2 above. Apply water-soluble lubricant to disposable probe. *Lubricant makes insertion easier and minimizes risk of damaging the anus.*

7. Enlist the assistance of another staff member. *Restraint may be necessary and will decrease the risk of injury.*

8. Retract buttocks and insert the probe no deeper than $1/2$ inch for the infant and 1 inch for the child. *Accurate body temperature is detected when the probe is placed near the large blood vessels in the anus. Risk for injury is minimized by paying attention to the depth of insertion.*

9. Leave the thermometer in place according to manufacturer's recommendations. *Most digital and electronic thermometers will signal completion with a beep.*

10. Follow step 4 above. *This will help prevent the spread of infection.*

SAMPLE DOCUMENTATION

(date) 0800   *(Note: Temperature portion only. This is a focused part of a complete documentation entry.)* Temperature 100.9°F AX. Reported to Dr. Phillips, orders received. _____ R. Copper, LPN

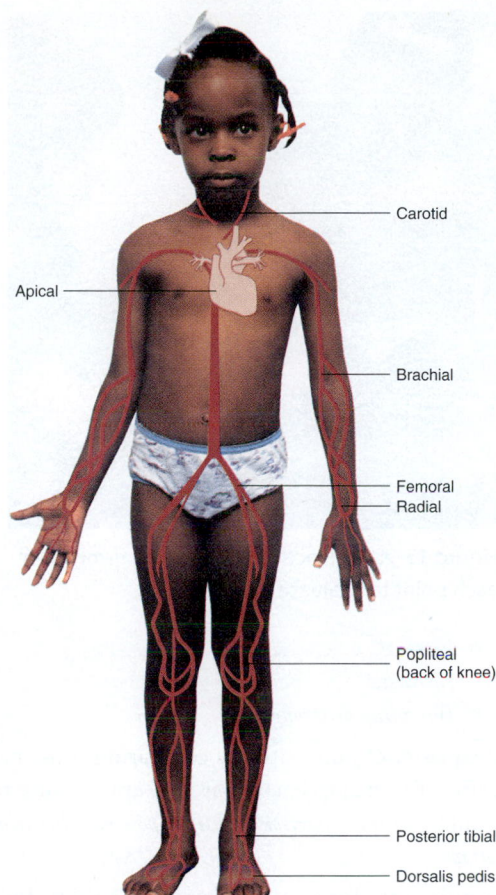

Carotid

Apical

Brachial

Femoral

Radial

Popliteal
(back of knee)

Posterior tibial

Dorsalis pedis

Figure 13-7. ■ The sites used to assess pulses in children.

Pulse

Due to fat distribution and small arteries, obtaining an accurate radial, carotid, popliteal, and pedal pulse may be difficult. Generally, an apical pulse, counted for 1 minute, is obtained on a child (Figure 13-7 ■). The pulse rate decreases with age until the normal adult range is reached by age 16 (see Table 13-2). Procedure 13-2 ■ provides information on obtaining pulse rates in children.

Respiration

Children use the diaphragm as the main muscle of breathing. (See Chapter 17 ⬭ for further information on the anatomy and physiology of respiration in the pediatric client.) Because the diaphragm is used, the nurse can observe or feel the abdominal movement to count the number of respirations per minute. The respiratory rate decreases with age until the normal adult range is reached by age 16 (see Table 13-2). Procedure 13-3 ■ supplies information on obtaining the respiratory rate in children.

clinical ALERT

If the respiratory rate is greater than 60, report this finding immediately to the nurse in charge and/or the doctor. At a respiratory rate of 60 or greater, little oxygen can get to the alveoli for gas exchange.

| PROCEDURE 13-2 | **Obtaining Pulse Rate** |

Purpose

■ To determine a child's pulse rate and compare to normal ranges
■ To identify variances in normal pulse rate
■ To report abnormal pulse rates, in a timely fashion, in an effort to facilitate treatment

Equipment

■ Clock or watch with second hand
■ Stethoscope

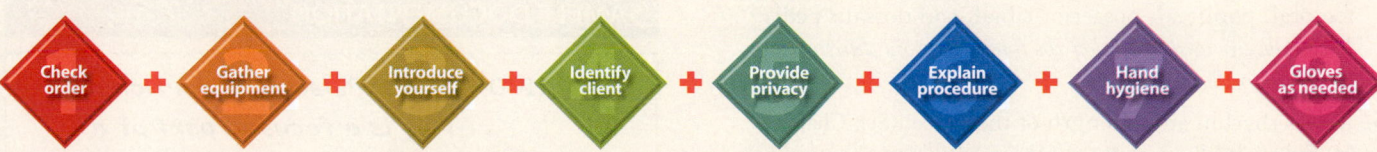

Interventions

1. Perform preparatory steps (see icon bar).
2. Determine client's normal pulse rate by reviewing the chart (see Table 13-2).

3. Position the infant in a supine position and the child in a supine or seated position. *This position allows adequate access for listening to pulse sounds.*

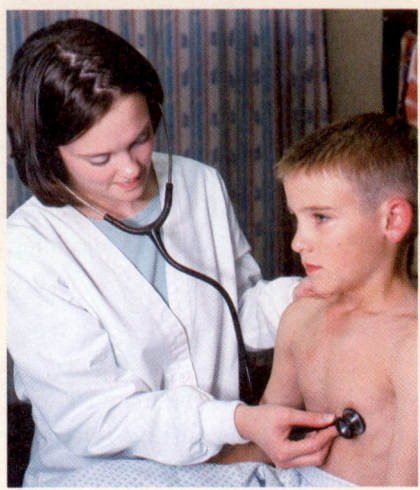

Figure 13-8. ■ Assessing the apical heart rate.

4. Determine the pulse and document any abnormalities. *Accurate readings provide a baseline for further care or give information about the client's change in status.*

AUSCULTATING AN APICAL PULSE

5. Choose a time to listen to the heart when the infant or small child is quiet or asleep. *An accurate pulse rate is difficult to assess when a child is crying.*

6. Place the diaphragm of the stethoscope over the apex of the heart (Figure 13-8 ■). Do not attempt to listen through the child's clothing. *The apex or **point of maximal impulse** (PMI) is the site where the heart rate can be best heard. Heart sounds can be muffled if assessed through clothing.*

7. Listen for two distinct heart sounds, lub-dub of rhythm. *The two heart sounds are S1 (closing of the AV valves) and S2 (closing of the semilunar valves). Together they make one heartbeat.*

8. Count the heartbeat for a full minute. *This provides the most accurate assessment of the apical pulse.*

PALPATING A PERIPHERAL PULSE

5. Use the fingertips to locate the child's pulse (Figure 13-9 ■). Peripheral pulse sites are brachial, radial, carotid, femoral, popliteal, posterior tibial, and dorsalis pedis. *Fingertips are used instead of the thumb to avoid detecting your own pulse in the thumb.*

6. Assess rhythm and strength of the pulse. (See Chapter 19 for more about pulse rhythms.) *Rhythm is assessed by determining the space between the beats and is described as regular or irregular. Strength is assessed by the amount of pressure exerted with each beat. Strength can be documented by using the following scale:*

- *0 = Absent*
- *1+ = Thready or weak*

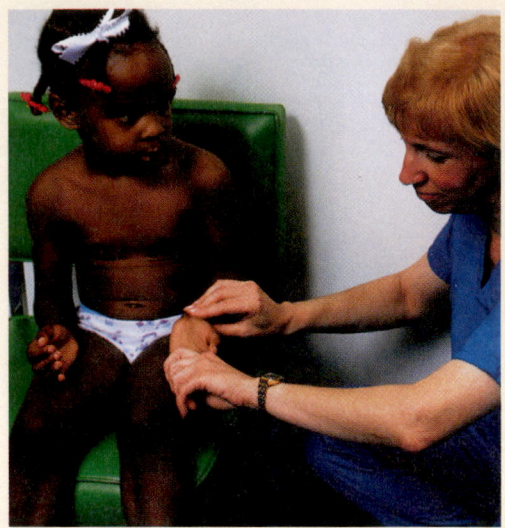

Figure 13-9. ■ Place the fingerpads firmly over each point to evaluate the pulsation.

- *2+ = Normal*
- *3+ = Increased*
- *4+ = Bounding or strong*

7. Assess equality of pulse sites by comparing proximal and distal sites. For example, compare the apical pulse to the radial pulse. *This comparison identifies possible alterations in circulation.*

8. Count pulse rate for a full minute. *This makes it easier to notice any irregularities and/or irregular pulse. Once the nurse is experienced at taking pulse rates, the pulse may be counted for 30 seconds and multiplied by 2 to calculate the beats per minute (bpm).*

clinical ALERT

Avoid pressing the carotid pulse, bilaterally, at the same time. This could stop blood flow to the brain.

9. Document pulse rate and report any abnormalities.

SAMPLE DOCUMENTATION

(date) 1100 (Note: Pulse rate portion only. This is a focused part of a complete documentation entry.) Radial P 68, 2+ equal bilaterally. _____
S. Brown, LVN

<table>
<tr><td>PROCEDURE 13-3</td><td># Obtaining Respiratory Rate</td></tr>
</table>

Purpose

- To determine a child's respiratory rate and compare to normal ranges
- To identify variances in normal respiratory rates
- To report abnormal respiratory rates, in a timely fashion, in an effort to facilitate treatment

Equipment

- Clock or watch with second hand

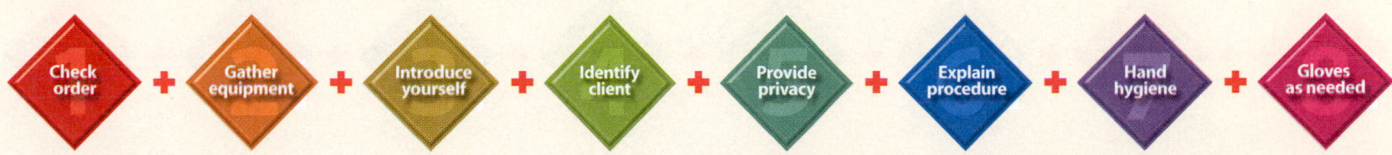

Interventions

1. Perform preparatory steps (see icon bar).
2. Determine client's normal range of respirations by reviewing the chart (see Table 13-2).
3. Position the infant or child in a supine position.
4. Observe the abdomen rise and fall in the infant and young child. Observe the chest rise and fall in the older child and adolescent. The nurse may need to place a hand on the chest or abdomen to feel the rise and fall. *Infants and young children breathe from their diaphragm; thus, the abdomen will rise and fall. Older children breathe more in the chest.*
5. Observe the depth, rhythm, and effort required for respirations.
   - *Depth describes the volume of air exchanged and may be documented as "deep" or "shallow."*
   - *Rhythm refers to the spacing of the respirations and may be described as "regular" or" irregular."*
   - *Effort refers to the energy expended during respirations and may be described as "with effort" or "without effort" or as "labored" or "unlabored."*
6. Count respirations. Document respiratory rate and report any abnormalities. *One respiration consists of an inspiration (inhalation) and an expiration (exhalation).*

SAMPLE DOCUMENTATION

(date) 1400   *(Note: Respiratory rate portion only. This is a focused part of a complete documentation entry.)*
R 24, shallow and irregular, c/o difficulty breathing. HOB raised.
_____ I. Mullins, LPN

Blood Pressure

The procedure for obtaining a blood pressure is the same as for adults (Procedure 13-4 ■). It is important to explain the procedure to the child using age-appropriate language. Reassure small children that the cuff will not pinch for long. Some clinical agencies require blood pressure to be measured only on older children or on the extremely ill younger child. Blood pressure readings on small children and infants are generally done with Doppler ultrasound equipment.

Although using the upper arm and brachial artery is most common for obtaining blood pressures, using the thigh and popliteal artery or calf and posterior tibial artery is also common in infants and small children. To obtain an accurate measurement, the correct cuff size must be used. The cuff should cover two-thirds of the upper arm, thigh, or calf. If the cuff is too large, the blood pressure will read a false low. If the cuff is too small, the blood pressure will read a false high. The blood pressure in children is lower than adults and gradually increases until the normal blood pressure ranges are reached by age 16 (see Table 13-2).

Pain, the Fifth Vital Sign

Pain is considered the fifth vital sign, and the Joint Commission on Accreditation of Healthcare Organizations (JCAHO) requires regular assessment and documentation

Blood pressure

PROCEDURE 13-4   Measuring Blood Pressure

Purpose

- To determine a child's blood pressure and compare to normal ranges
- To identify variances in normal blood pressure
- To report abnormal blood pressure findings, in a timely fashion, in an effort to facilitate treatment

Equipment

- Variety of sizes of blood pressure cuffs (Figure 13-10 ■)
- Electronic blood pressure monitor, or sphygmomanometer and stethoscope

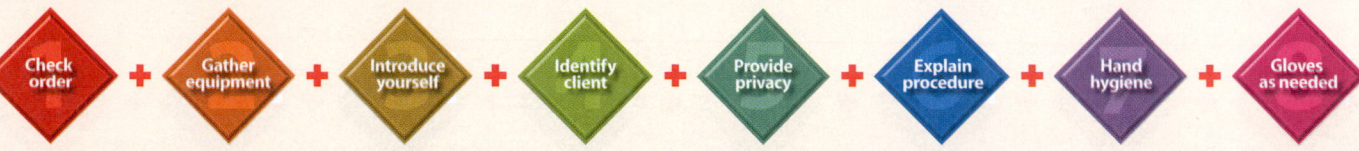

Check order + Gather equipment + Introduce yourself + Identify client + Provide privacy + Explain procedure + Hand hygiene + Gloves as needed

Interventions

1. Perform preparatory steps (see icon bar).

2. Determine client's normal blood pressure range (see Table 13-2).

3. Discuss the fact that the arm will be squeezed tightly for a short period of time. *The client will be more compliant when the procedure is explained beforehand.*

4. Position the client in a seated or recumbent position.

5. Wrap the proper size cuff 1 in. above the antecubital space for an upper arm blood pressure or 1 in. above the popliteal artery for a thigh blood pressure. *If the cuff is too large, the blood pressure equipment will give a false low reading. If the cuff is too small, the blood pressure equipment will give a false high reading.*

ELECTRONIC BP ASSESSMENT

6. Turn the power switch on.

7. Position the extremity at the level of the heart. *The blood pressure will be higher than normal if the extremity is lower than the heart.*

8. Press the start button and wait for a reading.

9. Record the digital BP reading and report abnormalities.

MANUAL BP ASSESSMENT

6. Close the valve of the sphygmomanometer.

7. Palpate the brachial artery. *This identifies the proper stethoscope placement.*

8. Place the bell or diaphragm of the stethoscope against the artery with the dominant hand (Figure 13-11 ■).

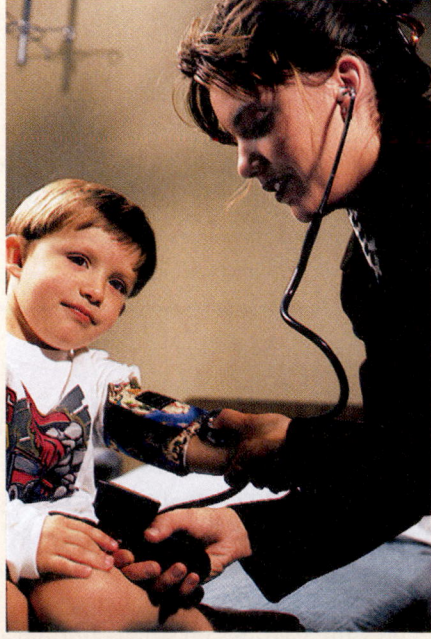

Figure 13-11. ■ With the cuff snugly wrapped around the arm, hold the arm with the cubital fossa at the level of the heart and place the stethoscope against the artery with the dominant hand.

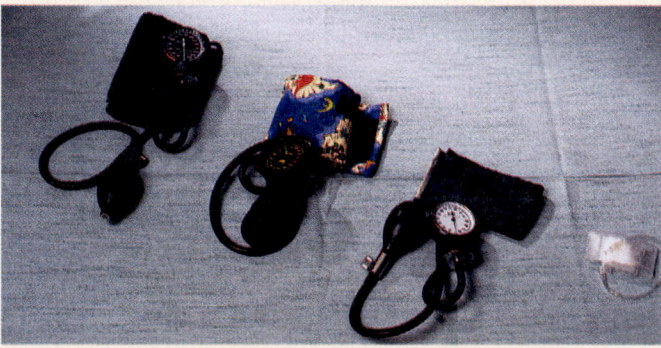

Figure 13-10. ■ Blood pressure cuffs are available in various types and sizes for pediatric clients.

With the nondominant hand, inflate the bulb of the sphygmomanometer 30 mm Hg above the client's normal systolic blood pressure. *This provides enough pressure to observe a reading at the first sound.*

9. Slowly release the valve of the bulb of the sphygmomanometer at a rate of 2 to 3 mm Hg/second. Observe the number on the dial corresponding with the presence of the first sound. *This is the systolic pressure.*

10. Continue releasing the air in the bulb at the same rate. Observe the number on the dial corresponding with the disappearance of the pulse. *This is the diastolic pressure.*

11. Release the remainder of the air in the bulb quickly and remove the cuff.

12. Document blood pressure and report any abnormalities.

clinical ALERT

In children younger than 12 years of age, the diastolic pressure is noted as a muffling of the pulse and not as a disappearance of the sound.

SAMPLE DOCUMENTATION

(date) 1800 *(Note: Blood pressure portion only. This is a focused part of a complete documentation entry.)* BP 112/66 L arm, seated position.
_____ F. Darnell, LVN

---

of it. Pain is subjective; therefore, it exists when the client says it does. The assessment of the pediatric client with regard to pain may be difficult. The infant and small child may not be able to verbalize pain (see Health Promotion Issue on pages 404 and 405). The difficulty of assessing pain in children contributes to inadequate pain control. Physiologic responses to pain (e.g., tachycardia, tachypnea, pupil dilation, pallor) may last only a short time. The nurse must look at other indicators of pain, such as restlessness, short attention span, facial grimacing, moaning, crying, posturing or splinting, anorexia, and sleep disturbances (insomnia, drowsiness, or constantly sleeping). The nurse should keep in mind that the child who has had surgery or an injury is likely to be in pain to some degree. Special pain assessment tools have been developed to assist with the evaluation of pain in children (Figure 13-12 ■). Pain assessment is further addressed in Procedure 13-5 ■ on page 406.

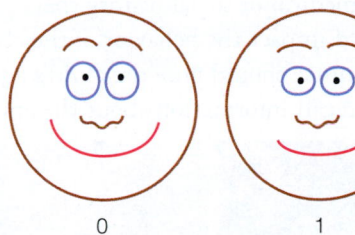 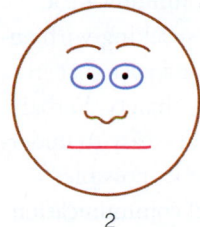 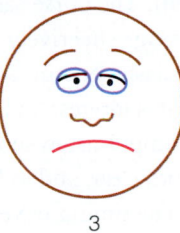 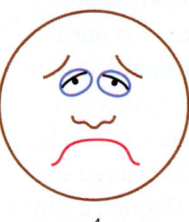 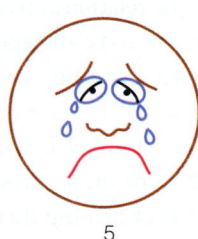

| 0 | 1 | 2 | 3 | 4 | 5 |

1. Explain to the child that each face is for a person who feels happy because he or she has no pain (hurt, or whatever word the child uses) or feels sad because he or she has some or a lot of pain.

2. Point to the appropriate face and state, "This face..." :
   0—"is very happy because he (or she) doesn't hurt at all."
   1—"hurts just a little bit."
   2—"hurts a little more."
   3—"hurts even more."
   4—"hurts a whole lot."
   5—"hurts as much as you can imagine, although you don't have to be crying to feel this bad."

3. Ask the child to choose the face that best describes how he or she feels. Be specific about which pain (e.g., "shot" or incision) and what time (e.g., Now? Earlier before lunch?)

Figure 13-12. ■ Wong-Baker Pain Rating Scale for children 3 to 7 years. (From Hockenberry, M. J. [2005]. *Wong's essentials of pediatric nursing.* [7th ed.]. St. Louis: Mosby, p. 1301. Copyright by Mosby Inc. Reprinted by permission.)

(Text continues on p. 406.)

DEVELOPING A THERAPEUTIC RELATIONSHIP WITH A PEDIATRIC CLIENT

The LPN/LVN working in a pediatrician's office is approached by a recently hired LPN/LVN. Her past nursing experience has been with adult clients in an acute-care setting. She states that she has never worked with children before and is having some difficulty relating to them. She is most distressed that the children seem afraid of her. The children will not open up to her and talk to her about issues related to their health care. She is concerned that these factors will affect the type of nursing care she is able to give and ultimately affect the child's health care. She wants some assistance in performing her nursing tasks without scaring the children.

DISCUSSION

For the nurse to assist the child to become healthy, a positive nurse-client relationship must be established. This relationship develops over time, demonstrates respect and confidentiality, is client focused and not nurse focused, and has respect and mutual trust as its basis.

For the relationship between a child and a nurse to be therapeutic, the nurse must display caring behaviors mixed with a professional attitude that conveys competence. Trust develops when children believe that the nurse cares about them and is capable of helping them through a situation. Trust develops as the nurse:

- Listens attentively to what the child says, even if the child is talking about cartoons or toys.
- Displays empathy. Empathy includes recognizing the child's needs, acknowledging the child as real, and showing the child that the nurse is working diligently to meet expressed needs.
- Is honest with the child. Children can see through dishonesty. They need straight, simple responses or an honest "I don't know."
- Is genuine. Caring cannot be contrived. Caring for a child requires knowledge of their developmental levels, of their emotional status, and of their social history. The genuine nurse displays spontaneous behaviors that seek to restore and protect the child.

As the nurse communicates with children, she must recognize that this is accomplished both verbally and nonverbally. Although many people think that spoken words convey our message, in actuality nonverbal communication conveys more than 80% of our message. Nonverbal communication includes our personal appearance. It is said that an opinion of us is formed by other individuals within the first 3 seconds of our first encounter. This opinion is developed before we ever say a word and is largely based on our dress, our posture, our facial expressions, and our gait.

Verbal communication is more than the words we say; it is also how we say them. The nurse can communicate a message effectively by speaking with enthusiasm, energy, and at a pace that indicates interest and not anxiety. Verbal communication should be easy to understand, clear, and as brief as possible.

The timing of verbal communication is also important. The message can go unheard if the child is not ready or willing to listen.

Children learn in different ways. Some must hear the information, whereas others must see it. Still others need to use their hands (e.g., write information or handle a stethoscope) before they can learn.

Developmental levels also influence how a child learns. For instance, a preschooler enjoys learning by trial and error. An adolescent needs to learn independently.

The nurse must consider the child's vocabulary, education, psychomotor abilities, emotional status, societal values, and attention span when developing a teaching plan.

It is also important to choose an appropriate teaching strategy. The nurse can use demonstration to teach a skill and then ask the child to return demonstration. The nurse could also model specific behaviors. Teaching aids may assist the nurse in communicating the proper information. Written materials, posters, anatomic models, games, videos, computers, or dolls may be used in both formal teaching and informal teaching.

PLANNING AND IMPLEMENTATION

Development of a Nurse-Client Relationship

Prior to the child's appointment, the nurse reviews the child's chart, noting any medical or social history that would impact the behavior of the child. The nurse should note the child's age and recall information about the appro-

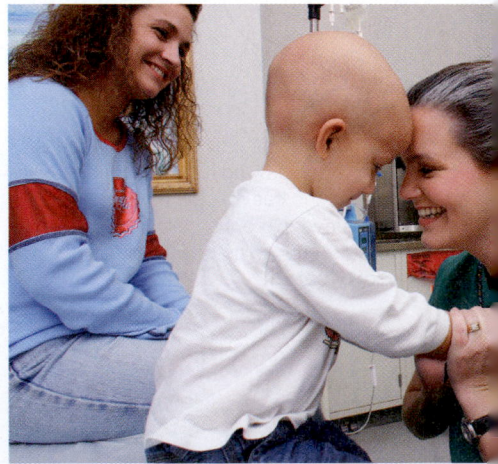

(George Dobson\Pearson Education/PH Colle

priate developmental age. The nurse should practice pronouncing the child's name and note any special likes or dislikes that are noted in the chart. For example, if the child likes a certain cartoon character, the nurse might be able to find a Band-Aid with that character on it or place the child in an exam room decorated with this character. Be sure to include this documentation in the child's chart and update as needed.

Social interaction at the beginning of the appointment is necessary to help ease the child's anxiety and to develop a trusting relationship. The nurse should be at eye level with the child when speaking directly to him or her (see Figure 13-1). Initially, the nurse should avoid touching the child until trust is established.

As the appointment progresses and the nurse seeks to understand the health care needs of the child, listening becomes vital. Active listening requires much energy and is vital in achieving trust. Listening behaviors include eye contact and body language that suggests a willingness to listen (e.g., relaxed body parts, a face-to-face position, a slight leaning toward the child). Listening also requires silence on the nurse's part. As the child speaks, the nurse must actively consider the child's words and not try to develop a wise or witty comeback while the child is speaking. Only after gathering all subjective and objective data can the nurse develop a plan of action. Plans developed before data collection is complete are likely to be ineffective.

Appropriate Communication Techniques

Pediatric nurses often choose bright-colored uniforms that will appeal to children. Hair should be neat. Makeup should look natural, so as not to distract or frighten the child. Posture should be erect but not tense.

Children can read the thoughts of the nurse through the nurse's facial expressions. It is important for nurses to learn to control feelings of disgust, impatience, or boredom. The nurse's face needs to display interest, enthusiasm, and energy. If a child confides that he or she has been abused by an adult, the nurse must not express horror or anger. The nurse's face should convey interest and concern so the child will continue to share information.

When communicating verbally with children, the nurse should speak to the child in language and terms that he or she can understand. The nurse should use open-ended questions when trying to obtain information from a child. Questions such as "Tell me how your tummy feels" or "What happened to your leg?" will elicit more information than a question that can simply be answered "yes" or "no."

Appropriate Teaching Methods

The nurse needs to have a variety of teaching aids available in order to conduct formal or informal teaching for the child. A simple drawing of the body can help the nurse describe a disease, procedure, or surgery. Dolls or puppets appeal to preschoolers.

In school settings, videos are often a way of providing information. If videos are used, the dialogue should be appropriate for the age group. Slides or photographs should also be age appropriate. For example, photographs of genitalia should not be shown in a classroom of mixed genders. The nurse should carefully assess readiness to learn and evaluate learning following the teaching session.

With diligence and continued effort, the nurse should be able to relate to the pediatric client and provide effective care.

SELF-REFLECTION

When a child reacts negatively to you, what feelings do you have? If a child has never acted negatively to you, imagine what the scenario might look like. Be honest about your feelings. When you encounter a strange environment, what factors make you feel more uncomfortable? What factors make you feel more comfortable? What do you need to change in your nursing practice to help develop trust with your clients? To communicate better with your pediatric clients? To be more effective in providing them with teaching as it relates to their health care?

SUGGESTED RESOURCES

For the Nurse

www.ChildbirthGraphics.com The catalog available at this website can provide the nurse with posters, pamphlets, three-dimensional models, and videos to assist in health care teaching.

Blackwell, P., & Baker, B. (2002). Estimating communication competence of infants and toddlers. *Journal of Pediatric Health Care, 16*(1), 19–35.

Humphries, J. (2002). The school health nurse and health education in the classroom. *Nursing Standard, 16*(17), 42–45.

Sydnor-Greenberg, N., & Dokken, D. (2001). Communication in healthcare: Thoughts on the child's perspective. *Journal of Child and Family Nursing, 4*(3), 225–230.

PROCEDURE 13-5   Pain Assessment

Purpose

- To assess the nature of the child's pain to include location and intensity
- To report findings to the appropriate personnel in an effort to assist in the relief of the child's pain

Equipment

- Variety of pain assessment scales that are appropriate for the child's age

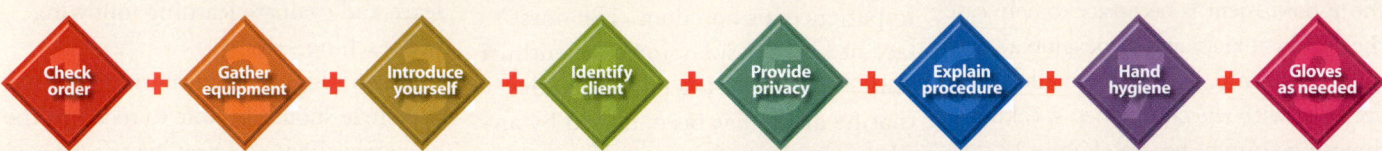

Interventions

1. Perform preparatory steps (see icon bar).

2. Observe the child for manifestations of pain. *Objective data related to pain may be obtained through observation.*

3. If the child is verbal, ask him or her to describe the location and intensity of pain. *The verbal child should be able to assist the nurse by indicating the location and severity of the pain, according to a numeric scale.*

4. If the child is young but able to communicate, the nurse uses the scale to determine a pain level using nonverbal cues. *The child can point to the face that most resembles the pain he or she feels, or to the part of the body that hurts the most.*

5. Document objective and subjective data gathered.

SAMPLE DOCUMENTATION

(date) 2200   *(Note: Pain portion only. This is a focused part of a complete documentation entry.)* 9-year-old boy crying, moaning. States "my head really hurts." Rates headache as 8 on a scale of 10. Shades closed. TV turned off. Cool cloth applied. Report given to charge nurse. _____
E. Gorden, LPN

GROWTH MEASUREMENTS

Growth measurements can be taken in U.S. or metric units, depending on facility policy. Box 13-3 ■ provides some commonly needed conversions (inches to centimeters, etc.). See Appendix V for more common conversions and lab values.

Height

With the infant or child lying supine, use a tape measure, measuring stick, or measurement mat to measure the child's length. Length is assessed from crown to heel. Once the child is able to stand, the height measurement can be obtained with the child standing against the measuring stick. Procedure 13-6 ■ provides more information on measuring height and length.

BOX 13-3

Some Common Conversions in U.S. and Metric Measurements

1 g = 1 mL (used when weighing diaper to determine fluid output)

1 grain = 60 mg

15 grains = 1 g

1 oz = 30 mL

2.2 lb = 1 kg (used when recording in metric or computing body mass index [BMI])

1 in. = 2.5 cm (used when recording in metric)

39 in. = 1 yd 3 in. = 1 m (used when recording in metric)

Measuring Height and Length

Purpose

- To obtain an accurate measure of the client's height or length
- To report abnormal findings in a timely fashion, in an effort to facilitate treatment; abnormal findings might include lack of growth in height between yearly well-child visits

Equipment

- Tape measure, yard stick, meter stick, or measuring mat
- Stadiometer
- Platform scale with stature-measuring device

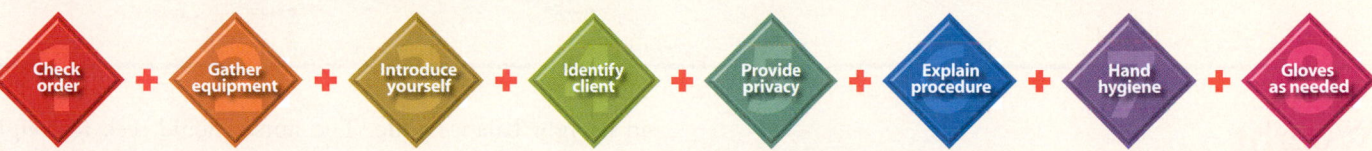

Check order + Gather equipment + Introduce yourself + Identify client + Provide privacy + Explain procedure + Hand hygiene + Gloves as needed

Interventions

1. Perform preparatory steps (see icon bar).

FOR INFANTS

2. Place the infant in a supine position.

3. Place the infant's head against a flat surface. Extend legs until the knee is straight.

4. Use a tape measure, measuring stick, or measuring mat to measure from the crown to the heel (Figure 13-13 ■). Note the length in inches or centimeters.

5. Plot the measurement on a standardized growth chart. *Note:* Appendix II 🔗 shows growth charts from infancy to age 18.

FOR CHILD

2. Have the child stand erect, without shoes and with the head level, with the back of the head against the measuring device (Figure 13-14 ■).

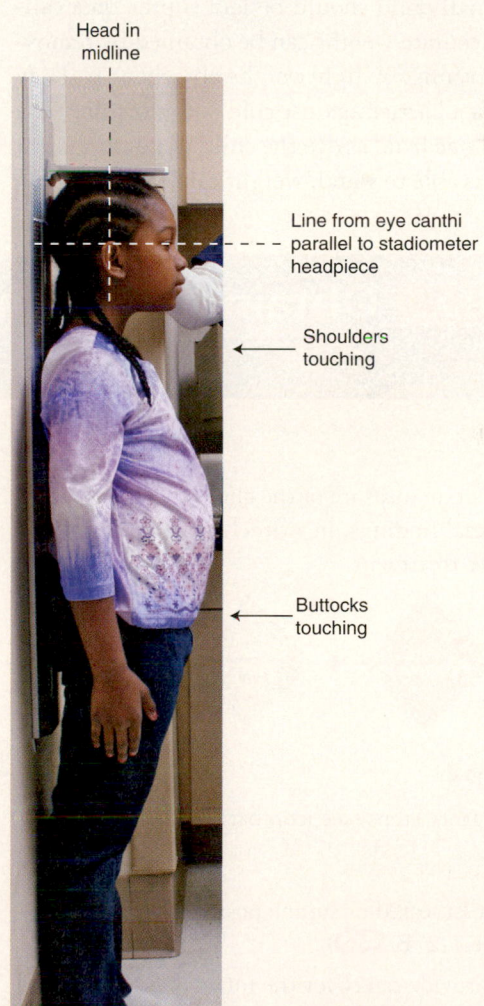

Head in midline

Line from eye canthi parallel to stadiometer headpiece

Shoulders touching

Buttocks touching

Heels touching and together

Figure 13-14. ■ Standing height measurements are taken routinely at each well-child visit to assess the child's rate of growth. Position the head in an erect and midline position while the shoulders, buttocks, and heels touch the wall. Move the headpiece down to touch the crown. Measure the height reading to the nearest 0.5 cm or ¼ in.

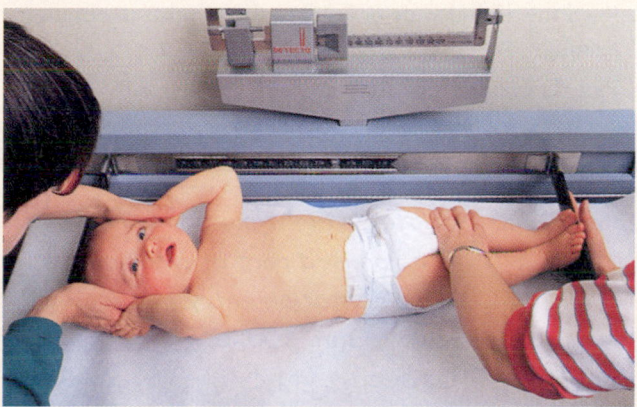

Figure 13-13. ■ Measure an infant's length carefully from the crown of the head to the heel.

3. Place the headpiece onto the child's crown.
4. Note the height in inches or centimeters.
5. Plot the measurement on a standardized growth chart.

SAMPLE DOCUMENTATION

(date 0800)   *(Note: Height portion only. This is a focused part of a complete documentation entry.)* Male infant, 3 hours old, 18 in. Spine intact. Arms and legs without visible defect. _____
B. Marty, LVN

Weight

The infant and small child should be laid supine on a calibrated scale. An accurate weight can be obtained by removing the child's clothing. A lightweight absorbent pad can be used to serve as a barrier against cold and moisture. The nurse should hold one hand above the child to guard against a fall. If the child is able to stand, weight can be obtained on an upright balance scale. The nurse should seek to weigh the child similarly at each visit. For instance, the child should always be with or without shoes, fully clothed, or in underclothing only. The child's privacy and modesty should be protected. See Box 13-3 for pound–kilogram conversion and Procedure 13-7 ■ for more information on obtaining weight.

PROCEDURE 13-7 **Obtaining Weight**

Purpose

■ To obtain an accurate measure of the client's weight
■ To report abnormal findings, in a timely fashion, in an effort to facilitate treatment

Equipment

■ Infant scale, calibrated
■ Floor scale, calibrated

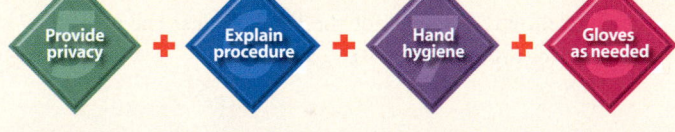
Check order + Gather equipment + Introduce yourself + Identify client + Provide privacy + Explain procedure + Hand hygiene + Gloves as needed

Interventions

1. Perform preparatory steps (see icon bar).

FOR INFANTS

2. Place the infant in seated or supine position on the infant scale (see Figure 7-27B 🔗).
3. Stand close to provide safety for the infant.
4. Read the scale when the infant is still.
5. Plot the weight on a standardized growth chart.

FOR CHILD

2. Ask the child to stand on the scale without shoes.

3. Read the digital scale or balance the weights to obtain reading.
4. Plot the weight on a standardized growth chart.

SAMPLE DOCUMENTATION

(date) 0900   *(Note: Weight portion only. This is a focused part of a complete documentation entry.)* 11-year-old male, 48 in., 100 lb. _____
D. Deen, LVN

Body Mass Index

The body mass index (BMI) is used differently in children and adults. The BMI for children is gender and age specific, and called the BMI-for-age. It can be used for children age 2 through adolescence. The BMI is derived by calculating the weight in kilograms divided by height in meters squared (Procedure 13-8 ■). This measurement can indicate whether a child is underweight, overweight, or at risk for becoming overweight. However, it should be remembered that children's body fat changes as they grow and also according to their gender.

Head Circumference

Using a tape measure, the head circumference is measured from slightly above the eyebrows, above the pinna of the ear, and around the occiput (Procedure 13-9 ■). Head circumference should be obtained on all children younger than 36 months of age and any child with a neurologic defect.

PROCEDURE 13-8   Calculating Body Mass Index

Purpose

- To determine a child's risk of being underweight or overweight

Equipment

- BMI-for-age chart

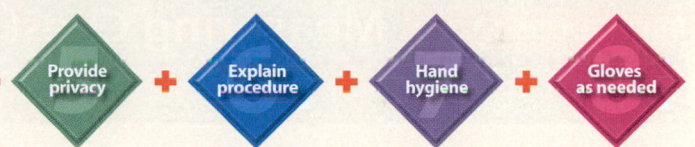

Interventions

1. Perform preparatory steps (see icon bar).
2. Plot the child's weight and height in relation to gender.
3. Obtain BMI. Calculate the BMI by dividing the child's weight in kilograms by the height in meters squared. For example, if a 17-year-old boy weighs 180 lb and is 78 in. tall:

   180 lb divided by 2.2 lb/kg = 81.8 kg
   78 in. divided by 39 in./m = 2 m
   81.8 kg divided by 2 × 2 = 81.8 kg divided by
      4 m^2 = 20.45 is BMI

   This boy would have a BMI a bit lower than the 50th percentile for his age (Ball, 2006).
4. Report findings to appropriate personnel.

SAMPLE DOCUMENTATION

(date) 1300   *(Note: BMI portion only. This is a focused part of a complete documentation entry.)* 11-year-old male, 48 in., 100 lb. BMI 30.6. Report given to C. Cox, CRNP. ____
L. April, LPN

PROCEDURE 13-9   Measuring Head Circumference

Purpose

- To determine normalcy of the infant's head circumference in relation to chest circumference

Equipment

- Tape measure

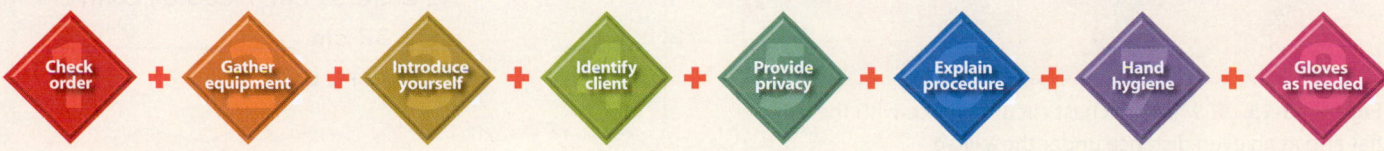

Interventions

1. Perform preparatory steps (see icon bar).
2. Position the infant in a supine position.
3. Place the tape measure slightly above the eyebrows, above the pinna of the ear, and around the occiput (see Figure 7-27C 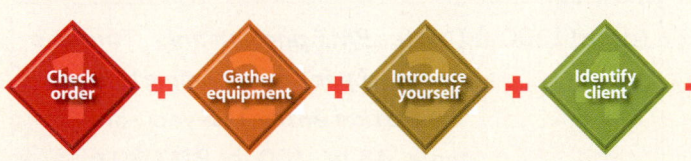). *This is the largest diameter of the infant's head.*
4. Document the head circumference in inches or centimeters. The nurse may also document the amount of *molding* (shaping of the head during the birth process). *Documentation provides information for later comparison.*
5. Compare to chest circumference. *Head circumference is equal to or 2 cm greater than chest circumference until age 2.*
6. Plot the measurement on a standardized growth chart.

PROCEDURE 13-10   # Measuring Chest Circumference

Purpose

- To determine normalcy of the infant's chest circumference in relation to head circumference

Equipment

- Tape measure

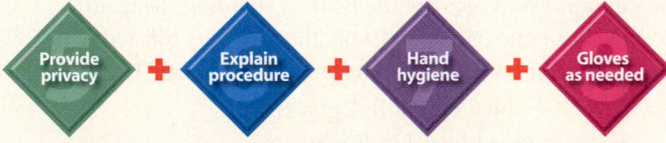

Interventions

1. Perform preparatory steps (see icon bar).
2. Position the infant in a supine position.
3. Encircle the chest with the measuring tape. Place the tape measure against the bare skin of the infant's chest, at the nipple line, under the axillae (Figure 13-15 ■). *This is the largest diameter of the infant's chest.*
4. Document the chest circumference in inches or centimeters.
5. Compare to head circumference. *Head circumference is equal to or 2 cm greater than chest circumference until age 2.*
6. Plot the measurement on a standardized growth chart.

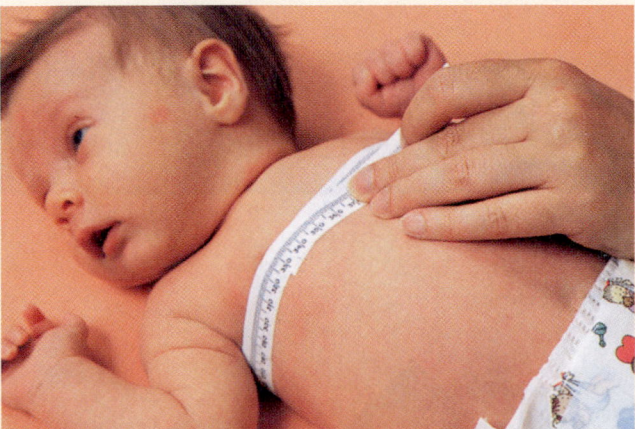

Figure 13-15. ■ Measure chest circumference with the tape flat and at an even distance under the axillae.

Chest Circumference

Using a tape measure, the chest circumference is measured from under the axillae, across the nipples, and around the back (Procedure 13-10 ■). The normal height, weight, and head and chest circumference measurements can be found on growth charts in Appendix II ⚭. The abdomen may also be measured, as described in Procedure 13-11 ■.

CARE OF THE CHILD DURING DIAGNOSTIC PROCEDURES

Diagnostic procedures are often necessary to determine treatment for the pediatric client. These procedures are often frightening to children. The nurse must be able to communicate in an age-appropriate manner to the child. There are, however, times when a child must be restrained to ensure safety. If possible, the parent should be allowed to accompany the child during procedures.

clinical ALERT

For procedures in a hospital, it is important that the child be taken to an examination room. If painful procedures are performed in the child's room, the child may become fearful of going to sleep or of being left alone in the room.

Restraining the Child

At times, children must be restrained during procedures to protect their safety. Procedures such as medication administration by injection, initiating intravenous access, lumbar puncture, or using an otoscope require some form of restraint. It is important to use the least restrictive type of restraint for the shortest period of time to reach the desired goal. The child's age, size, condition, and the needed procedure are taken into account when deciding on a type of restraint. Parents should be present if possible. However, to prevent feelings of mistrust, avoid requiring the parent to restrain the child.

PROCEDURE 13-11 **Measuring Abdominal Girth**

Purpose

■ To determine normalcy of the infant's or child's abdominal girth
■ To check for abnormal findings such as umbilical and inguinal hernias, bowel obstructions, ascites, constipation, and organ enlargement

Equipment

■ Tape measure

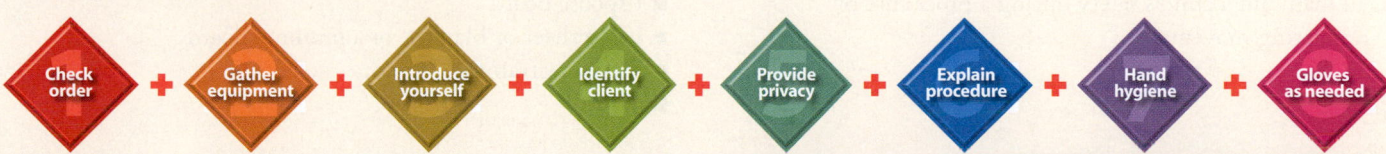

Interventions

1. Perform preparatory steps (see icon bar).
2. Position the child in a supine position.
3. Place the tape measure against the bare skin of the child's abdomen, at the umbilicus. *This is the largest diameter of the abdomen.*
4. Document the abdominal circumference in inches or centimeters.

SAMPLE DOCUMENTATION

(date) 0930   *(Note: Abdominal girth portion only. This is a focused part of a complete documentation entry.)* Male infant weighed after breastfeeding, 7 lb 7 oz (3.38 kg). Abdominal girth 33 cm.
_____ M. Kay, LPN

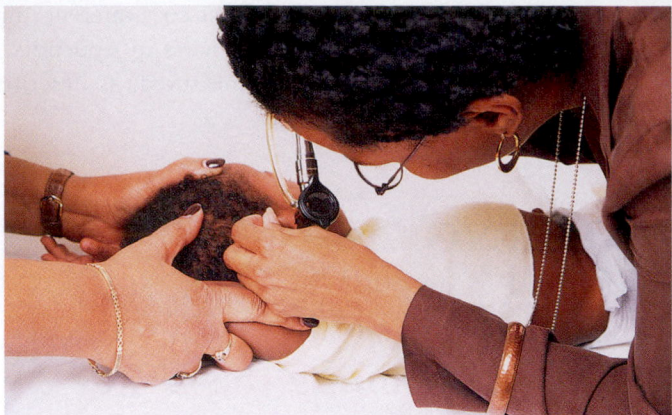

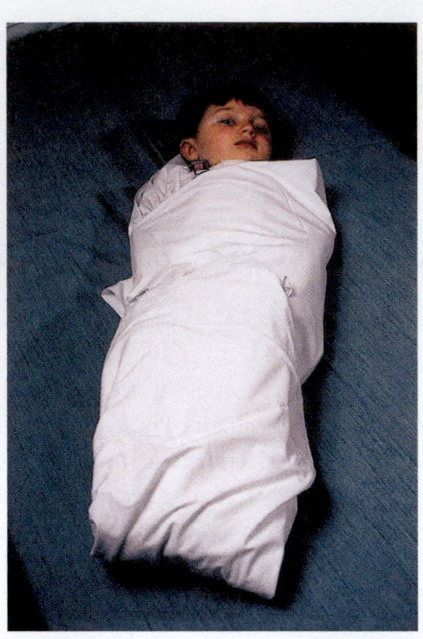

A

Figure 13-16. ■ To restrain an uncooperative child, place the child supine on the examining table. (**A**) Have an assistant hold the child's arms next to the head to restrain the child's head movements. Restrain the child's body movements by lying across the child's body. (**B**) A mummy restraint is an alternative method of restraining all but the head of a child.

B

Often, infants can be restrained by holding them in position (Figure 13-16A ■). Larger children may require a mummy wrap in a sheet (Figure 13-16B). Restraint sleeves can be used to keep a young child from bending the arms. This type of restraint is useful to prevent the child from playing with tubes or dressings applied to the arms, head, or chest. Mittens or socks can be put over the hand and pinned to the long sleeve of a shirt to keep the child from grasping and pulling. Procedure 13-12 ■ discusses steps in restraining a child.

PROCEDURE 13-12 **Restraining the Child**

Purpose
■ To maintain a child's safety during a procedure by restricting movement

Equipment
■ Papoose board
■ Large sheet or blanket, or a mummy board
■ Elbow restraints
■ Tape

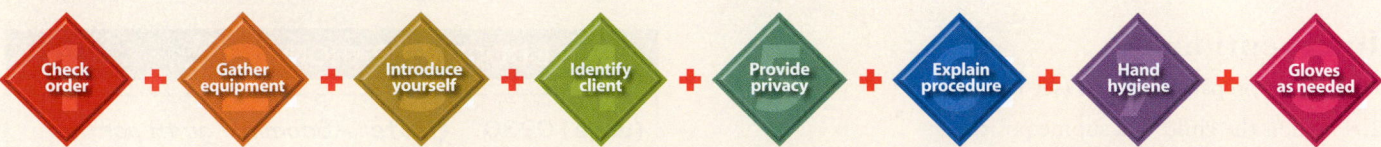

Interventions

1. Perform preparatory steps (see icon bar).

2. Obtain an order from the physician to apply restraints. If the child's safety is compromised and restraints must be applied prior to receiving the order, obtain the order within 1 hour. *Legally, the nurse must have a physician's order to apply restraints. Safety of the child is the priority.*

3. Discuss procedure with the child or the parents. *Except for small children, clients will be more compliant when the procedure is explained beforehand.*

4. Solicit the assistance of a coworker. *This will prevent injury to the child.*

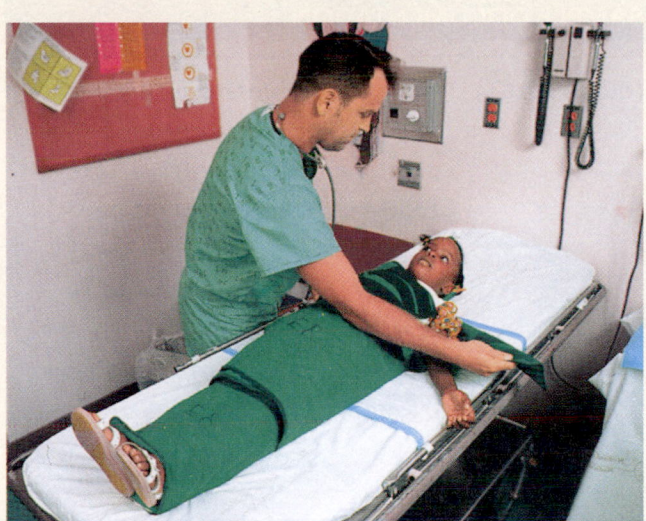

Figure 13-17. ■ Child on a papoose restraint board.

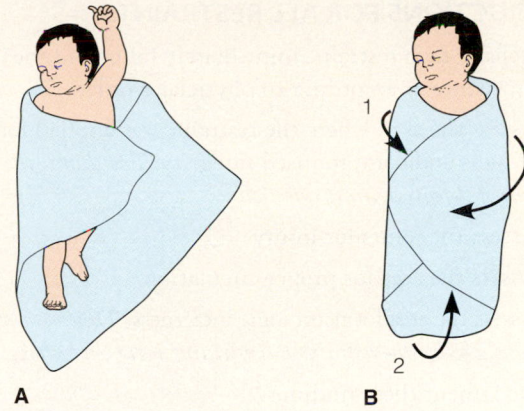

A   **B**

Figure 13-18. ■ Making a mummy restraint.

APPLYING PAPOOSE RESTRAINTS

5. Place the child in a supine position on the papoose board, which has been padded with a towel or blanket.

6. Wrap the fabric around the child according to manufacturer's recommendations (Figure 13-17 ■). Secure with Velcro, paying special attention to securing the joints. *This prevents the child from bending the joint(s) and sustaining injury.*

APPLYING MUMMY RESTRAINTS

For the Infant

5. Place the blanket on a hard surface. Position it in a diamond shape.

6. Fold down the top corner. Lay the infant in a supine position with the neck on the folded edge (Figure 13-18A ■).

7. Wrap the blanket around one arm and across the body (Figure 13-18A).

8. Weave this same part of the blanket under and over the opposite arm and tuck it under the back.

9. Fold the bottom corner of the blanket up over the infant's abdomen and tuck (Figure 13-18B). *These steps ensure a secure hold without injury*

10. Take the other side of the blanket and bring it over the infant's abdomen and then tuck it under the body (Figure 13-18B).

For the Child

5. Place the blanket on a hard surface. Position it in a diamond shape.

6. Fold down the top corner. Lay the child in a supine position with the shoulders on the folded edge.

7. Wrap one edge of the blanket to hold the arm, close to the body (as for the infant). Tuck it under the arm and under the back.

8. Take the other side of the blanket and bring it over the child's abdomen and then tuck it under the back and legs. *These steps ensure a secure hold without injury.*

APPLYING ELBOW RESTRAINTS

5. Place the elbow restraints on the child's arm. Secure the restraint according to manufacturer's recommendations. This may be with pins, ties, or Velcro. Most models are positioned from wrist to axilla (Figure 13-19 ■). *This device will not allow the child to bend the arm, and prevents the child from reaching and grabbing.*

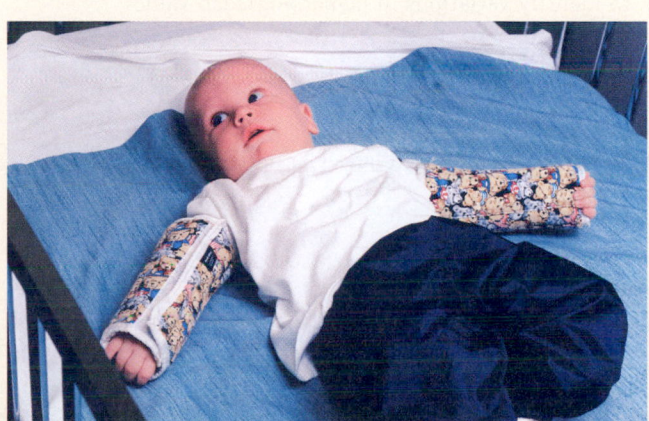

Figure 13-19. ■ Infant with elbow restraints.

INSTRUCTIONS FOR ALL RESTRAINTS

5. Release each restraint immediately following the procedure or according to physician's order.

6. Assess the skin where the restraint was applied for redness and compromised integrity. *The skin is the first line of defense against infection.*

7. Assess the joints for injury.

8. Assess the area for proper circulation.

9. Assess the area for neurologic intactness. *These measures determine whether the restraint is constricting nerve conduction.*

10. Document these findings.

SAMPLE DOCUMENTATION

(date) 1000 *(Note: Restraints portion only. This is a focused part of a complete documentation entry.)* Elbow restraints applied per policy following initiation of IV therapy. No redness noted to hand. Nail beds blanch with immediate return of blood flow. C. Rome, LPN

SPECIMEN COLLECTION

There are many specimens that may need to be obtained for effective treatment of a child. These specimens include blood, urine, stool, wound drainage, sputum, spinal fluid, and throat. Throat cultures are unpleasant for the child and often stimulate the gag reflex, resulting in vomiting. Care must be taken to prevent trauma to the oral pharynx. The head should be held still while the mouth is opened and the pharynx is swabbed.

Collecting urine and stool specimens is a particular challenge with children. Older children may be embarrassed at the thought. Age-specific instruction is essential, and the nurse may obtain assistance from the parent. Stool specimens can be collected directly from the diaper with a tongue blade. To collect a urine specimen from infants and non–toilet-trained children, a urine collection bag is used. It is important to check the bag frequently for leakage and skin irritation. Methods for collecting specimens are provided in Procedures 13-13 ■ to 13-18 ■.

PROCEDURE 13-13 **Obtaining Blood Specimens**

Purpose

■ To identify variations in hematologic lab values

Equipment

Capillary test:

■ Lancet
■ Automatic pen to hold lancet, if desired
■ Alcohol swab
■ Collection card
■ Reagent strip
■ Capillary tube
■ Glucometer

Venous and blood cultures:

■ Tourniquet
■ 20- to 27-gauge needle
■ **Vacutainer**® (a hollow, plastic device with a shielded or blunted needle on one end and a sharp needle on the other end that enters the vein) (Figure 13-20 ■); facilitates the collection of blood specimens
■ Variety of collection tubes or culture media collection bottles
■ Gloves (clean for capillary and venipuncture, sterile for blood culture collection)

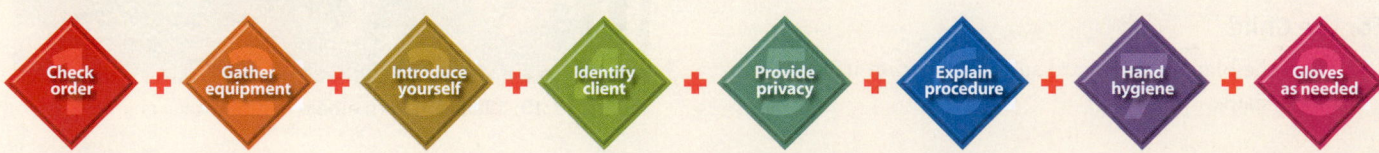

Check order + Gather equipment + Introduce yourself + Identify client + Provide privacy + Explain procedure + Hand hygiene + Gloves as needed

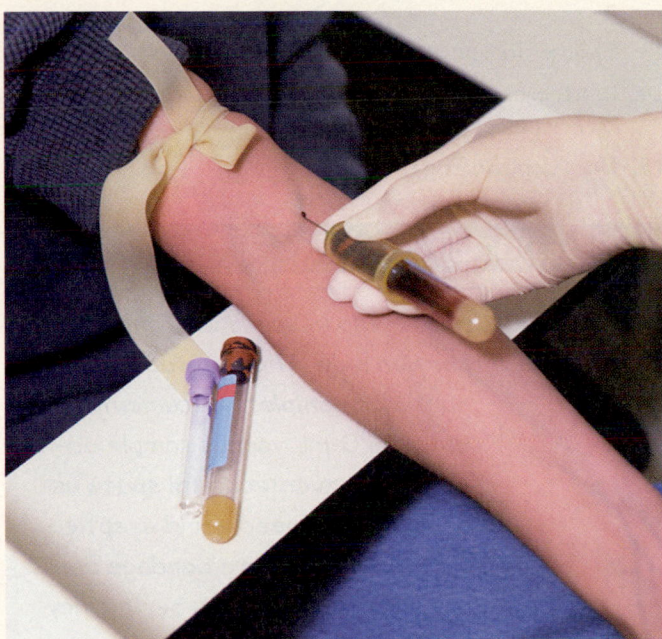

Figure 13-20. ■ Vacutainer® is used in collecting blood specimens.
(Getty Images Photodisc)

Interventions

1. Perform preparatory steps (see icon bar).
2. *Note:* ALWAYS work within the nursing practice acts of your state and within facility guidelines.
3. Solicit the assistance of a coworker. *This will help prevent injury to the child.*

CAPILLARY SPECIMENS

4. Cleanse site (fingertip or heel) with alcohol or soap and water. *Repeated exposure to alcohol may make the site tough and inappropriate for future collection of specimens.*
5. Puncture the site using the lancet. Obtain at least one drop of blood.

6. Collect specimen onto desired source (collection card, reagent strip, or collection tube).
7. If obtaining a specimen for glucose monitoring, insert reagent into glucometer and proceed according to manufacturer's recommendations.

VENOUS SPECIMENS (FIGURE 13-21A–C ■)

4. Apply a tourniquet proximal to the intended site for venipuncture. *Restricting blood flow to the site allows venous pooling at the site, dilating the vein for easier access.*
5. Determine the appropriate site for specimen collection, using inspection and palpation.
6. Cleanse the site with alcohol or povidone-iodine (according to agency policy). *Be sure to verify that the child is not allergic to povidone-iodine.* Use firm pressure beginning at the center of the site, creating a circular pattern. *This technique will reduce the likelihood of transferring harmful bacteria to the puncture site (Figure 13-21B).*
7. Steady the site by using the nondominant hand to displace the skin just below the site. Be careful not to touch the previously cleansed site. *This maintains the sterile site and aids insertion of the needle.*
8. Hold the needle with attached Vacutainer, bevel up, at a 15- to 20-degree angle above the previously cleansed site. Insert the needle. Advance until blood return occurs (Figure 13-21C).
9. Insert desired collection tube(s).
10. Release tourniquet. *This lessens the pressure, slowing blood flow.*
11. Carefully remove needle and apply pressure to the site. *This ensures that bleeding has ceased.*
12. Cleanse site and apply bandage if necessary. Allow the child to select the type of Band-Aid. *Band-Aids often give the child ownership of the procedure, provide a distraction, and serve as a source of pride for bravery during the procedure.*

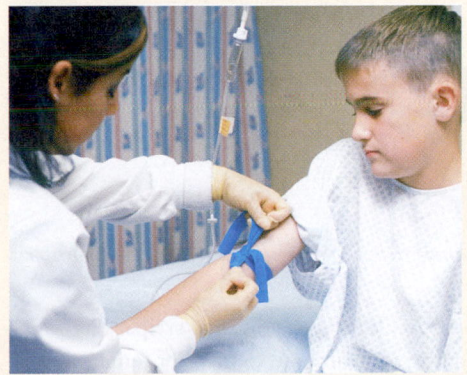
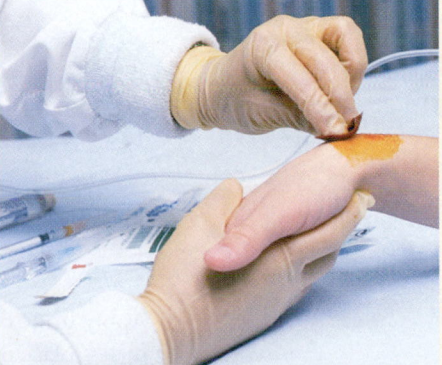
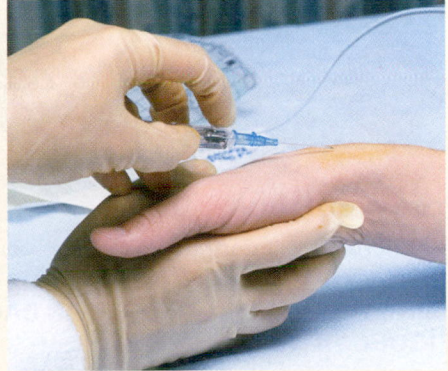

A   **B**   **C**

Figure 13-21. ■ Venipuncture procedure. **(A)** The tourniquet is applied to restrict venous blood flow. **(B)** The area for venipuncture is cleaned by the nurse with Betadine and alcohol solutions and dried with a cotton ball. **(C)** The needle is placed with the bevel up and gently inserted into the identified vein.

13. Label, package, and transport specimen according to agency policy.

BLOOD CULTURES

4. Apply sterile gloves.

5. Proceed as outlined previously for venipuncture, using needle with attached syringe.

6. Withdraw approximately 20 mL of blood.

7. Carefully remove contaminated needle.

8. Discard used needle or syringe and replace with sterile needle using sterile technique.

9. Cleanse top of each collection bottle with an antimicrobial agent.

10. Insert blood specimen in collection bottle. Gently mix. *The blood specimen needs to be mixed with the culture medium to obtain reliable test results.*

11. As ordered, repeat the procedure at desired intervals using another peripheral site and sterile needle for each venipuncture.

12. Apply pressure to site. *This ensures that bleeding has ceased.*

13. Cleanse site and apply bandage if necessary.

14. Label, package, and transport specimen according to agency policy.

15. Document findings.

SAMPLE DOCUMENTATION

(date) 1500   *(Note: Blood specimen collection portion only. This is a focused part of a complete documentation entry.)* 20-mL venous sample obtained from antecubital space using 20-gauge needle and aseptic technique. Pressure bandage applied. Specimen to lab per agency policy for basic metabolic panel.
_____ N. Thomas, LVN

PROCEDURE 13-14   Obtaining Urine Specimens

Purpose

■ To obtain information concerning chemical composition of the urine sample
■ To determine the presence of harmful bacteria or blood in the urine specimen

Equipment

■ Infant collection bag or sterile collection container
■ Soap, sterile water, and sterile cotton swabs or prepackaged antiseptic wipes
■ Alcohol wipes
■ Sterile needle with 20-mL syringe (from indwelling catheter only)

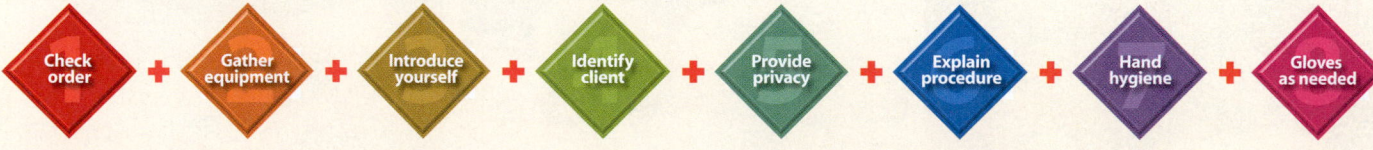

Check order ✛ Gather equipment ✛ Introduce yourself ✛ Identify client ✛ Provide privacy ✛ Explain procedure ✛ Hand hygiene ✛ Gloves as needed

Interventions

1. Perform preparatory steps (see icon bar).

USING AN INFANT COLLECTION BAG (FIGURE 13-22 ■)

2. Cleanse the perineum. Wipe with soap, water, and cotton ball from tip of penis to scrotum for males and clitoris to anus for females. Discard cotton ball. Repeat twice. Rinse with sterile water. *Cleansing removes*

micro-organisms and foreign matter that might alter laboratory results.

3. Apply urine collection bag with adhesive strips. For males, place over the scrotum and penis. For females, place over entire labia majora (Figure 13-22A).

4. Apply diaper over the urine collection bag to secure. *The diaper will support the device and prevent the infant from handling the collection bag.*

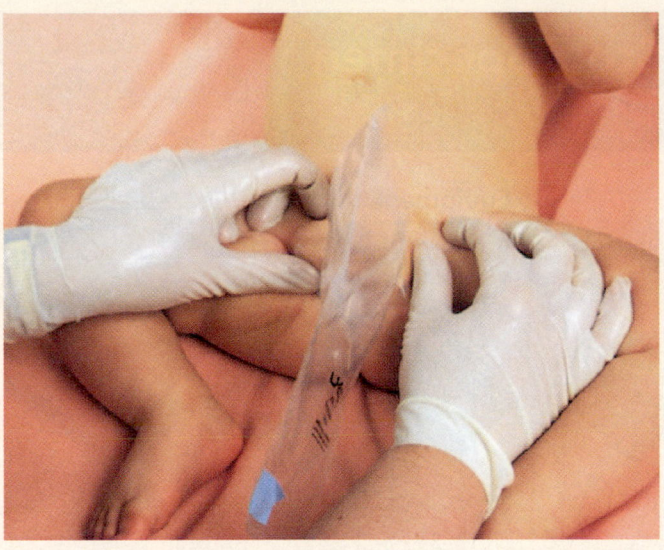
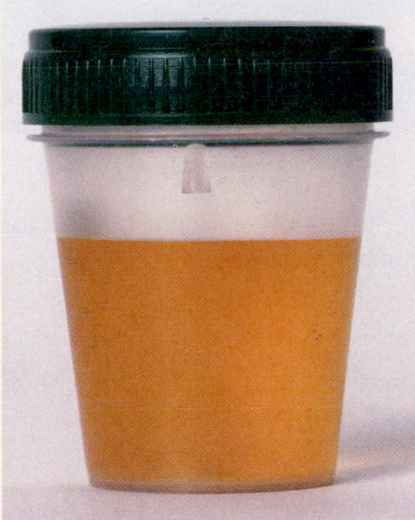

Figure 13-22. ■ **(A)** Attaching the urine collection bag. **(B)** Urine cup. (© Dorling Kindersley Media Library)

5. When specimen is obtained, remove gently from the infant's skin.

6. Place entire bag in sterile specimen container.

7. Label, package, and transport specimen according to agency policy.

OBTAINING A CLEAN CATCH SPECIMEN

2. Instruct the child to cleanse the perineum. The LPN/LVN may need to assist in this process, using clean gloves, if the child is unable. For a male, use a cleansing swab or soap and water to cleanse the head of the penis in a circular pattern beginning at the tip of the penis and moving outward. *Note:* If the male has foreskin, it should be retracted. For a female, separate the labia and cleanse from the clitoris to the anus. *Note:* Three cleansing swabs should be used. *This technique lessens the likelihood of carrying bacteria toward the urinary meatus. Separate swabs prevent reinfection.*

3. Ask the child to initiate urination.

4. If possible, have the child stop the stream, place the sterile urine container (Figure 13-22B), and begin flow again.

5. Remove container. Instruct child to finish emptying the bladder.

6. Label, package, and transport specimen according to agency policy.

OBTAINING A STERILE URINE SPECIMEN FROM AN INDWELLING CATHETER

2. Clamp the catheter for a few minutes to obtain a specimen.

3. Cleanse the catheter port with an alcohol swab. *This minimizes contamination of specimen with bacteria.*

4. Insert sterile needle with attached syringe into port.

5. Withdraw specimen.

6. Inject specimen into sterile specimen container without touching the sides of the container with the needle or syringe.

7. Unclamp the catheter.

8. Label, package, and transport specimen according to agency policy.

SAMPLE DOCUMENTATION

(date) 1300 (*Note: Urine specimen portion only. This is a focused part of a complete documentation entry.*) Urine collection bag attached to male infant according to agency policy. 30 mL clear, yellow urine obtained. Transferred to sterile specimen container and sent to lab for urinalysis. _____
B. Brockway, LVN

PROCEDURE 13-15 | **Obtaining a Stool Specimen**

Purpose

- To determine the presence of harmful bacteria, parasites, or blood in the stool specimen

Equipment

- Tongue blade or cotton swabs
- Stool specimen container
- Guaiac card and solution for occult blood

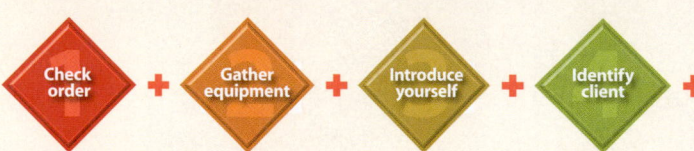

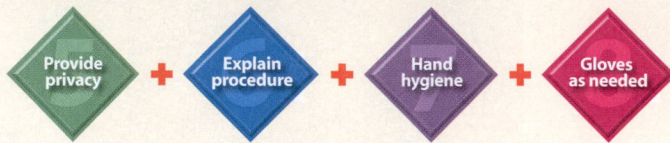

Interventions

1. Perform preparatory steps (see icon bar).

2. Obtain stool specimen from diaper, bedpan, or commode.

3. Remove amount of specimen needed for particular test with tongue blades or cotton swabs. (Some tests require 2 tsp. Others require the entire specimen.)

4. Place specimen in stool specimen container (Figure 13-23 ■).

5. Label, package, and transport specimen according to agency policy.

TESTING FOR OCCULT BLOOD

3. Smear a thin layer of stool onto the guaiac card.

4. Apply test solution according to manufacturer's instructions.

5. Read results. Document negative or positive findings. Report positive findings.

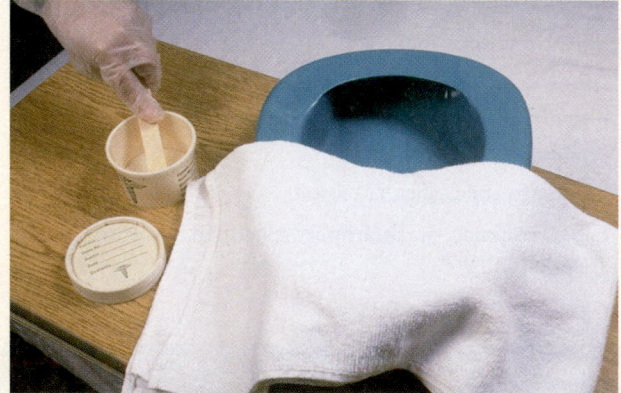

Figure 13-23. ■ Equipment for a stool specimen. In the case of an infant or toddler, the specimen could be collected from a soiled diaper. (George Dodson/Pearson Education/PH College)

SAMPLE DOCUMENTATION

(date) 0745 *(Note: Stool specimen portion only. This is a focused part of a complete documentation entry.)* Stool specimen obtained from infant's diaper. Sent to lab for culture. _____
K. David, LPN

PROCEDURE 13-16 | **Obtaining Sample for Wound or Throat Culture**

Purpose

- To assist in the detection of harmful bacteria that may be present in wounds, body cavities, or throat

Equipment

- Sterile swab
- Culturette with preserving medium
- Penlight

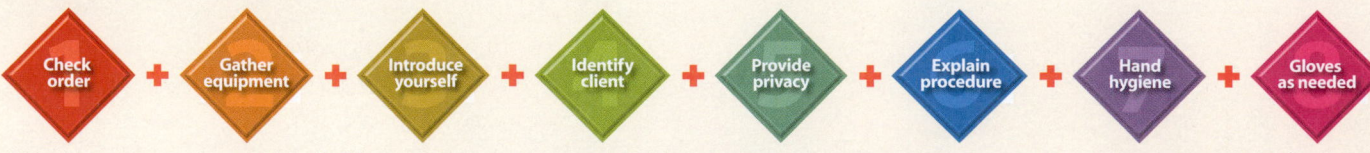

Interventions

1. Perform preparatory steps (see icon bar).
2. Gently swab the area to be cultured (Figure 13-24 ■).

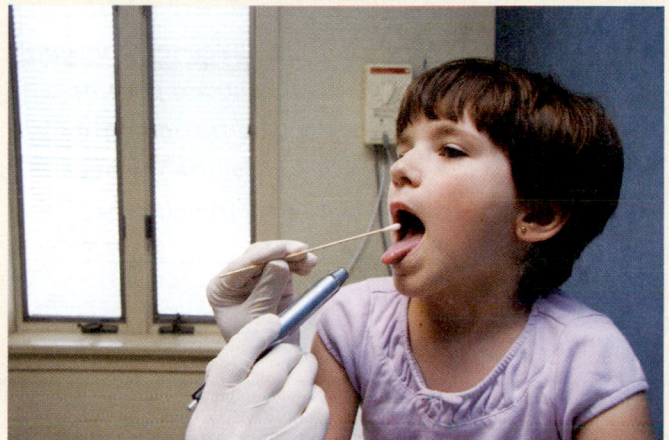

Figure 13-24. ■ A long cotton-tipped applicator can be used as a throat swab or wound swab.
(Molly Schlachter/Pearson Education/PH College)

3. Carefully place swab into preserving medium without touching the sides of the tube. *This ensures that bacteria is transferred to the medium and does not adhere to the tube.*
4. Label, package, and transport specimen to lab according to agency policy.

SAMPLE DOCUMENTATION

(date) 1630   *(Note: Wound specimen portion only. This is a focused part of a complete documentation entry.)* Specimen obtained from abdominal incision. Thick, green exudate noted. _____

B. Smartt, LPN

PROCEDURE 13-17 # Obtaining a Sputum Specimen

Purpose

■ To assist in the detection of harmful bacteria that may be present in respiratory secretions

Equipment

■ Sterile suction catheter with attached suction trap
■ Sterile saline
■ Sterile specimen container

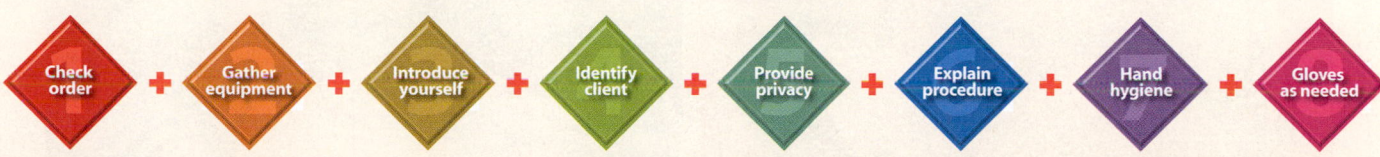

Check order + Gather equipment + Introduce yourself + Identify client + Provide privacy + Explain procedure + Hand hygiene + Gloves as needed

Interventions

1. Perform preparatory steps (see icon bar).

FROM AN INFANT

2. Attach the suction tubing to low suction.
3. Place the catheter in the infant's nose.
4. Clear secretions from tubing with sterile saline (see Procedure 13-25).

5. Label, package, and transport specimen to lab according to agency policy.

FROM A CHILD

2. Place the child in a seated position.
3. Instruct the child to take several deep breaths. *This will help cause the client to cough deeply.*

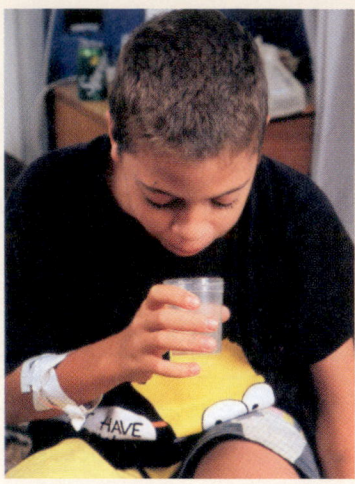

Figure 13-25. ■ Child supplying a sputum specimen.

4. Ask the child to spit sputum into the sterile specimen container (Figure 13-25 ■).
5. Label, package, and transport specimen to lab according to agency policy.

SAMPLE DOCUMENTATION

(date) 1000   (*Note: Sputum specimen portion only. This is a focused part of a complete documentation entry.*) Small amount of white, viscous sputum obtained for culture. Specimen to lab. _____
A. Evans, LVN

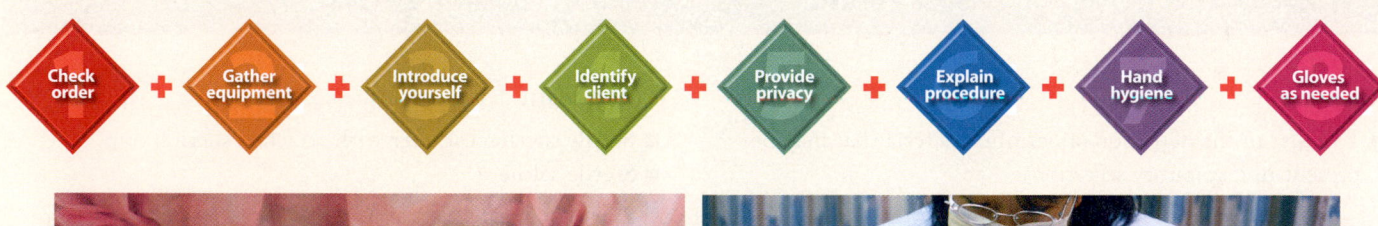

PROCEDURE 13-18 Positioning a Child for Lumbar Puncture

Purpose
- To provide safety during the lumbar puncture
- To assist the practitioner in obtaining a spinal fluid specimen

Equipment
- Clean gloves
- Light source

Check order + Gather equipment + Introduce yourself + Identify client + Provide privacy + Explain procedure + Hand hygiene + Gloves as needed

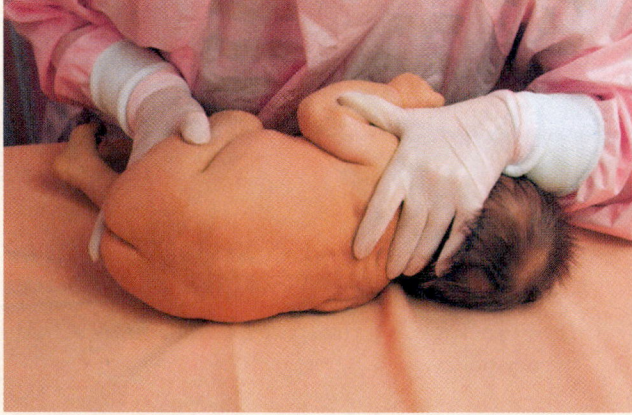

A

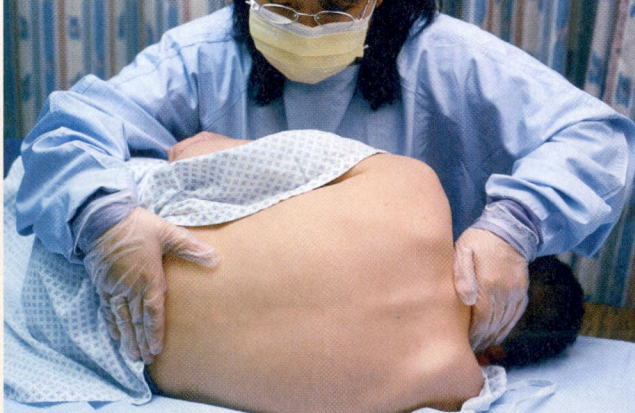

B

Figure 13-26. ■ (**A**) Infant positioned for a lumbar puncture. (**B**) Child positioned for a lumbar puncture.

Interventions

1. Perform preparatory steps (see icon bar).

2. Solicit the assistance of a coworker. *This will help prevent injury to the child.*

3. Position the infant in a lateral position (Figure 13-26A ■). Hold the infant by placing one hand behind the neck and one hand around the thighs, maintaining a curve in the spine.

4. Position child in a lateral position (Figure 13-26B). Ask the child to flex both the neck and the knees. Hold the child by placing one hand behind the neck and one hand around the hips.

5. Talk quietly and gently to the child during the procedure. *This serves to lower anxiety levels and increase compliance.*

SAMPLE DOCUMENTATION

(date) 0900   *(Note: Positioning portion only. This is a focused part of a complete documentation entry.)* Assisted child into lateral position, knees and neck flexed. Position secured during lumbar puncture. No complaints voiced following procedure. _____ A. McIntire, LPN

ASSISTING WITH NUTRITION

Feeding a Child

There are occasions when the nurse may need to feed a child orally (Procedure 13-19 ■). A child who has had surgery and is in pain may need assistance with nutrition. The visually impaired child may also need help. If increased calories are essential to the child's health, it may be necessary for the nurse to be present at all meals and to encourage increased food intake. Mealtime should be pleasant and stress free. Forcing a child to eat puts the child at risk for aspiration because of crying or struggling.

Often, giving the child choices will reinforce independence and protect dignity.

TUBE FEEDING

There are several types of tubes through which a liquid food may be introduced to the client for hydration or nourishment. In gavage feeding, the stomach tube is inserted through the nares, pharynx, and esophagus, and into the stomach. Care must be taken to ensure that the tube is in the stomach before the liquid nourishment is introduced (discussed in Proce-

PROCEDURE 13-19 Feeding a Child Orally

Purpose

■ To encourage the child in obtaining adequate nutritional intake

Equipment

■ Child-size utensils
■ Straws
■ Divided plates to keep food separate

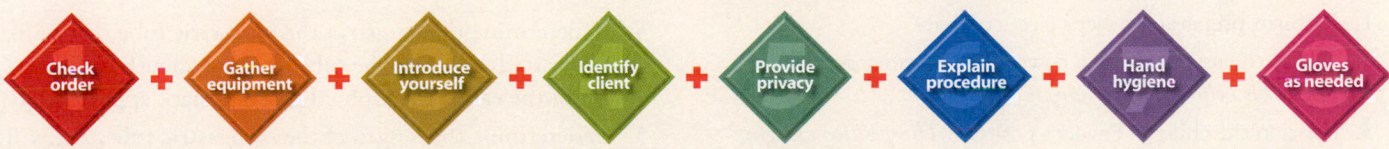

Interventions

1. Perform preparatory steps (see icon bar).
2. Create an environment conducive to eating. Limit distractions. Remove items with strong odors. Consider feeding child in an area other than the hospital room.
3. Cut food into bite-size pieces. *This will help prevent choking.*
4. Offer the child's favorite foods if they are allowable to prescribed diet. *This encourages compliance.*
5. Use straw in a covered drink container. *This will avoid spills.*
6. Use praise only and avoid negative comments. *This will make mealtime pleasant and encourage the child to eat.*
7. Document the percentage of meal eaten.

---

dures 13-20 ■ and 13-21 ■). After the fluid is instilled or after the tube feeding is finished, the tube is removed. It is reinserted for the next feeding. In some agencies, introduction of the feeding tube in a small infant is not an LPN/LVN function. However, gastric suction may be performed by the LPN/LVN in most facilities (Procedure 13-22 ■).

If tube feeding is expected to be a long-term necessity, the physician may insert a gastric tube or jejunostomy tube.

Liquid nourishment can then be introduced. The tube remains in place between feedings. Skin care around the tube is important to prevent skin breakdown and infection. At times, the tube needs to be replaced. Once the stoma has healed, the gastric or jejunostomy tube can be replaced by the LPN/LVN according to state Board of Nursing rules and agency policy.

PROCEDURE 13-20   Inserting and Removing an Orogastric and Nasogastric Tube

Purpose

- To provide nutritional supplementation or medications
- To remove stomach contents

Equipment

- Orogastric or nasogastric tubes in a variety of sizes
- Suction equipment
- Litmus paper
- Water-soluble lubricant
- 20-mL syringe

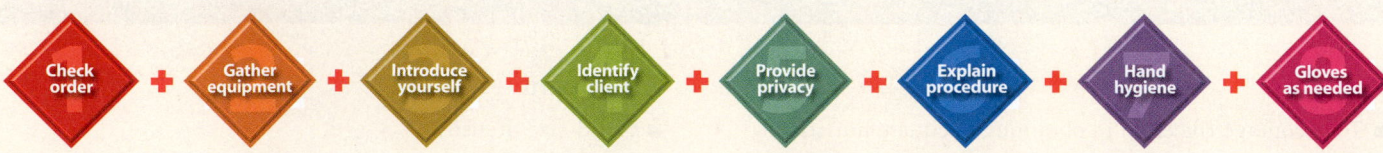

Check order + Gather equipment + Introduce yourself + Identify client + Provide privacy + Explain procedure + Hand hygiene + Gloves as needed

Interventions

1. Perform preparatory steps (see icon bar).
2. Solicit the assistance of a coworker. Consider restraints prn. *This helps prevent injury to the child.*
3. Position the child in Fowler's position. *This position uses gravity when inserting the tube and helps minimize aspiration of fluid.*
4. To determine the length of the orogastric tube that will be inserted, measure the tube from the mouth to the tragus of the ear to the xiphoid process. Mark appropriately.
5. To determine the length of the nasogastric tube that will be inserted, measure the tube from the tip of the nose to

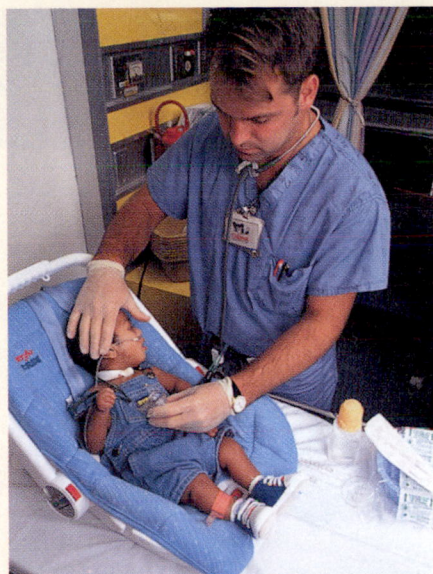

A

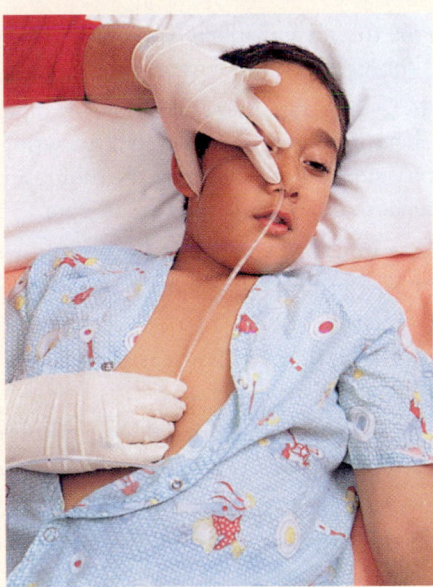

B

Figure 13-27. ■ Measuring for nasogastric tube placement. (**A**) Infant. (**B**) Child. (A similar technique is used in measuring for orogastric tube insertion.)

the tragus of the ear to the xiphoid process (Figure 13-27 ■). Mark appropriately.

6. Apply lubricant to the tip of the tube for easier insertion.

7. For the orogastric tube, insert the tube into the child's mouth with the neck hyperextended and advance it toward back of the throat. Continue advancing until mark is reached.

8. For the nasogastric tube, insert the tube into the child's nares with the neck hyperextended and advance it straight. If resistance is met, increase pressure slightly or rotate the tube. Continue advancing until mark is reached.

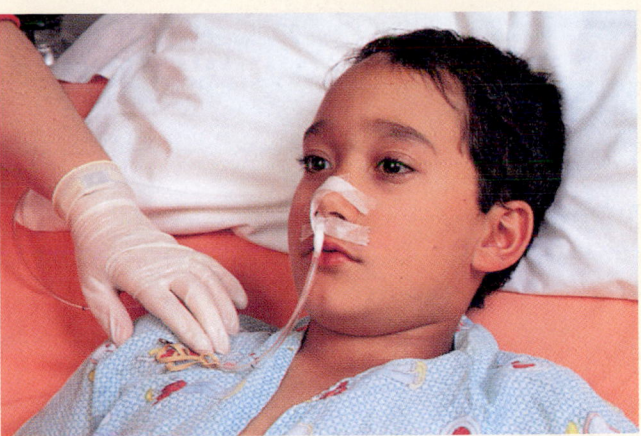

Figure 13-28. ■ Nasogastric tube taped securely in place.

9. Use the syringe to aspirate a small amount of gastric content. Test the pH of the gastric contents using the litmus paper. *A pH of 3 or less indicates gastric contents and, therefore, proper placement.*

10. Secure the tube with tape or (if available) a manufactured product that holds nasogastric tubes in place (Figure 13-28 ■). *It is important to secure the tube to prevent it from dislodging.*

TUBE REMOVAL

11. Position the child in Fowler's position to avoid aspiration if gagging occurs.

12. Cover the child's chest with a towel. *Secretions sometimes drip off the tube when it is removed.*

13. Put 10 to 20 mL of air into the tube to remove secretions in tube.

14. Remove tape, ask the child to hold his or her breath and close the eyes. Then clamp and gently withdraw the tube. *This prevents secretions from getting in the eyes.*

15. Suction prn.

SAMPLE DOCUMENTATION

(date) 1600   (Note: Nasogastric tube portion only. This is a focused part of a complete documentation entry.) NG tube inserted per agency policy. Aspiration of gastric contents reveals pH 2. Low suction attached. No nausea or GI distress noted. ___ J. Baker, LPN

Gavage tube

MediaLink

PROCEDURE 13-21 Administering a Gavage/Tube Feeding

Purpose

■ To provide nutritional support when the child is unable to obtain adequate calories orally

Equipment

■ Nutritional supplementation
■ Tap water
■ 20-mL syringe
■ Clean towel

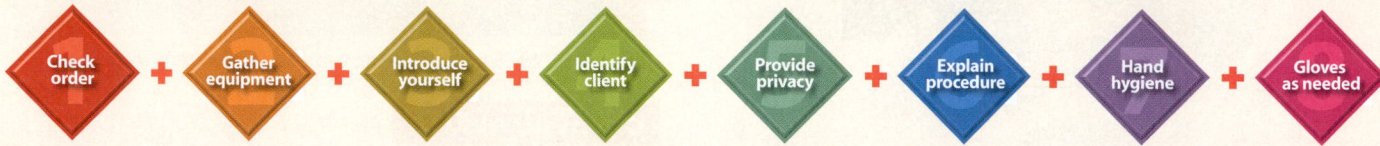

Check order + Gather equipment + Introduce yourself + Identify client + Provide privacy + Explain procedure + Hand hygiene + Gloves as needed

Interventions

1. Perform preparatory steps (see icon bar).

2. Allow nutritional supplement to reach room temperature. *This will prevent cramping.*

3. Position the child in a Fowler's or high Fowler's position. Place a towel across the child's abdomen. *This position prevents aspiration, and the towel helps keep the child's clothing free of soiling.*

4. Check placement (see Procedure 13-20).

5. Assess residual gastric volume. *The feeding should be withheld if the residual volume is too great because this indicates that digestion may be altered. The agency may designate this volume, and the physician may include the residual volume in the original order.*

6. Flush the tubing with tap water. *This is necessary to clear the tubing of gastric contents.*

7. Clamp the tubing and attach barrel of syringe or primed tubing for continuous feeding.

8. For bolus feeding, raise barrel of syringe no more than 18 inches above the child's abdomen. Fill the syringe with nutritional supplement. Unclamp the tubing and allow supplement to flow slowly into tube (Figure 13-29 ■).

9. Watch the infusion carefully and do not allow air into the tube. Clamp the tubing. *Air could cause the child to have gas.*

10. Maintain the child in the Fowler's position for 1 to 2 hours. *This will prevent aspiration.*

11. Follow the bolus feeding with a flush of tap water. *The amount of the flush will typically be ordered by the physician.*

12. For continuous feeding, label the bag with date and time. Set the rate as prescribed and monitor it closely.

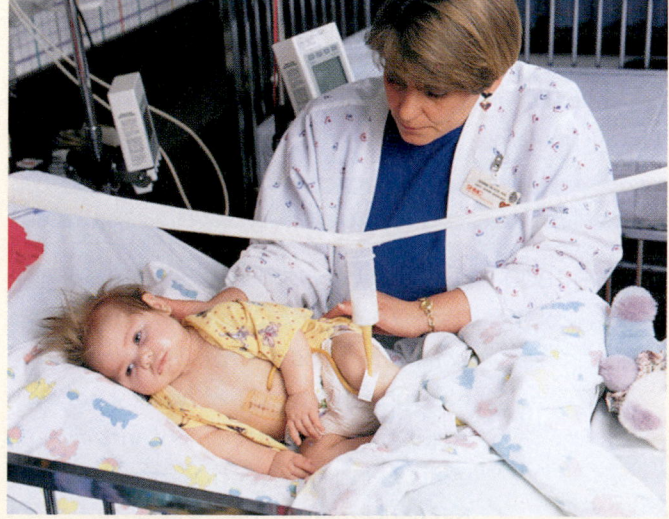

Figure 13-29. ■ Gravity assists the flow of a gavage feeding to this hospitalized infant.

SAMPLE DOCUMENTATION

(date) 0845 *(Note: Gavage/tube feeding portion only. This is a focused part of a complete documentation entry.)* No gastric residual obtained. Orogastric tube flushed with 10 mL tap water. 30 mL Enfamil with iron given bolus via orogastric tube. 30 mL tap water flushed following feeding. HOB at 45 degrees. _____ A. David, LPN

PROCEDURE 13-22 Performing Gastric Suction

Purpose
■ To remove gastric contents for further evaluation or decompression

Equipment
■ Suction equipment
■ Litmus paper

Check order + **Gather equipment** + **Introduce yourself** + **Identify client** + **Provide privacy** + **Explain procedure** + **Hand hygiene** + **Gloves as needed**

Interventions
1. Perform preparatory steps (see icon bar).
2. Check for proper tube placement (see Procedure 13-20).
3. Attach gastric tube to suction equipment.
4. Suction according to physician order.
5. Document color, consistency, and amount of gastric contents suctioned.

SAMPLE DOCUMENTATION

(date) 1515 1350   (Note: Gastric suction portion only. This is a focused part of a complete documentation entry.) 10 mL thin, green gastric contents suctioned from nasogastric tube. No distress noted. _____
C. Tolbert, LVN

There are many commercially prepared tube feeding formulas. The specific formula to meet the nutritional needs of the child is ordered by the doctor. All opened containers should be stored in the refrigerator. The liquid nourishment must be administered at room temperature to avoid stomach cramping.

Giving small amounts of tube feeding frequently is safer than introducing large quantities that might overdistend the stomach and cause vomiting or aspiration. At times, feedings are introduced by an intermittent bolus. At other times, feedings are by slow continuous infusion. It is important to assess the amount of residual tube feeding fluid periodically to determine if the feeding is being digested. **Residual volume** is the amount of the feeding that remains in the client's stomach. It is obtained by aspirating and measuring gastric contents before the feeding is begun. If the residual volume is equal to or greater than the amount of feeding being given per hour, stop the feeding and re-evaluate in 1 hour. If the residual volume continues to be high, it is an indication that the child is not digesting the nourishment properly. If this finding is assessed, the supervising nurse and/or physician should be notified. Most facilities have their own protocols for handling tube feedings and residual volumes.

ASSISTING WITH ELIMINATION

The nurse can assist in promoting normal elimination patterns by encouraging a diet adequate in fiber and fluids, as well as regular exercise. If the child becomes constipated, oral medication, suppositories, or an enema might be ordered (Figure 13-30 ■). The administration of a suppository or enema is an invasive procedure, so age-specific instructions are essential. To ensure the child's safety during these procedures, a second nurse may be needed to help restrain the child. Procedure 13-23 ■ provides information on assisting with bowel elimination.

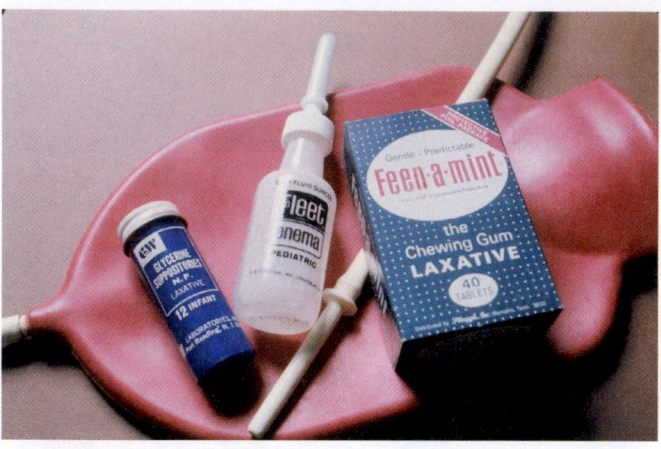

Figure 13-30. ■ Enema equipment, suppositories, and laxatives.
(Pearson Education/PH College)

Enema

Administer the solution ordered by the physician. Commercially prepared solutions are available in pediatric dosage. The solution should be isotonic to prevent fluid shift into or out of the cells. A smaller volume of solution, administered with less pressure, is needed for children. The following volumes are given unless other volumes are ordered by the physician:

Infant = 40–100 mL
Toddler = 100–200 mL
Preschooler = 200–300 mL
School age = 300–500 mL
Adolescent = 500–700 mL

PROCEDURE 13-23 Administering an Enema

Purpose
■ To clear the bowel of feces, relieving constipation
■ To prepare the bowel for a procedure

Equipment
■ Solution ordered

■ Enema container or bag with attached tubing. For the infant, syringe with bulb or size 10 to 12 French rectal tube. For the child, size 14 to 18 French rectal tube.
■ Water-soluble lubricant
■ Waterproof pads
■ Bedpan, bedside commode, or accessible bathroom

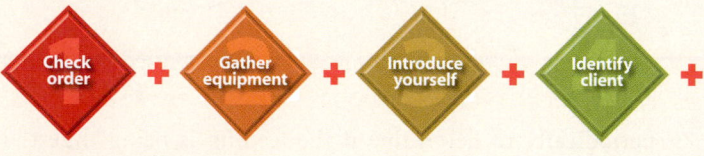

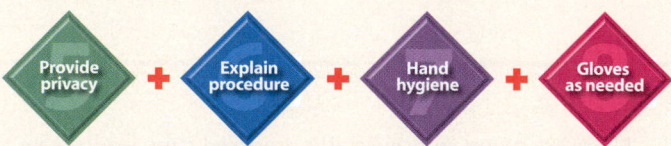

Interventions

1. Perform preparatory steps (see icon bar).
2. Solicit the assistance of a coworker. *This will help prevent injury to the child.*
3. Prepare equipment. Prime the tubing. Ensure appropriate temperature.
4. Position the child in a left lateral position, knees flexed. Place waterproof pad underneath the child.
5. Lubricate tip of rectal tube with water-soluble lubricant.
6. Insert the rectal tube. For the infant, 1 to 1.5 inches. For the child, 2 to 3 inches.
7. Raise the container above the child's hips. Avoid raising it higher than 12 to 18 inches. *Raising the container higher than the recommended height will cause an increased pressure gradient on the colon. This could cause colon damage.*
8. Open the clamp and allow fluid to infuse slowly over 10 to 15 minutes.
9. Gently remove rectal tube, asking the child to hold the fluid for the prescribed amount of time. For the infant, the buttocks are held together.
10. Assist the child on the bedpan or to the bedside commode or bathroom to expel the contents of the enema.
11. Assist the child with hygiene measures.

SAMPLE DOCUMENTATION

(date) 0630 (*Note: Enema portion only. This is a focused part of a complete documentation entry.*) 100-mL soap suds enema given. _____ M. McCune, LPN

(date) 0640 Assisted to BR to expel enema. _____ M. McCune, LPN

(date) 0655 Approximately 100 mL enema expelled. Assisted with perineal and anal hygiene. _____ M. McCune, LPN

PROCEDURE 13-24 **Inserting an Indwelling Catheter**

Purpose

■ To provide continuous decompression of the bladder

Equipment

■ Disposable catheterization tray containing the appropriate size catheter and sterile equipment for cleansing the perineum
■ Tape
■ Light source

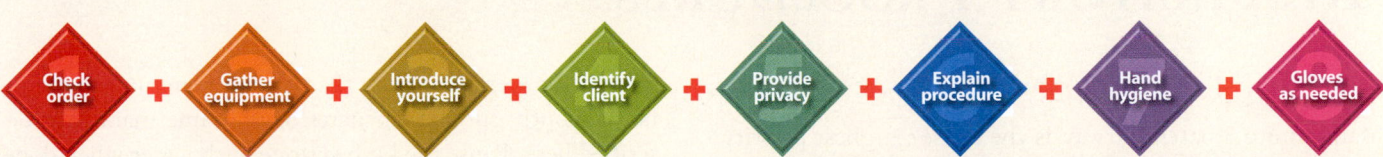

Check order + Gather equipment + Introduce yourself + Identify client + Provide privacy + Explain procedure + Hand hygiene + Gloves as needed

Interventions

1. Perform preparatory steps (see icon bar).
2. Solicit the assistance of a coworker. *This will help prevent injury to the child.*
3. Provide for the child's privacy.
4. Position the child in a supine position with knees flexed and abducted.
5. Apply sterile gloves.
6. Prepare the equipment: Pour antiseptic solution in reservoir; test the bulb for patency by injecting the syringe filled with sterile water (leaving this syringe attached to the tubing); lubricate the tip of the catheter.
7. Drape the perineum with the provided drape.
8. With the dominant hand, dredge cotton balls in antiseptic solution by holding them with forceps.
9. For the female child, separate the labia of the female child with the nondominant hand. Clean the perineum, from front to back, laterally. Discard cotton ball. Repeat on other side. Wipe midline, from urethral meatus to anus. Discard.
10. For the male child, with the nondominant hand, retracting the foreskin if necessary, grasp the penis, separate meatus with thumb and forefinger. With the dominant hand, use a circular motion to clean from the meatus outward. Discard cotton ball and repeat until head of penis has been cleansed entirely. Recommended practice is three times.
11. Use the dominant hand to pick up the lubricated catheter.
12. Insert catheter into the meatus until urine is returned or seen in tubing.
    - For the female: 2 to 3 inches plus 1 inch following presence of urine

    - For the male: 4 to 5 inches plus 1 inch following presence of urine

clinical ALERT

Do not advance the catheter using force if resistance is felt. Encourage the child to relax the perineal muscles by taking deep breaths in through the nose and out through the mouth. If this is unsuccessful, remove the catheter and obtain a size smaller. Attempt catheterization again.

13. Hold the catheter with the nondominant hand. Use the dominant hand to inflate the bulb with the attached sterile water-filled syringe.
14. Pull back gently on the catheter until resistance is met. *This documents proper placement of the bulb in the bladder.*
15. Secure the catheter by taping tubing to the child's leg.
16. Perform hygiene to remove antiseptic solution. *Antiseptic solution may cause irritation.*

SAMPLE DOCUMENTATION

(date) 1245   *(Note: Catheter portion only. This is a focused part of a complete documentation entry.)* Urinary catheter #10 inserted per sterile technique with return of clear, yellow urine. Tubing secured to leg with tape. No complaints voiced. _____
L. Lynn, LVN

Urinary Elimination

The nurse can assist in promoting normal urinary elimination by encouraging an adequate fluid intake and regular emptying of the bladder. If the child's bladder becomes distended, the nurse should encourage emptying of the bladder by assisting the child to the bathroom, providing privacy, placing the child's hand in warm water, and providing water to drink. If the child is unable to empty the bladder, urinary catheterization may be necessary (see Procedure 13-24 on p. 427).

Urinary catheterization may cause anxiety and discomfort for the child. The nurse should thoroughly explain the procedure to both the parent and the child, using a kind, soft tone when communicating with the child. Choosing the smallest size catheter and lubricating the catheter well can reduce discomfort for the child.

RESPIRATORY PROCEDURES

Airway Clearance

Maintaining a patent airway is the nurse's highest priority in client care. The nurse must be familiar with various types of suctioning equipment and be able to use them properly. A bulb syringe may be used to remove secretions from the nose and mouth of infants. This piece of equipment has the advantage of being small and portable.

Compress the bulb and insert the tip into the mouth (Figure 13-31 ■). Releasing the bulb will draw secretions into the bulb tip. Empty the bulb syringe by covering the tip with a tissue or cloth and then squeezing bulb again, forcing the secretions from the tip. After suctioning the infant's mouth, suction the nares in the same manner as described here. Rinse the bulb syringe with water when done.

Suctioning the airway of an infant or child is the same as for adults, except that a smaller size suction catheter is used. Due to the small air passages in the nose, it may be difficult to insert a suction catheter. The suction catheter can be introduced into the mouth and advanced into the pharynx. Suction is then applied to remove secretions. However, when suction is applied, air is pulled out of the lungs. For this reason, preoxygenation is important, and the *maximum* amount of time suction is applied is 5 to 10 seconds. Table 13-3 ■

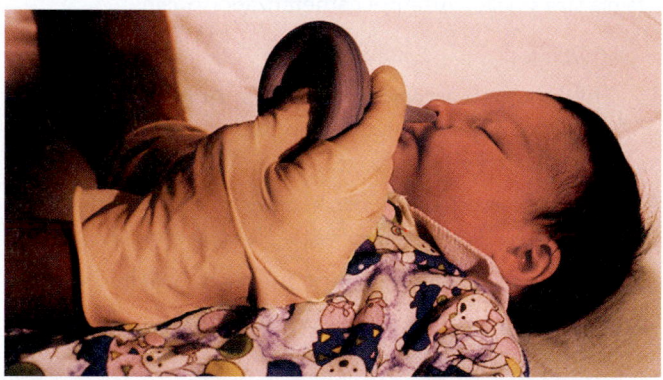

A

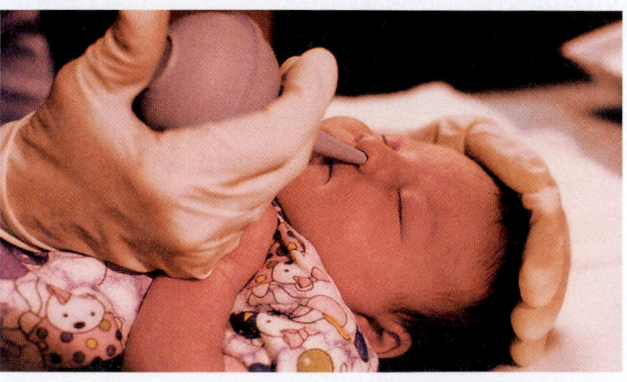

B

Figure 13-31. ■ (A) Insertion of a deflated tube bulb syringe. **(B)** Removal of a reinflated bulb syringe.

TABLE 13-3		
Suggested Endotracheal Tube and Suction Catheter Size for Children		
AGE	ENDOTRACHEAL TUBE SIZE (mm)	SUCTION CATHETER SIZE (FRENCH)
Premature newborn	2.0–2.5	5
Newborn	3.0–3.5	6–8
6 months	3.5	8
12–18 months	4.0	8
3 years	4.5	8
5 years	5.0	10
6 years	5.5	10
8 years	6.0	10
12 years	6.5	10
16 years	7.0–8.0	12

Source: Bindler, R. C., Ball, J. W., London, M. L., & Ladewig, P. W. (2003). *Clinical skills manual for maternal–newborn & child nursing.* Upper Saddle River, NJ: Prentice Hall.

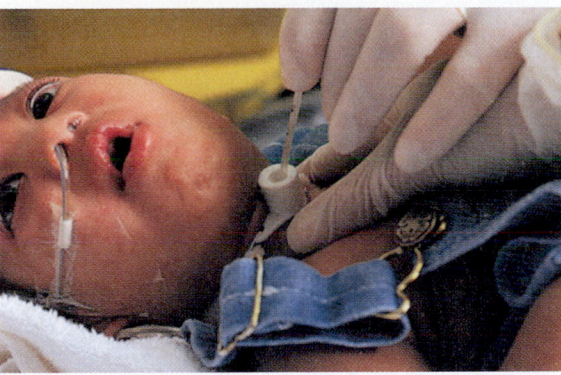

Figure 13-32. ■ Tracheostomy tube suctioning.

lists suggested endotracheal tube and suction catheter sizes.

An infant or child may have an endotracheal or tracheostomy tube for airway maintenance. Suctioning through these devices requires care and practice. The nurse, if authorized, can insert a suction catheter through the endotracheal or tracheostomy tube to remove secretions (Figure 13-32 ■). At times, the oral/pharyngeal catheter is advanced into the trachea. Follow facility policy regarding tracheal suction by an LPN/LVN. Procedure 13-25 ■ describes steps for several types of suctioning.

PROCEDURE 13-25 | # Suctioning a Child

Purpose

- To remove respiratory secretions to assist ventilation
- To obtain a specimen in order to detect harmful bacteria

Equipment

- Bulb syringe
- Normal saline
- Suction catheter, variety of sizes
- Oxygen source, resuscitation bag and mask
- Tracheostomy tubes

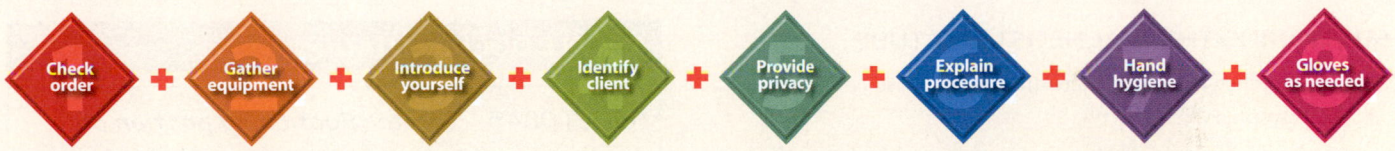

Interventions

1. Perform preparatory steps (see icon bar).
2. Solicit the assistance of a coworker. *This will help prevent injury to the child.*
3. Prior to the procedure, assess the child's breath sounds, respiratory rate and effort, and patency of airway. *This provides data for evaluating the effectiveness of the procedure.*
4. After suctioning, assess respiratory status.

USING THE BULB SYRINGE

5. Position the infant in a supine position. The older child may be in a seated position.
6. Clean the oral cavity by depressing the bulb and inserting the tip of the syringe into the left buccal cavity of the child's mouth. Repeat in the right buccal cavity. *Placing the syringe into the buccal cavity avoids eliciting the gag reflex.*
7. Depress the bulb into a tissue or towel to clear the bulb syringe.
8. Depress the bulb and place the tip of the syringe into the nares. *If the bulb is not depressed prior to insertion, air could force the secretions into the nasopharynx.*

9. Release the bulb and withdraw secretions.
10. Wipe tip of bulb to remove debris.
11. Rinse the bulb syringe by depressing it into a cup of water and flushing it out. Repeat until clean.

SUCTIONING A CONSCIOUS CHILD

5. Place child in a semi-Fowler's position with neck hyperextended.
6. Attach suction tubing to source of suction. See Table 13-3 for selecting the size of the suction catheter and the endotracheal tube. Use settings as ordered by physician or according to agency policy.
7. Apply sterile gloves. *This prevents exposure to and spread of micro-organisms.*
8. Insert the suction catheter into the nares. Close the suction port with the thumb to initiate suction. Limit suctioning to 5 to 10 seconds. Repeat in other nares.
9. Suction the mouth in the same manner.

SUCTIONING A CHILD WITH DECREASED LEVEL OF CONSCIOUSNESS

5. Administer oxygen by face mask. *Preoxygenating the child avoids hypoxia during suctioning.*

6. Position the child in a lateral position. *The lateral position can prevent aspiration because it prevents the tongue from falling back and blocking the oropharynx. It allows gravity to assist in the drainage of secretions.*

7. Apply sterile gloves.

8. Moisten the catheter with water and insert the suction catheter into the nares. *Moistening the catheter eases insertion.*

9. Close suction port with thumb to initiate suction. Limit suctioning to 5 to 10 seconds.

10. Apply oxygen mask. *This improves oxygenation.*

11. Repeat in other nares.

12. Apply oxygen mask.

13. Suction the mouth in the same manner.

14. Apply oxygen mask.

15. To remove secretions beyond the hypopharynx and trachea, advance the catheter further. Apply suction by occluding the suction port. Rotate gently upon withdrawal. *This removes secretions attached to the walls of the trachea. Rotation also prevents suction equipment from adhering to one spot.*

SUCTIONING THE TRACHEOSTOMY TUBE

5. Inform the child that suctioning may cause coughing and dyspnea.

6. Position the child in a supine position with the head of bed raised 30 degrees to prevent aspiration.

7. Attach oxygen source to resuscitation bag.

8. Apply sterile gloves.

9. Using the nondominant hand, remove the humidity source from tracheostomy tube.

10. Preoxygenate the child as ordered.

11. With the dominant hand, insert suction catheter into the tube without suction. Advance the catheter no farther than 0.5 cm below the opening of the tracheostomy tube (see Figure 13-32).

12. Apply intermittent suction, rotating the catheter during withdrawal to remove the maximum amount of secretions. Do not suction for longer than 5 to 10 seconds.

13. Withdraw the catheter completely and apply oxygen. *Suction removes both oxygen and secretions.*

SUCTIONING THE ENDOTRACHEAL TUBE

5. Position the child in a supine position with head of bed raised 30 degrees to prevent aspiration.

6. Attach oxygen source to resuscitation bag.

7. Apply sterile gloves.

8. Have assistant disconnect the ventilator.

9. Preoxygenate the child as ordered to prevent hypoxia.

10. With the dominant hand, insert the suction catheter into the tube without suction. Advance the catheter no farther than 0.5 cm below the opening of the ET tube.

11. Apply intermittent suction, rotating the catheter during withdrawal. Do not suction for longer than 5 to 10 seconds. *Rotation ensures greater removal of secretions. It also prevents suction from adhering to one spot.*

12. Withdraw the catheter completely and apply oxygen.

13. Reconnect ventilator.

14. Repeat prn.

15. Clear the suction catheter using sterile saline.

SAMPLE DOCUMENTATION

(date) 0845   *(Note: Suctioning portion only. This is a focused part of a complete documentation entry.)* R 32, uneven and labored. Cough ineffective. Rhonchi auscultated bilaterally. Sterile oral/pharyngeal suctioning performed according to policy. Moderate amount of thick, white secretions obtained. Breathing less labored, R 22. _____

J. Edward, LPN

Oxygen Administration

Oxygen can be administered to an infant or child by cannula, catheter, mask, hood, or tent (Figure 13-33 ■; Procedure 13-26 ■). The method of administration is determined by the amount of oxygen required and the client's tolerance. High concentrations of oxygen given over a long period of time can be damaging to some body tissues. Retinal damage and lung disorders from oxygen administration are discussed in Chapter 18 of this text. Frequent assessment of blood oxygen concentration

(Text continues on p. 432.)

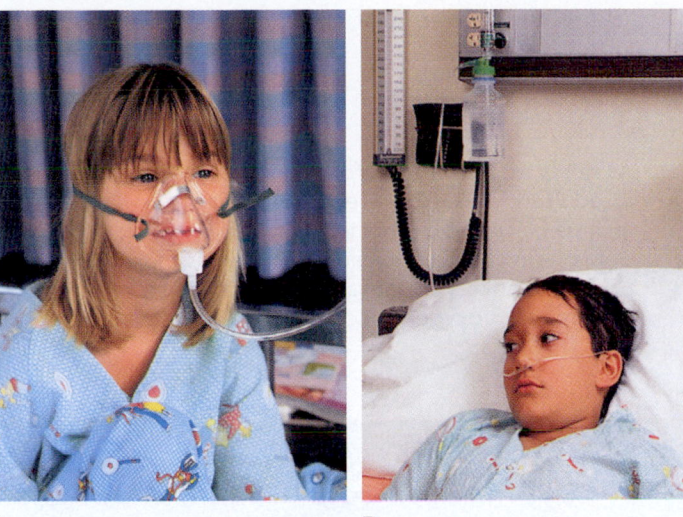 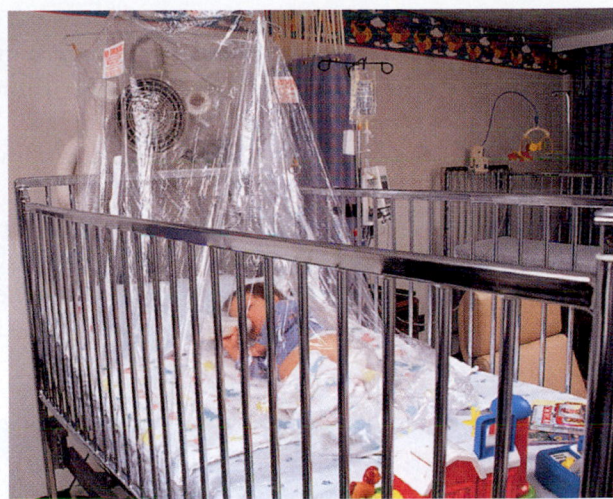

A   **B**   **C**

Figure 13-33. ■ (**A**) Simple face mask. (**B**) Nasal cannula. (**C**) Oxygen tent.

Administering Oxygen to Children

Purpose

■ To provide the prescribed concentration of oxygen to the child

Equipment

■ Oxygen supply, including a flowmeter
■ Device to humidify the oxygen
■ Nasal cannula, face masks, or oxygen tent
■ Oxygen tubing

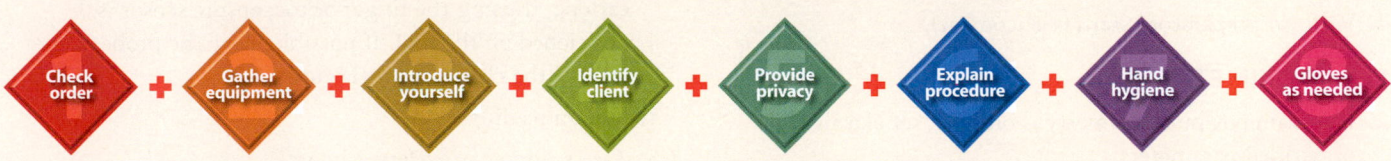

Check order + Gather equipment + Introduce yourself + Identify client + Provide privacy + Explain procedure + Hand hygiene + Gloves as needed

Interventions

1. Perform preparatory steps (see icon bar).
2. Set up oxygen delivery method, including humidification.
3. Turn on oxygen to prescribed flow rate.
4. Place the face mask over the bridge of the child's nose to the cleft of the chin (see Figure 13-33). OR

   Place the nasal cannula into the anterior nares and put an elastic band around the child's head. OR

   Surround the child in the hospital bed with the oxygen tent. Secure the edges of the tent to deliver prescribed oxygen dosage and prevent escape of oxygen.

SAMPLE DOCUMENTATION

(date) 0700   *(Note: Oxygenation portion only. This is a focused part of a complete documentation entry.)*
O_2 per nasal cannula at 2 L/ minute applied. Band secured around head. _____
K. Coffey, LPN

is essential to prevent tissue damage (Procedure 13-27 ■). Arterial blood gas analysis is most accurate, but measuring blood oxygen tension through the skin via pulse oximetry is an acceptable noninvasive method of assessment. The recording should be obtained as close to the child's head as possible.

Oxygen is a dry gas and may need to be humidified prior to administration. Humidifier reservoirs can be a host for growth of micro-organisms and a source of infection. Facility policy should be followed regarding the use and cleaning of humidifiers and humidifying equipment.

clinical ALERT

All safety measures used for administration of oxygen to an adult should be followed with children as well. These include placing "No Smoking; Oxygen in Use" signs on doors; removal of static-causing materials, including wool or nylon blankets and toys; and instructing clients and visitors about oxygen precautions.

PROCEDURE 13-27 | # Monitoring Oxygen Status

Purpose

- The pulse oximetry is used to measure oxygen saturation of the blood.
- The apnea monitor is used to measure breathing patterns.
- The peak expiratory flow rate (PEFR) meter is used to measure pulmonary function in the child.

Equipment

- Pulse oximeter, variety of sizes
- Apnea monitor, electrodes, alcohol swabs
- PEFR meter

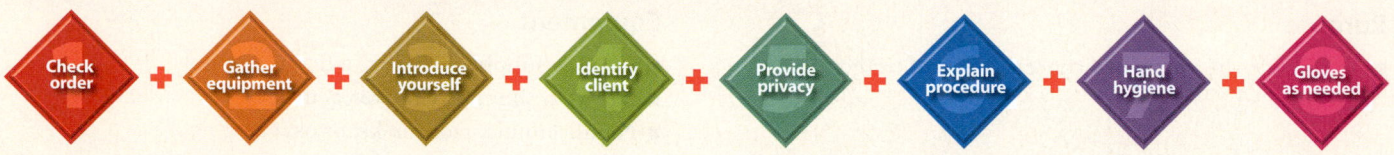

Check order + Gather equipment + Introduce yourself + Identify client + Provide privacy + Explain procedure + Hand hygiene + Gloves as needed

Interventions

1. Perform preparatory steps (see icon bar).

PULSE OXIMETRY

2. If continuous pulse oximetry is ordered, set alarms at prescribed parameters.

3. Apply the sensor to the index finger, the large toe, or the earlobe. If using the finger or toe, ensure sensor is positioned on the nail. If possible, have the probe at the level of the child's heart (Figure 13-34 ■).

4. Obtain readings.

5. Assess skin at site every 2 hours.

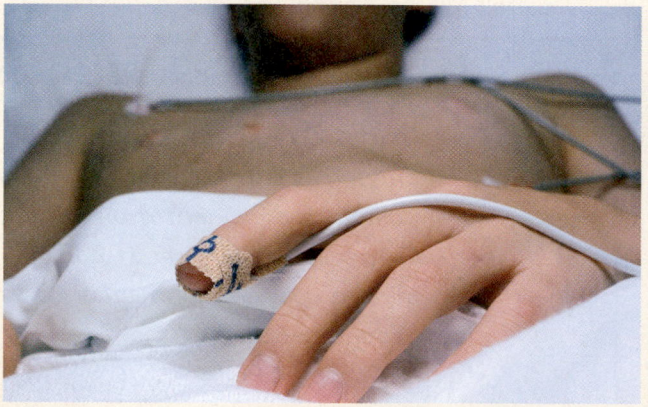
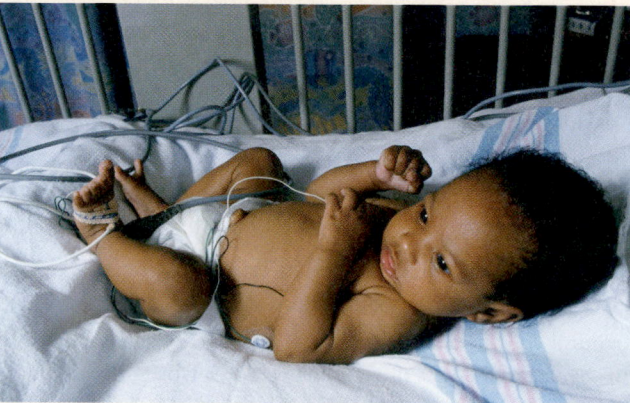

A   **B**

Figure 13-34. ■ **(A)** Pulse oximeter on finger. **(B)** Pulse oximeter on infant's foot.

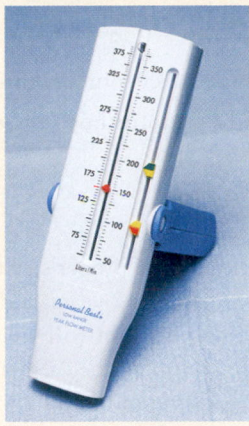

A

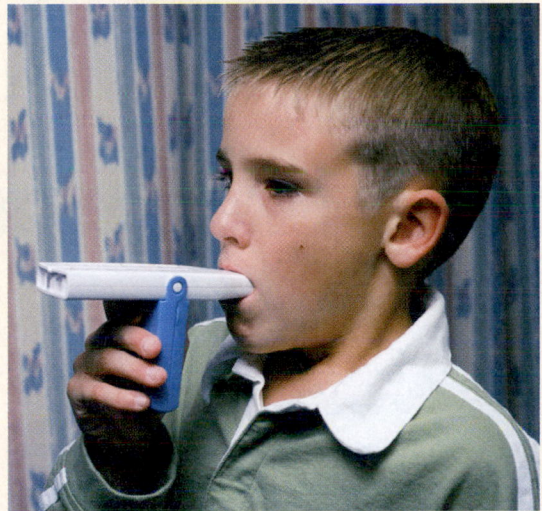

B

Figure 13-35. ■ **(A)** Peak expiratory flow rate (PERF) meter. **(B)** Child using PEFR meter.

APNEA MONITOR

2. Set alarms at prescribed parameters.

3. Apply alcohol to electrode sites. Allow to dry. *This removes body oils and will ensure more effective attachment of electrodes.*

4. Apply electrodes in the following pattern: one on the right side, one on the left side, and one on the lateral side of the abdomen.

5. Assess respiratory rate and pulse if alarm sounds.

PEFR MONITOR (Figure 13-35A)

2. Set the PEFR monitor according to the child's previous scores.

3. Instruct the child to put the mouthpiece in the mouth (Figure 13-35B ■). The child should then take a deep breath and blow as hard as possible into the meter.

4. Observe the score shown on the meter.

5. Repeat two to three times. Average the scores.

6. Compare the scores with previous scores.

7. Administer prescribed treatment, prn.

SAMPLE DOCUMENTATION

(date) 1430   *(Note: Oxygen monitoring portion only. This is a focused part of a complete documentation entry.)*
R 77. Pulse oximetry applied to infant's earlobe. 88%. O_2 applied via face mask at 4 L/minute per order.
_____ S. Locke, LVN

PROCEDURE 13-28   Assisting with Airway Insertion

Purpose

■ To assist the practitioner in inserting an artificial airway in an effort to maintain an airway of the conscious or unconscious child

Equipment

■ Oropharyngeal airways, variety of sizes
■ Nasopharyngeal airways, variety of sizes
■ Endotracheal tubes, variety of sizes, including stylet
■ Suction equipment, including resuscitation bag
■ Water-soluble lubricant
■ Tape
■ Laryngoscope, variety of blade sizes

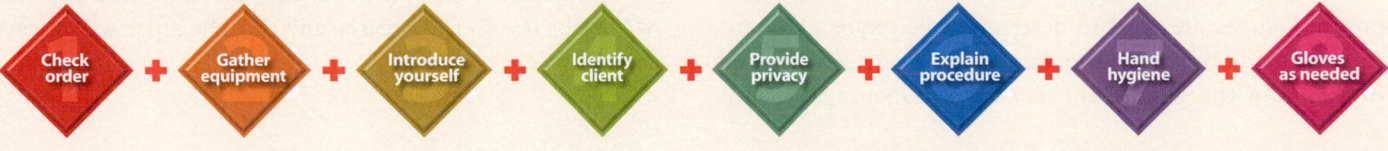

Interventions

1. Perform preparatory steps (see icon bar).

OROPHARYNGEAL

2. Assist in the selection of the proper size tube (see Table 13-3). The front flange should be at the level of the central incisors, and the distal end should reach to the angle of the jaw (Figure 13-36A ■).

3. Hold the child's head midline. Avoid flexion or extension. *This position ensures proper alignment of the trachea.*

NASOPHARYNGEAL

2. Assist in the selection of the proper size tube. Measure from the tip of the nose to the tragus of the ear (Figure 13-36B).

3. Lubricate airway with water-soluble lubricant.

4. Position the child in a supine position with HOB elevated.

ENDOTRACHEAL TUBE

2. Assist in the selection of the proper size tube (see Table 13-3). For a child older than 2 years, add 16 to the age in years and divide by 4. This sum will yield the size of ET tube necessary. Also, compare the diameter of the child's fifth finger to the diameter of the ET tube to select the proper size.

3. Position the child in a supine position and hyperflex the neck.

4. Secure the tube with tape after insertion. Assess the child's respiratory status.

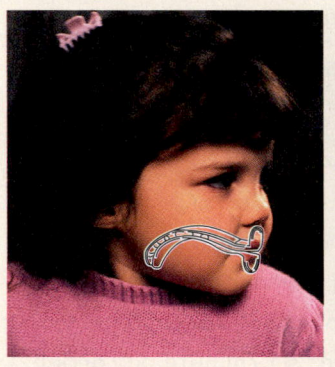 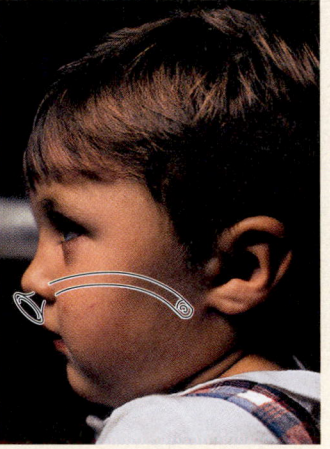

A

B

Figure 13-36 . ■ **(A)** Estimating the size of an oropharyngeal airway. **(B)** Estimating the size of a nasopharyngeal airway.

SAMPLE DOCUMENTATION

(date) 0815 (*Note: Airway insertion portion only. This is a focused part of a complete documentation entry.*) Nasopharyngeal airway inserted. Tube taped in place. Positioned child in left lateral position. R 32 and even. _____

H. Payne, LPN

Often, the best method of administering humidified oxygen to children is by tent. The tent is usually set up by the respiratory therapy department, but the nurse must be able to set up and monitor the equipment's functioning. Follow facility policy and manufacturer's recommendations on use of the equipment.

Generally, the tent consists of a frame that is suspended over the bed or crib (see Figure 13-33C). Plastic "roof and walls" are draped over the frame and tucked under the mattress. Humidified oxygen is forced into the tent by a pump. Gauges are used to determine the oxygen concentration inside the tent. The amount of oxygen is adjusted to maintain the desired concentration. Opening the tent lowers the oxygen concentration. Therefore, it is important to plan and implement care to decrease the amount of time the tent is open.

The high humidity level inside the tent causes condensation on everything inside the tent. The cool, moist air can cause the child to chill. The bed linen and client clothing should be changed to keep the child warm and dry. Nonabsorbent toys should be placed in the tent to entertain the child. The nurse can help decrease the child's anxiety about being inside the tent by reassuring the child that the tent will make it easier to breathe and that the nurse will always be available.

PHARMACOLOGY AND MEDICATION ADMINISTRATION TO CHILDREN

The administration of medications to children carries great responsibility. Extensive research must be conducted on the use, long-term effects, and dosage of medications for children. Absorption, metabolism, and excretion of drugs differ from those actions in adults because children have body systems that may be immature (Table 13-4 ■). Allergic reactions, toxic effects, or other adverse reactions may be dramatic and more severe in children. Drug literature must be read carefully and followed for client safety.

All dosage calculations and measurements must be checked for accuracy. Some facilities require dosages of certain drugs to be checked by two nurses. Some examples are Lanoxin, insulin, heparin, and chemotherapy agents. In some facilities, the LPN/LVN is not permitted to calculate

---

TABLE 13-4

Effects of Medications on Children versus Adults

BODY COMPONENT OR SYSTEM	VARIATION	ABSORPTION RATE VARIABLES	NURSING IMPLICATIONS
Muscle mass 　Infancy 　10–11 year 　Adult	 25% 40% 50%	Decrease in absorption due to erratic blood flow to muscle tissue	Less muscle tissue available in children for injections
Body fat 　Infant 　1 year 　4 year 　10–11 year 　Adult	 16% 22–24% 12% 18–20% 15%	Some drugs are dependent on the amount of fat tissue.	Blood levels increase with fat saturation effects. Different variable in percentage of fat may lead to different milligram-per-kilogram dosage to achieve therapeutic blood levels.
Body fluid 　Infant 　1 year 　4 year 　10–11 year 　Adult	 70–80% 58–60% 60% 60% 50–60%	Dehydrated state can alter the needed dosage and response to medication.	Greater milligram-per-kilogram dosage of water-soluble drugs is needed in young children.
Skin 　Children 　Adult	 Thin dermis and epidermis Relatively inactive sebaceous glands before puberty Larger surface	Affects the absorption of topical medication	Prone to skin irritations and allergies
Gastrointestinal system 　Infant 　2 year 　Adult	 Gastric emptying time: 6–8 hours Peristalsis is irregular in infants Gastric emptying time: 2 hours Gastrointestinal tract long in proportion to body size	Erratic absorption of oral medication, especially in newborns and infants Infant and young child's pH level affects acidic drugs; basic drugs are more readily absorbed.	Infant having a lower gastric pH level will not metabolize medications effectively.
Liver	Less developed in infants and young children Lower levels of liver enzymes	Maternal hormones, free and fatty acids compete with the neonate plasma protein-binding sites. They decrease the biotransformation rates, causing toxic effects of some drugs to be reached more readily.	Drugs that bind to plasma proteins are needed in smaller doses. Monitor the infant's and young child's blood levels. Monitor for side effects.

(continued)

TABLE 13-4

Effects of Medications on Children versus Adults (continued)

BODY COMPONENT OR SYSTEM	VARIATION	ABSORPTION RATE VARIABLES	NURSING IMPLICATIONS
Cardiovascular system	Infants have a poorly developed peripheral circulation.	May cause intramuscular and subcutaneous injections to absorb erratically	
Endocrine system	Increased levels of sex steroids in adolescents Sexual maturity Genetic makeup Male adolescents	May compete for enzymes necessary for drug metabolism May affect the rate of elimination May influence the metabolism and elimination of certain drugs May increase binding in certain drugs	
Neurologic system	Blood–brain barrier is not mature in children younger than age 2.	Central nervous system stimulants and depressants often cause unpredictable results	
Renal system	Glomerular filtration rate in infants is 30–50% that of an adult. Mature rates are reached within 6 months. Infants have lower tubular secretions. Newborn urinary pH contains a higher amount of acid (more acidic). Children and adults have a higher amount at night.	Longer half-life in infants for drugs excreted by glomerular filtration and by tubular secretion Increased reabsorption of acidic drugs	Can lead to an increase in dehydration and overhydration Observe closely for drug toxicity.
Immune system	Immature	Allergies are more common, especially in skin and respiratory systems.	Carefully record any drug reaction.
Respiratory system	Infants' alveoli are immature and not fully functional. Infants breathe almost totally through the nose. Children have proportionally smaller lungs and shorter and narrower upper and lower respiratory passages.	They have a higher metabolic rate.	Respiratory rate is higher.

fractional dosages. State Board of Nursing regulations and facility policy must be followed. Box 13-4 ■ illustrates some dosage problems.

Pediatric doses are smaller than adult doses. Orders are usually written for milligrams of the drug per body weight of the child per 24 hours, as well as the number of doses the child is to receive per day. The nurse must calculate the number of milligrams per dose the child is to receive. Before administering medication to a child, the nurse should verify the dose is within the recommended amount allowed for the size of the child. If a dose is questionable, the physician, pharmacist, or nurse supervisor should be consulted.

Oral Administration

The oral route of administration of medication may be preferred in children because it is less invasive and has a slower absorption rate (Procedure 13-29 ■). However, at times it is a challenge to get the infant or small child to swallow the oral medication. Children younger than 5 years of age may have difficulty swallowing pills or capsules. Medication may have a bitter taste and should be mixed in a pleasant-tasting medium. Mixing medication in common foods such as orange juice, applesauce, or pudding may cause the child to develop a dislike for those foods. Consult the pharmacist before

BOX 13-4

Pharmacology: Dosage Problems

1. Calculate the dosage for the following medication orders. The recommended dosage of Ceclor is 20 mg/kg/day in three divided doses. How many milligrams should a child weighing 20 kg receive per day?
   Answer: Multiply 20 mg by 20 kg. This equals 400 mg/day, which is the recommended dosage of Ceclor per day for a child weighing 20 kg.

2. The physician orders Demerol 0.5 mg/lb IM. A child weighs 27 lb. How many milligrams should the child receive? You have a syringe of Demerol 50 mg/1 mL. How many milliliters should the child receive?
   Answer: Multiply 0.5 mg by 27 lb. This equals 13.5 mg and is the ordered dosage of Demerol. The next step is to work

the problem using the formula D/H × Q. In this scenario you would use 13.5/50 × 1 = 0.27 mL. The nurse would draw 0.27 mL of Demerol into the syringe and administer the medication intramuscularly.

3. The doctor orders 35 mg of Demerol every 3 hours prn for pain. The child weighs 10 kg. The package insert states that the recommended dosage for pain relief in children is 0.5 mg/lb to 0.8 mg/lb. Is it safe to give the 35 mg ordered?
   Answer: Convert kilogram to pounds. Multiply 10 kg by 2.2. This equals 22 lb. Next multiply the lower end of the range and the upper end of the range by the child's weight in pounds. 0.5 × 22 = 11 mg and 0.8 × 22 = 17.6 mg. Therefore, a child weighing 22 lb should receive a dose of Demerol between 11 and 17.6 mg. This dose is too high for this child. The medication should not be given, and the physician should be contacted.

PROCEDURE 13-29   Administering Oral Medications

Purpose

- To provide medication that has been ordered to a child who requires treatment of a medical condition

Equipment

- Measuring device: medicine cup, eye dropper, syringe, spoon
- Mortar and pestle
- Prescribed medication
- Food or beverage of the child's choice

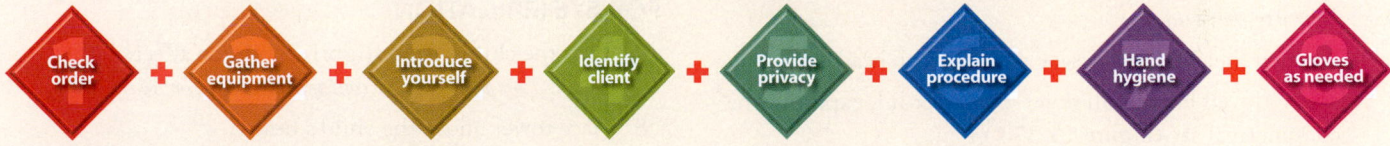

Check order + Gather equipment + Introduce yourself + Identify client + Provide privacy + Explain procedure + Hand hygiene + Gloves as needed

Interventions

1. Perform preparatory steps (see icon bar).

2. Prepare medication appropriately. Crush medications if permitted. Do not crush enteric-coated medications, time-released capsules, or other capsules.

3. Mix crushed medication in food or beverage of the child's choice. Be sure it is not the child's favorite food. *If the favorite food is used and the medication flavor is unpleasant to the child, the child may develop a dislike for the food as well.*

4. Measure carefully. *Pediatric doses must be extremely accurate.*

5. For the infant, place in a supine position. Use an eyedropper. Squeeze a small amount in the buccal area of the infant's mouth. Allow the infant to swallow, and repeat until medication is consumed. *This method should be used to prevent aspiration.*

6. For the child, place in a semi-Fowler's position. Children can sit if conditions permit. Administer the

medication, small portions at a time, with a syringe or medicine cup.

7. Avoid administering oral medications while the child is crying. *This will prevent aspiration.*

SAMPLE DOCUMENTATION

(date) 1545   *(Note: Oral medication administration portion only. This is a focused part of a complete documentation entry.)* 40 mg acetaminophen given PO as ordered. Medication crushed and mixed with strawberry gelatin.
_____ H. Hurley, LVN

opening capsules or crushing tablets to ensure that the action of the drug will not be altered. Generally, enteric-coated tablets and time-released capsules cannot be crushed.

Liquid medication must be measured accurately in a medicine cup, oral syringe, or medicine dropper. Medication may be given directly from the syringe or dropper into the buccal pocket of the mouth. Give small amounts at a time to avoid choking. Older children may drink the liquid from the medicine cup. The nurse may need to restrain the child to administer the proper dosage. A crying, struggling child may spill or aspirate medication.

EAR, EYE, OR NOSE DROPS

When administering medications in the eye (Procedure 13-30 ■), ear (Procedure 13-31 ■), or nose (Procedure 13-32 ■), the child may need to be restrained for the

(Text continues on p. 440.)

PROCEDURE 13-30

Administering Ophthalmic Medications

Purpose

- To provide prescribed medications to the eye safely
- To remove debris from the eye

Equipment

- Prescribed medication, drops, or ointment
- Sterile gloves
- Tissues
- For irrigation: prescribed irrigation solution and tubing or syringe, basin, towels

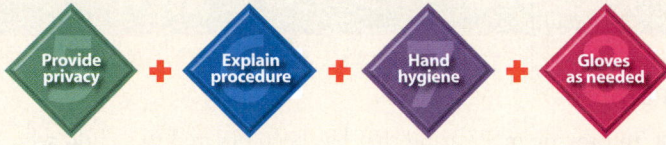

Check order + Gather equipment + Introduce yourself + Identify client + Provide privacy + Explain procedure + Hand hygiene + Gloves as needed

Interventions

1. Perform preparatory steps (see icon bar).
2. Solicit the assistance of a coworker. *This will help prevent injury to the child.*
3. Position the child in a supine position with head extended.
4. With gloved hand, pull down the lower lid, exposing the conjunctival sac (Figure 13-37 ■).
5. Place the prescribed drops or ointment in the center of the conjunctival sac. *This will prevent placement of medication directly onto the cornea.*

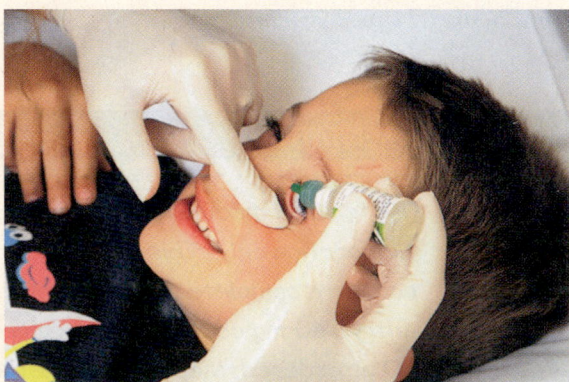

Figure 13-37. ■ Administering an ophthalmic medication. The child is instructed to close his eye and pretend to look up toward his head. The nurse then gently retracts the lower lid and inserts the medication.

6. Have the child close the eyes for 30 seconds and keep the head midline. *This will prevent the medication from running out of the eyes and promotes absorption.*

FOR EYE IRRIGATION

7. Turn the child's head slightly, with the affected eye down. *This will prevent contamination of the unaffected eye.*
8. Place towel under the child's head.
9. If using tubing, prime the line first.
10. Gently separate the upper and lower eyelids with thumb and forefinger of dominant hand.
11. Open the clamp on the tubing and allow fluid to flood the eye. Turn the flow off periodically to allow the child to close the eye.

SAMPLE DOCUMENTATION

(date) 0725 (Note: Ophthalmic medication administration portion only. This is a focused part of a complete documentation entry.) 0.2-in. ribbon of Illytocin applied to both eyes. No redness or exudate noted. ___
_____ M. Martin, LPN

PROCEDURE 13-31 Administering Otic Medications

Purpose

- To provide prescribed medications safely to the ear
- To remove debris from the ear

Equipment

- Prescribed otic medication equipped with dropper
- Cotton ball
- For irrigation: prescribed solution, otoscope, syringe with tubing, emesis basin, towels

Check order + Gather equipment + Introduce yourself + Identify client + Provide privacy + Explain procedure + Hand hygiene + Gloves as needed

Interventions

1. Perform preparatory steps (see icon bar).
2. Solicit the assistance of a coworker. *This will help prevent injury to the child.*
3. Correctly identify the child with the identification band.
4. Position the child in a supine position with head turned to the side and the affected ear up (Figure 13-38 ■).
5. Pull the pinna in the appropriate direction according to the child's age (see Figure 13-2A and B).
6. Hold the dropper above the ear and instill prescribed number of drops. Never occlude the ear canal completely. *Occlusion can create a pressure change and damage the eardrum.*
7. Place a cotton ball loosely in the opening of the ear.
8. Have the child lay in this position for 5 to 10 minutes. *This will give the medication time to be absorbed.*

ASSISTING WITH IRRIGATION OF THE EAR CANAL

9. Warm prescribed solution to body temperature. *Solution below body temperature may cause nausea and vertigo.*
10. Hand the practitioner the otoscope. *The tympanic membrane should be seen as intact with the otoscope to avoid further damage.*
11. Position the child in a supine position with the head turned and the affected ear up.
12. Place the emesis basin under the affected ear. Place a towel over the child's neck and shoulders. *This will prevent clothing from becoming saturated.*
13. Draw up 20 mL of solution in syringe with attached tubing.
14. Repeat as necessary.

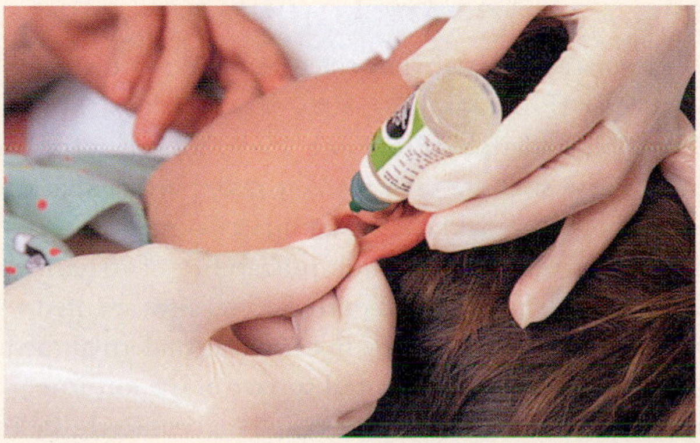

Figure 13-38. ■ Administering an otic medication.

SAMPLE DOCUMENTATION

(date) 0945 (*Note: Otic portion only. This is a focused part of a complete documentation entry.*) Left ear irrigated with 40 mL of normal saline. Return of 40 mL yellow-tinged fluid. _____
R. Love, LVN

PROCEDURE 13-32 **Administering Nasal and Inhaled Medications**

Purpose

- To provide prescribed medications to the nasal cavity safely

Equipment

- Prescribed medication, drops, or aerosol
- Delivery device, dropper for nasal and nebulizer for aerosol medications

Check order + Gather equipment + Introduce yourself + Identify client + Provide privacy + Explain procedure + Hand hygiene + Gloves as needed

Interventions

1. Perform preparatory steps (see icon bar).
2. Solicit the assistance of a coworker. *This will help prevent injury to the child.*

NASAL MEDICATIONS

3. Position the child in a supine position with the head hyperextended.
4. Administer medication into narse as ordered.
5. Have the child maintain the position for 5 minutes. *This will give the medication time to absorb.*

AEROSOL MEDICATIONS

See Chapter 18 for further discussion on the use of aerosol medications in the treatment of asthma.

3. Position the child in a semi-Fowler's position. *This position enables easier lung expansion than the supine position.*

4. Instruct the child to place the tubing in the mouth and breathe deeply for approximately 10 minutes. Observe for understanding of instructions.

SAMPLE DOCUMENTATION

(date) 1130   *(Note: Nasal/inhaled medication administration portion only. This is a focused part of a complete documentation entry.)* 0.05% naphazoline hydrochloride, two sprays, administered in both nostrils. ____
_____ C. Wellman, LPN

---

procedure. This will help prevent injury to the child. For children younger than 3 years, it is important to pull (see Figure 13-2A) the pinna of a child down and back. For the child older than 3 years, pull the pinna up and back (see Figure 13-2B). This will straighten the ear canal and allow the medication to be administered properly. Table 13-5 ■ discusses routes of medication administration in children.

Rectal Suppository

Rectal suppository is a common route of administration for pediatric drugs when the child is unable to take oral medications (Procedure 13-33 ■). The child may need to be restrained for the procedure. Insert the suppository into the anus. Using the small finger, push the suppository into the rectum approximately 1 inch ($1/2$ inch for the infant).

Medications by Injection

Medications administered by the parenteral route include intramuscular (Procedure 13-34 ■), subcutaneous (Procedure 13-35 ■), intradermal (Procedure 13-36 ■), and intravenous routes. These sites are used when it is important that drugs are metabolized quickly. Also, an injection may be preferred when drugs would have a high probability of irritating the child's stomach if given by mouth. Several sites are used when administering medication by injection. Intradermal medications can be given on the ventral surface of the forearm or the scapula. Subcutaneous injections can be given in the deltoid, abdomen, lower back, scapula, and thigh. Intramuscular injections are given to the infant in the vastus lateralis muscle. To the child who has walked for 1 year, they are given in the ventrogluteal muscle. The deltoid site can also be used for the child who has appropriate muscle mass and when small amounts of medication are to be given (Figure 13-40A–C ■).

TABLE 13-5

Routes of Drug Administration by Age in Children

AGE	ORAL LIQUID	SUBLINGUAL	INTRAMUSCULAR INJECTION OR SUBCUTANEOUS INJECTION	INTRAVENOUS
Infant	Preferred route; may be administered by dropper into buccal sac	Generally avoided due to their inability to keep pill under tongue	Vastus lateralis used. Many sites are not well developed enough for IM injection.	Veins are very small. Scalp, wrist, or ankle veins may be used for IV administration. Armboard and restraints required to maintain site.
Toddler and preschooler	Preferred route of administration Administered by syringe or cup Greater predictability of the drug action by this route	Carefully assess the child's ability to swallow.	Few possible sites because of low muscle mass. Gluteus maximus used as site after toddler has been walking for 1 year.	Access difficult because of vein size; armboard and restraints required to maintain site. Greater predictability of the drug action by this route
School-age child	Preferred route of administration Administered by syringe or cup Greater predictability of the drug action by this route	Carefully assess the child's ability to swallow.	Sites as for adult	Greater predictability of the drug action by this route
Adolescent	Preferred route of administration Administered as liquid, tablet, or capsule Greater predictability of the drug action by this route	Same as for adult	Sites as for adult	Greater predictability of the drug action by this route

PROCEDURE 13-33 Administering Rectal Suppositories

Purpose

- To provide prescribed medications in the rectal canal safely

Equipment

- Prescribed medication, stored in the refrigerator
- Water-soluble lubricant
- Gloves

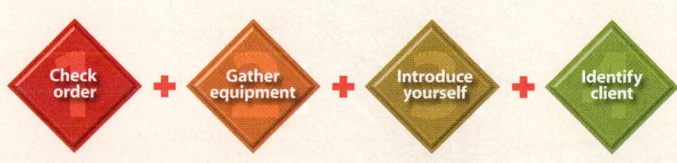 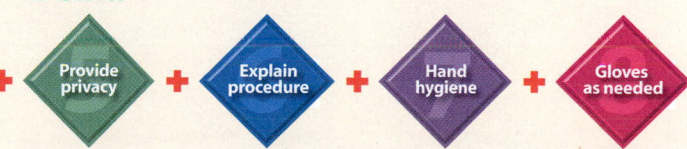

Check order + Gather equipment + Introduce yourself + Identify client + Provide privacy + Explain procedure + Hand hygiene + Gloves as needed

Interventions

1. Perform preparatory steps (see icon bar).
2. Solicit the assistance of a coworker. *This will help prevent injury to the child.*
3. Correctly identify the child with the identification band.
4. Place the child in the left lateral position.
5. Lubricate the suppository with water-soluble lubricant. *This allows for easier insertion.*

6. For infants and toddlers, the nurse uses the little finger and carefully inserts the suppository just beyond the internal sphincter (about ½ in. or 1.25 cm) (Figure 13-39 ■).
7. For the older child, use the index finger and carefully insert the suppository just beyond the internal sphincter (about 1 in. or 2.5 cm).
8. Have the child maintain this position for 5 to 10 minutes. The nurse may also need to hold the buttocks together for

about 1 minute. *This will facilitate absorption of the medication and prevents the medication from being expelled.*

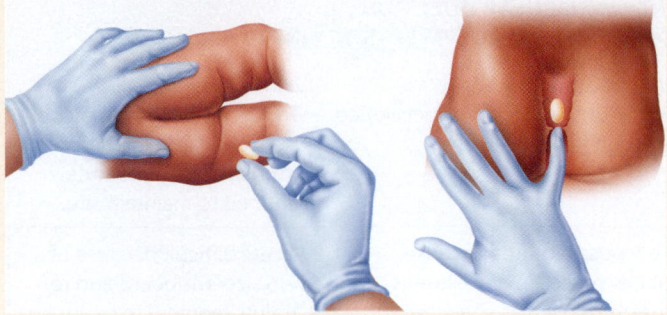

Figure 13-39. ■ The suppository is inserted gently just past the internal sphincter (about 1 in. or 2.5 cm in children; about ½ in. or 1.25 cm in infants). In infants, the little finger may be used instead of the index finger to insert the suppository. (Network Graphics\Pearson Education/PH College)

SAMPLE DOCUMENTATION

(date) 0900   *(Note: Rectal medication administration portion only. This is a focused part of a complete documentation entry.)* T 101.9°F; 325 mg acetaminophen given rectally. R. Ress, LPN

(date) 1000   T 99.9°F; resting without complaint. _____ R. Ress, LPN

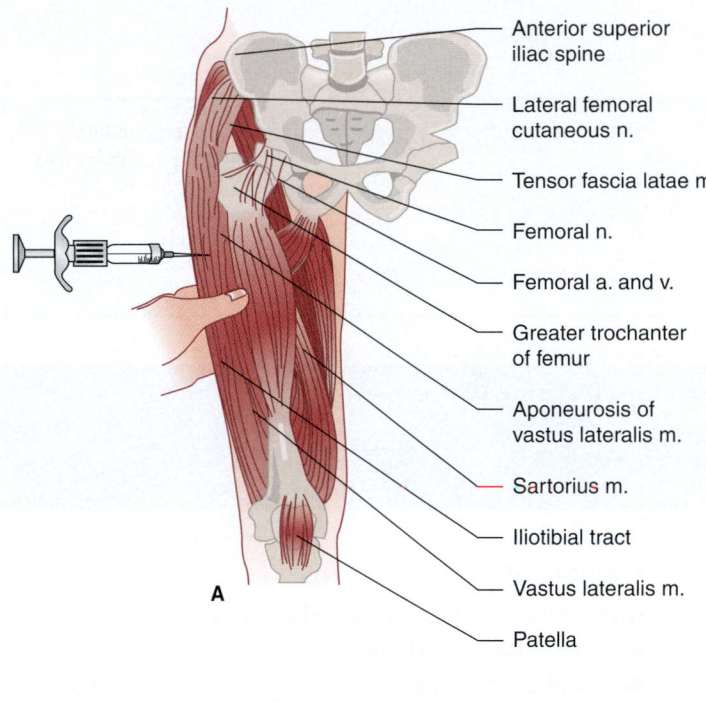

Anterior superior iliac spine
Lateral femoral cutaneous n.
Tensor fascia latae m.
Femoral n.
Femoral a. and v.
Greater trochanter of femur
Aponeurosis of vastus lateralis m.
Sartorius m.
Iliotibial tract
Vastus lateralis m.
Patella

A

Tubercle of iliac crest
Gluteus medius m.
Anterior superior iliac spine
Branches of superior gluteal a. and v.
Branch of superior gluteal n.
Gluteus minimus m.
Tensor fascia latae m.
Greater trochanter of femur
Gluteus maximus m.

B

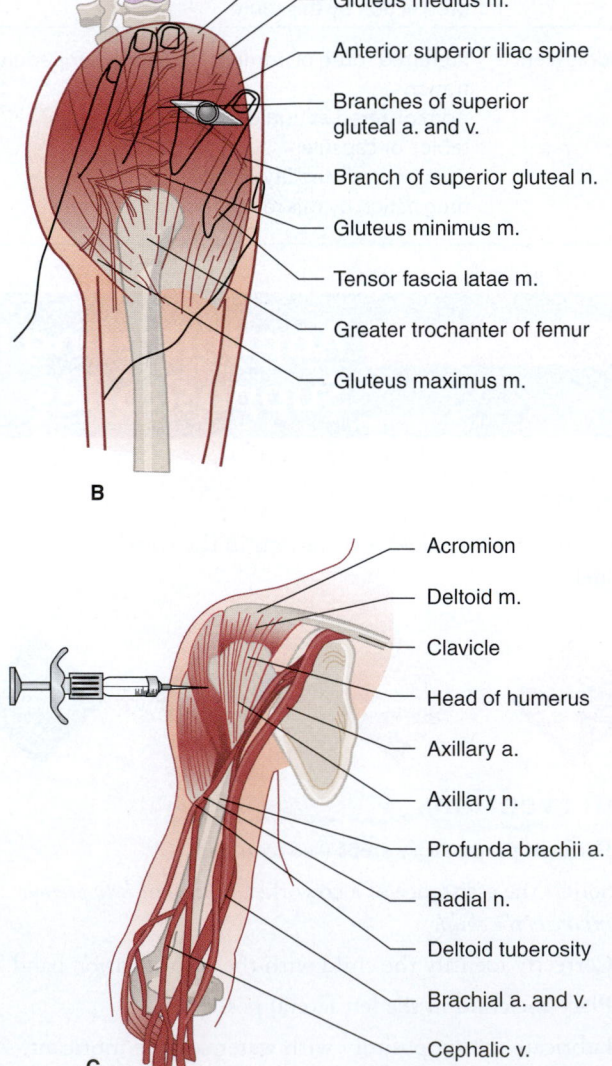

Acromion
Deltoid m.
Clavicle
Head of humerus
Axillary a.
Axillary n.
Profunda brachii a.
Radial n.
Deltoid tuberosity
Brachial a. and v.
Cephalic v.

C

Figure 13-40. ■ Intramuscular injection sites. (**A**) Vastus lateralis (**B**) Ventrogluteal. (**C**) Deltoid. (Adapted from Bindler, R., & Howry, L. [1997]. *Pediatric drugs and nursing implications* [2nd ed.]. Stamford, CT: Appleton & Lange, pp. 39–42.)

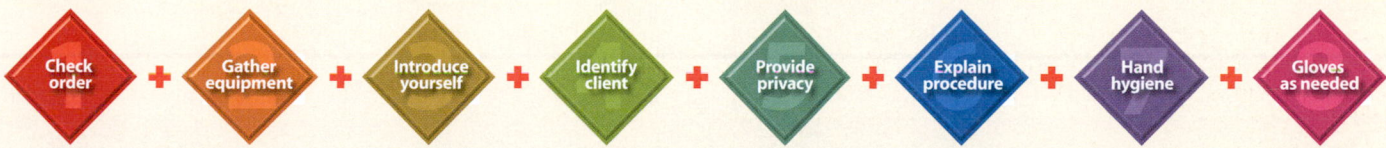

PROCEDURE 13-34 ## Administering Intramuscular (IM) Injection

Purpose

■ To provide prescribed medications intramuscularly in a safe manner

Equipment

■ Prescribed medication
■ 21- to 25-gauge needle with lengths 0.5 to 1 in.
■ 1- to 3-mL syringe
■ Alcohol swab
■ Adhesive bandage

Check order + Gather equipment + Introduce yourself + Identify client + Provide privacy + Explain procedure + Hand hygiene + Gloves as needed

Interventions

1. Perform preparatory steps (see icon bar).

2. Solicit the assistance of a coworker. *This will help prevent injury to the child.*

3. Correctly identify the child with the identification band.

4. Ensure that the amount of medication is appropriate for the child's age and the muscle chosen as the site (Table 13-6 ■).

5. Choose the correct site for administering a medication intramuscularly. *For the infant, the vastus lateralis (see Figure 13-40A) is used. For the toddler who has been walking for 1 year or more, the ventrogluteal (see Figure 13-40B) can be used, but is still not preferred until the child has been walking for several years.*

6. Choose the correct size needle. *A smaller-gauge needle should be used for injections into the smaller muscles such as the deltoid. The child's muscle mass and body weight should also be taken into consideration.*

7. Position the child according to the site chosen (see Figure 13-40C). *For the deltoid site, place the child in the lateral position. This restrains one arm on the surface under the child so the arm receiving the injection can be restrained by the nurse. For the vastus lateralis, place the child in the supine position or seated on the parent's lap with the parent restraining the arms (Figure 13-41 ■). For the ventrogluteal position, place the child in the prone position.*

8. Cleanse the site with alcohol from the center outward.

9. Insert the needle quickly at a 90-degree angle with the dominant hand.

10. Using the nondominant hand, pull back on the plunger slightly, observing for the return of blood. Be careful not to move the needle because this can cause additional discomfort.

TABLE 13-6

Appropriate Volumes for IM Administration by Age

AGE	MAXIMUM AMOUNTS
Infant	Avoid volumes greater than 0.5 mL.
Toddler	Avoid volumes greater than 1 mL.
Older child and adolescent	Deltoid: Avoid volumes greater than 1 mL. Vastus lateralis: Avoid volumes greater than 2 mL. Gluteal: Avoid volumes greater than 3 mL.

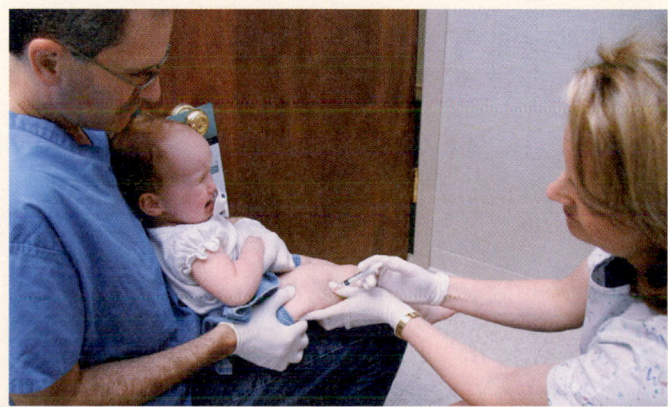

Figure 13-41. ■ The child is restrained by staff while an injection is being administered. The vastus lateralis is the appropriate site for a child of this age. (M. C. Schlachter Photography)

11. If there is no blood, inject the medication slowly, remove the needle, and massage the site.

12. If there is blood in the syringe, withdraw the needle without injecting the medication. *Blood indicates that the needle is in a blood vessel. Injecting the medication at this point would mean the medication is administered intravascularly.*

13. Needles cannot be recapped. Dispose of needle and syringe in the proper container. *The equipment used for an intramuscular injection is considered to be contaminated and poses the threat of transmitting harmful substances.*

PROCEDURE 13-35 # Administering Subcutaneous (SQ) Injection

Purpose

■ To administer prescribed medications subcutaneously in a safe manner

Equipment

■ Prescribed medication
■ 25- to 26-gauge needle with lengths ⅜ to ⅝ in.
■ 1- to 3-mL syringe
■ Alcohol swab
■ Adhesive bandage

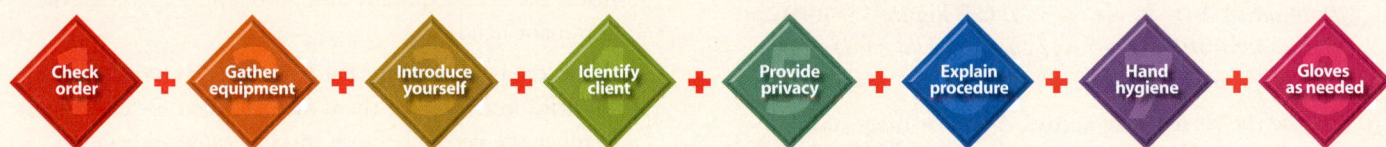

Check order + Gather equipment + Introduce yourself + Identify client + Provide privacy + Explain procedure + Hand hygiene + Gloves as needed

Interventions

1. Perform preparatory steps (see icon bar).

2. Solicit the assistance of a coworker. *This will help prevent injury to the child.*

3. Choose the correct site for administering a medication subcutaneously. *Sites available for subcutaneous injections include the deltoid, the abdomen, the thighs, the lower back, and the scapula.*

4. Position the child according to the site chosen. *For the deltoid site, place the child in the lateral position. This restrains one arm on the surface under the child so the arm receiving the injection can be restrained by the nurse. For the abdomen, place the child in the supine position. For*

the lower back or scapula, position the child in the prone position.

5. Cleanse the site with alcohol from the center outward.

6. Insert the needle quickly at a 45-degree angle with the dominant hand.

7. Using the nondominant hand, pull back on the plunger slightly, observing for the return of blood. Be careful not to move the needle because this can cause additional discomfort.

8. If there is no blood, inject the medication slowly, remove the needle, and massage the site, unless administering

heparin or insulin. *The effect of these two medications may be altered if massage occurs after injection.*

9. If there is blood in the syringe, withdraw the needle without injecting the medication. *Blood indicates that the needle is in a blood vessel. Injecting the medication at this point would mean the medication would be administered intravascularly.*

10. Never recap a needle. Dispose of needle and syringe in the proper container. *The equipment used for a subcutaneous injection is considered to be contaminated and poses the threat of transmitting harmful substances.*

SAMPLE DOCUMENTATION

(date) 0730   *(Note: Subcutaneous injection portion only. This is a focused part of a complete documentation entry.)* Two units regular insulin administered SQ in RUQ. _____
A. Page, LVN

PROCEDURE 13-36 # Administering Intradermal (ID) Injection

Purpose

■ To inject prescribed medication intradermally in a safe manner

Equipment

■ Prescribed medication
■ 27-gauge needle with lengths ¼ to ⅜ in.
■ 1-mL syringe
■ Alcohol swab
■ Adhesive bandage

Check order + Gather equipment + Introduce yourself + Identify client + Provide privacy + Explain procedure + Hand hygiene + Gloves as needed

Interventions

1. Perform preparatory steps (see icon bar).

2. Solicit the assistance of a coworker. *This will help prevent injury to the child.*

3. Choose the correct site for administering a medication subcutaneously. *Sites available for intradermal injections include the ventral surface of the forearm and the scapula.*

4. Position the child according to the site chosen. *For the forearm, place the child in a semi-Fowler's position. The older child who is able to understand the importance of holding still may be seated for this injection. For the scapula, position the child in the prone position.*

5. Cleanse the site with alcohol from the center outward.

6. Insert the needle quickly at a 15-degree angle with the dominant hand.

7. Do not aspirate.

8. Inject the medication slowly, creating a wheal or blister. *This verifies placement of the medication in the dermis.*

9. Withdraw needle and do not massage. *It is important for the medication to stay at the site.*

10. Mark site with a permanent marker for future assessment.

11. Needles cannot be recapped. Dispose of needle and syringe in the proper container. *The equipment used for an intradermal injection is considered to be contaminated and poses the threat of transmitting harmful substances.*

SAMPLE DOCUMENTATION

(date) 1430   *(Note: Intradermal injection portion only. This is a focused part of a complete documentation entry.)* 0.1 mL purified protein derivative antigen given ID in right ventral forearm. Wheal marked with permanent marker. Parent instructed to return to clinic in 48 hours. ___
T. Thomas, LPN

Intravenous (IV) Administration

The intravenous route is routinely used to administer pediatric medications (Procedures 13-37 ■ and 13-38 ■). It is generally less traumatic to the child than intramuscular injection every few hours. Care must be taken to ensure proper dilution of the medication. Infusion pumps are predominantly used to regulate the rate of administration. The site must be assessed for infiltration and patency before administration of each dose of medication. Many drugs are irritating to tissues, and if infiltration occurs, the physician must be notified. In some areas, the administration of pediatric medications by the intravenous route is not an LPN/LVN function. State Board of Nursing regulation and facility policy must be followed.

PROCEDURE 13-37 | **Initiating Intravenous Access to Administer Intravenous Fluid**

Purpose

■ To initiate intravenous access properly
■ To infuse prescribed intravenous fluid in a safe manner

Equipment

■ Tourniquet or rubber band if accessing a scalp vein
■ Antiseptic solution, alcohol, or povidone-iodine
■ IV catheter:
  • For infants, 24 gauge
  • For toddlers to school-age children, 20 to 22 gauge
  • For adolescents, 18 to 20 gauge
  • Butterfly needles, which are 22 to 25 gauge, can be used in temporary situations
■ T-connector, flushed
■ Saline-filled and/or heparin-filled syringe
■ Prescribed IV solution
■ Appropriate tubing
■ Armboard, variety of sizes
■ Tape
■ For saline or heparin lock, needleless catheter cap
■ Rate-controlling device such as a pump, Buretrol (Figure 13-42 ■), Soluset, or Metriset
■ Gloves

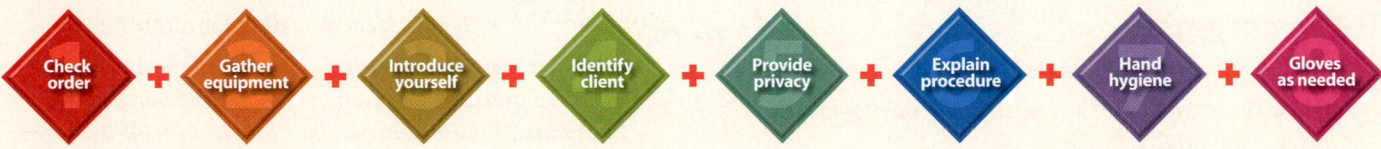

Interventions

1. Perform preparatory steps (see icon bar).
2. Solicit the assistance of a coworker. *This will help prevent injury to the child.*
3. Attach the tubing to the IV bag and prime.
4. If using a rate-controlling chamber device, attach to the IV bag. Fill chamber with 50 mL of IV fluid.
5. Position the child in a supine position. Restrain as necessary.
6. Apply tourniquet.
7. Use inspection and palpation to locate an appropriate vein (see Figure 15-8 ⬀ for pediatric venous access sites).
8. Release tourniquet.
9. Apply armboard to location chosen (Figure 13-43 ■).
10. Reapply tourniquet.
11. Cleanse the site with antiseptic solution as outlined in facility policy. Use a circular pattern, beginning at the desired puncture site and moving outward. *This pattern of cleansing the site moves bacteria away from the injection site.*
12. Carefully insert the catheter at a 15-degree angle, bevel up. As blood appears in the catheter, carefully advance the catheter. Remove needle. Apply pressure at the end of the catheter and release tourniquet.
13. Quickly attach T-connector and flush with saline-filled syringe.
14. Attach prescribed IV solution and set to infuse at the prescribed rate per pump or by gravity.
15. Tape the catheter securely.

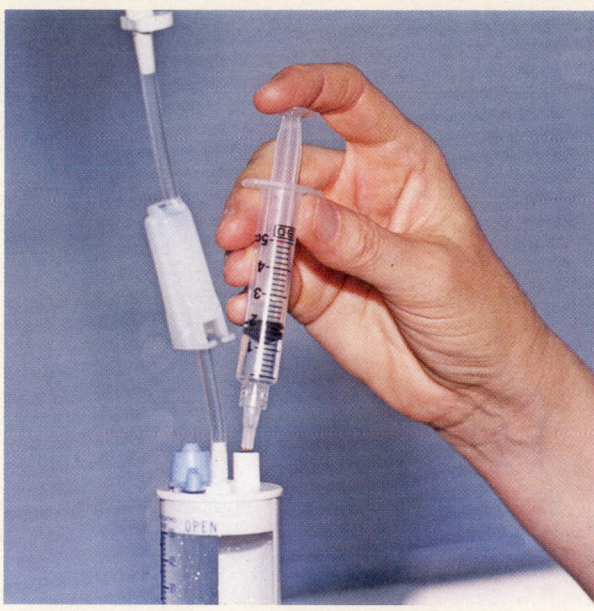

A

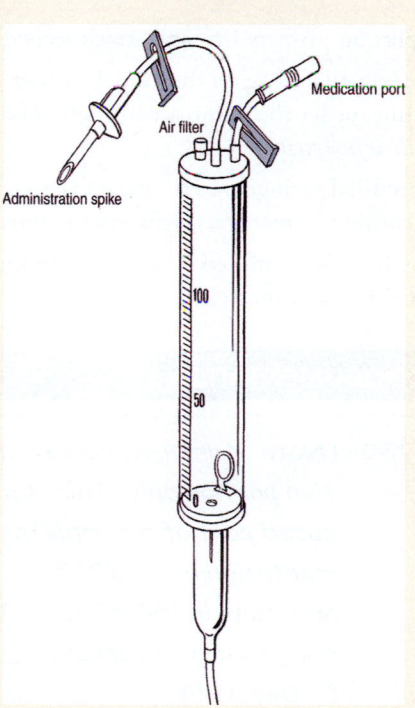

B

Figure 13-42. ■ Buretrol device. (**A**) Adding medication to the volume-control device. (Elena Dorfman/Pearson Education/PH College) (**B**) Parts of the volume-control infusion set.

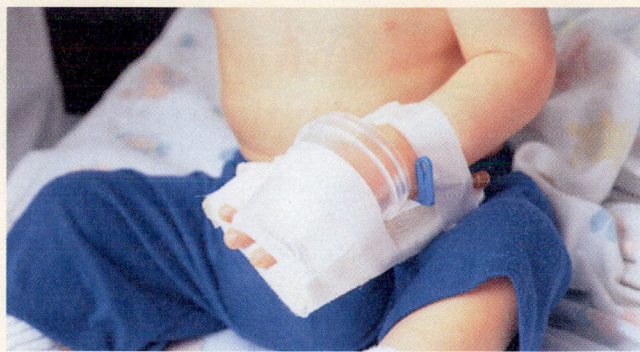

Figure 13-43. ■ This intravenous site on a hand has been placed on an armboard, securely wrapped, and covered with part of a plastic cup to prevent the child from disrupting the line.

CONVERTING IV TO SALINE OR HEPARIN LOCK

16. Prime needleless cap with the saline- or heparin-filled syringe.

17. Clamp the T-connecter. *This prevents loss of blood through the catheter.*

18. Discontinue IV tubing from the catheter hub and quickly insert the needleless cap.

19. Open the clamp. Attach and inject the saline or heparin slowly to flush the needleless cap. *Heparin keeps the site patent by preventing clots at the site.*

20. Remove the syringe and clamp the T-connector.

21. Secure the site according to agency policy.

SAMPLE DOCUMENTATION

(date) 1330   (Note: Initiating IV portion only. This is a focused part of a complete documentation entry.) IV of 250 mL D51/2 NS started with 22-gauge catheter into R antecubital space after cleansing with antiseptic solution. Rate set per pump at 50 mL/hour. ___ K. Adams, LPN

Storage of Medication

Safe storage of medicines is essential. In an acute- or long-term care facility, medications are kept locked in storage cupboards or drawers for safety. Medication cannot be left at the bedside. Intravenous infusion pumps must be locked so the rate of administration cannot be adjusted by clients or visitors. In the home, medication should be safely stored out of reach of the child.

PROCEDURE 13-38 # Administration of Intravenous Medications

Purpose

■ To infuse prescribed medication intravenously in a safe manner

Equipment

■ Prescribed medication
■ Syringe and needle or needleless system
■ Appropriate tubing
■ Alcohol swabs
■ Gloves

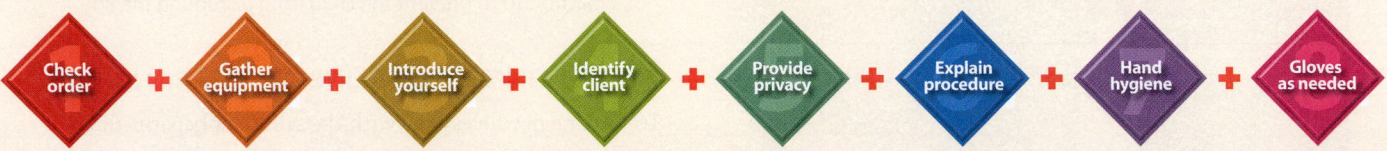

Check order + Gather equipment + Introduce yourself + Identify client + Provide privacy + Explain procedure + Hand hygiene + Gloves as needed

Interventions

1. Perform preparatory steps (see icon bar).

BOLUS ADMINISTRATION

2. Prepare prescribed amount of medication for bolus.

3. Assess the IV line for patency. *Line must be clear and open for medication to infuse properly.*

4. Cleanse the access port with alcohol.

5. Insert needle or needleless syringe into the cleansed port.

6. Inject medication slowly, observing closely for changes in the child's condition. *IV medications go directly into the bloodstream and so take effect quickly.*

7. Increase the intravenous fluid rate for several minutes to flush the medication from the tubing. *This ensures that all medication is delivered to the client.*

INITIATING A SECONDARY INFUSION

2. Obtain the prescribed medication from the pharmacy in either a 50-mL or a 250-mL bag of fluid or a prefilled syringe (5 mL or 60 mL).

3. Attach secondary tubing.

4. Cleanse port on primary line and attach secondary tubing.

5. Hang the secondary bag on the IV pole, lower than the primary line, or set the pump accordingly. *The bag that is highest will infuse first.*

6. For the prefilled syringe, insert into infuser and set to infuse according to manufacturer's instructions.

7. When medication is infused, discontinue secondary line and resume primary infusion.

SAMPLE DOCUMENTATION

(date) 0730   *(Note: Administering IV medication portion only. This is a focused part of a complete documentation entry.)* 363 mg ampicillin in 150 mL D_5W IVPB hung to infuse rapidly. _____
D. Day, LPN

NURSING CARE

PRIORITIES IN NURSING CARE

When caring for children before, during, and after procedures, the nurse must remember that the child is typically in a foreign environment, among strangers, and exposed to frightening instruments and situations. There is often pain associated with procedures, which only increases the child's fear. Adequate preparation for the procedure, as well as a kind, comforting, and gentle manner can assist the child in overcoming fear and anxiety.

ASSESSING

The nurse assesses the child's anxiety, fear, and stress before, during, and after procedures. Subjective statements related to the child's anxiety should be documented. The speaker (parent or child) should be identified. Younger children with verbal skills are likely to admit fear or anxiety before, during, or after the procedure. Older children and adolescents may want to project a brave attitude and often deny fear. Irritability, preoccupation, lack of eye contact, restlessness, trembling, GI distress, urinary frequency, confusion, and increased pulse, blood pressure, and respirations may all be objective signs of fear, anxiety, and stress related to procedures.

DIAGNOSING, PLANNING, AND IMPLEMENTING

Nursing diagnoses for a child who is required to have a procedure might include:

- Anxiety related to the situational crises of a procedure
- Fear related to threat of physical harm caused by the procedure
- Fear related to a lack of knowledge about the procedure
- Ineffective Coping related to the threat created by the procedure.

Some outcomes for a child who is required to have a procedure are as follows:

- The child will not demonstrate negative behaviors related to anxiety.
- The child will be able to manage fearful thoughts.
- The child will seek and express understanding of accurate information about the procedure.
- The child will take part in some forms of diversion, relaxation, or play.

The nurse's role in providing support to these clients includes the following:

- Teach the parent and child factual information about the procedure. *Increased knowledge helps reduce anxiety and fear.*
- Encourage the child to express anxiety verbally. *Expressing concerns relieves the child and allows the nurse to address the concerns.*
- Provide verbal and nonverbal support before, during, and after the procedure. The appropriateness of touch as a method of giving nonverbal support may vary among cultures (Box 13-5 ■). *The child should understand that the nurse respects feelings. Respect builds trust in the nurse-child relationship.*
- Arrange for the care of the child to be consistent. *Continuity of care builds trust and increases the child's comfort.*
- Allow the child to have a comfort item or parent present during the procedure. *Familiar items or family members increase the child's comfort level.*
- Give the child some choices in the procedure whenever possible. These choices could include which arm to start

---

BOX 13-5	CULTURAL PULSE POINTS

Use of Touch as Nonverbal Support

Most procedures require the nurse to use touch. Personal space and cultural norms must be taken into consideration when implementing procedures. Casual touch should be avoided in children of Asian or American descent. European cultures are more comfortable with casual touch. Permission should be obtained from the child and his or her family, regardless of culture, prior to the procedure. However, this is especially important when the child is uncomfortable with casual touch.

---

the IV, going to the procedure room or staying in the hospital room for the procedure, or what type of bandage they receive. *Choices allow the child to have ownership in the procedure and may help reduce fear.*
- Decrease the child's environmental stimulation before, during, and after the procedure. Lower the lights, turn off the TV, and close the door. *A quiet, calm environment is more comforting to the child.*

EVALUATING

Evaluating a child with anxiety or fear related to a procedure includes continually observing for manifestations of fear, anxiety, and inability to cope. The nurse should document these and report them appropriately. Remember to document interventions aimed at reducing anxiety and fear prior to using restraints during procedures.

NURSING PROCESS CARE PLAN
Client with Fractured Arm

Keri is 3 years old. She sustained a broken left arm and facial cuts in an automobile crash. Her fractured arm required an open reduction and internal fixation. The facial lacerations required sutures. Keri's dad is at her bedside, but her mother was injured in the incident and is currently in surgery. Upon return from surgery, Keri is grimacing and crying softly. Her vital signs are T 98.6, P 144, R 35, and BP 100/60.

Assessment
- Grimacing, crying softly
- Elevated pulse, respiration, and blood pressure
- Facial wounds with sutures
- Left arm post open reduction and internal fixation

Nursing Diagnosis. The following important nursing diagnosis (among others) is established for this client:

Acute pain related to surgical and facial wounds

Expected Outcomes. Expected outcomes for Keri are:

■ Will adequately express pain.
■ Will be able to express a pain level.
■ Will not experience unresolved pain.

Planning and Implementation

■ Administer medication as ordered. *Medications relieve pain and pain perception.*

■ Teach child and parent signs and symptoms of pain, especially nonverbal symptoms. Use a pain scale with facial expressions to assist a child with limited vocabulary. *Parent and child need instruction in recognizing pain and reporting it promptly in order to initiate pain relief methods quickly.*

■ Allow the child to "assist" in medication administration. For example, give her a clean empty syringe (no needle, no medication) to play with while the nurse is administering the medication. *This gives the child a feeling of control and provides a method of distraction as well.*

■ Implement nonpharmacologic pain relief methods such as positioning, use of cold or heat application, or playing soothing music to relax the child between medication administrations. *Nonpharmacologic pain relief methods complement pharmacologic methods and may extend their effectiveness.*

These nonpharmacologic methods (see Box 14-3 ∞) may also allow the client to be weaned sooner from the use of pharmacologic methods of relieving pain.

■ Monitor medication effectiveness. *Adequate assessment of medication effectiveness allows the nurse to respond quickly when the medication is ineffective.*

Evaluation. Prompt evaluation of pain management provides the nurse with an avenue to provide client-specific pain relief measures.

Critical Thinking in The Nursing Process

1. What distraction activities would be appropriate for Keri?
2. What response should the nurse give Keri when she asks where her mommy is?
3. Based on Keri's age, how might she express pain?

Note: Discussion of Critical Thinking questions appears in Appendix I.

Note: The references and resources for this and all chapters have been compiled at the back of the book.

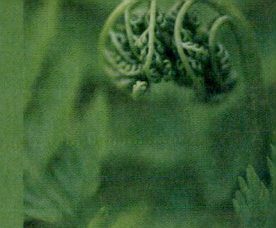

Chapter Review

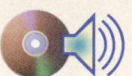 **KEY TERMS** by Topics

Use the audio glossary feature of either the CD-ROM or the Companion Website to hear the correct pronunciation of the following key terms.

Pulse
point of maximal impulse

Specimen Collection
Vacutainer®

Feeding a Child
residual volume

KEY Points

- Most procedures are the same for children as for adults, but modifications might be necessary.

- Children often feel safer if the nurse makes a self-intro-duction to the parent first, and then to the child.

- The order of assessment in children is organized so the least comfortable or most invasive parts are done last.

- Children are generally fearful of procedures, especially in-vasive ones. The nurse provides teaching and emotional support to alleviate fear.

- Older children and adolescents generally cooperate bet-ter if they are informed about a procedure ahead of time. Small children may cooperate less. Inform parents ahead of time, and give limited information to the small child di-rectly before the procedure.

- Parents need factual information: the reason for the proce-dure, the steps in the procedure, the results expected, any risks associated with the procedure, and follow-up measures.

- Doppler is the preferred equipment for blood pressure readings on small children.

- The child's safety during procedures is the nurse's pri-mary responsibility. Perform the procedure correctly, re-strain the child when necessary, and observe the child's well-being following the procedure.

- Correct documentation of the procedure is vital: date and time, objective information about the procedure, results of the procedure, condition of the child following the procedure, any further nursing measures that were nec-essary, and any reports given.

- Restraints should be used as a last resort to ensure the safety of the child during procedures. Use of restraints should be temporary, and the nurse must observe for haz-ardous symptoms during their use.

- Use appropriate-sized equipment for procedures involv-ing pediatric clients (needles, BP cuffs).

- Children younger than 3 years should have IM injections in the vastus lateralis; gluteal muscles are not developed adequately.

- In infants and toddlers, enema tubing or suppositories should be inserted to ½ in. (1.25 cm), not to 1 in. (2.5 cm)

as is done with older children. The little finger can be used instead of the index finger to insert a suppository.

- Fluid overload is a significant complication for pediatric clients receiving IV infusion. Assess rate of infusion, condi-tion of the IV site, and systemic effects of the infusion.

- Be constantly aware of the child's airway and oxygena-tion. Employ proper positioning and feeding methods. Administer oxygen correctly by nasal cannula, face mask, or oxygen hood.

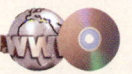 **EXPLORE Media**Link

Additional interactive resources for this chapter can be found on the Companion Website at www.prenhall.com/towle.

Click on Chapter 13 and "Begin" to select the activities for this chapter.

For chapter-related NCLEX-style questions and an audio glossary, access the accompanying CD-ROM in this book.

Animations

Child physical assessment	Tracheostomy
Blood pressure	Metered dose inhaler
Capillary pressure	Applying a mummy wrap
Client pain assessment	Gavage tube
Pluse oximeter	Ostomy care
Throat culture	

FOR FURTHER Study

For a photo showing an infant being weighed, see Figure 7-27.

For an illustration of pediatric venous access sites, see Figure 15-8.

For further discussion on the use of aerosol medications in the treatment of asthma, see Chapter 18.

For more about heart sounds, see Chapter 19.

For standardized growth charts, see Appendix II.

For common conversions and lab values, see Appendix V.

Critical Thinking Care Map

Caring for a Child Requiring Restraints
NCLEX-PN® Focus Area: Safe and Effective Care Environment

Case Study: Casey, an 18-month-old male, needs to have a nasogastric tube inserted for persistent vomiting. Casey is crying and kicking as the nurse takes him to the procedure room. He is yelling, "No, no, no." The nurse decides that in order to do the procedure safely, she needs assistance from a colleague and will need to restrain Casey during the procedure.

Nursing Diagnosis: Risk for Injury related to nasogastric tube insertion

COLLECT DATA

Subjective	Objective
_____	_____
_____	_____
_____	_____
_____	_____
_____	_____
_____	_____
_____	_____

Would you report this? Yes/No

If yes, to: _____

Nursing Care

_____
_____
_____
_____
_____
_____
_____
_____
_____
_____
_____
_____
_____
_____

How would you document this? _____
_____
_____
_____

Compare your documentation to the sample provided in Appendix I.

Collect Data
(use those that apply)

- Crying
- Kicking and screaming
- Yelling "no, no, no"
- Face red
- Carotid pulse 120 bpm
- 50 mL green vomitus
- 100 mL yellow urine
- Phenergan 12.5 mg, rectal suppository inserted

Nursing Interventions
(use those that apply; list in priority order)

- Administer Phenergan 12.5 mg, rectally.
- Measure urine output every shift.
- Obtain physician's order for mummy restraints.
- Provide emotional care during and after procedure.
- Enlist assistance of a colleague during procedure.
- Remove restraints immediately after procedure.
- Assess restraints every 15 minutes.

1 For which of the following children would it be appropriate for the nurse to measure head circumference? Choose all that apply.

1. 6 months
2. 1 year
3. 6 years
4. 2 years
5. 3 years
6. 5 years

2 What is the best method the nurse can use to measure urine output in the infant?

1. inserting an indwelling catheter
2. weighing the diapers
3. applying an external collection bag
4. weighing the infant after each voiding

3 The most appropriate nursing intervention for a child in an oxygen tent is:

1. changing linens frequently.
2. allowing the child to enter and exit the tent at will.
3. providing several stuffed animals for the child to play with.
4. providing the child with a fan to assist with lowering the temperature.

4 The nurse needs to give an infant an intramuscular injection of hepatitis B vaccine. Where should the injection be given?

1. deltoid
2. dorsogluteal
3. rectus femoris
4. vastus lateralis

5 An infant, shortly after birth, is coughing, and the nurse hears a moist sound on inspiration. Which of the following nursing interventions is most appropriate?

1. Suction the mouth, then the nose.
2. Insert an endotracheal tube and attach to continuous suction.
3. Insert a feeding tube and attach to continuous suction.
4. Suction the nose, and then the mouth.

6 In which of the following situations can the nurse apply restraints? Choose all that apply.

1. on all children in the hospital
2. only when other methods of restraint fail
3. as the first choice of restraint
4. to keep the arm immobilized during injections
5. to prevent the child from pulling bandage

7 The nurse needs to insert a rectal suppository in a 6-month-old infant. Choose the appropriate method(s).

1. Insert using the index finger.
2. Insert $1/2$ in. into the rectum.
3. Both a and b.
4. Never given.

8 Which of the following vital signs, obtained from a 2-year-old male, would require the nurse to report the findings?

1. P 150, R 50
2. P 120, R 35
3. P 125, R 38
4. P 140, R 40

9 Which of the following vital signs, obtained from a 15-year-old female, would require the nurse to report the findings?

1. P 100, BP 130/90
2. P 70, BP 119/80
3. P 60, BP 110/78
4. P 90, BP 115/70

10 When choosing an assessment method, which of the following is appropriate for a child experiencing pain?

1. Assess head to toe so no areas are forgotten.
2. Assess only physical symptoms.
3. Put the child on bed or table.
4. Assess areas that are painful last.

Answers for Review Questions, as well as discussion of Care Plan and Critical Thinking Care Map questions, appear in Appendix I.

Chapter 14

Care of the Hospitalized or Chronically Ill Child

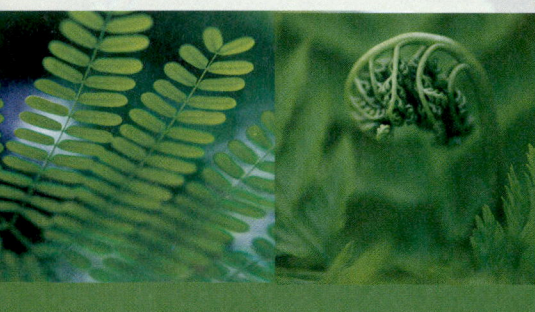

NURSING PROCESS CARE PLAN: The Child Undergoing Hospitalization for Surgery

HEALTH PROMOTION ISSUE: Unlicensed Personnel Administering Medications at School

CRITICAL THINKING CARE MAP: Caring for a Child with Bilateral Hip Splints on a Rehabilitation Unit

BRIEF Outline

Role of the LPN/LVN

HOSPITALIZED CHILD

Age-Specific Preparation for Hospitalization

Admission Process

Preparation for Procedures

Care of the Child Before and After Surgery

Preparation for Discharge

Nursing Care

CHRONICALLY ILL CHILD

Care at Home

Care at School

Rehabilitation

Long-Term Care

Care of the Caregivers

Nursing Care

LEARNING Outcomes

After completing this chapter, you will be able to:

- Describe how to prepare children for hospitalization.
- Describe how to prepare parents for their child's hospitalization.
- Describe the preoperative and postoperative care of children.
- Describe how to prepare parents and children for discharge.
- Describe important aspects of care for the chronically ill child and the family.
- Describe the role of the LPN/LVN in caring for children with acute or chronic disorders.
- Discuss how to care for children in the home or in long-term care settings.

Community-based nursing practice involves caring for the client and family in any setting. It is generally agreed that the home is the ideal place to care for a child with an **illness** (state of disease or sickness). Illness may be physical or psychological. It may be characterized as **acute** (having rapid onset, severe symptoms, and a short course), **chronic** (long-lasting, slowly progressing), or **terminal** (final, fatal). However, sometimes we find a child who is ill in other settings. For example, a child might be healthy when he or she goes to school but becomes ill during the day. The child might have a chronic condition like asthma that does not prevent him or her from attending school but that may require care while at school. A child with an acute disorder may require hospitalization. Some children with complex illnesses may not be able to leave home or might be placed in a long-term care setting away from home. The nurse must be prepared to work with other professionals to plan and implement the best care possible for the child and family in any environment.

A child with a minor illness or injury is commonly cared for at home. Parents recall their own upbringing and apply the concepts they learned to care for their own children. For example, if their mother provided them with chicken noodle soup and ginger ale when they had an upset stomach, parents will probably fix these same foods for their children who are ill. If a child has a fever, parents will provide an over-the-counter antipyretic medication, encourage fluid intake, and allow the child to rest.

If the symptoms become worse or do not improve in a reasonable period of time, the parents might seek additional medical attention. Unless the child's condition warrants hospitalization, the child will return home to be cared for by the parents, who must administer medication and other prescribed treatment.

When parents have sought medical attention, the nurse should provide detailed instructions about the illness and medical treatment. These instructions generally involve cleanliness, nutrition and fluids, rest, and medications. Symptoms of complications and follow-up care also need to be discussed.

If the child's illness is serious or acute, it may be necessary to admit him or her to the hospital. Admitting a child to the hospital is a stressful event for the child, as well as for the parents and siblings. Usually the best place for the child to recover is at home. However, the severity of the child's illness might require that the child be admitted for emergency or diagnostic procedures, treatment, surgery, and rehabilitation. The more prepared the child and family are for the hospitalization, the less stress they will experience. This chapter addresses the key issues in caring for the child who is acutely or chronically ill in a variety of settings.

Role of the LPN/LVN

The LPN/LVN's role is to assist in the care of the child. For example, in the office or clinic, the LPN/LVN collects data about the child and family (see Chapter 3 ⚭), assists with diagnostic procedures, and provides instructions for home care or upcoming hospitalization. At school, the LPN/LVN assists with health screening such as vision or scoliosis detection, administers prescribed medications, cares for the ill child until parents arrive, and provides health teaching, such as hand washing, in the classroom. In the hospital, the LPN/LVN provides direct care by assisting with activities of daily living (ADLs) and administers medications within the legal scope of practice. A pediatric admission form provides information about the developmental level of the child and can be used to maintain the child's daily patterns and preferences (Figure 14-1 ■). The nurse can help the child through **therapeutic play** (play that allows the individual to deal with fears associated with the health care experience). The nurse can also reinforce rehabilitation therapies and encourage health promotion activities. The LPN/LVN provides verbal and written explanations about plans for discharge.

HOSPITALIZED CHILD

Hospitalization of a child causes stress for clients and families. It is the responsibility of the nurse to lessen the stress to the extent possible. When a child is hospitalized, the nursing responsibility seems greater. It is difficult to provide detailed instruction to children who, due to their age, are unable to fully comprehend, or participate in, their care.

Parents might have feelings of fear, guilt, or anger about their child's hospitalization. The two parents may not agree on treatment. Parents may experience conflict between the need to continue working and the need to be with their child who is ill. Siblings are curious about what is happening to their brother or sister. They might feel responsible for the illness or be fearful that their sibling might die.

Family patterns, structure, culture, and ethnicity (see Chapter 3 ⚭) may affect family functioning when a child is to be hospitalized. Some families may be heavily involved in their child's care (Figure 14-2 ■; Box 14-1 ■). Others may insist that siblings stay away from a hospitalized child.

Sensory deficits, especially deafness, can affect a child who is hospitalized. For a child who is deaf, the family home may be the only place where communication is understood easily. The hospital may take special measures to provide an interpreter who knows sign (see sign language

Infancy (Birth To 1 Year)		School Age (6 To 11 Years) And Adolescent (12 To 16 Years)	

Infancy (Birth To 1 Year)

Motor / Sensory
- ☐ Follows objects 180°
- ☐ Reaches for objects
- ☐ Smiles / laughs
- ☐ Passes hand to hand
- ☐ Rolls over
- ☐ Sits
- ☐ Crawls
- ☐ Stands
- ☐ Walks

Nutrition
- ☐ Breast-fed
- ☐ Bottle
- ☐ Cup
- ☐ Cereal
- ☐ Baby food

Frequency of feeding _____

- ☐ Other _____

_____

Sleep
- ☐ Crib   ☐ Sleeps alone
- ☐ Bed   ☐ With parent
- ☐ Naps
- ☐ Sleeping pattern _____

Habits
- ☐ Sucks thumb
- ☐ Favorite toy or blanket?

Elimination   Last void _____ Last B.M. _____

Other _____ No of B.M.'s a day? _____

Assessment appropriate for age? ☐ Yes ☐ No

Comments _____

Toddler Through Pre-School (13 Months To 5 Years)

Motor / Sensory
- ☐ Walks
- ☐ Climbs steps
- ☐ Vocalizes
- ☐ Dresses self
- ☐ Bathes self
- ☐ Brushes teeth
- ☐ Combs hair
- ☐ Ties a bow

Nutrition
Does child feed self? ☐ Yes ☐ No
- ☐ Finger foods   ☐ Spoon
- ☐ Fork   ☐ Knife
Does child drink from?
- ☐ Bottle ☐ Cup
Frequency   ☐ Three meals a day
- ☐ Nap and/or bed time snacks
Diet   ☐ Regular
- ☐ Other _____

_____

Play Habits   ☐ Nursery school ☐ Baby-sitter ☐ Home

Favorite games, toys, etc. _____ ☐ Pet

Assessment appropriate for age?   ☐ Yes   ☐ No

Sleep
- ☐ Crib   ☐ Sleeps alone
- ☐ With parent
- ☐ Other _____

Has child slept away
from home?
- ☐ Often
- ☐ Rarely
- ☐ Never
- ☐ Sleeping pattern _____

_____

Elimination
- ☐ Is child toilet trained?
  - ☐ Bowel
- ☐ Bladder
  - ☐ Partially
  - ☐ Toilet
  - ☐ Potty chair

Last void? _____

Last B.M.? _____

Frequency of B.M? _____

Developmental Section
Pediatric Admission Assessment Record

School Age (6 To 11 Years) And Adolescent (12 To 16 Years)

Motor / Sensory
- ☐ Ambulates well
- ☐ Other _____

Sleep

Bedtime? _____

Arise? _____

Bed-wetting? _____

Nightmares? _____

Education

Grade level? _____

Learning disability? _____

_____

Academics
- ☐ Above   ☐ Average
- ☐ Below

Habits
- ☐ Smoking   ☐ Thumbsucking
- ☐ Alcohol   ☐ Tantrums
- ☐ Drugs   ☐ Other _____

Socialization Relationship to?

Parent? ☐ Good   ☐ Poor

Peers? ☐ Good   ☐ Poor

Hobbies   Athletic? ☐ Yes ☐ No
- ☐ Other _____

Assessment appropriate for age? ☐ Yes   ☐ No

Nutrition

Diet _____

Frequency? _____

Snacks? _____

Likes/dislikes? _____

Dental visits? ☐ Yes ☐ No

Condition of teeth?
- ☐ Poor   ☐ Good
- ☐ Appliances
- ☐ Comments _____

Elimination

Last Void? _____

Last B.M.? _____

Frequency? _____

Comments _____

Menses

Age started _____

Last period _____

Problems _____

Vaginal discharge? _____

Sexually active ☐ Yes ☐ No

Oral contraceptives? _____

Exposed to disease? _____

Is there a possibility you could be

pregnant? _____

NURSE'S SIGNATURE

DATE

CLIENT IDENTIFICATION

Figure 14-1. ■ Portion of a pediatric admission form showing developmental level and habits of children.

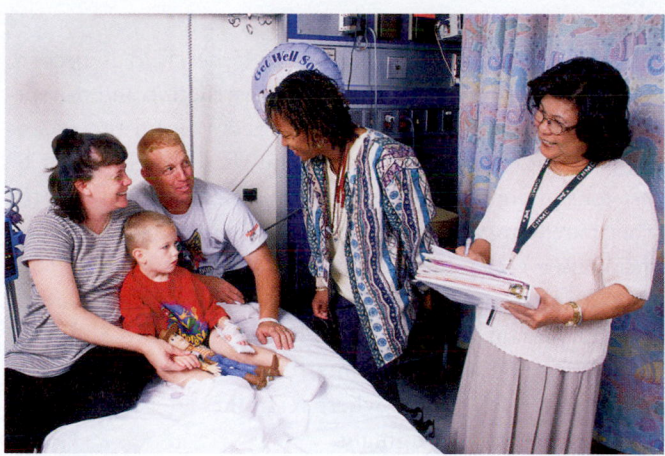

Figure 14-2. ■ Children and their families need to be actively involved in decisions about care when appropriate. Here, the family and staff come together to discuss the child's care in a positive and honest manner.

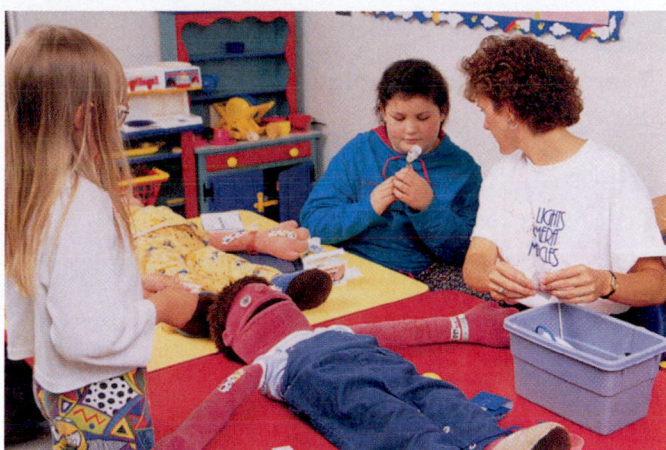

Figure 14-3. ■ A child specialist works with children being treated for cancer. Special dolls are used to familiarize children with the procedures they will undergo.

in Appendix VI), but the interpreter is likely to participate only when decisions and plans are being made. Nurses need to be creative to prevent children who are deaf from feeling isolated. Quality nursing care requires that nurses understand the importance of families, cultures, and special needs.

Many larger hospitals have special units designed to care for the pediatric client and the family. These might include special pediatric intensive care units (PICU); preoperative and postoperative care units, pediatric oncology, pediatric orthopedics, pediatric burn units, and pediatric rehabilitation units. They may also have overnight facilities (e.g., the Ronald McDonald House) where families can stay during the child's hospitalization. Nurses with expertise in the care of children team with respiratory therapists and physical therapists. A **child life specialist** (trained professional who plans therapeutic activities for the hospitalized child) may be available to plan age-

appropriate activities to assist children in working through their feelings about hospitalization, their specific illness, and surgery (Figure 14-3 ■). If the school-age child will be hospitalized for more than a few days, schoolwork may need to be completed in order for the child to keep up with the class.

Smaller hospitals may not have the luxury of these special units. In small hospitals, children are generally admitted to a private room and cared for by the same nurses and staff as the adult clients. There might be days or weeks when the small hospital has no inpatient pediatric client. Nurses must have adequate resources available to meet the needs of the pediatric client, without interfering with the care of adult clients. If a child life specialist is not available, the LPN/LVN may assist with therapeutic play techniques (Figure 14-4 ■). Table 14-1 ■ identifies some therapeutic play techniques that might be used.

BOX 14-1   CULTURAL PULSE POINTS

Mexican American Family Support System

The Mexican American family is a strong support system. Although the father is the spokesperson for the family, extended family members may be present during hospitalization. The nurse should include them in explanations about health care.

With every family, it is important for the nurse to try to answer certain questions:

- Who is the decision maker?
- Is the family expressive or stoic about their feelings?
- What kind of physical presence does the family expect or want to have with the hospitalized child?

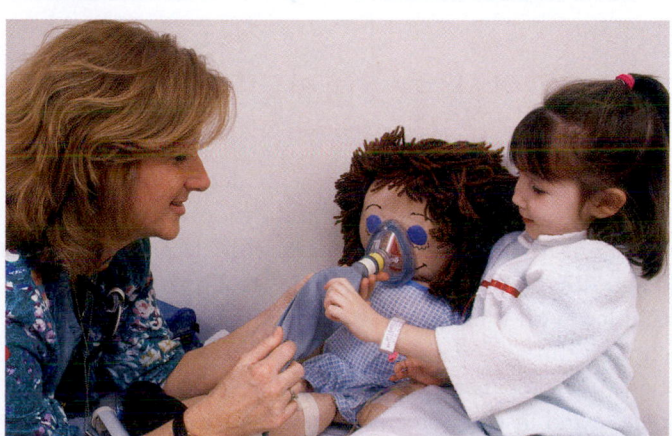

Figure 14-4. ■ Role-playing is one type of therapeutic play. Putting a mask on her doll gives this child some mastery over her coming surgical experience. It is important for children to see and touch medical equipment in order to reduce their fear of the unknown.

TABLE 14-1

Therapeutic Play Techniques

TECHNIQUE	INTERVENTION
Drawing	■ Use a simple gender-specific picture and have the child draw what he or she thinks is his or her medical problem. ■ Use drawings to explain care, procedures, and surgery. ■ Say to the child, "Tell me about your picture." Be alert for the child's emotions such as fear, sadness, etc.
Music	■ Encourage family to bring tapes/CDs of favorite music. ■ Use music to relax and reduce stress. ■ If family is unable to visit, have them tape messages to the child. ■ Play time could include musical instruments and singing.
Pets	■ Animals foster relaxation. Safety rules must be followed, and pets must be approved inside the facility.
Puppets	■ Use a puppet to ask the child questions. Children may answer a puppet instead of person. ■ Perform skits to teach child necessary care.
Role Playing	■ Provide dolls and medical equipment. Help child role-play procedures and/or surgery. ■ Use toys that foster expression of emotions. Dolls with disabilities similar to the child's are available.
Stories	■ Read or make up stories to explain procedure, surgery, or specific illness. ■ Have child make up a story about a picture. ■ Talk about the child's feelings identified in the story.

Age-Specific Preparation for Hospitalization

The reason for hospitalization helps determine guidelines for preparing families for hospitalization activities. If the hospitalization will be for a short-term elective surgery or diagnostic procedure, written and verbal teaching might be coupled with a facility tour. If the hospitalization is for a chronic illness and the client has a history of hospitalizations, the preparation might include a review of past experiences and instruction on any new experiences. In an emergency situation, little time is available, so preparation might be limited to verbal instruction given under stress. In part, the age of the child also determines the method and amount of preparation.

INFANT

In early infancy, little preparation of the child is needed. Parents and siblings, however, need instruction and reassurance. It is difficult for them to witness painful procedures (e.g., IV sticks) being performed on the baby. It might be best for only one parent to remain with the infant and the other parent to wait with siblings at this time. The nurse must observe the parents for signs that they might faint (pale, diaphoretic skin, and light-headedness) if they are allowed to remain with the infant during these times. A chair should be provided for parents to prevent falls. Following procedures or treatments where restraints are used, the parent should comfort the infant.

The infant needs close supervision while in the hospital. Unless the infant is sleeping, family or trained hospital personnel should be in attendance at all times.

Separation Anxiety

At about 6 months of age and older, the infant is able to identify primary caregivers and develops anxiety when separated from them. **Separation anxiety** is apprehension due to the removal of significant persons or items from the environment. The infant or toddler progresses through three stages of separation: protest, despair, and detachment.

PROTEST STAGE. When the primary caregiver leaves the child, he or she feels alone and abandoned. The child expresses his or her feelings of being abandoned by loud protests, including screaming and crying. The approach of a nurse or other stranger may result in increased protest. The child may be labeled as "bad."

DESPAIR STAGE. The crying gradually stops, and the child enters the second stage of separation anxiety, despair. The child may fall asleep for a short time. When awake, the child may appear sad and depressed, and lie quietly, not playing with toys. The child may be labeled as "adjusting." When the parents return, the child may regress to loud protests.

DETACHMENT STAGE. In the third stage, detachment, the child becomes more interested in the surroundings, playing and behaving as "usual," but becoming disinterested in parents and significant others. The child appears to have adjusted to the separation. However, the nurse must understand that the child is using a defense mechanism to cope with the pain of separation. If the child remains in the detachment stage, long-term and often permanent disruption of parent-child bonding may occur. In this case, professional help is needed to heal the parent-child relationship.

Promoting a Sense of Security

It is important to encourage as much parental involvement as possible. If parents are unable to remain with the child, other familiar adults may help reduce separation anxiety. Leaving the child with a favorite toy or blanket may help ensure a feeling of security. If the parents will be absent for some time, leaving a picture can help the child feel connected to the parents. Parents should be encouraged to talk to the child about leaving them for a short time, indicating that they will return. Even though the child may not understand the situation, honest communication from the parents helps develop trust. Parents should be discouraged from "slipping away when the child is distracted" because this can break the trust bond.

TODDLER

The toddler is beginning to understand that people get sick and that, in a short time, they get better. Toddlers have no understanding of cause and effect and may think that something they said or did caused the illness. The toddler is beginning to identify body parts and can point to "where it hurts."

Remember that toddlers use magical thinking in their mental processing. Seeing other children with tubes, dressings, or IVs, toddlers might think something bad or mysterious has happened to the children and become afraid it will happen to them as well. It is important to tell toddlers that the treatments they (or others) are having will fix their body and "make it better." Instruction needs to be brief and given just prior to the procedure. If the procedure will be painful, toddlers need to be told that it will hurt but that holding still will help. If possible, a parent should be present to support the child.

Toddlers are very attached to their parents, and separation still causes extreme anxiety. Parents should be encouraged to be present as much as possible and to participate in care. Besides pictures of parents, it may be helpful to have audiotapes or other reminders left with children when the parents are absent. A favorite toy or blanket should be brought with the toddler.

Unless they are sleeping, toddlers require one-to-one supervision. This can be provided by the parents, family, volunteers, assistive personnel, or nurses. It is critical for safe care that staffing be provided to allow for this level of supervision.

PRESCHOOLER

The preschooler is learning about safety and daily practices to keep healthy. To the extent possible, following routine practices in the hospital should be encouraged. Preschoolers are beginning to think about cause and effect but may not be correct in the association. Preschoolers might think that something they did caused the illness. For example, if a preschooler did not pick up his toys as his mother instructed and then later threw up, he might think he was sick because he had not done what his mother had told him to do. Preschoolers need reassurance that the illness or injury is not their fault.

Although preschoolers can be away from parents for a brief period of time, they are easily frightened by new people and experiences. Parents should be encouraged to participate in care and reinforce instructions provided by the

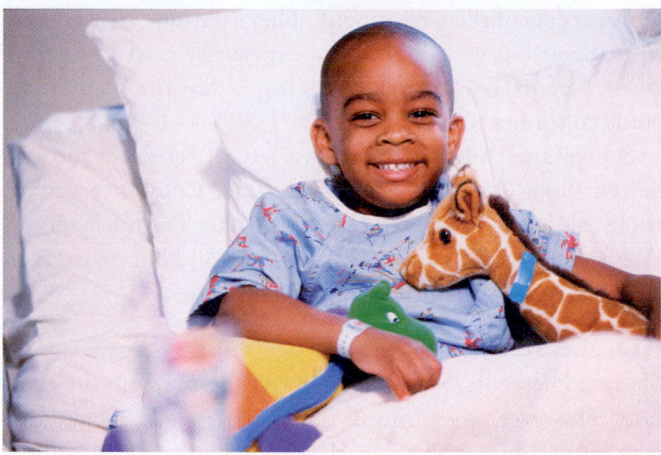

Figure 14-5. ■ This child has brought a favorite toy from home to make the hospital environment feel more secure and familiar. (Ken Chernus/Getty Images, Inc./Taxi)

nurse. Preschoolers may be left unattended for a few minutes but generally should be supervised at all times. Familiar objects (Figure 14-5 ■) continue to provide a sense of security for the preschooler. Rituals and family routines should continue as much as possible.

SCHOOL-AGE CHILD

School-age children can actively participate in their care and treatment (Figure 14-6 ■). They can understand written and verbal instructions, ask questions, and be responsible for

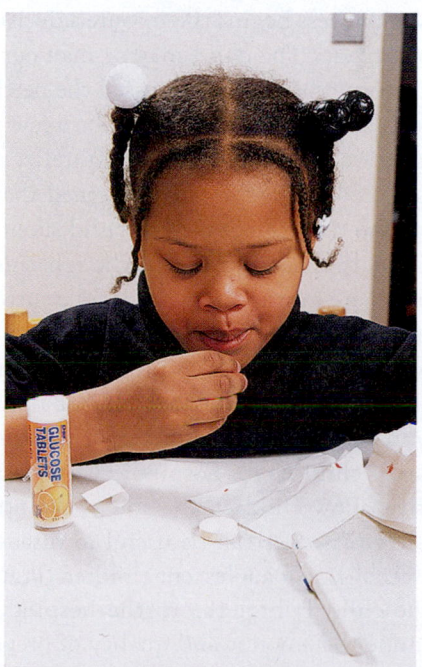

Figure 14-6. ■ This child is old enough to understand the need to take glucose tablets or another form of rapidly absorbed sugar when her blood glucose level is low.

some aspects of their treatment. They continue to need parent support but generally do not experience extreme anxiety when parents are absent. Bringing a favorite item from home continues to offer comfort.

School-age children enjoy a variety of activities and can be left alone for brief periods of time. Computer games, books, and movies can be used to fill time. The nurse should interact frequently with the school-age child but may not be required to remain in the room all the time.

ADOLESCENT

Many adolescents want to be active participants in their care. However, they might be embarrassed, modest, or uncomfortable about their changing bodies. They might have participated in activities that put them at risk for illness or injury without their parent's consent. Adolescents need reassurance that their modesty and privacy will be protected. The nurse needs to provide instructions directly to the adolescent and encourage questions.

Some adolescents want parents present during procedures; others prefer parents to stay in the waiting room. Many adolescents will have frequent visits from their friends. The nurse must maintain control of the environment to ensure that the adolescent has adequate rest and has privacy during treatments. The nurse may request that friends limit their visits to ensure adequate time for nursing care.

Admission Process

The admission process begins the minute a decision for hospitalization is made. The child may or may not have been present at the time the doctor discussed the need for hospitalization with the parents. There may be a few minutes or several days between the decision to hospitalize and the actual admission. Some parents are concerned that the child will be fearful, so they do not tell the child about the hospitalization until the last minute. Although this approach may be appropriate for the young child, the surprise of hospitalization may bring additional stress and fear. Other parents use a variety of resources to prepare the entire family. Children's books are available that present hospitalization and surgery in a positive light. These stories may be helpful when preparing children for hospitalization (Table 14-2 ■). Drawings that allow children to show their interpretation of the disease or disorder can be useful in discussing treatment with school-age or adolescent children (Figure 14-7 ■).

When the child is brought to the hospital, the nurse must determine the amount and quality of preparation the child and family have received. It is important to establish a positive relationship with the child and family, answer questions, and reduce fear and anxiety as much as possible. Remember that even though parents may have a general understanding of hospital equipment and routines, the

experiences will be new for the child. Time must be allowed for adequate explanation, orientation to the environment, and emotional support.

The admission procedure for children is similar to that for adults. The child and family must be oriented to the environment, including the location of the bathroom, use of nurses' call light, and instructions on how to raise and lower the head of the bed. A toddler or young child may be placed in a crib with a hard bubble top to prevent him or her from climbing out (Figure 14-8 ■).

clinical ALERT

For safety, the mattress must fit securely in the crib. The distance between the slats should be no greater than 2⅜ in. (6 cm). If the child is capable of climbing, a hard bubble top should be secured to the crib.

Hospital routines should be discussed, including meal time, unit security, and visiting hours. The child will be asked to put on hospital pajamas, and the nurse will complete and document an assessment. Although the focus of the assessment will be the child's presenting medical condition, the nurse should also evaluate the child's level of growth and development. The child's height and weight should be obtained (see procedures in Chapter 13 ⬭). The nurse should observe the child's behavior and question the child and parents to determine if the child has met developmental milestones. The charge nurse will determine client problems and begin the nursing care plan.

Preparation for Procedures

To some extent, preparing the child and family for procedures is no different than preparing an adult for the same procedure. Providing instruction, obtaining informed consent, giving medication, assessing health status, and documenting care are the same. However, more time needs to be spent in preparing the child for procedures. Some children will need a brief explanation immediately before the procedure, while others will need detailed information several days ahead of time. If too much time is allowed between instruction and the procedure, some children might forget the instructions; in contrast, others might become upset, worrying about what is ahead. Parents are instrumental in preparing the child. See Table 14-2 for some resources that can be used to prepare children for hospitalization and procedures.

Children like to dress up as part of play. Fear of the unknown can be decreased by helping children dress like a doctor or nurse, play with a doll, and use equipment similar to that used in the procedure. This therapeutic play can be used one to one with the child, or in small groups of siblings or children experiencing similar procedures.

TABLE 14-2

Books for Hospitalized Children

TITLE AND AUTHOR	READING LEVEL	PUBLISHER AND PUBLICATION DATE	DESCRIPTION
Chemo Girl: Saving the World One Treatment at a Time (Paperback) by Christina Richmond	All ages	Jones & Bartlett; 1st ed., 1996	Describes chemotherapy and cancer treatment through superhero Chemo Girl
Doctor Maisy (Paperback) by Lucy Cousins	Baby–preschool	Candlewick; 2001	Maisy and Tallulah play hospital; Poor Panda is sick but feels much better with Doctor Maisy in charge; when it's Maisy's turn to need help, Nurse Tallulah comes to the rescue
My Friend the Doctor (Hardcover) by Joanna Cole	Baby–preschool	HarperCollins; 2005	A reassuring, cheery book about going to the doctor
Kevin Goes to the Hospital (The On My Way Books) (Hardcover) by Liesbet Slegers	Baby–preschool	Kane/Miller; 2002	A book that will explain, comfort, and make less scary the experience of going to the hospital
The Hospital (Talk-about-Books No. 15) (Board book) by Debbie Bailey	Baby–preschool	Annick Press; 2000	Explores in a positive and realistic fashion what children can expect if they go to a hospital
How Do Dinosaurs Get Well Soon? (Hardcover) by Jane Yolen	Ages 4–8	Blue Sky Press; 2003	Playful read-aloud verse and wonderfully amusing pictures relieve children's fears about being sick
What Is Cancer Anyway?: Explaining Cancer to Children of All Ages (Paperback) by Karen L. Carney	Ages 4–8	Dragonfly; 1998	This book provides basic, essential information when someone in the family has cancer
Kathy's Hats: A Story of Hope (Hardcover) by Trudy B. Krisher	Ages 4–8	Albert Whitman & Company; reprint ed., 1992	A story about chemotherapy treatments and hair loss
A Day With Dr. Waddle (Paperback) by Center for Basic Cancer Research	Ages 4–8	KSU Center for Basic Cancer Research; 1988	A coloring workbook educates children about cancers, and addresses fears and misconceptions
Why, Charlie Brown, Why?: A Story About What Happens When a Friend Is Very Ill (Hardcover) by Charles M. Schulz	Ages 4–8	Ballantine Books; 2002	*Peanuts* gang faces leukemia in a good friend; a story of a child dealing with great challenges and profound questions
Henry and the White Wolf (Hardcover) by Tim Karu	Ages 4–8	Workman; 2000	Storybook and allegory drawn from teenager's own feelings of being in the hospital
A Night without Stars (Paperback) by James Howe	Ages 9–12	Aladdin; 1996	Girl about to undergo open heart surgery meets patient who answers questions and becomes a friend
Jamie Drum's Massive Recovery (Paperback) by Paul Davies	Ages 9–12	Element Books Ltd.; 1998	Entertaining, inspirational, and funny book about a 13-year-old boy in the hospital
Let Him Live (One Last Wish) (Paperback) by Lurlene Mcdaniel	Ages 9–12	Laurel Leaf; 1993	17-year-old boy awaiting a liver transplant; his "one last wish" money is used to build a center for terminally ill kids

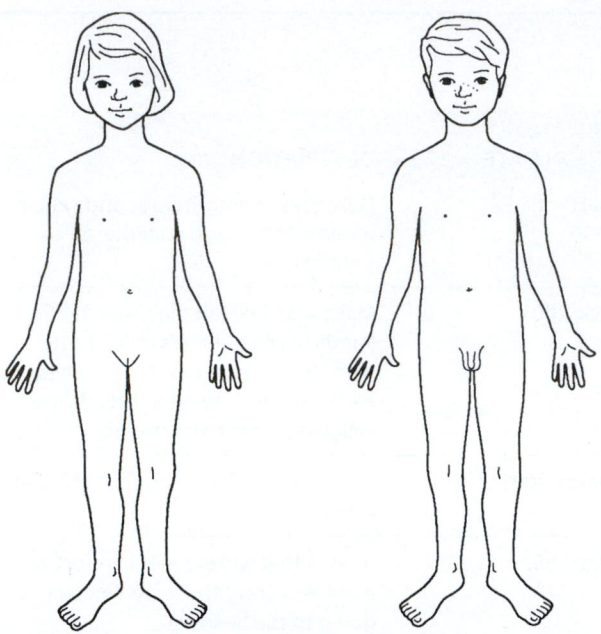

Figure 14-7. ■ The nurse can use a simple gender-specific drawing of a child's body to encourage children to draw what they think about their medical problems. Such drawings reveal the child's interpretation, which the nurse can work with to provide appropriate care.

In most cases, the actual procedure will be the same as for an adult. However, conscious sedation may be used to keep the child calm, provide for the child's safety, and limit the child's memory of the experience. Conscious sedation is discussed later in this chapter.

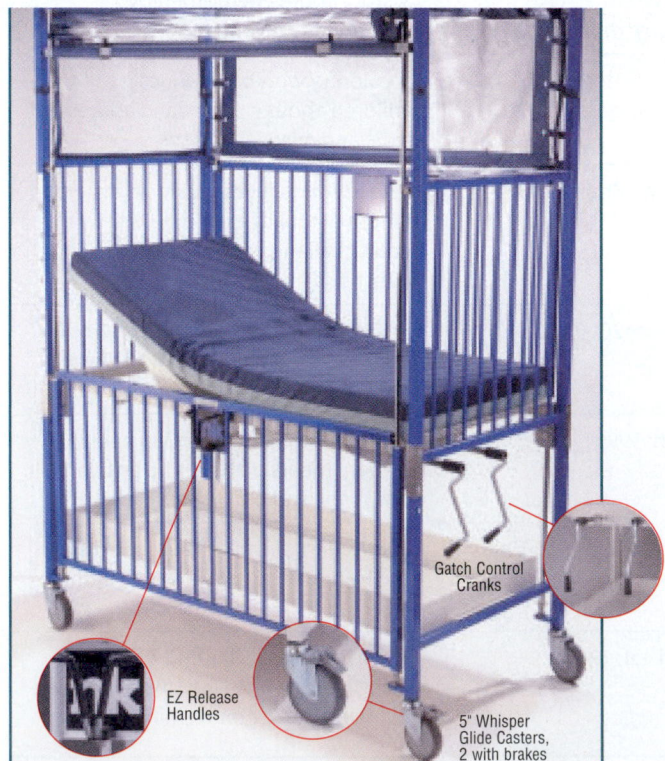

Gatch Control Cranks

EZ Release Handles

5" Whisper Glide Casters, 2 with brakes

Figure 14-8. ■ A hard bubble-top crib protects a climbing child from injury. (Courtesy of nk Medical Products.)

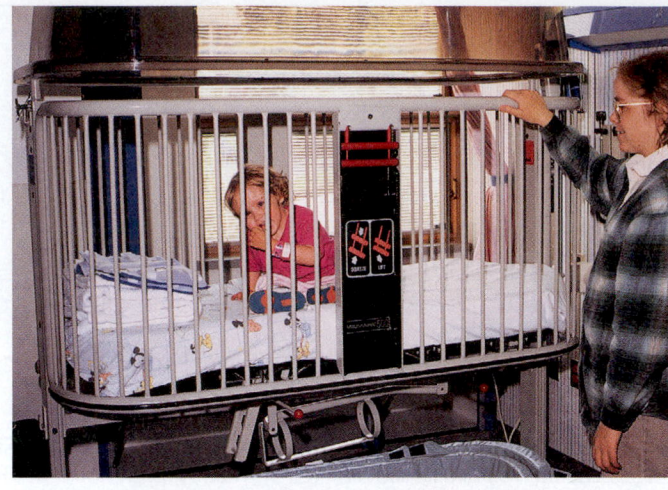

A

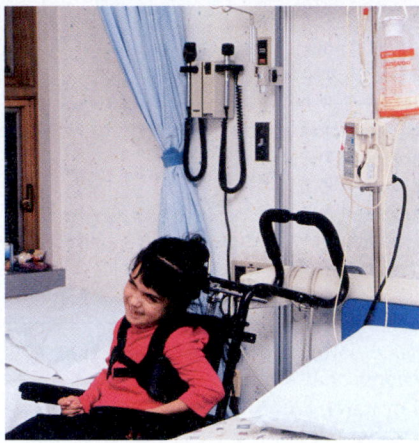

B

Figure 14-9. ■ (**A**) Infants and toddlers are transferred in high-topped cribs. (**B**) This child, who is getting tube feedings or other infusions during the day, can be easily and safely transported in a wheelchair equipped with a safety harness. The tube feeding or infusion on the pole can be rolled with the child from place to place. Pumps can be attached to the pole to regulate infusion rates.

TRANSFER SAFETY

If the child is to be transported to another area of the hospital for the diagnostic exam or treatment, safety is an issue. The child should be transported in a crib with high sides, a youth bed, or a wheelchair with a safety harness, or on a stretcher (Figure 14-9 ■). The child should be lying down with the side rails raised. A safety belt may be fastened across the child's abdomen to prevent the child from falling off the stretcher. Children should not be left unattended.

Care of the Child Before and After Surgery

BEFORE SURGERY

The care of the child before and after surgery is similar to the care of the adult. In all clients, psychological preparation helps relieve fear of the unknown. Children need to

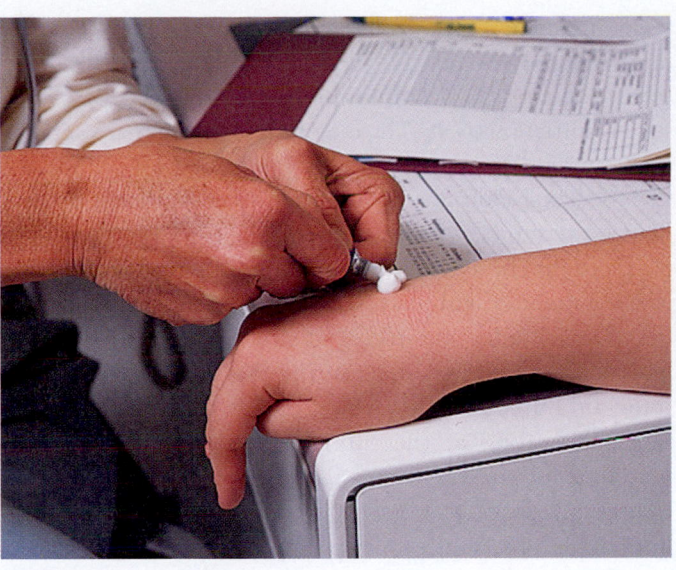

A

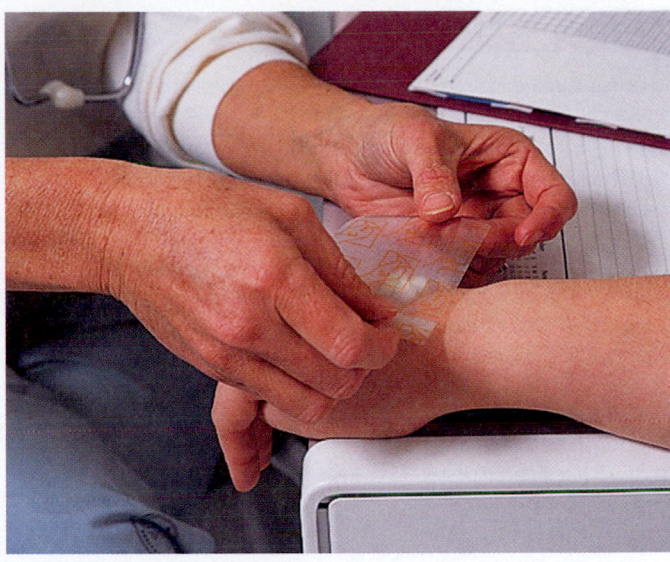

B

Figure 14-10. ■ When painful procedures are planned, use EMLA cream to anesthetize the skin where the painful stick will be made. **(A)** A thick layer of cream is applied over intact skin (½ of a 5-g tube). **(B)** The cream is covered with a transparent adhesive dressing, sealing all the sides. The cream anesthetizes the dermal surface in 45 to 60 minutes.

be reassured that parents will be able to remain with them as long as possible and will be there shortly after they wake up. They should be introduced to key operating room personnel and be shown surgical attire. For example, the anesthesiologist wearing surgical scrubs and a surgical hat should meet the child and talk briefly about how he or she will observe the child during the surgery. The anesthesiologist should put on a surgical mask in front of the child and explain that everyone in the operating room will be wearing masks. When time allows, the child should have the opportunity to play with anatomically correct dolls, drawings, and surgical attire in order to learn about the surgical experience.

The physical preparation of the child preoperatively is the same as that for adults. A parent or legal guardian must sign the informed consent. (Teenage children may also sign a consent form, and in some states, their consent is sufficient to perform certain procedures. See Chapter 2 ⚭ for discussion of legal and ethical issues related to children. The nurse needs to be familiar with legal practices within the state.) Preparation includes nothing by mouth (NPO) for several hours, emptying the bladder, initiating an IV infusion, and administering preoperative medication. Local or topical anesthetics may be used for painful procedures such as IV infusions. Figure 14-10 ■ illustrates the application of eutectic mixture of local anesthetics (EMLA) cream.

PCA Pump Instructions

Older children may be trained in the use of a patient-controlled analgesia (PCA) device. The **PCA pump** (Figure 14-11 ■) is a device attached to an IV line that allows the client to

release pain medication as needed. It is often used as a short-term treatment method after surgery. It is also used in clients who are terminally ill as a way of providing palliative care. After a loading dose of pain medication is administered to initiate pain relief, the client may push a button to obtain more medication as pain intensifies. The pump can be programmed to deliver medication at certain intervals (e.g., during the night) when the client is asleep. It also has a "lockout interval" that prevents too much medication from being administered too quickly.

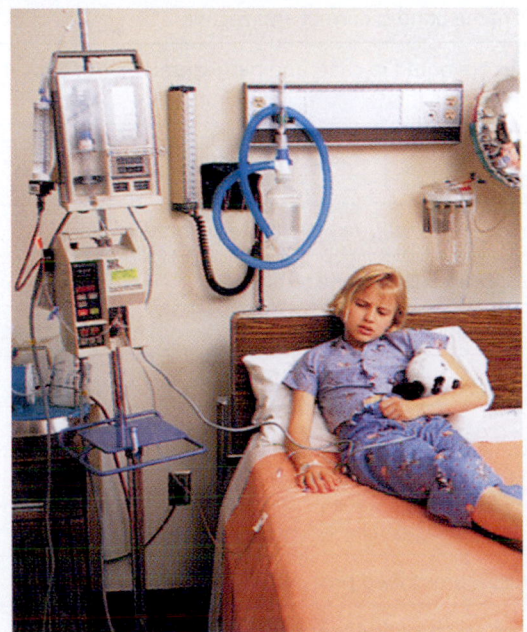

Figure 14-11. ■ The older child is able to regulate a PCA pump.

The nurse must ensure that safeguards are in place to protect clients from accidental overdose with PCA pumps:

- The nurse checks the medication order and computes the maximum 24-hour dose to be sure it does not exceed the safe maximum dose for the child (see Procedure 13-38 ⚭).
- The nurse checks the "lockout interval" of the pump to prevent the child from receiving the entire amount of pain medication too quickly.
- The nurse ensures that the pump is locked so changes to the drip rate or amount can only be made by qualified personnel.
- All pump settings are double checked and documented by two licensed nurses.

The PCA pump is useful because it allows the client control over pain relief measures, thus reducing anxiety. There is no significant difference between the amount of analgesic medication used with this and other methods (Smith, 2004).

Preoperative check sheets are used to ensure that all care has been completed. Table 14-3 ■ provides a sample preoperative checklist.

AFTER SURGERY

Following surgery, the child will be taken to a recovery room where routine postoperative care begins. The airway is maintained, level of consciousness is assessed, vital signs are recorded frequently, surgical dressings and drainage tubes are assessed, IV fluids are monitored, and pain control is initiated. (*Note:* The major discussion of pain appears in Chapter 16 ⚭ . Also, see Figure 13-12 ⚭ for the Wong-Baker Pain Rating Scale.) In some facilities, parents are allowed to be with the child in the recovery room.

Once the child is stable, he or she might be transferred to the inpatient or ambulatory care room. Routine postoperative care includes monitoring of airway, breathing, and circulation; managing pain; ensuring that elimination occurs; providing fluids and advancing diet as tolerated; monitoring the healing of the surgical incision; and providing teaching for the client and family as preparation for discharge (see Boxes 23-1 and 23-5 ⚭). The nurse may teach (or reinforce teaching) about postoperative exercises, such as deep breathing, coughing, and use of the incentive spirometer (IS). Procedure 14-1 ■ describes proper use of the IS.

The LPN/LVN provides input into the individualized care plan and assists in the implementation and evaluation of care. A postoperative checklist for the nurse is provided in Box 14-2 ■.

CARE OF THE CHILD UNDERGOING CONSCIOUS SEDATION

Conscious sedation is the administration of IV medication to produce an impaired level of consciousness. The child will be able to maintain a patent airway, protective reflexes, and response to physical and verbal stimuli. Conscious sedation is used outside the operating room when sedation is required to perform therapeutic or diagnostic procedures safely. In contrast, **deep sedation** is a

TABLE 14-3
Preoperative Checklist
Consent forms are signed, witnessed, and in chart.
Child's name band is correct and secure.
Allergies are noted in chart and highlighted on front cover of chart.
All prosthetic devices are removed, including orthodontic appliances.
Loose teeth and tongue piercings are noted in chart.
Eyeglasses and jewelry are removed.
Skin preparation and preop bath are completed if ordered.
Clean hospital gown; allow child to wear underwear.
All ordered tests are completed and reports are on chart.
Child should void before surgery.
Keep child NPO (usually 4–6 hours preoperatively).
Administer prescribed preoperative medication.
Transport to operating room on stretcher (or in crib).

BOX 14-2	**NURSING CARE CHECKLIST**

Caring for a Child After Surgery

Care of the child after surgery includes both physical and emotional interventions.

- ☑ Monitor vital signs and compare them to baseline.
- ☑ Assess for pain.
- ☑ Provide pain relief and comfort measures.
- ☑ Support effective airway clearance and monitor for signs of respiratory depression or distress.
- ☑ Maintain a complete intake and output record, including fluid loss through dressings, tubes, or vomiting.
- ☑ Check IV status regularly.
- ☑ Monitor the child's level of consciousness.
- ☑ Monitor wound site and dressings for signs of complications.
- ☑ Change dressings as ordered.
- ☑ Provide or reinforce instructions to family and caregivers.

PROCEDURE 14-1 | Teaching Use of the Incentive Spirometer

Purpose

■ To assist lung expansion during the postoperative period

Equipment

■ Incentive spirometer
■ Tissue or paper towel for cleared secretions

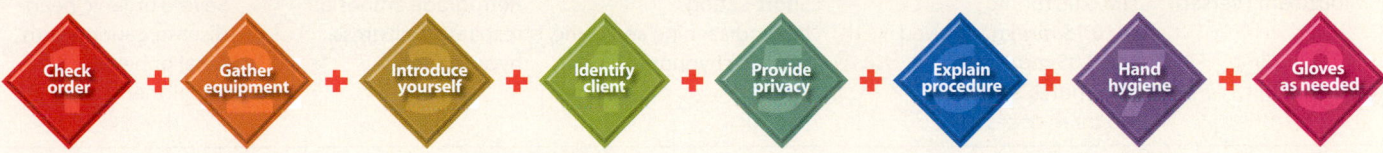

Check order + Gather equipment + Introduce yourself + Identify client + Provide privacy + Explain procedure + Hand hygiene + Gloves as needed

Interventions

1. Explain to parents and child why the spirometer is used. *Lung expansion promotes oxygenation of tissue and clearing of secretions in the airway.*

2. Allow the child to examine the equipment as you describe its use. Point out the elements inside the spirometer tubes (Figure 14-12 ■) and describe how they work. *Having the child handle and feel ownership of the spirometer will encourage compliance.*

3. Indicate the measurements that show how much air the child is inhaling. Tell the child you will mark the highest amount the child can reach. *Having the child focus on the greatest goal possible encourages good results. If there is a presurgical baseline, mark this on the side of the container.*

4. If necessary, show the child how to splint an incision while performing this exercise. *Splinting an abdominal wound will reduce the child's discomfort while performing the exercise.*

5. Instruct the child to exhale as much breath as possible, to close the lips around the mouthpiece of the spirometer, and to slowly inhale. The inside balls or tubes will rise to indicate the amount of air the child is inhaling. Have the child hold the breath for a few seconds and then exhale slowly through pursed lips. *A slow steady breath will fill lungs most completely. Sustained exhalation will concentrate secretions and allow the child to cough them up more easily.*

6. Have the child repeat the procedure two or three times at several points in the day. *This will promote a healthy airway and help in removal of mucus secretions that might otherwise pool in the respiratory tract.*

7. Encourage the child to try to move the balls or tubes higher with each attempt. *Making the exercise into a game encourages repetition and can help promote compliance.*

Note: If an incentive spirometer is not available or is too complicated for the child to use, the child may be given a pinwheel to spin. The child would be encouraged to spin the pinwheel for increasing lengths of time.

Figure 14-12. ■ The incentive spirometer is an excellent method of promoting lung expansion in school-age and older children. (Pearson Education/PH College)

SAMPLE DOCUMENTATION

(date, time)   IS used every 2 hours with maximum inhalation of two balls. Productive cough of white mucus following IS. _____
J. Seege, LPN

controlled state of depressed consciousness or unconsciousness in which the child is unable to maintain protective reflexes. Deep sedation, used during surgical procedures, is administered and maintained by an anesthesiologist or nurse anesthetist.

The medication used for conscious sedation is administered by a skilled RN in an environment where emergency resuscitation equipment and medication are available. Common drugs used for conscious sedation are included in Table 14-4 ■.

TABLE 14-4

Pharmacology: Drugs Used for Conscious Sedation

DRUG	USUAL ROUTE/DOSE	CLASSIFICATION	SELECTED SIDE EFFECTS	DON'T GIVE IF
Diazepam (Valium)	IM/IV less than 5 years, 0.2–0.5 mg slowly every 2–5 minutes up to 5 mg; more than 5 years, 1 mg; every 5 minutes up to 10 mg	Anxiolytic, anticonvulsant	Drowsiness, dizziness, hypotension, respiratory distress	Other drugs are being administered (do not mix)
Midazolam (Versed)	IM 0.08 mg/kg IV 0.15 mg/kg followed by 0.05 mg/kg every 2 minutes × one to three doses	Short-acting benzodiazepine anxiolytic, sedative hypnotic	Retrograde amnesia, respiratory distress, hypotension	Severe organic heart disease; caution with renal or hepatic impairment
Lorazepam (Ativan)	PO, IV, IM 0.05 mg/kg	Benzodiazepine anxiolytic, sedative hypnotic	Drowsiness, sedation, respiratory distress	Child is younger than 12 years

Following the procedure, one-to-one observation and care are required until the child has stable vital signs, age-appropriate verbal and physical response, adequate hydration, and presedation orientation. Parents are instructed regarding diet, fluids, home care, and follow-up as appropriate for the specific procedure.

Preparation for Discharge

Preparation for discharge begins at time of admission. Through use of the nursing process, client and family needs for discharge are identified and plans are made. An RN is responsible for discharge planning, including establishment of the complete teaching plan, follow-up appointment schedules, home health referrals, equipment rental, etc. The LPN/LVN helps with routine teaching, making telephone calls, answering questions, and completing documentation. If the child is going home, all those who will participate in care at home need to be taught proper technique. If the child will be returning to school, the school nurse, teacher, and office personnel must be made aware of the child's health needs, including medication that needs to be given at school. If the child is going to another care facility, communication with the nursing personnel at that facility is critical for a smooth transition. Documentation should include a detailed description of the condition of the child, the instruction provided to the child and family, and verification that all belongings were sent home with the family.

NURSING CARE

PRIORITIES IN NURSING CARE

Besides meeting the biologic needs of airway, breathing, and circulation, the priority of care for a child who is being hospitalized is to make the child feel safe and secure. Hospitaliza-

tion can be frightening to the child and family, and care must be taken to alleviate fear to the greatest extent possible.

ASSESSING

Besides normal pre- or postoperative assessments (vital signs, pain, wound drainage, intake and output (I&O), etc.), observe the child and family for signs of anxiety and fear.

- Is the child "hiding" behind a parent? Does the child hang on to the parent? *These are signs that the child is scared and seeking the protection of the parent.*
- Does the child talk with parents, family, and nurse (if age appropriate)? *If the child is fearful, he or she may talk only with parents or family and avoid answering the nurse's questions.*
- Is the child crying, screaming, or running away from the nurse? *These are common reactions in the fearful child.*
- Do the parents show any unusual or extreme signs of anxiety, fear, or physical reaction to the situation or procedure? *Parents who are extremely anxious will not be able to adequately support the needs of the child. This observation should be reported to the charge nurse.*

DIAGNOSING, PLANNING, AND IMPLEMENTING

The plan of care is based on the specific medical problem. Because children may not have an accurate understanding of their condition and their environment, hospitalization causes fear of the unknown. One nursing diagnosis for every hospitalized child should be:

- Fear related to hospitalization.

  Expected outcomes would include:

- The child will rest quietly in bed.
- The child will express less fear, either verbally or nonverbally.
- The child will interact appropriately with the nurse.

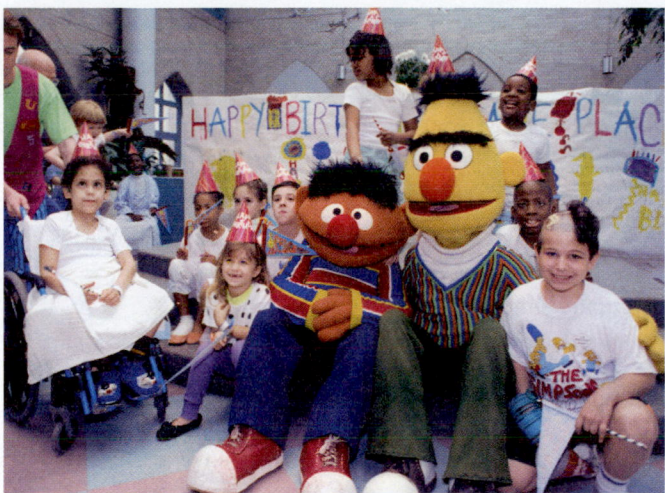

Figure 14-13. ■ Play areas can give the child a welcome diversion from the hospital room. They can also provide space for special events that coincide with hospitalization. (AP Wide World Photo)

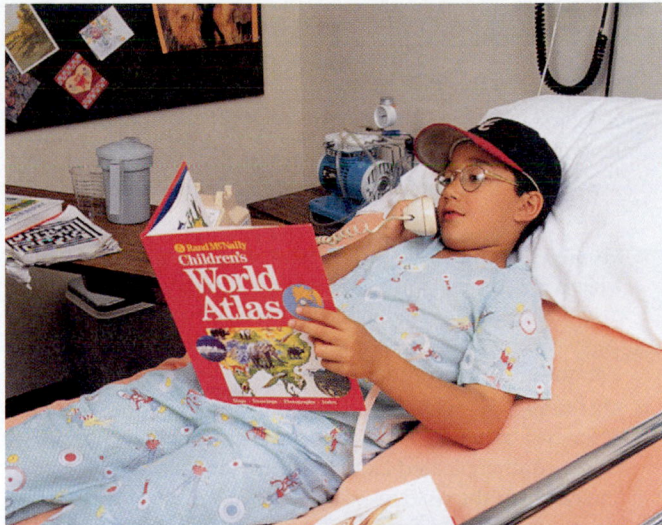

Figure 14-14. ■ It important that the hospitalized child does not fall behind in schoolwork. As soon as the child is able, schoolwork should be resumed. If the child is unable to get out of bed, all necessary study materials should be brought to the child. The child can consult with teachers or classmates on the phone or via computer.

Nursing interventions might include the following.

- Approach child with a smile and introduce self by first name. Avoid bringing equipment to the bedside during the introductory phase of relationship. *The child is fearful in a new environment. A friendly face can help alleviate fear. Additional equipment will only increase the fear of the unknown.*
- Allow a parent or guardian to remain with child. *Family is reassuring to the child.*
- Allow child to hold a favorite toy or blanket. *The familiarity of a favorite toy or blanket provides security to the frightened child.*
- Provide a tour of the hospital and pediatric unit, including introduction of staff when possible. Allow children to play in the playroom before going to their room (Figure 14-13 ■). *Seeing the environment and staff ahead of time can decrease fear of the unknown.*
- Avoid having the child see other children who are very sick or who have a lot of equipment. *Seeing other children who are very sick or who have a lot of equipment may increase the child's fear. The child's imagination can lead him or her to believe that he or she will become extremely sick.*
- Allow child to see and touch equipment before procedures. Use play therapy when providing instructions. *When a child is allowed to see, touch, and "play" with equipment, procedures and hospital routine are not as frightening.*
- Encourage developmentally appropriate activities when possible. *School-age children may find distraction in books or schoolwork* (Figure 14-14 ■).
- In addition to typical postsurgical care, consider alternative measures that may provide comfort (Box 14-3 ■).
- When possible, assign the same nurses to the child on consecutive days. *The child is able to cope better when familiar staff provide care.*
- Review expected events with parents and answer questions as needed. *Reminders about what is to come can reassure the*

overwhelmed parent that things are "under control." Providing answers as soon as possible prevents anxiety from building. A calm parent can be more effective in reassuring and calming a child.

- Encourage parents to provide comfort measures as often as possible (Figure 14-15 ■). *When a child is scared or in pain, the physical presence of the parent can be soothing.*

EVALUATING

The evaluation of the child's level of fear must be made with each interaction. Children need consistency and security in order to rest and heal. Every effort must be made to provide an environment within the hospital that meets this need.

NURSING PROCESS CARE PLAN
The Child Undergoing Hospitalization for Surgery

Five-year-old Timmy is being admitted to the pediatric unit for surgical repair of an umbilical hernia. This is his first hospitalization. His parents told him yesterday of the upcoming surgery.

Assessment

- Timmy appears shy, avoids eye contact, and holds on to his father's hand.
- Timmy answers questions in one or two words, in a whisper.
- Timmy's mother rapidly answers all admission questions.
- Timmy's mother asks numerous questions about all the equipment in the room, and about postoperative care.

BOX 14-3   COMPLEMENTARY THERAPIES

Postoperative Care

After surgery, the child will need physical and pharmacologic interventions as he or she progresses toward recovery. Along the way, alternative therapies may also be of use. Techniques such as the following may be useful.

- **Music Therapy:** Soft music can be played in the background while a child is resting or sleeping; lively, "happy" music can help draw a child's attention away from pain or worry. A recording of ocean waves or even "white noise" created by a fan can override small background sounds and allow deeper sleep.

- **Massage:** A gentle hand or foot massage, or gentle stroking of the hair or head, can be done in almost any body position unless contraindicated. Light massage can relieve some pain and can help the child relax. Rocking, if allowed, provides some muscle stimulation, as well as warmth and security. See also Box 9-3 🔗.

- **Imaging and Relaxation Techniques:** A "let's imagine" game or (for older children) a more directed form of guided imagery can help the child focus attention on a place of comfort and happiness. Flexing and releasing portions of the body not affected by surgery (a hand, a foot, etc.) can improve circulation and increase the child's overall comfort.

- **Hydrotherapy, Heat and Cold Applications:** Hydrotherapy, heat applications, and cold applications may be administered as ordered. However, remember that extra caution is needed with young children, whose skin is thinner than an adult's.

- **Play Therapy:** A variety of play therapy techniques (see Table 14-1) can offer mental relief and diversion to the hospitalized child.

- **Diversion:** In some hospitals, parents may bring video game units from home and connect them to the television in the hospital room. Children may also bring small electronic devices, such as Gameboys, CD players, or MP3 players. Video and DVD players are available for watching favorite movies.

- **TENS:** Transelectrical nerve stimulation (TENS) provides low-voltage electrical stimulation to pain areas or areas that innervate a painful area. Cutaneous stimulation provides pain relief to many clients.

Note: Aromatherapy should not be used in the presence of nausea because it could increase nausea and stimulate emesis. Some aromas can also cause respiratory irritation and distress.

Nursing Diagnosis. The following important nursing diagnosis (among others) is established for this client:

- Anxiety (Child and Family) related to hospitalization, equipment, and surgical outcome.

Expected Outcomes

- The child and his family will show behavior indicating decreased anxiety.

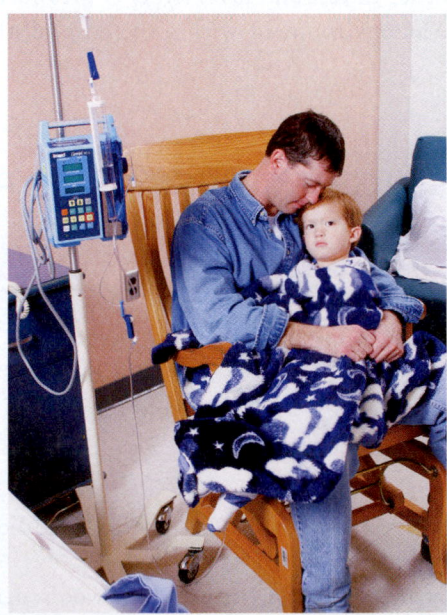

Figure 14-15. ■ The presence of the parent is an important part of pain management.

- The child and his family will verbalize understanding of equipment and events related to hospitalization and surgical outcome.

Planning and Implementation

- Orient the child and family to the hospital setting. *Familiarity with the environment decreases anxiety.*
- Encourage parents to support the child. *Parents have a better understanding of the hospital environment and routines and can be a valuable support for the child.*
- Ask questions of the parent and child about surgery. *Baseline data directs client and family teaching.*
- Teach about preoperative and postoperative events using age-appropriate techniques such as dolls, drawings, and stories. *Allowing children to play "surgery" with dolls helps identify their understanding of what is happening to them. It also is a good way to identify areas for routine preoperative and postoperative teaching.*
- Reinforce the information the family has about the purpose of surgery. *Reinforcing information helps ensure that family members will remember information accurately for future use.*

Evaluation. Observe the child and family for signs of decreased anxiety including increased eye contact, normal speech patterns and tone of voice, and relaxed posture. In-depth preoperative teaching should wait until the child and family become comfortable with the hospital environment. Table 14-5 ■ illustrates a more in-depth care plan for this child in a format that resembles those used in clinical agencies.

(*Care plan questions appear on p. 471.*)

TABLE 14-5

Nursing Process for a Child Undergoing Hospitalization for Surgery

NURSING DIAGNOSIS	GOALS/ OUTCOMES	INTERVENTIONS	RATIONALES
Deficient Knowledge related to preoperative and postoperative events	The child and family will verbalize procedures and events related to the operation. The child and family can demonstrate skills needed in the postoperative period.	■ Ask questions of the parent and child about surgery. ■ Teach about preoperative and postoperative events using age-appropriate techniques such as dolls, drawings, and stories. ■ Reinforce information the family has received about the purpose of surgery. ■ Have the child demonstrate postoperative events pertaining to his or her case (i.e., deep breathing, coughing, putting bandage on doll). ■ Allow parents and child to ask questions.	■ Prior knowledge and understanding can be reinforced and used to guide presentation. ■ Developmental level determines the cognitive approach that works best for teaching. ■ The physician may have explained the surgery. ■ Concrete experience promotes learning. ■ Learners must have the opportunity to ask questions.
Anxiety related to pre- and postoperative events	The child and family will show decreased behavior indicating anxiety. Parents support the child for traumatic procedures.	■ Question the child about expectations of hospitalization and previous experiences. ■ Orient the child to the hospital setting. ■ Institute age-appropriate play and interactions. ■ Explain procedures and prepare for those that might cause trauma. ■ Encourage parents to support the child. ■ Allow the parents and child to ask questions.	■ Previous experiences can influence a client's present anxiety level. ■ Familiarity with the setting and people can decrease anxiety by removing unknown factors. ■ Play can increase the trust level and decrease anxiety. ■ The child is more likely to trust caregivers if they are truthful. ■ The child is more likely to be relaxed if parents are present. ■ Questioning provides an opportunity to explain the unknown, which decreases anxiety.
Risk for Infection related to surgical procedure and intravenous lines	The child will show no signs of infection.	■ Monitor vital signs per hospital routine. Record and report changes from baseline. ■ Monitor surgical dressing and drains every hour. ■ Change or reinforce dressings when wet. ■ Check the IV site every hour for redness, swelling, pain, or pallor.	■ Changes in vital signs, especially increased temperature and pulse, can indicate infection. ■ Excess drainage may indicate infection. ■ Wet dressings can allow organisms to come in contact with surgical wound. ■ IV lines may become infected or infiltrated.
Risk for Injury r/t medications	The child will remain free from injury.	■ Keep side rails up after sedating medications are given. ■ Maintain NPO status while ordered. ■ Inspect skin and respiratory status at least each shift. ■ Monitor IV site for signs of infiltration, infection, and inflammation. ■ Transport child safely secured.	■ Medication can lower level of consciousness. ■ NPO status prevents aspiration. ■ Skin lesions, adventitious breath sounds, and nasal drainage can indicate infection. ■ IV lines may become infiltrated, infected, or cause thrombophlebitis. ■ The child will not fall from bed/stretcher.
Constipation related to surgical procedure and medications	The child will achieve and maintain normal bowel functioning by third postoperative day.	■ Auscultate bowel sounds every 4 hours. Offer liquids only when bowel sounds are present. Assess abdomen for distention. ■ Document the character and frequency of bowel movements. ■ Advance the diet as tolerated. ■ Increase activity as ordered and tolerated.	■ Restricting fluids avoids distention if peristalsis is not normal. ■ Knowledge of bowel status ensures early identification of constipation. ■ Fluids and roughage promote normal bowel function. ■ Physical activity promotes peristalsis.

(continued)

TABLE 14-5

Nursing Process for a Child Undergoing Hospitalization for Surgery (continued)

NURSING DIAGNOSIS	GOALS/ OUTCOMES	INTERVENTIONS	RATIONALES
Imbalanced Fluid Volume (excess/deficit) related to intravenous infusion and NPO status	The child will achieve and maintain proper circulating volume. The child will tolerate oral intake when started, with no nausea, vomiting, or dehydration present.	■ Monitor vital signs per hospital routine. ■ Record intake and output. Be alert for fluid loss via dressings and watery stools. Evaluate hydration status by skin turgor and mucous membranes. ■ Monitor laboratory values of hematocrit and hemoglobin. ■ Begin oral intake after assessment of bowel sounds. Record vomiting. Administer antiemetics as indicated.	■ Changes in vital signs, especially pulse and blood pressure, can indicate fluid imbalance. ■ Intake and output are roughly equivalent. Urinary retention may occur as a result of anesthesia. Good skin turgor and moist mucous membranes indicate fluid balance. ■ Change in lab values indicate dehydration or overhydration. ■ Vomiting can cause fluid loss.
Ineffective Airway Clearance related to anesthetics and pain	The child will maintain adequate ventilation with no respiratory impairment.	■ Auscultate lungs every 2 hours. Record rate, rhythm, and quality of respiration. Evaluate respiratory rate after analgesics. ■ Administer oxygen if ordered. ■ Turn, cough, and deep breathe every 2 hours. Use incentive spirometer, pinwheels, or other appropriate blow toys. Suction airway as needed. ■ Ensure proper intake and output.	■ Early identification of respiratory difficulty aids early treatment. Analgesics, especially narcotics, slow respiratory rate. ■ Oxygen may facilitate breathing. ■ Repositioning and deep breathing ensures expansion of all lung fields. Coughing facilitates removal of mucus from airways. ■ Fluid balance ensures liquification of secretions.
Pain related to surgical procedure	The child will maintain an adequate comfort level.	■ Assess behavioral cues (e.g., crying, movement, guarding). ■ Use an appropriate pain scale with verbal children. ■ Administer prescribed pain medication on a regular basis. ■ Use age-appropriate nonpharmacologic methods of pain control (e.g., distraction, repositioning).	■ Behavior of preverbal children provides clues to pain experience. ■ Pain scales allow children to quantify the amount of pain. ■ Narcotic and nonnarcotic analgesics alter pain perception. ■ Nonpharmacologic interventions interfere with pain perception.
Risk for Impaired Skin Integrity related to limited mobility after surgery	The child's skin will remain intact. The wound heals without complications.	■ Turn and reposition every 2 hours. ■ Keep linens clean and dry. ■ Check pressure areas when turning and gently rub red areas with lotion. ■ Get the child up and ambulating when ordered. ■ Check the incision for drainage, redness, and intactness every 4 to 8 hours. Change wet dressings as ordered.	■ Repositioning takes pressure off the skin and allows increased circulation. ■ Clean linens decrease the chance of skin breakdown. ■ Gently rubbing increases circulation. ■ Movement decreases pressure on skin. ■ Early detection of infection or problems with wound healing can ensure fast treatment. Dry dressings prevent skin breakdown around wound.
Anxiety (Child and Family) related to equipment and surgical outcome	The child and family will demonstrate coping skills to deal with hospitalization.	■ Explain monitors, drains, dressings, IV lines, other equipment, and procedures. ■ Reassure the child and family that anxiety is a normal response to the stressful event of surgery. ■ Encourage parental presence and care of the child.	■ Knowledge of purpose decreases anxiety. ■ Knowledge of what is expected decreases anxiety. ■ The child's anxiety decreases with parental presence.
Deficient Knowledge related to home care.	The child and family will verbalize self-care required at home.	■ Provide oral and written home care instructions regarding surgical wound care, medications, activities, diet, and signs of complications. ■ Provide a number to call for questions or concerns. Instruct on follow-up visits.	■ Teaching regarding home care is necessary early in hospitalization. Written instruction provides a reference when at home. ■ Parents need to know emergency information and that follow-up care is required.

Critical Thinking in the Nursing Process

1. Timmy asks when he can play T-ball again. How should the nurse respond?

2. Timmy's parents ask if the umbilical hernia can come back in the future. How should the nurse respond?

3. What would be some indications that surgery should not take place?

Note: Discussion of Critical Thinking questions appears in Appendix I.

CHRONICALLY ILL CHILD

Some children with chronic illness have a **hereditary condition** (genetic inheritance from a parent or parents). Others have a **congenital condition** (condition present at birth) that results in a chronic disorder. Some of these children, using adaptive equipment, lead a relatively normal life. They go to school, church, and stores, and participate in individual or group activities, including sports. However, other children have more difficulty adapting and spend their life at home with limited outside activities. Parents need direction and support from nurses in learning to care for these children. Details about specific illnesses are discussed in later chapters of this book.

Care at Home

Caring for a child who is chronically ill at home can be physically, emotionally, and financially draining. Depending on the condition of the child, special equipment might be needed, including beds, ventilators, IV infusion pumps, and wheelchairs (Figure 14-16 ■). Parents either purchase or lease this equipment. The house might need some remodeling to accommodate the equipment. Time and resources are needed for this adjustment. The child might be cared for in a rehabilitation facility or placed in a long-term care facility while the adjustments to the home are being made.

Many children with chronic illness need 24-hour care or supervision. For example, if the child's illness involves the respiratory system and requires the child to be on a ventilator, a care provider needs to be present to suction the airway or respond to an emergency. Parents who must work outside the home and care for other children may not be able to provide this 24-hour care. As the child grows, the parent may not be physically able to provide all the care the child needs.

Parents of these children are on an emotional roller-coaster. At times, they feel guilt about the condition of their child and their ability (or inability) to provide care. They might blame each other or themselves because they are unable, either physically or financially, to meet the demands the child places on the family. They might be angry with the ill child for "robbing" them of a "normal" family life. Although they love the child, they might sometimes want the child to die so the burden of caring for him or her would be lifted.

The nurse has several roles in such situations. To assist the child and family, the nurse not only provides care and uses

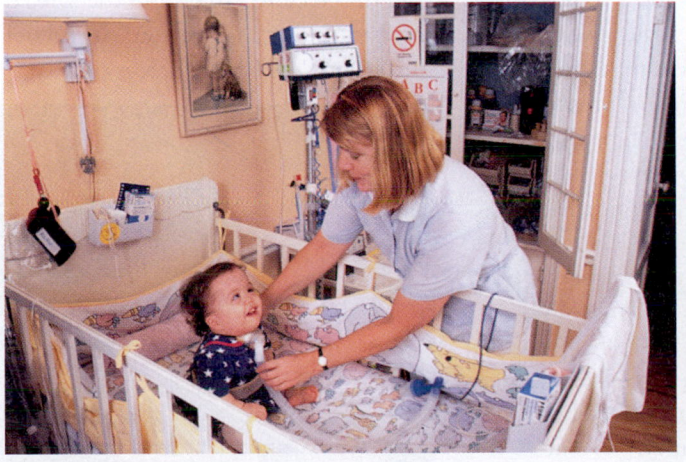
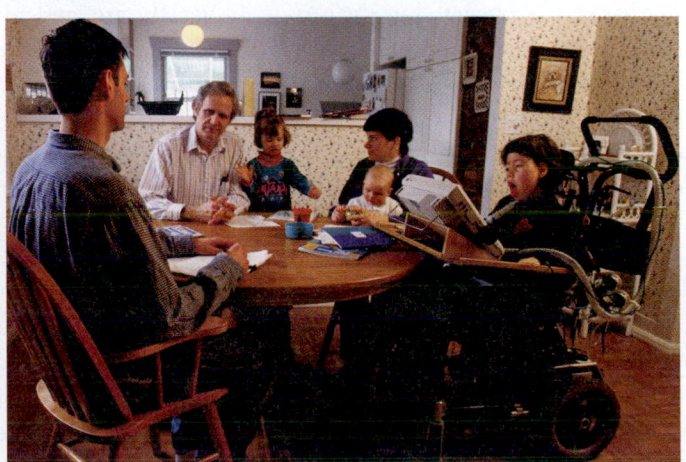

A   B

Figure 14-16. ■ **(A)** It is often desirable from a family and cost perspective to provide health care in the home, and advances in technology have made this possible. **(B)** Daily caregiving demands of the child who is medically fragile continue 24 hours a day, 7 days a week. Parents need to identify ways to share the care of the child and other family care management. When the child lives with a single parent, additional health care resources are needed so the parent can sleep.

MediaLink   Tracheostomy

therapeutic communication to help explore feelings, but also assists the family in finding additional resources. The LPN/LVN can assist with direct care, provide respite to family members, and monitor the child's condition.

Care at School

The staff in school have a responsibility to provide care for children if they become ill or injured. This responsibility includes care of the child riding to and from school on a bus, care of the child on the playground, and care of the child during field trips and during extracurricular activities. Some school districts are able to have an RN in each school to care for students who are ill or injured (Figure 14-17 ■). In other school districts, an RN must travel among several schools. An LPN/LVN might be hired to assist the RN. In the absence of a licensed nurse, the counselor, teacher, or office personnel will be required to assist a child who is ill or injured until a parent or guardian can be called. It is important to

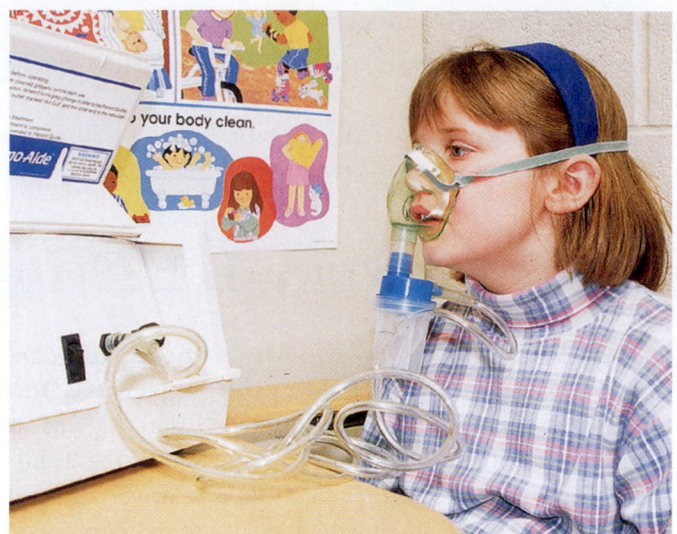

Figure 14-17. ■ This child requires use of a nebulizer during school hours. The nurse or trained school personnel must administer medication on a regular basis. (Photo: © Chris Lowe/Phototake/All rights reserved)

HEALTH PROMOTION ISSUE

UNLICENSED PERSONNEL ADMINISTERING MEDICATIONS AT SCHOOL

Jane, an 8-year-old second-grader, was recently diagnosed with chronic asthma. The doctor ordered medication by inhaler to control bronchospasms. Jane will need to have medication available for use at school if she needs it. Jane's school district has an RN on staff, but she is responsible for children in three grade schools and therefore may not be present to administer the medication. The office secretary will be responsible for administering the medication when necessary.

DISCUSSION

The administration of medications has been one of the major duties of RNs and LPNs. This duty was specifically identified in state nurse practice acts as being within the scope of licensed nurse practice. The standard was that any individual who administered medication to anyone except immediate

family without RN or LPN licensure could be accused of practicing nursing without a license.

In recent years, many changes in nursing practice have resulted from nursing shortages, the rising costs of health care, and advances in medical science. Today, in a variety of settings, unlicensed personnel are responsible for the administration of prescribed and over-the-counter medications. Some states have approved courses to prepare unlicensed persons to administer medications safely. These courses cover the administration process, but they do not address pharmacology or pathophysiology. It is the responsibility of licensed nurses to ensure these medications are administered safely and to evaluate their effectiveness.

The administration of medication by the office secretary is an example of this

issue. Many children with chronic disorders are required to take prescribed medication several times a day. If a dose is due while the child is at school, an adult school employee must be responsible for giving the medication to the child. To ensure the safe administration of medication, the school nurse must follow the delegation

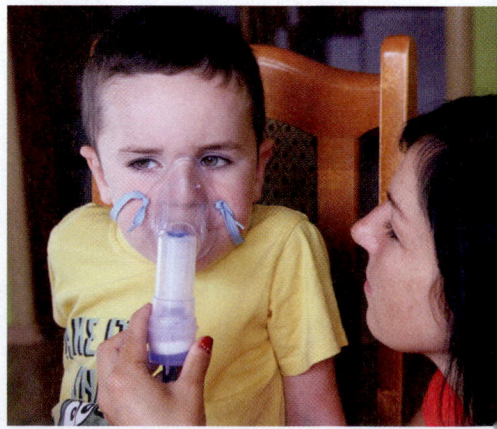

(greenland/Alamy)

teach the school personnel to care for the child who is ill or injured. Teaching would include basic first aid, cardiopulmonary resuscitation (CPR), and administration of medications. See Health Promotion Issue below.

Most children who become ill at school have a respiratory or gastrointestinal infection. They need to be removed from contact with other children while waiting for parents or guardians. To prevent spread of infection, anyone caring for these children must wash their hands before having contact with others.

Children at school could also get injured on the playground. These injuries include falls, broken bones, or cuts and scrapes. Basic first aid is needed in most cases. If the injury appears severe, emergency medical personnel should be called.

Some common chronic conditions affect children but do not prevent them from attending school. An **individualized education plan (IEP)** is an interdisciplinary plan that pinpoints the special educational needs of a particular student and establishes a plan for meeting them. The IEP may need to be established and may include home tutors, specialized services from speech therapists, transport of the child with disabilities to school, and provisions for specialized medical care as needed. When this is the case, the school nurse works with parents and school personnel to ensure that the health needs of the child are met. Examples of these conditions include asthma, diabetes, cerebral palsy, muscular dystrophy, spinal cord injuries, Down syndrome, and attention deficit disorder. These children might need assistance with blood testing, administration of insulin, and diet monitoring. Medication and counseling for children with behavior problems must be provided. Special equipment, such as walkers and wheelchairs, might be needed. Classrooms might need to be altered to make room for this equipment. The child with spinal cord injury might need respiratory support and airway clearance. The child might need help using the bathroom or eating lunch. Often, an individual is hired to provide this one-to-one care while the child is at school. The nurse should meet with school personnel and parents to assess health needs and to plan, implement, and evaluate care.

process in assessing, teaching, and supervising the unlicensed school personnel. (Review the delegation process in Chapter 1 ⚭.)

To supervise unlicensed school personnel in the safe administration of medication, the nurse must:

- Assess the child and parents. The nurse must meet with the parents to obtain information about the child's disorder, the prescribed medication, and the child's usual reaction to the medication. The nurse should receive consents, the medication, and a copy of the physician's orders from the parents.
- Meet with the appropriate school personnel to obtain information about their knowledge and experience in the administration of medication to children.

PLANNING AND IMPLEMENTATION

Once the nurse has obtained information from the child, parents, and school personnel, plans for administering the medication can be made. These plans should include:

- Teaching the school personnel about the medication, how to give and document the medication, when not to give the medication, and when to call the school nurse.
- Indicating when and where the medication will be given, and how the child will get there.
- Indicating when, where, and how the nurse will provide supervision.

The nurse should watch the unlicensed person administer the medication until consistent safe administration can be documented. The nurse should be available in person or by telephone to answer questions.

SELF REFLECTION

What would your feelings be about having your child receive medication while at school? In what circumstances do you think an unlicensed person would need to call the nurse? What information must the nurse give to the unlicensed person in order to ensure safe administration of medication?

SUGGESTED RESOURCES

For the Nurse

- Bindler, R., & Howry, L. (2005). *Pediatric drug guide with nursing implications.* Upper Saddle River, NJ: Prentice Hall.

- Newacheck, P. A., McManus, M., Fix, H. B., Hung, Y. Y., & Halfon, N. (2000). Access to health care for children with special health needs. *Pediatrics, 105*(4), 760–766.

Even in the absence of illness or injury, the school nurse is instrumental in collecting health-related data for all school children. Vision testing, hearing testing, and keeping records related to growth and immunizations are but a few examples. Sometimes there might be an outbreak of head lice or infectious disease such as whooping cough. The school nurse must work with other public health department personnel to assess, treat, and evaluate children and to assist in teaching parents.

Rehabilitation

Some children with chronic conditions can benefit from rehabilitation. For example, a 10-year-old with *Legg–Calvé–Perthes disease* (a disorder characterized by degeneration of the femoral head) will need extensive rehabilitation to learn to walk with leg braces and to regain normal use of the legs once the braces are removed (Figure 14-18 ■; see Chapter 17 ⚭). During the rehabilitation process, the child may be admitted to a pediatric rehabilitation unit or a general rehabilitation center. When planning and implementing physical care for the pediatric client, the nurse must also take care to meet the child's growth and development needs (see Figure 14-18B). School-age children and adolescents may need a tutor to keep up with schoolwork.

Long-Term Care

Some children have chronic conditions that prevent them from attending school or, because of family conditions, that prevent them from living at home. These children might be placed in a long-term care facility. Some communities may have a long-term care facility, such as a state school and hospital, that is designed for children with extensive physical and mental disabilities (Figure 14-19 ■). Other communities have only long-term care facilities that have been designed for the elderly. Although placing children with disabilities and clients who are elderly together can promote a special bond, these facilities may not be prepared to deal with the care necessary to stimulate the development of the child. Admitting a child to these facilities poses a challenge for the nurses and staff; it also places an emotional and financial drain on the family.

The physical care of the child with chronic disabilities may be similar to that of the dependent adult; however, it has different challenges. With the proper attention, many children with major disabilities can remain stable or make progress. Progress may or may not allow them to live independently, but it may allow them to enjoy life in a different way. Activities need to be planned that provide age-specific physical, mental, and occupational therapy. Because pro-

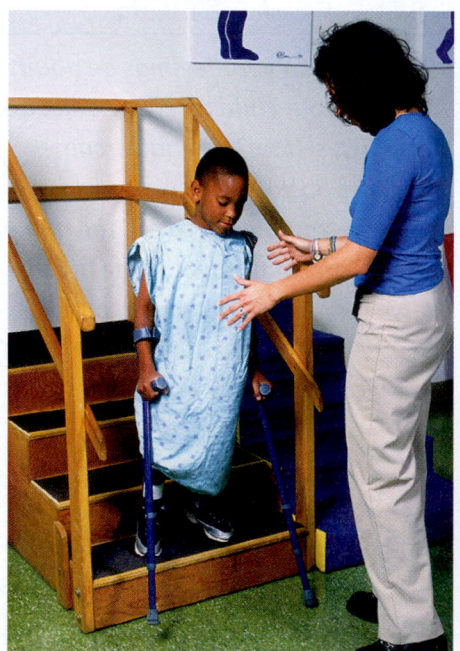
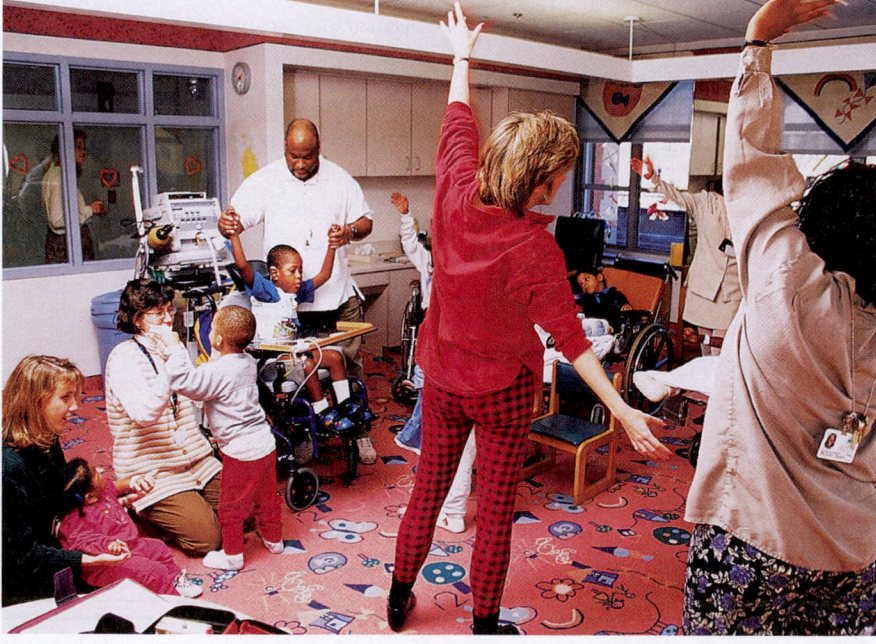

A   B

Figure 14-18. ■ (A) Rehabilitation units provide an opportunity for the child to relearn such tasks as walking and climbing stairs. They provide an important transition from hospital to home and community. (B) The nurse can help the child and family accept and adjust to new circumstances. Encouraging a child in a wheelchair to participate in group activities can help build self-esteem, goal attainment, personal satisfaction, and general health.

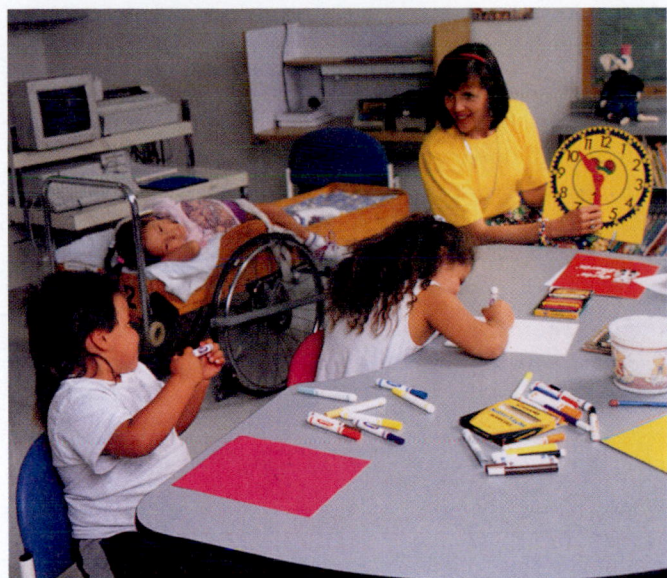

Figure 14-19. ■ Shriner's Hospital in Spokane, Washington, has a special room and teachers for children undergoing lengthy hospital stays, enabling them to remain current with their schoolwork.

gress might be slow, it is important to provide the child with consistent daily therapy for many years.

The nurse needs to work closely with other professionals who have received education specific to the child with a disability in a long-term care facility. Programs of physical therapy, behavioral therapy, and occupational therapy must be designed to meet the needs of each child. Caregivers and therapists must be consistent in their approach to the child. It can be the responsibility of the LPN/LVN to assist in the plan development, supervise unlicensed caregivers, and document changes. Care of these children must be through an interdisciplinary team approach. LPNs and LVNs can be important members of that team.

Care of the Caregivers

Providing care on a daily basis for the child who is chronically ill or disabled is extremely challenging and stressful. The entire family is affected by the amount of attention the child requires. If the child needs close supervision 24 hours a day, parents may take turns monitoring the child at night while the other parent sleeps. Over time, the caregivers become physically and mentally tired. They can begin to feel trapped. They suffer from burnout. The marriage relationship suffers, and divorce is common.

Siblings in a family with a child who is chronically ill may believe that they must compete for parental attention. They may become jealous of the sibling or angry that the sibling takes so much of their parents' time and financial resources. At school or on the playground, they may be put in a situation of defending their sibling. If they are old enough, they may be asked by the parents to help with the physical care of the child with a disability. These issues place additional stress on family relationships.

It is important for the nurse to address caregiver strain. The nurse can be instrumental in helping the family explore their feelings and develop a plan to prevent burnout. The plan might include a respite support system, taking time for each other and the other members of the family. Sometimes the family needs to discuss obtaining additional help or admitting the child to a long-term care facility. Resources might include extended family, friends, clergy, support groups, and social services.

NURSING CARE

PRIORITIES IN NURSING CARE

The priorities in providing care for the child who is chronically ill or disabled include:

- Providing a safe environment for the child
- Providing activities that promote healing
- Providing activities that promote growth and development in the child
- Providing for caregiver support.

ASSESSING

An assessment of the environment where the child will live and develop must be made in advance of the child's arrival. The environmental assessment must include the following questions:

- What is the functional level of the child?
- What assistive devices are needed for the child?
- Can the child access the bathroom, dining area, and bedroom?
- Are the rooms large enough to accommodate any necessary equipment?
- Is the environment safe for the child?
- Is appropriate care available 24 hours a day?
- Is transportation available for the child to attend school, church, and clinic visits?
- What is the child's current developmental level?
- Are the care activities and household duties shared by members of the family?
- Is a support system available to provide respite for the caregivers?

DIAGNOSING, PLANNING, AND IMPLEMENTING

In addition to nursing diagnoses for the specific disorder, other nursing diagnoses might include:

- Self-Care Deficit (specific to the individual child)
- Delayed Growth and Development
- Compromised Family Coping
- Risk for Caregiver Role Strain.

Expected outcomes for these diagnoses include:

- The child will provide as much self-care as possible in a safe environment.
- The child will maintain or show progress in growth and development.
- The caregivers will verbalize stress at an acceptable level.

The nurse would perform the following interventions to assist children who are chronically ill and their families:

- Help parents provide a safe environment for the child, taking into account any needed equipment or accommodation. *The home of a child who is chronically ill may need many adjustments in order for a safe environment to exist.*
- Encourage the child to care for self as much as possible. *Self-care aids the child's development and supports self-esteem.*
- Encourage parents to allow child to care for self as much as possible. *The parents may want to do things "for" their child. Remind them that they are showing love when they allow the child to do all he or she can.*
- Teach caregivers to provide necessary care. *All caregivers must receive instruction so safe and adequate care can be provided.*
- Encourage caregivers to verbalize feelings. *Teach caregivers that verbalizing feelings will allow them to look at the situation honestly and work together for solutions.*
- Encourage caregivers to make a plan to minimize stress. *Planning time for self and for activities that minimize stress will allow the caregiver to return refreshed to continue giving care.*
- Provide written referrals for the child and family. *Resources and support groups can help the child and family cope more effectively.*

EVALUATING

Evaluation must be an ongoing process. Once a safe environment has been established, changes will only need to be made if the child's condition changes. The child's growth and development should be evaluated every 3 to 6 months and the plans updated. Caregiver strain should be evaluated with each nursing contact.

Note: The references and resources for this and all chapters have been compiled at the back of the book.

Chapter Review

 ## KEY TERMS by Topic

Use the audio glossary feature of either the CD-ROM or the Companion Website to hear the correct pronunciation of the following key terms.

Introduction
illness, acute, chronic, terminal

Role of the LPN/LVN
therapeutic play

Hospitalized Child
child life specialist

Age-Specific Preparation for Hospitalization
separation anxiety

Care of the Child Before and After Surgery
PCA pump, conscious sedation, deep sedation

Chronically Ill Child
hereditary condition, congenital condition, individualized education plan (IEP)

KEY Points

- The needs of the individual child and family must be assessed, and an interdisciplinary plan must be developed.
- Teaching must be provided to the child, parents, and members of the community who will be responsible for aspects of care.
- The child's limited understanding of what is occurring produces anxiety over hospitalization and diagnostic and therapeutic procedures.
- It is important for the nurse to help relieve stress by providing age-specific preparation for hospitalization and for every procedure the child will experience.
- The child who is chronically ill or disabled may require care at school, at home, or in a rehabilitation center or long-term care facility. Nurses in these areas must be prepared to meet the child's physical and developmental needs.
- Caregivers need support to prevent fatigue and burnout.

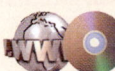 ## EXPLORE MediaLink

Additional interactive resources for this chapter can be found on the Companion Website at www.prenhall.com/towle.

Click on Chapter 14 and "Begin" to select the activities for this chapter.

For chapter-related NCLEX-style questions and an audio glossary, access the accompanying CD-ROM in this book.

Animations

Client pain assessment

Tracheostomy

FOR FURTHER Study

See Chapter 2 for discussion of legal and ethical issues related to children.

Information about culture, ethnicity, and family is discussed in Chapter 3.

Procedures for child's height and weight and for intravenous medications are in Chapter 13.

The Wong-Baker Pain Rating Scale is shown in Figure 13-12.

The major discussion of pain is provided in Chapter 16.

Musculosketal rehabilitation is discussed in Chapter 17.

Details about specific illnesses are discussed in the body systems chapters (16 to 25) of this book.

See Boxes 23-1 and 23-5 for more nursing care after surgery.

Critical Thinking Care Map

Caring for a Child with Bilateral Hip Splints on a Rehabilitation Unit

NCLEX-PN® Focus Area: Physiologic Integrity

Case Study: Andrew Paulson, a 10-year-old with Legg–Calvé–Perthes disease, has been admitted to the rehabilitation unit of a children's hospital. Andrew's disease has been stabilized, and he has been fitted with bilateral hip splints. He will be on the rehabilitation unit for a minimum of 1 month before he is discharged.

Nursing Diagnosis: Risk for Delayed Development related to prolonged rehabilitation

COLLECT DATA

Subjective	Objective
_____	_____
_____	_____
_____	_____
_____	_____
_____	_____
_____	_____
_____	_____

Would you report this? Yes/No

If yes, to: _____

Nursing Care

_____
_____
_____
_____
_____
_____
_____
_____
_____
_____
_____
_____
_____

How would you document this? _____
_____
_____
_____

Compare your documentation to the sample provided in Appendix I.

Data Collected
(use those that apply)

- BP 108/62
- Is in fourth grade
- Does not like school
- Weight 89 lb
- Enjoys reading fiction stories
- States pain in both hips
- States he misses playing football
- Good strength in upper extremities

Nursing Interventions
(use those that apply; list in priority order)

- Tell him he must attend classes to keep up with his schoolwork.
- Limit extra reading until schoolwork is completed.
- Orient to environment and facility routine.
- Insist he participate in physical therapy activities.
- Administer pain medication as ordered.
- Insist he perform ADLs with minimal assistance.
- Contact teacher to obtain information about school assignments.

NCLEX-PN® Exam Preparation

TEST-TAKING TIP When answering questions about care of children, use any information about age or developmental stage to help determine the appropriate response.

1 Ten-month-old Susie was admitted to the pediatric unit with newly diagnosed cystic fibrosis. The nurse would expect Susie to respond to the staff with which of the following behaviors:

1. outward hostility
2. fear of strangers
3. frequent negativism
4. occasional jealousy

2 A child with cystic fibrosis is to be treated with a mist tent while in bed at home. Before discharge, which of the following is most important for the discharge planner to evaluate?

1. the size of the child's bedroom
2. the child's respiratory rate while sleeping
3. who will provide care for the child at school
4. the relationship of the parents

3 An 8-year-old has been prescribed antibiotic tablets every 6 hours. One dose is due during school hours. The parents should be advised to:

1. keep her home from school until the antibiotics are gone.
2. have her skip the dose while at school.
3. have school personnel administer the dose.
4. have her double the next dose.

4 When caring for a 3-year-old child in the hospital, it is important to keep the routine as close as possible to _____.

5 A Native American 4-year-old girl has been admitted for surgery tomorrow. Her family requests that the medicine man be allowed to burn incense and dance around her before surgery. The nurse should respond:

1. "Modern medicine will make her better. Those primitive measures are of no use."
2. "I will provide space and privacy for you. Please keep any music or chanting to a low volume to avoid disturbing other clients."
3. "That is not allowed within the hospital environment."
4. "Because of hospital policy, I cannot allow you to burn anything."

6 Joan is a pediatric client who is severely disabled and who is being cared for at home. When the home health nurse arrives, Joan's mother is pale, weak, and tearful. She states she has

not slept for several nights because Joan has been having diarrhea. The nurse should respond to the mother:

1. "The diarrhea is probably caused by Joan's antibiotics."
2. "I will make arrangements for Joan to be admitted to the nursing home."
3. "Can you tell me how you are feeling right now?"
4. "I will let the doctor know about Joan's diarrhea."

7 When discussing home care for a 5-year-old client who is paraplegic, the nurse should question the family about all of the following. Place them in priority order.

1. plans for the client to attend kindergarten
2. how the client will be bathed
3. transferring the client from bed to wheelchair
4. evacuation plan in case of fire

8 How should a 9-month-old infant be transported to surgery?

1. in a crib with the side rails up
2. on a stretcher with the safety belt fastened
3. in his mother's arms
4. on a youth bed with the side rails up

9 A 3-year-old child is being admitted to a nursing home for long-term care following a severe brain injury acquired in a car accident where both parents were killed. In planning care for this child, the nurse should consider which of the following?

1. a private room to allow for the equipment
2. a semiprivate room with an elderly roommate
3. a room away from the nurses' station to avoid disrupting the child's sleep
4. refusing to admit the child because a nursing home is for the elderly

10 A 16-year-old is admitted to the hospital for knee surgery following a football injury. In providing preoperative teaching, the nurse should:

1. provide brief instruction immediately before surgery to lessen anxiety.
2. provide detailed instruction to the client with a parent present.
3. provide instruction only to the parents so they can sign the consent form.
4. question the client about the use of illicit drugs when the parents are out of the room.

Answers for Review Questions, as well as discussion of Care Plan and Critical Thinking Care Map questions, appear in Appendix I.

Chapter 15

Care of the Child with Fluid, Electrolyte, and Acid-Base Disorders

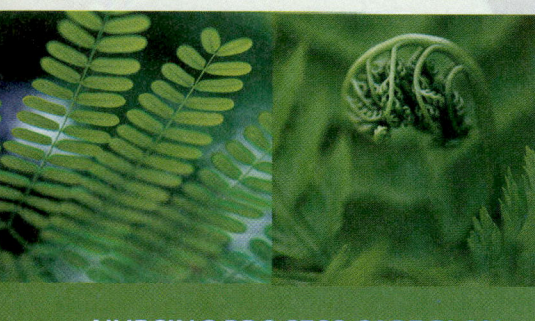

NURSING PROCESS CARE PLAN:
Client with Diarrhea

HEALTH PROMOTION ISSUE:
Self-Asphyxiation as a Game

CRITICAL THINKING CARE MAP:
Caring for a Client with
Fluid Volume Excess

BRIEF Outline

LEARNING Outcomes

After completing this chapter, you will be able to:

- Discuss fluid and electrolyte balance in children.
- Discuss acid-base balance in children.
- Identify alterations in fluid and electrolyte and acid-base balance in children.
- Describe appropriate assessment and interventions related to fluid and electrolyte and acid-base imbalances.

A finer line exists between fluid balance and imbalance in children than in adults. The percent of water in the body varies with age (Figure 15-1 ■). In adults, the percent of water ranges from 50% (females) to 55% (males). Approximately 50% of a child's weight consists of water. In infants, water comprises 60% of body weight. In the newborn, 75% of the weight is water. Because of this high percentage of water, fluid and electrolyte imbalances are much more dangerous in pediatric clients than in adults.

Principles Related to Fluids and Electrolytes

To provide the best nursing care to children with fluid and electrolyte disorders, the nurse must recall foundational principles related to the body's fluids and electrolytes. Health is maintained when fluids and electrolytes are balanced within the body. This state of balance is called **homeostasis.**

FLUIDS

The largest component of the body is water. Body fluids are distributed in two distinct compartments: intracellular and extracellular. Intracellular fluid is found within the body cells. Extracellular fluid is found outside the body cells. Extracellular fluid can be further distinguished as **plasma** (the fluid portion of circulating blood) and interstitial fluid (Figure 15-2 ■). (**Interstitial** relates to spaces within a structure, such as the spaces within a tissue or an organ.)

Before discussing how this fluid moves within the child's body, it is necessary to review certain terms. Fluids consist of liquids and solids. A **solute** is a substance that is dissolved in a solution or fluid. The liquid in which a substance or solute is dissolved is called a **solvent.** A **solution** is formed when one or more solutes are dissolved in a solvent.

The solution of fluids and electrolytes constantly moves across the cell membrane to maintain the work of oxygenation, metabolism, excretion, and other body processes. This movement is accomplished by four methods: osmosis, diffusion, filtration, and active transport (Figure 15-3 ■).

Osmosis is the movement of fluid, the solvent, across the cell membrane from an area of lesser solute concentration to an area of greater solute concentration. Osmosis causes the concentration of solutes on both sides of the cell membrane to become equal.

Through the process of **diffusion,** solutes move across the cell membrane from an area of higher concentration to an area of lower concentration.

Filtration is a process by which solvents and solutes are pushed across a cell membrane from an area of higher pressure to an area of lower pressure. This pressure is called *hydrostatic pressure* or *capillary blood pressure.*

The movement of solutes across the cell membrane by means of metabolic activity and carrier cells is called **active transport.** Active transport uses energy to carry a solute from an area of lower concentration into an area of higher concentration. For example, normally, sodium is most abundant outside the cell and potassium is most abundant inside the cell. To maintain balance of these electrolytes, the

MediaLink

Fluid

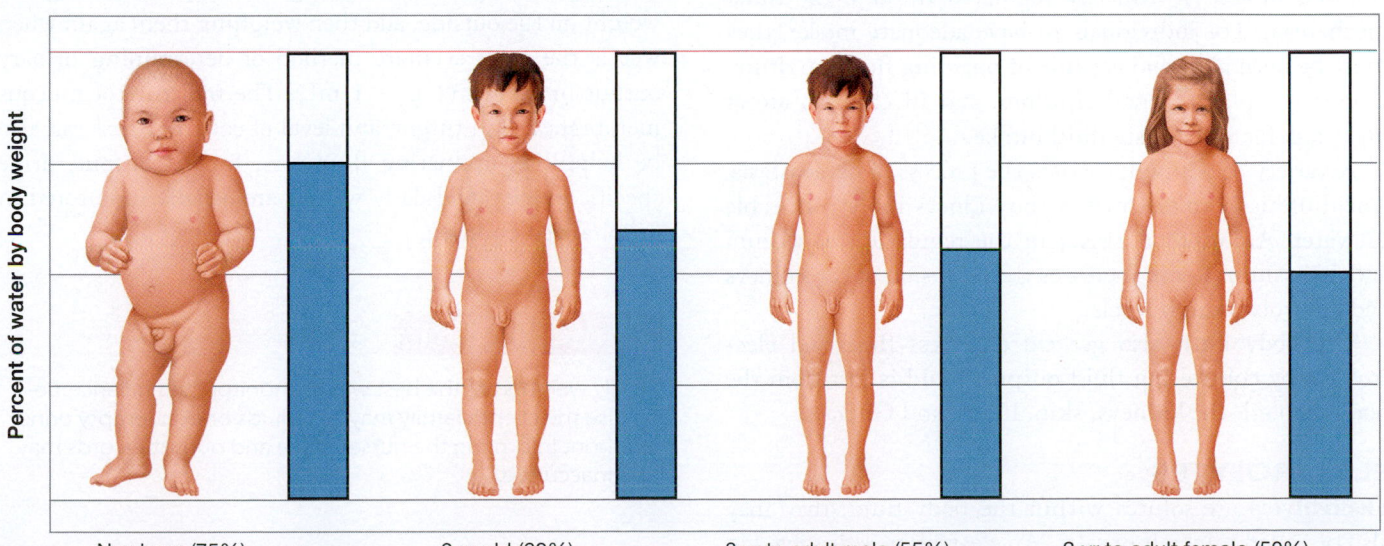

Newborn (75%)   2 yr old (60%)   3 yr to adult male (55%)   3 yr to adult female (50%)

Figure 15-1. ■ Percentage of water by body weight changes dramatically from 75% in infants to about 50% to 55% in adults. The greater percentage of water in infants makes them highly susceptible to fluid imbalance.

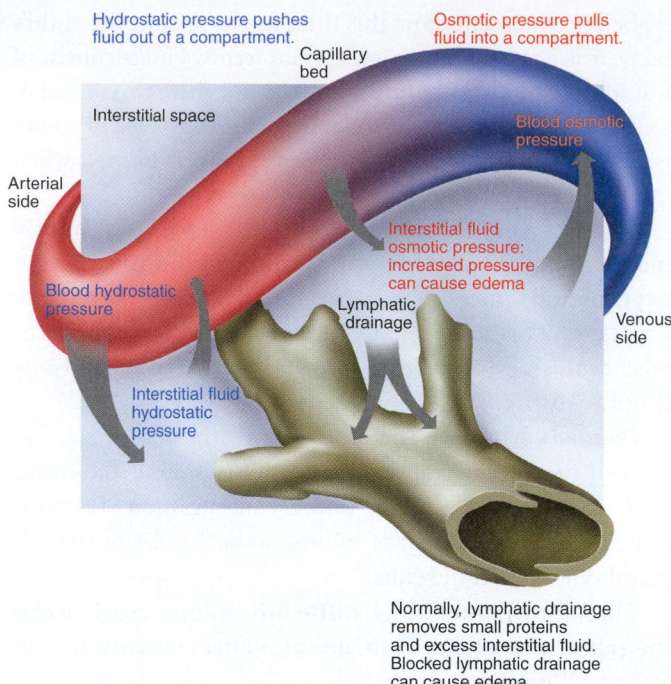

Hydrostatic pressure pushes fluid out of a compartment.

Osmotic pressure pulls fluid into a compartment.

Capillary bed

Interstitial space

Blood osmotic pressure

Arterial side

Blood hydrostatic pressure

Interstitial fluid osmotic pressure: increased pressure can cause edema

Lymphatic drainage

Venous side

Interstitial fluid hydrostatic pressure

Normally, lymphatic drainage removes small proteins and excess interstitial fluid. Blocked lymphatic drainage can cause edema.

Figure 15-2. ■ When fluid is inside the body's arteries, veins, and capillaries (*vasculature*), it is plasma. When fluid moves across the *space* from circulatory structures to cells, it is interstitial fluid. Once it moves into cell structures, it is called intracellular fluid.

sodium-potassium pump assists in the process. The pump works by employing carrier or transport cells to assist movement across the cell membrane.

The movement of fluids and electrolytes assists the body in maintaining homeostasis. Homeostasis is also affected by fluid intake, hormonal regulation, and fluid output.

Fluid intake is primarily regulated through the thirst mechanism. For individuals to have adequate intake, they must be both alert and capable of pursuing fluids to drink. Therefore, infants, small children, and ill children are at great risk for inadequate fluid intake.

A variety of hormones assists the process of homeostasis. Antidiuretic hormone makes the kidneys more permeable to water. Aldosterone assists in the regulation of sodium and potassium. Renin increases the perfusion of the kidneys and controls sodium levels.

The body must also get rid of excess fluid and electrolytes by controlling fluid output. Fluid is lost from the body through the kidneys, skin, lungs, and GI tract.

ELECTROLYTES

Electrolytes are solutes within the body fluid; they may also be called minerals or salts. An electrolyte is dissolved in a solvent and is broken down into ions. These ions carry an electrical charge (hence the name). Electrolytes are measured in milliequivalents per liter (mEq/L). Milliequivalents

represent the number of grams of the electrolyte dissolved in a liter of plasma.

Cations are positively charged electrolytes. Potassium (K^+), sodium (Na^+), and calcium (Ca^+) are common cations. Sodium is the body's most abundant electrolyte. It controls the balance of the body's water. It is regulated mainly through dietary intake and aldosterone. Potassium is found mostly in the intracellular space. Its main function is to control muscle contractions. Potassium is regulated by dietary intake and renal excretion. Calcium is stored in the bones, plasma, and body cells. The chief functions of calcium are to maintain bones and teeth and to assist in blood clotting. Calcium is mainly regulated by protein albumin.

Anions are negatively charged electrolytes. Chloride (Cl^-), bicarbonate (HCO_3^-), and sulfate (SO_4^-) are common anions. Chloride is found in the extracellular fluid. It functions in conjunction with sodium and is regulated by dietary intake and the kidneys. Bicarbonate is found in the extracellular and intracellular fluid. Its primary function is to maintain acid-base balance. Bicarbonate is regulated by the kidneys. Acid-base balance is discussed later in the chapter.

Brief Assessment Overview

In the child who is ill, the assessment of fluid balance is essential. Vomiting and diarrhea lead quickly to fluid and electrolyte loss (see Figure 15-1), and could lead to hypovolemic shock (see Chapter 20 ⬤⬤). Measuring output might be difficult because the child may not be able to follow directions of vomiting into a basin or collecting stool in the proper receptacle. Weighing dry diapers, writing the weight on the outside, and then weighing them again when wet is the most accurate method of determining urinary output in infants (1 g = 1 mL). The moisture of mucous membranes, skin turgor, and level of consciousness can also be helpful in evaluating fluid loss. Intake, output, urine specific gravity, and daily weight are usually monitored in hospitalized children.

clinical ALERT

Daily weights are the best way to monitor fluid balance. Because the client's family may give fluids or even empty urine without informing the nurse, intake and output records may be inaccurate.

Table 15-1 ■ provides information about assessing fluid and electrolyte status in infants and children. Procedure 15-1 ■ reviews intake and output measurement.

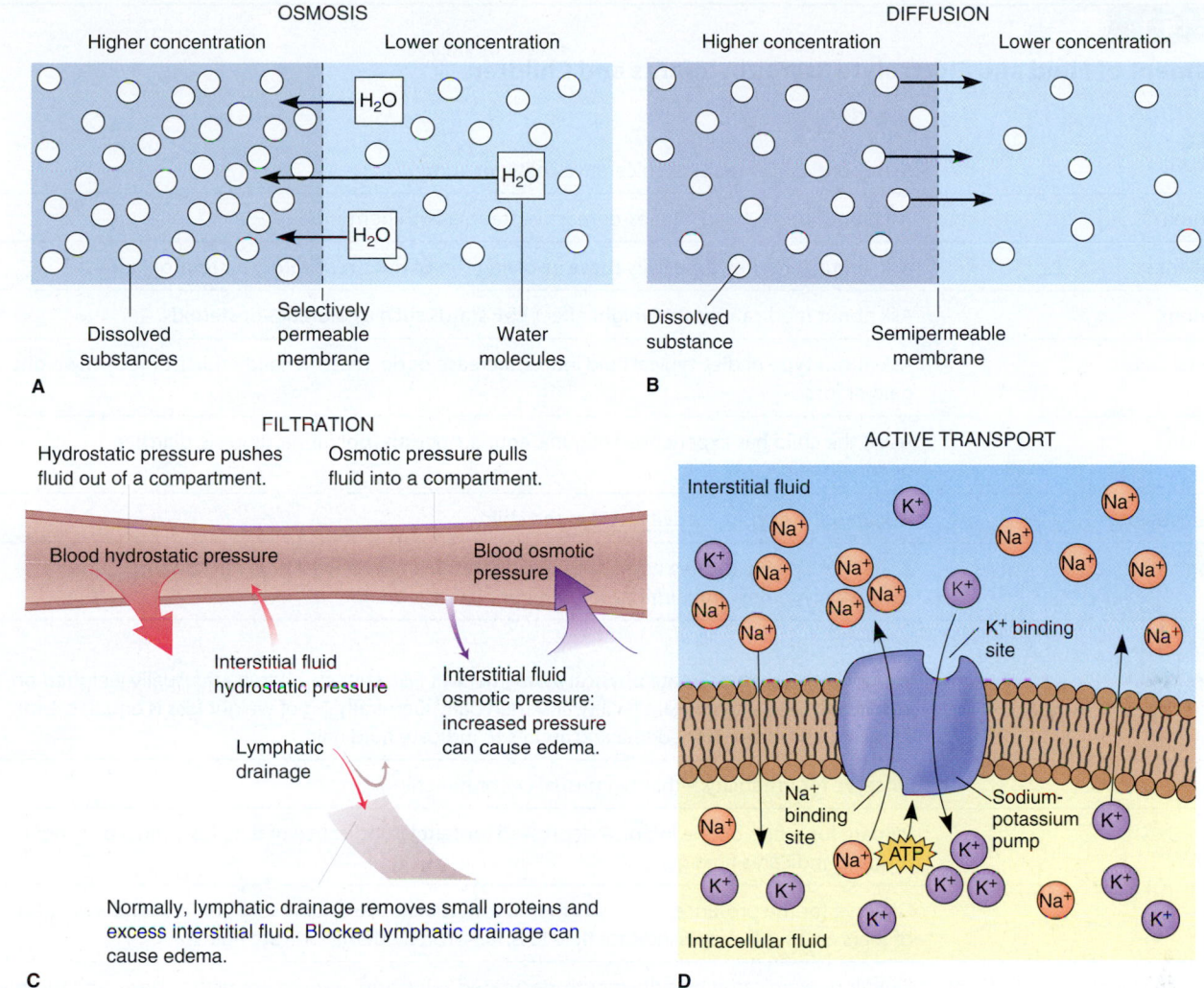

Figure 15-3. ■ **(A)** Osmosis. Water moves across a selective permeable membrane into an area of higher solute concentration and out of the area of lower solute concentration. **(B)** Diffusion. Molecules move across a semipermeable membrane from an area of higher solute concentration to an area of lower solute concentration. **(C)** Filtration is the process by which water and solutes move across capillary membranes driven by fluid pressure. The pumping action of the heart and gravity push water and solutes into the interstitial space. Note that water is returned into the vascular space by osmosis. **(D)** Active transport. The movement of sodium and potassium ions across cell membranes against their concentration gradients.

FLUID AND ELECTROLYTE DISORDERS

Recall that homeostasis is maintained when the child's intake and output are balanced. In states of illness, body fluids and the electrolytes contained within them may become unbalanced. Both fluid loss (e.g., through diarrhea, vomiting, or burns) and fluid gain (e.g., from IV fluid overload or cardiac and kidney disease) can create these imbalances in fluids and electrolytes.

Deficient Fluid Volume (Dehydration)

Dehydration is a condition of deficient fluid volume in the intravascular and interstitial fluid compartments. Dehydra-

tion is often accompanied by imbalances in sodium. This disease process can be classified as isotonic, hypotonic, or hypertonic.

- The most common type of dehydration in children is **isotonic dehydration.** This is a loss of fluid and sodium in equal proportions (as from vomiting). Sodium levels are normal, and most of the fluid lost is from the extracellular compartment.
- **Hypotonic dehydration** is fluid and sodium loss in which relatively more sodium than fluid is lost (as in renal disease). Less salt than normal remains in the body. As sodium levels fall below normal range, fluid shifts into the intracellular space from the extracellular space.

TABLE 15-1

Assessment of Fluid and Electrolyte Status in Infants and Children

HISTORY	
Chronic diseases	Ask about cancer, diabetes, ulcerative colitis, or anorexia.
Past trauma	Ask about burns, head injuries, or massive trauma with hemorrhage.
Past surgeries	Ask about surgeries, especially those involving the GI tract, respiratory system, or kidneys.
Medications	Ask about medications that might affect F&E status such as diuretics or steroids.
Nutritional status	Ask about type of diet, typical fluid intake, increase or decrease in child's thirst, or recent weight gain or loss.
Elimination	Ask if the child has experienced oliguria, anuria, nocturia, polyurina, diuresis, diarrhea, or constipation.
Exercise/activity	Ask about the typical activity level of the child.
Neurologic status	Ask about any headaches, numbness, disorientation, muscle weakness or cramping, tremors, confusion, memory impairment, lethargy, or blurred vision.
PHYSICAL	
Weight	Weight is the most accurate physical assessment of F&E status. Children are usually weighed on admission to the health care facility and then daily. Generally 1 g of weight loss is equal to 1 mL of fluid loss. Observe for edema and ascites to indicate fluid gain.
General appearance	Observe for irritability, lethargy, unusual cry, or twitching.
Head	Palpate fontanels on the infant. A depressed fontanel is indicative of fluid loss, and a bulging fontanel indicates fluid gain.
Eyes	Observe for the presence of tears. Remember that tears are not present until 4 months of age. Lack of tears and sunken eyes indicate fluid loss. Periorbital edema indicate fluid gain.
Throat and mouth	Fluid loss is indicated by a dry mouth, decreased salivation, cracked lips with fissures, and furrows on the tongue. Fluid gain may be marked by increased mucous production, and edema of the tongue may leave impressions of the teeth on the child's tongue.
Cardiovascular	Observe jugular vein. A flat vein may indicate fluid loss, while a distended vein indicates fluid gain. A weak pulse rate greater than 160 in infants and greater than 120 in children may be related to fluid loss. The blood pressure may also be decreased in severe fluid loss. A full and bounding pulse and increased blood pressure are associated with fluid gain. A third heart sound may also be heard with fluid gain. ECG changes occur with potassium and acid-base imbalances.
Gastrointestinal/urinary	Observe the abdomen. It may be sunken in fluid loss, distended in malnutrition, and fluid filled with ascites. Auscultate bowel sounds. In early fluid loss, there will be hyperactive bowel sounds. In later fluid loss, the sounds may be hypoactive. Describe and measure stools, vomitus, and urinary output.
Respiratory	Observe the respiratory rate and effort. Fluid gain and acid-base imbalances may cause a change in rate and effort. Auscultate the lung sounds. Moist sounds may be heard in fluid gain.
Neurologic	Assess muscle tone. Tone is likely to be increased with hypocalcemia and decreased with hypokalemia and hypercalcemia. Assess DTRs. In hypocalcemia, they are increased, and in hypercalcemia, they are decreased or absent.
Integumentary	Assess the skin's appearance. In fluid loss, it may be pale, gray, or mottled. In fluid gain, it may be red or shiny. Assess skin temperature. Skin temperature is typically decreased in fluid loss and increased in fluid gain. Assess the degree of pitting edema, if present. This is a sign of fluid gain. Assess skin turgor. Poor skin turgor is indicative of fluid loss.

Measuring Intake and Output

Purpose

- To contribute to the assessment of a child's fluid and electrolyte balance

Equipment

- Chart form
- Specimen pan
- Measuring cup

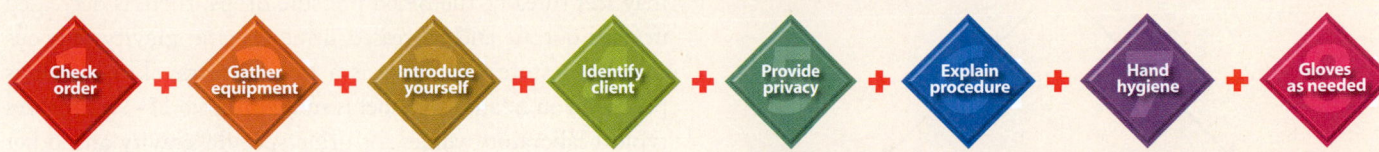

Check order + Gather equipment + Introduce yourself + Identify client + Provide privacy + Explain procedure + Hand hygiene + Gloves as needed

Interventions

1. Perform preparatory steps (see icon bar).

2. Instruct parent and child to measure and record all intake and output (Figure 15-4 ■).

3. Carefully measure all oral intake such as gelatin, ice chips, ice cream, soup, juice, and water. Include fluids obtained through feeding tubes. Intake also includes IV fluids and medications, tube feedings, and blood products. *Fluid requirements for children are calculated by weight (see Chapter 13 ⚭). Fluid deficit or overload can easily be identified by calculating daily intake. Children weighing 2.2 to 22 pounds (1–10 kg) should receive 100 mL/kg of fluid per day. Children weighing 22 to 44 pounds (10–20 kg) should receive 1,000 mL plus 50 mL/kg over 10 kg per day. Children weighing more than 44 pounds (20 kg) should receive 1,500 mL plus 20 mL/kg over 20 kg per day.*

4. Carefully measure all output, including urine (Figure 15-5 ■), diarrhea, vomitus, gastric suction, and drainage from wounds

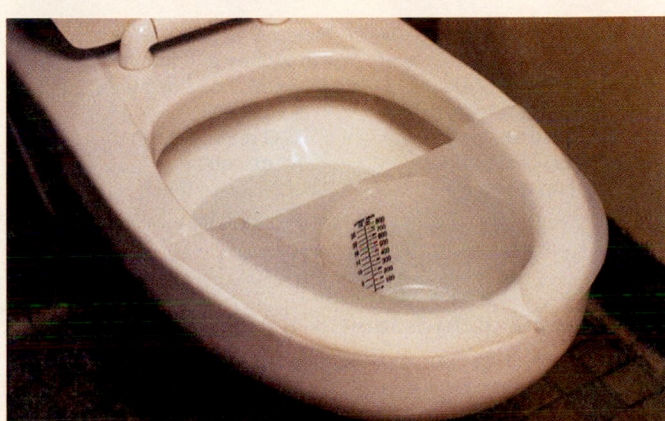

Figure 15-5. ■ A urine collection device can be placed in the toilet for children who are out of diapers.

or tubes. For children in diapers, weigh diapers. One gram equals 1 mL of urine. *Fluid deficit or overload can be identified by calculating daily output. Urine output for infants and toddlers is more than 2 to 3 mL/kg/hour; for preschoolers and younger school-age children, it is more than 1 to 2 mL/kg/hour; and for older school-age children and adolescents, it is more than 0.5 mL/kg/hour.*

5. Total the intake and output for the entire shift and record on the chart form in the child's permanent record. *Comparing the daily intake and output record can identify trends related to fluid and electrolyte imbalances.*

			PATIENT LABEL
Intake and Output Record			
INTAKE	0600-1800	1800-0600	TOTAL
Oral			
Tube feeding			
IV (primary)			
IV Meds			
TPN			
Blood			
TOTAL			24-Hour Total
OUTPUT	0600-1800	1800-0600	TOTAL
Urine			
Emesis			
G.I. Suction			
Stool			
TOTAL			24-Hour Total

Figure 15-4. ■ The intake–output chart is an important tool for monitoring fluid status.

SAMPLE DOCUMENTATION

(date) 1500 *(Note: I&O portion of documentation only)* 10-year-old boy 3 days postsurgery for appendicitis. Consumed 50% of breakfast tray, 100 mL apple juice, and 25 mL whole milk. Voided 55 mL clear, yellow urine. ___ M. Manning, LPN

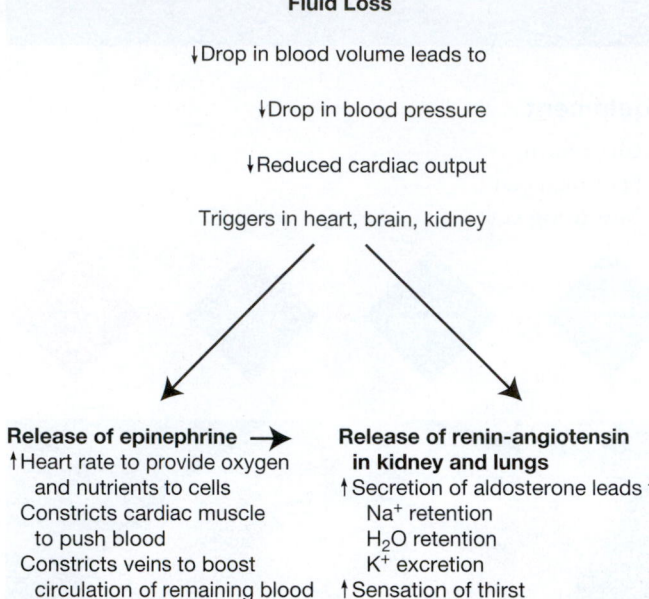

Fluid Loss

↓Drop in blood volume leads to

↓Drop in blood pressure

↓Reduced cardiac output

Triggers in heart, brain, kidney

Release of epinephrine →
↑Heart rate to provide oxygen
 and nutrients to cells
Constricts cardiac muscle
 to push blood
Constricts veins to boost
 circulation of remaining blood

**Release of renin-angiotensin
in kidney and lungs**
↑Secretion of aldosterone leads to
 Na⁺ retention
 H₂O retention
 K⁺ excretion
↑Sensation of thirst

Figure 15-6. ■ The body's response to fluid loss involves several body systems.

■ **Hypertonic dehydration** is fluid and sodium loss in which relatively more fluid than sodium is lost (as in diabetes). An excess of salt remains in the body. Fluid shifts from the intracellular space into the intravascular space.

As fluid is lost within the child's body, there is a loss of circulating fluid volume, which lowers cardiac output and blood pressure. The body tries to compensate for lack of fluid (Figure 15-6 ■). As the blood pressure lowers, triggers in the heart, kidneys, and brain increase cardiac output and sodium and water retention. These triggers also release epinephrine, which increases the heart rate, cardiac contractility, and venous constriction, increasing the circulating rate of the remaining blood volume.

Blood volume is increased through the release of renin-angiotensin (which causes the kidneys to decrease urine production). Sensors also stimulate the thirst mechanism and water retention. However, these compensatory mechanisms will fail if the dehydration is not treated promptly.

Dehydration (fluid volume deficit) leads to about 10% of pediatric hospitalizations (Figure 15-7 ■). Isotonic dehydration is caused by vomiting and diarrhea; it can also occur during periods of food and fluid restriction, such as before and after surgery. Hypotonic dehydration is caused by gastroenteritis, burns, renal diseases, nasogastric suctioning, and inappropriate IV fluid replacement without electrolytes. (See Chapter 24 ◯◯ for more discussion on burns in children.) Hypertonic dehydration is caused by diabetes or IV fluid replacement containing high concentrations of electrolytes. All forms of dehydration require attention. Some cultures have periods of fasting that may conflict with rehydration needs (Box 15-1 ■). In most cases, medical conditions exempt a person from following strict fasts.

Manifestations

Dehydration is classified by the percentage of body weight lost. Symptoms increase in severity as weight loss increases (Table 15-2 ■). In general, the child's pulse becomes rapid and may feel thready, the blood pressure drops, there is decreased urinary output and increased urine specific gravity, mucous membranes are dry, there is a lack of tears, skin turgor is poor, and an infant's fontanel is sunken. Table 15-3 ■ provides typical laboratory values for urine specific gravity and other common indicators of fluid or electrolyte imbalance.

clinical ALERT

The nurse must be aware of impending signs of shock, including a mottled, cyanotic appearance; dropping blood pressure; behavior from expressionless to restless; increasing respiratory rate with shallow breaths; and increasing blood urea nitrogen (BUN) levels.

Diagnosis

A careful history of the symptoms leading up to dehydration is essential in making a diagnosis. The nurse can also assist in gathering physical data related to dehydration. Weight loss is the most accurate physical assessment used to determine dehydration and the degree of dehydration. The weight of a pediatric client should be assessed upon admission to the health care facility and then daily thereafter. Procedure 15-2 ■ describes how to calculate weight loss. See Procedure 13-2 ◯◯ for more about obtaining weights.

Laboratory data are also used in the diagnosis of dehydration. Loss of fluid causes concentration of the solutes within the plasma, so hemoglobin, hematocrit, glucose, BUN, creatinine, and protein levels are elevated in dehydration. The urine specific gravity is also found to be elevated.

Treatment

Treatment of dehydration is based on the degree of dehydration. Fluid and electrolyte replacement is essential. The underlying cause must also be treated. Fluid replacement can occur orally or intravenously.

ORAL FLUID REPLACEMENT. Teach parents the importance of maintaining oral hydration in children. On warm days, children may lose enough fluid through the skin and respiration to become dehydrated. Due to limited communication skills, they may have difficulty knowing they are thirsty or requesting a drink of water. Parents should develop a habit of offering water hourly, especially on hot days.

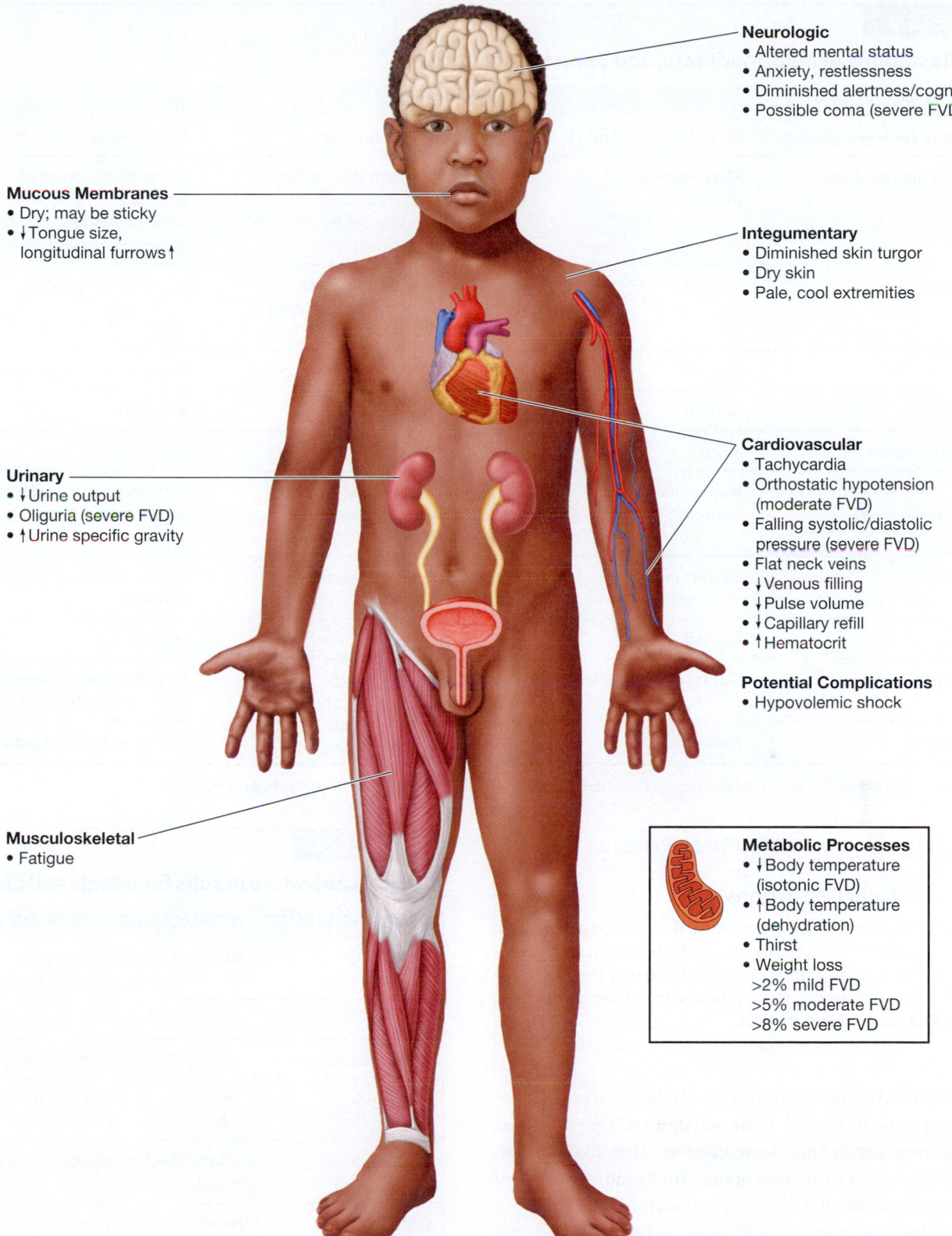

Neurologic
- Altered mental status
- Anxiety, restlessness
- Diminished alertness/cognition
- Possible coma (severe FVD)

Mucous Membranes
- Dry; may be sticky
- ↓Tongue size, longitudinal furrows↑

Integumentary
- Diminished skin turgor
- Dry skin
- Pale, cool extremities

Urinary
- ↓Urine output
- Oliguria (severe FVD)
- ↑Urine specific gravity

Cardiovascular
- Tachycardia
- Orthostatic hypotension (moderate FVD)
- Falling systolic/diastolic pressure (severe FVD)
- Flat neck veins
- ↓Venous filling
- ↓Pulse volume
- ↓Capillary refill
- ↑Hematocrit

Potential Complications
- Hypovolemic shock

Musculoskeletal
- Fatigue

Metabolic Processes
- ↓Body temperature (isotonic FVD)
- ↑Body temperature (dehydration)
- Thirst
- Weight loss
  >2% mild FVD
  >5% moderate FVD
  >8% severe FVD

Figure 15-7. ■ Multisystem effects of fluid volume deficit (FVD).

TABLE 15-2

Manifestations of Mild, Moderate, and Severe Dehydration

CLINICAL ASSESSMENT	MILD	MODERATE	SEVERE
Percent of body weight lost	Up to 5% (40–50 mL/kg)	6–9% (60–90 mL/kg)	10% or more (100 + mL/kg)
Level of consciousness	Alert, restless, thirsty	Irritable or lethargic (infants and very young children); thirsty, restless (older children and adolescents)	Lethargic to comatose (infants and young children); often conscious, apprehensive (older children and adolescents)
Blood pressure	Normal	Normal or low; postural hypotension (older children and adolescents)	Low to undetectable
Pulse	Normal	Rapid	Rapid, weak to palpable
Skin turgor	Normal	Poor	Very poor
Mucus membranes	Moist	Dry	Parched
Urine	May appear normal	Decreased output (less than 1 mL/kg/hour), dark color; increased specific gravity	Very decreased or absent output
Thirst	Slightly increased	Moderately increased	Greatly increased unless lethargic
Fontanel	Normal	Sunken	Sunken
Extremities	Warm; normal capillary refill	Delayed capillary refill (greater than 2 seconds)	Cool, discolored; delayed capillary refill (greater than 3–4 seconds)
Respirations	Normal	Normal or rapid	Changing rate and pattern

Source: Ball, J. W., & Bindler, R. C. (2003). *Pediatric nursing: Caring for children* (3rd ed.). Upper Saddle River, NJ: Prentice Hall, p. 314.

BOX 15-1   **CULTURAL PULSE POINTS**

Voluntary Fluid Restrictions

Muslim families require fasting or restriction of food and beverage from sunrise to sunset in the holy month of Ramadan. When a child requires oral rehydration, this tradition may become flexible. However, the devout Muslim family may have some concerns about disregarding this fast.

If it has been determined the child is dehydrated, fluid replacement must be started. Oral rehydration is ideal because it is the most natural and least invasive. Box 15-2 ■ highlights important information about fluid requirements and oral rehydration amounts by different weights in children.

The nurse and parents will need to be creative in administering oral fluids. Children often prefer sweetened flavored solutions such as Popsicles, gelatin, decarbonated cola, or ginger ale. However, these can make diarrhea worse due to the osmotic effect of the sugar. When used, they should be diluted by 50%. Commercially prepared oral replacement solutions are preferred because they contain necessary electrolytes and less sugar. Some choices are

(*Text continues on p. 490.*)

TABLE 15-3

Typical Laboratory Results for Infants and Children

COMPONENT TESTED	NORMAL LABORATORY VALUES
Hematocrit	Newborn: 44–65%; 1 to 3 years old: 29–40%; 4 to 10 years old: 31–43%
Urine specific gravity	Newborn: 1.001–1.020; Child: 1.005–1.030
Blood urea nitrogen	Infant: 5–15 mg/dL; Child: 5–20 mg/dL
Potassium	Infant: 3.6–5.8 mEq/L; Child: 3.5–5.5 mEq/L
Sodium	Infant: 134–150 mEq/L; Child: 135–145 mEq/L
Calcium	Newborn: 3.7–7.0 mEq/L or 7.4–14.0 mg/dL; Infant: 5.0–6.0 mEq/L or 10–12 mg/dL; Child: 4.5–5.8 mEq/L or 9–11.5 mg/dL
Blood gases pH PaCO$_2$ HCO$_3$	 Child: 7.36–7.44 Child: 35–45 mm Hg Child: 22–26 mEq/L

Note: Lab values may vary. Consult the laboratory at your health care agency.

Calculating Weight Loss

Purpose

- To contribute to the assessment of a child's fluid and electrolyte imbalance, particularly fluid loss

Equipment

- Calibrated scale
- Documentation of child's previous weight

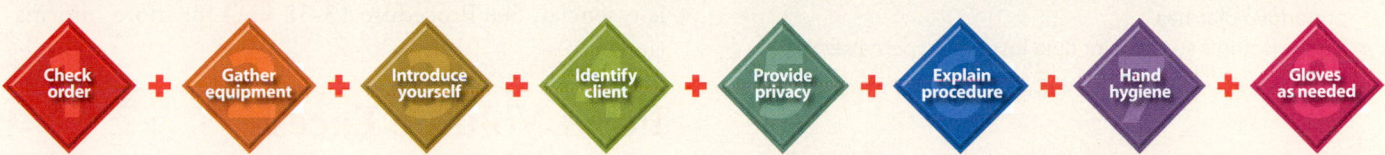

Interventions

1. Perform preparatory steps (see icon bar).
2. Review documentation of the child's previous weight.
3. Weigh the child on a calibrated scale in the same manner as the child was weighed previously (e.g., without shoes or with clothes; before or after meals; and using the same scale if available). *Changing these variables can give a false reading about changes in weight.*
4. Subtract the child's current weight from the previous weight.
5. Divide this value by the child's previous weight to obtain the percentage of weight loss. For example:

Previous weight: 25 lb
Current weight: 20 lb

$25 - 20 = 5$
Weight loss: 5 lb
$5/25 = .20 = 20\%$
Percent weight loss: 20%

SAMPLE DOCUMENTATION

(date) 0800   5-year-old male child. Admission weight 40 lb. Current weight, day 5 of hospitalization, 38 lb. Percent weight loss = 5%. _____
W. Smartt, LVN

BOX 15-2

Fluid Requirements in Children and Oral Rehydration

Fluid Requirements

- Fluid requirements for children are calculated by weight (see Chapter 13 ⭕⭕).
- Children weighing 2.2 to 22 pounds (1–10 kg) should receive 100 mL/kg of fluid daily.
- Children weighing 22 to 44 pounds (10–20 kg) should receive 1,000 mL plus 50 mL/kg over 10 kg per day.
- Children weighing more than 44 pounds (20 kg) should receive 1,500 mL plus 20 mL/kg over 20 kg per day.

Oral Rehydration Amounts

- Fluids are given by mouth in small amounts frequently, for example, 1 to 2 tsp (5–10 mL) every 10 to 15 min-utes. Continue giving oral fluids even if the child vomits because some of the fluid might be absorbed.
- For mild dehydration, the child should be given almost 1 fluid ounce per pound (50 mL/kg) of body weight every 4 hours, plus the amount of fluid lost by vomiting and/or diarrhea during the same time.
- For moderate dehydration, the child should be given about 2 fluid ounces per pound (100 mL/kg) of body weight every 4 hours plus the amount lost through emesis and/or stool.
- For severe dehydration, the child is hospitalized, and fluids are given intravenously.

Commercial Rehydration Agents

Oral Agents

- Pedialyte, Rehydralyte, Infalyte, Oral Maintenance Solution—for mild to moderate dehydration

Intravenous Agents

- Normal saline—isotonic solution for restoring water and sodium
- Lactated Ringer's—isotonic solution for burns, bleeding, and prolonged diarrhea
- D_5W—isotonic solution for fluid loss and hypernatremia

listed in Box 15-3 ■. If the child's condition worsens or does not improve after 4 hours of oral fluid replacement, the doctor should be consulted.

INTRAVENOUS FLUID REPLACEMENT.   When severe dehydration has occurred, the child should be hospitalized and IV fluid administered. Because children have small veins, inserting an IV needle can be a challenge. Figure 15-8 ■ shows alternative pediatric IV sites. In some areas, the initiation of IV therapy is not an LPN/LVN function. However, assisting with the monitoring of the infusion might be required. The nurse must know and follow the state's nurse practice act and facility policy.

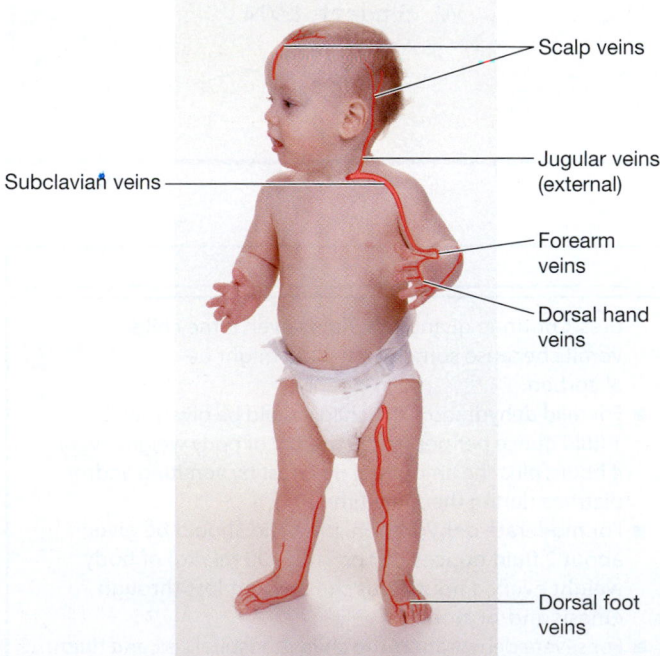

Figure 15-8. ■ Pediatric access sites are more difficult to use because of the small size of the veins.

The needle is protected to prevent infiltration and the need to change sites. Padded limb boards and limb restraints may be needed to protect the child and prevent the needle from becoming dislodged (see Figure 13-43 ⚭). An IV infusion control device is used to prevent too rapid administration of fluids. This device should be locked to prevent accidental adjustment of the rate of infusion. Usually the rate is most rapid for the first few hours and then the rate is decreased. Careful frequent monitoring of the rate, site, and reaction to the therapy is essential. See Procedure 13-38 ⚭ for more information.

Fluid Volume Excess (Hypervolemia)

Fluid volume excess (FVE) occurs when there is retention of fluid and, in some cases, sodium in the extracellular compartment. It may also be called **hypervolemia.** FVE may arise due to cardiac disorders such as congestive heart failure and renal disorders. The affected child may also be taking glucocorticoids. FVE may also be caused by an overload of IV fluids, particularly those containing sodium (Figure 15-9 ■). Low protein intake and high sodium intake might also cause FVE.

Manifestations

Symptoms of FVE include acute weight gain and edema. Edema is usually generalized in infants and *dependent* (occurring in lower legs, feet, or other areas affected by gravity) in children. The child's vital signs change. The pulse becomes fast and bounding. The blood pressure and respiratory rate increase. The child may also become dyspneic. Upon auscultation to the chest, crackles are heard. Urine output may also increase.

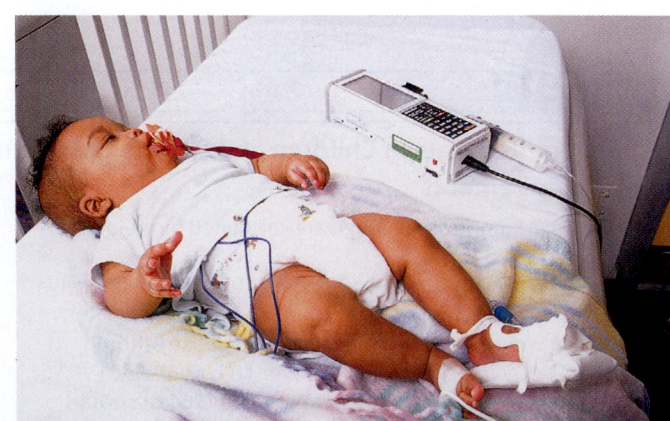

Figure 15-9. ■ If isotonic fluid containing sodium is given too rapidly or in too large an amount, an extracellular fluid volume excess will develop. It is important to monitor fluid intake, excretion, and retention in infants and children.

Diagnosis

Diagnosis of FVE is usually made by symptom recognition, especially weight gain. The following lab results may also be associated with FVE:

- Decreased hematocrit (HCT)
- Decreased urine specific gravity
- Decreased BUN.

The lab values are due to hemodilution. Fluid may be seen in the lungs upon x-ray.

Treatment

Medical treatment of hypervolemia is primarily focused on treating the cause of the condition. Other treatments may include sodium and fluid restriction, as well as diuretic administration to promote fluid loss. In severe cases, hemodialysis may be required.

Nursing Considerations

Accurate measure of daily weight and careful documentation of the child's intake and output are important nursing interventions. The nurse must carefully explain and monitor fluid and sodium restrictions. Foods containing sodium must be discussed with the parent and child. Edematous tissue is fragile; therefore, careful nursing attention should be given to promoting skin integrity. If the child is dyspneic, the nurse can promote breathing by elevating the head of the bed (HOB) to 30 degrees, loosening restrictive clothing, and administering oxygen as ordered.

clinical ALERT

Hypervolemia can progress to pulmonary edema. The nurse needs to be alert and must quickly recognize symptoms of pulmonary edema. These include restlessness, tachypnea, labored breathing, a full and bounding pulse or a weak and thready pulse, possible crackles on lung auscultation, and profuse diaphoresis. This condition is considered to be a medical emergency. The nurse must position the child to facilitate breathing and contact the physician promptly. Narcotics, diuretics, and bronchodilators may be ordered. Careful attention must be given to avoid complicating the child's condition with an overload of IV fluid. (See more on listening to the heart in Chapter 13, Procedure 13-2, and Chapter 19 ⚭ . See more on lung conditions in Chapter 18 ⚭ .)

Sodium Imbalance

Sodium is found in high levels in extracellular fluid and in lower levels in intracellular fluid. Each cell is equipped with a sodium-potassium pump (see Figure 15-3D) that maintains sodium concentrations. Otherwise, the laws of diffusion would cause movement of the sodium outside the cell into the area of lower concentration (inside the cell).

HYPONATREMIA

Hyponatremia is a state of sodium deficit related to the body's water. It is caused by excessive water gain or excessive sodium loss. Excessive water intake can occur in:

- IV fluid overload, especially with hypotonic solutions
- Children with congestive heart failure
- Overuse of tap-water enemas
- Oral ingestion of excessive tap water; infants are particularly at risk for hyponatremia if parents are diluting formula incorrectly and because their thirst mechanism is not developed fully.

Excessive sodium loss can occur in diarrhea, vomiting, cystic fibrosis, burns, and renal disease.

Manifestations

Hyponatremia is manifested as headaches, lethargy, confusion, muscle weakness, and decreased deep tendon reflexes. In severe cases the child may develop seizures, and lethargy may progress to coma.

Diagnosis

Lab values related to hyponatremia are sodium levels below normal limits for the age group, decreased urine specific gravity, and serum osmolality greater than 280 mOsm/kg.

Treatment

Mild hyponatremia is treated by fluid restriction, oral sodium supplements, isotonic IV solutions, and a diet high in sodium. More severe cases require a hypertonic IV solution, diuretics, and admission to the intensive care unit.

Nursing Considerations

Children with hyponatremia are at risk for injury due to muscle weakness and possible seizure activity. The nurse must provide a safe environment and watch carefully for seizures. Parents and children need to be taught about fluid restriction (Procedure 15-3 ■). Monitoring and documentation of vital signs, intake and output, and lab values are important interventions for the child with hyponatremia.

HYPERNATREMIA

Hypernatremia is a state of sodium excess related to the body's water. The thirst mechanism is the body's best line of defense against hypernatremia. Infants or children who cannot react to thirst are vulnerable.

Hypernatremia can be caused by excessive administration of a hypertonic IV solution. Excessive water losses from diarrhea, burns, and pulmonary infections also cause hypernatremia.

Manifestations

Symptoms of hypernatremia are most commonly thirst and neurologic symptoms. Restlessness, confusion, stupor, seizures, and coma may occur. The child may also have dry mucous membranes, a low-grade fever, oliguria, and flushed skin.

PROCEDURE 15-3   Assisting with Fluid Restriction

Purpose

■ To assist children who have excesses in fluid volume to limit oral intake

Equipment

■ Measuring cups

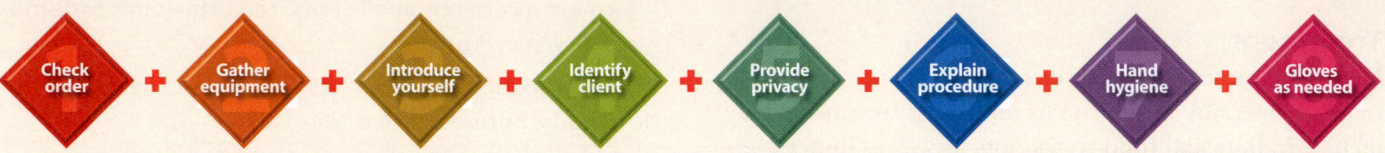

Interventions

1. Perform preparatory steps (see icon bar).

2. Explain the rationale for the restriction to the child and the parent. *Compliance can be increased when a connection can be made between the restriction and the restoration of health.*

3. State clearly the amount of fluid, if any, permissible in a 24-hour period. Post signs in the child's room to alert other health care personnel.

4. Inform the child and parent that ice chips, gelatin, ice cream, and broth are considered to be fluid intake.

5. Develop a plan that will allow the child to have fluids throughout the day. Consult the child and parent when devising this plan. Be sure to include oral intake required to swallow medications and brush the teeth. *Children are typically more active between 7:00 A.M. and 3:00 P.M., so more oral intake is needed during these hours.*

6. Monitor oral hygiene carefully. *Limited fluid intake or the restriction of fluid intake dries the mucous membranes and puts the child at risk for cracking and drying of the lips and mouth.*

7. Provide distraction activities. *A child who is not busy may focus on the desire for oral intake. Distraction activities such as group games, videos, or special toys may assist the child in managing fluid restrictions.*

8. Record fluid intake. *Documenting the oral intake improves patient compliance and assists health care personnel in appropriately managing oral intake.*

SAMPLE DOCUMENTATION

(date) 0700   Fluid restriction of 1,000 mL ordered. Discussed fluid restriction with child and parent. Plan of care developed: 240 mL breakfast, 100 mL midmorning snack, 240 mL lunch, 100 mL afternoon snack, 20 mL medication administration, 240 mL dinner, 20 mL medication administration, 40 mL bedtime snack. Signs posted above bed and on client's door.
_____ L. Lowman, LPN

Diagnosis

Lab values include serum sodium levels greater than expected for the age group and increased or decreased urine specific gravity, depending on the cause.

Treatment

Medical management of hypernatremia includes oral and IV rehydration. This must occur gradually to avoid a rapid shifting of water into the brain cells, causing cerebral edema. The child may be placed on a low sodium diet, and diuretics may be administered.

Nursing Considerations

Assist the child and the parents with oral rehydration by providing a variety of fluids and encouraging them to set a schedule for oral intake. The nurse can assist the child in making appropriate low-sodium diet choices. Oral hygiene and moisturizer for the child's mouth should be provided frequently because of dry mucous membranes. The nurse should observe closely for symptoms of fluid overload. Seizure precautions and other safety measures are necessary when the child's neurologic status is compromised.

Potassium Imbalance

HYPOKALEMIA

Hypokalemia occurs when there is a decrease in serum potassium levels to below normal range. Potassium loss can be caused by increased excretion, decreased intake, a shift into the cells from the extracellular fluid, and loss of potassium by vomiting or nasogastric suctioning. Hypokalemia is also related to inappropriate use of diuretics, diarrhea, alkalosis, anorexia nervosa, bulimia, and hypomagnesemia. Children who have ingested large amounts of black licorice may be at risk for hypokalemia because the candy increases renal excretion of potassium.

Manifestations

Clinical manifestations of hypokalemia include weakness, fatigue, intestinal distention, polyuria, and cardiac irregularities (Figure 15-10 ■). Serum potassium levels will be decreased according to the child's age (see Table 15-3).

Diagnosis

Diagnosis of hypokalemia is made by reviewing symptoms and laboratory values of potassium.

Treatment

Medical management of hypokalemia is focused on treating the causative factor. Potassium is replaced orally or intravenously. Prompt management of hypokalemia will avoid life-threatening complications.

Nursing Considerations

Priority nursing interventions will include replacing potassium, as ordered, either orally or intravenously. Table 15-4 ■ provides more information about potassium supplementation. Children and their parents will also need to be taught about increasing potassium in the diet. The nurse teaches about foods containing potassium and ways to incorporate them into the diet (Box 15-4 ■).

Because potassium imbalances have the potential to affect cardiac and respiratory status, the nurse must vigilantly monitor the child's pulse and respiratory rate and rhythm. If electrocardiogram (ECG) monitoring is ordered, it must be observed closely as well.

The nurse must also keep strict intake and output records. Imbalances should be reported promptly. The effects of hypokalemia may cause the child to be at risk for injury. Safety measures should be implemented.

HYPERKALEMIA

Hyperkalemia occurs when there is an increase above normal range in serum potassium levels. Hyperkalemia is associated with renal dysfunction and failure, burns, sickle cell anemia, blood transfusions, prematurity, severe

HYPOKALEMIA

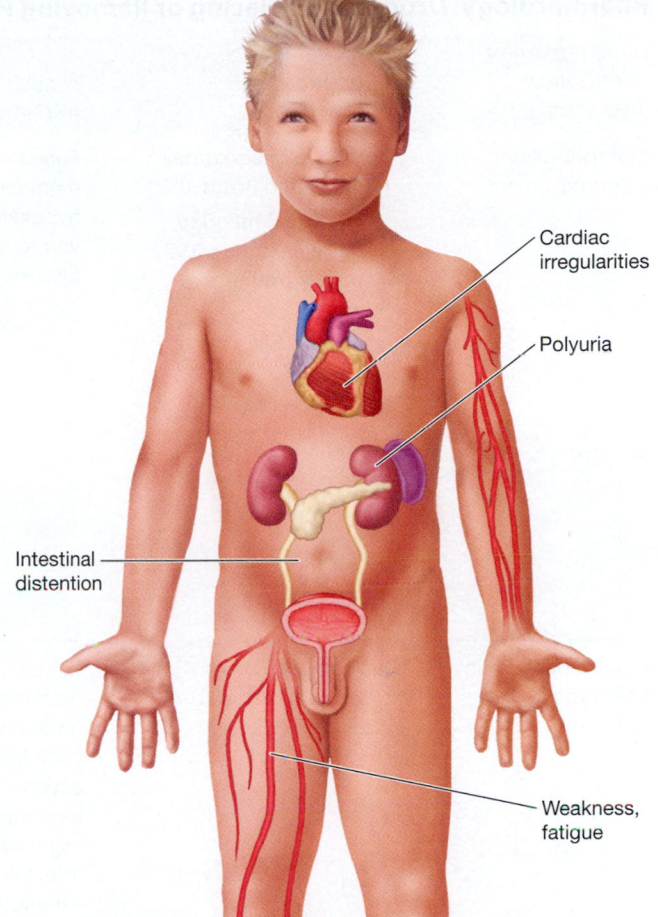

Cardiac irregularities

Polyuria

Intestinal distention

Weakness, fatigue

Figure 15-10. ■ Multisystem effects of hypokalemia.

hypovolemia, lead poisoning, and acidosis. It can also be the result of an excessive IV infusion of potassium supplementation.

Manifestations

Clinical manifestations for hyperkalemia include anxiety, hypotension, dysrhythmias, diarrhea, weakness, and cardiac arrhythmias progressing to cardiac arrest.

Diagnosis

Serum potassium levels will be increased according to the child's age (see Table 15-3). Diagnosis of hyperkalemia is

MediaLink

Hyperkalemia

TABLE 15-4

Pharmacology: Drugs for Replacing or Removing Potassium

DRUG (COMMON BRAND NAME AND GENERIC)	USUAL ROUTE/DOSE	CLASSIFICATION AND PURPOSE	SELECTED SIDE EFFECTS	DO NOT GIVE IF
Klor (potassium chloride)	PO: 1–3 mEq/kg/day in divided doses IV: up to 3 mEq/kg/day at less than 0.02 mEq/kg/minute	Potassium supplement used to treat hypokalemia due to vomiting, diarrhea, diuresis	Nausea, vomiting, ECG changes	Urine output is not within normal limits for age group. PO: Dilute in water or juice; instruct child not to crush or chew. IV: Never give IV push. Dilute carefully before administering. Mix well. Any signs of blood vessel irritation occur. Stop infusion immediately with recognition of symptoms.
Kayexalate (sodium polystyrene sulfonate)	PO 1 g/kg every 6 hours PR 1 g/kg every 2–6 hours	Sulfonic cation-exchange resin that removes potassium from body by exchange of sodium ion for potassium, especially in large intestine; resin is excreted	May cause gastric upset, sodium retention, hypocalcemia, hypokalemia, hypomagnesemia	Child shows clinical signs of hypokalemia. Child has hypersensitivity to the drug. Client cannot tolerate even a small increase in sodium load (e.g., congestive heart failure).

BOX 15-4   NUTRITION THERAPY

Foods High in Potassium

Apricots

Bananas

Cantaloupe

Carrots

Dates

Fish

Meat

Milk and milk products

Oranges

Peas

Potatoes

Raisins

Spinach

Tomatoes

made by reviewing symptoms and laboratory values of potassium.

Treatment

Medical management for hyperkalemia includes restricting intake of potassium. Kayexalate may be given to promote excretion of potassium. Peritoneal dialysis may also be necessary. IV calcium gluconate may be given to decrease cardiac effects. Insulin and glucose or sodium bicarbonate may be ordered to promote shifting of potassium into the cells.

Nursing Considerations

When caring for a child with hyperkalemia, the nurse will closely monitor serum potassium values and report imbalances promptly. Because potassium imbalances have the potential to affect cardiac and respiratory status, the nurse must vigilantly monitor the child's pulse and respiratory rate and rhythm. If ECG monitoring is ordered, it must be closely observed as well.

Kayexalate causes bowel excretion of potassium. Frequent hygiene must become a priority nursing action. This will facilitate the child's comfort and protect skin integrity.

Calcium Imbalance

HYPOCALCEMIA

Hypocalcemia is characterized by decreased serum calcium levels below normal levels. The condition may be caused by poor dietary intake of calcium accompanied by lack of vitamin D intake, lack of exposure to sunlight, surgical removal of the parathyroid, acute pancreatitis, and steatorrhea. The child who receives multiple blood transfusions is at risk for hypocalcemia. This is because citrate, which is a preservative in the blood, competes for calcium-binding sites; it causes calcium to be flushed through the body without being metabolized. Medications associated with hypocalcemia include overuse of antacids and laxatives, anticonvulsants, antineoplastics, and phosphate-containing preparations. Table 15-5 ■ provides a comparison of the causes of hypo- and hypercalcemia.

Manifestations

Clinical manifestations of hypocalcemia include numbness and tingling in the fingers and around the mouth, muscle cramps, pathologic fractures, and increased deep tendon reflexes (DTRs) (Figure 15-11 ■). The newborn with hypocalcemia may develop congestive heart failure.

Diagnosis

Serum calcium levels will be decreased for the child's age (see Table 15-3).

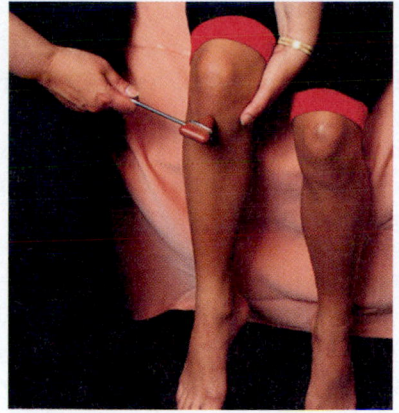

Figure 15-11. ■ The child with hypocalcemia may exhibit increased deep tendon reflexes.

Treatment

Medical management of hypocalcemia includes administering calcium supplementation orally or intravenously. Vitamin D supplementation may also be prescribed. The child should also have a diet high in calcium.

Nursing Considerations

The nurse should slowly administer calcium gluconate diluted in D_5W. Rapid IV infusion may cause dizziness, hypotension, and cardiac arrhythmias. Monitor the child's IV site carefully for infiltration, which can cause tissue sloughing and necrosis. In an effort to decrease GI upset, the nurse should give PO calcium at least 1 hour after meals or administer it with milk. Vital signs, including cardiac monitoring, should be observed closely. Safety measures and seizure precautions are important to implement.

MediaLink

Evaluate deep tendon reflex

TABLE 15-5

Causes of Hypocalcemia and Hypercalcemia

RELATED FACTOR	HYPOCALCEMIA	HYPERCALCEMIA
Vitamin D	Lack of dietary calcium and vitamin D	Overdose
Endocrine imbalance	Hypoparathyroidism	Hyperparathyroidism
Disease or disorder	Malabsorption Chronic renal insufficiency Chronic diarrhea Alkalosis	Bone tumors and other cancers
Medications/drugs	Laxative abuse	Thiazide diuretics
Medical procedure	Rapid infusion of plasma expanders Large blood transfusion (citrated blood)	—
Congenital basis	—	Familial hypercalcemia

HYPERCALCEMIA

Hypercalcemia is a condition characterized by an increase in serum calcium above normal levels. The condition may be caused by hyperparathyroidism, prolonged immobilization, leukemia, bone tumors, and intake of excessive calcium, including total parenteral nutrition with excessive calcium content.

Manifestations

Clinical manifestations of hypercalcemia include decreased muscle tone, nausea, vomiting, weakness, decreased level of consciousness (LOC), renal calculi, cardiac arrhythmias, and possible cardiac arrest.

Diagnosis

Serum calcium levels will be increased according to the child's age (see Table 15-3).

Treatment

Medical management of hypercalcemia includes hydration to encourage excretion of calcium through diuresis. Diuretics may also be administered. Glucocorticoids may be used to decrease intestinal absorption of calcium and bone resorption. Dialysis may be necessary to facilitate removal of calcium.

Nursing Considerations

The nurse caring for a child with hypercalcemia should promote adequate fluid intake to keep urine dilute and to prevent constipation. It may be necessary to strain urine for calculi. The child with hypercalcemia is at risk for falls due to weakness. The nurse should ambulate the child with care and promote safety measures.

NURSING CARE

PRIORITIES IN NURSING CARE

When caring for a child with fluid and electrolyte imbalances, priority must be given to monitoring daily weight, intake and output, and lab values. Even slight variations in these objective findings could be significant in children. The nurse will need to report variations immediately to the health care provider in order for the child to receive prompt care.

ASSESSING

The nurse needs to obtain adequate baseline vital signs, weight, and physical assessment data. These findings are then compared to data obtained throughout the course of the illness. Closely monitor changes in skin turgor, edema, moisture in mucous membranes, and lung sounds. Review the child's hematocrit, hemoglobin, urine specific gravity, BUN, creatinine, and electrolyte studies. Once treatment has begun, an improvement in these values should be demonstrated.

DIAGNOSING, PLANNING, AND IMPLEMENTING

Nursing diagnoses for fluid and electrolyte imbalances might include:

- Deficient Fluid Volume related to excessive GI loss
- Excess Fluid Volume related to excessive accumulation of fluid
- Imbalanced Nutrition: Less than Body Requirements related to inadequate intake
- Impaired Skin Integrity related to irritation caused by diarrhea.

Some outcomes for fluid and electrolyte imbalances are as follows. The child will:

- Exhibit symptoms of adequate hydration
- Be free of symptoms of fluid volume excess
- Maintain adequate nutritional intake, appropriate for weight and age
- Maintain intact skin.

The nurse's role in providing support to these clients would include the following nursing interventions:

- Administer oral rehydration as ordered. *Oral fluids replace fluid losses but must be given slowly, in small amounts, to children with vomiting and diarrhea.*
- Assist with IV rehydration as ordered (see Procedure 13-22 ⬲). *IV rehydration allows for more rapid fluid replacement when the child is severely dehydrated.*
- Monitor IV infusion closely. *Fluid overload could occur with rapid infusion of IV fluids.*
- Teach parents how to recognize signs and symptoms of fluid loss. *Timely recognition of symptoms will facilitate treatment.*
- Teach parents the appropriate method of oral rehydration (see Box 15-2). *Parents who recognize early symptoms of fluid loss can initiate rehydration early and possibly avoid severe imbalances.*
- Assist the child and the parents in restricting fluids, if ordered. *Compliance will be improved if the child assists in planning for fluid restriction.*
- Administer diuretics as ordered. *Diuretics assist in removing excess fluid.*
- Ensure that the child changes position every 2 hours. *Edematous skin tears easily. Position changes will prevent skin breakdown.*
- Advance diet slowly, as ordered. *Food needs to be reintroduced slowly to avoid GI distress. Initial foods should be low in fiber and bland.*

- Encourage breastfeeding mothers to resume feedings. *Breast milk reduces the severity of the imbalance.*
- In infants with diarrhea, change the diaper frequently. *The diarrhea stool may contain excessive acid and irritate the skin.*
- Use a mild soap and water to cleanse the perineal area with each diaper change. *Soaps with high alcohol content and fragrances or commercial baby wipes may further irritate the skin.*
- Apply protective ointment as ordered. *Ointments can provide a moisture barrier to protect the skin.*

EVALUATING

Expected outcomes for a client with fluid and electrolyte imbalance include return of adequate hydration, weight gain or weight loss, and intact skin. The nurse can accurately evaluate these outcomes by monitoring vital signs, intake and output, lab values, and symptoms related to the imbalances. Documentation should include response to client teaching, tolerance to rehydration and diet changes, physical findings related to the imbalance, daily intake and output, daily weight, and lab values. Lack of response to treatment and worsening of symptoms must be reported to the charge nurse or physician promptly.

NURSING PROCESS CARE PLAN
Client with Diarrhea

Wesley is a 3-month-old infant who is formula fed. He is typically a pleasant child who has regular bowel habits. His big brother, Mark, has been home from school with a stomach virus this week. Today, after his morning bottle, Wesley has had several loose stools and is irritable when awake. His mother calls the pediatrician's office for advice.

Assessment. The nurse should gather the following data during the phone call:

- Changes in diet by obtaining a 24-hour diet history
- Onset of diarrhea
- Color, consistency, frequency, amount, and odor of stools
- The presence of mucus in the stools
- Associated symptoms such as vomiting, fever, and lethargy.

When the child is seen in the pediatrician's office, gather the following data:

- Current weight
- Vital signs
- Skin turgor and texture
- Presence of skin breakdown in diaper area
- Bowel sounds

- Abdominal distension (by measuring abdominal circumference).

Nursing Diagnosis. The following important nursing diagnosis (among others) is established for this client:

- Deficient Fluid Volume related to excessive diarrhea

Expected Outcomes

- The child will have balanced intake and output in the next 24 hours.
- The child will have adequate hydration, as evidenced by moist mucous membranes, good skin turgor, lab values, and vital signs within normal limits.

Planning and Implementation

- Obtain daily weight.
- Maintain strict record of intake and output during each shift.
- Document and review vital signs as ordered. Report abnormal values promptly.
- Review serum electrolytes, urine specific gravity, BUN, creatinine, and hematocrit lab values during each shift. Report abnormal values promptly.
- Carefully administer oral and IV fluids, as ordered.
- Provide frequent perineal hygiene.
- Provide frequent oral hygiene.
- Instruct parent in recognition of symptoms of fluid volume deficit and management techniques (see Table 15-2 and Box 15-2).

Evaluation. The child's intake and output are balanced. Return of hydration is evident in mucous membranes, skin turgor, lab values, and vital signs. The child's bowel and bladder habits return to normal.

Critical Thinking in the Nursing Process

1. A dangerous risk of diarrhea in a child is hypovolemic shock. How would the nurse recognize hypovolemic shock?
2. Wesley's mothers asks if the formula caused her son's diarrhea. She wants to know if she should change formulas. What is the most appropriate nursing response?
3. Wesley's mother wonders if his brother gave him the stomach virus. She does not understand how this could have happened because they do not share eating utensils. What does she need to be taught about the spread of infectious diarrhea?

Note: Discussion of Critical Thinking questions appears in Appendix I.

ACID-BASE DISORDERS

Principles Related to Acid-Base Disorders

The principle of homeostasis, or balance, also applies to the balance of hydrogen ion concentration within the body. The concentration has 1 part carbonic acid (H_2CO_3) to 20 parts bicarbonate (HCO_3^-) (Figure 15-12 ■). Homeostasis of the hydrogen ion is measured by determining the pH of the blood. Normal blood pH for a child is 7.36 to 7.44. The condition of **acidosis** develops when there is an increase of hydrogen ion concentration. In acidosis, the body's pH will be less than 7.36. The condition of **alkalosis** develops when there is a decrease of hydrogen ion concentration. In alkalosis, the body's pH will be greater than 7.44.

When pH levels become abnormal, certain body mechanisms are initiated in an effort to correct the abnormal value and restore the child's acid-base balance. There are three body mechanisms that compensate for abnormal pH levels: the buffer system, the respiratory system, and the renal system.

BUFFER SYSTEM

The buffer system is activated within seconds of detecting the abnormal value. The buffer system uses various chemicals such as bicarbonate, phosphate, hemoglobin, and protein to compensate for imbalances. Chemical reactions either rid the body of excess hydrogen ion or seek to conserve hydrogen ion when there is a hydrogen deficit (Figure 15-13 ■).

RESPIRATORY SYSTEM

The respiratory system is activated next, usually within minutes of a detectable imbalance. Normal respiration in-

volves breathing in oxygen and breathing out carbon dioxide (CO_2) and water. CO_2 is continuously formed in the body. It moves out of the cells and into the interstitial fluids, then into the intravascular fluid. It is transported through the venous system to the lungs and is exhaled from the body.

If CO_2 becomes excessive, the CO_2 combines with body water and forms an acid. This chemical reaction causes a decrease in the body's pH. The body recognizes the imbalance and stimulates the respiratory system to increase the rate and depth of respirations to "blow off" excess CO_2.

If CO_2 is deficient, there is less than normal CO_2 to mix with water and form the acid the body needs. In this case, the body's pH increases. The body recognizes the imbalance and decreases the rate and depth of respirations, conserving CO_2.

RENAL SYSTEM

The final compensation method to occur takes place in the renal system. It may take several days for this method to be initiated. When a person is healthy, the kidneys excrete more hydrogen ion and conserve bicarbonate (hydroxide). A normal, healthy person's urine has a pH of 6.

However, when there is too much hydrogen ion in the blood, the body will increase urinary output. When this oc-

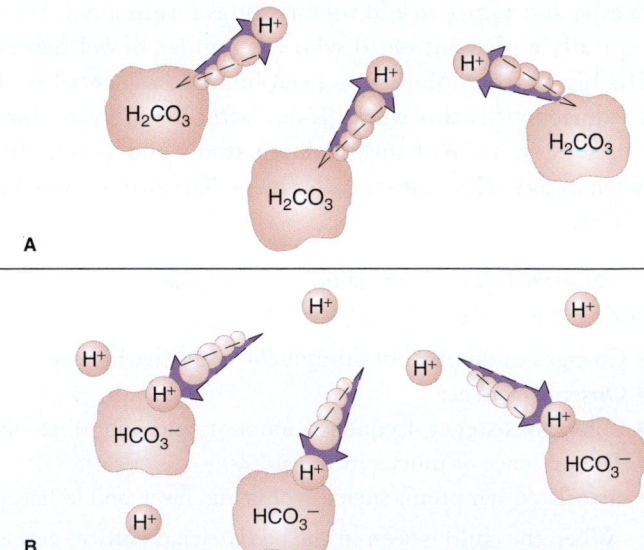

Figure 15-13. ■ Buffer response to acid-base. (**A**) The way in which buffers respond to an excess of base. If the blood has too much base, the acid portion of a buffer pair (e.g., H_2CO_3 of the bicarbonate buffer system) releases hydrogen ions (H^+) to help return the pH to normal. (**B**) The way in which buffers respond to an excess of acid. If the blood has too much acid, the base portion of a buffer pair (e.g., HCO_3^-) of the bicarbonate buffer system) takes up hydrogen ions (H^+) to help return the pH to normal.

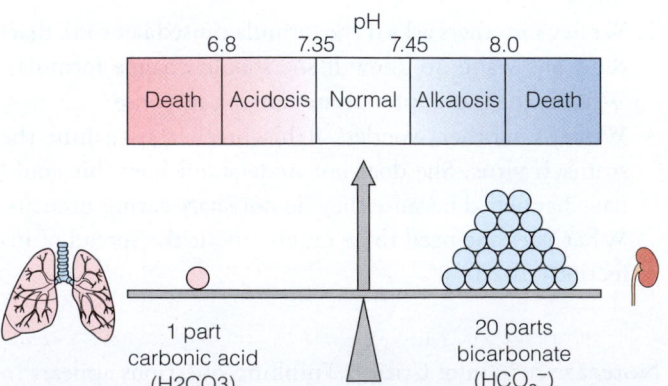

Figure 15-12. ■ The normal ratio of bicarbonate to carbonic acid is 20:1. As long as this ratio is maintained, the pH remains within the normal range of 7.36 to 7.44 (child) or 7.35 to 7.45 (adult).

curs, there is more hydrogen ion in the urine than normal, making the urine pH less than 6. When there is too little hydrogen ion in the blood, the body will decrease urinary output. In this case, there is less hydrogen ion in the urine than normal, making the urine pH increased, or greater than 6.

ARTERIAL BLOOD GAS ANALYSIS

Arterial blood gas (ABG) analysis is an essential part of the data used to assess acid-base imbalances. ABG actually determines the functioning of the respiratory system. The nurse needs to understand the analysis process and be able to detect imbalances so they can be reported promptly.

ABG specimens may be obtained by an RN, lab technician, or respiratory technician. They are usually drawn from an arterial site such as the radial, brachial, or femoral artery. A heparinized syringe is used to avoid clotting of the specimen. Care must be taken not to allow air to enter the syringe. If air in the environment mixed with the blood specimen, it would alter the gas content of the blood. To reduce metabolism of the cells, the syringe containing the specimen is submerged in crushed ice and is taken to the lab immediately.

To analyze ABG results accurately, memorize the following principles:

- pH measures the hydrogen ion concentration of the specimen.
- $PaCO_2$ measures the partial pressure of the CO_2 in arterial blood. This is an indication of the effectiveness of ventilation.
- HCO_3^- measures the metabolic content of the arterial blood.
- The pH and $PaCO_2$ values move in opposite directions when the client has a respiratory condition. For example, pH 7.33 and $PaCO_2$ 51 indicates respiratory acidosis.
- The pH and HCO_3^- values move in the same direction when the client has a metabolic condition. For example, pH 7.51 and HCO_3^- 28 indicates metabolic alkalosis.

Box 15-5 ■ provides steps for reviewing ABG lab results.

Practice in ABG Analysis

Here are five examples of ABG results. *After reading Box 15-5, test your knowledge by covering the answers with a book or paper and writing the condition after each set of data.*

1. pH 7.34, $PaCO_2$ 50, HCO_3^- 22 _____
2. pH 7.33, $PaCO_2$ 44, HCO_3^- 20 _____
3. pH 7.46, $PaCO_2$ 45, HCO_3^- 30 _____
4. pH 7.47, $PaCO_2$ 33, HCO_3^- 25 _____
5. pH 7.33, $PaCO_2$ 50, HCO_3^- 30 _____

Answers

1. respiratory acidosis
2. metabolic acidosis
3. metabolic alkalosis

BOX 15-5	NURSING CARE CHECKLIST

Reviewing ABG Results

Follow these steps when reviewing ABG results:

☑ Review the pH to determine acidosis or alkalosis. A pH less than 7.36 indicates acidosis; a pH greater than 7.44 indicates alkalosis.

☑ Review the $PaCO_2$. Is it normal? Remember the principle: The pH and $PaCO_2$ values move in opposite directions when the client has a respiratory condition. For example, a respiratory condition is indicated when the pH is increased and the $PaCO_2$ is decreased *or* when the pH is decreased and the $PaCO_2$ is increased.

☑ Review the HCO_3^-. Is it normal? Remember the principle: The pH and HCO_3^- values move in the same direction when the client has a metabolic condition. For example, a metabolic condition is indicated when the pH and HCO_3^- are both increased *or* when the pH and HCO_3^- are both decreased.

☑ If all three values are abnormal, the body is compensating for the imbalance.

4. respiratory alkalosis
5. respiratory acidosis with compensation

Respiratory Acidosis

Respiratory acidosis is an accumulation of CO_2 caused by states of hypoventilation, altered perfusion, or inadequate respiratory diffusion. In children, respiratory acidosis can be caused by airway obstruction resulting in CO_2 retention. As CO_2 builds, the pH decreases. The body seeks to compensate for this imbalance by increasing the rate and depth of respiration. The kidneys also conserve bicarbonate in an effort to raise the body's pH.

Respiratory acidosis is associated with diseases that impair the child's ability to breathe normally. These diseases include severe pneumonia, pneumothorax, cystic fibrosis, and croup (see Chapter 18 ⊂⊃). Central nervous system (CNS) injuries also compromise the child's ability to ventilate properly. These injuries include brain tumors, head injuries, and spinal cord injuries. Respiratory acidosis can also occur with the use of anesthetics, sedatives, and narcotics that impair the respiratory effort.

Manifestations

Acidosis, a lowering of the body's pH, results in CNS depression characterized by disorientation, lethargy, and headaches. CNS depression can also progress to unconsciousness. Cardiac symptoms of respiratory acidosis include tachycardia, hypotension, and ventricular fibrillation. The child may have muscle weakness or convulsions, depending on the cause of the imbalance. Respirations are rapid and shallow.

Diagnosis

ABG findings, along with clinical manifestations, assist in the diagnosis of this imbalance. Serum pH is decreased, P_{CO_2} is increased, and the bicarbonate is normal unless compensation is occurring, at which time the bicarbonate increases. During compensation, the urine pH is decreased.

Treatment

Medical management of respiratory acidosis involves improving ventilatory status. The cause of the imbalance must be corrected. All avenues should be explored to determine the cause (see Health Promotion Issue on pages 502 and 503). Treatment often includes administration of bronchodilators, oxygen, and antibiotics; chest physiotherapy; mechanical ventilation; and removal of foreign objects that are obstructing the airway.

Nursing Considerations

Nursing care for the child with respiratory acidosis is focused on restoring adequate ventilation. A simple nursing measure is to raise the head of the bed and to avoid positioning that would allow chest compression or slumping to the side (Figure 15-14 ■). Emergency methods may be necessary to remove objects obstructing the airway. See Chapter 12 ⚭ for more information about preventing airway obstruction. The child may require temporary ventilatory

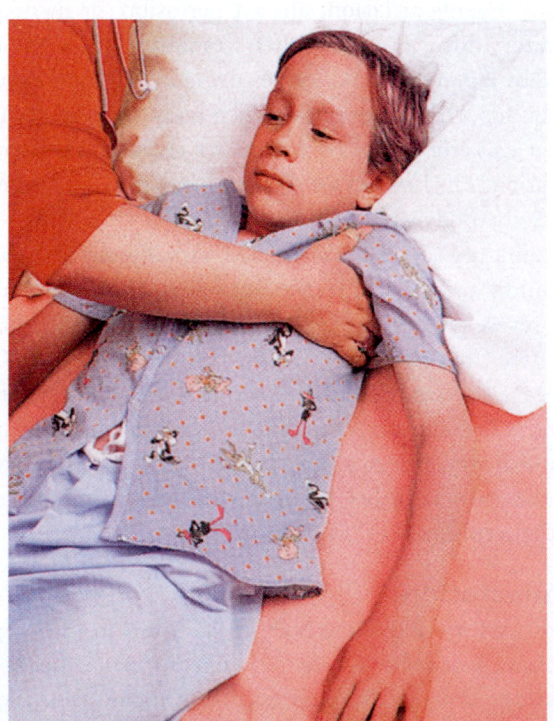

Figure 15-14. ■ Positioning to facilitate chest expansion. Positioning the child to avoid chest compression or slumping to the side will help correct respiratory acidosis.

support. See Chapter 18 ⚭ for more information on nursing care related to ventilators.

Safety is also a consideration for children with respiratory acidosis. Environmental hazards need to be assessed and removed if present. Sedation should be avoided to promote safety and to avoid further depressing the CNS. Parents will need reassurance and support.

Respiratory Alkalosis

Respiratory alkalosis, commonly known as hyperventilation, is a condition characterized by a low level of CO_2 in the blood.

Lack of CO_2 causes the serum pH to increase. In children, the most common cause of respiratory alkalosis is anxiety, fear, or panic. These emotional states cause the child to breathe rapidly and deeply. Other causes of respiratory alkalosis include pain, salicylate poisoning, altitude sickness, meningitis (see Chapter 16 ⚭), septicemia, and mechanical overventilation (see Chapter 18 ⚭).

Manifestations

The earliest symptom of this imbalance is tingling of the fingers and toes with a rapid, deep respiratory rate. Because the CNS is stimulated in alkalosis, the child may become light-headed, confused, anxious, and unable to concentrate. Other clinical manifestations include tachycardia, dysrhythmias, tetany, numbness, and hyperreflexia.

Diagnosis

ABG values show an increased serum pH, decreased P_{CO_2}, bicarbonate within normal limits without compensation, and a decreased bicarbonate when compensation is occurring.

Treatment

Medical treatment seeks to correct the cause of respiratory alkalosis and restore CO_2 levels to within normal limits. Oxygen therapy is ordered for acute hypoxemia. Sedatives and antianxiety agents are used for children expressing anxiety, fear, pain, or panic.

Nursing Considerations

The simplest corrective action for early respiratory alkalosis is to encourage rebreathing of the child's own expiratory CO_2 by asking the child to breathe into a paper bag or cupped hands. Ensure that proper ventilation is promoted and mechanical ventilation is functioning properly.

The nurse also instructs the child in anxiety-reducing techniques and attends to the emotional needs of the child. Pharmacologic and nonpharmacologic pain relief methods are indicated for children experiencing pain.

Metabolic Acidosis

Metabolic acidosis is a condition involving an excess of acids in the body. It results from the process of metabolism or a loss of bicarbonate through urine or gastrointestinal (GI) fluids. When the body produces an abundance of ketone bodies, metabolic acidosis may result.

Metabolic acidosis, called **ketoacidosis,** occurs when glucose storage is depleted and fat storage must be used for energy needs.

Manifestations

Metabolic acidosis may also occur due to starvation, anorexia nervosa, bulimia, severe diarrhea, intestinal malabsorption, drug toxicity, draining GI fistulas, diabetes, and renal failure. Children who ingest aspirin or toxic chemicals such as antifreeze may develop metabolic acidosis (Figure 15-15 ■). The child may manifest symptoms of hyperventilation. **Kussmaul** (rapid and deep) respirations may be present. The CNS is depressed, and the child may exhibit general malaise that progresses to unconsciousness. Hypotension, ventricular fibrillation, a dull headache, muscle weakness, nausea, vomiting, and abdominal pain may also occur.

Diagnosis

Diagnosis is accomplished by observing for symptoms and evaluating ABG values. Serum pH levels and bicarbonate will be decreased. The P_{CO_2} will be within normal limits if uncompensated and decreased if compensation is occurring. Urine pH levels will be decreased if compensation is occurring.

Treatment

Medical treatment seeks to correct the cause of metabolic acidosis. Insulin will be administered to correct ketoacidosis. Severe metabolic acidosis will be treated with IV sodium

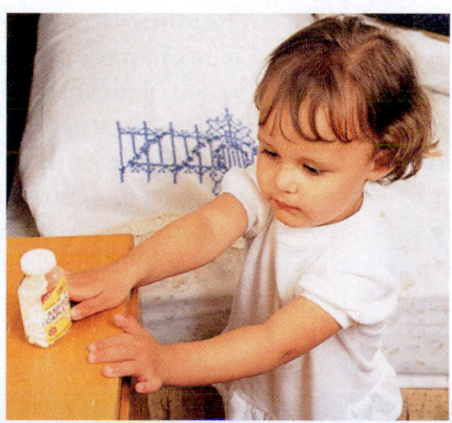

Figure 15-15. ■ Teaching parents to use safety latches on cabinets to keep aspirin away from small children can prevent one cause of metabolic acidosis.

bicarbonate. For the renal client or child with an overdose, dialysis may be required. Antidiarrheal drugs may be used to treat diarrhea.

Nursing Considerations

The nurse closely monitors the child with metabolic acidosis for progressive respiratory, neurologic, and cardiac symptoms. Worsening symptoms must be reported promptly to the charge nurse and physician. Ventilation should be facilitated by proper positioning.

Oral hygiene should be provided for children with vomiting and rapid respirations. The child's lips also become dry due to rapid respiration. Lip balm should be applied as needed. Prompt attention is necessary to protect the skin from irritation due to diarrhea. The nurse may need to assist the child in conserving energy if muscle weakness and malaise are present.

Diabetic clients and their families need teaching on symptom recognition for ketoacidosis. They will also need instruction on management techniques for this condition. Children who have overdosed, accidentally or purposefully, need to understand how to prevent this hazard. Referral to behavioral medicine units may be appropriate.

Metabolic Alkalosis

Metabolic alkalosis is a condition that results from a loss of metabolic acid or an excess of bicarbonate.

Loss of metabolic acids occurs due to vomiting, nasogastric suction, cystic fibrosis, inappropriate use of diuretics, and hypokalemia. Excess bicarbonate may occur:

- When the child ingests baking soda or an overdose of antacids
- Following blood transfusions with multiple units of blood
- In increased renal absorption.

Manifestations

Clinical manifestations of metabolic alkalosis includes abdominal distention, constipation, cardiac arrhythmias, polyuria, decreased rate and depth of respirations, tetany, seizures, weakness, confusion, lethargy, and coma.

Diagnosis

Lab work from a child with metabolic alkalosis reveals increased serum pH, increased HCO_3, normal P_{CO_2} when uncompensated, and increased P_{CO_2} when compensation is occurring.

Treatment

Medical management is focused on treating the causative factor. Treatment will include IV infusion with normal saline and administration of acetazolamide to facilitate renal excretion of bicarbonate.

(Text continues on p. 504.)

HEALTH PROMOTION ISSUE

SELF-ASPHYXIATION AS A GAME

The LPN works for the local school system and frequently visits several middle schools with an RN to provide health screenings, administer medications, and provide wellness information to students. One week a month, the nurses have lunch in each school in an effort to get to know the students better. This lunchtime visit also provides an opportunity for the students to learn to trust the nurses.

Recently, the nurses overheard a group of eighth-grade students planning a gasp party. The students appeared to be familiar with the nature of this type of party and only interested in obtaining information about the party particulars, such as time, date, and location.

When the crowd began to disperse for class, the LPN/LVN approached a female student whom she had previously befriended. The LPN/LVN asked the student for more information about the nature of a gasp party. The nurse was careful not to appear overly concerned and anxious. The student, who was not involved in the planning of this party, was willing to give the nurse information because she too was concerned about the health risks of this activity.

The LPN/LVN and the RN met with representatives from the school to discuss

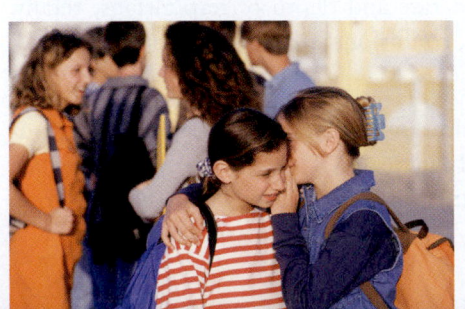

what might be done to protect the students from this dangerous activity. This group's first action item was to discover more information about this game.

DISCUSSION

In alarming numbers, preteen and early teens are engaging in an asphyxiation game that momentarily alters consciousness and causes a 10- to 20-second "high" or "rush." The game can be played in groups or alone. When played in groups, a child's chest or neck is compressed to arrest the blood flow, and therefore the oxygen flow, to the brain. The resulting hypoxia induces feelings of light-headedness, numbness, or tingling. There is a distinct possibility of loss of consciousness during this time. Children report feelings of euphoria, timelessness, and peace during this stage. Next, the pressure to the chest or neck is released, causing the blood to coarse quickly through the carotid arteries on its way to the brain, returning consciousness. This provides a "rush" sensation.

When the "choking game" is played alone, the child loses consciousness and is likely to be unable to loosen the constriction around his or her own neck. Hypoxia quickly proceeds to anoxia. Death can result in just a few minutes.

The game is believed to be addictive, and there have been reports of children playing the game for many hours in a row. During these marathon sessions, a child may actually lose consciousness several times.

The game is known by names other than the choking game. Some of the most common names are gasp, the American Dream game, space monkey, black out, pass out, space cowboy, rising sun, airplaning, funky chicken, flat liner, tingling and suffocation roulette, the fainting game, ghost, and the something dreaming game.

The choking game is most popular among middle school children ages 9 to 14. These children are usually popular in school and in their communities, and are seemingly well adjusted. Their families state that they are close and maintain habits of functional families, such as eating meals together, taking vacations together, and keeping regular schedules. These children rarely cause trouble at home or school and are found to make good grades.

It is difficult to gather exact figures on how many children are participating in this dangerous activity. Often, when the child is found dead, hanging from a rope or belt, the medical examiner determines the death a suicide instead of an accident due to the choking game.

Health risks associated with asphyxiation activities include injuries. They can be minor lacerations or sprained joints to more serious neck injuries causing permanent disability. Retinal damage has also been reported. The choking game may cause episodes of syncope. Ventricular arrhythmia can also be associated with the choking game. Brain damage and death, of course, are the most serious risks of the choking game.

PLANNING AND IMPLEMENTATION

The nurses and school staff developed a plan to raise awareness about this game. They also wanted to provide information to students, parents, and school officials about the health dangers associated with the choking game. First, they developed an informational pamphlet to be mailed to the homes of all middle school children. The pamphlet contained a detailed description of this game and the health risks associated with it. Warning signs and symptoms were also listed. These included:

- Linear abrasions or areas of ecchymosis on the neck
- Petechiae found on the face, eyelids, or conjunctiva
- Intermittent hoarseness when the child does not have a cold, sinus problems, or allergies
- Dog leashes, choke collars, bungee cords, ropes, belts, cords, or even wire clothes hangers draped in an unexplained manner over door frames or closet rods
- Frequent choice of high-necked shirts or turtlenecks, even in warmer months
- Frequent headaches
- A sudden increase in the amount of time spent alone in the child's bedroom.

The pamphlet concluded with a plan for discussing these dangers with children. It was suggested that parents include the choking game in their discussion of other dangerous activities such as smoking, alcohol, drugs, and sexual activity. They were encouraged to ask the child to consider the consequences of the decision to play this game. Parents were advised to cite specific incidences in which children lost their life to this activity. Parents were also encouraged to check the history and activity of a child's computer to determine if they are engaging in chat rooms where the game is discussed or visiting how-to websites related to the choking game. A contact number was given for more information and assistance.

The second intervention aimed at reducing the incidence of this game among middle school children was random health screening in the school setting for symptoms related to the choking game. Children would be given a questionnaire to determine their knowledge and involvement in the game. Children considered at risk would be referred to the school counselor.

The third intervention was a forum to discuss the issues with all school officials, including teachers, administrators, and support staff. Because this activity is often practiced on school grounds, school officials were encouraged to consider security cameras that would allow them to monitor for the activity.

School officials were also encouraged to be diligent in offering exciting alternatives to this type of risk-taking behavior. A variety of safe activities that appeal to a child's sense of adventure were encouraged.

SELF-REFLECTION

Consider the risk-taking activities you may have engaged in during your middle school and high school years. Did you have conversations with strangers who could have harmed you? Did you walk alone in wooded areas without someone knowing where you were? Did you drive recklessly? Were you in a car when your friend played "chicken" with oncoming traffic? Think carefully about what caused you to engage in these behaviors. What could have prevented your participation in these activities? How can you incorporate these findings into your own practice with children?

SUGGESTED RESOURCES

For the Nurse

- Le, D., & Macnab, A. J. (2001). Self strangulation by hanging from cloth towel dispensers in Canadian schools. *Injury Prevention, 7(3)*, 231–233.

For the Client

- Shapiro, L. (2004). *The secret language of children: How to understand what your kids are really saying.* Naperville, IL: Sourcebooks. This book gives parents the tools to communicate more effectively with their children.

- http://teenchokinggame.com This website publishes a newsletter that includes case histories, news articles, resource directory, links, and publications related to the choking game.

- www.stop-the-choking-game.com This website is dedicated to providing information about the choking game in an effort to educate parents. The site also displays biographic information about victims of this deadly game.

Nursing Considerations

Nursing care for children with metabolic alkalosis includes assisting the child to breathe effectively and monitoring neurologic status closely. Measures must be implemented to keep safe the child who has an altered LOC.

Strict monitoring of intake and output for the child who is vomiting is essential to the nursing care plan. The child who is vomiting frequently also needs regular oral hygiene.

NURSING CARE

PRIORITIES IN NURSING CARE

Children experiencing an acid-base imbalance are at risk for ventilation and oxygenation difficulties. The nurse must be diligent in monitoring ventilation and oxygenation and in recognizing changes in these processes. The nurse should also prevent further compromise in these processes by positioning the child to facilitate ventilation, minimizing administration of narcotic pain relief, and keeping the airway free of obstruction through oral suctioning as necessary.

ASSESSING

In respiratory and metabolic acid-base imbalances, the nurse must give priority to assessing patency of the airway. Monitor respiratory rate, rhythm, and effort. Other vital signs, pulse, and blood pressure may also change in response to the imbalance and must be monitored closely. The child's neurologic status and cardiac function may indicate worsening of the condition. ABG values and pulse oximetry findings are assessed frequently.

DIAGNOSING, PLANNING, AND IMPLEMENTING

Nursing diagnoses for acid-base imbalances might include:

- Ineffective Breathing Pattern related to hyperventilation
- Impaired Gas Exchange related to hypoventilation
- Risk for Injury related to central nervous system stimulation
- Disturbed Thought Process related to central nervous system depression.

Some outcomes for acid-base imbalances might include that the child will:

- Demonstrate effective breathing pattern as evidenced by rate, rhythm, and effort of respirations within normal range
- Demonstrate improved ventilation and oxygenation
- Avoid injury until acid-base balance is restored
- Regain usual thought process appropriate for age.

The nurse's role in providing support to these clients would include the following:

- Position the child to facilitate breathing. *Positions that promote lung expansion will improve breathing.*
- Encourage slow, deep breathing for respiratory acidosis. *Correcting hypoventilation is a priority goal.*
- Encourage rebreathing of CO_2 for respiratory alkalosis. *Respiratory alkalosis is marked by hyperventilation and CO_2 deficits.*
- Aspirate oral secretions as needed (prn). *Maintaining a patent airway might require assisting the child in removing oral secretions.*
- Administer humidified oxygen or carbon dioxide as ordered. *Oxygen administration prevents hypoxemia. Humidified oxygen assists in the thinning of secretions. Carbon dioxide replacement may be necessary in respiratory alkalosis.*
- Administer IV solutions as ordered. *Corrects acidosis.*
- Administer sedation medications carefully. *In respiratory acidosis, sedation may be contraindicated because respiratory depression may occur. Sedation may reduce anxiety in respiratory alkalosis.*
- Create a safe environment for the child. Keep the bed in the lowest position. Keep the floor free of safety hazards. Assist the child to ambulate. *Muscle weakness and risk for seizure activity create a safety hazard for the child with an acid-base imbalance.*
- Encourage parents to monitor the child's muscle strength and neurologic status and to report noticeable changes. *Parents can often observe more subtle changes in the child's physical status. Early reporting of symptoms can lead to more effective treatment.*
- Provide brief and concise reorientation to reality. *Challenging the child's thinking would frustrate them. It is, however, important to present reality rather than agreeing with the child's distorted thinking.*
- Assure parents that distorted thinking is part of the acid-base imbalance. *This information relieves the parents' anxiety about the distorted thinking.*

EVALUATING

Expected outcomes for a client with acid-base imbalances include return of ABG values to normal limits, improved neurologic status, improved respiratory function, and improved cardiac function. Lack of response to treatment and worsening of symptoms must be reported to the charge nurse or physician promptly.

Note: The references and resources for this and all chapters have been compiled at the back of the book.

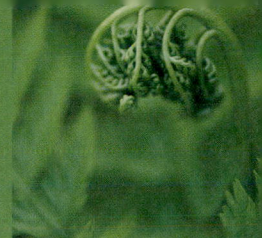

Chapter Review

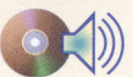

KEY TERMS by Topic

Use the audio glossary feature of either the CD-ROM or the Companion Website to hear the correct pronunciation of the following key terms.

Principles Related to Fluids and Electrolytes
homeostasis, plasma, interstitial, solute, solvent, solution, osmosis, diffusion, filtration, active transport, electrolytes, cations, anions

Deficient Fluid Volume (Dehydration)
dehydration, isotonic dehydration, hypotonic dehydration, hypertonic dehydration

Fluid Volume Excess (Hypovolemia)
hypovolemia

Sodium Imbalance
hyponatremia, hypernatremia

Potassium Imbalance
hypokalemia, hyperkalemia

Calcium Imbalance
hypocalcemia, hypercalcemia

Principles Related to Acid-Base Disorders
acidosis, alkalosis, respiratory acidosis, respiratory alkalosis, metabolic acidosis, ketoacidosis, Kussmaul, metabolic alkalosis

KEY Points

- Children have a high percentage of water; therefore, fluid and electrolyte imbalances are much more dangerous in pediatric clients than in adults.

- Homeostasis is achieved by balance of fluid, electrolytes, acids, and bases.

- Careful measuring of intake and output is essential to detecting fluid and electrolyte imbalances.

- Obtaining accurate measurement of the child's weight can assist the nurse in correctly identifying imbalances in fluid and electrolytes.

- The treatment of dehydration requires rehydration. This may be accomplished with oral or IV fluids based on the degree of dehydration.

- Fluid restriction is a necessary treatment for some fluid and electrolyte imbalances. Younger children will have difficulty understanding why they cannot have oral fluids. The nurse must take care to explain the fluid restriction in terms the child can understand. It is also important, when developing a plan for spacing the allotted fluid throughout the day, to involve the child and his or her parents.

- Acidosis develops when there is an increase of hydrogen ion concentration. Alkalosis develops when there is a decrease of hydrogen ion concentration.

- Three body mechanisms that compensate for abnormal pH levels leading to acidosis or alkalosis are the buffer system, the respiratory system, and the renal system.

- The nurse must be able to analyze ABG results accurately by reviewing pH, CO_2, and HCO_3 values.

- Children experiencing an acid-base imbalance are at risk for ventilation and oxygenation difficulties.

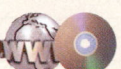

EXPLORE MediaLink

Additional interactive resources for this chapter can be found on the Companion Website at www.prenhall.com/towle.

Click on Chapter 15 and "Begin" to select the activities for this chapter.

For chapter-related NCLEX-style questions and an audio glossary, access the accompanying CD-ROM in this book.

Animations

Fluid

Acid

Evaluate deep tendon reflexes

Hyperkalemia

FOR FURTHER Study

See Chapter 12 for more information about preventing airway obstruction.

For information about obtaining vital signs, taking weights, and providing IV medications, see Chapter 13.

For a discussion of meningitis, see Chapter 16.

For a discussion of mechanical ventilation, pneumonia, pneumothorax, cystic fibrosis, croup, and other respiratory disorders, see Chapter 18.

For more on hypovolemic shock, see Chapter 20.

See Chapter 24 for more discussion on burns in children.

Critical Thinking Care Map

Caring for a Client with Fluid Volume Excess
NCLEX-PN® Focus Area: Physiologic adaptation

Case Study: Jayden, 3 days old, developed hyperbilirubinemia. The physician ordered placement of the newborn under phototherapy lights (bililights) and initiation of IV fluids to maintain adequate hydration. Following initiation of this therapy, the LPN noticed the IV rate infusing was greater than the rate ordered.

<table>
<tr><td colspan="2">Nursing Diagnosis: Fluid Volume Excess</td></tr>
</table>

COLLECT DATA

Subjective	Objective
_____	_____
_____	_____
_____	_____
_____	_____
_____	_____
_____	_____

Would you report this? Yes/No

If yes, to: _____

Nursing Care

_____
_____
_____
_____
_____
_____
_____
_____
_____
_____
_____
_____
_____
_____

How would you document this? _____
_____
_____
_____

Data Collected
(use those that apply)

- Flat fontanel
- Moist lung sounds
- Urine output 1 mL/kg/hour
- LPN states, "This rate is twice the rate ordered by the physician."
- Generalized edema
- Poor skin turgor
- Hemoglobin 30 g/dL
- Hematocrit 40%
- Urine specific gravity 1.000
- Sodium 133 mEq/L
- Pulse 110 bpm, bounding
- BUN 17 mg/dL

Nursing Interventions
(use those that apply; list in priority order)

- Turn infant every 30 minutes.
- Monitor vital signs.
- Observe for edema of the extremities, face, and neck.
- Monitor and document intake and output.
- Weigh the infant daily and document.
- Hold feedings until approved by charge nurse.
- Monitor IV fluid rate.
- Observe closely for symptoms of pulmonary edema, including restlessness, tachypnea, labored breathing, a full and bounding or weak and thready pulse, possible crackles on lung auscultation, and profuse diaphoresis. Position the child to facilitate breathing, and notify the physician immediately if symptoms are present.
- Monitor lab values and report imbalances.
- Remove child from bililights until edema has resolved.

Compare your documentation to the sample provided in Appendix I.

NCLEX-PN® Exam Preparation

1 A nurse is caring for a 2-year-old with a diagnosis of fluid volume excess (FVE). The nurse knows that with FVE, certain clinical findings may be present. Which of the laboratory report findings reflect the diagnosis?

1. urine specific gravity 1.019
2. BUN 15 mg/dL
3. Hematocrit 27%
4. Sodium 137

2 A 2-year-old client has had diarrhea for 1 week and now has hypernatremia. The nurse monitors the client for which of the following signs and symptoms of this disorder?

1. thirst and neurologic symptoms
2. anemia and other hematologic symptoms
3. anorexia and other dietary symptoms
4. constipation and other digestive symptoms

3 A nurse is assigned to a child with a diagnosis of hyperkalemia. The nurse prepares to care for the client and plans to do which of the following?

1. Monitor pulse, respiratory rate, and rhythm.
2. Monitor blood glucose levels every 3 to 4 hours.
3. Monitor for dependent edema every hour.
4. Monitor urine output hourly.

4 An infant is admitted with a diagnosis of hyponatremia. The nurse knows to monitor the client for _____, a common sign of a worsening condition with this diagnosis.

5 A pediatric client with hypercalcemia has just been admitted to the hospital. The child is weak and vomiting. Which of the following orders written by the physician should the nurse caring for this client complete first?

1. Strain all urine.
2. Monitor for decreased LOC.
3. Monitor for weakness.
4. Administer diuretics as ordered.

6 The nurse has just finished giving instructions to the parents of a 3-year-old client with dehydration. The nurse realizes that the parents need more instruction about intake and output when they say:

1. "We don't have to worry about noting if Susie vomits."
2. "We will weigh Susie's diapers."
3. "We will record all fluids Susie takes."
4. "We know we have to record if Susie has diarrhea and estimate the amount."

7 A pediatric client has just been admitted with a diagnosis of dehydration. The nurse anticipates all but one of the following written orders by the physician:

1. Obtain daily weight.
2. Maintain strict intake and output.
3. Take vital signs as ordered.
4. Provide fluids as wanted.

8 A 4-year-old pediatric client has suspected respiratory alkalosis. When reviewing the laboratory report, the nurse knows which of the following is most likely indicative of this diagnosis?

1. pH 7.40
2. Pco_2 25 mm Hg
3. Na^+ 140
4. K^+ 4.0

9 The nurse assesses a child and suspects the child is dehydrated. The nurse's suspicions are confirmed when she observes the following:

1. bounding, strong pulse
2. increased blood pressure
3. weak, thready pulse
4. edematous tongue

10 Calculate the following percentage of weight loss. The infant's birth weight was 7 lb 12 oz. At 3 days after birth, the infant weighs 7 lb 8 oz. _____

Answers for Review Questions, as well as discussion of Care Plan and Critical Thinking Care Map questions, appear in Appendix I.

Chapter 16

Care of the Child with Neurologic and Sensory Disorders

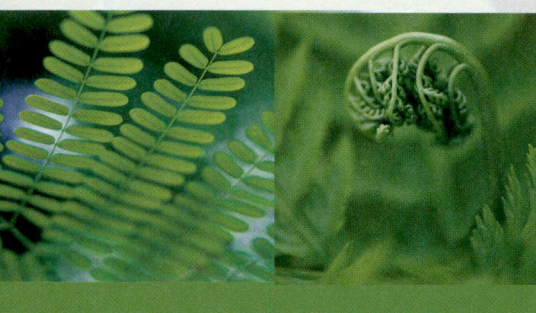

HEALTH PROMOTION ISSUE:
Amyotrophic Lateral Sclerosis (ALS) in a Teen

NURSING PROCESS CARE PLAN:
Child with Cerebral Palsy

CRITICAL THINKING CARE MAP:
Caring for a Client with Meningitis

BRIEF Outline

Anatomy and Physiology
Brief Assessment Overview
Pain
NEUROLOGIC DISORDERS
Congenital Neurologic Defects
Nervous System Disorders
Nervous System Infections
Neurologic Trauma
Brain Tumors
Mental Retardation

SENSORY DISORDERS
Eye Disorders
Eye Conditions
Eye Injuries
Visual Impairment
Ear Disorders
Ear Conditions
Hearing Acuity Screening
Nursing Care

LEARNING Outcomes

After completing this chapter, you will be able to:

- Discuss the anatomy and physiology of the pediatric neurologic system.
- Describe neurologic disorders to include seizures, cerebral palsy, meningitis, spina bifida, hydrocephalus, and Guillain–Barré syndrome.
- Explain appropriate nursing interventions for children with neurologic disorders.
- Describe disorders of the eye and ear in children.
- Explain appropriate nursing interventions for children with disorders of the eye and ear.
- Discuss clinical manifestations, diagnostic procedures, medical management, and nursing interventions related to neurologic trauma.

Anatomy and Physiology

The nervous system can be divided into two parts: the central nervous system (CNS) and the peripheral nervous system (PNS). The CNS includes the brain and the spinal cord. The PNS includes the nerves, **ganglia** (groups of nerve cell bodies located in the PNS), and sensory receptors.

CENTRAL NERVOUS SYSTEM

Neurons are the nerve cells that transmit impulses from one part of the body to another. Each neuron contains three parts: the cell body, the axon, and the dendrite. The **axon** is a fiber carrying the impulse away from the **cell body** (the part of the cell that contains the nucleus and cytoplasm). The **dendrite** conducts the electrical impulses toward the cell body (Figure 16-1 ▪). At birth, the infant has the same number of neurons as an adult, but the infant does not have the connecting axons and dendrites until later in childhood (Figure 16-2 ▪).

At birth, the axons in a child's body are lacking myelination, and this allows for the presence of newborn reflexes. The **myelin sheath** is the lipoprotein covering of the axon. As the infant ages, myelination develops in a cephalocaudal direction. The process of myelination allows more voluntary control of the muscles, enabling the child to develop fine and gross motor skills and coordination.

Brain

Fetal development of the brain and spinal cord begins in the third week of pregnancy. The nervous system is most vulnerable to harmful substances such as drugs, alcohol, cigarettes, chemicals, and infection during the period of **organogenesis** (formation of organs, days 15 to 60 of pregnancy).

The developing brain is an intricate, delicate structure composed of many structures (Figure 16-3 ▪). There are four main regions of the brain: the cerebrum, the diencephalon, the brainstem, and the cerebellum (Figure 16-4 ▪). It is important to understand the functions of each region.

At birth, the bony structure or **cranium** surrounding the brain is not fully fused, which allows for growth of the brain. Two sites of connective tissue joining the bones of the

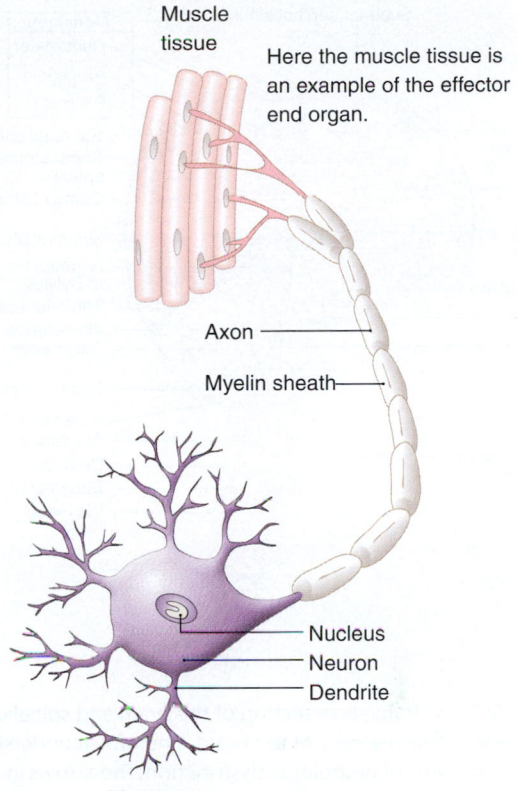

Figure 16-1. ▪ Structures of the neuron. The dendrites bring information to the nucleus. The axon carries messages away from the nerve cell.

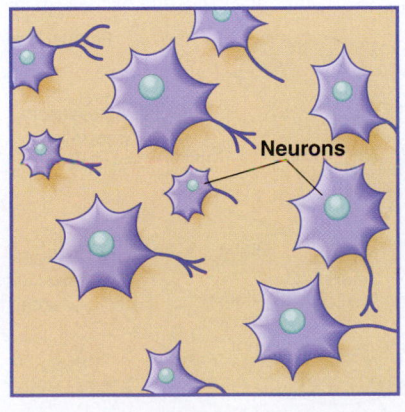
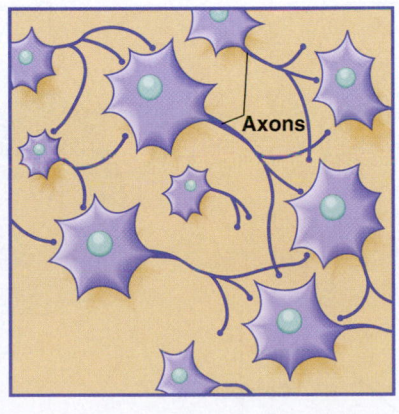
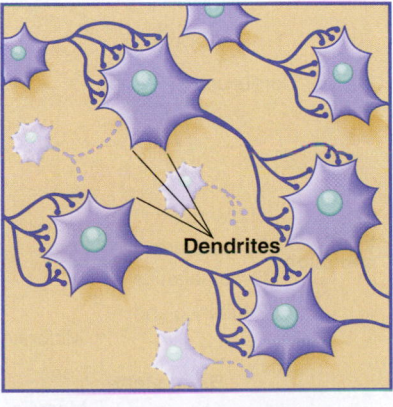

A   B   C

Figure 16-2. ▪ The developing brain. (**A**) At birth, the infant's brain has a complete set of neurons but relatively few synaptic connections. (**B**) During the first year, the axons grow longer, the dendrites increase in number, and a surplus of new connections is formed. (**C**) Over the next few years, active connections are strengthened, while unused connections atrophy. (Reprinted from Kassin, S. [2001]. *Psychology* [3rd ed.]. Upper Saddle River, NJ: Prentice Hall.)

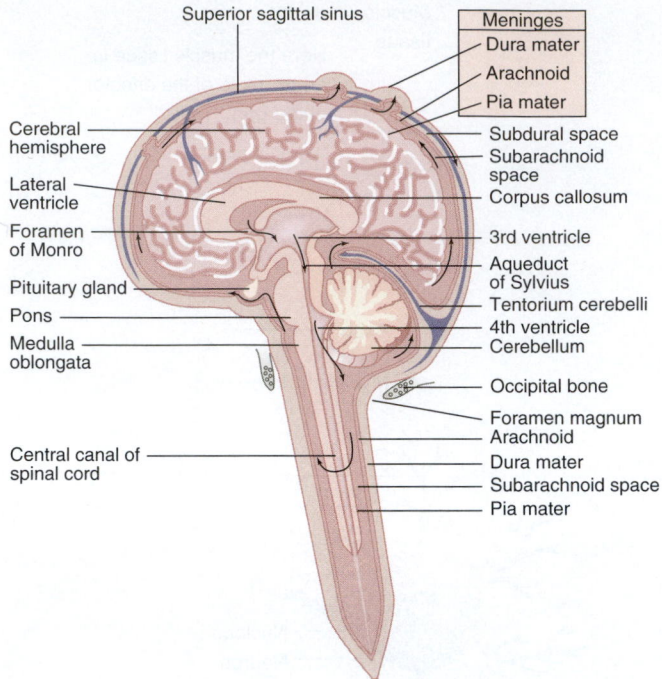

Figure 16-3. ■ Transverse section of the brain and spinal cord. Knowledge of the anatomy of the brain is helpful in understanding the symptoms of neurologic dysfunction. The arrows in the illustration indicate flow of cerebrospinal fluid.

cranium are the anterior fontanel and the posterior fontanel (see Figure 9-16 ⬭). The anterior fontanel closes when the child is between 18 and 24 months. The posterior fontanel closes around 2 months. The bones of the cranium are fully developed by age 12. Until then, risk of injury to the head and brain is greater.

Spinal Cord

The spinal cord is the structure extending from the brainstem to the lumbar region. It is surrounded and protected by the vertebrae. It supplies nerve impulses to the brain along the ascending and descending pathways. The ascending pathways transmit sensory impulses, and the descending pathways transmit motor impulses. Review Figure 16-5 ■ to understand the areas governed by each section of the spinal cord.

Physical sensation and stimulation are important to development. Children who are deprived of normal amounts of physical stimulation may develop broad developmental or emotional deficits (Box 16-1 ■). Likewise, overstimulation can have dramatic negative effects, especially in premature infants. Nursing care must take into account the importance of stimulation in the health and healing of infants and children (Box 16-2 ■).

Cerebral spinal fluid (CSF) transports nutrients and removes waste. CSF is the clear, colorless fluid that nourishes and cushions the brain and spinal cord. (See Figure 16-3 to note the circulation pattern of CSF.) CSF is formed in the choroid plexus and contains protein, vitamin C, glucose, and a few blood cells. In infancy, the child produces 100 mL of CSF/day. In adulthood, 500 mL are produced daily. CSF provides a cushion surrounding the brain and spinal cord and, therefore, protects these organs from trauma.

Intracranial Pressure

Intracranial pressure (ICP) is defined as the force exerted within the cranial cavity by the brain, blood, and CSF. Normal pressure is 0 to 12 mm Hg. Until closure of the

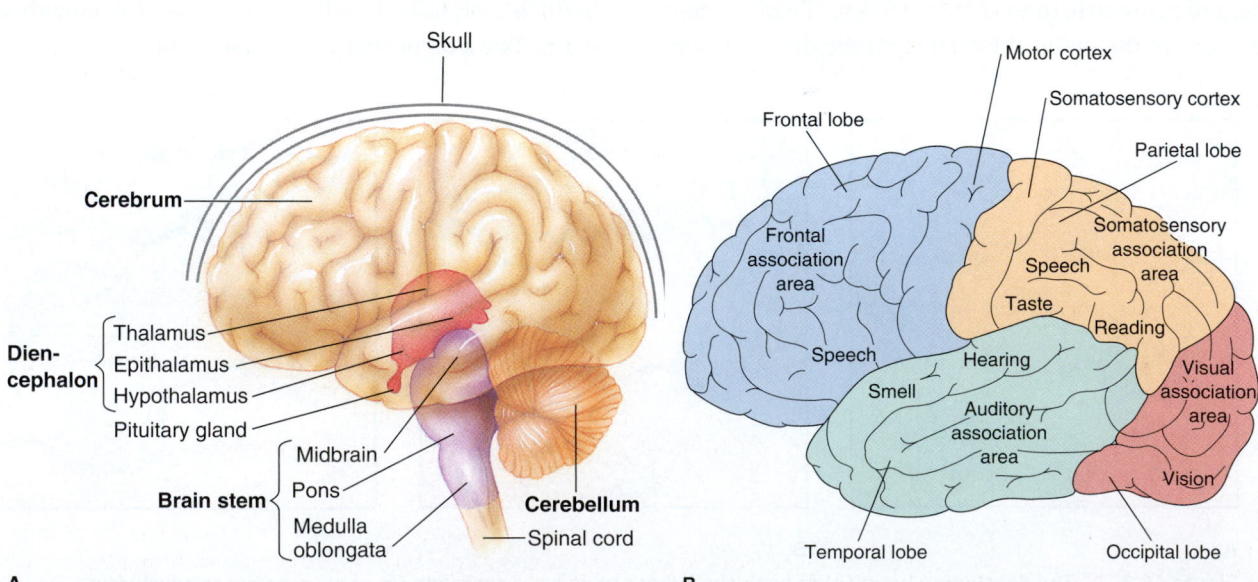

Figure 16-4. ■ (A) The four major regions of the brain: cerebrum, cerebellum, diencephalon, and brainstem. (B) Lobes of the cerebrum and functional areas of the cerebral cortex. The illustration shows what areas of the cerebrum are associated with what senses.

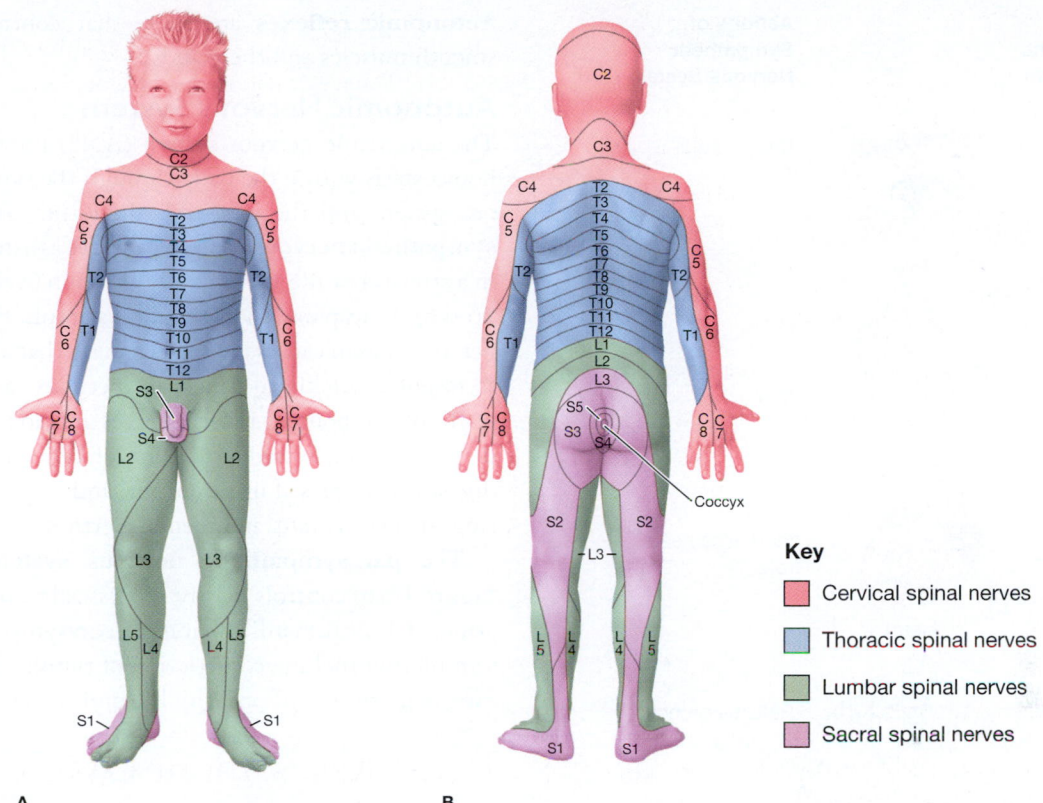

Key

■ Cervical spinal nerves

■ Thoracic spinal nerves

■ Lumbar spinal nerves

■ Sacral spinal nerves

Figure 16-5. ■ (A) Anterior dermatomes of the body. **(B)** Posterior dermatomes of the body.

fontanels, the infant can adapt more easily to ICP changes. The body compensates for increased ICP by *shunting* (diverting) CSF and reducing cerebral blood flow. Early signs of increased ICP are headache, vomiting, level of consciousness changes, asymmetric pupils, and seizures. In the infant, a high-pitched cry, bulging fontanels, dilated scalp veins, and irritability may be noted. Later signs include significant changes in level of consciousness (LOC), respiratory distress, bradycardia, increased systolic blood pressure, fixed and dilated pupils, and death.

PERIPHERAL NERVOUS SYSTEM

The PNS consists of 31 pairs of spinal nerves, 12 pairs of cranial nerves, and somatic and autonomic reflexes. **Somatic reflexes** are those that control skeletal muscle contractions.

BOX 16-1   CLIENT TEACHING

Importance of Emotional and Physical Care

Researchers (Wismer Fries et. al., 2005) studied 18 four-years-olds who had lived in Eastern European orphanages for an average of 16.6 months. These children were adopted into American families. After living with these families for an average of 34.6 months, the researchers studied hormone levels and compared them with 21 children of similar age who lived with biologic parents.

The hormone levels of oxytocin and arginine vasopressin were found to be lower in the children who had come from the orphanages. These hormones have been linked to the ability to form social bonds. This study raises the question of the long-term effects of neglect early in life. Nurses can use this study to develop teaching plans that can encourage parents to provide both emotional and physical care to their children.

BOX 16-2   COMPLEMENTARY THERAPIES

Music as an Aid in the NICU

Premature infants in the neonatal intensive care unit (NICU) are often bombarded with sounds, lights, and other excessive stimuli. This excessive stimuli can have negative effects on the improvement of the infant's condition. Simple positive changes in the environment of the NICU can have positive effects on the premature infant. One of these changes is using music therapy. Music therapy is defined as healing with music, voice, or sound. Several research studies have found music therapy to be effective in the NICU. Infants, after being exposed to calming music, were less likely to experience high arousal states, had shorter hospital stays, and weighed more than infants who were not exposed to music.

Olson (1998) provided six principles essential to the effective use of music therapy. (1) Music is a method of demonstrating caring. (2) Music has emotional and physical effects and can facilitate the healing process. (3) Music can bring a human approach to a clinical environment. (4) Music is a method of individualizing client care. (5) Tone, rhythm, pitch, and volume of music can create a peaceful environment. (6) Music of the child's religious faith provides spiritual care to the client.

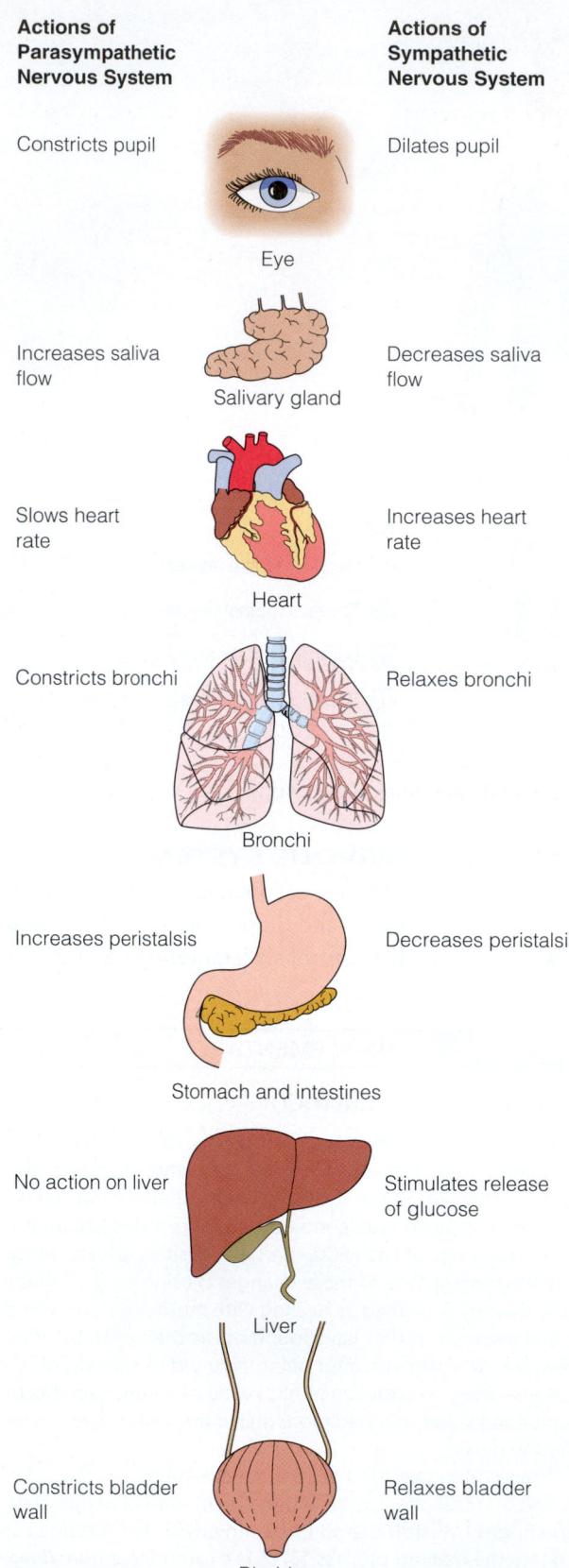

Actions of Parasympathetic Nervous System		Actions of Sympathetic Nervous System
Constricts pupil	**Eye**	Dilates pupil
Increases saliva flow	**Salivary gland**	Decreases saliva flow
Slows heart rate	**Heart**	Increases heart rate
Constricts bronchi	**Bronchi**	Relaxes bronchi
Increases peristalsis	**Stomach and intestines**	Decreases peristalsis
No action on liver	**Liver**	Stimulates release of glucose
Constricts bladder wall	**Bladder**	Relaxes bladder wall

Figure 16-6. ■ Autonomic nervous system and the organs it affects. The *left side* shows the actions of the parasympathetic nervous system. The *right side* shows the actions of the sympathetic nervous system.

Autonomic reflexes are those that control cardiac and smooth muscles and the glands.

Autonomic Nervous System

The autonomic nervous system (ANS) provides control of homeostasis within the body through the sympathetic nervous system and the parasympathetic nervous system. The **sympathetic nervous system** provides assistance to a person in a stressful or life-threatening situation (*right side* of Figure 16-6 ■). In response to frightening stimuli, the sympathetic nervous system causes physical changes that allow the person to respond quickly to danger (sometimes called the "fight-or-flight" response). These changes include dilated pupils; diaphoresis; tachycardia; dilation of bronchioles; decreased digestion; decreased urine output; and increased blood clotting, metabolic rate, and mental alertness.

The **parasympathetic nervous system** (*left side* of Figure 16-6) controls bodily processes in nonstressful situations. Clinical manifestations of parasympathetic nervous stimulation include constriction of pupils, decreased heart rate, constriction of bronchioles, and increased peristalsis.

Brief Assessment Overview

HISTORY

All Children

Because neurologic disorders in children could be the result of incidents occurring during fetal development, obtaining a history of the pregnancy is an important aspect of assessment. The nurse should ask about drug use, infections, birth trauma, and complications in the immediate postpartum period. (See also Apgar score in Chapter 7 ◉◉.) The birth weight of the child could indicate prematurity or nutritional status. By assessing the mental status and intellectual ability of both parents, the nurse can gain information that will be useful in planning and implementing care for the child.

Infants

To assess the history of the infant, the nurse will need to obtain information from the parents. The nurse should ask about tremors, unusual movements, irritability, and difficulties sucking or swallowing. Sometimes neurologic disorders are evidenced by problems in other body systems. The nurse should ask about intestinal cramps or colic.

Toddlers and Preschoolers

As the child grows and develops, the nurse should obtain information from both the child and the parents. The nurse should assess the child's ability to communicate, both verbally and nonverbally, and compare the child's ability with the expected ability for his or her age and developmental level. The nurse should ask about headaches or seizure activity and obtain as detailed a description as possible. The nurse should ask about the child's behavior, including fears, concerns, aggressive behaviors, and attention span. Any signs of abuse or suspected abuse should be reported to the charge nurse. (See legal information in Chapter 2 ⬮ and discussion of abuse in Chapter 27 ⬮.)

School-Age Children and Adolescents

The school-age child and adolescent can provide a lot of information about their own neurologic status. These clients may be reluctant to discuss some aspects of their behavior with parents present. The nurse should provide privacy and maintain confidentiality within legal requirements and facility policy. The nurse should compare the child's responses with those of the parents. The nurse should ask about general mood or noticeable changes in behavior, as well as headaches, seizure activity, and alcohol or drug consumption. The nurse will note general behavior, such as responsiveness and activity level. (See more about behavior and thought process disorders in Chapter 27 ⬮.)

PHYSICAL

Infants

The physical assessment of the infant's neurologic status provides information about growth and development and also identifies areas of concern. The nurse should measure head circumference and compare the measurements with the normal range for the age of the child. The spine should be palpated for intactness, and the nurse should observe the infant's posture. Although a spinal check was done at the time of delivery, small spinal defects may not be apparent until the child grows. The nurse should test the infant's reflexes and reaction to stimuli as described in Chapter 9 ⬮. To assess LOC, the Glasgow Coma Scale can be used. See Procedure 16-1 ■.

Toddlers, Preschoolers, School-Age Children, and Adolescents

As the child grows and develops, more detail can be added to the objective data. The nurse should test balance, coordination, and accuracy related to motor skills. Sensations of touch, temperature, and pain should be assessed, especially in areas of the body of concern. Many reflexes change as the child grows and should be tested. The child's memory should be assessed, keeping in mind that the memory of young children may not be accurate because of the developmental level, not necessarily because of pathology.

Pain

PHYSIOLOGY

Pain in children can be a result of ischemia, tissue pressure, injury, or tension created by air or fluid filling a body cavity. A pain impulse stimulates the nociceptor, causing

transduction of pain sensation. The **nociceptors** are sensory receptors that detect and differentiate pain sensation. Following transduction, the pain impulse is transmitted along peripheral sensory nerves to the spinal cord and brain.

PERCEPTION

Pain perception occurs as the pain impulse reaches the brain. Depending on which sensory receptor is stimulated, the child may perceive dull, burning, sharp, localized, cutaneous, somatic, visceral, or chronic pain. The child may express the pain verbally or nonverbally. Verbal expressions of pain include crying, moaning, groaning, or screaming. Nonverbal expressions of pain include facial grimacing, posturing, splinting, restlessness, and sleep disturbances. Box 16-3 ■ provides one mnemonic for assessing pain. See the Pain Assessment section of Chapter 13 ⬮ for more nursing information about assessing the child in pain.

PAIN THEORIES

The gate control theory (Figure 16-7 ■), developed by Melzack and Wall in 1965, is the most commonly used theory of pain and pain management. The gate control theory proposes that certain actions, if employed, can block pain transduction at the spinal cord before it reaches the brain. These behaviors include touch, distraction, and breathing and relaxation techniques.

PAIN MANAGEMENT

Treatment of Pain

The medical management of pain includes the use of narcotic and nonnarcotic medication. (Refer to Chapter 13 ⬮ for discussion of pain as the "fifth vital sign" and for pain assessment, Procedure 13-5 ⬮.) When possible, the oral route of administration is preferred for children. Careful dosage calculation is essential in preventing an overdose. If narcotics are used, monitoring the respiratory status is vital because narcotics can depress respiration. In cases of severe or prolonged pain, a PCA pump may be used (see Figure 14-11 ⬮).

Other nursing measures may be effective in the control of pain. Distraction or involving the child in other activities and play can reduce anxiety and the awareness of pain. Massaging or rubbing the area or rocking and holding the child provide a stimulus to compete with pain receptors and therefore decrease transmission of pain. The application of heat or cold may reduce swelling, inflammation, and muscle spasm causing the pain. Care must be taken to avoid damage to the skin with either heat or cold.

Pain can be associated with disorders of the neurologic system and also with conditions associated with the eye and ear. Neurologic disorders include congenital defects, infections, trauma, and disorders such as seizures, cerebral palsy, and fibromyalgia.

(*Text continues on p. 516.*)

PROCEDURE 16-1 Glasgow Coma Scale

Purpose

- To provide a score related to level of consciousness
- To allow health care providers a benchmark assessment that will allow them to document either improvement or deterioration of the child's neurologic condition

Equipment

- Glasgow Coma Scale (Table 16-1 ■)

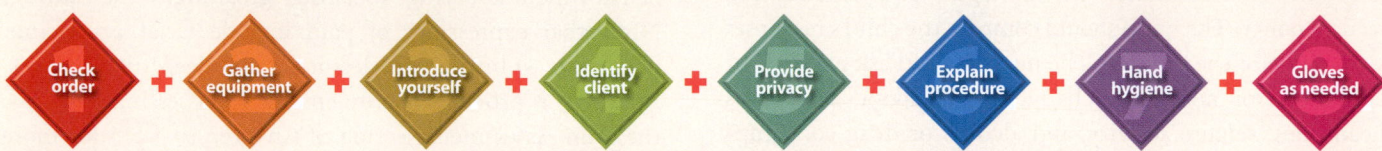

Check order + Gather equipment + Introduce yourself + Identify client + Provide privacy + Explain procedure + Hand hygiene + Gloves as needed

Interventions

1. Perform preparatory steps (see icon bar).

2. Use the Glasgow Coma Scale to assess the child with a neurologic injury or disorder. Assign a score, based on the criteria outlined, for eye opening, motor response, and verbal response.

3. A total score of 15 indicates adequate neurologic function. A total score of 3 indicates neurologic unresponsiveness.

4. Document results and report scores below 15 to the charge nurse.

5. Repeat the Glasgow Coma Scale as necessary.

SAMPLE DOCUMENTATION

(date) 1500   4-year-old male admitted to pediatric intensive care following closed head injury due to 6-foot fall from tree. Glasgow Coma Scale score 5. Score reported to charge nurse. R. Roberts, LPN

TABLE 16-1

Glasgow Coma Scale

FACULTY MEASURED	RESPONSE	SCORE
Eye opening	Spontaneous	4
	To verbal command	3
	To pain	2
	No response	1
Motor response	To verbal command	6
	To localized pain	5
	Flexes and withdraws	4
	Flexes abnormally	3
	Extends abnormally	2
	No response	1
Verbal response	Oriented, converses	5
	Disoriented, converses	4
	Uses inappropriate words	3
	Makes incomprehensible sounds	2
	No response	1

Note: 15 points = alert and oriented; 8 or less = comatose; totally unresponsive = 3 or less.

BOX 16-3   ASSESSMENT

Pain in Children

Here is a quick way to remember how to assess for pain in children. Use the abbreviation PQRST:

P Precipitating Factors—What caused the pain?

Q Quality and Quantity—Describe the pain. Is it steady, or does it come and go?

R Region, Radiation, and Related Symptoms—Describe the exact location of the pain. Does it radiate to other parts of the body? What symptoms are associated with the pain?

S Severity—Rate the pain as to its impact (e.g., Can you walk during the pain? Can you continue talking during the pain?).

T Timing—What time of the day or night does the pain occur? Does it occur every day? Is it associated with other activities, such as breathing, lying down, walking, etc.?

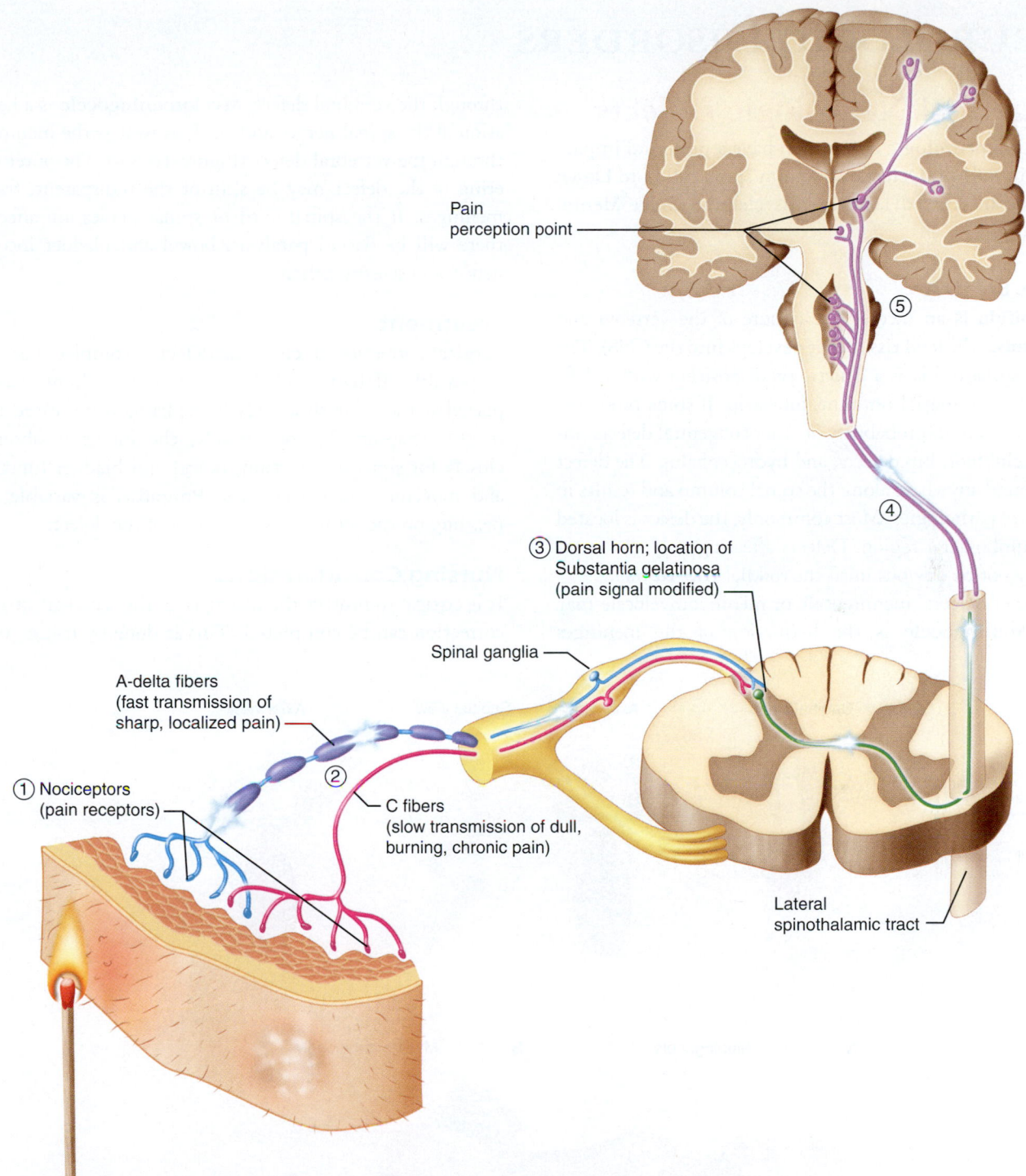

Figure 16-7. ■ Gate control theory of pain perception. Nociceptors (free nerve endings at the site of tissue damage) transmit information by specialized nerve fibers to the spinal cord. Nociceptors are stimulated by mechanical, thermal, and chemical injury. Biochemical mediators, produced in response to tissue damage, activate the nerve response or sensitize nerve endings. C fibers slowly transmit dull, burning, diffuse pain, as well as chronic pain. A-delta fibers quickly transmit sharp, well-localized pain. The pain signal may be modified at the dorsal horn of the spinal cord *(lower right)*, depending on other stimuli from the brain or the periphery. The pain signal is then transmitted to the brain, where perception occurs. Once the sensation reaches the brain, the emotional responses may increase or decrease the intensity of the pain perceived.

NEUROLOGIC DISORDERS

Congenital Neurologic Defects

Congenital neurologic defects can have a profound impact on quality of life. Defects vary from spina bifida to Down syndrome (discussed later in this chapter under Mental Retardation).

SPINA BIFIDA

Spina bifida is an incomplete closure of the vertebra and **neural tube** (the fetal tissue that develops into the CNS). The cause of spina bifida is a genetic predisposition with a deficiency of the essential nutrient, folic acid. If spina bifida exists, there is a high probability of other congenital defects, including clubfoot, hip defects, and hydrocephalus. The defect can be found anywhere along the spinal column and results in a variety of pathologies. Most commonly, the defect is located in the lumbosacral region. Defects affecting only the vertebrae may not be obvious until the toddler tries to walk.

In larger defects, meningocele or meningomyelocele may result. **Meningocele** is the herniation of the meninges through the vertebral defect. **Myelomeningocele** is a herniation of the spinal nerves and cord, as well as the meninges, through the vertebral defect (Figure 16-8 ■). The outer covering of the defect may be skin or the transparent, fragile meninges. If the spinal cord or spinal nerves are affected, there will be flaccid paralysis, bowel and bladder incontinence, and sensory deficits.

Treatment

Surgical correction to close the defect is completed as soon as possible. If hydrocephalus is present, a shunt may be placed at the same time. (Hydrocephalus is discussed later in this chapter.) Postoperatively, the infant is observed closely for signs of infection, bowel and bladder function, and movement of extremities. Prognosis is variable, depending on the location and severity of the defect.

Nursing Considerations

It is critical to protect the integrity of the sac until surgical correction can be completed. This is done by using sterile

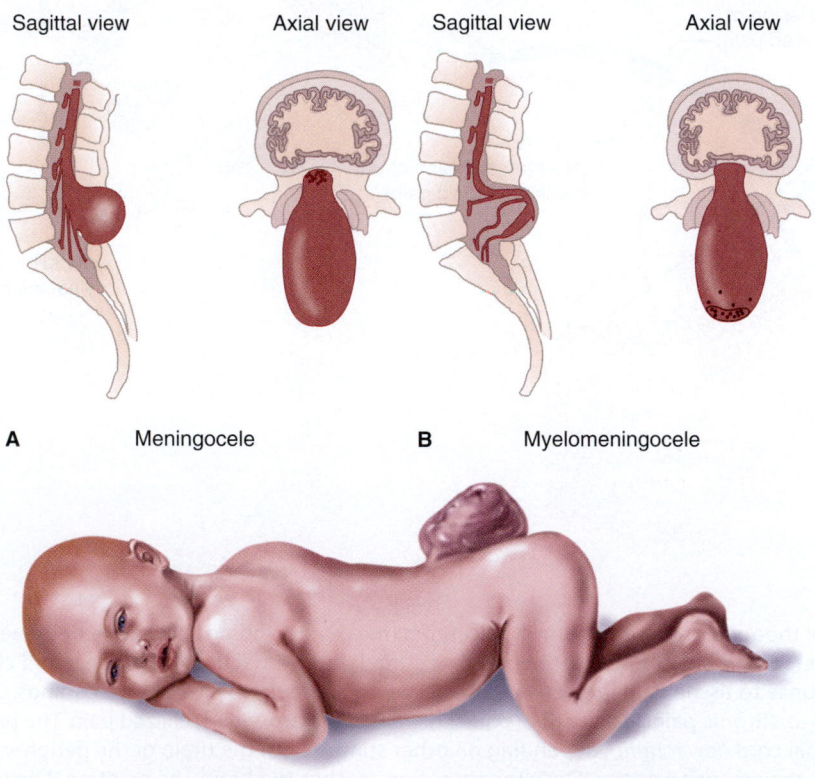

Sagittal view   Axial view   Sagittal view   Axial view

A   Meningocele   **B**   Myelomeningocele

C

Figure 16-8. ■ (A) Meningocele. A saclike protrusion through the bony defect in the spinal column containing meninges and cerebrospinal fluid. Sac may be transparent or membranous. **(B)** Myelomeningocele. Saclike herniation through the defect holding meninges, cerebrospinal fluid, and a portion of spinal cord or nerve root. Fluid leakage may occur because the lesion may be poorly covered. This defect is more common than the meningocele; 99% of children with this defect are disabled. **(C)** The infant with a myelomeningocele is placed prone or in a side-lying position, and the exposed sac is protected carefully and kept moist.

gloves and linens to cover the defect. The linens covering the sac are kept moist with saline. The infant must be positioned so as not to exert pressure on the meninges (see Figure 16-8C). A prone position is typically used. The nurse must monitor carefully for symptoms of infection. The infant should be kept warm. An isolette is appropriate to avoid placing heavy covers over the sac.

Emotional care and tactile stimulation are still vital for this infant. Encourage parents to hold their baby's hand and talk gently to him or her. For feeding, the baby may need to be placed on the parent's lap in a prone position with the head turned to one side. Parents will need assistance from the nurse to accomplish feeding because the baby cannot be held in typical feeding positions.

Postoperatively, the nurse will observe the child for signs of infection, changes in vital signs, and neurologic changes. Observe the skin closely to prevent breakdown from bony prominences of the pelvis as the child lies in the prone position. Change the child's position to side-lying or hold the child upright. Passive range-of-motion exercises are important to prevent contractures. The nurse should observe the infant for urinary and bowel retention because this disorder often causes sensory loss and loss of sphincter control. Older children and adolescents with spina bifida will be taught to perform clean intermittent catheterization to maintain urinary health.

HYDROCEPHALUS

Hydrocephalus results from increased production, decreased absorption, or blockage of the flow of CSF. Blockage can be caused by a variety of pathologies, including infections, ventricular hemorrhages, tumors, cysts, or malformations. Malformations include:

- *Chiari II malformation* (downward displacement of the cerebellum, brainstem, and fourth ventricle, along with herniation through the foramen magnum into the cervical spaces)
- Stenosis of the aqueduct of Sylvius, a recessive X-linked disorder
- *Dandy-Walker syndrome* (a disruption of fetal brain development in which the fourth ventricle enlarges into a cyst).

Manifestations

Sometimes hydrocephalus is obvious at birth, but more commonly it develops over time. The classic symptoms of hydrocephalus include the child's head circumference being greater than normal, with the forehead and top of the head being out of proportion to the face (Figure 16-9 ■). The anterior fontanel bulges with the increasing ICP. The sclera of the eyes often can be seen above the iris giving a "setting sun" appearance to the eyes. The child may be irritable or lethargic and experience nausea and vomiting because of increased ICP.

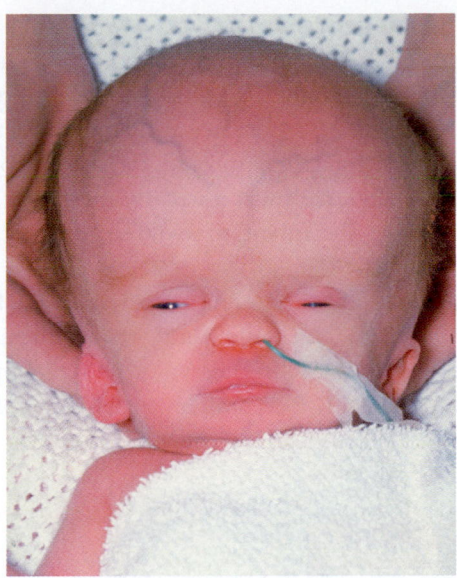

A

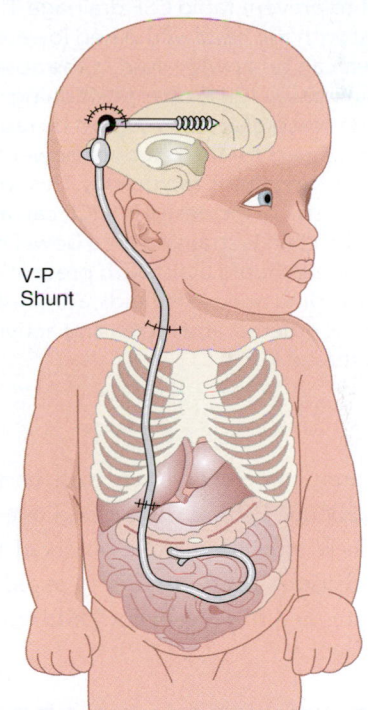

V-P Shunt

B

Figure 16-9. ■ **(A)** Infant with hydrocephalus. **(B)** A ventriculoperitoneal shunt, which allows fluid to leave the cranial cavity and so reduces intracranial pressure, is usually placed at 3 to 4 months of age. (A. M. A. Ansary/Custom Medical Stock Photo, Inc.)

Treatment

Surgical placement of a ventriculoperitoneal shunt (Figure 16-9B) can relieve the increasing ICP. As the child grows, a longer shunt may need to replace the initial shunt. If the blockage is caused by a tumor or cyst, surgical removal of the growth may correct the hydrocephalus. See Chapter 9 ⦿ for more about congenital anomalies.

Nursing Considerations

Nursing strategies for the child with hydrocephalus include measuring the child's head circumference regularly (see Procedure 13-9 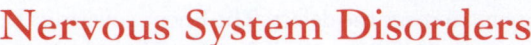). Before and after corrective surgery, the child must be monitored for symptoms of increased ICP. The nurse must carefully support the head when transferring the infant to avoid strain on the neck muscles.

Because the skin of the cranium is stretched and thin in hydrocephalus, the nurse should handle the infant gently and be careful to prevent skin breakdown on the cranium. Vomiting due to increased ICP is common with hydrocephalus, so feedings should be frequent and small in amount.

clinical ALERT

In the immediate postoperative period, the infant will need to lie flat to prevent rapid CSF drainage. The supine position is best with the head of the bed lowered. The head of the bed can be slowly raised in the absence of symptoms of increased ICP. Proper positioning should prevent tears in the cerebral arteries caused by rapid drainage of CSF. Assess for the return of bowel sounds, and avoid introducing fluids too quickly. This will prevent vomiting and the risk of increased ICP. ICP can also be increased while the child is straining for a bowel movement. Therefore, the nurse should assist with prevention of constipation by providing adequate fluids, administering stool softeners as ordered, and increasing activity in the absence of increased ICP.

Following shunt placement, there will be two surgical sites—most likely one behind the ear and one in the chest or abdomen. These sites need to be observed for integrity and signs of infection. Teach parents to avoid pressure on these incision sites and to prevent the child from "playing" with them.

AMYOTROPHIC LATERAL SCLEROSIS

Although rare in children, amyotrophic lateral sclerosis (ALS) may appear as a familial disorder linked to chromosome 21 defects. ALS (sometimes called *Lou Gehrig disease*) is a progressive, degenerative neurologic disease in which muscle weakness and wasting progress from the extremities to the core. In about 50% of cases, death results 2 to 5 years after the onset of symptoms, usually as a result of respiratory failure. In clients with such severe degenerative disorders, much special care is needed (see Health Promotion Issue on pages 520 and 521). Referrals are crucial for support for family and caregivers. Refer to a medical–surgical book for in-depth information on diagnosis and treatment.

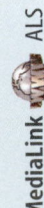

Nervous System Disorders

SEIZURES

Seizures are periods of sudden discharge of electrical activity in the brain that cause involuntary muscle activity, change in LOC, or altered behavior and sensory manifestation. Seizures may be the result of genetic factors; pathologic conditions such as tumors, trauma, infection, and toxins; or a rapid elevation in temperature above 102°F (39°C) called febrile seizures.

Febrile Seizures

A febrile seizure is a generalized seizure that usually occurs when a child's temperature rises rapidly to above 102°F (39°C). The seizures in children involve general tonic–clonic movements lasting less than 15 minutes (usually 1–2 minutes). Rarely, the seizure may be complex, lasting longer than 15 minutes and recurring within 24 hours. In newborns, seizures may present as rhythmic repetitive movement of an extremity; repetitive blinking, lip smacking, sucking, or tongue thrusting; or horizontal deviation of the eyes (Ball & Bindler, 2006). Febrile seizures in small children are often seen by nurses.

Seizures are quite frightening to parents. Anticonvulsants may be prescribed to prevent recurrence of seizures for the remainder of a febrile illness. However, the American Academy of Pediatrics (AAP; 1999) does not recommend long-term anticonvulsant therapy for febrile seizures. Instead, parents are taught methods of lowering fevers, such as administering nonaspirin antipyretic medication, dressing the child who has fever in light clothing, and cooling the body with tepid compresses or baths. (*Note:* Alcohol compresses or baths are no longer recommended for use in children with high fevers.) Parents must also be taught safety measures to protect a child who is having a seizure (see Nursing Considerations section).

Epilepsy

Epilepsy is a chronic disorder characterized by repeated seizure activity. **Status epilepticus** is a continuous seizure for more than 30 minutes accompanied by loss of consciousness. Status epilepticus can also occur sequentially.

Manifestations

Partial or **focal seizures** are caused by abnormal electrical activity in a specific area of the brain, most commonly in the temporal, frontal, or parietal lobes of the cerebrum. Common symptoms include a momentary blank stare, facial movement, or report of hearing abnormal sounds. There is no loss of consciousness with focal seizures.

Generalized seizures result from diffuse electrical activity that begins in one area of the brain and spreads to involve the entire cerebral cortex and brainstem. General seizures begin with a *tonic phase* in which the child loses consciousness and has continuous muscle contractions. This

TABLE 16-2

Pharmacology: Drugs Used to Prevent Seizures

DRUG (COMMON BRAND NAME AND GENERIC)	USUAL ROUTE/DOSE	CLASSIFICATION AND PURPOSE	SELECTED SIDE EFFECTS	DON'T GIVE IF
Dilantin (phenytoin)	PO 15–20 mg/kg loading dose, then 5 mg/kg in two to three divided doses	Anticonvulsant for seizure prevention	Drowsiness, hypotension, gingival hyperplasia	Bradycardia
Tegretol (carbamazepine)	Children less than 6 years: PO 10–35 mg/kg/day in three to four divided doses Children 6–12 years: PO 100–800 mg/day in three to four divided doses	Anticonvulsant for seizure prevention	Leukopenia, vomiting, fatigue	Children less than 6 months
Barbital (phenobarbital)	Neonate: PO or IV 3–4 mg/kg/day Child: PO or IV 3–8 mg/kg/day	Anticonvulsant for seizure prevention	Drowsiness, hypotension, vomiting	Serum concentration greater than 50 mcg/mL In liquid form, do not give without shaking bottle thoroughly; shaking ensures accurate dosage

is followed by a *clonic phase* characterized by alternating muscle contraction and relaxation. Some seizures are preceded by an **aura** (a recognizable sensation that signals a seizure is about to occur). A **postictal** period (period following a seizure) of confusion, sleepiness, slurred speech, poor coordination, or headache is common following a generalized seizure. Due to the limited communication ability of the infant, an aura may be impossible to detect. Older children, however, may be able to describe this activity in detail.

Treatment

Anticonvulsants may be prescribed for the child to prevent further seizure activity (Table 16-2 ■). Depending on the cause and number of seizures, medication may be prescribed long term. It is important to administer medication on time to maintain therapeutic levels of medication. The child should be observed closely for repeated seizure activity until therapeutic levels of medications are established. Periodic or routine blood tests may be ordered to evaluate these therapeutic levels.

Nursing Considerations

Seizure precautions, including padding side rails and having suction equipment available, should be implemented for all children who have a history of seizures or who are at risk for seizures. These precautions will help prevent injury to the child during a seizure.

In the event of a seizure, the first priority is to establish a safe environment for the child (Figure 16-10 ■). The child should not be restrained, but the head and extremities should be protected from hitting furniture, side rails, or the floor. Nothing should be put into the child's mouth during a seizure. Because the child does not breathe during the tonic phase of the seizure, circumoral cyanosis is common (LeMone & Burke, 2004). Note where the seizure began,

(*Text continues on p. 522.*)

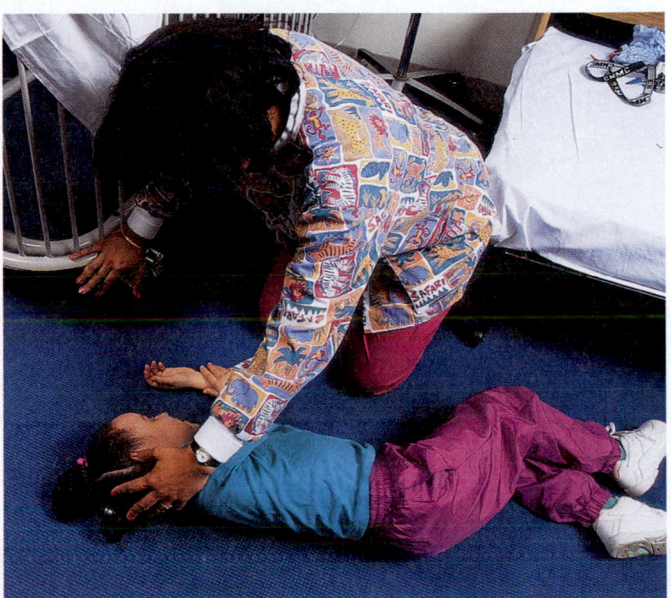

Figure 16-10. ■ A child who has a seizure when standing should be gently assisted to the floor and placed in a side-lying position. The area around the child should be cleared of any objects that might injure the child.

HEALTH PROMOTION ISSUE

AMYOTROPHIC LATERAL SCLEROSIS (ALS) IN A TEEN

Jamie, an 18-year-old Caucasian male, was diagnosed with amyotrophic lateral sclerosis (ALS) 3 years ago. His muscle weakness has progressively gotten worse until his speech, swallowing, chewing, and finally his breathing have been affected. He has a feeding tube and is on oxygen. Jamie is in and out of the hospital frequently. His parents provide his care at home, although they have a home health nurse who provides a weekly assessment of his status. Jamie and his family developed a living will shortly after his initial diagnosis that includes Jamie's request not to be placed on a respirator should his breathing be compromised.

Jamie's physician discussed the rapid progression of his disease and encouraged the family to make some decisions about end-of-life care. The physician suggested contracting with a hospice agency to provide Jamie's care. After the physician leaves the exam room, Jamie's mother breaks down and sobs to the nurse. She states that she just cannot call hospice because that would mean she is giving up and will give Jamie the message that they have no hope. She also states that she does not know what hospice can do that she and her husband and the home health nurse are not already doing for Jamie.

DISCUSSION

Empowering the dying client by allowing a say in how and where death occurs can facilitate emotional acceptance of the eventual death. Because saying good-bye to a loved one is difficult, providing physical care to the dying client may become overwhelming to the caregivers. Answers for many clients and their families come from health care agencies that focus on providing dignity in the last days by giving the client control and relieving stress on the family.

One agency that provides this type of care is the hospice agency. Hospice provides palliative nursing and medical care, including nutrition, comfort measures, and pain management. The hospice caregiver also provides supportive social, emotional, and spiritual services. This care is most often given in the client's home. Care can be provided weekly, daily, or 24 hours/day. If the client has to be admitted to the hospital, the hospice caregiver is available to continue care during the time of hospitalization. In all states, it is required that the hospice agency be certified to provide health care services. Many state boards of health require that the agency also be licensed.

Hospice Services

A physician coordinates the care given to the client who has contracted the services of hospice. Registered nurses and licensed practical nurses provide hygiene, wound care, medication administration, nutritional support, pain management, and other services as necessary. A social worker may be assigned to assist the family in taking advantage of community resources. Aids or volunteers can assist the family with meal preparation, grooming, laundry services, running errands, car pooling, or babysitting. The agency may also offer physical, occupational, or speech therapies provided by a professional. Grief counseling is a standard of care for hospice agencies. The agencies assess the grief of the client and the family, and continue this assessment and care following the death of the client.

MediaLink   Palliative care

(© Ragnar Schmuck/zefa/Corbis)

Costs

To be eligible for third-party reimbursement, a physician must provide documentation that the client may live less than 6 months. Medicare, Medicaid, and private health insurance policies can be used to pay for the services of hospice. Clients may also pay for the services, and hospice agencies frequently provide care free of charge when other resources are not available.

PLANNING AND IMPLEMENTATION

The nurse provides Jamie's mother with emotional comfort measures. She also uses therapeutic communication techniques to discover more about the feelings Jamie's mother has about his illness and probable death in the near future.

The nurse understands that in order for Jamie and his family to move to the acceptance phase of grief, they must acknowledge that Jamie's illness is incurable. The nurse also understands that Jamie's mom equates hospice care with Jamie's death. As long as Jamie was receiving treatment, there was a shred of hope that a cure could be found.

The nurse also interviews Jamie's father and Jamie individually to ascertain their feelings regarding Jamie's illness, impending death, and hospice care. The nurse understands that in order for hospice care to be effective for the family, each member must believe that the care provided is necessary and can contribute to their well-being.

The nurse asks Jamie and his parents for permission to tell them more about hospice. She also provides them with literature for further study. She has secured a list of clients within the practice who have benefited from hospice care. She encourages Jamie and his family to call these families to discuss their experiences with hospice.

The nurse schedules a home visit with Jamie and his family several days later to continue the discussion about hospice. During this visit, Jamie and his family tell the nurse they are ready to begin hospice care in their home. Jamie's mother thanks the nurse for helping them make the decision. She is especially grateful for the client referrals. She found them both helpful and encouraging.

The nurse and Jamie's family discuss the process for selecting a hospice agency. They call several agencies and set up in-home interviews.

In 1 week, the nurse telephones Jamie's family and learns that the hospice agency is already providing care, and that the family is quite satisfied with the care. In 1 month, Jamie dies at home in the presence of his family and the hospice nurse. Several weeks later, the nurse receives a thank you note from the family expressing their gratefulness to the nurse for encouraging them to seek hospice care.

SELF-REFLECTION

Imagine that you have a terminal illness. What would be important to you related to your final days? Where would you like to be? Who would you like to be around you? What type of care do you want to ensure that you have? What type of care do you want to avoid? Communicate these wishes and desires to a trusted individual or, better yet, record them officially in a living will.

SUGGESTED RESOURCES

For the Nurse

- www.alsa.org This is the national website for the Amyotrophic Lateral Sclerosis (ALS) Association.

- www.hpna.org This is the website for the Hospice and Palliative Nurses Association. Included on this site are Professional Competencies for the LPN/LVN and Scope and Standards of Nursing Practice for the LPN/LVN.

- www.aacn.nche.edu/elnec This website provides continuing education opportunities for nurses related to palliative care.

- www.palliativecarenursing.net This website provides helpful information to nurses caring for clients who are dying.

For the Client

- www.dyingwell.org

- www.nhpco.org This is the website for the National Hospice and Palliative Care Organization.

the specific movements or behavior, eye movements, and pupil response.

Immediately following the seizure, position the child on his or her side, remove mucus and drainage from the airway, and assess for airway patency. Oxygen may be needed if SpO$_2$ levels are less than 95%. The child may have been incontinent of urine and stool, so skin care may be needed. After the seizure, check neurologic function, including LOC, pupil response, equal bilateral movement and strength of extremities, and signs of injury if a fall occurred during the seizure. Remain with the child until consciousness returns and the airway is patent.

Seizure activity can be frightening for the parents and family. The nurse should remain calm during the child's seizure to inspire confidence and provide support to the family. Parents should be taught how to care for the child at home, during and after a seizure, as well as administration and side effects of medications. Parents, fearful for their child's safety, may become overprotective. With proper diagnosis and treatment, most children can have an active life. Parents should be encouraged to help their child reach developmental milestones.

CEREBRAL PALSY

Cerebral palsy (CP) is a disorder affecting motor function and posture. CP develops secondary to lesions or anomalies of the brain, hypoxic damage, or birth trauma to the motor center of the brain. The damage can occur during the prenatal, perinatal, or postnatal periods and up to 2 to 3 years of age. Neonatal infections (e.g., meningitis), as well as *kernicterus* (a condition associated with infantile hyperbilirubinemia), can result in CP. CP occurs more often in children born in the occipitoposterior position than in children born in the occipitoanterior position (see Figure 7-10 in Chapter 7 ⚭). CP occurs most frequently in very low-birth-weight and small-for-gestational-age infants. Some children may have a condition that mimics it (Box 16-4 ▪).

Manifestations

Cerebral palsy is characterized by abnormal muscle tone and lack of coordination. Children with CP are frequently delayed in meeting growth and development milestones. Other neurologic problems may also be present, including hearing loss, visual defects such as nystagmus or strabismus, speech delay or impediment, seizures, or mental retardation.

Characteristic signs of CP, which may be present shortly after birth, include weak or absent sucking or swallowing, jitteriness, and slow or absent reflexes. Children with CP are at risk for notable delays in reaching developmental milestones. Infants may exhibit an abnormal or asymmetric crawl. Spastic movements may be noted. If the child learns to walk, a scissor gait and toe walking are common.

Diagnosis

CP is diagnosed by documentation of clinical manifestations.

Treatment

The focus of treatment for the child with CP is to improve motor function and communication skills. CP does not have a cure. Devices that assist with motor function, such as braces, walkers, and wheelchairs, enable the child to achieve a level of independence (Figure 16-11 ▪). Physical, occupational, and speech therapists are used to assist the child.

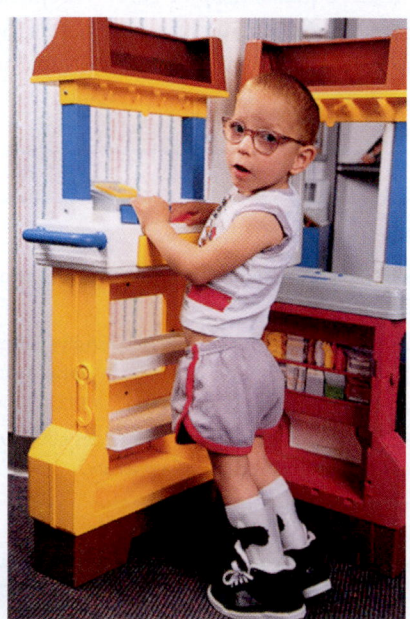

Figure 16-11. ▪ A child with cerebral palsy has abnormal muscle tone and lack of physical coordination. Muscles can be strengthened by periods of standing with support.

Several surgical procedures may also be necessary to improve motor function in the child with CP. The Achilles tendon can be lengthened, the hamstring can be released, hip adduction can be improved, and the feet can be repositioned to improve the child's gait. Medications can also be administered to control muscle spasms and seizures.

Nursing Considerations

It is important for the nurse to teach the parents and family members how to care for the child with cerebral palsy. The child with CP will need long-term physical therapy to maintain joint mobility and prevent contractures. Parents should be referred to the appropriate resources to obtain adaptive appliances such as customized wheelchairs, braces, and eating utensils. Parents should be taught the importance of safety belts and helmets to prevent injury.

The child with CP may not be intellectually disabled. Use terminology for the developmental stage of the child. The nurse teaches the parents how to encourage and support the child in order to foster positive self-esteem. Due to the long-term nature of the disorder, the child and parents should be referred to appropriate counseling and support groups. Parents may need financial assistance to provide the needed care.

FIBROMYALGIA

Fibromyalgia is a disorder characterized by widespread musculoskeletal pain and fatigue. It may also be accompanied by irritable bowel syndrome, chronic headaches, temporomandibular joint dysfunction, PMS in the adolescent, skin sensitivities, and impaired coordination. The child with fibromyalgia will be treated for pain and fatigue. Exercise, such as water therapy, has been shown to be beneficial. The nurse can assist children and parents to modify the child's lifestyle to conserve energy and minimize pain.

Nervous System Infections

MENINGITIS AND ENCEPHALITIS

Meningitis is an inflammation of the meninges by either bacteria or a virus (Figure 16-12 ■). The majority of cases of meningitis in children occur before the age of 5 years. Bacterial meningitis is the more serious of the two types, causing

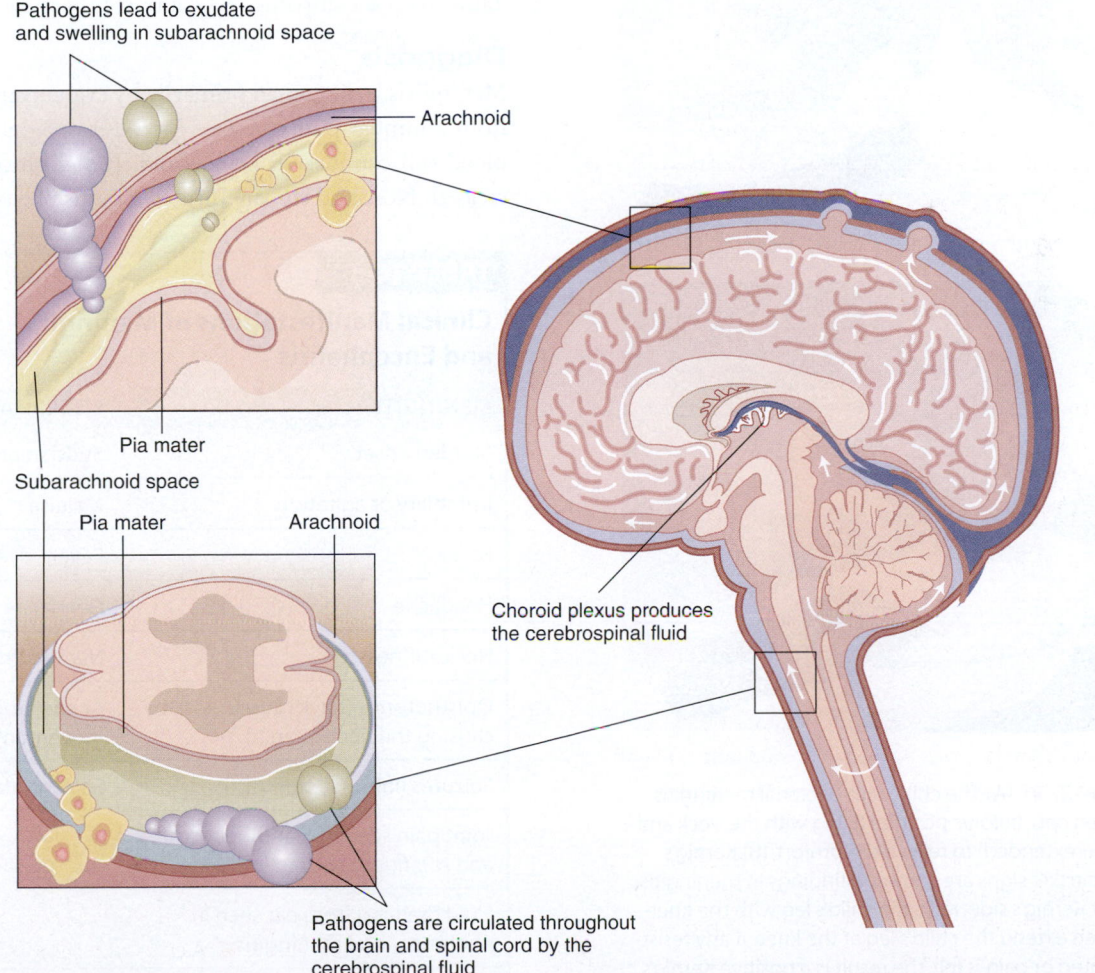

Figure 16-12. ■ Central nervous system infections. After a virus or bacteria reach the central nervous system, the pia mater, the arachnoid, and the cerebrospinal fluid–filled subarachnoid space all become infected. The cerebrospinal fluid then circulates the pathogens throughout the brain and spinal cord.

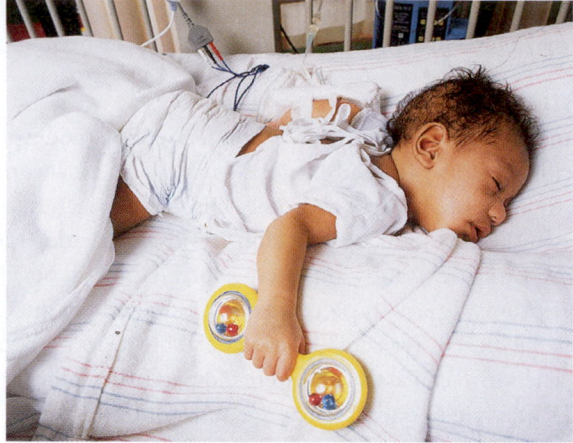

A

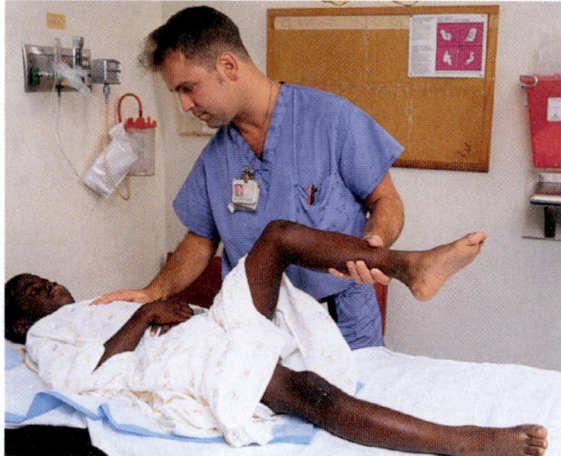

B

C

Figure 16-13. ■ **(A)** The child with bacterial meningitis assumes an *opisthotonic* position (lying with the neck and head hyperextended) to relieve discomfort. **(B)** Kernig's and Brudzinski's signs are common findings in meningitis. To test for Kernig's sign, raise the child's leg with the knee flexed. Then extend the child's leg at the knee. If any resistance is noted or pain is felt, the result is a positive Kernig's sign. **(C)** To test for Brudzinski's sign, flex the child's head while the child is supine. If this action makes the knees or hips flex involuntarily, a positive Brudzinski's sign is present.

neurologic damage and possible death. Causative agents of bacterial meningitis include *Haemophilus influenzae*, *Streptococcus pneumoniae* (causes pneumococcal meningitis), *Neisseria meningitides* (causes meningococcal meningitis), and *Escherichia coli*. Viral meningitis can be cause by enterovirus, adenovirus, mumps, and arbovirus. See Chapter 26 🔗 for further discussion of communicable diseases.

Manifestations

Symptoms of bacterial or viral meningitis include fever, change in appetite, vomiting, and diarrhea. These may occur suddenly or progress over a week, depending on the causative organism. The child may be lethargic or extremely irritable. Rocking or cuddling, which usually calms the child, may make the child more irritable. The child may also have headache, photophobia, nuchal rigidity, or a stiff neck. The child is comfortable only when lying on his or her side with the neck hyperextended and may have a positive Kernig's or Brudzinski's sign or both (Figure 16-13 ■). A hemorrhagic rash beginning as petechiae and progressing to larger lesions may be seen with meningococcal meningitis. Meningitis and encephalitis may sometimes be confused. Table 16-3 ■ compares and contrasts these two disorders.

Diagnosis

Meningitis is diagnosed primarily by evaluating CSF obtained from a lumbar puncture (see Procedure 13-18 🔗). White blood cell counts will be elevated. Blood glucose can be decreased. Nose and throat cultures may also be obtained.

TABLE 16-3	
Clinical Manifestations of Meningitis and Encephalitis	
MENINGITIS	**ENCEPHALITIS**
Sudden onset	Sudden or gradual onset
Irritability or agitation	Malaise
Fever	Fever
Headache	Headache
Neck stiffness	Neck stiffness
Opisthotonos (back muscle spasms causing the back to arch)	Ataxia (uncoordinated movement)
Seizures (initial symptom)	Seizures (later symptom)
Joint pain seen in meningococcal and *H. influenzae*	
Fluid draining from ear seen in pneumococcal meningitis	
Petechial rash seen in meningococcal meningitis	

Treatment

Oral fluids are provided to the child with meningitis if the child is responsive and able to swallow. Otherwise, fluids may be given intravenously to prevent dehydration. Broad-spectrum antibiotics may also be administered intravenously until the bacteria is identified from the lumbar puncture.

To control the fever and alleviate pain, nonsteroidal anti-inflammatory drugs are administered. If the fever is extreme, tepid baths or a cooling blanket may be needed.

Parents should be encouraged to verbalize their feelings and concerns. Involving them in the care of their child can help relieve their fears. Because bacterial meningitis can damage the nervous system, long-term rehabilitation may be needed. Referral to social workers or clergy may be necessary.

Nursing Considerations

The nurse will be responsible for frequent monitoring of vital signs and LOC. Measure and record head circumference daily due to the potential for ICP. The child with meningitis is at increased risk for seizures. Monitor for signs of sensory and/or movement deficiencies. For example, the child may lose the ability to hold the bottle, drink, or manage oral secretions. The child could develop respiratory distress, including periods of apnea due to cerebral edema, electrolyte imbalances, or other neurologic changes.

The child with meningitis should be placed in a private room to prevent spread of the infection to others. Keep the room dark and quiet to prevent photophobia and to decrease the risk of seizures because increased activity can induce seizures. Until the causative agent is determined, the child should be placed in respiratory precautions. All individuals entering the room should wear gown, gloves, and mask.

Encephalitis is inflammation of the brain, most often caused by a viral infection. Common causative organisms include St. Louis encephalitis virus, West Nile virus, eastern and western equine virus transmitted by ticks and mosquitoes, herpes simplex virus, or rabies virus. It may also occur after vaccination with measles, mumps, or rubella vaccines.

Herpes simplex type I is the most common cause of encephalitis after the newborn period. It is associated with a high mortality rate. Surviving children often have significant neurologic deficits (cognitive, auditory, motor, or visual). The cardiovascular system, as well as the lungs or liver, may be affected.

clinical ALERT

Younger children generally have more serious illness and greater residual effects from this disorder.

REYE'S SYNDROME

Reye's syndrome is a complication of viral infection. It is an acute encephalitis characterized by an onset of symptoms 1 to 3 weeks following a viral infection. Because the syndrome seems to be associated with salicylate use during viral infections, parents should be taught to avoid giving the child products containing salicylate for pain or fever relief during a viral infection. (See Chapter 26 ⚭ for Reye's syndrome and communicable diseases.)

clinical ALERT

Teach parents to avoid products containing *salicylate* (aspirin). Inform them of the following over-the-counter products that contain salicylate: Pepto-Bismol, Triaminicin, Coricidin, and Alka-Seltzer.

GUILLAIN–BARRÉ SYNDROME

Guillain–Barré syndrome (postinfectious polyneuritis) is a relatively rare disorder characterized by ascending and then descending paralysis. It can be an acute viral infection (most commonly *Campylobacter jejuni*), cytomegalovirus, or Epstein–Barr virus. It has also been associated with administration of vaccines. Although Guillain–Barré syndrome can affect anyone at any age, it is most commonly seen in children between 4 and 9 years of age.

Manifestations

Typically, Guillain–Barré syndrome begins with pain and weakness in the lower extremities. The muscle weakness and paralysis can progress upward to involve the abdomen, chest, upper extremities, and possibly the entire body. The paralysis can stop at any point and recede. Respiratory efforts may be compromised. The child may have difficulty talking, chewing, and swallowing. Dysfunction of the autonomic nervous system may cause hypertension, postural hypotension, cardiac arrhythmias, diaphoresis, and urinary and bowel incontinence.

Diagnosis

The syndrome is diagnosed by the presence of symptoms, lumbar puncture (see Figure 13-26 ⚭ for positioning), and CSF evaluation and electroconduction tests.

Treatment

Medical and nursing care is supportive until the paralysis resolves in 2 to 4 weeks.

Nursing Considerations

The focus of nursing care for Guillain–Barré syndrome is maintaining respiratory function, preventing malnutrition, preventing complications associated with immobility, providing emotional support, and teaching the family to care for the child at home.

The child's respiratory function must be continuously monitored in the early phase of the disease. Signs of labored breathing, color changes, fatigue, and low oxygen saturation indicate the need for medical intervention. The child may be intubated and placed on mechanical ventilation until the paralysis subsides.

The child's ability to swallow should be evaluated frequently, especially before feeding. If the child drools instead of swallowing saliva, oral liquid or food should not be given due to the risk of aspiration. To meet nutritional requirements, the child will need IV supplements or enteral feedings.

Within a few days of onset of the disease, the child will become either partially or totally immobile. The child can develop complications of immobility, such as constipation and skin breakdown. The concepts of basic nursing care should be followed and taught to the family. These include turning and maintaining proper alignment every 2 hours, active and passive range of motion, skin care, bowel care, and diversion activities.

The entire family will need support to deal with the sudden life-threatening disorder that may have long-term effects on the child. Referral should be made to a home care nurse, social worker, and rehabilitation specialist. With aggressive rehabilitation, children usually recover with few permanent deficits.

Neurologic Trauma

Neurologic trauma is defined as any injury to the head or spinal cord due to force, anoxia, or penetration. **Closed head injury** is a result of head trauma, either from an external force such as a blow to the head or an internal force, such as shaking the infant hard enough for the brain to strike the inside of the skull (called *shaken-baby syndrome*; see Chapter 27 🔗). Head injuries are the most common serious injury in childhood. The younger the child, the greater the risk of head trauma because the head is proportionately larger and heavier than the rest of the body.

HEMATOMA

The impact of the head injury can cause several types of hematomas, or blood trapped within the brain tissue. These hematomas can be subdural, epidural, or intracerebral. Subdural hematomas (Figure 16-14A ▪), bleeding between the dura and the brain, are caused by falls, motor vehicle

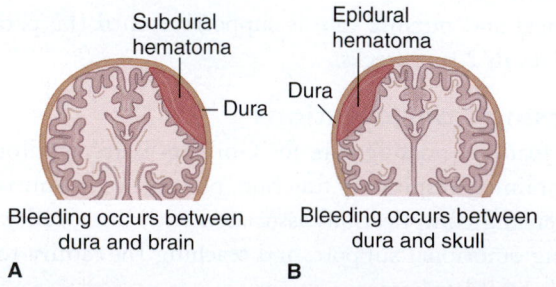

Figure 16-14. ▪ Intracranial hematomas. (**A**) In subdural hematoma (which literally means under the dura), bleeding occurs between the dura and the brain. (**B**) In epidural hematoma, bleeding occurs between the dura and car

crashes, and shaken-baby syndrome. Epidural hematomas, bleeding between the dura and the skull, are caused by blunt traumas such as an injury from a baseball. Bleeding within the cerebrum is called an intracerebral hematoma. This type of hematoma is caused by deep contusions or penetrating injuries to the skull.

Spinal cord injury can result from hyperflexion, lateral flexion, and extension or compression of the vertebrae. The specific trauma and area of injury determines the type of damage. The injury could be a bruising to partial or complete laceration of the spinal cord. At the time of injury, the child becomes flaccid below the injury. Cervical injuries are the most common due to the weight of the head and flexibility of the neck, and they are the most serious due to respiratory complications.

Manifestations

The signs of head trauma depend on the severity of the injury. The child may lose consciousness, have amnesia, have a headache, or be nauseous and vomiting. The child may have signs of increased ICP, including decreasing LOC, fixed dilated pupils, decorticate or decerebrate posturing (Figure 16-15 ▪), alteration in reflexes, and seizures. Hypoxic or anoxic neurologic trauma may result from drowning, carbon monoxide poisoning, or aspiration.

Diagnosis

Evaluating the head injury or spinal cord injury includes data gathered in the history and physical. The neurologic assessment is critical. To determine specific injuries, the health care provider will order x-rays, computed tomography (CT) scan, and/or magnetic resonance imaging (MRI).

Treatment

Treatment of head injuries may be extensive and require intensive and long-term care. In some cases, oxygenation is facilitated by intubation. ICP must be controlled by the use of diuretics, sedation, and environmental control to decrease stimuli.

Nursing Considerations

It is important for the nurse to determine the exact time of the injury, the events surrounding the injury, the exact location of the injury, and whether the child lost consciousness. Nursing care begins with airway management. Evaluation of ICP is essential. Skin integrity becomes an issue if the child is immobilized for long periods of time.

Parents of a child with neurologic injury need to be able to vent their feelings. Care must be provided in a nonjudgmental manner. Parents may need help deciding whether to take a comatose child home or place the child in a long-term care facility. The nurse should assist the family as needed.

Prevention of neurologic trauma is an essential component of client and family teaching, including the use of car

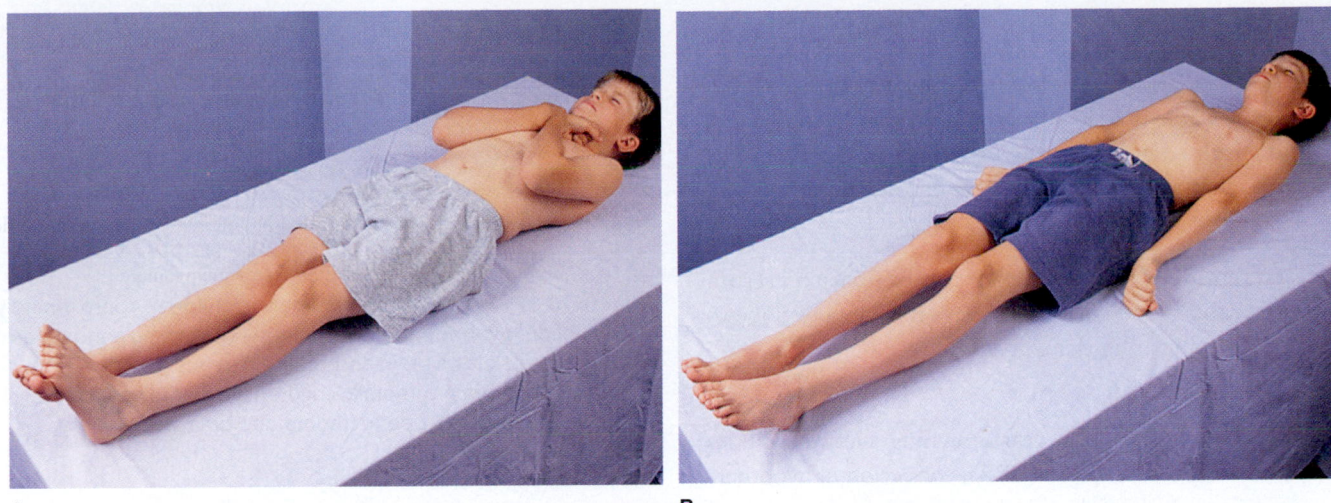

A   **B**

Figure 16-15. ■ **(A)** Decorticate posturing, characterized by rigid flexion, is associated with lesions above the brainstem in the corticospinal tracts. **(B)** Decerebrate posturing, distinguished by rigid extension, is associated with lesions of the brainstem.

seats, bicycle (and other) helmets, and firearm safety. Caregivers must be taught not to shake infants in order to prevent shaken-baby syndrome, a potentially lethal form of closed head injury. (Shaken-baby syndrome is discussed in Chapters 10 🔗 and 27 🔗.) The nurse needs to be aware of the possibility of parental abuse as a cause of trauma.

CONCUSSION

A **concussion** is an injury that causes temporary neurologic impairment but no permanent damage to brain tissue. It may be caused by blunt injury to the head or by shaking an infant or child. A concussion is caused by stretching, compressing, or tearing the nerve fibers near the brain.

Manifestations

Clinical manifestations of a concussion include altered mental status or loss of consciousness, nausea, vomiting, headache, dizziness, and amnesia.

Diagnosis and Treatment

An x-ray will be ordered to rule out skull fracture. The child should also be observed closely for 24 hours following the injury for decreasing LOC and disorientation. The child with a concussion may have difficulty staying awake because of the trauma/swelling to the brain. The child can be allowed to sleep following a concussion but must be awakened frequently (every 1 to 2 hours) to check LOC. (Review the Glasgow Coma Scale in Procedure 16-1.) The child should receive no analgesics or sedatives while under observation.

DROWNING OR NEAR-DROWNING

Drowning, loss of life within 24 hours following submersion in water or other liquid, is the second leading cause of injury-related death for children ages 1 to 14. **Near-drowning** is defined as suffocation from submersion in liquid that is survived in the first 24 hours following the incident. Children lose consciousness within 3 to 5 minutes. Neurologic and circulatory impairment occurs within 5 to 10 minutes following submersion. Asphyxia and aspiration are the physical conditions most often associated with near-drowning.

Manifestations

Clinical manifestations of near-drowning include restlessness, loss of consciousness, vomiting, cyanosis, tachypnea, tachycardia, hypotension, and hypothermia. The child is at risk for pneumonia if bacteria and debris were ingested. Children who have had a near-drowning experience in saltwater are at risk of severe electrolyte imbalance that may cause death (Figure 16-16 ■).

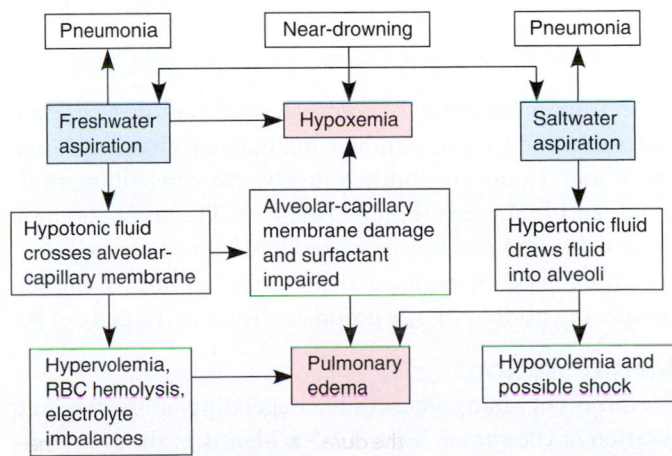

Figure 16-16. ■ Flowchart of near-drowning in fresh- or saltwater. Note the electrolyte imbalances that can occur.

Adequate information about the near-drowning incident must be obtained in order to treat the child appropriately. It is important to ask how long the child was under water, what type of water it was, what the temperature was, what the child's immediate response was when pulled from the water, and what rescue methods were employed.

Diagnosis

Lab tests required include blood gas evaluation, serum chemistries, and blood cultures. X-rays may also be done to observe for head or lung damage.

Treatment

Immediate treatment of the near-drowning victim includes cardiopulmonary resuscitation (CPR), correction of hypothermia, correction of electrolyte imbalance, and prevention of hyper- or hypovolemic shock. Neurologic dysfunctions such as increased ICP, cerebral edema, and seizures may need to be managed. Oxygen is given by nonrebreather face mask. Positive end-expiratory pressure (PEEP) can be used to keep the alveoli open. Administration of vasopressor medication may be necessary to maintain the child's blood pressure. Antibiotics are administered to children who develop pneumonia.

Nursing Considerations

Nursing care is focused on improving neurologic function, providing oxygenation, and decreasing the risk of infection. The child who has survived a drowning accident may develop a fear of water. The nurse can encourage the child to verbalize fears and to develop strategies for resolving these fears.

Drowning can be prevented by promoting community education and by encouraging environmental changes such as the use of fences and pool alarms. Pools should be surrounded with fences taller than 5 feet that are difficult for a child to climb. Buckets should be kept empty when not in use, and children should be supervised when near pools, at the beach, or in the bathtub. Families with pools should be encouraged to keep a phone near the pool and to learn CPR techniques.

Brain Tumors

Brain tumors are the most common solid tumor in children and the second most common malignancy after leukemia. Most brain tumors in children involve the cerebellum, midbrain, and brainstem (Figure 16-17 ■). The most common brain tumors in children are medulloblastoma, cerebellar astrocytoma, ependymoma, and brainstem glioma. Common tumors in children by age group are listed in Table 16-4 ■.

Manifestations

Symptoms of brain tumors differ, depending on the type and location of the tumor. Table 16-5 ■ identifies the symptoms and medical treatment of the four common brain tumors in children. The nurse must be alert for atypical, nonspecific symptoms. These include slight behavior change, poor

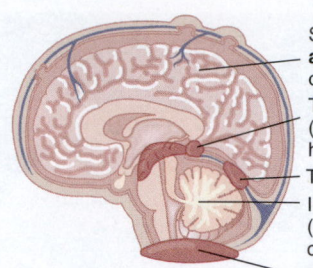

Supratentorial tumors (**cerebral astrocytoma, ependymoma,** optic nerve gliomas)
Tentorial notch tumors (pineal region tumors, hypothalamic glioma)
Tentorial tumors
Infratentorial tumors (**brainstem gliomas, medulloblastoma,** cerebellar astrocytoma, ependymoma)
Foramen magnum tumors

Figure 16-17. ■ Sites of brain tumors in children. Approximately 1,500 children younger than 15 years are diagnosed annually as having tumors of the brain and central nervous system. The four most common brain tumors in children are medulloblastoma, cerebral astrocytoma, ependymoma, and brainstem glioma.

school performance, and change in coordination. Tumors in the area of the hypothalamus or pituitary gland can induce diabetes insipidus and growth abnormalities caused by excess excretion of hormones.

Diagnosis

Ask the parents if the symptoms developed slowly or quickly in a matter of a few weeks. This can help determine the tumor growth rate.

To determine type and location of the tumor, CT scans, MRIs, positron emission tomography scans, and single-

TABLE 16-4

Tumor Sites by Age Group

	UP TO 5 YEARS	5–9 YEARS	10–14 YEARS	15–19 YEARS
Leukemia	36%	31%	18%	12%
Brain	13%	25%	18%	10%
Lymphoma	10%	16%	25%	27%
Kidney	10%	5%	N/A	N/A
Eye	6%	2%	N/A	4%
Soft tissue	7%	5%	5%	5%
Bone	13%	3%	11%	7%
Ovary/testis	2%	N/A	3%	11%
Neuroblastoma	7%	3%	N/A	N/A
Thyroid	N/A	N/A	4%	8%
Skin	N/A	N/A	N/A	6%
Other	2%	10%	16%	10%

Source: Data from Crist, W. M. (2000). Neoplastic disease and tumors. In R. E. Behrman, R. M. Kliegman, & H. B. Jenson (Eds.), *Nelson textbook of pediatrics* (16th ed.). Philadelphia: Saunders, p. 1531. Reprinted with permission from Elsevier.

TABLE 16-5			
Manifestations and Treatment of Brain Tumors			
TUMOR	**ETIOLOGY**	**CLINICAL MANIFESTATIONS**	**CLINICAL THERAPY**
Medulloblastoma	External layer of cerebellum	Headache, vomiting, ataxia	Surgery; chemotherapy with lomustine, vincristine, prednisone, cisplatin; radiation
Astrocytoma	Glial cells, supratentorial of infratentorial	Seizures, visual disturbances, increased intracranial pressure, vomiting	Surgery; chemotherapy with vincristine, dactinomycin; radiation
Ependymoma	Fourth ventricle, posterior fossa	Hydrocephalus	Surgery, radiation
Brainstem glioma	Pons	Cranial nerve (VI + VII) tract signs: nystagmus, ataxia, motor symptoms	Surgery, radiation

photon emission computed tomography scans are used. Lumbar punctures are used to identify malignant cells in the CSF. Bone marrow aspiration and bone scans detect metastasis to other areas of the body (Ball & Bindler, 2006).

Treatment

Medical treatment of brain tumors includes surgery, radiation, chemotherapy, or a combination of these treatments. The goal of treatment is to destroy as much of the tumor as possible, with a minimum of complications. Laser surgery is used when tumors are located close to vital tissue or blood vessels. The use of radiation and improved chemotherapeutic agents have improved the prognosis of many types of brain cancer such as medulloblastoma and ependymoma. Complications of radiation and chemotherapy include infection, seizure activity, hydrocephalus, growth problems, and neurologic deficits.

Nursing Considerations

Nursing care requires a multidisciplinary approach. The oncologist and neurosurgeon work closely with the pediatrician in providing medical treatment. The nurse coordinates with the dietitian, social worker, and physical and occupational therapist in managing complications of treatment. Parents can be taught to provide home care, including the administration of medication, physical exercises, and the need for follow-up examinations. The child and family members need support when the child has permanent deficits.

Mental Retardation

Mental retardation (MR) is defined by the American Association of Mental Retardation (2002) as "a disability characterized by significant limitations both in intellectual functioning and in adaptive behavior as expressed in conceptual, social, and practical adaptive skills. This disability originates before age 18." Specific limitations include communication, social skills, activities of daily living, schoolwork, and employment. Intelligence quotient (IQ) tests of individuals with MR are typically less than 70 to 75. The child with

mild MR has an IQ between 50 and 70. For moderate MR, the IQ is between 35 and 50. For severe MR, the IQ is between 20 and 35. Profound retardation is characterized by an IQ of less than 20.

Mental retardation is associated with other conditions such as Down syndrome (see also Chapter 9), fetal alcohol syndrome (discussed in Chapter 27), and maternal infections passed on to the child prenatally, such as rubella and cytomegalovirus (see Table 8-4). Other causes of MR include hypoxia, infections such as meningitis or encephalitis, neurologic trauma, and ingestion of poisons such as lead.

Clinical Manifestations

Infants with MR appear unresponsive to contact. They do not maintain eye contact during feeding. They are often irritable and take longer periods of time to feed. As these children age, they will exhibit developmental delays in language, social skills, cognitive skills, and motor skills. Learning is difficult for the child with MR, and he or she often does not do well in school.

Diagnosis

A careful history and physical examination are important in determining both the cause and the extent of MR. Laboratory tests may help determine the cause of MR. These tests include chromosomal analyses, blood enzyme levels, toxicology screens, and cranial imaging. A standardized test used to screen for developmental delays is the Denver Developmental Screening Test II (see Appendix IV). A test used to screen for the child's cognitive functioning is the Stanford–Binet Intelligence Scale. This can be found in a child development text.

Treatment

Because the degree of MR varies, each child will require a specific plan to help him or her function at the highest level achievable. The child's family, physician, nurse, social worker, physical therapist, teachers, and school administrators all play a significant role in managing the care of the child with MR. Education programs must be adapted to accommodate the needs of the child with MR. The infant needs increased visual and physical stimulation. The preschooler needs a learning environment where the teacher can devote the necessary time to help the child learn. The school-age child can benefit from special education programs and perhaps progress to a regular classroom. The adolescent with an IQ in the higher range of MR will require job training. Families may need assistance finding alternative living options for the child with MR.

Nursing Considerations

Families with children who are diagnosed with MR often experience grief and have difficulty coping. The nurse can play an important role in helping the family work through these emotions. Providing referrals to agencies that can assist the family in caring for the child with MR is a much-needed nursing strategy.

Children with MR do not have sound judgment. Because their safety may be compromised, they often require close supervision. The nurse can provide teaching to help the child avoid physical harm and assist the parents in removing environmental hazards.

Parents should be encouraged to allow the child to perform as many activities of daily living as possible. This will require patience and kindness. Children with MR benefit from being able to care for their needs, including dressing themselves, brushing their own teeth, and feeding themselves.

The nurse should discuss issues of sexuality and living apart from their parents with the adolescent with mental retardation. These issues include safety, birth control, prevention of sexually transmitted infections, money management, and responsibility. The nurse can refer the family to community resources to assist in dealing with these issues.

DOWN SYNDROME

Down syndrome is the most common chromosomal abnormality seen in infants to cause moderate to severe MR. It occurs when there are three chromosomes at position 21 (see Figure 4-2C ⬤⬤) and is also called *trisomy 21*. The frequency of Down syndrome increases with maternal age.

Manifestations

The infant with Down syndrome presents with a short head (*bradycephaly*), flat forehead, short limbs, and a short, wide neck (Figure 16-18 ■). The tongue may be protruding due to a high-arched palate. Epicanthal folds (a fold of skin over the inner canthus of the eye) are common. Hands are short and wide with a **simian crease** (a horizontal crease extending across the entire palm). There is a wide space between the great and second toe. Moro reflex is absent, and the newborn exhibits sluggish reflexes (*hypotonia*). The eyes may have **Brushfield spots** (white speckles on the edge of the iris).

The child with Down syndrome has an increased risk for congenital heart defect, diabetes, leukemia, and hearing loss.

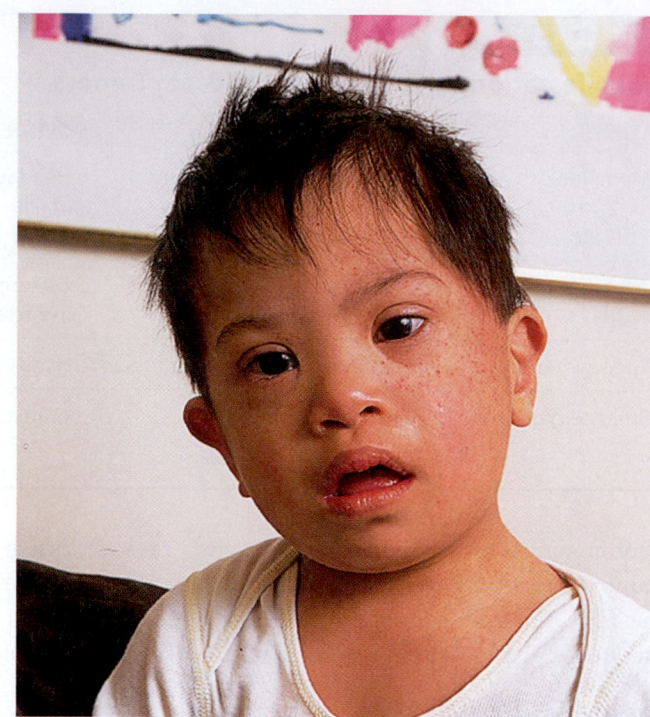

Figure 16-18. ■ This child with Down syndrome has typical characteristics, including Mongolian slant, short wide neck, and a protruding tongue.

The degree of mental retardation varies among children with Down syndrome and is not able to be assessed at birth.

Down syndrome alone would not necessitate keeping the newborn in the neonatal intensive care unit (NICU). However, the newborn with Down syndrome may be hospitalized for some time after birth to allow time for the parents to adjust to the diagnosis and to learn any special care that might be necessary.

Diagnosis

Initial diagnosis is by clinical findings most often evident at birth. Cardiac defects may be diagnosed by x-ray or ultrasound. Definitive diagnosis is by chromosomal analysis.

Treatment

The need for medical treatment of a congenital heart disorder (discussed in Chapter 19 ⬤⬤) will be a priority intervention. Surgery may be necessary to correct cardiac, gastrointestinal, or cranial deformities. A team approach will be instituted to assist the parents in coping with the child's physical and mental condition and in obtaining help through community resources.

Nursing Considerations

Parents of children with Down syndrome will need emotional support in coping with the new infant. There will be grief over the loss of their "perfect child." Nurses can model a loving and positive response to the neonate. They may need to repeat information that was provided because the parents may be overwhelmed at the thought of caring for a child with this disorder. Children with Down syndrome require lifelong assistance. With support, many children with Down syndrome are "mainstreamed" in schools and live in group homes as adults. Before discharge, the nurse must ensure that the parents are provided with information about the disorder and any necessary referrals.

SENSORY DISORDERS

Eye Disorders

ANATOMY AND PHYSIOLOGY

A child's eye is composed of external and internal structures. Figure 16-19 ■ reviews the eye's anatomy. Six muscles are responsible for the eye's movement. Vision occurs as light comes into the eye by way of the clear cornea. It then passes through the lens and is focused by the ciliary muscles onto the retina. The rods and cones relay the light impulses via the optic nerve to the occipital region of the brain.

BRIEF ASSESSMENT OVERVIEW

History

Ask about loss of vision, eye pain, *diplopia* (double vision), excessive or deficient tearing, drainage, and blurred vision. In a young child, the nurse may have to phrase questions to explain what is meant. For example, to check for double vision, the nurse may hold up one finger and ask, "How many fingers do you see?" The nurse would inquire about corrective lenses or glasses. Ask the parent for any behavior that would suggest the child is having difficulty seeing.

Physical

Observe for anatomic variations of the eye and the surrounding adnexa. Inspect the conjunctivae, sclerae, iris, and pupils.

Use the pen light to determine **PERRLA** (pupils equally round and react to light and accommodation).

Later in this chapter Procedures 16-2 ■ and 16-3 ■ describe visual acuity testing with eye charts.

Eye Conditions

ACUTE CONJUNCTIVITIS

Acute conjunctivitis is commonly called *pinkeye* (Figure 16-20 ■). It is the inflammation of the conjunctiva caused by allergies, bacteria, or viruses. Bacterial and viral conjunctivitis are contagious and easily transmitted among children.

Manifestations

Children with acute conjunctivitis can present with eye irritation, photophobia, redness, inflammation, and drainage, which may be purulent or watery. Conjunctivitis caused by an allergen will usually be accompanied by pruritus.

Diagnosis

Cultures of the drainage can assist in the differentiation between bacterial and viral conjunctivitis.

Treatment

Treatment for acute bacterial conjunctivitis includes ophthalmic antibiotics in the form of drops or ointment. Antiviral agents are available for viral conditions. Comfort measures for children with conjunctivitis caused by an allergen include cool compresses and antihistamines.

Nursing Considerations

The nurse should assist parents with the child's eye hygiene. To prevent transferring the harmful organism to others, the nurse can teach the child and parents to practice frequent hand washing, practice proper ophthalmic administration, change linens frequently, and avoid rubbing the eyes. The child should not go to school or day care while the infection is present.

> **clinical ALERT**
>
> It is best to place an infant in a quiet, dim environment to encourage him or her to open the eyes for examination or administration of ocular medications. Forcibly prying the eyelids open may cause trauma to the delicate tissues of the eye.

STYE

A stye is an infection of a sebaceous gland or oil gland of the eye lid. *Staphylococcus* is the most common causative agent. The child with a stye may have pain, redness, and edema of the eyelid. The preauricular lymph nodes may also be enlarged. Styes are treated with ophthalmic antibiotic ointment and warm, moist compresses to relieve discomfort.

PERIORBITAL CELLULITIS

Periorbital cellulitis (Figure 16-21 ■) is an inflammation of the subcutaneous tissue of the eyelid. It may be caused by a pre-existing infection, insect bites, or trauma.

Manifestations

The early symptoms of periorbital cellulitis often mimic those of acute conjunctivitis. The child may also have a fever, elevated white blood cells, malaise, and decreased visual acuity.

Treatment

The child will be hospitalized to administer IV antibiotics. Prompt treatment prevents damage to the optic nerve.

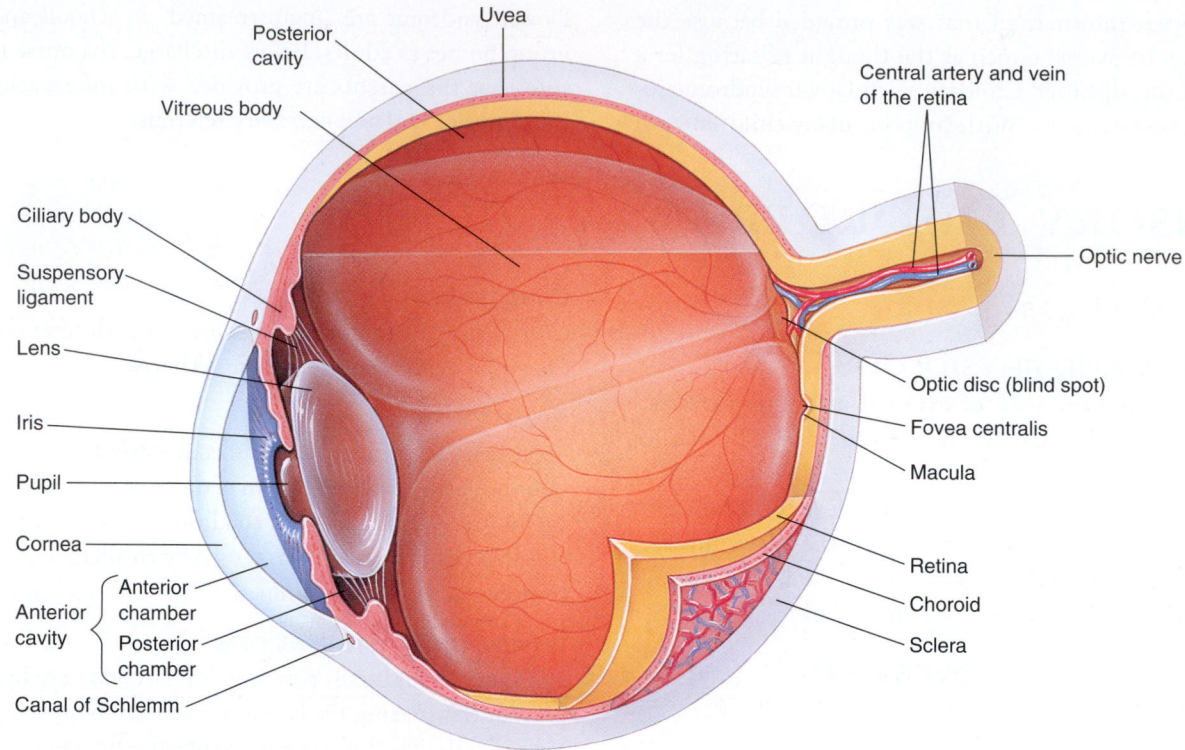

A

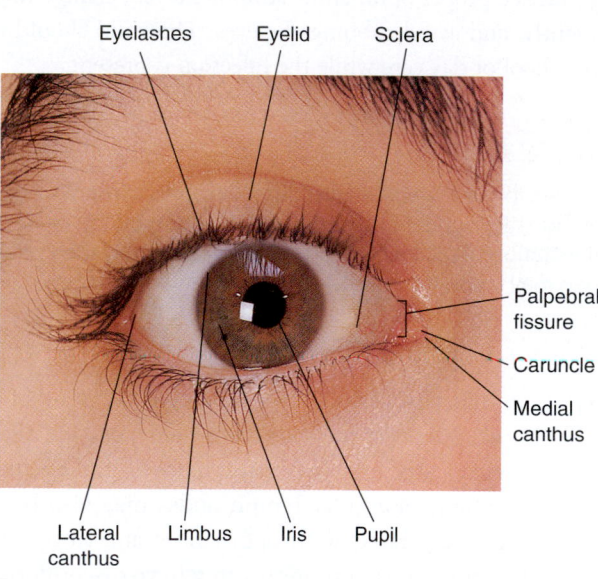

B

Figure 16-19. ■ (**A**) Internal structure of the eye. (**B**) External structure of the eye.

Eye Injuries

The cornea of the infant and young child is proportionally larger than that of an adult. The structures of the eye are not protected as well, especially from the side. Eye injuries cause the child intense pain, excessive tearing, light sensitivity, and changes in vision. Eye injuries are classified as penetrating or nonpenetrating. Prompt treatment of any eye injury is of utmost importance.

PENETRATING INJURIES

Penetrating injuries to children's eyes are typically caused by toys, glass, pencils, and other sharp objects. The object, if it remains in the eye, should not be removed until the child is sedated and an ophthalmologist or eye surgeon is available. Ophthalmic antibiotics are administered, the affected eye patched, and a tetanus booster administered if necessary.

NONPENETRATING INJURIES

Nonpenetrating eye injuries include corneal abrasion; foreign object trauma that does not penetrate the eye, such as trauma from air bags or baseball bats; hyphema; and chemical burns.

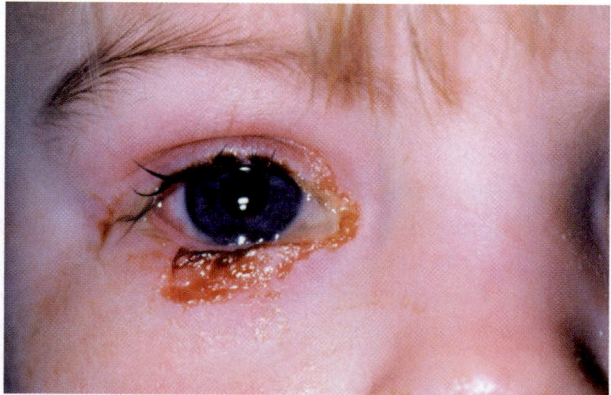

Figure 16-20. ■ Acute conjunctivitis. The discharge from bacterial conjunctivitis is purulent discharge and may cause crusting. The discharge from viral conjunctivitis is *serous* (watery). Allergic conjunctivitis produces watery to thick drainage and is characterized by itching. (Dr. P. Marazzi\Photo Researchers, Inc.)

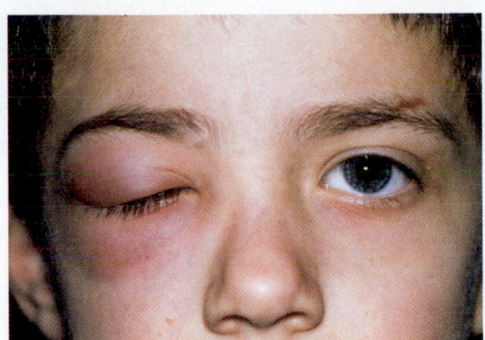

Figure 16-21. ■ Periorbital cellulitis is an infection of the eyelid and surrounding tissues, not of the eye itself. It is a serious bacterial infection that can spread to the optic nerve if not treated promptly with intravenous antibiotics. (Dr. P. Marazzi/Photo Researchers, Inc.)

To remove a superficial foreign object from the eye, grasp the eyelashes of the upper eyelid and stretch downward. Place a cotton-tipped applicator in the center of the eyelid, and pull the eyelid up and over the applicator (Figure 16-22 ■). Observe for the foreign object. If it is not embedded, it will be gently removed with another moist, cotton-tipped applicator. An ophthalmic antibiotic ointment will be prescribed. Water or saline eye irrigation in copious amounts is used for a chemical burn to the eye to flush out as much of the causative agent as possible.

HYPHEMA

Hyphema is a hemorrhage into the anterior chamber of the eye. Both of the child's eyes are patched. The child is placed on bed rest to prevent an increase in intraocular pressure and to allow for the reabsorption of the blood in the anterior chamber.

Visual Impairment

Several conditions can occur that interfere with a child's vision. Visual impairment can cause learning difficulties. Visual acuity screenings are available to determine light refraction disorders such as **hyperopia** (farsightedness), **myopia** (nearsightedness), and **astigmatism** (an uneven focusing of light resulting in blurred images) (Figure 16-23 ■). See Procedures 16-2 and 16-3. Lenses may be needed to correct the child's visual deficiencies.

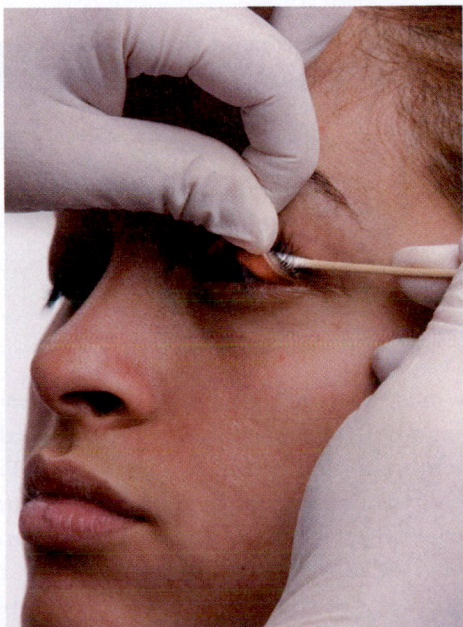

Figure 16-22. ■ Small pieces of debris or foreign objects can be visualized more readily by rolling the eyelid up over a cotton swab. (Patrick Watson\Pearson Education/PH College)

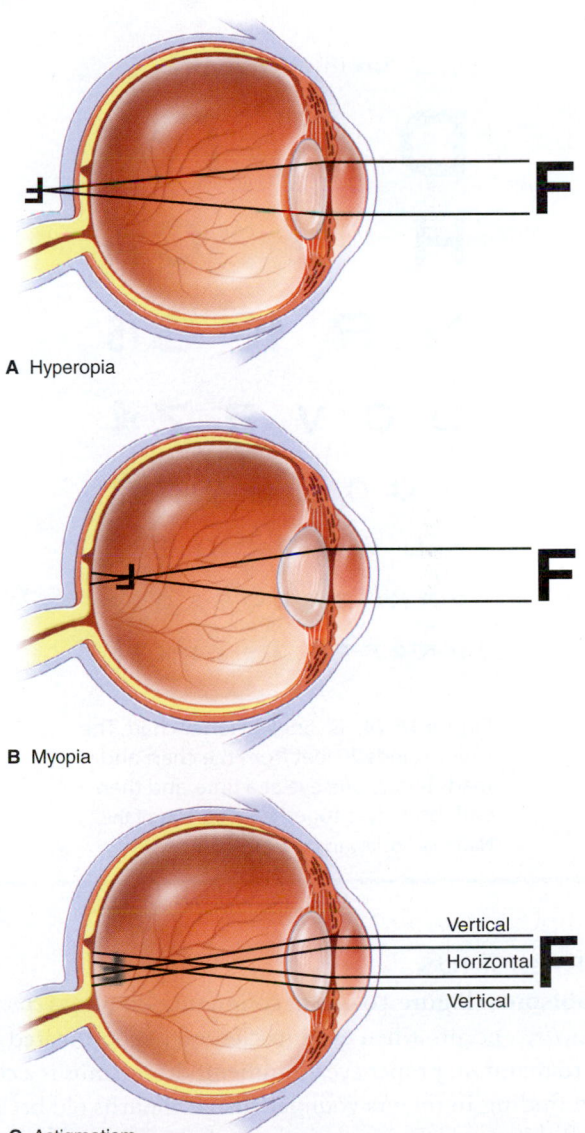

A Hyperopia

B Myopia

C Astigmatism

Figure 16-23. ■ (A) Hyperopia. In hyperopia, light rays focus behind the retina, making it difficult to focus on objects at close range. (B) Myopia. In myopia, light rays focus in front of the retina, making it difficult to focus on objects that are far away. (C) Astigmatism. In astigmatism, light rays do not uniformly focus on the eye due to abnormal curvature of cornea or lens.

PROCEDURE 16-2 ## Snellen Letter Chart

Purpose

■ To determine visual acuity for the child who can read the alphabet

Equipment

■ Snellen letter chart (Figure 16-24 ■)

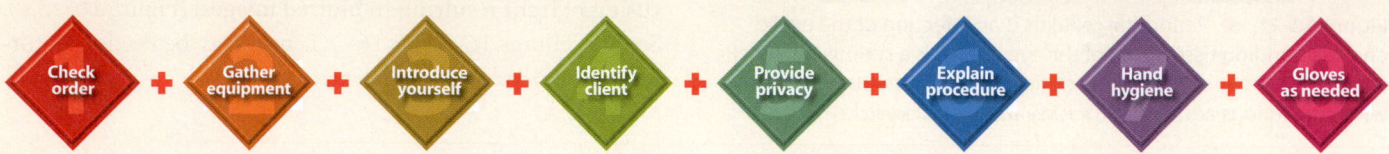

Interventions

1. Position the child 20 feet from the chart.

2. To test the right eye, cover the left eye completely, and ask the child to read the line on the chart indicated.

3. To test the left eye, repeat as above, except cover the right eye completely.

4. Interpret the findings. *If the child can read the line marked 20 feet, his or her vision is considered to be 20/20. If, however, the child can only read lines labeled 40 to 200 feet, his or her vision is considered to be 20/40 to 20/200. Note: Charts are available using a distance of 10 feet. Appropriate visual acuity in children older than 3 years is 20/20.*

5. Report visual acuity findings to charge nurse.

6. Document findings.

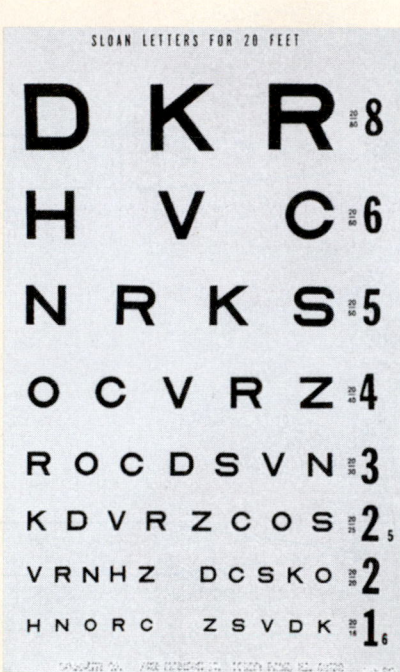

Figure 16-24. ■ Snellen letter chart. The client stands 20 feet from the chart and reads letters one eye at a time, and then with both eyes together. (Courtesy of the National Society to Prevent Blindness.)

SAMPLE DOCUMENTATION

(date) 0800   Snellen letter chart used. Right eye 20/20. Left eye 20/20. _____
B. Darnell, LVN

STRABISMUS

Strabismus (Figure 16-26 ■), commonly known as *cross-eye* or *walleye*, occurs when eye muscles are uncoordinated and fail to maintain proper eye alignment. Strabismus is a common finding in infants younger than 2 months old because the child is trying to focus and muscles are immature. **Esotropia** is the turning of the eye inward. **Exotropia** is the turning of the eye outward. **Hypertropia,** also called *anoopsia*, is a vertical deviation of one eye.

The child with strabismus has difficulty seeing objects clearly and may be clumsy. The child may close one eye frequently in an effort to see better. The cover test may be used to diagnose strabismus. In the cover test, the nurse gives the child an object with which to play. The nurse covers one of the child's eyes and observes the movement of the uncovered eye. Inward movement, outward movement, or vertical deviation of at least one eye indicates that the eye was not fixed on the toy and strabismus is present. Strabismus can be treated with corrective lenses, patching, **orthoptics** (eye exercises to correct coordination), or miotic medications to improve muscle function, or by surgery.

PROCEDURE 16-3	Snellen E or Picture Chart

Purpose

- To determine visual acuity for the child who cannot read the alphabet

Equipment

- Snellen E chart (also called tumbling E chart) or Snellen picture chart (Figure 16-25 ■)

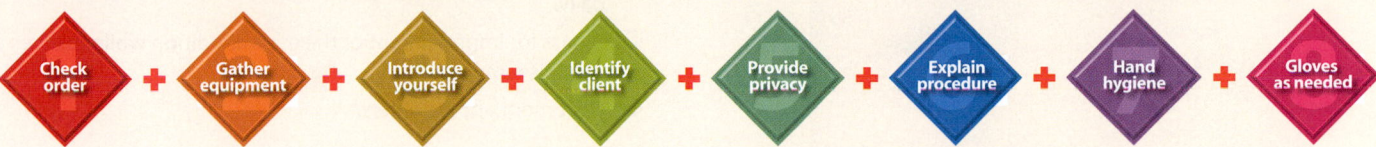

Interventions

1. Position the child 20 feet from the chart.

2. Start with the right eye.

3. Snellen E chart: Cover one eye, and point to the direction the legs of the letter are pointing. The child can also be given a card with a letter E on it. Ask the child to turn the card to match what he or she sees on the chart. Repeat with the other eye.

   Snellen picture chart: Cover one eye, and identify the pictures on the chart in order. Repeat with other eye.

4. Record the findings. *If the child can read the line marked 20 feet, his or her vision is considered to be 20/20. If, however, only lines labeled 40 to 200 feet can be read, his or her vision is considered to be 20/40 to 20/200. Note: Charts are also available using a distance of 10 feet.*

5. Report visual acuity findings to charge nurse.

6. Document finding in the chart.

SAMPLE DOCUMENTATION

(date) 1000   Visual acuity assessed with Snellen picture chart. Right eye 20/20. Left eye 20/20. _____
V. Gates, LPN

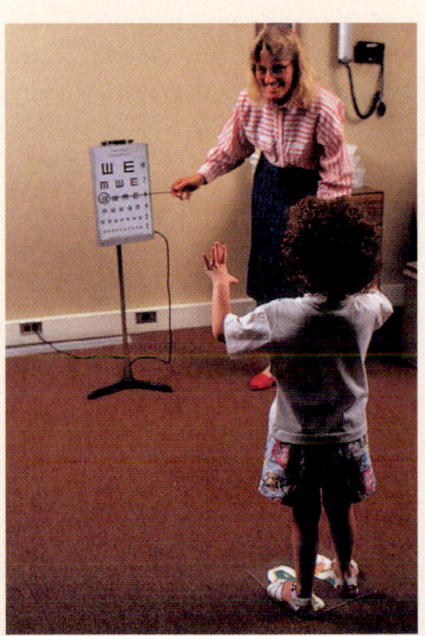

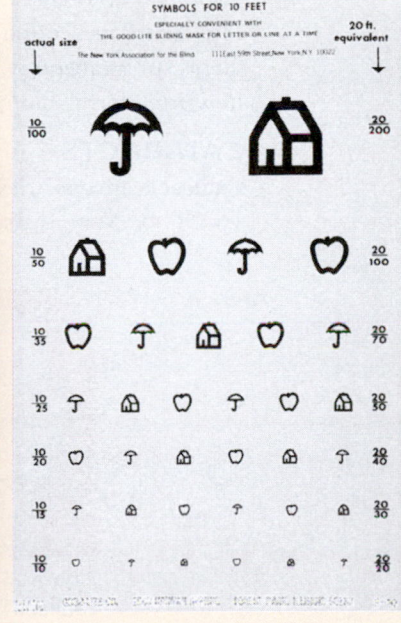

Figure 16-25. ■ (A) The Snellen E chart is often used for young school-age children. (B) The Snellen picture chart is used for very young children who can talk. (Courtesy of the National Society to Prevent Blindness.)

A

B

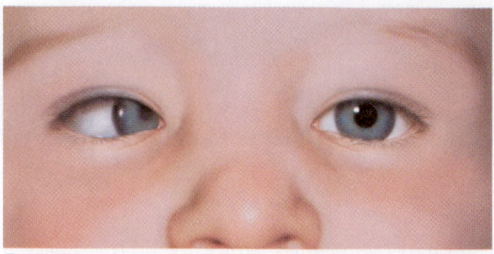

Esotropia

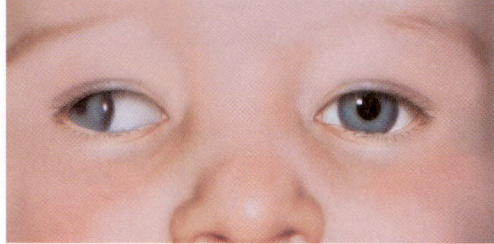

Exotropia

Figure 16-26. ■ Strabismus. In strabismus, the muscles of the eyes are not coordinated. (Pearson Education/PH College)

AMBLYOPIA

Amblyopia, or *lazy eye,* is a reduction of vision in one eye. Without treatment, the child may lose vision in the eye. Strabismus may lead to amblyopia. However, the child may also not have any symptoms. The condition can be detected in routine visual screening. Referral to an ophthalmologist or optometrist is important. Amblyopia can be

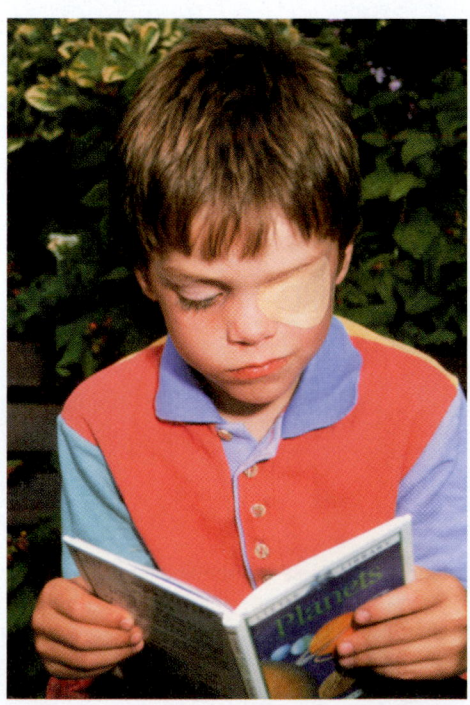

Figure 16-27. ■ An eye patch is used with nystagmus ("lazy eye") to strengthen the weaker eye. (Mark Clarke/Photo Researchers Inc.)

BOX 16-5	NURSING CARE CHECKLIST

Guidelines for a Child with Amblyopia

☑ Male children, in particular, may enjoy pretending to be a pirate with an eye patch. This may also encourage them to be compliant with care.

☑ Secure patch with adhesive underneath the patch, tape over the patch, and/or a bandage or elastic band around the head.

☑ Use restraints only if necessary.

☑ Ensure that the child has the patch removed at least 2 hours daily.

☑ Assess for improvement of the eye's condition while the patch is removed.

☑ Document appropriately.

treated with corrective lenses, patching (Figure 16-27 ■), or orthoptics. Treatment should be initiated by ages 5 to 6 for the best chance of success. Some nursing interventions for children with amblyopia are provided in Box 16-5 ■. Nurses can teach parents these guidelines as well.

DYSLEXIA

Dyslexia is a specific, common learning disability that is neurologic in origin (International Dyslexia Association, 2002). Children with dyslexia often see mirror images of letters, numbers, and symbols. This condition makes speaking, writing, memorizing, working math problems, reading, and spelling difficult. Although the child may have other visual impairments, dyslexia is not treated by correcting the vision. Children with dyslexia (or other neurologic-based learning disorders) need specialized assistance with learning. Learning techniques often involve stimulating several of the senses simultaneously, such as providing the material orally, in written form, and by three-dimensional model.

CATARACTS

Cataracts are opacities of the lens of one or both eyes (Figure 16-28 ■). Very dense cataracts may prevent light from

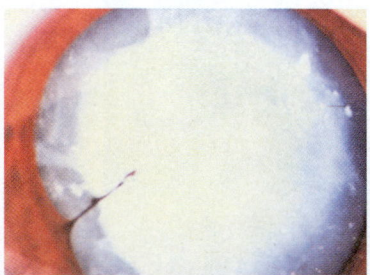

Figure 16-28. ■ Congenital cataract. The cataract reduces or prevents light from reaching the retina. (From Vaughan, D., Asbury, T., & Riordan-Eva, P. [1992]. *General ophthalmology* [13th ed.]. New York: McGraw-Hill, p. 172.)

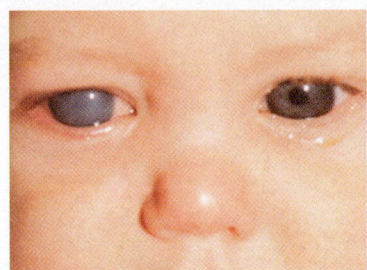

Figure 16-29. ■ Congenital glaucoma can be seen in this child's right eye as a cloudy film. (From Vaughan, D., Asbury, T., & Riordan-Eva, P. [1992]. *General ophthalmology* [13th ed.]. New York: McGraw-Hill, p. 172.)

reaching the retina. Cataracts can be acquired or congenital. Acquired cataracts are due to infections during pregnancy, trauma, or other disease processes. Congenital cataracts can be caused by an inherited autosomal dominant trait.

The nurse may be able to observe severe cataracts with the naked eye. The normal red reflex (the reflection of light off the retina when using an ophthalmoscope) may also be distorted or absent. An infant may not be able to focus on close objects or may demonstrate **nystagmus** (involuntary movement of the eyes). The older child may report blurred vision. Cataracts are removed surgically to restore the child's vision. Corrective lenses or artificial lens implants will be necessary to restore vision. Surgery is necessary before age 2 months in the infant with severe cataracts in an effort to prevent permanent visual impairment.

GLAUCOMA

Glaucoma is a condition caused by increased intraocular pressure (IOP) due to inadequate drainage of the aqueous humor (Figure 16-29 ■). Increased IOP from the anterior chamber of the eye has the potential to cause retinal damage, compression of the optic disc tissue, and eventually visual field defects or blindness.

Glaucoma in the pediatric client can be congenital or acquired. The child with congenital glaucoma may have increased tearing (called **epiphora**), eyelid spasms, enlargement of the eyeball (called **buphthalmos**), and sensitivity to light (called **photophobia**). The child with acquired glaucoma, if able to walk, may bump into objects because he or she has difficulty seeing objects in his or her peripheral vision due to visual field defects. The child may also report seeing halos around objects.

IOP is measured by a **tonometer.** In children, this procedure may require anesthesia because the device must be placed against the anterior eye globe. Normal IOP is 12 to 20 mm Hg. Increased IOP, above 30 mm Hg pressure, may require prompt surgical correction. One surgical technique is called a

goniotomy. During a goniotomy, the flow of aqueous humor is increased from the anterior chamber. More than one surgery may be necessary to reduce the IOP to a level at which the risk of damage is reduced.

Ear Disorders

ANATOMY AND PHYSIOLOGY

The ear is composed of three sections: the external ear, the middle ear, and the inner ear (Figure 16-30 ■). The auricle, tympanic membrane, and external ear canal are parts of the *external ear*. The eustachian tube, malleus, incus, and stapes are parts of the *middle ear*. The semicircular canals, cochlea, and cranial nerve VIII are parts of the inner ear.

The most important thing for the nurse to understand when assessing a child's hearing is the difference in the anatomic shape of the eustachian tube of young children (see Figure 16-30B). The eustachian tube of the young child is shorter, wider, more horizontal, and more flaccid. This shape increases the risk for otitis media because fluid and harmful bacteria more easily accumulate in it.

BRIEF ASSESSMENT OVERVIEW

History

Ask about hearing loss, vertigo, **tinnitus** (ringing or other sound in the ears), drainage, and ear pain.

Physical

Observe for placement of the ear on the head (Figure 16-31 ■). (Low-set ears are often associated with renal disorders.) Inspect the external ear for symmetry, proportion, and color. Inspect the external ear canal for drainage, color, and the presence of wax (*cerumen*). Test for pain and tenderness by pulling on the auricle (down and back) and by palpating the mastoid process directly behind the ear. Assess for hearing acuity. (Hearing acuity testing is addressed later in this section.)

Ear Conditions

HEARING IMPAIRMENT

Sound is received through the external auditory canal and directed toward the tympanic membrane, causing it to vibrate (see Figure 16-30A). This vibration conducts the sound waves to the malleus, incus, and stapes, and then to the nerve endings in the cochlea. The cochlea transmits sound waves to the brain, where the child perceives the sound.

Hearing impairment can occur from birth or be acquired later in childhood. Hearing impairment can range from a slight hearing loss to total deafness. Three of every 1,000 babies are born with a hearing loss (Peck, 2005b). Causes of hearing loss include autosomal dominant inherited diseases;

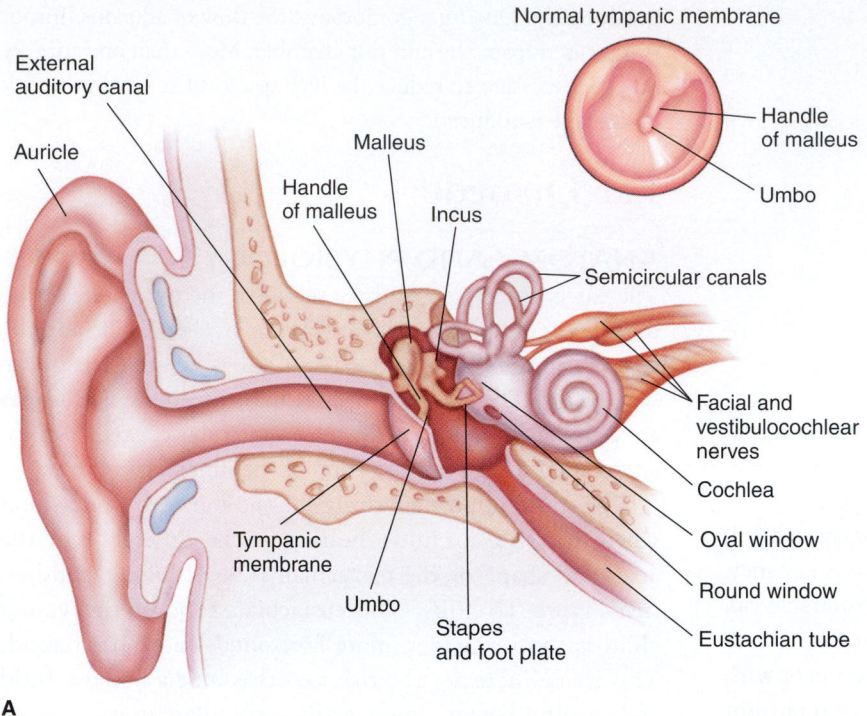

Normal tympanic membrane

Handle of malleus

Umbo

External auditory canal

Auricle

Malleus

Handle of malleus

Incus

Semicircular canals

Facial and vestibulocochlear nerves

Cochlea

Oval window

Round window

Eustachian tube

Tympanic membrane

Umbo

Stapes and foot plate

A

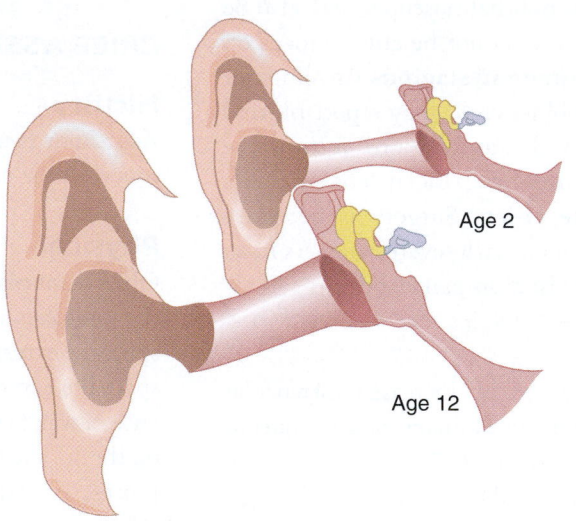

Position of eustachian tube is at less of an angle (more horizontal) in the young child, resulting in decreased drainage.

Age 2

End of eustachian tube in nasal pharynx opens during sucking.

Age 12

Eustachian tube equalizes air pressure between the middle ear and the outside environment and allows for drainage of secretions from middle ear mucosa.

Figure 16-30. ■ (**A**) Ear anatomy. (**B**) Difference in the eustachian tube between an infant and an adult.

B

prenatal infections such as rubella and toxoplasmosis; perinatal asphyxia and anoxia caused by birth trauma; ototoxic drugs; radiation; childhood infections such as measles, mumps, and otitis media; head trauma; and excessive environmental noise (Figure 16-32 ■). Table 16-6 ■ provides information about degrees of hearing loss.

Manifestations

Clinical manifestations of hearing impairment differ according to a child's age. The infant may not startle at loud noises or may fail to be soothed by his or her mother's voice. The older infant may not imitate sounds. Calling the name of a toddler may not elicit a response. The sound of a train

approaching may go unnoticed. The toddler may also use nonverbal language instead of attempting to communicate verbally. The preschooler looks curious when given instructions or frequently asks for them to be repeated. The preschooler also may need to watch a person's lips in order to understand what is being said.

Diagnosis

See Hearing Acuity Screening section on page 541.

Treatment

A child with a hearing impairment may benefit from speech therapy or from learning to read lips or use sign language. (Some basic sign language is provided in Appendix VI ▣▣).

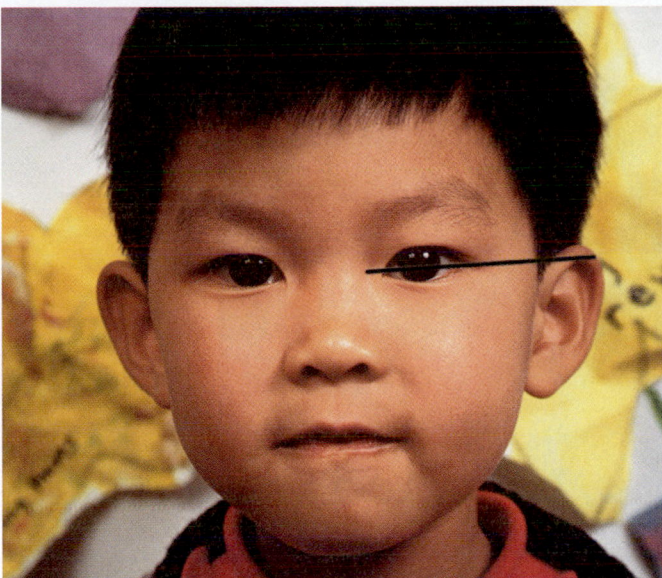

Figure 16-31. ■ The correct placement of the external ears is found by drawing an imaginary line through the medial and lateral canthi of the eye toward the ear. This line normally passes through the upper portion of the pinna. The pinna is considered "low set" when the top lies completely below the imaginary line. Low-set ears are often associated with renal disorders.

A hearing aid may be necessary for the child to develop language skills. Infants younger than 6 months may be fitted for hearing aids. A hearing aid uses a microphone to convert sound waves into electrical impulses. These impulses are then broadcast across the tympanic membrane. The hearing aid is battery operated and fits into the child's ear. It requires a transmitter that fits behind the ear, on the child's glasses, or at the waist. Hearing aids can be costly, and it is likely that health insurance will not cover the expense.

COCHLEAR IMPLANTS.   **Cochlear implants** are devices that can assist children who are deaf to hear (Figure 16-33 ■). In cochlear implant surgery, an electrode is implanted behind the ear with a wire leading to the cochlea. The child wears a headpiece behind the ear that contains a transmitter that transfers sound. The headpiece also contains a microphone to amplify sound. The speech processor is worn at the waist.

FOREIGN OBJECT IN EAR

Hearing may also be temporarily impaired by the presence of a foreign object in the ear. Curious children may take small objects and place them in the external ear canal. Upon otoscopic examination by the health care practitioner, the foreign object may be visualized. The nurse may assist in irrigation of the ear to remove the foreign object (see Procedure 13-31 ⚭). The health care practitioner may use sterile forceps to remove the foreign object if irrigation is unsuccessful. Caution parents against attempting to remove the foreign object themselves. This may force the object further into the ear canal.

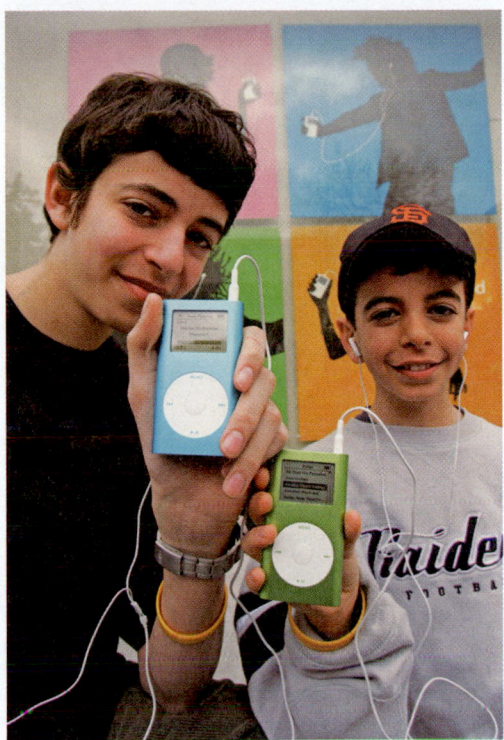

Figure 16-32. ■ Listening to loud music with headphones or at rock concerts is a frequent cause of hearing loss among teenagers and young adults. Children need guidelines about this activity. (AP Wide World Photos.)

OTITIS MEDIA

Otitis media is inflammation of the middle ear that may be accompanied by fluid in the middle ear. Increased incidence of otitis media is seen in children with upper respiratory infections, cleft palate, and immunodeficiencies. Otitis media

TABLE 16-6	
Degree of Hearing Loss	
TYPE OF LOSS	**IMPAIRMENT**
Slight	Cannot hear whispers, no speech impairment, compensates by leaning forward and speaking loudly
Mild	Slight speech impairment, tries to face person to read lips
Moderate	Speech impairment present, difficulty with normal conversations, schoolwork is affected, may need a hearing aid
Severe	Hearing aid is needed for all sounds, speech therapy required
Profound	Sounds are not heard, severe speech deficits

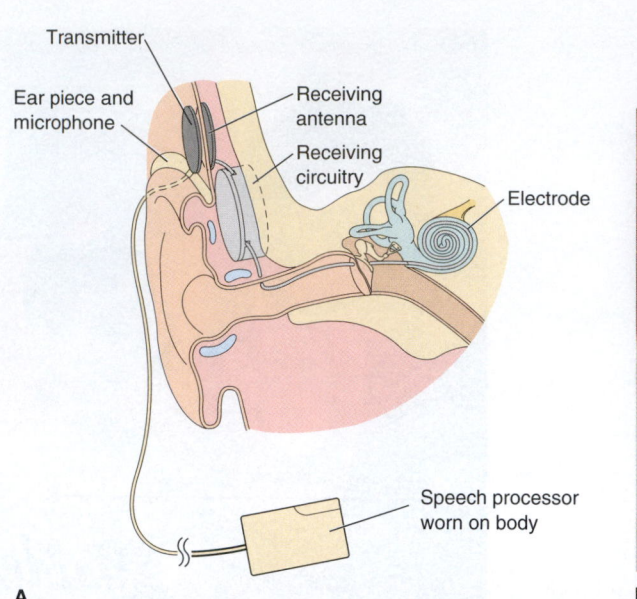

Transmitter

Ear piece and microphone

Receiving antenna

Receiving circuitry

Electrode

Speech processor worn on body

A

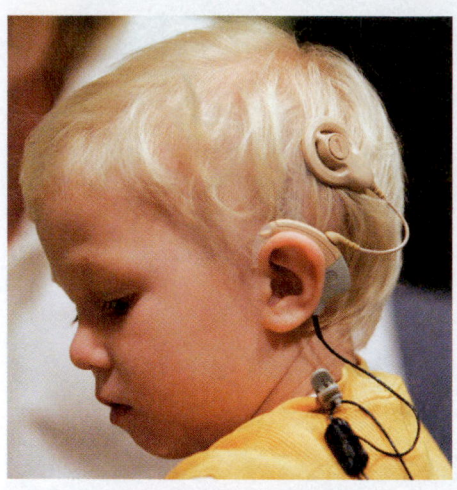

B

Figure 16-33. ■ **(A)** Structure and positioning of cochlear implant. **(B)** Child with cochlear implant. Success with this surgery is greatest when the child is young. (AP Wide World Photos)

is also seen more commonly in children who are bottle fed, who use a pacifier, and who are exposed to cigarette smoke. Bottle-propping, which leads to formula pooling in the eustachian tube, provides a medium for bacterial growth. Pacifier use raises the soft palate and alters the direction of the eustachian tube. This provides an entry point for harmful bacteria from the nasopharynx (Ball & Bindler, 2006). Children exposed to second-hand smoke are at greater risk for respiratory infections that can lead to otitis media. During the winter and spring of the year, when upper respiratory infections are common, more children will develop otitis media.

Manifestations

Clinical manifestations of otitis media include symptoms of an upper respiratory infection accompanied by fever and **otalgia** (ear pain). Although the older child can report pain, the infant and toddler may be observed pulling at the ear in an attempt to relieve the pain (Figure 16-34). Irritability, vomiting, and diarrhea may also accompany otitis media because of accompanying illness, cold, or flu.

clinical ALERT

Because of the connection of the eustachian tube with the pharynx, the child with an ear infection may also have a throat infection.

Diagnosis

Diagnosis of otitis media includes recognition of symptoms and ophthalmic examination of the tympanic membrane by the health care practitioner. The tympanic membrane is normally a pearl gray color with a light reflex. In otitis

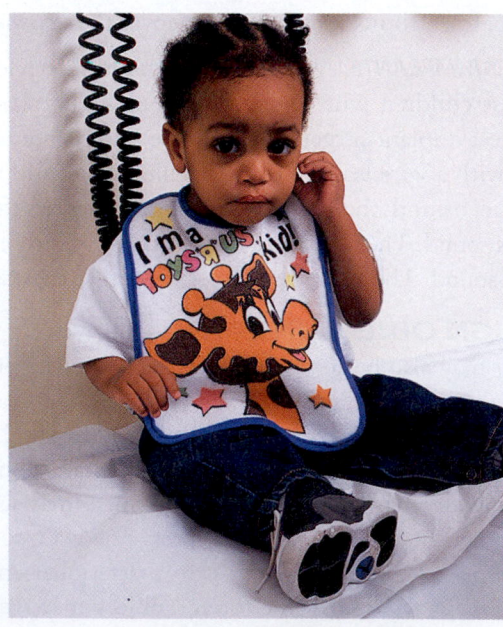

Figure 16-34. ■ This young child is pulling at an ear and acting fussy, two important signs of otitis media.

MediaLink Otitis media

media, the tympanic membrane appears red and bulging, and the light reflex is diminished or absent (see Figure 16-34B).

Treatment

Otitis media is treated with broad-spectrum antibiotics, decongestants, analgesics, and antipyretics. Parents need to understand that hearing can be diminished for up to 6 months following treatment. Recurrent otitis media may require a surgical procedure called a **myringotomy.** During the myringotomy, a small plastic tube is inserted through the tympanic membrane to facilitate drainage of fluid and ventilation of the middle ear. This procedure can be done on an outpatient basis with local anesthesia. The tubes are usually effective for 6 to 12 months and may fall out naturally or be removed by the health care practitioner.

Nursing Considerations

Hospitalization is rare for the child with otitis media. Most of the care provided to this child will be in an outpatient setting or in the home. The child with otitis media can experience a significant amount of pain. The nurse should provide information to parents on the proper administration of analgesics, including topical anesthetic ear drops. Remember to teach parents how to straighten the ear canal for proper administration of otic medication in infants or older children (see Figure 13-38).

Prevention methods should be discussed with the child's family. Smoking cessation should be discussed with the parents because exposure to second-hand smoke challenges the respiratory system and is associated with an increased incidence of otitis media. Pacifier use should be discouraged at bedtime in infants with prior infection because it may also increase incidence (Niemela et al., 2000). Parents of children who are in day care and who have frequent episodes of otitis media should consider alternative forms of child care to avoid exposure to pathogens.

> **clinical ALERT**
>
> The nurse must teach the parents about care of the child while the tubes are in place. Parents should be cautioned against allowing water to enter the child's ears. During bathing, showering, swimming, or other water activities, ear plugs should be used to prevent infection from outside micro-organisms.

Hearing Acuity Screening

Delayed speech and language development may be the result of poor hearing acuity. It is important to perform hearing acuity screening to identify hearing impairment from an early age. The American Academy of Pediatrics (AAP)

has endorsed universal newborn hearing screening in birthing units as the standard of care (Johnson, 2002). Currently the goal is to screen all infants by 1 month of age and to provide early treatment interventions before 6 months to all affected children (AAP & American College of Obstetricians and Gynecologists [ACOG], 2002). Periodic screening is done at schools and in pediatrician's offices. Procedures 16-4 ■ and 16-5 ■ describe hearing screening tests.

NURSING CARE

PRIORITIES IN NURSING CARE

The priorities in assessing a child with a neurologic impairment are determined by the type and degree of impairment. In general, the nurse ensures that the child has a patent airway and is well oxygenated. These children need protection from injury due to their altered mobility or their cognitive impairment. The nurse should perform a neurologic assessment every 2 hours to include level of consciousness, verbal responses, and motor responses.

ASSESSING

Children with nervous system disorders should be assessed for changes in LOC, reaction to stimuli, and ability to respond to stimuli. The nurse must monitor closely for signs of seizures, increased intracranial pressure (ICP), changes in LOC, and poor oxygenation.

> **clinical ALERT**
>
> Neurologic deterioration can occur rapidly in infants and young children. Changes in baseline vital signs and LOC must be recorded and reported immediately.

DIAGNOSING, PLANNING, AND IMPLEMENTING

The following nursing diagnoses may apply to the infant with a nervous system disorder:

- Ineffective Airway Clearance, related to excessive mucus
- Risk for Deficient Fluid Volume, related to imbalance of fluids and electrolytes
- Anticipatory Grieving (Parent), related to potential loss of neurological function
- Risk for Injury, related to neurologic deficit
- Impaired Verbal Communication, related to hearing impairment

(Text continues on p. 544.)

PROCEDURE 16-4 Pure Tone Audiometry

Purpose

- To determine the auditory acuity of a child older than 3 years

Equipment

- Private room, free of distractions
- Calibrated audiometer, including earphones
- Alcohol pads

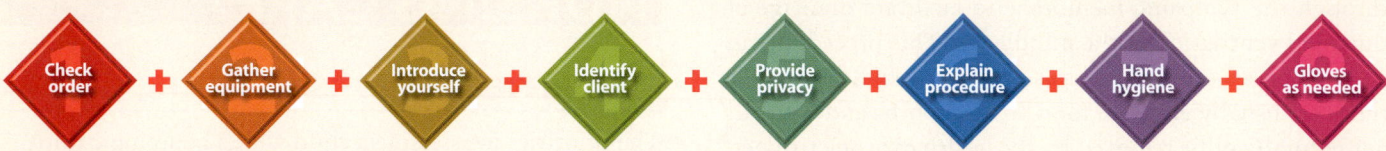

Interventions

1. This test is usually performed in the clinic setting.
2. Clean the earphones with alcohol pads. *Harmful bacteria could be transmitted via the earphones.*
3. Explain the procedure thoroughly to the child and parent.
4. Demonstrate the equipment, sounds, and method used to test hearing. *The usual method for testing hearing is to have the child raise a hand on the side where the sound is heard.*
5. Have the child return demonstration of hand signals. *Do not proceed until proper understanding is determined.*
6. Position the child with the back toward the machine. *This ensures that the child cannot see the machine or the examiner and thus cannot receive visual cues about sounds heard.*
7. Place the earphones on the child and deliver sounds randomly to both ears. Each ear should be tested with the following pitches: 500, 1,000, 2,000, and 4,000 Hz.

8. Interpret the findings. *Passing auditory acuity findings are 20 to 25 decibels (db) for 500, 1,000, and 2,000 Hz and 25 db for 4,000 Hz.*
9. Report findings to the charge nurse and document them in the chart.
10. Repeat the test in 2 weeks if the child does not pass the test. If the second test is also unsuccessful, further evaluation is necessary.

SAMPLE DOCUMENTATION

(date) 0900   Pure tone audiometry indicates 20 db at 500 and 1,000 Hz; 25 db at 2,000 and 4,000 Hz in both ears. D. Bryant, LPN

PROCEDURE 16-5 Tympanometry

Purpose

- To determine an estimate of middle ear pressure and tympanic membrane movement in older infants and children

Equipment

- Calibrated tympanometer
- Disposable probe
- Graph paper

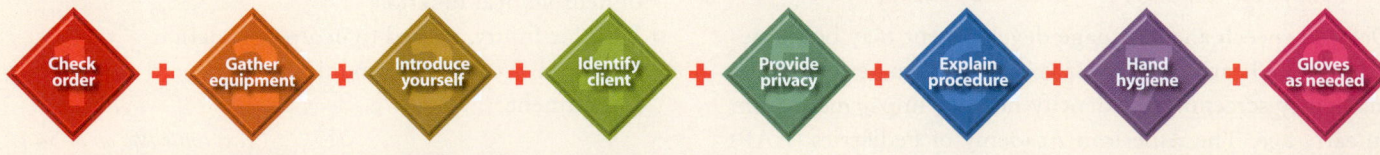

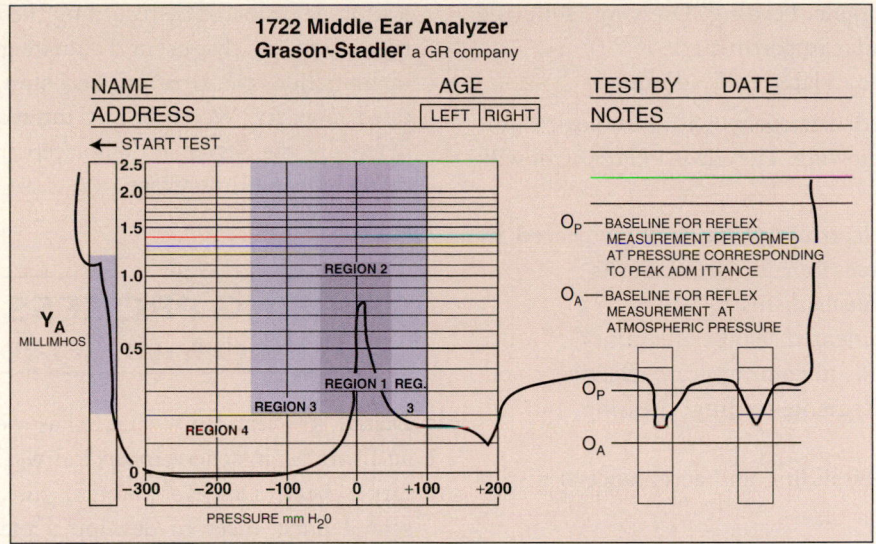

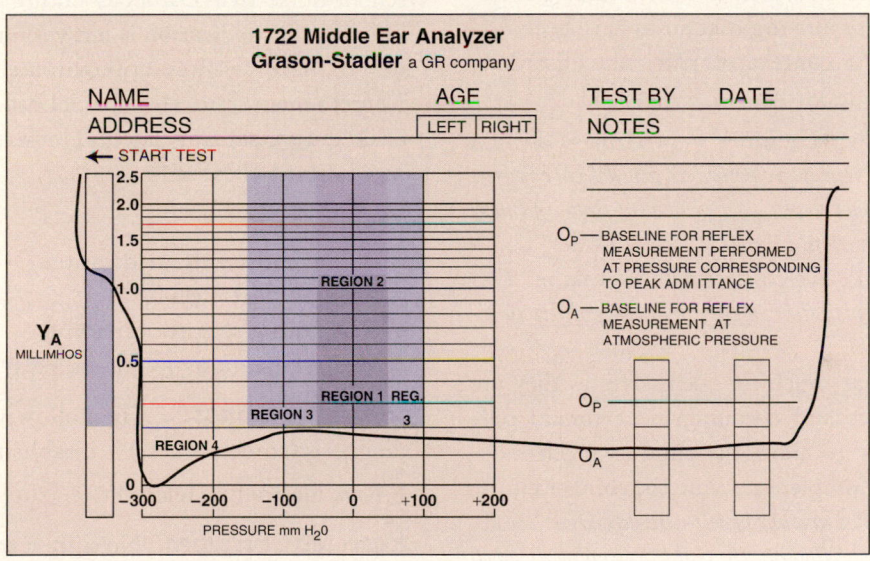

Figure 16-35. ■ **(A)** This tympanogram demonstrates normal hearing as evidenced by the curve showing the tympanic membrane's movement when a sound wave is emitted into the ear canal. Mobility is between 0.2 and 1.0 mL, the normal range. **(B)** In contrast, note the flat pattern in the second tympanogram, which shows restricted mobility of the tympanic membrane in response to sound.

Interventions

1. Explain the procedure and the importance of remaining still to the child and his or her parents. *The risk of pain and injury to the auditory canal from the earpiece is reduced.*

2. Insert the earpiece covered with the disposable probe into the auditory canal. Ensure a seal. *The tight seal will provide an accurate measurement.*

3. Provide a tone from the tympanometer.

4. Repeat on the other ear.

5. Interpret findings plotted on graph paper (Figure 16-35 ■).

6. Report findings to charge nurse and document them in the chart.

SAMPLE DOCUMENTATION

(date) 1400   Tympanometry indicates fluid accumulation or pressure changes in the middle ear. Findings reported to charge nurse. _____
                T. Edward, LVN

- Self-Care Deficit: Hygiene, Feeding, Dressing, Toileting related to neuromuscular impairment
- Disturbed Body Image, related to head injury

Some outcomes for pediatric clients with neurologic disorders might include the following. The client and/or parent will:

- Have a patent airway
- Maintain fluid and electrolyte balance as evidenced by vital signs and lab values within normal limits
- Demonstrate coping mechanisms
- Provide a safe environment that prevents injury
- Learn alternate methods to communicate effectively
- Accept assistance in hygiene, feeding, dressing, and toileting
- Demonstrate an understanding and acceptance of disfigurement.

The following nursing interventions are appropriate for children with neurologic impairment. (*Note:* Nursing interventions for some of these nursing diagnoses have been discussed previously in the context of particular disorders. They are not repeated here.)

- Adapt communication techniques for cognitive ability, not chronologic age. *Neurologic disorders can delay or regress cognitive ability. Sometimes cognitive development stops and may never show normal progression.*
- Face the child and make eye contact when speaking. *This allows the child with a visual or moderate hearing defect to receive nonverbal cues.*
- Allow children to do as much for themselves as they are able. Provide assistance and encouragement toward self-care. Encourage family to allow the child as much independence as possible. Complete any care the child or family is unable to perform. *The amount of self-care depends on the degree of neurologic damage. Allowing the child to complete as much self-care as possible fosters independence and self-esteem.*
- Provide factual information to the child and family to assist in dealing with disturbed body image. Allow the young child expression of feeling through puppet play. Include other specialists such as physical therapist, occupational therapist, and speech therapist as needed. *Young children may not perceive disfigurement to the same extent as family members. Nursing care should focus on the family as the primary support for the child.*
- Reinforce teaching about the condition, and provide written materials and referrals as needed. *Parents may need information repeated so they can cope with the necessary adjustments at home, learn about the disorder, and follow up appropriately.*

EVALUATING

Evaluate airway patency by assessing the child's color, oxygen saturation, and respirations. The effectiveness of seizure medications is evaluated by recording the number, frequency, and type of seizures that occur. Evaluate for respiratory infection, malnutrition, constipation, and skin breakdown due to altered mobility. Watch family interaction with the child to determine the degree of their acceptance of the child's physical and mental limitations.

NURSING PROCESS CARE PLAN
Child with Cerebral Palsy

Daniel, a 9-year-old with CP, has moved to a different city and will begin school in several weeks at a public elementary school. Daniel's parents, his pediatrician, and the school nurse meet to develop a plan to manage Daniel's health care while he is at school. The pediatrician tells the school nurse that Daniel is taking antiseizure medication but that the medication is not yet regulated. Daniel continues to have seizures approximately two times a week. Daniel's mom states that Daniel has fallen out of his wheelchair during seizures lately. However, he has not been injured during these falls.

Assessment
- Taking antiseizure medication
- Seizures twice weekly
- Falls during seizure activity
- Medical diagnosis—cerebral palsy

Nursing Diagnosis. The following important nursing diagnosis (among others) is established for this client:

- Risk for Trauma related to seizure activity

Expected Outcomes. No sign of trauma following seizure activity.

Planning and Implementation
- Teach school staff to recognize and manage seizures. *Daniel's safety will increase if all staff have proper training in management of seizure activity.*
- Have oxygen and suction equipment available. *Seizures may cause hypoxia and/or airway obstruction.*
- Administer antiseizure medications as prescribed. *Proper administration of medication will assist in preventing seizure activity.*
- Teach Daniel to report aural warning promptly. *Aural warning may predict seizure activity and allow staff to better manage the seizure.*
- Consider protective headgear for Daniel. *The headgear may protect Daniel's head from injury.*
- Emphasize to the staff the importance of remaining with Daniel during the entire seizure. *Physical safety can be managed better, and documentation of events can be achieved.*

- Avoid restraining Daniel during the seizure. *Restraint may cause physical injury.*
- If necessary, use a chin-lift maneuver to open Daniel's airway during the seizure. *This maneuver maintains patent airway and prevents hypoxia.*
- Following the seizure, reassure Daniel and monitor neurologic status. *Return to expected neurologic status indicates that the seizure is over.*
- Clearly document the seizure activity. *Management of the seizure activity is facilitated with correct documentation of aura, type and duration of movement, changes in level of consciousness, eye movement, pupil size, bowel and bladder incontinence, and teeth clenching.*

Evaluation. In children with seizure activity, evaluate orientation and LOC regularly. Slight changes in these findings should be reported promptly. The nurse can evaluate the child's environment to determine the safety risk and make suggestions for improving the environment.

Critical Thinking Questions

1. What other physical challenges would the school nurse have in managing Daniel's case?
2. What social challenges will Daniel meet as he enters a new school with a disability?
3. What can the school nurse do to help Daniel overcome these social challenges?

Note: Discussion of Critical Thinking questions appears in Appendix I.

Note: The references and resources for this and all chapters have been compiled at the back of the book.

Chapter Review

 **KEY TERMS** by Topic

Use the audio glossary feature of either the CD-ROM or the Companion Website to hear the correct pronunciation of the following key terms.

Anatomy and Physiology
ganglia, neurons, axon, cell body, dendrite, myelin sheath, organogenesis, cranium, somatic reflexes, autonomic reflexes, sympathetic nervous system, parasympathetic nervous system

Pain
nociceptors

Congenital Neurologic Defects
spina bifida, neural tube, meningocele, myelomeningocele

Nervous System Disorders
seizures, epilepsy, status epilepticus, focal seizures, generalized seizures, aura, postictal, fibromyalgia

Nervous System Infections
meningitis, encephalitis, Reye's syndrome, Guillain–Barré syndrome (postinfectious polyneuritis)

Neurologic Trauma
closed head injury, concussion, drowning, near-drowning

Mental Retardation
mental retardation, simian crease, Brushfield spots

Eye Disorders
PERRLA, acute conjunctivitis

Eye Injuries
hyphema

Visual Impairment
hyperopia, myopia, astigmatism, strabismus, esotropia, exotropia, hypertropia, orthoptics, amblyopia, dyslexia, cataracts, nystagmus, glaucoma, epiphora, buphthalmos, photophobia, tonometer, goniotomy

Ear Disorders
tinnitus, cochlear implants, otitis media, otalgia, myringotomy

KEY Points

- Neurologic assessments include assessing for level of consciousness (LOC) and verbal and motor response to stimuli.

- Early signs of increased ICP are headache, vomiting, LOC changes, asymmetric pupils, and seizures. In the infant, a high-pitched cry, bulging fontanels, dilated scalp veins, and irritability may be noted. Later signs include significant changes in LOC, respiratory distress, bradycardia, increased systolic blood pressure, fixed and dilated pupils, and death.

- In the child verbal expressions of pain include crying, moaning, groaning, or screaming. Nonverbal expressions include facial grimacing, posturing, splinting, restlessness, and sleep disturbances.

- During a seizure, the first priority is to establish a safe environment for the child. Immediately following the seizure, position the child on the side, remove mucus and drainage from the airway, and assess for airway patency.

- The Snellen letter chart, picture chart, and E chart are available to screen for visual acuity.

Animations

Otitis media	Child's ear
Culture of deafness	Adolescent ear
Trauma	Middle ear
Conjunctivitis	Down syndrome

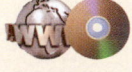 FOR FURTHER Study

See Chapter 2 for legal information.

See Figure 4-2C for trisomy 21, also called Down syndrome.

Information on the Apgar score is provided in Chapter 7; the Apgar scoring system is shown in Table 7-4; Figure 7-10 illustrates birth positions.

See Table 8-4 for a description of maternal infections that can be passed on to the fetus prenatally.

See Chapter 9 for more on congenital anomalies; Figure 9-16 illustrates neonatal fontanels.

Shaken-baby syndrome is discussed in Chapters 10 and 27.

See Chapter 13 for procedures for pain assessment, head circumference, irrigating eye and ear, and positioning for lumbar puncture.

A PCA pump is illustrated in Figure 14-11.

Congenital heart disorders are discussed in Chapter 19.

Chapter 26 discusses communicable diseases and Reye's syndrome.

Chapter 27 discusses thought process disorders, fetal alcohol syndrome, child abuse, and shaken-baby syndrome.

The Health Promotion Issue in Chapter 28 discusses organ donation in a dying child.

Denver Developmental Screening Test II is Appendix IV, and basic sign language is in Appendix VI.

EXPLORE MediaLink

Additional interactive resources for this chapter can be found on the Companion Website at www.prenhall.com/towle.

Click on Chapter 16 and "Begin" to select the activities for this chapter.

For chapter-related NCLEX-style questions and an audio glossary, access the accompanying CD-ROM in this book.

Caring for a Client with Meningitis

NCLEX-PN® Focus Area: Safety

Case Study: Jessie is a 4-year-old female who developed a fever, anorexia, and vomiting, and complains of pain in her neck. Jessie attends day care Monday through Friday while her mother works at the bank. Several of the children in her class have been ill. Her big brother is in second grade. Jessie's mom calls the pediatrician's office to ask for advice on caring for her child.

Nursing Diagnosis: Risk for Infection

COLLECT DATA

Subjective	Objective
_____	_____
_____	_____
_____	_____
_____	_____
_____	_____

Would you report this? Yes/No

If yes, to: _____

Nursing Care

_____
_____
_____
_____
_____
_____
_____
_____
_____
_____
_____
_____

How would you document this? _____
_____
_____
_____

Compare your documentation to the sample provided in Appendix I.

Data Collected
(use those that apply)

- Vital signs: T 101.4, P 70, R 12, BP 90/60
- Pain level: 8 using Oucher scale
- Jessie states, "My tummy hurts right here."
- Positive Brudzinski's sign
- Weight: 29 lb
- Mom states, "She is very irritable."
- 24-hour diet history: two crackers, 50 mL Pedialyte
- Emesis: 30 mL green vomitus ×1
- Mom states, "Several children in her class at day care are sick with the same thing."
- Positive Kernig's sign

Nursing Interventions
(use those that apply; list in priority order)

- Teach mom signs and symptoms of infection and when to seek medical attention.
- Record intake and output.
- Monitor CBC values for signs of infection.
- Review immunization record.
- Assess for Kernig's and Brudzinski's signs.
- Monitor pain levels for changes.
- Identify comfort measures that decrease the child's pain level.
- Administer pain medications as ordered.
- Discuss ways to prevent transmission of bacteria, including hand washing techniques and isolating the child from other sick children.
- Monitor vital signs for subtle changes.

NCLEX-PN® Exam Preparation

1 A 10-month-old is admitted to the hospital with possible meningitis. An IV has been started in her left forearm, and a restraint is being used to prevent interference with the IV infusion. Her aunt has come to stay with her for the afternoon and asks if the restraint can be removed. The nurse's best response is:

1. "It can only be removed with a doctor's order."
2. "It can be removed only if you are staying in the room."
3. "It needs to be kept on at all times."
4. "It can be removed only if the nurse is in the room."

2 A child has an order for acetaminophen (Tylenol) 240 mg PO. The label on the bottle reads 160 mg/5 mL. How many milliliter should be administered to the child?

3 Seeing his son with spina bifida for the first time, a father exclaims, "What is that on his back!" An appropriate response would be:

1. completely describing the condition, including long-term complications.
2. defining the term "spina bifida" and providing a simple explanation of the anomaly.
3. directing his attention away from the defect.
4. saying, "I don't know. I'll have the doctor call you."

4 The nurse is assessing the infant for signs and symptoms of pain following circumcision. Choose all of the following symptoms that could be indicators of pain.

1. facial grimacing, tachycardia
2. bradypnea, flushing
3. pupil dilation, restlessness
4. tachypnea, anorexia
5. sleepiness, bradycardia

5 The physician orders phenobarbital IV 20 mg/kg/day for the infant with status epilepticus. Available is phenobarbital 30 mg/mL. How many total milliliter will the nurse give for the infant who weighs 7 lb 5 oz?

6 The nurse is preparing to test the visual acuity of a 2-year-old female client using a Snellen chart. The nurse performs the test knowing that which of the following identifies the accurate procedure for this type of visual acuity testing for 2-year-olds?

1. The child is held by her mother at approximately 40 ft from the chart.
2. Both eyes are tested at the same time, and then the left eye is tested first followed by the right eye.

3. The child is held by her mother at approximately 30 ft from the chart and asked to identify the characters on the chart that can be read from 200 ft away.
4. The right eye is tested first, then the left eye, and then both eyes are tested together.

7 A nurse is caring for a client with Reye's syndrome. The nurse realizes the client's father understands the teaching about this syndrome when he makes the following comment:

1. "I am going to give my son Pepto-Bismol if he has an upset stomach."
2. "I realize I will have to check labels to make sure we don't give our son anything containing aspirin or aspirin-like products."
3. "I understand that Reye's syndrome was caused by a bacteria."
4. "I will give my son Triaminicin for his next cold."

8 The nurse is helping with a lumbar puncture for a 6-year-old client with suspected Guillain–Barré syndrome. The nurse places the client in which of the following positions?

1. prone knee-chest position
2. supine
3. lateral position, with the knees flexed up to the abdomen, back bowed at the edge of the bed, and chin resting on the chest
4. immobilized, with the client on a spinal backboard to prevent movement during the procedure

9 The nurse is instituting seizure precautions for a 3-year-old client being admitted from the emergency department with a closed head injury and suspected concussion. Which of the following nursing interventions would the nurse avoid in planning for this client's safety?

1. keeping airway, suction and oxygen equipment at the bedside
2. taping a padded tongue blade at the head of the bed
3. padding the side rails of the bed
4. having IV equipment ready for quick insertion of an IV line

10 The nurse is caring for a client newly diagnosed with cerebral palsy (CP). The parents are overwhelmed and ask the nurse about CP. The nurse responds to the parents based on the understanding that CP is:

1. an infection of the central nervous system.
2. a virus that causes an inflammation of the brain.
3. a congenital condition resulting in severe mental retardation.
4. a chronic disability that is characterized by difficulty in controlling muscles.

Answers for Review Questions, as well as discussion of Care Plan and Critical Thinking Care Map questions, appear in Appendix I.

Chapter 17

Care of the Child with Musculoskeletal Disorders

BRIEF Outline

Anatomy and Physiology
Brief Assessment Overview
Congenital Skeletal Defects
Musculoskeletal Disorders

Musculoskeletal Trauma
Musculoskeletal Infection
Musculoskeletal Tumors
Nursing Care

LEARNING Outcomes

After completing this chapter, you will be able to:

- Discuss the anatomy and physiology of the pediatric musculoskeletal system.
- Describe musculoskeletal disorders to include developmental hip dysplasia, scoliosis, muscular dystrophy, osteomyelitis, osteosarcoma, and musculoskeletal injuries.
- Discuss clinical manifestations, diagnostic procedures, and medical management related to musculoskeletal disorders.
- Explain appropriate nursing interventions for children with musculoskeletal disorders.

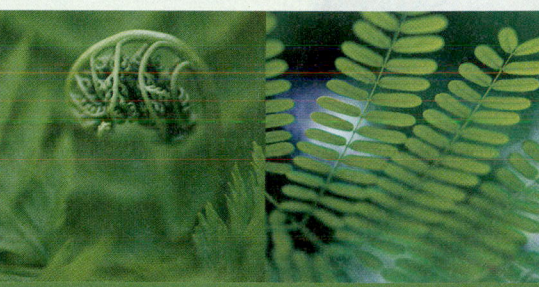

HEALTH PROMOTION ISSUE:
Children and Body Building

NURSING PROCESS CARE PLAN:
The Child with an Amputation

CRITICAL THINKING CARE MAP:
Caring for a Child with a Fracture

The muscular system at birth is essentially complete, except for the growth in length and circumference of muscle that occurs as the child ages. Skeletal growth, however, is extensive during the period of childhood and adolescence. For example, Figure 17-1 ■ illustrates changes in the hand from infant to adult.

Anatomy and Physiology

MUSCLES

There are three types of muscles in the body: cardiac, smooth, and skeletal. Skeletal muscles are typically voluntary and striated. These striated muscles assist in movement and maintaining posture. Tendons attach bones to muscles and also continue to grow in length as the child ages. The focus in this chapter is skeletal muscles.

SKELETON

Ossification or bone formation is almost complete at birth. Fontanels connect the cranial bones at birth (see Chapter 9 ⊙⊙). However, the long bones of a child's body continue to grow until he or she reaches adulthood at age 20 or 21.

The three sections of the long bone (Figure 17-2 ■) are the epiphysis, metaphysis, and diaphysis. The **epiphysis** is the attachment site for muscles and the site for ossification. The **epiphyseal plate** or *growth plate* remains open until late adolescence. Injuries to this area during childhood may affect the growth of the bone. This tissue can also be affected by nutrition and hormone levels, particularly growth hormone. There are some variations in bone mass and density related to race (Box 17-1 ■).

The **metaphysis** is responsible for converting new cartilage into bone. The **diaphysis** contains the medullary cavity, where **hematopoiesis** (production of blood cells) occurs. Fat is also stored in the medullary or *marrow*).

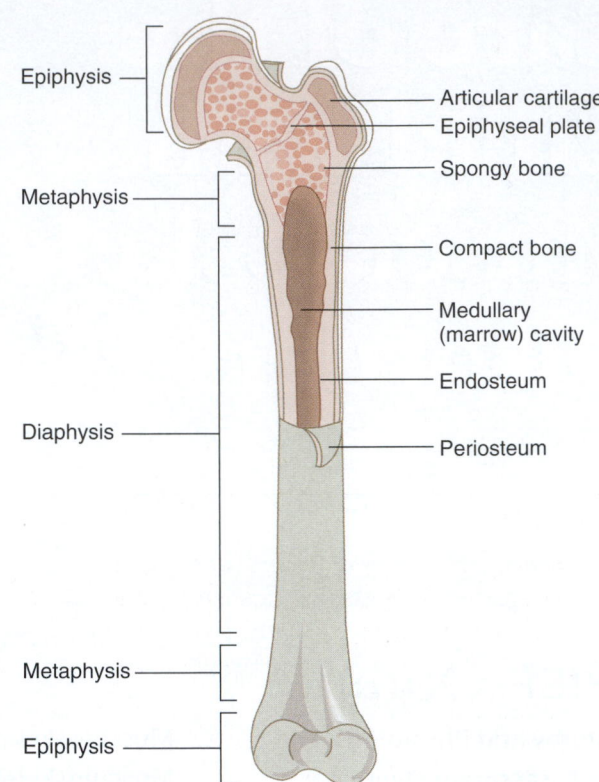

Figure 17-2. ■ The three sections of the long bone are the epiphysis, metaphysis, and diaphysis. Note the *growth plate* or *epiphyseal plate* near the top of the illustration.

Long bones in children are porous and less dense than in adults. Injuries to the long bone can therefore result in a bend or buckle in addition to a break. The bending or buckling of a long bone is called a **greenstick fracture** (discussed later in this chapter). During periods of rapid growth of long bones, the child may complain of aching or pain in the bones. Commonly called *growing pains,* this discomfort is the result of the stretching of muscles as the bone is growing.

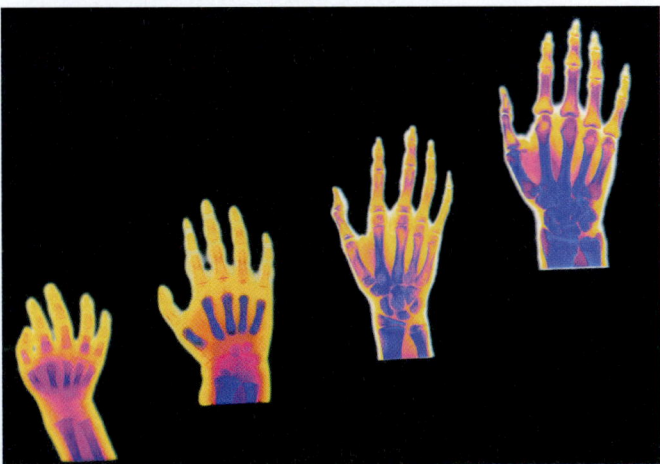

Figure 17-1. ■ These images show the remarkable development of bone as children grow. (Photo: © Salisbury District Hospital/Science Photo Library/Photo Researchers, Inc.)

BOX 17-1	CULTURAL PULSE POINTS

Variations in Musculoskeletal System by Ethnicity or Race

Children of Hindu heritage are at risk for osteomalacia. This disease is typically the result of calcium and vitamin D deficiency. In contrast, children of African heritage tend to have greater bone density.

Indians, as well as Ethiopians and Algerians, are at risk for a disease called lathyrism. *Lathyrism* (Stedman, 1997) is a disorder associated with a diet high in certain plants (vetches, khasari, and allied species). Its manifestations include paralysis of the leg muscles, rendering the child crippled.

Localized and inbred populations of Amish (a religious community) are at risk for *dwarfism* (the condition of being abnormally undersized).

MediaLink   ● Skeleton

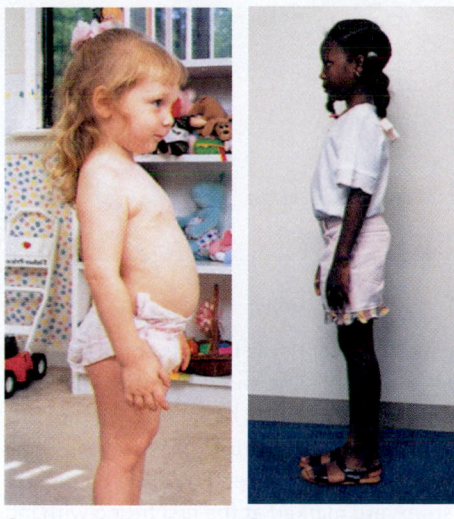

A   **B**

Figure 17-3. ■ Posture. (**A**) The infant's posture changes from a straight spine at about 10 to 15 months to the protruding abdomen and lumbar lordosis shown here in a toddler. (**B**) The school-age child has two curves in the spine that balance each other: thoracic (convex) and lumbar (concave) curves.

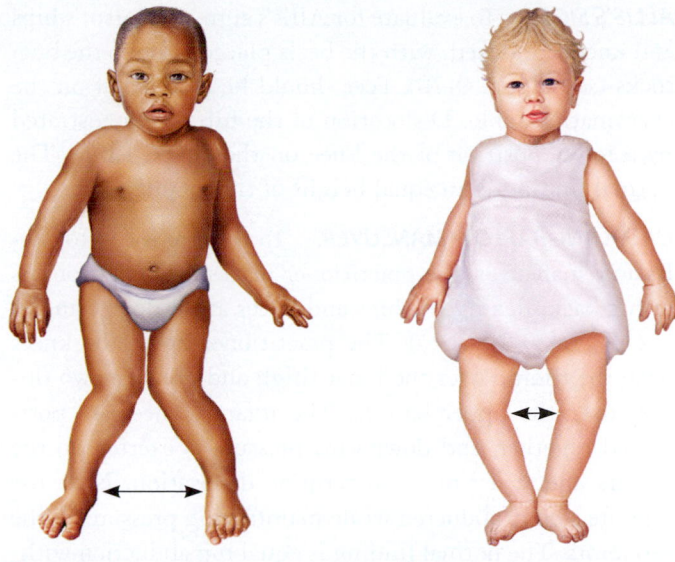

A   **B**

Figure 17-4. ■ (**A**) Genu valgum, or knock-knees. Note that the ankles are far apart while the knees are together. (**B**) Genu varum, or bowlegs. The legs are bowed so the knees are far apart as the child stands. This second condition is often associated with vitamin D deficiency (rickets) or Blount's disease if the genu varum persists beyond 2 years of age.

Postural changes occur as the child ages (Figure 17-3 ■). Prior to birth, the thoracic and sacral areas of the spine are convex curves. When the infant can hold his or her head up, the cervical area becomes concave. Then as the child learns to stand, the lumbar area also becomes concave.

The arch of a newborn's foot is absent. It normally develops gradually during the preschool years. The child may appear to have knock-knees (**genu valgum**) (Figure 17-4 ■). This condition usually resolves by late childhood or early adolescence. Infants may appear to have bow legs (**genu varum**). Yet, this usually resolves as the child begins to walk. Further evaluation would be needed if these conditions do not resolve within the expected time frame.

Brief Assessment Overview

HISTORY

- With infants, review the history of birth. A child who experienced trauma or hypoxia during the birthing process may develop musculoskeletal difficulties.
- Obtain information on injuries to bones and muscles, such as the nature of the injury and treatment.
- Inquire about deformities of limbs, spine, and fingers or toes.
- Determine the child's activity level, including participation in sports activities.
- Inquire about developmental delays.

PHYSICAL

- Inspect posture and gait.
- Note symmetry of shoulders and hips and any unusual curvature of the spine.
- Assess for full range of motion (ROM) of joints.
- Assess muscle strength.

Congenital Skeletal Defects

Skeletal defects can be minor and easy to correct, or they can be major malformations requiring long-term therapy. These defects are rarely life threatening. However, they require correction, if possible, in order for normal support and movement to occur. Two common defects are discussed here: developmental dysplasia of the hip (DDH) and clubfoot.

DEVELOPMENTAL DYSPLASIA OF THE HIP

DDH is a developmental abnormality of the femoral head (ball), acetabulum (socket), or both.

Manifestations

DDH is displayed by partial or complete dislocation of the hip joint. This results in shortening of the femur, uneven thigh and gluteal folds, and limited abduction on the affected side.

Diagnosis

DDH is usually diagnosed by physical exam during the newborn assessment, but at times it may be identified later. These assessments include Allis's sign and the Ortolani–Barlow maneuver.

ALLIS'S SIGN. To evaluate for Allis's sign, the infant's hips and knees are flexed, with the heels placed close to the buttocks (see Figure 9-20). Feet should be placed flat on the examination table. Dislocation of the hip is demonstrated by a lower position of the knee on the affected side. The normal finding is an equal height of the infant's knees.

ORTOLANI–BARLOW MANEUVER. To perform the Ortolani–Barlow maneuver, the practitioner places the infant on his or her back, flexing the hips and knees at 90-degree angles (see Figure 9-20 ⚭). The practitioner holds the knees with the thumb over the inner thigh and the first two fingers over the upper femurs. The infant's knees are positioned together, and downward pressure is exerted on the femurs one at a time to determine dislocation. Next the hips are slowly abducted while maintaining pressure on the hip joints. The normal finding is equal hip abduction without resistance. Resistance or a clunking sound or movement indicates hip dislocation. LPNs/LVNs may be trained in this maneuver. If the LPN/LVN notices a hip click, the practitioner should be informed.

If the child is ambulatory, a notable limp is present. Box 17-2 ■ identifies signs of DDH. Symptoms and prognosis worsen when left untreated.

Treatment

Treatment of DDH should begin as soon as possible. If only a small amount of abnormality is present, triple diapering is used to support the hip in abduction, until ligaments are strong enough to maintain hip alignment permanently. If more support is needed, a Pavlik harness (Figure 17-5 ■) is commonly used for 3 to 4 months. Skin traction is used for older children. If the harness is unsuccessful, surgery followed by a **hip spica cast** (a cast covering the upper thighs and lower torso) may be necessary.

Nursing Considerations

The nursing care of children with DDH includes maintaining traction through triple diapering, the Pavlik harness, or skin traction, and providing cast care. Procedures for these nursing actions appear later in this chapter in the Musculoskeletal Trauma section.

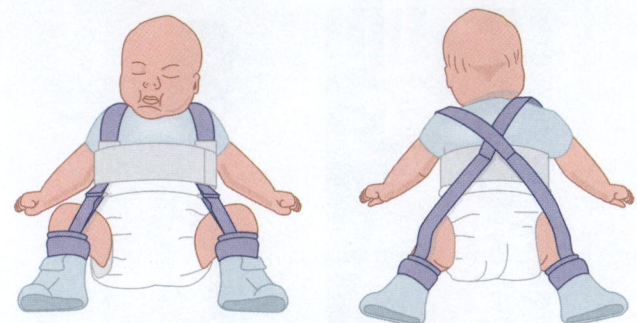

Figure 17-5. ■ Steps for Pavlik harness application. (1) Position the chest halter at nipple line and fasten with Velcro. (2) Position the legs and feet in the stirrups, being sure the hips are flexed and abducted. Fasten with Velcro. (3) Connect the chest halter and leg straps in front. (4) Connect the chest halter and leg straps in back. All straps are marked at the first fitting with indelible ink so they can be reattached easily after the harness is rinsed and dried.

Immobility and the resulting complications are a hazard to children with DDH. The nurse should frequently assess lung sounds, neurovascular symptoms, and skin. Children with a cast should change positions at least every 2 hours. Pillows can assist in positioning the child comfortably. Covering rough edges of the cast with moleskin or tape (called *petaling*) can protect the child's skin from injury. To enhance the child's bladder and bowel function, the nurse should encourage a diet high in fiber with adequate intake of fluids.

TALIPES (CLUBFOOT)

Talipes or clubfoot is a congenital, unilateral or bilateral twisting of the foot, usually inward (Figure 17-6 ■).

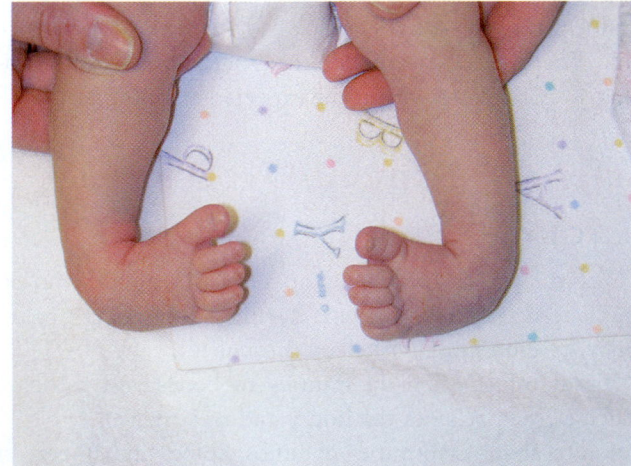

Figure 17-6. ■ Clubfoot, with the midfoot directed downward, the hindfoot turned inward, and the forefoot curled toward the heel and upward. This condition is corrected surgically.
(Shea, MD/Custom Medical Stock Photo, Inc.)

BOX 17-2	ASSESSMENT

Developmental Dysplasia of the Hip

The following are signs of developmental dysplasia of the hip:

- Hip click with abduction (Ortolani–Barlow maneuver)
- Asymmetric thigh folds
- Uneven knee level (Allis's sign)
- Limited hip abduction

Manifestations

The foot cannot easily be moved into alignment due to deformity in three areas of the foot:

- The equines or midfoot is directed downward.
- The varus or hindfoot turns inward.
- The forefoot curls toward the heel and upward.

The clubfoot is usually smaller than the other foot, and the child has a shortened Achilles tendon. The muscles of the lower leg are atrophied.

Diagnosis

Talipes is diagnosed by observation of symptoms and confirmed by x-ray.

Treatment

Nonsurgical treatment involves moving the foot into correct alignment and applying a cast to hold the foot in the corrected position. The cast is changed every 1 to 2 weeks for about 3 months until alignment is achieved. Failure to achieve alignment could result in the need for surgical correction.

clinical ALERT

Infants can be frightened by the noise of a cast cutter. Thus, the nurse, in consultation with the physician, can suggest that the parents remove a plaster cast prior to the office visit when indicated. The cast can be removed easily by soaking it in a warm bath until it disintegrates. Encourage the parents to bathe the skin thoroughly after the cast is removed. Note that cast removal must be approved by the physician.

A bottle, pacifier, or familiar toy can provide distraction during cast application. Depending on the age of the child, earphones to a battery-operated CD or MP3 player may be provided to listen to music while the cast is being removed. (Regular radios should never be used in proximity to water because of the risk of electrocution.)

Nursing Considerations

The nurse is responsible for assisting with cast application (see description in the Musculoskeletal Trauma section of this chapter). Proper cast care is taught to the parents. If the child has surgery, the nurse is responsible for pain management. Observation for drainage and bleeding from the surgical site is also essential.

Musculoskeletal Disorders

Musculoskeletal disorders are some of the most common disorders affecting the older child. Their frequency is due partly to changes in bone structure during periods of rapid growth and partly to accidents as the child interacts with the environment.

MUSCULAR DYSTROPHY

Muscular dystrophy (MD) is a group of inherited diseases that cause muscle degeneration and wasting. There are several kinds of MD, but the most common form affecting children is Duchenne's muscular dystrophy. This sex-linked recessive disorder is carried by mothers and passed to their sons.

Manifestations

The onset of symptoms occurs in the first 3 to 4 years of life. The child with MD generally appears normal for the first year, but walking may be delayed. The child gradually gains enough muscle strength to walk but tires easily, especially when running or climbing. As muscles degenerate over time, the child trips and falls frequently, develops a waddling gait, and may walk on the toes. A classic symptom is a positive Gower's maneuver, in which the child uses the upper extremities to lift up from the floor. Figure 17-7 ■ illustrates a positive *Gower's maneuver*. Most children are wheelchair bound by age 12, and death from respiratory paralysis occurs during adolescence.

In examining the child with MD, the calf muscles appear to hypertrophy, but they are actually enlarged due to increased fatty tissue. As the chest muscles waste, the child will develop scoliosis, respiratory difficulty, and the inability to sit upright. Swallowing may be affected, leading to respiratory infection and malnutrition.

Diagnosis

Diagnosis of MD is made by observation of clinical manifestations. Serum creatine kinase will be elevated. A muscle biopsy is used to measure levels of dystrophin, which will be low. Electromyography, which measures electrical activity of skeletal muscles at rest and during voluntary muscle contractions, will show activity at rest and increased voluntary muscle contractions.

Treatment

There is no cure for muscular dystrophy. Deformities of the chest, including scoliosis, may need to be corrected surgically to promote adequate respiration. Respiratory infections must also be treated promptly. Physical therapy is implemented to maintain ROM. However, the use of braces and wheelchairs may be necessary.

Nursing Considerations

The goals of nursing care are to prevent complications, promote independence for as long as possible, and support the family in dealing with this progressive, incapacitating, and ultimately fatal disease. Nursing interventions may include

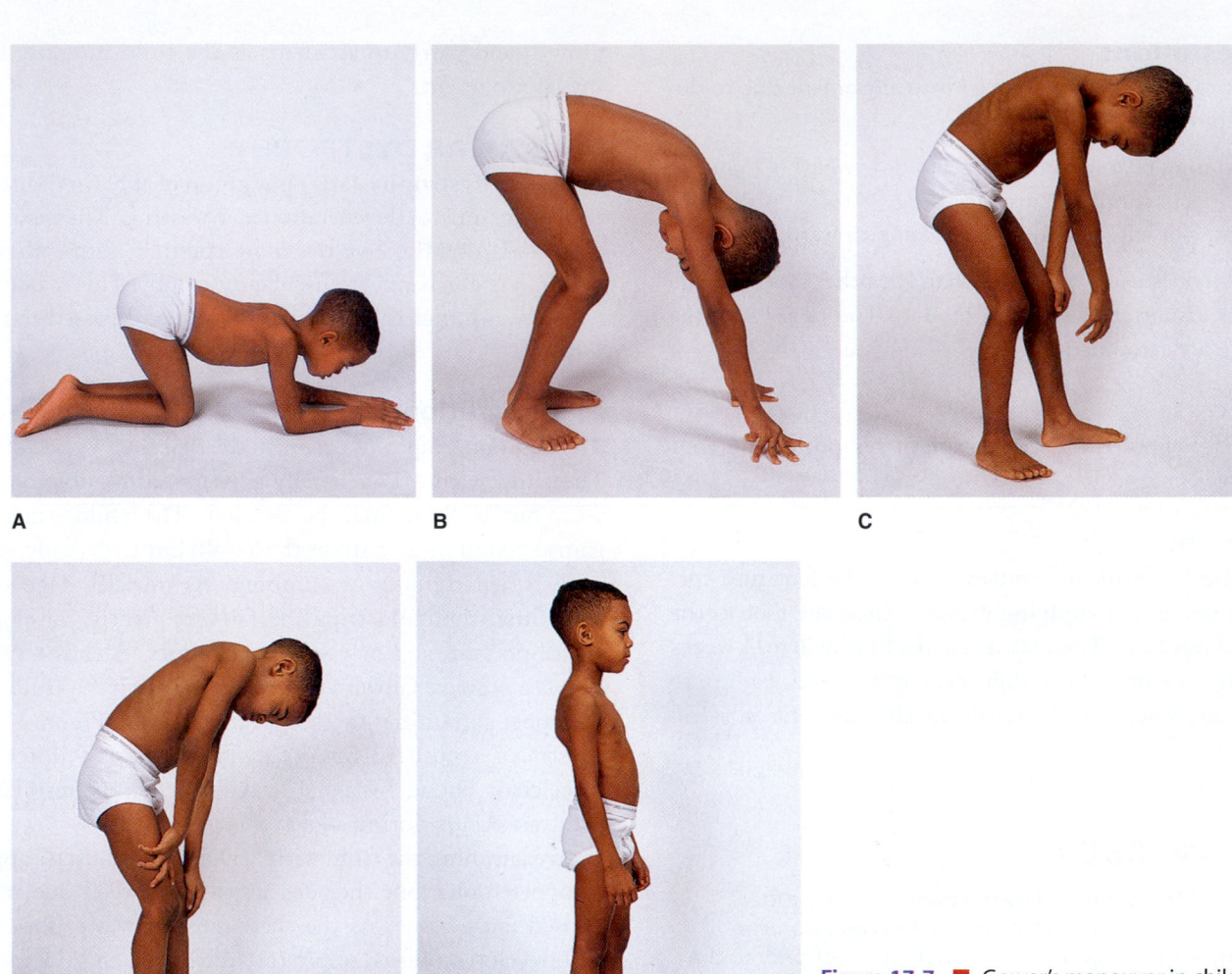

Figure 17-7. ■ Gower's maneuver in child with muscular dystrophy. (**A** and **B**) The child first maneuvers to a position supported by arms and legs. (**C**) The child pushes off the floor and rests one hand on the knee. (**D** and **E**) The child pushes the body up straight.

oxygen administration, respiratory therapy, administration of medications, tube feeding, monitoring for signs of infection, and preventing skin breakdown. Parents will need a lot of support and will need to be taught how to offer support to their child. The nurse can help the child and family design a plan of active and passive ROM exercise. They can be taught the advantages of controlling weight gain within the normal limits with a low-calorie, high-protein, and high-fiber diet, and they can be taught to drink plenty of fluids to prevent constipation. It also is important to refer the family to appropriate resources and support groups.

The child's development should be assessed periodically. Parents, teachers, therapists, and nurses should meet to devise plans to meet the child's learning and developmental needs. The focus should be on what the child *can do* instead of what the child *cannot do.*

LEGG–CALVÉ–PERTHES DISEASE

Legg–Calvé–Perthes disease is a self-limiting condition in which the circulation to the femoral head is interrupted. The femoral head dies from lack of blood supply, which gradually returns as healing occurs. The necrotic bone is reabsorbed and replaced with vascularized granulation tissue. In approximately 3 years, ossification occurs, forming a new femoral head.

The cause of Legg–Calvé–Perthes disease is unknown, but it is believed to occur following mild trauma. The disorder could be unilateral or bilateral. Boys between the ages of 4 and 8 are most commonly affected (Figure 17-8 ■). People of African and Chinese descent have a lower incidence of the disease.

Manifestations

Symptoms may be present for several months before the parents seek medical assistance. Early symptoms include

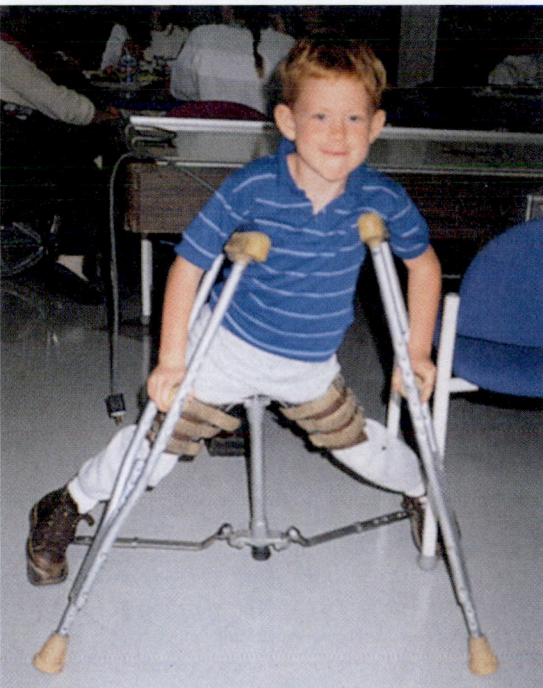

Figure 17-8. ■ Toronto brace used for Legg–Calvé–Perthes disease. This young boy needs to use crutches to be able to walk in the Toronto brace for treatment of Perthes disease.

BOX 17-3	CLIENT TEACHING

School-Age Children with Braces

School-age children are energetic and industrious. It is important to promote these developmental characteristics in children who must wear a brace. The nurse must ensure that the child is able to move and ambulate before discharge from the health care facility. Use the following suggestions when teaching children and their parents how to redirect the child's energy.

Fine Motor Skills

- Encourage journaling about the experience of this disease.
- Teach the child a new craft, such as beaded jewelry.
- Supply the child with art supplies and encourage drawing or painting.

Gross Motor Skills

- Teach the child to ride a horse.
- Join the YMCA and go swimming several times a week.
- Encourage the child to learn to play Ping-Pong or pool.

Cognitive Activities

- Supply the child with educational computer activities.
- Encourage reading or listening to books on tape.
- Challenge the child to competitions such as learning the capitals of the 50 states, memorizing the presidents in order, or memorizing Bible verses.

mild hip and anterior thigh pain and a limp. The symptoms are worse with activity and relieved by rest. The child favors the leg and limits movement to decrease the pain. As the disease progresses, muscle wasting and decreased mobility occur. The affected thigh will be 2 to 3 cm smaller in diameter than the unaffected thigh.

Diagnosis

Diagnosis is made by reviewing symptoms, x-rays, bone scans, and magnetic resonance imaging (MRI) scans.

Treatment

The medical treatment is directed at relieving pain, and holding the femoral head in place while healing occurs. The femoral head is held abducted with internal rotation by use of a Toronto (see Figure 17-8) or a Scottish-Rite brace. These braces hold the hip in place and support the weight of the child on the ischium. The child should wear the braces for 23 hours a day.

Nursing Considerations

Nurses are involved in teaching parents how to apply the braces, monitoring for signs of skin breakdown under the braces, and providing skin care to prevent skin breakdown. The child will learn to ambulate with the braces but may need crutches to help with balance.

Helping the child and family deal with the long-term nature of the treatment may be a challenge for the nurse.

Because the disease occurs at an age when the child is very active, the limitations of the brace cause stress to the child and family. Parents should be given suggestions to help direct the child's energy within the limitations of the brace (Box 17-3 ■). The child should return to school as soon as possible.

Follow-up visits are arranged at regular intervals to evaluate the healing process and make adjustments to the brace as the child grows. Toward the end of treatment, the child may be allowed periods of limited exercise without the brace. Activities such as swimming can increase muscle strength without stressing the growing bone. Prognosis is good as long as the femoral head is contained. If treatment is delayed or the child and family are noncompliant with the treatment plan, there is a high probability of permanent deformity and arthritis later in life.

SCOLIOSIS

Scoliosis is a lateral S- or C-shaped curve of the spine, with rotation of the spine and ribs. Scoliosis is more common in girls between 10 and 13 years of age than in other groups. It is also associated with other musculoskeletal and nervous system deformities. Most commonly, there is a right-sided thoracic curve and a left-sided lumbar curve.

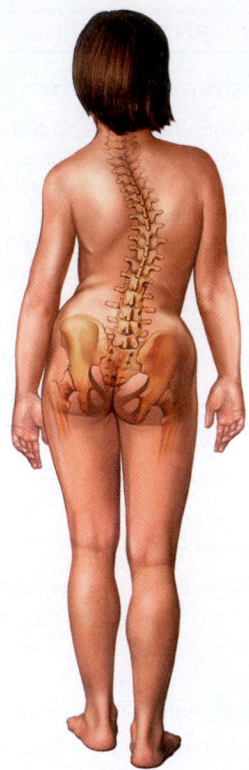

Figure 17-9. ■ Scoliosis, showing deviation of the spine to the left. (Nucleus Medical Art, Inc./Alamy)

Manifestations

Symptoms of scoliosis develop slowly and without pain. In assessing the back, the shoulders and hips are different heights (Figure 17-9 ■), causing the clothing to hang unevenly. Rotation of the vertebrae and ribs causes a one-sided rib hump and a prominent scapula. The assessment includes comparing the level of the right and left hip and shoulders. The child is also asked to bend forward, and the posterior chest is inspected for symmetry. The school nurse routinely assesses many children for scoliosis.

Diagnosis

Moire photography—wavelike patterns projected onto the client's back to highlight asymmetry of bony landmarks—can be used to document the degree of asymmetry in the spine. If scoliosis is suspected, the child is referred for spinal x-ray and follow-up care.

Treatment

The goal of treatment is to limit or stop the progression of spinal deformity. The method of treatment depends on the degree of curvature. Mild scoliosis can be treated with exercise to increase muscle tone and flexibility and to improve posture. See Health Promotion Issue on pages 558 and 559. Chiropractic adjustments may be used to realign vertebrae if there is a mild degree of curvature

(Box 17-4 ■). A Boston or Milwaukee brace is used to treat moderate scoliosis. These braces are custom fit for the child and should be worn 23 hours a day. During the hour without the brace, the child may bathe, shower, or take part in activities that the brace would restrict. Unless otherwise instructed by the physician, the child is not prohibited from participating in sports activities (Hart, 2003).

Severe scoliosis requires surgery to fuse the spine and insert rods or wires to straighten the spine. A halo brace (Figure 17-10 ■) may be used after surgery to hold the body in

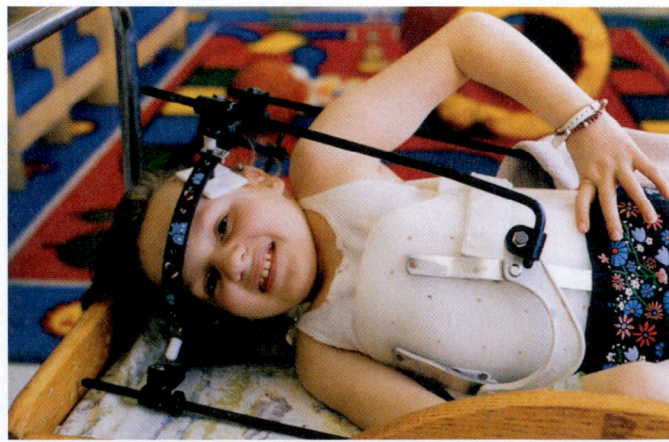

Figure 17-10. ■ In severe scoliosis, the child may wear a halo brace, shown here, to hold the body in position after surgery.

TABLE 17-1

Spinal Curvatures

CONDITION	DIAGNOSIS AND TREATMENT	NURSING INTERVENTIONS
Lordosis: excessive concave curvature of the lumbar spine	Diagnosis: Look at child from side. Observe lumbar curve. Confirm with spinal x-ray. Treatment: Exercises and postural awareness. Chiropractic therapy.	Encourage physical conditioning exercises. Reassure family that condition may be outgrown as child matures.
Kyphosis: excessive convex curvature of thoracic spine	Diagnosis: Have child bend forward at waist. Look at thoracic spine at level of scapula. Confirm with x-ray. Treatment: Mild condition requires exercise, moderate condition requires bracing, severe condition requires surgery. Chiropractic therapy.	Encourage strengthening exercises and posture awareness. Teach brace application and postoperative care. Help deal with altered body image.
Scoliosis: "S" curve of the spine, often with rotation of spine and hips	Diagnosis: Observe back for deformity, uneven scapula and hips, uneven rib cage. Confirmed with x-ray. Treatment: Mild condition (10–20 degrees) requires exercise, chiropractic therapy. Moderate condition (20–40 degrees) requires bracing in addition to exercise. Severe condition (40 degrees or more) requires surgery with spinal fusion.	Promote compliance with treatment plan. Encourage diligence with exercise plan. Provide emotional support for child and family. Teach brace application and care. Teach postoperative care.
Torticollis: tilt of the head caused by rotation of the cervical spine	Diagnosis: Observe position of head and rotation of cervical spine. Treatment: Surgery, heat application, immobilization of the neck in the correct position.	Encourage physical conditioning exercises. Provide emotional support for child and family. Instruct in proper use of the immobilization device.

alignment. The surgery consists of spinal fusion, possible bone grafting, and insertion of permanent wires to stabilize the spine. Some surgeons may perform the surgery laparoscopically.

Postoperatively, the child will remain on bed rest during recovery. Once the child is able to get up, a plastic anterior and posterior shell is used to stabilize the back until healing is complete. The rod permanently immobilizes the spine, preventing the child from bending forward.

Scoliosis screening is routinely completed when the child is in the fifth and seventh grades. Any indication of scoliosis is discussed with the parents. If scoliosis is detected, treatment should begin immediately to slow or stop the progression. Follow-up evaluations would be made at regular intervals.

OTHER SPINAL CURVATURES

Three other spinal curvatures warrant mention. **Kyphosis,** excessive convex curvature of the thoracic spine, is also know as *hunchback.* **Lordosis,** or *sway back,* is an excessive concave curvature of the lumbar spine. Frequently, these abnormal curvatures are found together. **Torticollis,** or wry neck, is a tilt of the head caused by rotation of the cervical spine. Injury to the sternocleidomastoid muscle is typically the cause. This injury occurs most commonly at birth. Table 17-1 ■ identifies the type and degree of curvature, the recommended treatment, and nursing interventions.

JUVENILE RHEUMATOID ARTHRITIS

Juvenile rheumatoid arthritis (JRA or Still's disease) is an autoimmune inflammatory disease that affects children 2 to 5 years of age and 9 to 12 years of age. The cause of JRA is unknown. The diagnosis is made on the basis of history and clinical symptoms. Discussion of this condition appears in Chapter 21.

HEALTH PROMOTION ISSUE

CHILDREN AND BODY BUILDING

Ten-year-old Michael has been playing baseball since he was 3 years old. He pitches for his community team, and the coach has placed him as lead-off batter. He enjoys playing baseball and talks often about playing professionally. Michael's father played professional baseball until a shoulder injury ended his career. Because Michael's father wants Michael to avoid such injuries, he has hired a trainer and pitching coach to work with Michael several times a week. Recently, the trainer has suggested that Michael begin a weight training regimen to strengthen his muscles. This concerns his mother who is worried about the injuries Michael could sustain lifting heavy weights. She calls the pediatrician's office for information about the safety of weight training in children.

DISCUSSION

A study done in 1978 measured the muscle strength of preadolescent and adolescent boys following an 8-week resistance training program. The adolescent boys gained muscle strength while the preadolescent boys did not. Then, in 1988, another study reported that 12-year-old boys could not benefit from strength training that occurred three times a week for 4 to 6 weeks. Unfortunately, these studies were based on low resistance and only one or two sets of exercises per session. In 1983, the American Academy of Pediatrics (AAP) even published a

statement that said preadolescent boys could not significantly improve strength or muscle mass following weight training.

More recent studies with better methods of testing muscle strength have found different results. Muscle strength has been demonstrated to improve with resistance training in preadolescent boys. Other studies have found improvement in muscle coordination and greater flexibility. One study even reported that parents found children who participated in strength training to be more willing to do household chores and homework. There have, however, been no studies that can link weight training with improved sports performance.

Many of the studies that do link injuries with weight lifting are actually associated with weight lifting as a sport and not strength training or weight training. Strength training is defined as muscle conditioning using resistance in the form of free weights, weight machines, or resistance bands. Weight lifting and power lifting are competitive sports using a weighted barbell that is lifted from the ground to overhead.

In 2001, the AAP published a revised statement related to children and weight training. It reads, "Studies have shown that strength training, when properly structured with regard to frequency, mode (type of lifting), intensity, and duration of program, can increase strength

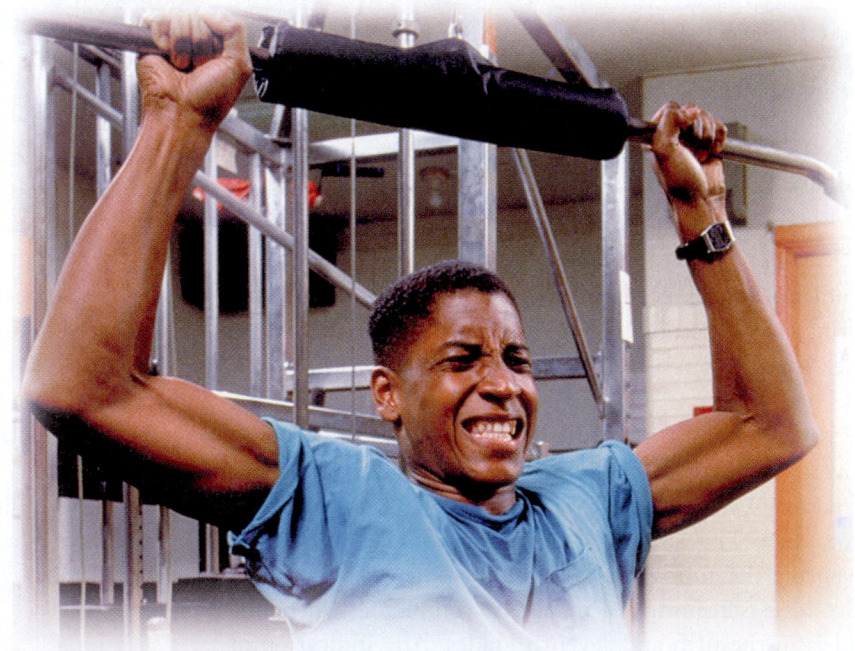

(Richard Hutchings\PhotoEdit, Inc.)

Musculoskeletal Trauma

Musculoskeletal trauma can occur in the form of muscle strains and sprains or fractures of the bones. A **sprain** occurs when the ligament associated with a joint is torn fol-

lowing trauma to the joint. Sprains are immobilized for the first 24 to 36 hours. Parents can be taught the RICE acronym for treatment of a sprain—**r**est, **i**ce, **c**ompression, and **e**levation. Nonsteroidal anti-inflammatory drugs (NSAIDs) may be prescribed to help reduce inflammation in preadolescents and adolescents" (p. 1472). The American College of Sports Medicine (ACSM) has also stated that strength training programs that are properly designed and supervised can enhance motor fitness skills and sports performance. The ACSM also states that strength training encourages healthy lifestyles, builds confidence, increases lean body mass, improves cholesterol levels, improves cardiac fitness and respiratory fitness, and improves bone fitness, self-image, and self-esteem.

PLANNING AND IMPLEMENTATION

The pediatric nurse should help Michael's mother understand the previous information, encouraging her that if Michael's plan includes supervision, a well-thought-out program, and proper technique, he should benefit from weight training.

Supervision of the weight training program is a must. The nurse should suggest that the adult supervisor be trained and certified as a fitness expert. The supervisor should have experience working with children. He or she should also remain with Michael during the entire training session and provide proper spotting of the weights during

lifts. Suggest to Michael's parents that the trainer have no more than 10 students to supervise at any given time.

Michael's parents should be encouraged to find a gym that is clean, safe, and spacious. The equipment should be child sized and have weight increments of 1 to 5 lb. Another important aspect is appropriate clothing and appropriate shoes. Clothing should not be large and baggy. Ill-fitting clothes can prove hazardous if they get caught on the weight machines. Shoes should provide foot and ankle stability and have adequate traction. The nurse should also suggest proper nutrition and hydration during the training period.

For Michael to achieve maximum benefit from weight training, proper technique must be implemented. Training should occur two to three times per week with 1 day off between training sessions. Experts suggest that every weight training session begin with time for stretching and aerobic activity. Each session should also end with a time for stretching. Weight can be increased when 15 repetitions become too easy, but should not be increased until Michael can do three sets of 15 repetitions of an exercise on three consecutive sessions.

Although the nurse may not be qualified to develop a specific workout plan for Michael, showing Michael's parents a sample weight training plan will assist them in approving an appropriate plan for Michael. Following is a sample plan for a preadolescent:

- 10 minutes stretching and brisk walk on the treadmill
- Shoulder exercises: 10 to 15 repetitions on deltoids, internal rotators, and external rotators
- Upper back exercises: 10 to 15 repetitions of bent-over lateral raises, bench rows, and latissumus pull-downs
- Lower back and abdomen exercises: 10 to 15 repetitions of crunches and reverse sit-ups
- 15 minutes of stretching and two laps around the track to cool down.

SELF-REFLECTION

Motivation for activities may arise from the child or from the parent. What are your feelings regarding parents encouraging or coercing a child to participate in a physical activity? Where should the line be drawn between helping the child develop discipline and requiring participation in physical activities?

SUGGESTED RESOURCES

For the Nurse

- American Academy of Pediatrics. (2001). Strength training by children and adolescent. *Pediatrics, 107*(6), 1470–1472.
- Benjamin H., & Glow, K. (2003). Strength training for children and adolescents: What can physicians recommend? *The Physician and Sportsmedicine, 3*(9).

For the Client

- Homeier, B. Strength training and your child. Accessed March 2006 at **http://kidshealth.org**.
- Robson, D. Weight training for children. Accessed March 2006 at **www.bodybuilding.com**.

and pain (Table 17-2 ■). After 36 hours, the child should gradually begin weight-bearing activities.

A **strain** is a more minor injury to the muscle or tendon. It can be caused by everyday activity, such as carrying a heavy backpack to school (Box 17-5 ■). A period of rest and

support is needed for the muscle or tendon to heal before returning to weight-bearing activities.

A **fracture** results from an injury and causes the continuity of the bone to be altered. Osgood–Schlatter disease is also a cause of musculoskeletal trauma.

TABLE 17-2

Pharmacology: Drugs Used to Reduce Inflammation (Nonsteroidal Anti-Inflammatory Drugs or NSAIDs)

DRUG (COMMON BRAND NAME AND GENERIC)	USUAL ROUTE/DOSE	CLASSIFICATION AND PURPOSE	SELECTED SIDE EFFECTS	DON'T GIVE IF
Naprosyn (naproxen)	For inflammation: 10–15 mg/kg/day PO, children greater than 2 years For pain: 5–7 mg/kg every 8–12 hours PO, children greater than 2 years	NSAID for inflammation and pain	Headache, drowsiness, dizziness, anorexia, heartburn, nausea	Child has GI irritation such as peptic ulcer
Indocin (indomethacin)	1–2 mg/kg/day or 150–200 mg/day PO	NSAID for juvenile rheumatoid arthritis	Dizziness, nausea, vomiting, headache	Child has an allergy to other NSAIDs or aspirin

BOX 17-5 | **CLIENT TEACHING**

Heavy Backpacks Cause Back Pain

Every day many children and teens strap on backpacks filled with lunch, textbooks, gym shoes and clothes, and numerous electronic devices. Many must walk to school, wait for the bus, or catch the subway with this weight straining their back. The backpacks can be 10% to 20% of the child's body weight. It is generally acknowledged that a child carrying more than 15 % of his or her body weight can suffer from severe back, neck and shoulder pain, headaches and other spinal discomfort.

A researcher at the University of California at San Diego developed a research project to measure the pressure exerted on a child's back when carrying a heavy backpack and to rate the pain this load causes (Macias, Murphy, Chambers, Hargens, 2005). He found that pressure exerted by the loaded backpacks was significantly greater than the pressure needed to occlude skin and muscle blood flow. Right shoulder pressures were also higher than left shoulder pressures. Back pain increased as the pressure that was exerted increased.

Parents and health care professionals need to develop methods of assisting children and teens to avoid added back strain from heavy backpacks. Health education programs can alert children and parents to the risks associated with carrying heavy backpacks and instruct children in proper body mechanics. Makers of backpacks have developed backpacks with wheels. Manufacturers should develop products that are appealing to the style-conscious child and yet are ergonomically correct.

Source: Data from Macias, B. R., Murthy, G., Chambers, H., and Hargens, A. (2005). High contact pressure beneath backpack straps of children contributes to pain. *Archives of Pediatrics and Adolescent Medicine, 159*(12), 1186–1187; Anrig, C. The backpack dilemma: Function vs. fashion. (2005). *Dynamic Chiropractic, 23*(18); and Sheir-Neiss, G. I., Kurse, R. W., Rahman, T., et al. (May, 2003). The association of backpack use and back pain in adolescents. *Spine, 28*(9), 922–930.

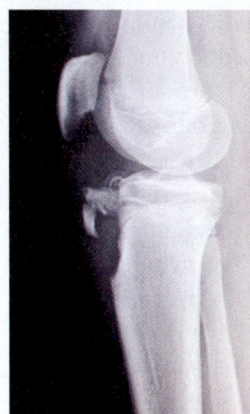

Figure 17-11. ■ Osgood–Schlatter disease often occurs in school-age children involved in running sports such as soccer. (Robert Destefano/Alamy)

OSGOOD–SCHLATTER DISEASE

Osgood–Schlatter disease (Figure 17-11 ■) is an overgrowth of the tibial epiphysis due primarily to recurring inflammatory episodes. The repeated pull of the quadriceps femoris as seen in athletic children is believed to cause the inflammation, new bone formation, and a bony prominence at the knee. The disease is most common in boys between 13 and 14 years and girls between 10 and 11 years (Box 17-6 ■). Treatment is aimed at resting the joint until healing occurs. Casting the knee may be necessary to relieve pain and swelling. Exercise to strengthen the muscles above and below the knee is sometimes helpful. Surgery is rarely needed.

FRACTURES

Fractures are a common occurrence in childhood due to the active nature of children. Injuries such as fractures, sprains, strains, and dislocations may result from sporting activities, play, or because the child is taking risks and not being careful.

BOX 17-6

Cheerleading: A Source of Musculoskeletal Injury

- Cheerleading is often not recognized by school officials as a sport. Therefore, training and certification for coaches may not be required. Without this training, students may not be taught safety measures to prevent injury.
- Cheerleading activities include acrobatics, pyramid building, and tosses. The flyer, or person being tossed or placed on top of the pyramid, is at greatest risk for a fall-related injury. The base, or person on the bottom of the pyramid, is at greatest risk for muscle strain and sprain or back injuries.
- A recent study found that between 1990 and 2002 more than 200,000 children ages 5 to 18 were treated in the emergency room for injuries related to cheerleading. U.S. Consumer Product Safety Commission reported nearly 25,000 cheerleading related injuries requiring emergency care in 2001 alone. Overall, cheerleading injuries have increased fivefold during the past 20 years. These injuries include strains, sprains, soft tissue injuries, fractures, dislocations, lacerations, concussions, and closed head injuries.

Source: Data from Shields, B. and Smith, G. (2006). Cheerleading related injuries to children 5 to 18 years of age: United States 1990–2002, *Pediatrics*, *117*:122–129; American Association of Cheerleading Coaches and Advisors. (2000). Position paper addressing the issue of cheerleading as a sport. National Center for Health Statistics (2001). Sports-related injuries cause 2.6 million visits annually by children and young adults to emergency rooms. Hyattsville, MD: Author.

BOX 17-7   ASSESSMENT

Possible Child Abuse

The nurse must consider physical child abuse when the following signs are noticed:

- Unexplained burns, bites, bruises, broken bones, or black eyes
- Fading bruises or other marks
- A child who is frightened of the parents and protests or cries when it is time to go home
- A child who shrinks at the approach of adults
- A child who reports injury by a parent or another adult caregiver.

Also consider the possibility of physical child abuse when the parent or other adult caregiver:

- Offers conflicting, unconvincing, or no explanation for the child's injury
- Describes the child as "evil," or in some other negative way
- Uses harsh physical discipline with the child
- Has a history of abuse as a child.

For more information about child abuse, see Chapter 2 🔗 for legal aspects and Chapter 27 🔗 for a detailed discussion of child abuse.

Source: Adapted from National Clearinghouse on Child Abuse and Neglect Information (DHHS). (2003). *Recognizing child abuse and neglect: Signs and symptoms.*

Manifestations

Signs of fracture vary, depending on the type of fracture and the location. Generally, pain, abnormal positioning, edema, discoloration, and abnormal movement characterize fractures. The common locations of fractures are clavicle, tibia, femur, radius, and ulna. X-ray is used to determine the exact location and type of fracture (Figure 17-12 ■). When assessing bruising and fracture, nurses must be alert to the possibility of child abuse (Box 17-7 ■).

When assessing the injured child, be alert for the possibility of fracture. The area should be immobilized prior to movement in order to prevent further injury. The child,

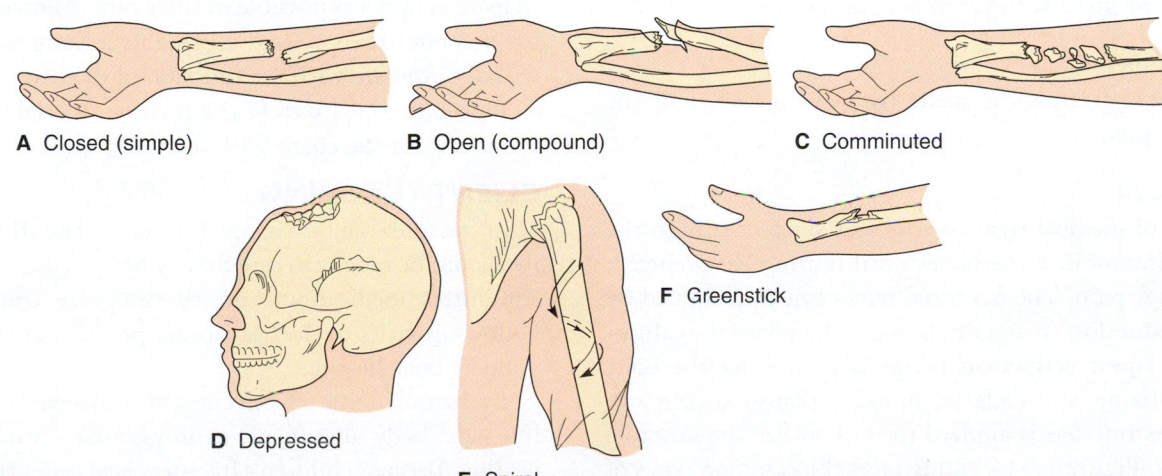

A Closed (simple)   **B** Open (compound)   **C** Comminuted

D Depressed   **E** Spiral   **F** Greenstick

Figure 17-12. ■ Fracture of the bone is defined as any disruption in the bone itself. It is classified as open or closed. (**A**) Closed (simple)—skin over the fracture remains intact. (**B**) Open (compound)—broken bone protrudes through the skin. (**C**) Comminuted—bone fragments into many pieces. (**D**) Depressed—broken bone is pressed inward (e.g., the skull). (**E**) Spiral—jagged break due to twisting force—often found in association with abuse. (**F**) Greenstick—incomplete break along the length of the bone (often found in young children).

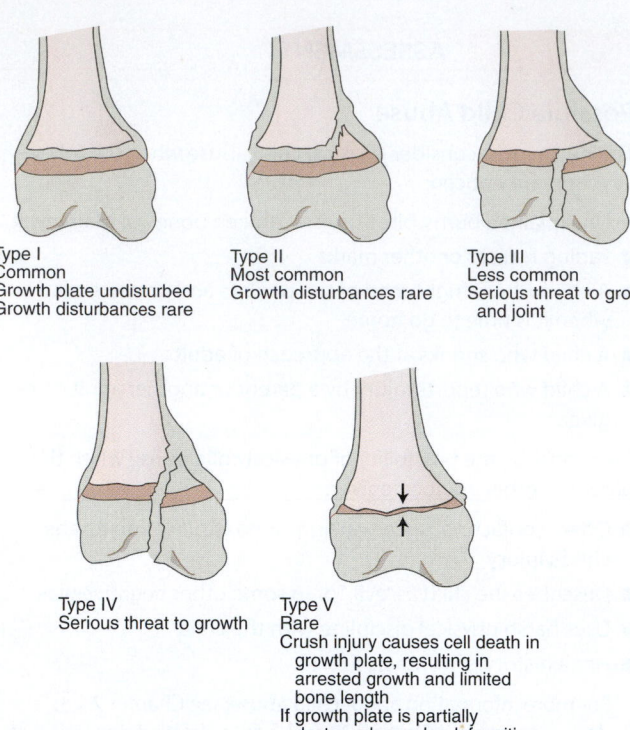

Type I
Common
Growth plate undisturbed
Growth disturbances rare

Type II
Most common
Growth disturbances rare

Type III
Less common
Serious threat to growth
and joint

Type IV
Serious threat to growth

Type V
Rare
Crush injury causes cell death in
growth plate, resulting in
arrested growth and limited
bone length
If growth plate is partially
destroyed, angular deformities
may result

Figure 17-13. ■ Salter–Harris classification system for fractures involving the epiphyses (growth plates).

parents, and family should be questioned to determine the cause of the injury.

The area of injury should be inspected for broken skin; circulation, including pulse and bleeding; and normal sensation. If the skin has been broken, bleeding should be controlled and sterile dressings applied.

When fractures involve the epiphysis, they can disrupt the growth process. Figure 17-13 ■ illustrates the Salter–Harris classification of fractures and shows which types of fracture can cause the greatest threat to normal growth.

Diagnosis

Diagnosis of fractures is made by viewing x-rays of the affected injury.

Treatment

The goal of medical treatment is to reduce or realign the fracture, immobilize the bones until healing has occurred, and manage pain. The fractured bones can be realigned by **closed reduction** (manually moving the bones into alignment) or **open reduction** (surgically aligning the bone and stabilizing the ends with nails, plates, or screws). Sometimes traction is applied to immobilize the unstable bone ends. Figure 17-14 ■ illustrates the common types of traction used for children. At other times, external fixators or stabilizers (Figure 17-14E and F) are used to immobilize the fracture while allowing the child more freedom of activity. A plaster or plastic cast may be used to immobilize

the fractured bone. Removable casts may be used for children because they are light and easy to apply and remove.

The care of the child in traction and external fixators is similar to that of an adult. The area should be assessed for circulation, movement, and sensation. Skin care must be given routinely to prevent breakdown. The weights used in traction should hang freely, and the child must be kept in proper alignment. This is a challenge with the young or uncooperative child who moves around in the bed. The skin around the pins of external fixative devices should be cleaned and dressed using sterile technique. However, pin care should only be done if it is specifically ordered.

The nurse must be alert for the development of compartment syndrome in the child with a cast. **Compartment syndrome** occurs when increased pressure in a limited space compromises circulation and nerve innervation, leading to possible necrosis.

clinical ALERT

Symptoms of compartment syndrome include:

Paresthesia

Pain/pressure

Pallor

Paralysis

Pulselessness

Deep pain unrelieved by analgesia, lack of sensation, and edema suggest compartment syndrome and should be reported immediately. The cast should be altered or removed promptly to prevent permanent damage to underlying tissue.

Children need special attention to deal with the anxiety related to orthopedic casts. They should be allowed to participate as much as possible in their care. Allowing children to "decorate" their casts is acceptable as long as decoration will not interfere with the function of the casts.

Procedures 17-1 ■ to 17-3 ■ review essential information about care for the client with fracture.

CLIENT TEACHING

Most fractures can be managed at home. The child and family should be taught to care for any orthopedic appliance, to administer medication, and to recognize complications. Follow-up visits to the health care provider are essential to evaluate bone healing.

Evaluation of the effectiveness of treatment includes skin integrity, body alignment, neurovascular status, and bone healing. Because children's fractures heal faster than adults', follow-up evaluation should occur every few weeks. Parents should be able to verbalize any modification that may be needed at home or school. The nurse should refer parents to home health nurses if indicated.

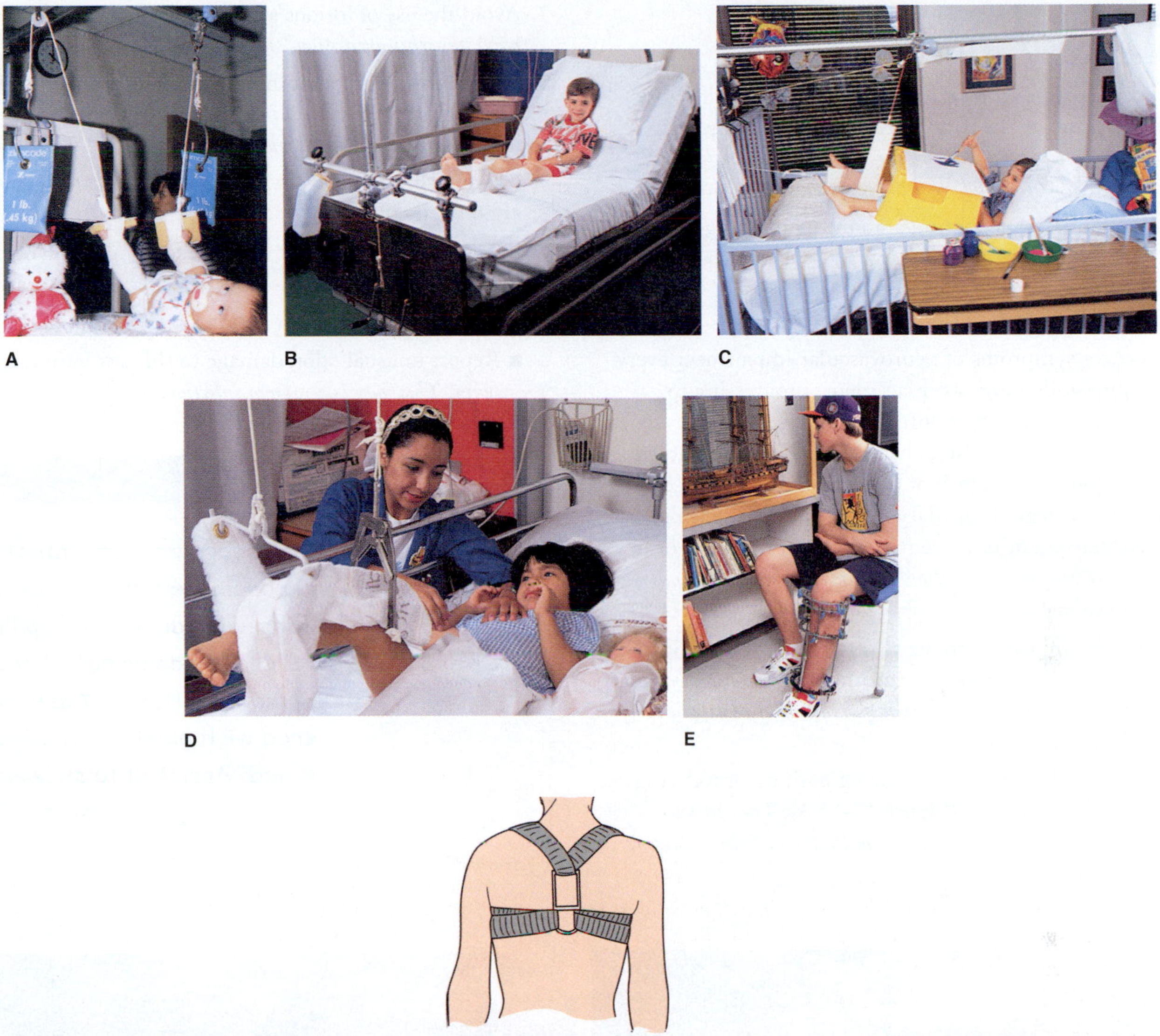

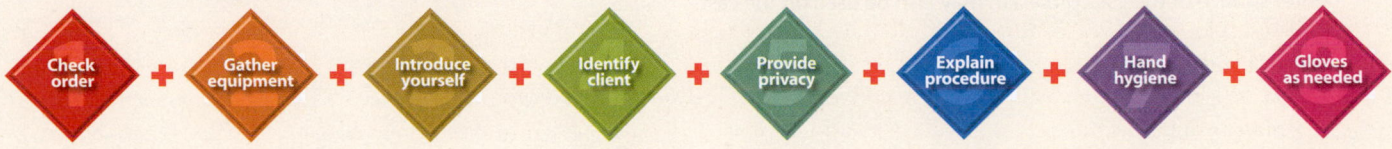

Figure 17-14. ■ Types of traction used for children. (**A**) Bryant traction. (**B**) Buck traction. (**C**) Russell traction. (**D**) 90–90 traction. (**E**) External traction (external fixator device). (**F**) Clavicle strap for stabilizing clavicle fracture.

PROCEDURE 17-1   Providing Cast Care

Purpose

- To note signs and symptoms of neurovascular impairment and report them promptly
- To maintain cast integrity, thus promoting healing

Equipment

- Pillows with waterproof covering
- Absorbent pads and protectors
- Plastic bag
- Permanent marker

Check order ✚ Gather equipment ✚ Introduce yourself ✚ Identify client ✚ Provide privacy ✚ Explain procedure ✚ Hand hygiene ✚ Gloves as needed

Interventions

1. Elevate recently casted limb. *This reduces edema.*

2. Inspect the damp cast for indentations and handle only with the palms of the hand until the cast is completely dry. *Damp casts move under pressure. Indentations indicate potential pressure areas where skin breakdown could occur.*

3. Observe for drainage, noting amount by marking the outline of the drainage area, date, and time on the cast with permanent marker. *Water-based marker could be removed by drainage or cleaning.*

4. Observe for symptoms of neurovascular impairment every 15 minutes following cast placement, progressing to every 2 hours. Report abnormal findings, such as decreased or absent pulses, change in color of skin above or below the cast, warmth of the extremity, decreased sensation, decreased capillary refill, increased edema, limited movement of extremity, or pain, burning, or tingling. *These measures allow the nurse to recognize and prevent complications.*

5. Instruct children and parents to observe for the previous findings as well and report accordingly. *Much of the healing time will be at home. The child and parents must be taught to recognize and report symptoms.*

6. Cover cast with a plastic bag during bathing or toileting to keep it dry and clean (Figure 17-15 ■). *The cast will disintegrate if it gets wet. It must remain dry in order to support proper healing.*

7. Avoid the use of lotions and powders under the cast. *These may cause skin irritation.*

8. Keep shirts or other clothing over the top edges of the cast on young children. *This helps keep the child from picking at the cast or putting small objects into the cast.*

9. Instruct children and their families about care of the cast at home, including:

   ■ The area under the cast and toes and fingers can be cleaned with alcohol and a cotton swab. Water should be avoided.

   ■ Use a cast shoe, sock, or sling to protect the cast.

   ■ Report unusual odor, damage to the cast, or unexplained fever. *This may be a sign of infection.*

SAMPLE DOCUMENTATION

(date and time)   Right forearm cast intact. No drainage noted. Fingers warm with adequate capillary refill. No edema noted. ROM without limitation. Cast covered with plastic and edges taped. Assisted to shower.
_____ L. Erskine, LPN

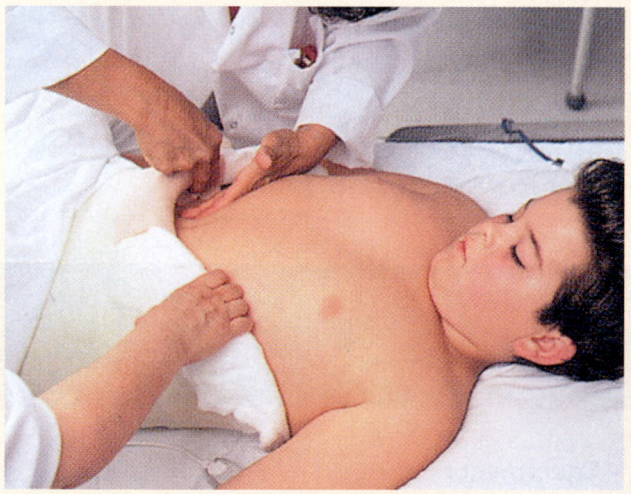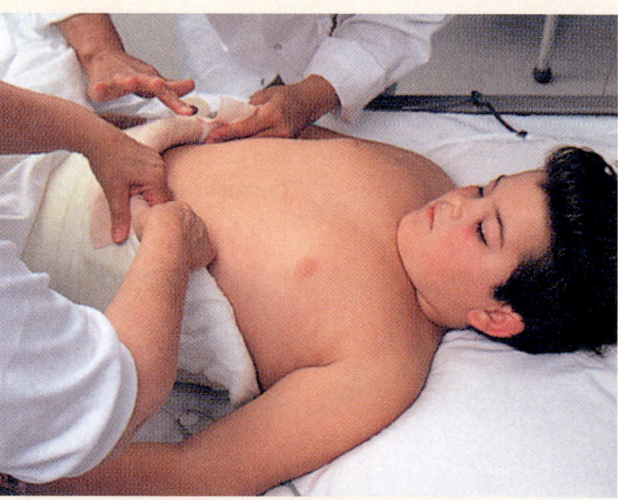

A   **B**

Figure 17-15. ■ Cast care. Plastic can be placed over the cast during bathing or toileting to keep materials dry and clean. (**A**) Nurses can protect children's skin from the rough edges of the cast by "petaling" it. (**B**) This is done by securing adhesive tape to the inside of the cast and pulling it over the edge, covering the jagged or broken pieces of plaster, and securing it to the outer surface of the cast. Moleskin may also be used on the cast.

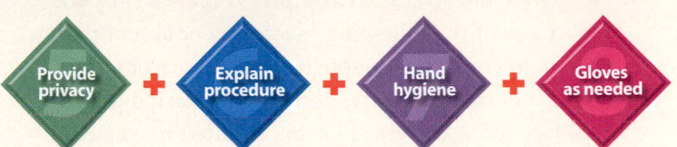

PROCEDURE 17-2 | # Setting Crutch Height

Purpose

- To ensure proper fit of crutches and facilitate ambulation

Equipment

- Crutches
- Measuring tape, if desired

Check order + Gather equipment + Introduce yourself + Identify client + Provide privacy + Explain procedure + Hand hygiene + Gloves as needed

Interventions

1. Have the child stand with elbows slightly and comfortably flexed.

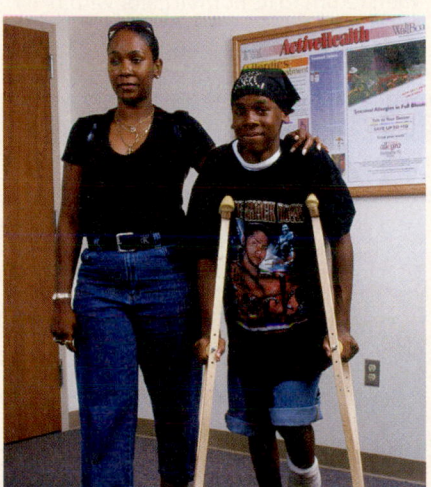

Figure 17-16. ■ Crutches should fit comfortably under the axillae so they do not rub against the skin. The child should not have to stoop to use the crutches.

2. Place the tip of the crutches 3 to 6 in. from the upper, outer border of the toes of each foot. *This provides a wider base of support for improved balance.*

3. Adjust the crutches to proper height, ensuring that the upper pad on the crutches is placed lightly under the child's axillae (Figure 17-16 ■). *The crutches should not put pressure on the axillae.*

4. Check the child's posture. The back or neck should not be flexed. *This would indicate that the crutches are too short.*

SAMPLE DOCUMENTATION

(date and time)   Crutches placed in axilla. Height adjusted. Correct posture and pad placement noted. Instructions on proper crutch walking given. Client verbalized understanding. ___ J. Ness, LVN

PROCEDURE 17-3 | # Applying Traction

Purpose

- To ensure appropriate traction is applied
- To ensure proper body alignment is maintained
- To maintain safety and prevent further injury

Equipment

- Poles, pulleys, rope, weight, pads as ordered
- Elastic wrap for external traction

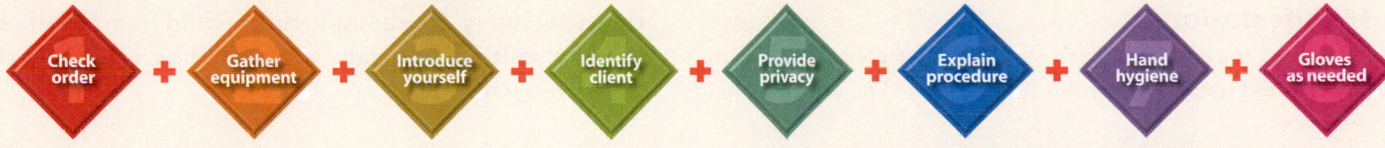

Check order + Gather equipment + Introduce yourself + Identify client + Provide privacy + Explain procedure + Hand hygiene + Gloves as needed

Interventions

1. Place weights as ordered.

2. Apply traction as ordered to affected extremity. *Proper weights and placement will ensure correct treatment.*

3. Make the following assessments every 30 minutes initially, and then every 1 to 2 hours when stable:
   - Proper position of traction
   - Proper body alignment
   - Neurovascular status of extremity (Figure 17-17 ■); report any of the following: decreased or absent pulses, change in color of skin above or below site of traction, warmth of the extremity, decreased sensation, decreased capillary refill, increased edema, limited movement of extremity, or pain, burning, or tingling

clinical ALERT

When assessing neurovascular status in a pediatric client with musculoskeletal injury, the nurse looks for **c**irculation, **m**ovement, and **s**ensation (CMS). Also, observe and document the five Ps: **p**aresthesia, **p**ain/pressure, **p**allor, **p**aralysis, and **p**ulselessness.

   - Condition of skin under and around traction application
   - Skin over bony prominences
   - Vital signs
   - Pain
   - Emotional state. *These assessments will ensure quality of care.*

4. Perform sterile pin care according to agency policy for internal traction or as ordered by physician. *Sterile cleansing is necessary to prevent introduction of micro-organisms to compromised skin.*

5. Provide teaching and evaluation of technique if the family will maintain traction at home. *Client teaching and return demonstration will provide the family with the knowledge and skills they need to support the healing process.*

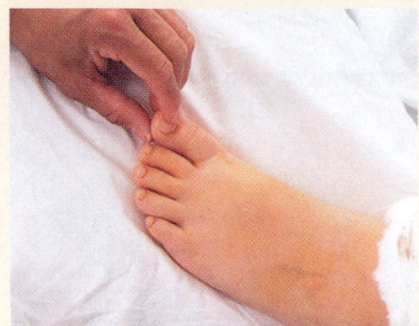

Figure 17-17. ■ The skin of the extremities should be warm. It should blanch when slight pressure is applied and then return to its normal color within 3 seconds.

SAMPLE DOCUMENTATION

(date and time)	Traction to left lower extremity applied per order. Toes warm, pink, with appropriate ROM. Client is without complaint at present. Verbalized understanding of plan of care. Video provided for distraction. Call bell within reach. _____ L. Atchley, LPN

Musculoskeletal Infection

OSTEOMYELITIS

Osteomyelitis (Figure 17-18 ■) is an infection of the bone that may spread to surrounding tissues.

The infection typically follows an injury or surgery and is the result of bacteria, virus, or fungi. The most common causative agent is *Staphylococcus aureus*. Children ages 1 to 12 years are most likely to have osteomyelitis, and boys are more likely to have it than girls.

Manifestations

The child may present with symptoms of constant pain in the affected area and surrounding tissues. The affected surrounding tissues may be edematous, and there may be decreased mobility of the joint. The child may refuse to use the affected limb or may limp. There may also be redness over the site of injury, and the child may have a fever.

Diagnosis

Diagnosis is made by a careful review of the child's history, including incidences of trauma. Laboratory results may indicate an increased white blood cell count and erythrocyte sedimentation rate. X-rays and bone scans are used to view the site of injury. Needle aspiration of fluid from the site allows the health care provider to culture the specimen for the causative agent.

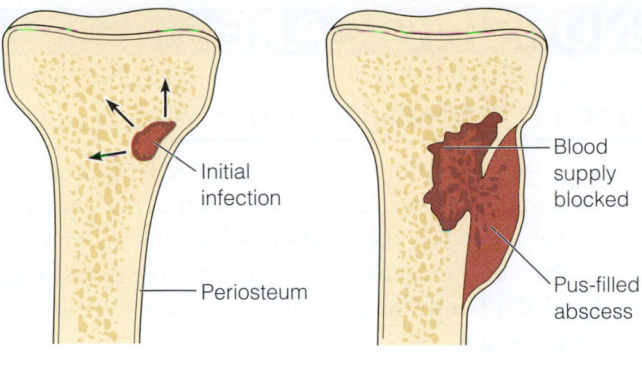

A Initial infection   **B** Acute phase

Figure 17-18. ■ Osteomyelitis. (**A**) Bacteria enters and multiplies in the bone. (**B**) The infection spreads to other parts of the bone, and the periosteum separates from the surface of the bone.

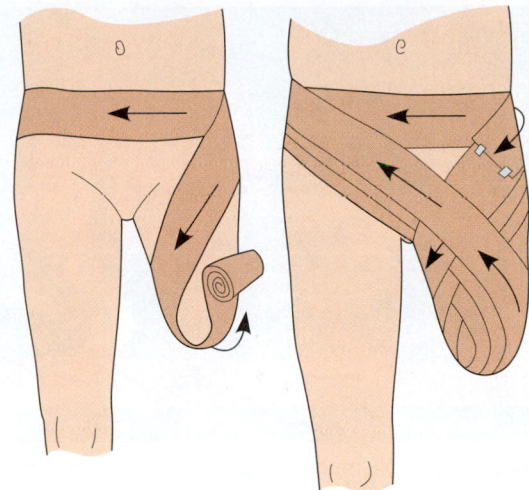

Figure 17-19. ■ With an above-the-knee amputation, a figure-eight bandage is wrapped around the waist, then brought down over the stump and back up around the hip.

Treatment

The child with osteomyelitis is hospitalized and administered IV antibiotics. Some form of antibiotic treatment is usually administered for 3 to 6 weeks. If the child is discharged from the hospital, antibiotic treatment will be continued at home either orally or intravenously. For the child who is discharged on IV antibiotics, a home health care nurse can assist in the administration and care of the IV site.

Musculoskeletal Tumors

OSTEOSARCOMA

Bone tumors are rare, but periods of rapid growth are the most common times for occurrence in adolescent boys. Bone tumors are usually found in the distal femur, proximal tibia, or proximal humerus.

Manifestations

Clinical manifestations include pain, swelling, and mobility or gait problems. Fever, elevated white blood cell count, and elevated erythrocyte sedimentation rate may be seen.

Diagnosis

X-ray, computed tomography (CT) or MRI scan, and tissue biopsy are used to reach a diagnosis of osteosarcoma.

Treatment

Treatment involves surgery and the use of chemotherapy and radiation. Depending on the extent of the tumor, limb-sparing surgery may be used to remove the tumor and surrounding bone. An internal prosthesis is then inserted. Amputation must be performed if the tumor is large or involves surrounding soft tissue, including nerves. Chemotherapy and radiation are given to treat nondetectable metastasis.

Nursing Considerations

Nursing management includes standard preoperative and postoperative care. Psychological assessment of the adolescent

and the family is necessary. Body image disturbances occur when a limb is lost. Signs of disturbed body image include:

- Refusal to look at or touch the altered body part
- Hiding the affected body part
- Preoccupation with the loss or change
- Overexposure of the body part
- Feelings of guilt, shame, or embarrassment.

Client and family support systems should be identified and contacted as soon as possible. The older child or adolescent will need to learn to care for the stump (Figure 17-19 ■ and Box 17-8 ■). Rehabilitation will be needed to help the

---

BOX 17-8   **NURSING CARE CHECKLIST**

Care of the Stump Following Amputation

☑ Carefully monitor vital signs and drainage from dressing.

☑ Keep a surgical tourniquet available to control bleeding if necessary.

☑ Observe strict sterile technique for dressing changes to prevent infection.

☑ Apply compression bandage as ordered (see Figure 17-19).

☑ Change bandages twice daily to observe for wound healing.

☑ Avoid hip flexion contractures by limiting time sitting in chair to less than 1 hour. Also avoid pillows under the limb.

☑ Explain phantom limb pain to the child and parents. Symptoms include coolness, heaviness, and pain.

☑ Administer pain medications as ordered to control the child's comfort.

☑ Assist with temporary prosthesis fitting.

☑ Assist with ROM exercises as ordered.

☑ Teach crutch walking with lower limb amputation as ordered.

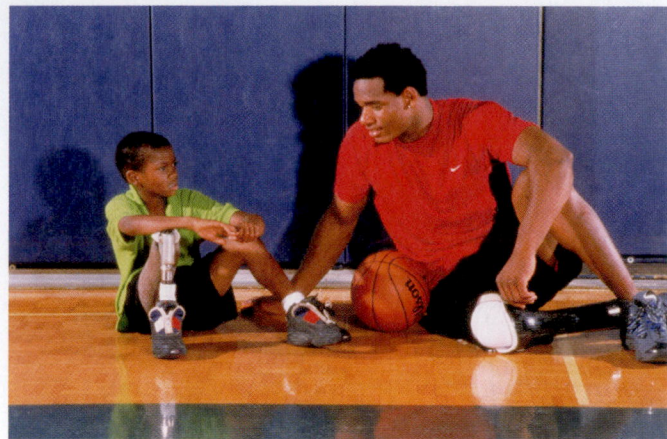

Figure 17-20. ■ A role model can provide support and encouragement to a child learning to adapt to life with a prosthetic limb. (Photo Researchers, Inc.)

child learn to use the prosthesis and adapt to the amputation (Figure 17-20 ■). With practice and at times with special devices, many children continue their involvement with sports.

Prosthetics can be expensive, and parents may need financial support beyond insurance. Referral to special hospitals such as the Shriner's Hospitals may be an option. The school should be contacted and plans made for the adolescent's return. Some adaptation may be needed to accommodate a wheelchair, crutches, or other appliances and to plan for emergency evacuation.

EWING'S SARCOMA

Ewing's sarcoma is a malignant tumor found most commonly on the femur, pelvis, tibia, fibula, ribs, humerus, scapula, and clavicle. Caucasians and Hispanics are most commonly affected. Children ages 10 to 20 years have the highest incidence of Ewing's sarcoma.

Manifestations

Clinical manifestations are similar to osteosarcoma. Fractures of the affected bone may occur.

Diagnosis

Diagnosis is made by biopsy of the tumor.

Treatment

Treatment includes chemotherapy to reduce the tumor size, followed by surgery to remove the bone. High-dose radiation may also be implemented. Chemotherapy typically follows surgery. Nursing care for children with Ewing's sarcoma is the same as outlined previously for osteosarcoma.

NURSING CARE

PRIORITIES IN NURSING CARE

When caring for children with musculoskeletal disorders, the nurse must promote independence of the child. Nursing care will also focus on the child's mobility and maintaining safety. The nurse must use available resources to assist the child and the family in getting support and establishing proper home care.

ASSESSING

Monitor cardiac, respiratory, urinary, and bowel function. Assess range of motion, mobility, posture, and muscle strength. Note any swelling or redness that may be associated with muscle sprain. If the child uses assistive devices, the nurse must assess the correct use of the devices and the effectiveness of the devices in aiding the child's mobility. For chronic disorders such as MD, the nurse collects data about the family's ability to care for the child long term in the home both physically and emotionally.

DIAGNOSING, PLANNING, AND IMPLEMENTING

The following nursing diagnoses may be used in planning nursing care for the child with a musculoskeletal disorder:

- Impaired Mobility related to musculoskeletal impairment
- Activity Intolerance related to weakness
- Risk for Injury related to altered mobility
- Compromised Family Coping related to caring for a child with a chronic condition.

Typical outcomes for the child or family with a musculoskeletal disorder might include these as well as others:

- Mobility will be restored through the use of assistive devices.
- Tolerance for activity will be demonstrated as evidenced by vital signs within normal limits.
- Family will create a safe environment.
- Family will participate effectively in developing a plan to care for the child.

Nursing interventions related to children with musculoskeletal disorders include:

- Teach client to use assistive devices. *Crutches, canes, braces, walkers, and wheelchairs require specific instruction to operate properly. Demonstration and return demonstration of the use of these devices will promote mobility.*
- Provide positive encouragement before, during, and after use of assistive devices. *Encouragement will promote well-being and the desire to continue working on using the devices properly.*

- Assist the family in planning daily activities to include periods of rest. *Adequate rest is essential for energy conservation.*
- Keep frequently used objects within easy reach. *Reducing the number of steps required to complete activities of daily living will assist in energy conservation.*
- Assist the parents in assessing their home environment for safety hazards. *Safety hazards must be identified in order to correct them.*
- Provide information about correcting identified hazards. *Instructing families in how to correct hazards will help them manage their environment correctly and prevent injury.*
- Discuss with the family the common responses to caring for a child with a musculoskeletal disorder. *The nurse can assist the family in identifying anxiety, fear, and depression as normal responses to families in their situation.*
- Provide the family with specific information on caring for their child with a musculoskeletal disorder. *Families can develop coping mechanisms when they are able to view the task before them and understand how it can be managed effectively.*

EVALUATING

The child is evaluated for mobility, tolerance to activity, and safety. The family can be evaluated for coping with the care of the child. These evaluations should be made on a regular basis because these criteria can change throughout the child's care.

NURSING PROCESS CARE PLAN
The Child with an Amputation

Jake is a 14-year-old who was admitted 1 week ago with a diagnosis of osteosarcoma and scheduled for surgery tomorrow. Jake's physician has informed Jake and his parents that Jake's leg may have to be amputated to ensure complete removal of the tumor. Jake has spent the last 5 years playing baseball and is "depressed" that he will no longer be able to play sports.

Assessment. The following data should be collected as soon as possible:

- Vital signs
- Condition of surgical site, preoperatively
- Client's and family's understanding of the disease process
- Client's and family's understanding of the treatment regimen
- Feelings and concerns about the possible amputation
- Client's understanding of the use of a prosthesis
- Level of familial support.

Nursing Diagnosis. The following important nursing diagnosis (among others) is established for this client:

- Disturbed Body Image related to surgical alteration of limb.

Expected Outcomes
- Will demonstrate a positive body image.
- Will express the desire to learn how to use a prosthesis.

Planning and Implementation
- Listen attentively to Jake's concerns in a nonjudgmental manner. *Therapeutic listening will provide a safe environment.*
- Encourage grief behaviors. *Dealing with emotions is part of healing.*
- Assist Jake and his family in developing coping mechanisms, using personal strengths.
- Encourage Jake to begin regular activities of daily living as soon as possible after surgery. *Independent self-care increases self-esteem.*
- Teach Jake's parents the importance of their responses related to his body changes. *Their modeling of acceptance and a positive attitude toward Jake's changed physical appearance will encourage similar changes in Jake.*
- Refer the family to social services for home care and follow-up. *Support services are essential in making this transition. Both parents and child may benefit from participation in a support group.*

Evaluation. Jake begins to care for his amputation shortly after surgery and readily accepts the duties related to stump and prosthesis care. He discusses life after amputation with a young girl who had an amputation 1 year ago. Upon discharge, he tells the nurse that he would love to learn more about playing sports with a prosthesis.

Critical Thinking in the Nursing Process

1. What competitive sporting activities could the nurse suggest for Jake to try?
2. Managing a prosthesis requires additional energy. What suggestions should the nurse make to assist Jake in having adequate energy?
3. List two caring responses to the following concern expressed by Jake: "I'm afraid people will stare at me when I walk by."

Note: Discussion of Critical Thinking questions appears in Appendix I.

Note: The references and resources for this and all chapters have been compiled at the back of the book.

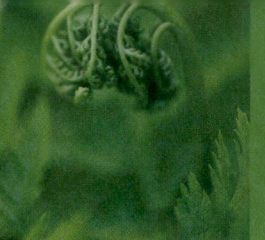

Chapter Review

 **KEY TERMS** by Topic

Use the audio glossary feature of either the CD-ROM or the Companion Website to hear the correct pronunciation of the following key terms.

Anatomy and Physiology
ossification, epiphysis, epiphyseal plate, metaphysis, diaphysis, hematopoiesis, greenstick fracture, genu valgum, genu varum

Congenital Skeletal Defects
hip spica cast, talipes

Musculoskeletal Disorders
muscular dystrophy (MD), kyphosis, lordosis, torticollis

Musculoskeletal Trauma
sprain, strain, fracture, closed reduction, open reduction, compartment syndrome

KEY Points

- Injuries to a child's bones may be due to the fact that the growth plate is still open and the child's long bones are less dense than an adult's. Children are also naturally curious and adventurous.

- A priority nursing role when caring for children with musculoskeletal disorders is to promote independence.

- An essential assessment for the nurse to make when caring for a child with a cast is observing for compartment syndrome, which occurs when increased pressure in a limited space compromises circulation and nerve innervation, leading to possible necrosis. Symptoms of compartment syndrome include paresthesia, pain/pressure, pallor, paralysis, and pulselessness.

- The nurse should teach the child and parents to prevent complications with a cast by teaching them to keep the cast dry and clean, avoid using powders or lotions, avoid sticking objects into the cast, and cover the cast to protect it from injury.

- When providing instruction to a child who is learning to walk with crutches, the nurse should ensure that the crutches are not pressing on the axillae and that the child is able to maintain a straight spine when walking.

- Besides physical care, children in traction need their emotional needs to be addressed.

- The nurse should observe the child with a musculoskeletal disorder for body image disturbance by recognizing the following signs: refusal to look at or touch the altered body part, hiding the affected body part, preoccupation with the loss or change, overexposure of the body part, and/or feelings of guilt, shame, or embarrassment.

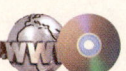 **EXPLORE MediaLink**

Additional interactive resources for this chapter can be found on the Companion Website at www.prenhall.com/towle.

Click on Chapter 17 and "Begin" to select the activities for this chapter.

For chapter-related NCLEX-style questions and an audio glossary, access the accompanying CD-ROM in this book.

Animations

Skeleton

Trauma

Importance of physical activity

FOR FURTHER Study

For more information about child abuse, see Chapter 2 for legal aspects and Chapter 27 for a detailed discussion of child abuse.

See Chapter 9 for additional information on fontanels and a complete discussion on developmental dysplasia of the hip; Figure 9-20 illustrates the Ortolani–Barlow maneuver.

For more information on juvenile rheumatoid arthritis, see Chapter 21.

Caring for a Child with a Fracture

NCLEX-PN® Focus Area: Physiologic Integrity

Case Study: Billy, an 8-year-old, is brought to the urgent care clinic for a possible fractured left lower leg. Billy had been rollerblading when he fell, twisting his left ankle. He is hopping on his right leg. He has been crying and states, "It hurts real bad."

Nursing Diagnosis: Impaired Physical Mobility

COLLECT DATA

Subjective	Objective
_____	_____
_____	_____
_____	_____
_____	_____
_____	_____
_____	_____

Would you report this? Yes/No

If yes, to: _____

Nursing Care

_____
_____
_____
_____
_____
_____
_____
_____
_____
_____
_____
_____
_____

How would you document this? _____
_____
_____

Compare your documentation to the sample provided in Appendix I.

Data Collected
(use those that apply)

- Pedal pulses present
- Crying
- States, "It hurts real bad."
- Ankle swollen, bruised
- Non–weight-bearing

Nursing Interventions
(use those that apply; list in priority order)

- Apply ice pack to ankle.
- Instruct not to put anything inside cast.
- Offer milk three times a day.
- Apply heat lamp to ankle.
- Instruct to support cast on pillows until dry.
- Teach crutch walking.
- Instruct regarding signs of impaired circulation.

NCLEX-PN® Exam Preparation

1 A 12-year-old asks, "Do I really have to wear this Milwaukee brace when I go to school? I look like a freak!" The nurse's best response would be:

1. "It is important that you wear the brace 23 hours a day."
2. "I know the brace does not look very stylish; let's see if we can find some pictures of cute shirts that may help."
3. "I will ask the doctor if you can wear another type of brace."
4. "I guess it will be all right for you to leave the brace off while you are at school."

2 The nurse is caring for a client with osteosarcoma. Which of the following symptoms would the nurse expect?

1. swelling in the area of the clavicle
2. difficulty using either hand
3. pain in the femur
4. frequently stiff back

3 A 17-year-old is 3 days postop below-the-knee amputation for osteosarcoma. The LPN is gathering data in a psychological assessment. Which of the following findings should be reported to the RN?

1. Client removed the bandage and looked at the wound.
2. Client discusses what it will be like without a leg.
3. Client keeps leg under the covers.
4. Client discusses the surgery with his best friend.

4 An infant was born with developmental dysplasia of the hip. His father states, "I am glad we will only have to triple his diaper for a few days. They look so uncomfortable." The nurse should reply:

1. "What did the doctor tell you about the infant's hip problem?"
2. "You are wrong, he will have to wear triple diapers for 3 to 4 months."
3. "You are right, he will only need triple diapers for a few days."
4. "Triple diapers are uncomfortable, so you will need to medicate your infant every 4 hours."

5 The nurse is providing instruction to parents about a synthetic cast applied to the child for treatment of clubfoot. Which of the following statements is true about synthetic casting?

1. "Make sure the cast is allowed to dry for 24 hours."
2. "Synthetic casts are stronger than plaster casts."
3. "This cast is heavier than a plaster cast."
4. "Synthetic casts allow greater mobility but are weaker than plaster."

6 The nurse is assisting the physician during an examination of an infant with a diagnosis of hip dysplasia. The physician is planning on performing an Ortolani–Barlow maneuver. The nurse understands that the physician is assessing the infant's hips for _____.

7 A nurse is taking care of a child in skeletal traction and avoids which action when caring for this child?

1. ensuring the weights are hanging freely
2. putting the bed linens on the traction ropes
3. making sure the weights are out of the child's reach
4. checking to ensure the weights are in the pulleys

8 The nurse is caring for a child with a right leg cast and is checking the capillary refill of the extremity. The nurse presses the nail bed of the great toe and it returns to the original color in 2 seconds. The nurse's next action is to:

1. document the findings.
2. prepare the child for immediate cast removal.
3. elevate the extremity on two pillows and recheck the capillary refill.
4. notify the physician.

9 A nurse is checking off instructions for the parents for care of a child with a newly applied cast to the right lower leg. Select all instructions that would be included on this list.

1. Observe the cast for drainage.
2. Contact the physician if the child complains of numbness or tingling in the leg.
3. Elevate the leg on pillows for the first 24 to 48 hours after the cast application.
4. Observe the toes for changes in color (blue color, pallor).
5. Cover cast with plastic bag during bathing.
6. Sprinkle powder inside the cast to keep the leg dry.

10 The nurse is providing instruction for the mother of an adolescent girl with scoliosis who has just been fitted for a Milwaukee brace. The nurse realizes additional instruction is needed when the mother states:

1. "I understand that the brace must be worn for 2 hours on and 2 hours off."
2. "I know I have to check around the brace for skin breakdown."
3. "I will provide skin care to prevent breakdown."
4. "I will work with my daughter so she can learn how to sit, stand, and walk with the brace."

Answers for Review Questions, as well as discussion of Care Plan and Critical Thinking Care Map questions, appear in Appendix I.

Chapter 18

Care of the Child with Respiratory Disorders

BRIEF Outline

Anatomy and Physiology
Mechanism of Respiration
Brief Assessment Overview
UPPER RESPIRATORY DISORDERS
Epistaxis
Upper Respiratory Infections

Foreign Body Obstructed Airway
LOWER RESPIRATORY DISORDERS
Congenital Respiratory Disorders
Lower Respiratory Infections
Additional Respiratory Disorders
Nursing Care

LEARNING Outcomes

After completing this chapter, you will be able to:

- Discuss the anatomy and physiology of the pediatric respiratory system.
- Describe respiratory disorders to include upper respiratory infections, tracheoesophageal fistula, cystic fibrosis, asthma, and lower respiratory infections.
- Explain appropriate nursing interventions for children with respiratory disorders.
- Discuss clinical manifestations, diagnostic procedures, medical management, and nursing interventions related to respiratory trauma.

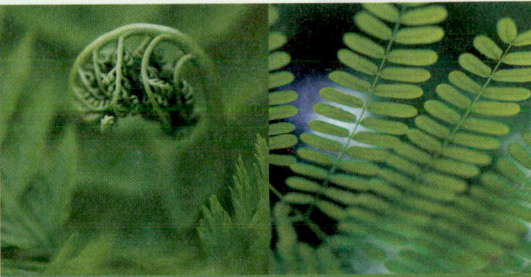

HEALTH PROMOTION ISSUE:
Tonsillectomy

NURSING PROCESS CARE PLAN:
Respiratory Syncytial Virus

NURSING PROCESS CARE PLAN:
Client with Asthma

CRITICAL THINKING CARE MAP:
Caring for a Client with
Respiratory Infection

Disorders of the respiratory system include congenital malformation, infections, and diseases resulting from chromosomal abnormalities or unknown causes.

Anatomy and Physiology

The respiratory system is divided into the upper respiratory system and the lower respiratory system. The upper respiratory system contains the nose, nasal sinuses, pharynx, and larynx. The lower respiratory system contains the trachea, bronchial tree, and alveoli inside the lungs. The right lung is divided into three lobes, and the left lung is divided into two lobes. The entire respiratory system is lined with a continuous mucous membrane that produces approximately 125 mL of mucus daily. The underlying epithelial cells of the lower respiratory system contain cilia, which are hairlike structures extending outward from the cell membrane. The cilia continuously move the mucus toward the pharynx. Figures 18-1 ■ and 18-2 ■ show the differences in upper respiratory structures between a child and an adult.

SINUSES

Air enters the nares or nostrils and flows through the nasal cavities. Protruding into the nasal cavity from the sides are three shelflike structures called **conchae.** These structures, covered with mucous membrane, increase the surface area for warming and humidifying the air and trapping foreign particles. The four pairs of nasal sinuses open into the nasal cavity. The frontal, sphenoidal, ethmoidal, and maxillary sinuses lighten the weight of the head, as well as warm and humidify the air. The openings of the sinuses into the nasal cavity are small and easily blocked by swelling of the mucous membrane. The lacrimal (tear) sacs also open into the nasal cavity.

PHARYNX

The pharynx or throat is made up of the nasal pharynx at the top, oral pharynx behind the mouth, and laryngopharynx above the larynx. The pharynx is simply a connection between the nasal cavity and the larynx and esophagus. Both air and food pass through this structure. The eustachian (auditory) canals from the middle ear open into the nasal pharynx. In infants, the eustachian tube is practically horizontal (see Figure 16-30B ∞); by age 12, it tilts diagonally down into the nasopharynx and so is less likely to promote middle ear infection.

Masses of lymphatic tissue or tonsils are embedded in the wall of the pharynx. The pharyngeal tonsils (adenoids) are

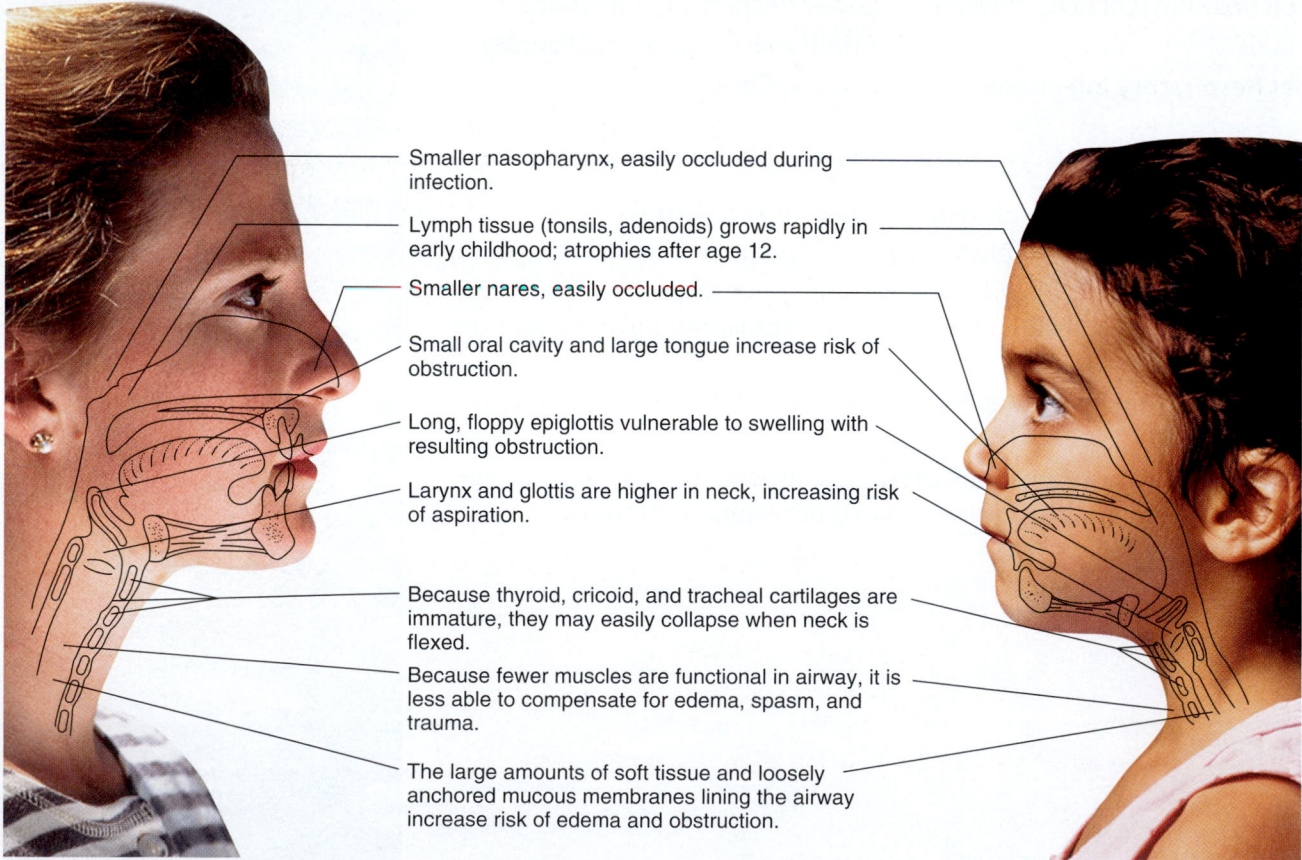

Smaller nasopharynx, easily occluded during infection.

Lymph tissue (tonsils, adenoids) grows rapidly in early childhood; atrophies after age 12.

Smaller nares, easily occluded.

Small oral cavity and large tongue increase risk of obstruction.

Long, floppy epiglottis vulnerable to swelling with resulting obstruction.

Larynx and glottis are higher in neck, increasing risk of aspiration.

Because thyroid, cricoid, and tracheal cartilages are immature, they may easily collapse when neck is flexed.

Because fewer muscles are functional in airway, it is less able to compensate for edema, spasm, and trauma.

The large amounts of soft tissue and loosely anchored mucous membranes lining the airway increase risk of edema and obstruction.

Figure 18-1. ■ The child's airway is clearly smaller and less developed that an adult's. Because of this, serious consequences may occur in the child with an upper respiratory tract infection, allergic reaction, or malpositioning of the head and neck during sleep. Swallowed objects pose a serious danger to the child.

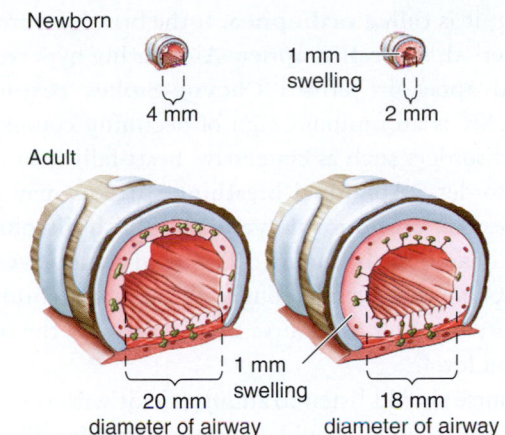

Figure 18-2. ■ The diameter of an infant's airway is approximately 4 mm; the adult's airway is 20 mm. An inflammation process that narrows the adult airway to 18 mm could easily narrow the infant's airway to 2 mm (see upper section of illustration).

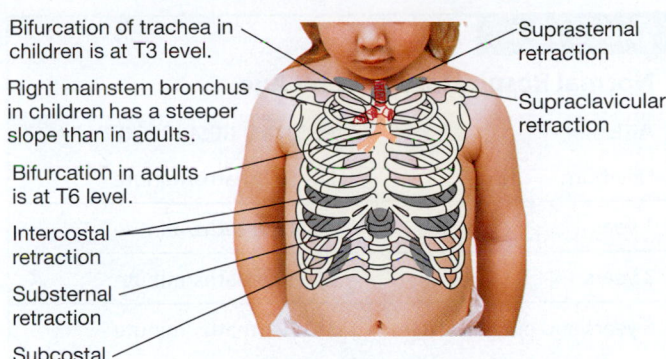

Figure 18-3. ■ In children, the trachea is shorter and the angle of the right bronchus at *bifurcation* (place where it splits in two) is more acute than in the adult. When you are resuscitating or suctioning, you must allow for the differences. *Note the shaded areas of retraction in the illustration.* Retractions may occur in the very young infant in the suprasternal area. In the older infant and child, retractions occur when the airway is severely obstructed, as in croup.

located in the nasal pharynx. The palatine tonsils are located on each side of the oral pharynx, and the lingual tonsils are located between the back of the tongue and the epiglottis. The tonsils begin to atrophy in midadolescence, so tonsillectomy and adenoidectomy are rarely performed after age 15. The epiglottis is a cartilage "door" that covers the larynx during swallowing in order to prevent food from entering the airway.

Besides a passageway for air to enter the lungs, the larynx contains the vocal cords. The larynx is surrounded by cartilage for protection. Muscles attached to the vocal cords control the pitch of the voice.

The trachea or windpipe extends from the larynx to the bronchi in the chest (Figure 18-3 ■). The trachea is held open by C-shaped rings of cartilage. The remainder of the respiratory tree is made up of branches of the trachea called bronchi and smaller bronchioles. Each bronchiole ends in an air sac or alveolus. The alveoli are surrounded by capillaries through which gas exchange takes place.

Although the structures of the respiratory system are the same for children as adults, the size of the organs is different. The small diameter of the airways makes obstruction more likely (see Figure 18-2). For example, the size of the child's trachea closely approximates the diameter of the little finger. Small toys, bits of food such as raisins, and hard candy can block the airway with serious consequences. A child's trachea is shorter than an adult's. Therefore, when suctioning the airway, the suction catheter does not need to be advanced as far (see Figure 18-3).

Mechanism of Respiration

The mechanism of breathing is a complex process of changing pressure. Inside the aorta and carotid arteries (the major

blood vessels leaving the left side of the heart) are specialized cells or chemoreceptors. When the carbon dioxide level in the blood rises, the chemoreceptors sense the elevation and send a message to the brain. The brain responds by stimulating a contraction of the **diaphragm** (the large muscle dividing the chest and abdominal cavities) and **intercostal muscles** (the muscles between the ribs). The contraction of these muscles causes the ribs to move outward and the diaphragm to flatten. The result is an increase in the size of the chest cavity, creating a vacuum that sucks air into the body. The pressure of oxygen inside the alveoli is greater than that in the blood, allowing oxygen to move into the capillary. The carbon dioxide level in the blood is greater than that in the alveoli, allowing carbon dioxide to move into the alveoli. The diaphragm and intercostal muscles relax, moving the ribs and diaphragm back to a resting state and pushing air out of the lungs. This cycle repeats 20 to 40 times a minute.

Brief Assessment Overview

Assessing the respiratory system of a child is the same as for an adult. However, because the child may not be able to tell you subjective information, observation of respiratory patterns and skin color are critical. The child should be quiet in order to assess breathing depth, regularity, and lung sounds accurately.

To assess respiratory rate and breathing patterns accurately, the child must be in a position with the chest exposed so the nurse can watch the chest rise and fall. Table 18-1 ■ identifies the normal respiratory rate by age. The child's respiratory rate gradually slows and, by age 6, approximates that of the adult.

TABLE 18-1

Normal Respiratory Rate by Age

AGE	RESTING RESPIRATORY RATE
Newborn	30–50 breaths/minute
1 year	20–40 breaths/minute
3 years	20–30 breaths/minute
6 years and older	16–22 breaths/minute

Up to approximately 6 months of age, the infant is a nose breather. After that time, the child will open the mouth to breathe when the nasal passages are congested. The normal breathing pattern (**eupnea**) is regular, with the client unaware of the breathing pattern. The newborn has an irregular breathing pattern, which gradually becomes regular over the first 3 to 4 months. **Hypoventilation** refers to slow shallow respirations that can indicate a depressed central nervous system function by drugs or other disorders. **Hyperventilation** refers to deep rapid respirations that occur from exercise, disorders that increase metabolism, or psychological stress. **Dyspnea** is difficulty breathing as evidenced by retractions or upward movement of the rib cage by contracting the neck muscles (see Figure 9-18). Areas of retraction are also shown as the shaded areas in Figure 18-3. If dyspnea is relieved by sitting or standing, it is called **orthopnea**. If the breathing stops for a brief period, it is called **apnea**. Alternating hyperventilation and apnea is termed **Cheyne–Stokes respiration (CSR)**. CSR is an ominous sign of declining condition in critical disorders such as congestive heart failure or neurologic disorders. Abnormal breathing patterns may be accompanied by **circumoral cyanosis** (bluish discoloration of the skin around the mouth). The child could have a productive or nonproductive cough. Whenever a child has a respiratory disorder, the nurse should monitor the oxygen saturation level.

The nurse should listen to all lung fields with the stethoscope. Lung sounds should be clear. **Crackles** (fine, dry sounds, formerly called rales), **rhonchi** (coarse, wet sounds), and wheezing are common sounds in the child with respiratory disorders. These sounds result when airways are partially obstructed by mucus or bronchial muscle spasms. Differentiating expiratory wheezes from inspiratory wheezes can be difficult due to the normally rapid respiratory rate. Occasionally, the child develops **stridor** (a high-pitched inspiratory crowing sound caused by severely narrowed airways).

clinical ALERT

When a child develops stridor, prompt medical attention is needed to prevent total airway obstruction.

UPPER RESPIRATORY DISORDERS

Epistaxis

Manifestations

Epistaxis or nosebleed is common in school-age children. The anterior nares, rich in blood vessels, are the usual source of bleeding. Blood vessels can be irritated by trauma, including nose picking, foreign bodies, and low humidity resulting in drying of the mucous membranes. Other causes could be allergies, forceful blowing of the nose, and infection.

Diagnosis

Diagnosis is made by obvious blood draining from the nares or down the throat. However, the location of the bleeding may be more difficult to determine. Most nosebleeds coming from the anterior septum stop in 10 minutes with treatment. The posterior septum can also be a source of nosebleeds. Posterior nosebleeds are usually more difficult to stop and may need medical attention. Posterior nosebleeds have a variety of causes that may include systemic conditions such as bleeding disorders, leukemia, and hypertension. If a nosebleed does not stop within 10 minutes or occurs frequently without identifiable cause, the child needs medical attention.

Treatment

First aid treatment of nosebleeds includes applying direct firm pressure to the bleeding nares where the nose attaches to the maxillary bone. By pushing the outer side of the nares against the nasal septum, blood supply is slowed and clot formation can begin. The child should hold the head slightly forward to prevent blood from going down the throat and into the stomach, which can cause nausea and vomiting. A cold cloth applied to the forehead and back of the neck can slow circulation to the nose and aid in clot formation. Once the nosebleed stops, the child should not blow the nose for several hours to prevent a second nosebleed.

Upper Respiratory Infections

Upper respiratory infections in young children are common. Infections stimulate the immune system to develop antibodies that will protect the young child in later life. However, if the immune system is immature or is overwhelmed by multiple infections or other disorders, the life of the child may be in danger. Upper respiratory system infections include bacterial and viral infections of the nasal and oral pharynx, tonsils, middle ear, and epiglottis.

NASOPHARYNGITIS

Manifestations

The most common infection in children, **nasopharyngitis**, also called **rhinitis, coryza,** or the "common cold," is inflammation of the nasal mucosa often caused by a viral infection (e.g., rhinovirus, coronavirus) or bacteria (especially group A *Streptococcus*). The classic symptoms include redness and swelling of the nasal and pharyngeal mucosa. Clear nasal discharge either through the nares or down the back of the throat is common. Tonsils may be enlarged, and vesicles may appear on the soft palate and the pharynx. Fever and irritability or general discomfort may occur. If the discharge becomes yellow or greenish, a bacterial infection should be suspected. Mouth breathing leads to drying of the mucous membranes, further irritation, and pain.

Diagnosis

Diagnosis is based on symptoms, nasal swabs, or throat culture.

Treatment

Nasopharyngitis usually resolves within 10 days. Parents may assist the child by providing humidified air when the child is sleeping. Saline nose drops can be administered every 3 to 4 hours and can be helpful to infants when given just prior to feeding. Older children may use drops or sprays. Decongestants or antihistamines may be prescribed. Parents should be taught to use over-the-counter medicines only if approved for use in children and only in the dosage recommended for the child's age and weight. Aspirin should be avoided because of its association with Reye's syndrome.

Between episodes, the child should be asymptomatic. If the infection persists or recurs frequently, the child should be evaluated by the primary care provider. Antibiotics, decongestants, and antihistamines may be prescribed. Persistent or recurring respiratory infections could indicate a bacterial infection or a more serious condition, such as leukemia or diabetes mellitus. Herbal remedies are sometimes employed to assist with symptoms (Box 18-1 ■). Teach parents to review home remedies with the care provider to ensure safety.

TONSILLITIS

Manifestations

Tonsillitis, inflammation of the palatine tonsils, commonly spreads from the nasopharynx through the drainage of lymphatic fluid. Tonsillitis may be caused by a virus or bacteria,

---

BOX 18-1	COMPLEMENTARY THERAPIES

Herbal Agents Used for Respiratory Disorders

Herbal remedies may be used to achieve balance in the body. Common herbs used to prevent or treat respiratory disorders are:

- Eucalyptus—Clears stuffy nose and congested sinuses; boil in water and breathe in steam.
- Garlic—Treats cough and may have some antibiotic effect when eaten raw.
- Mullein—Soothes and relaxes airway and relieves cough; mix with water and take orally.
- Echinacea—Boosts the immune system to help prevent infection.

---

and the condition tends to recur. The inflammation causes the tonsils to enlarge, resulting in pain, difficulty swallowing, and a risk for airway obstruction (Figure 18-4 ■). Frequently, the swelling of the mucous membrane narrows or closes the eustachian tubes, trapping fluid in the middle ear. Micro-organisms can be trapped in the middle ear as well, resulting in otitis media (see Chapter 16 ⬭).

clinical ALERT

Any child presenting with an upper respiratory infection should be evaluated for otitis media. Any child presenting with otitis media should be evaluated for an upper respiratory infection. These infections often occur simultaneously.

Diagnosis

When a child presents with a sore throat and swelling and infection of the tonsils, a culture is needed to determine the causative agent. The tympanic membranes are visualized and assessed for redness and fluid in the middle ear.

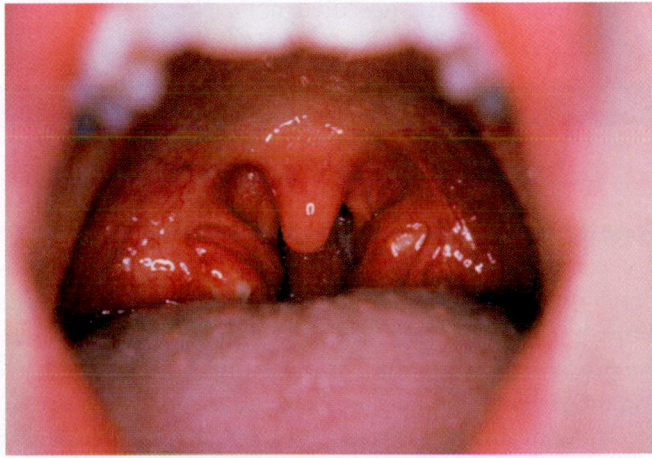

Figure 18-4. ■ Infected tonsils can swell and obstruct the airway. (DR P. MARAZZI / SCIENCE PHOTO LIBRARY\Custom Medical Stock Photo, Inc.)

HEALTH PROMOTION ISSUE

TONSILLECTOMY

Parents worry about their children's tonsils, either because the tonsils are large, making swallowing difficult and causing snoring, or because of frequent episodes of tonsillitis. Ear, nose, and throat specialists are reluctant to surgically remove the tonsils. When should tonsils be removed?

DISCUSSION

The *tonsils*, lymphatic tissue found in the posterior oral pharynx, function to drain the lymph from the nose and sinuses. The nasal passages are the first line of entry for airborne bacteria and viruses. The lymph from the nose may contain these bacteria or viruses. Once the lymph enters the tonsil tissue, the micro-organisms are destroyed by white blood cells. At times, the number of micro-organisms entering the nose or multiplying within the lymph is greater than the white blood cells can destroy. When this occurs, the tonsils become swollen, red, and painful. If tonsillitis is the result of a virus, the infection will usually resolve spontaneously in 10 days to 2 weeks. If tonsillitis is from a bacterial infection, the child may need antibiotics to help stop the infection. This is especially true when the causative organism is beta-

hemolytic *Streptococcus*, which can invade and damage heart tissue.

Two common indications for tonsillectomy are chronic tonsillitis, having continuous symptoms for more than 3 months, or recurrent tonsillitis, having at least five episodes of tonsillitis in a year. However, the American Academy of Otolaryngology recommends that children have a tonsillectomy if they have three or more episodes of tonsillitis in a year. In contrast, a study by Jack L. Paradise, MD (2002), reported that the modest benefit of a tonsillectomy in children who are moderately affected with sore throats (seven per year) does not seem to justify the risks, morbidity, or cost.

Sometimes the tonsils and adenoids become so enlarged that they cause obstructive sleep apnea (OSA). Children

with OSA snore, have labored breathing, observed apnea, restlessness, excessive daytime sleepiness, and behavior or learning problems, including attention deficit/hyperactivity disorder. Once the diagnosis of OSA is made, the child usually has both the tonsils and the adenoids removed (Marcus, C. L., Chapmen, D., Word, S. D., McColley, S. A., 2002).

Children with large tonsils can also have difficulty swallowing, resulting in feeding problems, failure to thrive, mouth breathing, and speech problems. As the child ages, the tonsils usually get smaller. If it is believed that the child will not outgrow the enlarged tonsils in a reasonable amount of time, or if the child is losing weight, a tonsillectomy may be performed.

The nurse collects data regarding the number of sore throats the child has

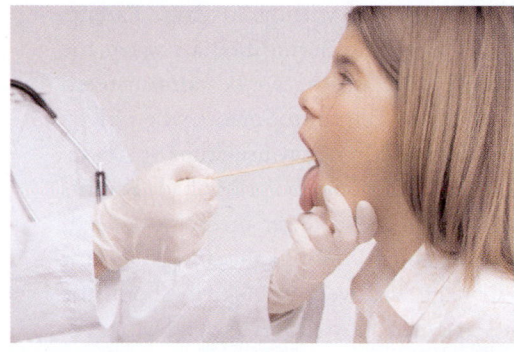

(Glow Wellness/Getty Images)

Treatment

When tonsillitis is caused by a virus, treatment is symptomatic until the infection resolves. Acetaminophen eases throat pain and reduces fever. Cold nonacidic liquids or frozen popsicles can soothe the throat and help prevent dehydration. A home humidifier can aid breathing during sleep. Teach parents to make a mild saltwater solution by dissolving ¼ tsp of common salt in 8 oz warm water. Parents may need to show the child how to gargle with this solution in order to wash and soothe the swollen tissue in the throat.

When tonsillitis is caused by bacteria, antibiotics are generally prescribed. Because some bacteria, such as beta-hemolytic *Streptococcus*, can cause more serious infections (e.g., rheumatic fever), it is important to encourage parents to obtain treatment in a timely manner.

If a child has frequent recurrent episodes of bacterial tonsillitis, consideration may be given to surgical removal of the tonsils (**tonsillectomy**). The Health Promotion Issue above discusses this topic.

had over time. It is important to obtain a throat culture to document the cause of the illness and to provide the correct medical treatment. Sore throat from postnasal drip does not count as an episode of tonsillitis unless the tonsils have pus on them. It is important for the nurse to question the child and parent regarding a current cold or sinus drainage. The severity of the symptoms should also be determined. If symptoms are so severe that the child misses a week of school with each episode of tonsillitis, a tonsillectomy may be warranted.

When a child presents with behavioral or attention problems, questions regarding sleep habits, snoring, and restlessness should be addressed. If the child is not growing at an acceptable rate or states dysphagia, the nurse should look in the throat to assess the size of the tonsils.

PLANNING AND IMPLEMENTATION

Parents need information about the child's specific disorder. If the child has recurrent or chronic tonsillitis, it is important for the nurse to teach the parents methods of preventing infection. Instruction must include hand washing, diet, adequate sleep, and avoiding infected persons. The nurse should answer questions about possible surgery, preoperative and postoperative care, and administration of antibiotics (including their side effects).

Even though the tonsils offer an important line of defense for the body, there are times when tonsillectomy is a necessary procedure. Continuous or recurrent tonsillitis can lead to more serious heart conditions and must be treated promptly. Sleep apnea is also a serious condition, and the parents should not wait for the child to outgrow the tonsil problems.

SELF-REFLECTION

Think of one time when you were out of breath from running or swimming. You may recall leaning forward over your knees (orthopneic position) and inhaling forcefully as you tried to "catch your breath." Gradually, your breathing returned to normal and your body relaxed. Knowing that in tonsillitis the child may experience restricted breathing, think of measures you can use to assist the child. Review both pharmacologic and nonpharmacologic measures.

SUGGESTED RESOURCES

For the Nurse

■ Aligne, C. A., Auinger, P., Byrd, R. S., & Weitzman, M. (2000). Risk factors for pediatric asthma. *American Journal of Respiratory and Critical Care Medicine, 162*(3), 873–877.

■ Baroi, M., Anderson, Y., & Mischler, E. (1997). Cystic fibrosis newborn screening: Impact of early screening results on parenting stress. *Pediatric Nursing, 23*(2), 143–151.

■ Marcus, C. L., Chapman, D., Ward, S. D., & McColley, S. A. (2002). Clinical practice guideline: Diagnosis and management of childhood obstructive sleep apnea syndrome. *Pediatrics, 109*(4), 704–712.

■ Paradise, J., L. (2002). Tonsillectomy and adenotonsillectomy for recurrent throat infection in moderately affected children. *Pediatrics, 110*(1), 7–15.

■ Ramilo, O., & Jafri, H. (2004). RSV can increase the risk of asthma. *Journal of Infectious Diseases, 198*(10), 1856–1865.

For the Client

■ www.everydaykidz.com This is a website for parents and caregivers of children with asthma-related breathing problems.

Nursing Considerations

When a tonsillectomy is planned, the nurse must provide preoperative teaching for the child and parents. The age and development of the child will influence the method of presenting information to the child. (See Chapters 12 and 14 ∞ for information about communicating with children.) Generally, routine preoperative care will be needed. This includes NPO for at least 4 hours, assessing the mouth for loose teeth, initiating an IV line, and giving sedation.

Postoperatively, the child's throat will be sore and the child may not want to swallow. Cold fluids such as popsicles may help relieve discomfort and increase fluids. Milk products are generally not given because they increase mucus production. Red fluids are also avoided so secretions do not appear to be blood. Liquid analgesics may be ordered.

The primary complication of a tonsillectomy is bleeding in the first 24 hours and again when the scab comes off around day 10. Excessive swallowing may indicate blood is draining down the back of the throat. The nurse must use a flashlight to look into the child's oral pharynx to assess for bleeding. The child may be discharged from the hospital within 24 hours after surgery. Parents should be taught to keep the child quiet for a few days, offer soft foods, and increase fluid intake. Bleeding will continue to be a concern until healing is complete in 7 to 14 days. Any trauma to the back of the throat will increase the risk of bleeding. For this reason, drinking straws should be avoided, and the child should be supervised while brushing the teeth. During the healing process, the dark scab will turn white and eventually slough off. Most commonly, the child will swallow the scab without noticing. Until healing is complete, the child's breath may have a strong foul odor. Gargling with mouthwash or saltwater is not recommended due to the increased risk of bleeding. The odor will subside once healing is complete. Teach parents to contact the doctor immediately if bleeding is noticed.

EPIGLOTTITIS

Manifestations

Epiglottitis is inflammation of the epiglottis caused by a bacterial infection of the pharynx and soft tissue of the larynx. As the epiglottis swells with inflammation, complete respiratory obstruction is possible. Therefore, epiglottitis is a potentially life-threatening condition. Typically, the child develops a sudden high fever (higher than 102°F or 39°C), a sore throat, muffled or hoarse voice (**dysphonia**), and difficulty swallowing (**dysphagia**). As swelling progresses, inspiratory stridor begins. Due to dysphagia, the child does not swallow saliva, resulting in drooling. Orthopnea is common.

clinicaL ALERT

The child might insist on sitting upright, leaning forward with the chin thrust forward, mouth open, and tongue protruding. This is called the **tripod position.** The child should be allowed to maintain this position because it helps keep the epiglottis from obstructing the airway.

Diagnosis

Diagnosis is based on symptoms. Visual inspection is contraindicated because of the danger of triggering laryngospasm and airway obstruction in the child. A lateral x-ray view of the neck may be taken. Culture is postponed until an endotracheal tube or tracheostomy is in place.

Treatment

Medical treatment includes the insertion of an endotracheal tube in order to maintain the airway (see Procedure 13-28 Assisting with Airway Insertion). IV antibiotics are given to treat the infection. Acetaminophen or ibuprofen may be used to reduce the fever and discomfort. The child with epiglottitis is often cared for in the intensive care unit (ICU).

Nursing Considerations

Nursing care consists of managing the airway, administering prescribed medications, maintaining hydration, and providing emotional support for the child and family. Crying stimulates the airway, increases oxygen consumption, causes the respiratory system to work harder, and could cause laryngospasm, which would totally occlude the airway. Provide a calm, quiet environment and a confident manner. The calmer the child is, the better. Avoid any painful or frightening procedure until after the airway is secured. At times, sedation may be needed.

clinicaL ALERT

Because of the life-threatening nature of epiglottitis, infants and toddlers who cannot ask for help must not be left alone during the acute phase of epiglottitis.

Difficulty swallowing, breathing, and speaking is frightening to the child and parents. The unfamiliar environment of the hospital creates additional stress. The nurse can reassure the child and family by remaining calm, explaining the various pieces of equipment, and providing care in a professional manner. Remaining in the room, or leaving for only a brief time, reassures the child and family that their needs will be met. Keep parents informed, and reassure them that any loss of voice is temporary.

Most children show rapid response to treatment with cool mist, fluids, and antibiotics. The endotracheal tube can usually be removed in 24 to 36 hours. Home care involves completing the antibiotics as ordered. Parents need instruction in medication administration and potential side effects of the specific medication.

Foreign Body Obstructed Airway

The airway can become obstructed when the child puts small objects in the mouth or chokes on food. Infants and young children must be watched closely while eating and be taught not to put small objects in the mouth. Even with appropriate care, foreign body obstruction of the

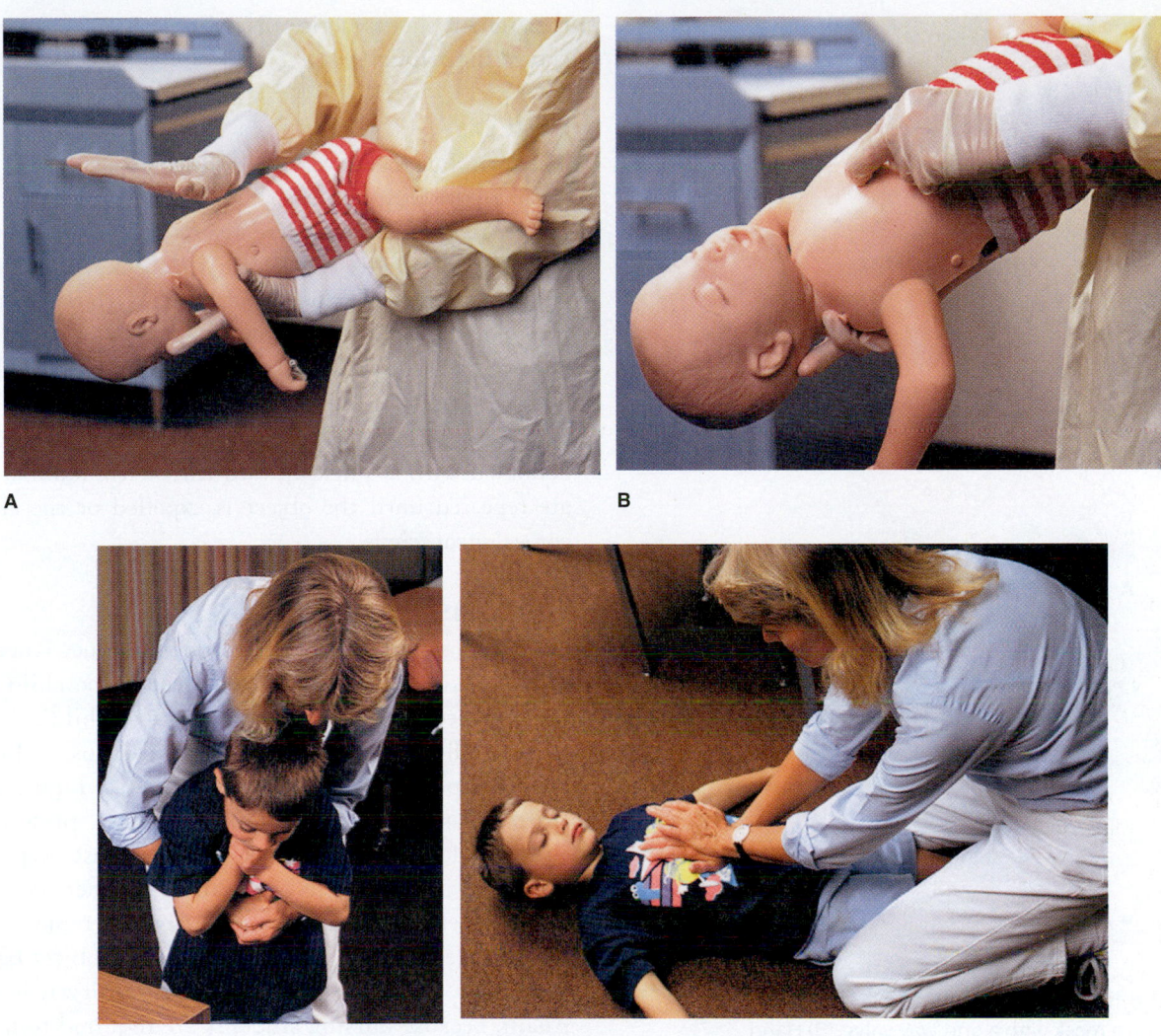

A

B

C

D

Figure 18-5. ■ Clearing a foreign object. (**A**) Back blows. (**B**) Chest thrusts on infant. (**C**) Standing thrusts (Heimlich maneuver) must be done more gently in a child than in an adult. (**D**) Chest thrusts on an unconscious child.

Medialink

Foreign body airway obstruction

airway can occur. In this emergency situation, the care provider must immediately open the airway. To determine if the airway is obstructed, observe the child's facial expression, ask the child if he or she can talk, and observe for respirations. If the object can be seen in the back of the throat, try to remove it with a finger sweep, taking care not to push it deeper into the airway. If the object cannot be removed, the Heimlich maneuver (Figure 18-5 ■) is the recommended procedure to clear an obstructed airway safely. The size of the child will determine the position and procedure used.

INFANT

To perform the Heimlich maneuver on an infant, the prone position is used with the baby's head lower than the trunk (see Figure 18-5A). Support the head and neck with one hand, with the torso on the forearm. Use the palm of the other hand to give five forceful back blows between the shoulder blades. After the back blows, the free hand is placed over the back of the neck sandwiching the infant between the hands. The infant is turned over maintaining the head-down position. Two fingers are placed on the middle of the sternum between the nipples. Five chest thrusts are given at a rate of one every 3 to 5 seconds. Abdominal thrusts are not used on infants due to the risk of damaging the internal organs. This procedure is repeated until the airway is cleared.

Cardiopulmonary resuscitation (CPR; Figure 18-6 ■) may be needed once the airway is open. (CPR training is not reviewed in detail in this text. Nurses often obtain training for CPR through the American Heart Association, local Red Cross, or their employing agency. Nurses may be expected or required to maintain current certification

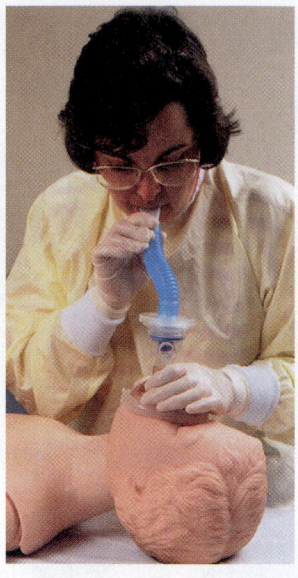

A

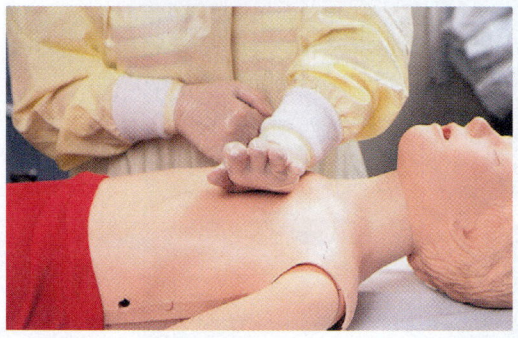

B

Figure 18-6. ■ CPR. (**A**) Mouth-to-mouth resuscitation using a mask with a one-way valve. (**B**) Hand position for chest compressions with a child.

throughout their practice.) Newborn resuscitation was discussed in Chapter 9 ⚭.

CHILD

The Heimlich maneuver is performed on a child the same as on an adult. However, the smaller the child, the more gently the abdominal thrusts are given. If the child is sitting or standing, grasp the child from the back with both arms wrapped around the child's abdomen. With one hand made into a fist, place the thumb side against the child's abdomen, slightly above the umbilicus and well below the xiphoid process of the sternum (see Figure 18-5C). The fist is grasped with the other hand and pressed into the child's abdomen with a quick upward thrust. Abdominal thrusts are repeated until the object is expelled or the child becomes unconscious.

UNCONSCIOUS CHILD

The unconscious child is positioned supine. Kneeling at the child's feet (standing at the feet if the child is on a table), place the heel of one hand on the child's abdomen, at the midline, slightly above the umbilicus, and well below the xiphoid process of the sternum (see Figure 18-5D). With the other hand on top of the first, press into the child's abdomen with a quick upward thrust. Repeat until the object is popped out of the airway. Sometimes, the object is expelled into the mouth and can be removed with a finger sweep, taking care not to push the object back into the airway. CPR may be needed once the airway is opened. Again, because nursing students are required to maintain CPR certification, the technique is not reviewed here.

LOWER RESPIRATORY DISORDERS

Congenital Respiratory Disorders

Tracheoesophageal fistula (TEF), a connection between the trachea and the esophagus, is the most common congenital anomaly affecting the respiratory system. TEF is associated with **esophageal atresia (EA)**, the esophagus ending in a blind pouch instead of connecting to the stomach. When the newborn takes breast milk or formula, the food will enter the trachea through the fistula, resulting in aspiration and pneumonia. There is a possibility that the baby could drown. Because the primary problem is with the esophagus, discussion is found in Chapter 22 ⚭.

CYSTIC FIBROSIS

Cystic fibrosis (CF) is an inherited recessive disorder of the exocrine glands affecting predominantly white chil-

dren. In CF, there is a defective chloride ion and water transport across the cell membranes of cells that secrete mucus, causing production of thick, tenacious mucus that obstructs all organs with mucous ducts. Electrolytes are lost through sweat saliva, and mucus secretions. The disease affects primarily the respiratory and gastrointestinal systems, but it has some effect on the integumentary, musculoskeletal, and reproductive systems as well (Figure 18-7 ■).

Manifestations

Presenting symptoms are usually meconium ileus (a small bowel obstruction) in the newborn, failure to thrive, or chronic recurrent respiratory infections. The child may be constipated often. The child will have a chronic, productive cough with thick, sticky mucus and

CYSTIC FIBROSIS

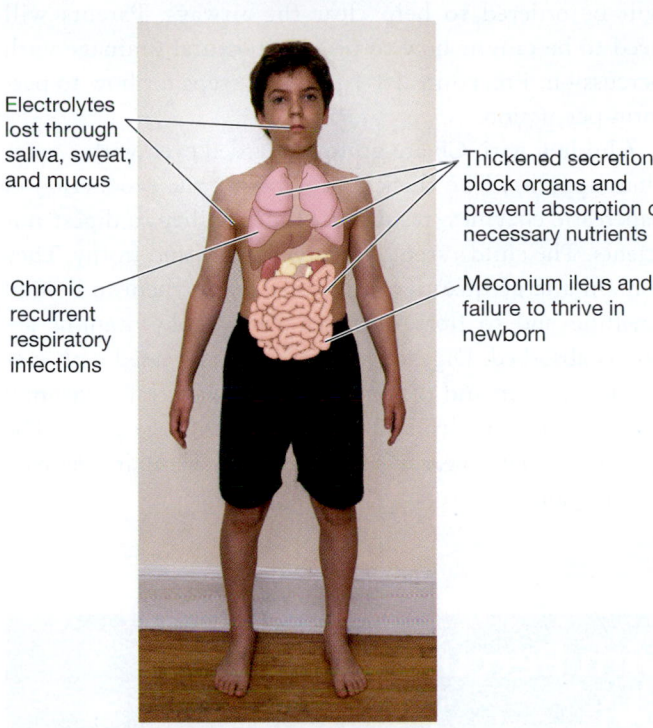

Electrolytes lost through saliva, sweat, and mucus

Thickened secretions block organs and prevent absorption of necessary nutrients

Chronic recurrent respiratory infections

Meconium ileus and failure to thrive in newborn

Figure 18-7. ■ Multisystem effects of cystic fibrosis.

MediaLink

Cystic fibrosis

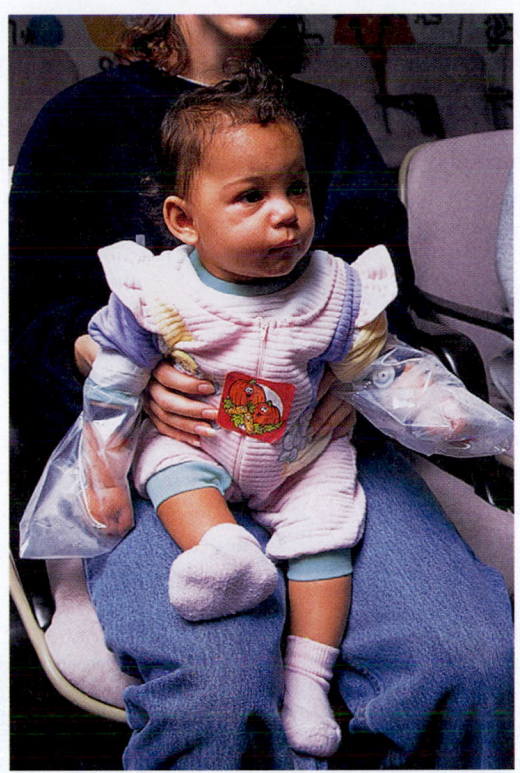

Figure 18-8. ■ Sweat test. The parent may hold and reassure the infant or small child being evaluated for cystic fibrosis with the sweat test. Sweat will be collected from the skin under the plastic wrappings for evaluation of sodium and chloride content. Note that sweat tests performed on infants younger than 4 weeks of age may not provide accurate results.

frequent respiratory infections. Despite a voracious appetite, children will have trouble gaining weight. There may be clubbing of fingers related to a reduction in oxygen reaching the tissues.

Diagnosis

Diagnosis is made by a positive sweat test (Figure 18-8 ■). Table 18-2 ■ describes this test. Diagnosis may be made before 1 year of age, but children with a mild form of the disease may not be diagnosed until adolescence. The disease is not generally terminal until adulthood.

Treatment

Medical treatment is aimed at maintaining maximum respiratory function and nutrition for as long as possible. Postural drainage (chest physiotherapy) is ordered to help the child eliminate respiratory secretions. Procedure 18-1 ■

TABLE 18-2				
Sweat Test for Cystic Fibrosis				
TEST	**PURPOSE**	**METHOD OF SPECIMEN COLLECTION**	**NORMAL FINDINGS**	**ABNORMAL FINDINGS**
Sweat test (pilocarpine iontophoresis)	To analyze sodium and chloride content	Two electrodes covered with special gel are placed on child's forearms. A small electric current is passed through electrode for 5 minutes. Some tingling may be noted. Electrodes are removed, and sweat collector is applied to same area. Sweat is collected for 30 to 45 minutes. Sweat collector is sent to laboratory for anaylsis.	Sodium: 10–30 mEq/L; Chloride: 10–35 mEq/L	Chloride: 50–60 mEq/L is suspicious More than 60 mEq/L with other signs is diagnostic

provides information on performing chest physiotherapy. Aggressive treatment of respiratory infections or allergies is required.

Pancreatic enzymes; vitamins A, D, E, and K; and a diet high in carbohydrates and protein are prescribed to manage the gastrointestinal complications of CF. On hot days, the child may need extra fluids and salt.

Nursing Considerations

When assessing a child with CF, pay close attention to respiratory function. Thick mucus can obstruct the bronchi, resulting in hypoxia and infection. The priority for assessment and intervention must be to open and maintain a patent airway (see Respiratory Procedures section in Chapter 13 ⦿). Children are frequently admitted to the hospital with an acute respiratory infection.

Respiratory therapy several times a day and antibiotics will be ordered to help clear the airways. Parents will need to be taught how to provide postural drainage with percussion. Procedure 18-1 provides steps for how to perform percussion.

Children with CF are growth retarded even with a voracious appetite. The thick mucus blocks the production of pancreatic enzymes, resulting in an inability to digest nutrients. The child's stools are large, bulky, and frothy. They contain a large quantity of fat that causes them to be foul smelling and to float in water. Fat-soluble vitamins are poorly absorbed. Digestive problems can be eased with special medication and diet modification. Pancreatic enzymes should be given with each meal and each large snack. The goal is to achieve near normal stools and maintain adequate weight gain.

PROCEDURE 18-1 # Postural Drainage with Percussion (Chest Physiotherapy)

Purpose

- To clear the airway of thick mucus

Equipment

- Bed or table for the child to lie on
- Pillows
- Hand towel

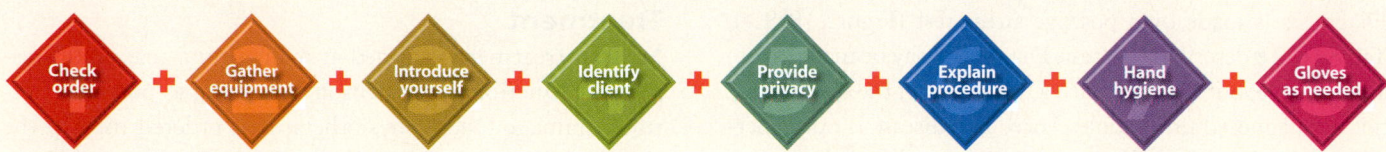

Check order + Gather equipment + Introduce yourself + Identify client + Provide privacy + Explain procedure + Hand hygiene + Gloves as needed

Interventions

1. Position the child on one side, usually with the head lower than the hips. (The various positions for chest physiotherapy are shown in Figure 18-9 ■.) The upper arm should be positioned over the head or across the anterior chest, exposing the lateral chest. Pillows may be used to support the child in position. *Positioning with the head down facilitates mucus moving from small bronchioles to larger bronchi by gravity.*

2. Place folded towel over the chest. *The towel protects the skin from trauma.*

3. With cupped hands (Figure 18-10 ■), gently clap on the lateral chest for 3 to 5 minutes. Turn the child to the abdomen to expose the back. Clap on the back over each lobe of the lung for 3 to 5 minutes each. Turn the child to

the opposite side and continue clapping over each lung field. *Clapping on the chest with cupped hands causes vibration inside the lung, moving mucus to larger airways.*

4. Sit the child up and have him or her deep breathe and cough. *Coughing helps expel mucus.*

5. With the child in a sitting position, clap over the upper chest to clear the right and left upper lobes. *The upper lobes are anterior to the main bronchus; therefore, the child must be sitting for gravity to pull the mucus toward the large airway.*

6. A mechanical vibrator can be purchased to provide percussion instead of clapping with the hands. The child's position will be the same. *Mechanical vibrators can be used with postural drainage to move mucus out of small airways.*

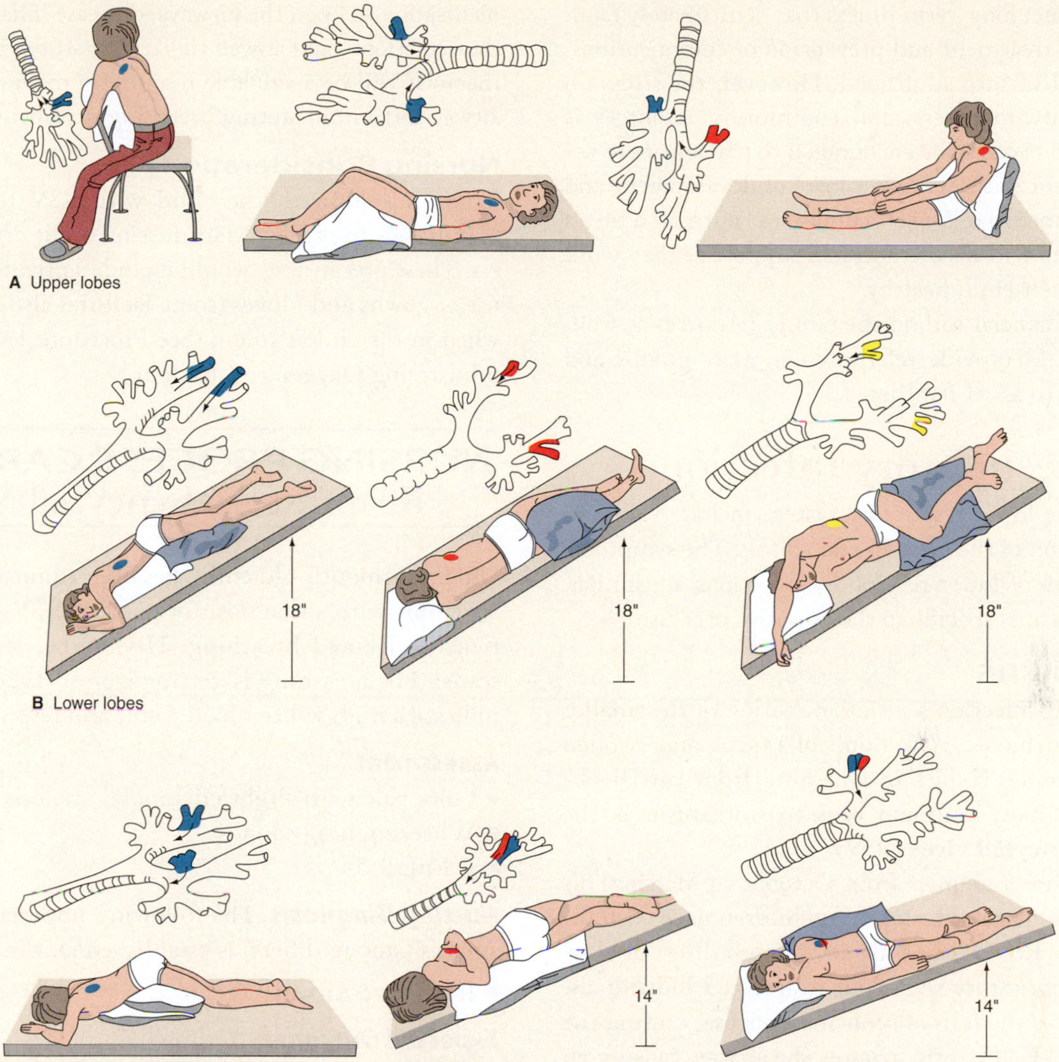

A Upper lobes

18"   18"   18"

B Lower lobes

14"   14"

C Lower Lobes (*continued*)   Right Middle Lobe   Left Upper Lobe

Figure 18-9. ■ Positions for postural drainage of different parts of the lung. The area of the lung to be drained is illustrated directly above the client's position. (Data from materials provided by Datalizer Slide Charts, Addison, IL)

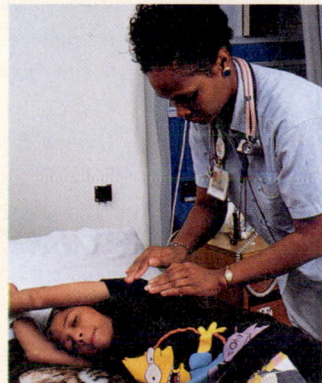

Figure 18-10. ■ The cupped-hand position is used to clap against the chest well over the segment to be drained. This creates a vibration that helps dislodge secretions. Various body positions are used, depending on the location of the obstruction. See Figure 18-9 for positions.

SAMPLE DOCUMENTATION

(date) 0730   Respirations labored, accessory muscles used with inspiration. Lung sounds diminished in right middle and lower lobes. Postural drainage with percussion to all lung fields performed by mother. Productive cough of a moderate amount of thick white mucus. Lung sounds clear bilaterally. Respirations less labored. _____
L. Hines, LPN

CF is a chronic, long-term illness that is ultimately fatal. With adequate treatment and prevention of complications, some children live into adulthood. However, the stress on the child, family members, and community resources is great. The child needs to be encouraged to participate in activities consistent with his or her level of development and physical endurance in order to maintain as "normal" a life as possible. Parents will need emotional support as they work daily to keep their child healthy.

CF takes a financial toll on the family resources as well. The nurse should provide referral to support groups and other resources to assist families.

Lower Respiratory Infections

Infections of the lower respiratory system include viral and bacterial infection of the bronchi and alveoli. The symptoms and nursing care of lower respiratory infections are similar. Medical treatment is specific to the causative organism.

BRONCHIOLITIS

Bronchiolitis is infection and inflammation of the smaller airways or bronchioles. A buildup of mucus and swollen mucous membranes results in wheezing from partial obstruction. The most common causative organism is the **respiratory syncytial virus (RSV)**.

RSV occurs in epidemics from October to March. This virus is easily transmitted, and most children have been infected by age 3. RSV is transmitted through direct or close contact with respiratory secretions of infected individuals. The virus invades the cells of bronchial mucosa, causing the cells to rupture. Cell debris irritates the airway, causing an increase in secretions that obstruct the bronchioles.

Manifestations

When the airways are partially obstructed, wheezing and crackles can be heard on auscultation. As the blockage continues, breath sounds diminish, causing impaired gas exchange and eventually leading to respiratory failure.

Symptoms of RSV begin with nasal stuffiness and fever, but within a few days they progress to frequent, deep cough; rapid, labored breathing; and respiratory distress, including retraction and nasal flaring. Parents report that the child appears sicker, refuses to eat, and is less playful. Labored lung sounds may diminish as airflow to the lungs decreases. The child may be dehydrated.

Diagnosis

Diagnosis is made by history, culturing nasopharyngeal secretions (e.g., with enzyme-linked immunosorbent assay or ELISA), and chest x-ray.

Treatment

The child with RSV will be hospitalized for treatment. The doctor will probably order IV fluids, humidified oxygen, and medication to open the airways, decrease inflammation, thin the secretions, and lower the temperature. The respiratory therapist will be a valuable resource in maintaining a patent airway and administering breathing treatments.

Nursing Considerations

When hospitalized, the child with RSV requires special precautions to prevent transmission of the organism to others. These precautions would include a private room and the use of gowns and gloves (some facilities also require masks) when in the child's room. (See Procedure 13-26 ⚭, Administering Oxygen to Children.)

NURSING PROCESS CARE PLAN
Respiratory Syncytial Virus

Omar, a 6-month-old child, has been admitted to the pediatric unit with a diagnosis of possible RSV. Omar is experiencing labored breathing. His mother states, "I am so scared. His breathing is getting worse." Laboratory reports indicate a high white blood count and respiratory acidosis.

Assessment
- Color pale with slight circumoral cyanosis
- Wheezing lung sounds
- P 150, R 54

Nursing Diagnosis.
The following important nursing diagnosis (among others) is established for this condition:
- Ineffective Airway Clearance.

Expected Outcome
- Airway will be clear within 48 hours.

Planning and Implementation
- Monitor vital signs every hour. *The child's condition can change rapidly and therefore must be closely monitored.*
- Monitor oxygen saturation continuously. *Continuous monitoring of oxygen saturation will alert the nurse if the child's condition deteriorates.*
- Administer oxygen as ordered. *Oxygen is administered to maintain oxygen saturation above 95%.*
- Anticipate worsening respiratory distress by monitoring breath sounds, respiratory effort, and level of consciousness. *Anticipating a worsening of the child's condition allows the nurse time to prepare for airway maintenance.*
- Reposition every ½ hour. *Frequent position changes facilitate drainage of respiratory mucus.*
- Administer IV fluids via appropriate equipment. *IV fluids are administered by infusion pump to prevent accidental fluid overload.*
- Administer medications with attention to dosage. *Pediatric dosage is individualized based on body weight. If dosage is not calculated carefully, overdose or underdose could occur. To maintain medication blood level in a therapeutic range, medications must be administered on time.*

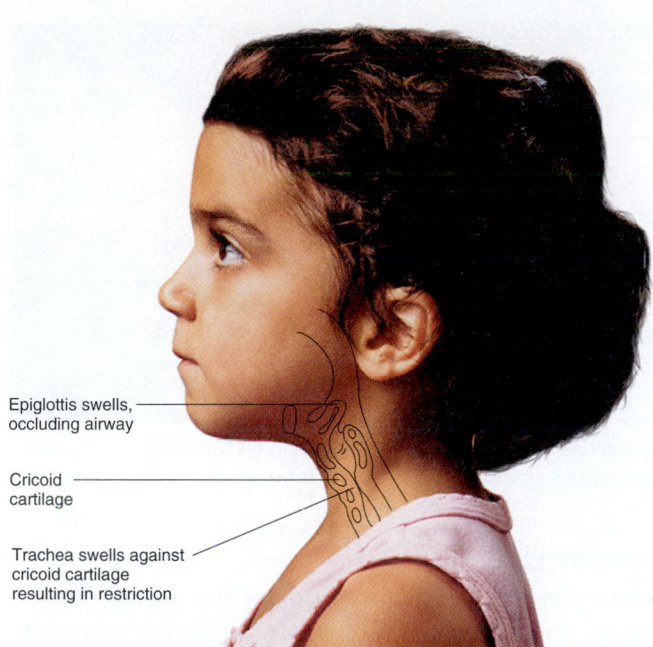

Figure 18-11. ■ In croup, the epiglottis swells and occludes the airway (*see inset*). The trachea swells against the cricoid cartilage, causing airway restriction.

Epiglottis swells, occluding airway

Cricoid cartilage

Trachea swells against cricoid cartilage resulting in restriction

Evaluation

- Lung sounds will be clear.
- Oxygen saturation will remain higher than 95%.

CROUP

Croup is a term used to represent a group of respiratory illnesses that results from inflammation and swelling of the larynx, trachea, and large bronchi (Figure 18-11 ■). The causative agent can be either viral or bacterial. Although laryngotracheobronchitis is the most common, epiglottitis (discussed previously) and bacterial tracheitis are the most serious. In these infections, swelling of the epiglottis occludes the larynx, and tracheal edema against the cricoid cartilage leads to obstruction.

(**Note:** infectious diseases such as pertussis—whooping cough—are discussed in Chapter 26. ⚭)

Manifestations

When a child has croup, inspiratory stridor will be present. A barking "seallike" cough and hoarseness are also present. The infant or child may have been ill for several days before the airway became partially obstructed and caused symptoms. Others may be healthy and develop severe symptoms in a matter of a few hours. Fever may or may not be present. The child may refuse to swallow saliva due to severe throat pain and swelling, resulting in drooling.

Diagnosis

Diagnosis is based on clinical findings. An x-ray may be taken to rule out foreign body obstruction. Pulse oximetry is used to detect hypoxemia.

Treatment

The goal of treatment is to reduce the swelling and open the airways. Cool mist administered by mask or tent (see Figure 13-33 and Procedures 13-25 to 13-28 ⚭) may be ordered. If a bacterial infection is present, appropriate antibiotic therapy will be prescribed. Endotracheal intubation may be needed to keep the airway open. Medications to reduce airway swelling may be ordered.

Nursing Considerations

As with other respiratory conditions, the child should be observed closely for airway patency, oxygen saturation, and retractions. It is important to deliver cool mist to the child in a quiet environment. The child should not be left alone because very young children may not be able to summon help. They should not cry because this can induce laryngospasm. Avoid probing the throat, including obtaining throat cultures, to prevent laryngospasm and complete obstruction.

Most children show rapid improvement once cool mist, oxygen, antibiotics, and fluids are started. The endotracheal tube, if used, can usually be removed in 24 to 36 hours. Discharge teaching includes the continued use of cool mist and administration of prescribed antibiotics, including side effects.

PNEUMONIA

Pneumonia is inflammation or infection of the bronchioles and alveoli in the lung (Figure 18-12 ■). Most common in

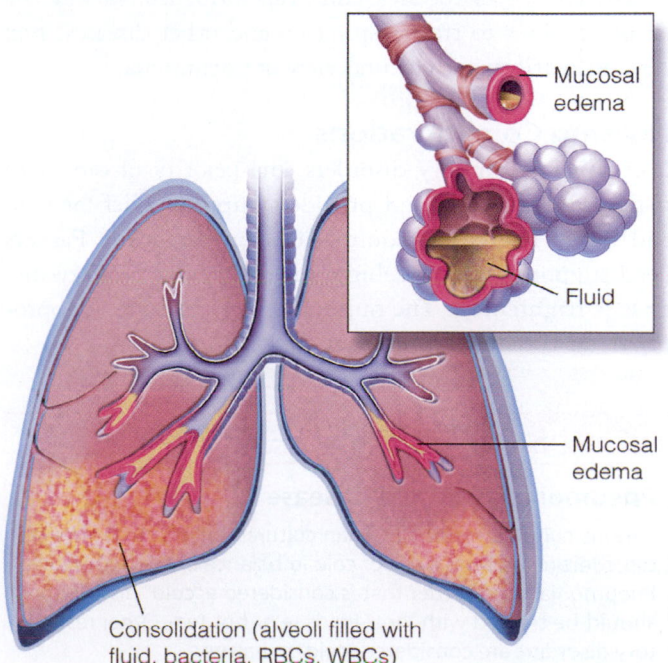

Mucosal edema

Fluid

Mucosal edema

Consolidation (alveoli filled with fluid, bacteria, RBCs, WBCs)

Figure 18-12. ■ Pneumonia in the lower lung lobes. The *inset* shows the buildup of fluid in the alveoli.

infants and young children, the causative organism is usually viral. In premature infants and older children, the causative agent is more commonly bacterial (*Pneumococcus*). Whether viral or bacterial in origin, the pathophysiology of pneumonia is the same. The infecting organism causes inflammation and swelling of the mucous membranes. Macrophages move to the area and engulf the organisms by phagocytosis. Thick mucus, dead cells, and other debris accumulate in the alveoli and small air passages where they block gas exchange. If the mucus remains in the small airways, it will consolidate and become more difficult to remove.

Manifestations

The child with lower respiratory infection will develop a fever, malaise, and a cough. Breath sounds may be wheezy, diminished, or absent in consolidated areas. Respirations will be fast (tachypnea) and labored. The child will be tired and want to sleep, but may be unable to rest due to dyspnea.

Diagnosis

Sputum cultures and chest x-rays are used to diagnose pneumonia.

Treatment

Medical treatment includes antibiotics (depending on the causative organism), fluids, cough suppressants, and antipyretics. If diagnosed early, the child may be treated at home. The hospitalized child will require oxygen (see Procedures 13-25 to 13-28), chest physiotherapy, and IV fluids. Most children recover in a short period of time.

The culture of the sick child can influence the way the family chooses to treat respiratory and other diseases. Box 18-2 ■ describes one cultural view of pneumonia.

Nursing Considerations

Like other respiratory disorders, the priority of care is to maintain the airway and provide symptom relief for pain and fever. The child requires constant attention. Parents need support because seeing their child in respiratory distress is frightening. The nurse provides teaching as appropriate for the situation and age of the child.

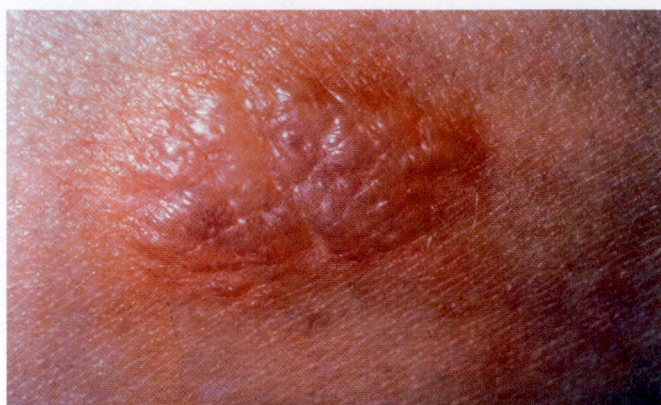

Figure 18-13. ■ Positive tuberculin skin test (Mantoux test), showing previous exposure to TB. (© BSIP/Custom Medical Stock Photo Inc.)

TUBERCULOSIS

Tuberculosis (TB) is an infection of the respiratory system by the acid-fast bacillus *Mycobacterium tuberculosis*. Most individuals with TB are immune compromised with disorders such as HIV/AIDS, leukemia, or other disorders affecting the white blood cells. When a child develops TB, it is most commonly due to close association with a TB-infected adult. If left untreated, the disease leads to lung damage and central nervous system involvement, including tuberculosis meningitis, coma, and death.

The organism enters the body by droplets from an infected individual. Once inside the lungs, the organism rapidly divides and spreads throughout the body via the lymphatic and circulatory systems. Granulomas develop around the site of primary exposure. The granulomas contain and destroy the bacteria, eventually scarring the lung tissue. Pockets of infection may survive the immune response and lay dormant for some time. A change in the body's internal environment can cause the disease to reactivate.

Diagnosis

Diagnosis is based on a combination of physical findings, positive purified protein derivative (PPD) skin tests (**Mantoux test**) (Figure 18-13 ■), x-rays, and laboratory isolation of *M. tuberculosis* in the sputum. In rare cases (Box 18-3 ■), the skin test may give a false-positive reading.

BOX 18-2 | **CULTURAL PULSE POINTS**

Pneumonia as a "Cold" Disease

Various cultures, especially Asian cultures, believe that physical disorders result from a hot or cold imbalance in the body fluids. Pneumonia is a disorder that is considered a "cold" disease that should be treated with "hot" fluids (e.g., hot tea). Other respiratory disorders are considered "cold" in nature.

BOX 18-3 | **CULTURAL PULSE POINTS**

Unusual Response to TB (Mantoux) Test

A false-positive tuberculin or Mantoux test can be expected from a child of Filipino heritage. This is due to the type of vaccine, bacille Calmette-Guérin, given to children of this country. To diagnose tuberculosis in these children, chest x-rays and sputum cultures are necessary.

TABLE 18-3

Pharmacology: Drugs Used to Treat Tuberculosis

DRUG (GENERIC AND COMMON BRAND NAME)	USUAL ROUTE/DOSE	CLASSIFICATION	SELECTED SIDE EFFECTS	DON'T GIVE IF
Isoniazid (INH)	10–15 mg/kg/day; give 1 hour before meals	Antituberculosis agent	Peripheral neuropathy, GI upset, weakness	Low BP (give with caution); liver damage
Rifampin (Rifadin)	10–20 mg/kg/day in divided dose every 12 hours	Antituberculosis agent	Dizziness, GI upset, colitis	Children younger than 5 years (use not determined)
Pyrazinamide (Tebrazid)	20–40 mg/kg/day in divided dose every 12 hours	Antituberculosis agent	Hemolytic anemia, difficulty urinating	Severe liver damage

Treatment

Medical treatment includes the administration of isoniazid, rifampin, and pyrazinamide for 2 months, followed by 6 months of isoniazid or rifampin. Table 18-3 ■ describes drugs used in the treatment of TB. The PPD test will be permanently positive. Chest x-ray will be required to determine the elimination or recurrence of the disease.

Nursing Considerations

Nursing care is centered on family education. Drug resistance to TB has increased dramatically in recent years, so parents must be taught the importance of adhering closely to the medical regimen and completing treatment. Teaching should include preventing the spread of the infection to others and stressing the necessity of taking the prescribed medication. All people who have come in contact with the infected child should be screened and treated as necessary.

Additional Respiratory Disorders

NEONATAL RESPIRATORY DISTRESS SYNDROME

Neonatal respiratory distress syndrome (RDS) is a condition commonly seen in premature infants. RDS is defined as an inadequate production of surfactant. (**Surfactant** is a mixture of phospholipids and apoproteins that attach to the internal surface of the alveoli, reducing the surface tension and improving the lungs' ability to remain inflated during exhalation.) Without adequate amounts of surfactant, the alveoli collapse (Figure 18-14 ■), and the infant must work hard to reinflate the alveoli with each breath.

Manifestations

The infant will exhibit signs of respiratory distress, including respirations greater than 60, retractions (see Figures 9-18 and 18-3 ◐◐), nasal flaring, and audible grunting. Lung sounds will be greatly decreased. Within a few minutes, symptoms can worsen.

Diagnosis and Treatment

Diagnosis, based on clinical symptoms, must be made rapidly in order to save the infant's life. Treatment includes oxygen and assisted mechanical ventilation (see Procedures 13-25 to 13-28 ◐◐). Synthetic surfactant, given within 24 hours, may be helpful in treating **atelectasis** (an airless state of the lung), but it does not prevent chronic inflammation.

Nursing Considerations

Children with RDS will be cared for in the ICU and will be monitored closely for oxygen and fluid levels. Infants will be placed in a warmer to maintain body temperature and reduce metabolic demands. Use of oxygen in premature infants can lead to bronchopulmonary dysplasia (discussed later) or blindness (called *retinopathy of prematurity*). Excess fluids can lead to pulmonary edema. The child may develop chronic lung disease.

Besides providing emergency treatment, the nurse must support the parents. The nurse may need to call clergy or family to be with the parents. Teaching about treatment can help alleviate the parents' fear of losing their child. Parents will need to learn CPR and oxygen administration. They may also need to learn how to use an apnea monitor or other equipment at home. Referral to a support group may be useful.

BRONCHOPULMONARY DYSPLASIA

Bronchopulmonary dysplasia (BPD) is a chronic lung disease that affects infants with RDS, congenital heart defects, meconium aspiration, or other conditions that result in assisted mechanical ventilation. Most infants with BPD have been on a mechanical ventilator for at least 3 days. The

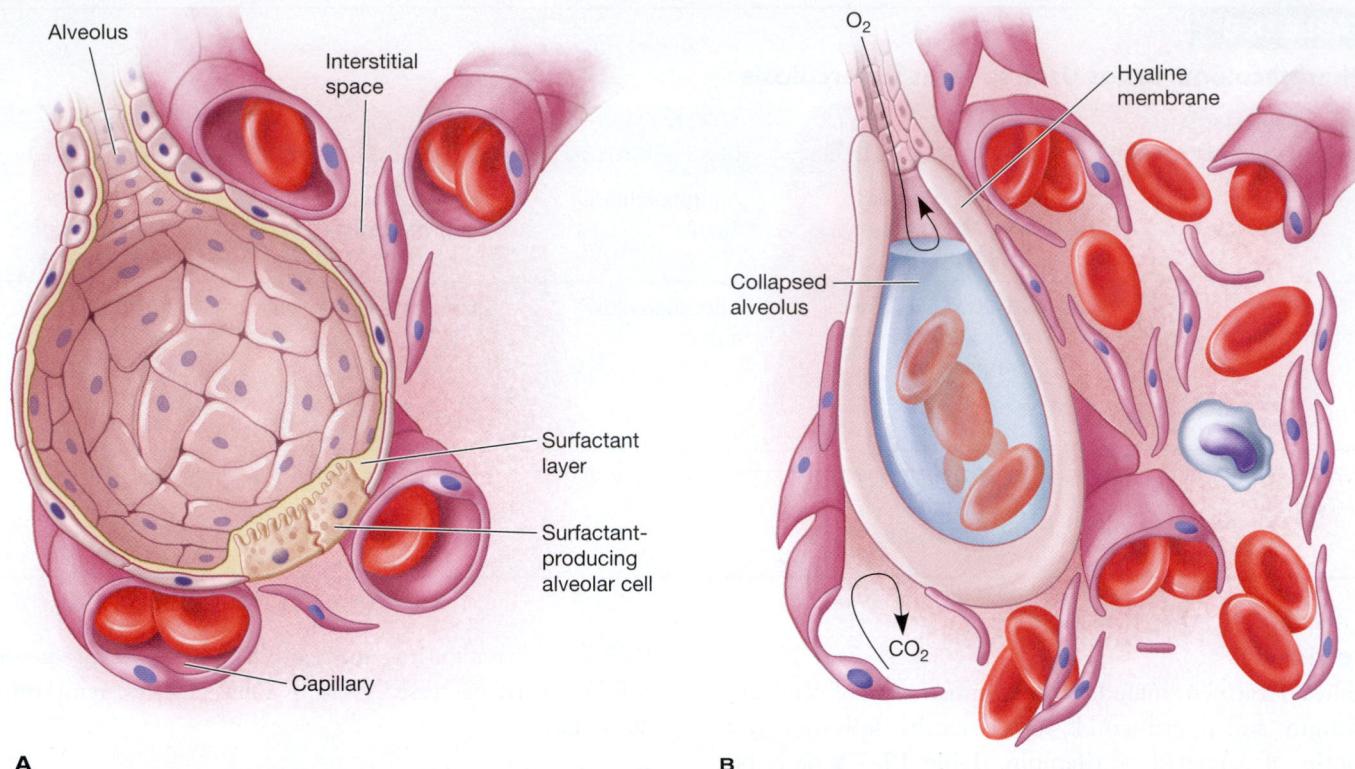

Figure 18-14. ■ Respiratory distress syndrome (RDS). When the newborn lung is lacking in surfactant, alveoli can collapse. **(A)** Healthy alveolus. **(B)** Collapsed alveolus.

immature lung becomes damaged from the high ventilator pressure and oxygen toxicity, resulting in pulmonary inflammation, cellular damage, and death of tissue.

Manifestations

The infant with BPD has persistent signs of respiratory failure due to bronchial edema and fibrosis of the lung tissue. There may be wheezing, crackles, retractions, nasal flaring, and grunting. Normal activities, such as feeding, place additional work on the respiratory system and may result in failure to thrive. Diagnosis is based on chest x-rays.

Treatment

Medical management involves supporting ventilation for weeks or months with progressive weaning from mechanical assistance, oxygen administration, nutrition, and anti-inflammatory medication. A tracheostomy is indicated for long-term mechanical ventilation. Long-term complications include asthma and recurrent pulmonary infections. Some infants require a gastrostomy tube for feeding in order to obtain adequate caloric intake to support growth.

Nursing Considerations

Nursing care focuses on promoting respiratory function and preparing the family for home care. The infant with BPD can become acutely ill with respiratory complications at any time, and parents must be alert for early symptoms. Parents must be

taught to administer feedings, oxygen, and medication. They must also learn to manage the required equipment. (See Figure 14-16 and respiratory Procedures 13-25 through 13-28 in Chapter 13 ⬯⬯.) At home, the infant may continue mechanical ventilation, oxygen, and medication. Parents who are fearful of assuming responsibility for their baby may require home nursing assistance. Referrals for respiratory supplies, medications, financial support, and follow-up care should be planned and coordinated before discharge.

SUDDEN INFANT DEATH SYNDROME

Sudden infant death syndrome (SIDS) is the sudden unexplained death of an infant younger than 1 year. SIDS most often strikes infants between 2 and 4 months of age and is more common in males. Other factors common in SIDS include Native American or African American descent, low birth weight, and multiple births (twins or triplets). SIDS is the leading cause of death of infants between 1 month and 1 year of age. Box 18-4 ■ identifies risk factors associated with SIDS.

Manifestations

When SIDS strikes, the infant is typically found not breathing, and emergency medical help is summoned. The infant is usually in a normal state of nutrition and hydration. In more than 50% of infants, blood-tinged frothy fluids are present in and around the mouth and nose. The diapers are filled with urine and stool. The infant may be clutching a blanket. There

BOX 18-4   ASSESSMENT

Risk Factors for SIDS

Infant

- Prematurity
- Low birth weight
- Twin or triplet birth
- Race (in decreasing order of frequency): most common in Native American infants, followed by African American, Hispanic, white, and Asian infants
- Gender: more common in males than females
- Age: most common in infants between 2 and 4 months of age
- Time of year: more prevalent in winter months
- Exposure to passive smoke
- History of cyanosis, respiratory distress, irritability, and poor feeding in the nursery
- Sleeping prone

Maternal and Familial

- Maternal age younger than 20 years
- History of smoking and illicit drug use (increases incidence 10 times)
- Anemia
- Multiple pregnancies, with short intervals between births
- History of sibling with SIDS (increases incidence four to five times)
- Low socioeconomic status; crowding
- Poor prenatal care, low birth weight gain

is no audible outcry at the time of death. Skin is a white ashen color, not the expected cyanotic blue found with respiratory distress. An autopsy will need to be performed to identify the cause of death.

Prevention and Treatment

Although infants who are at risk can be identified, SIDS remains unpredictable. The main preventive measure is to place infants on their back to sleep. If a child is found in respiratory arrest, CPR must be initiated immediately and emergency medical services called.

Nursing Considerations

The impact of SIDS on the family is one of extreme shock followed by extreme outrage. Family members commonly experience guilt, either self-blaming or projecting blame onto other family members or caregivers (e.g., a babysitter). Older children may fear SIDS will happen to them as well. Siblings may also believe that the infant died because of bad thoughts or desires they had toward their brother or sister.

The nurse has an important role in both supporting the family and educating the public. Recall that by 2 months infants are able to reposition their head to breathe. Ordinary bedding is incapable of causing hypoxia to the point of

suffocation. This knowledge can be used to help family members understand that the death was not their fault.

Although the need for support of parents and siblings is obvious, grandparents will need additional support. Grandparents will be experiencing grief at the loss of their grandchild, as well as extreme hurt at watching their own children suffer. Family members should be allowed to hold the infant, and receive handprints, footprints, and a lock of hair. Provide the family with information about local support groups.

ASTHMA

Asthma is a chronic inflammatory disorder of the tracheobronchial tree. Asthma attacks are influenced by a variety of triggers, including allergens, medication, fumes, exercise, or stress (Figure 18-15 ■). The stimulus that initiates the inflammatory process is specific to each individual. Before puberty, more boys have asthma, but by adulthood the disease is equally distributed between the genders.

Manifestations

As the lining of the tracheobronchial tree becomes irritated by an allergen, fumes, or dust, the cells release histamine.

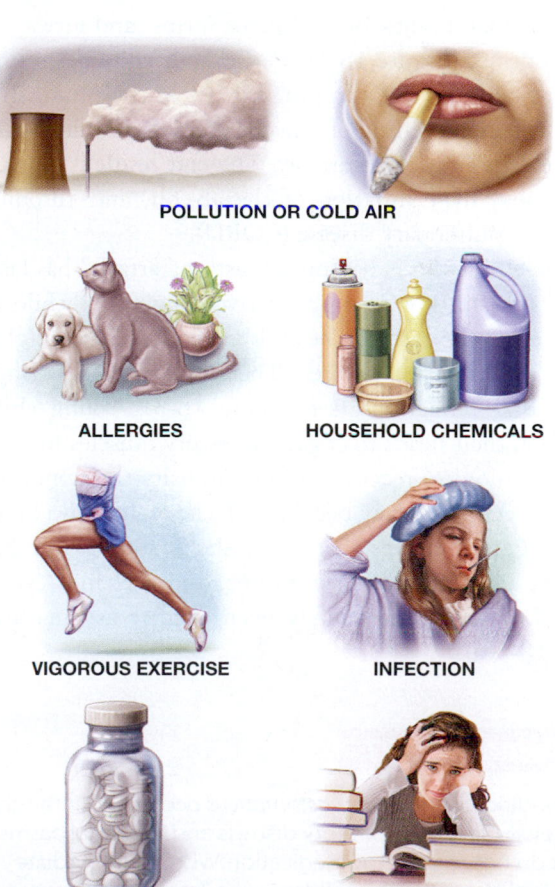

POLLUTION OR COLD AIR

ALLERGIES **HOUSEHOLD CHEMICALS**

VIGOROUS EXERCISE **INFECTION**

MEDICATIONS **STRESS**

Figure 18-15. ■ Some common triggers of asthma are shown above. Eliminating the child's exposure to potential asthma triggers requires significant lifestyle changes for the child and family, so be sensitive to the family's situation and needs.

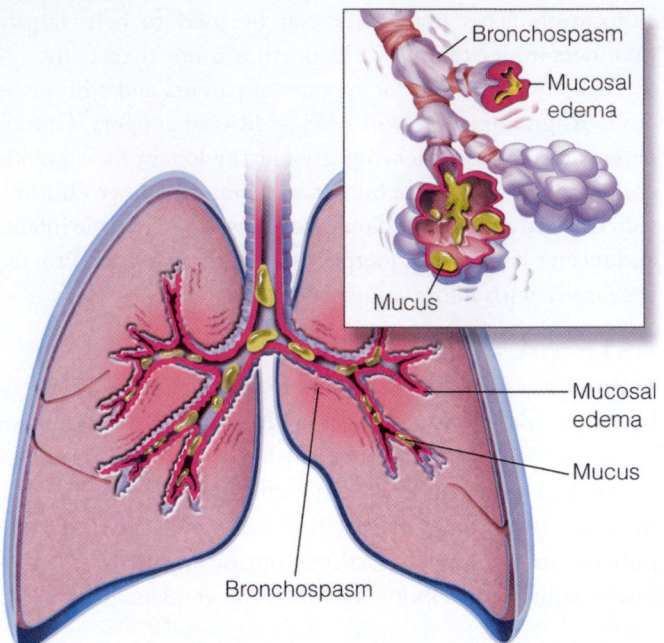

Figure 18-16. ■ When an asthma attack occurs, the bronchi constrict and spasm (see *inset*), and mucus obstructs the airway.
Patrick Watson\Pearson Education/PH College)

Mucous membranes swell, mucus forms, and airway muscles contract (Figure 18-16 ■). Copious amounts of mucus block small airways, trapping air below the plug. Chronic irritation and swelling of mucous membranes cause damage to the cells lining the airway. The end result is scar tissue formation, hyperinflation of the alveoli, and chronic obstructive pulmonary disease (COPD).

The child who is having an "asthma attack" has fast, labored breathing with a productive cough. The child often wheezes on expiration. The child may complain of tightness in the chest and appear tired. There may be nasal flaring and intercostal retractions (see Figure 18-3). Young children may bob their heads to engage accessory muscles to breathe.

Psychological reactions often intensify the symptoms of asthma. As the airway becomes blocked, the child becomes anxious and believes that he or she is suffocating. Severe anxiety intensifies the symptoms, and a vicious cycle ensues. Emotional stress may even trigger asthma attacks (Box 18-5 ■).

clinical ALERT

A condition called *status asthmaticus* occurs when the child develops severe respiratory distress and bronchospasms that do not respond to medication. Without immediate medical attention, the child may die. Treatment may involve airway intubation and ventilator support. The child will be admitted to the ICU. The role of the LPN/LVN is to assist the RN in providing care. The nurse would also observe for signs of anxiety in the child and family.

BOX 18-5	ASSESSMENT

Child with Acute Asthma: Focused Observations

The following provide important data for the assessment of a child with asthma:

- Is the child able to talk, or does respiratory distress prevent speech?
- Is the child wheezing?
- What is the child's color and heart rate?
- Is the child relaxed or fighting to breathe? Is the child crying?
- Does the child hold on to parents, or is he or she lying calmly on the bed?
- What is the family doing? Do they appear frightened? What is their tone of voice?
- Do the parents ask appropriate questions?

Diagnosis

Diagnosis of asthma is based on medical history, physical assessment, and pulmonary function tests. Peak expiratory flow rates (PEFRs) are used to determine the extent of damage. (See Chapter 13 ⊂⊃ for description and illustration of PEFR.) PEFR is the fastest speed at which air is exhaled. With asthma, airways collapse, trapping air in the alveoli and lowering the PEFR. Allergens can be identified by skin tests.

Treatment

Asthma management involves avoiding triggers, regulating medications, family teaching, and ongoing follow-up. Drug management depends on the severity and frequency of the child's symptoms. Short-acting bronchodilators, inhaled corticosteroids, and long-acting oral anti-asthmatics can be used alone or in combination. The newest class of drugs used to treat asthma is the luekotriene modifiers. These drugs prevent the bronchoconstrictive and anti-inflammatory action of leukotriene by blocking the receptor. Table 18-4 ■ lists common medications used in children with asthma.

Secondhand Smoke

Research has confirmed that secondhand cigarette smoke contributes significantly to asthma and other chronic respiratory problems in children of all ages. This fact should be stressed with parents. If a parent is not ready to quit smoking, he or she may be willing to smoke outside, at least keeping the inside of the home free of smoke.

Nursing Considerations

The child, with the help of the parents, may be able to avoid the specific allergens that trigger an asthma attack. Because exercise can bring on an acute asthma attack, the child should warm up well before exercising, avoid outdoor exercising in cold or dry air, and take prescribed medication 15 to 30 minutes before exercising.

TABLE 18-4

Pharmacology: Drugs Used to Treat Asthma

DRUG (GENERIC AND COMMON BRAND NAME)	USUAL ROUTE/DOSE	CLASSIFICATION	SELECTED SIDE EFFECTS	DON'T GIVE IF
Albuterol (Proventil, Vantolin)	PO: 2–6 years 0.1–0.2 mg/kg t.i.d. PO: 6–12 years 2 mg 3–4 times/day Inhaled: 6–12 years 1–2 inhalations every 4–6 hours	Beta-adrenergic agonist	Hypersensitivity, tremors, anxiety, blurred vision; call doctor if no relief	Epinephrine is being administered (possible additive effect)
Fluvoxamine (Flonase)	Inhaled: 1–2 inhalations bid	Anti-inflammatory	Candidal infection of oral-pharynx	Oral inhaler and nasal inhaler are not interchangeable
Prednisone, (Solumedrol, etc.)	*Acute asthma:* PO: 1–2 mg/kg in divided doses *Asthma:* PO: 10–40 mg every other day, depending on age	Glucocorticoid	Edema, muscle weakness, hyperglycemia, growth suppression	Do not stop or alter dose without consulting primary care provider
Montelukast (Singulair)	PO: 4–5 mg daily in evening	Bronchodilator (respiratory smooth muscle relaxant), leukotriene receptor	Fever, headache, nasal congestion	Monitor periodic live tests
Theophylline (Theo-dur)	PO/IV 0.4–0.8mg/ kg/hour	Xanthine bronchodilator	Irritability, headache, tachycardia	Wait 4–6 hour after IV dose before starting PO; check IV incompatibility
Levalbuterol (Xopenex)	Inhaled 0.31 mg tid	Autonomic nervous system agent, bronchodilator (respiratory smooth muscle relaxant)	Allergic reactions, anxiety, headache, dizziness, increased blood glucose, tachycardia	Past allergic reaction; not recommended for children younger than 6 years

Parents need to be taught to administer medication by metered-dose inhaler and by continuous nebulizer (see Procedure 13-32 ⬤⬤). Older children can be taught to perform their own respiratory treatments.

PEFR monitoring devices can be used in the home or at school to monitor the child's condition and response to treatment, as well as to detect deteriorating lung function. Parents, children, and school personnel should receive instruction on the proper use of the PEFR equipment. The use of the PEFR allows the family greater control over the management of asthma and decreases the need for hospitalization by alerting parents to the need for adjustments to prescribed therapy.

PNEUMOTHORAX

Pneumothorax, air in the chest cavity, can result from chest trauma or spontaneous rupturing of alveoli. When air enters the chest cavity, the normal negative pressure is lost and the lung cannot inflate (Figure 18-17 ■). Pressure from the intact lung can cause a shift of organs (*mediastinal shift;* see Figure 18-17B) that compresses the great vessels, leading to shock. If bloody fluid is in the chest cavity, the disorder is called a **hemothorax.**

Manifestations

Because air is unable to enter the bronchi, lung sounds will be absent. The child may complain of being unable to breathe. Oxygen saturation will decrease.

Diagnosis

Clinical findings, coupled with history of chest injury or chronic lung disease, will usually result in further investigation with a chest x-ray.

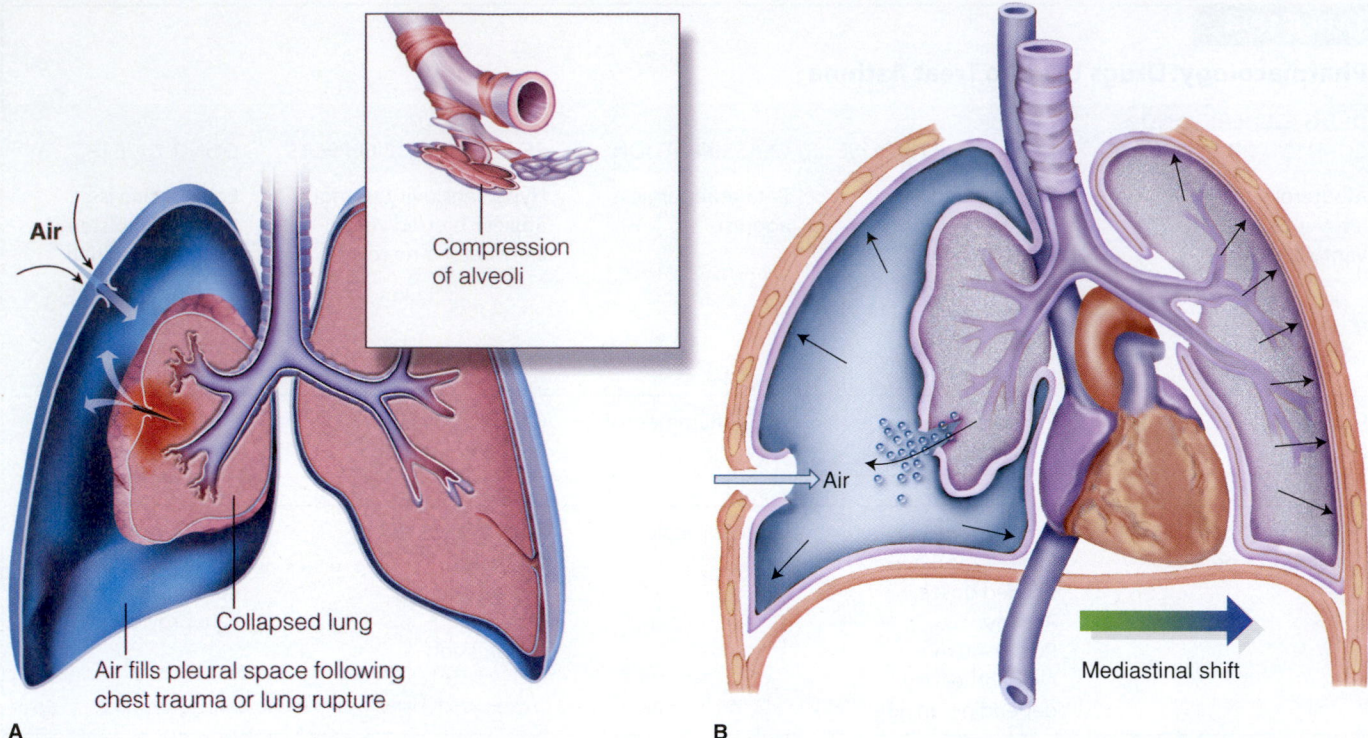

Figure 18-17. ■ **(A)** Pneumothorax. **(B)** Mediastinal shift caused by pneumothorax compresses the intact lung, further reducing the oxygen that can be provided to the body. Here compression of the great vessels occurs, leading to obstructive shock.

Treatment

Immediate treatment is required to reinstate normal lung functioning and prevent shock. To re-establish the negative pressure in the chest cavity, the primary care provider inserts a chest tube between two ribs and into the pleural space. If there is only air in the pleural space, the chest tube will generally be placed in the upper chest. If blood and fluid are in the pleural space (hemothorax), the chest tube will be placed low in the chest. The distal end of the chest tube is attached to an underwater seal (Pleurevac®) and suction.

Nursing Considerations

The management of the underwater seal is the same for children as for adults. Prior to insertion of the chest tube, the nurse must set up the Pleurevac following the package directions (Figure 18-18 ■). The water seal chamber and the section chamber are filled with sterile water. The suction tube is connected to continuous wall suction. Once the primary care provider has inserted the chest tube, it is attached to the client side of the Pleurevac. The suction is turned on to the prescribed level. The chest tube is sutured in place, and an occlusive dressing is applied. All tube connections are taped to prevent leaks. The tubes should be secured to the bed to establish straight drainage into the Pleurevac. The Pleurevac must be kept below the level of the chest tube. The nurse should observe the chest tube and Pleurevac frequently to maintain optimal function. The child's respiratory distress

should ease, and breath sounds should return in all lung fields. The chest tube can usually be removed in a few days.

Parents may be frightened to touch the child because of the chest tube. They should be reassured that the child can be touched, held, and played with as long as the chest tube is not pulled. Should an air leak occur, the chest tube should be clamped with large hemostats as close to the client as possible. The charge nurse and doctor should be notified immediately.

NURSING CARE

PRIORITIES IN NURSING CARE

The priorities of nursing care for children with respiratory disorders are to:

- Maintain patent airway
- Prevent infection
- Promote healing
- Prevent further respiratory damage.

ASSESSING

The infant or child with a respiratory disorder should be assessed for lung sounds bilaterally, oxygen saturation (see Figure 13-34 in Procedure 13-27 ⚭), elevated temperature, and stridor. If the throat is infected, the ears should be

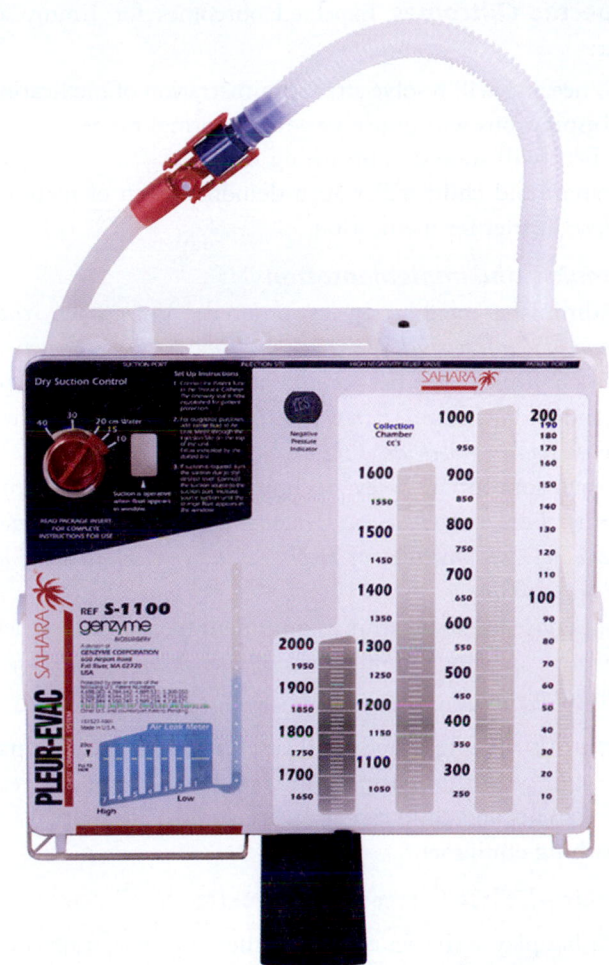

Figure 18-18. ■ Pleurevac®. A disposable chest drainage system. (Courtesy of Genzyme and Teleflex Medical.)

checked for signs of infection. Likewise, if the ears are infected, the throat should be assessed because of the communication between each through the eustachian tubes. Careful observation for signs of respiratory distress is critical. The airway of the infant is small and obstructs easily. The oxygen saturation should be monitored and reported to the supervising RN or physician if it falls below 90%. Many respiratory disorders affecting older children began in the younger years and continue into adolescence and adulthood. The older child should be assessed to determine if he or she is ready to assume some responsibility for the daily management of his or her respiratory condition.

DIAGNOSING, PLANNING, AND IMPLEMENTING

The following nursing diagnoses are common among pediatric clients with respiratory disorders and their families:

- Ineffective Airway Clearance
- Risk for Infection
- Deficient Fluid Volume

- Fear/Anxiety
- Deficient Knowledge.

The following outcomes may be used when caring for pediatric clients with respiratory disorders:

- Open airway
- No evidence of respiratory infections
- No evidence of fluid imbalance
- Client and family appear calm and relaxed
- Client and family verbalize understanding of respiratory disorder, medical treatment, and medication administration.

When planning and implementing care for the infant with severe respiratory disorders, the first priority is to establish and maintain an open airway. The nurse should ensure that artificial airways and suction equipment are available in case of airway obstruction.

- Take vital signs, including oxygen saturation measurements, at least every 2 hours in children with severe respiratory disorders. *The pediatric client condition may change rapidly, and the child may not be able to communicate this to the nurse.*
- Record intake and output if risk for deficient fluid volume exists. IV fluids may be administered. *The nurse must be alert for signs of dehydration, which can be life threatening.*
- Once the child is able to swallow, provide cool liquids. *Cool liquids can help decrease throat swelling, relieve discomfort, and maintain fluid balance.*
- Observe the child and the parents for signs of fear and anxiety. Remain with the child and family, and explain the need for the various pieces of equipment (Figure 18-19 ■). *Parents are fearful when the child is having difficulty breathing and has*

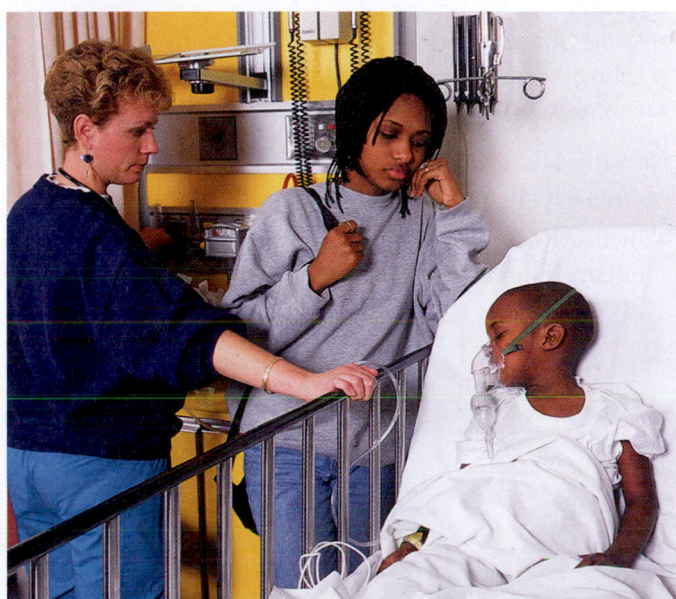

Figure 18-19. ■ Providing support to both the child and the parents is an important part of nursing care during acute episodes of asthma or other respiratory obstruction. This mother is exhausted after a sleepless night of caring for her son.

loss of voice. The hospital environment is frightening to the child and parents. The nurse's presence can be reassuring. Knowing about the equipment can reduce fear.

- Explain all procedures to the parents and encourage their participation in care of the child to the extent possible. *Infants and young children experience separation anxiety if the parents are not nearby. (See developmental stages in Chapter 11 and effects of hospitalization on children in Chapter 14.* ⚭*)*

- Promote age-appropriate activities to the extent possible. *Children with chronic respiratory conditions still need to progress developmentally. Encouraging children to do all they can will promote self-esteem.*

EVALUATING

Children with respiratory disorders are evaluated frequently for airway patency and oxygen saturation. An increase in urinary output indicates adequate fluid intake. Failure to complete ordered antibiotics can result in recurrence of the infection, so the importance of giving antibiotics as ordered must be emphasized with family members.

NURSING PROCESS CARE PLAN
Client with Asthma

Jimmy, a 7-year-old, is admitted to the pediatric unit with a diagnosis of acute asthma. His vital signs are T 98.4, P 112, R 36. He has high-pitched wheezing on expiration. The physician has ordered IV Solu-Medrol and breathing treatments.

Assessment
- Wheezing respirations
- Labored breathing
- Clings to mother

Nursing Diagnosis. The following important nursing diagnosis (among others) is established for this client:

- Ineffective Airway Clearance related to allergic response, inflamed bronchial tree.

Expected Outcomes. Expected outcomes for Jimmy are that:

- Wheezing will resolve after administration of medication.
- Respirations will return to within normal range.
- Client will state that breathing is easier.
- Parent and child will return demonstration of metered-dose inhaler for medication.

Planning and Implementation
- Administer medication as ordered. *Medications relieve bronchial inflammation, decrease swelling, and open airways.*
- Teach Jimmy and his parents how and when to use the handheld nebulizer. *Parent and child need instruction in technique and in proper use of the medication.*
- Teach appropriate "play" techniques to extend expiratory time. *Increasing expiratory pressure and extending expiratory time improves breathing by keeping airways open, allowing air to leave the lungs.*
- Supervise use of breathing equipment (e.g., inhalers, nebulizers, oxygen cannula/mask). *This ensures proper use of breathing equipment.*

Evaluation. Lung sounds will be clear, and breathing pattern will be within normal limits of 15 to 25 for a 7-year-old. Parents and child can verbalize and demonstrate use of breathing equipment.

Critical Thinking in the Nursing Process

1. What play activities could lengthen the exhalation time?
2. What questions should Jimmy and his parents be asked to help identify causative agents for the asthma attack?
3. What can the nurse do to help Jimmy express his feelings?

Note: Discussion of Critical Thinking questions appears in Appendix I.

Note: The references and resources for this and all chapters have been compiled at the back of the book.

Chapter Review

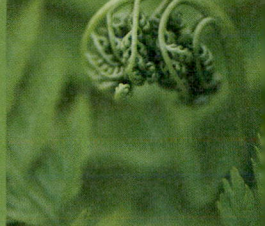

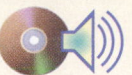 **KEY TERMS** by Topic

Use the audio glossary feature of either the CD-ROM or the Companion Website to hear the correct pronunciation of the following key terms.

Anatomy and Physiology
conchae

Mechanism of Respiration
diaphragm, intercostal muscles

Assessing the Respiratory System
eupnea, hypoventilation, hyperventilation, dyspnea, orthopnea, apnea, Cheyne–Stokes respirations (CSR), circumoral cyanosis, crackles, rhonchi, stridor

Epistaxis
epistaxis

Upper Respiratory Infections
nasopharyngitis, rhinitis, coryza, tonsillitis, tonsillectomy, epiglottitis, dysphonia, dysphagia

Congenital Respiratory Disorders
tracheoesophageal fistula (TEF), esophageal atresia (EA)

Lower Respiratory Disorders
bronchiolitis, respiratory syncytial virus (RSV), croup, pneumonia, tuberculosis (TB), Mantoux test

Additional Respiratory Disorders
neonatal respiratory distress syndrome (RDS), surfactant, atelectasis, bronchopulmonary dysplasia (BPD), asthma, pneumothorax, hemothorax

KEY Points

- Respiratory disorders are potentially life threatening and should not be taken lightly.

- Upper respiratory infections can spread to the lower organs.

- Viral infections should be treated with supportive care. Antibiotics should only be used for bacterial infections.

- Frequent swallowing after a tonsillectomy is the first sign of bleeding.

- Many respiratory disorders begin in early childhood and become chronic lifelong disorders.

- Pediatric clients can be taught to manage their chronic respiratory disorder.

- Management of asthma is focused on identifying and avoiding triggers, family education, medication administration, and follow-up care.

- Cystic fibrosis, an autosomal recessive trait, affects the child's respiratory and gastrointestinal systems. The life expectancy is 30 years.

- Health promotion activities, including immunizations, removing pollutants from the environment, and infection control measures, can help prevent or control pediatric respiratory disorders.

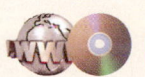 **EXPLORE Media**Link

Additional interactive resources for this chapter can be found on the Companion Website at www.prenhall.com/towle.

Click on Chapter 18 and "Begin" to select the activities for this chapter.

For chapter-related NCLEX-style questions and an audio glossary, access the accompanying CD-ROM in this book.

Animations

Foreign body airway obstruction

Pulse oximeter

Lung sounds

Pneumonia

Asthma

Cystic fibrosis

Epiglottitis

Interactivities: Match lung anatomy

FOR FURTHER Study

Newborn resuscitation was discussed in Chapter 9.

Review Chapter 11 for developmental levels of children as they relate to nursing care.

See Chapter 12 for information about communicating with children.

See Respiratory Procedures section in Chapter 13 and Procedures 13-25 to 13-28.

Review Chapter 14 for effects of hospitalization by age and development.

For additional information on otitis media, see Chapter 16.

Gastrointestinal disorders are discussed in Chapter 22.

Infectious diseases such as pertussis (whooping cough) are discussed in Chapter 26.

Critical Thinking Care Map

Caring for a Client with Respiratory Infection

NCLEX-PN® Focus Area: Physiologic Integrity

Case Study: Joseph, a 9-month-old infant, is admitted to the pediatric unit with a diagnosis of respiratory infection. He has a history of three episodes of bronchitis in the past 6 months. He has gained ½ lb since his last hospitalization 2 months ago. His mother states, "I don't know why he gets infections so easily."

Nursing Diagnosis: Ineffective Airway Clearance

COLLECT DATA

Subjective	Objective
_____	_____
_____	_____
_____	_____
_____	_____
_____	_____
_____	_____
_____	_____

Would you report this? Yes/No

If yes, to: _____

Nursing Care

_____
_____
_____
_____
_____
_____
_____
_____
_____
_____
_____
_____
_____

How would you document this? _____
_____
_____
_____

Compare your documentation to the sample provided in Appendix I.

Data Collected
(use those that apply)

- Lung sounds wheezy
- Crying
- T 103.2, P 148, R 40
- Mother reports not knowing cause of infection
- Nonproductive cough
- No eye contact
- Weight gain
- Labored breathing
- Withdrawn
- Circumoral cyanosis
- Jaundice
- Sleepy

Nursing Interventions
(use those that apply; list in priority order)

- Note mother-infant interaction.
- Offer 1,000 mL clear liquids.
- Offer milk four times a day.
- Administer IV medication as ordered.
- Provide mist tent.
- Administer expectorant cough syrup.
- Provide droplet precautions.
- Provide contact precautions.
- Suction airway every 2 hours.

1 An infant is in isolation for RSV. Which action by the nurse is most appropriate?
1. Wear sterile gloves when caring for the infant.
2. Double-bag soiled diapers.
3. Have the baby wear a mask when in the playroom.
4. Wear gown, mask, and gloves when feeding the infant.

2 A 6-month-old child is receiving oxygen in a mist tent. Which of the following is an important consideration in caring for this young child?
1. Change bedding and clothing frequently.
2. Remove child from the tent if restlessness occurs.
3. Keep all objects outside the tent to prevent fire hazard.
4. Open the mist tent every hour to decrease the temperature inside the tent.

3 The day an 8-year-old is discharged after an acute asthma attack, her mother asks the nurse to recommend a pet for her child. The most appropriate pet for the child would be a:
1. cat.
2. fish.
3. dog.
4. parakeet.

4 A 7-year-old with cystic fibrosis is admitted with bronchial pneumonia. The physician orders postural drainage, primarily to:
1. clear the lungs of mucus.
2. dilate the bronchi.
3. provide more room for lung expansion.
4. remove bacteria from the lungs.

5 A toddler is being admitted to the pediatric unit with a diagnosis of epiglottitis. In planning care for this child, the nurse should:
1. notify the respiratory therapist of the admission.
2. have tracheostomy equipment available.
3. make the child NPO.
4. have antibiotics prepared when the child is admitted.

6 A 5-year-old had a tonsillectomy yesterday. The nurse would be least concerned by:
1. halitosis.
2. increased pulse.
3. restlessness.
4. crying.

7 The second day after a tonsillectomy, a child is receiving a full liquid diet. Which should be avoided?
1. popsicles
2. jello
3. vanilla pudding
4. orange juice

8 A 10-year-old is admitted with an acute episode of asthma after playing soccer. All of the following interventions are needed prior to discharge. Place them in priority order.
1. Teach how to use prescribed inhalers.
2. Schedule follow-up appointment with primary care provider.
3. Stay with child to keep him calm.
4. Ask parents to identify triggers in the home environment.
5. Teach child the importance of warming up before playing soccer.

9 The nurse is teaching a mother how to administer 1 tsp of cough medicine to her 6-month-old child. The nurse should recommend which of the following?
1. household measuring spoon
2. silverware teaspoon
3. plastic medicine cup
4. plastic syringe (without needle) calibrated in milliliters

10 The doctor has ordered Albuterol liquid 0.2 mg/kg for a 43-lb child. Albuterol is supplied in 2 mg/5 mL. How many milliliters will be administered to this child?

Answers for Review Questions, as well as discussion of Care Plan and Critical Thinking Care Map questions, appear in Appendix I.

Chapter 19

Care of the Child with Cardiovascular Disorders

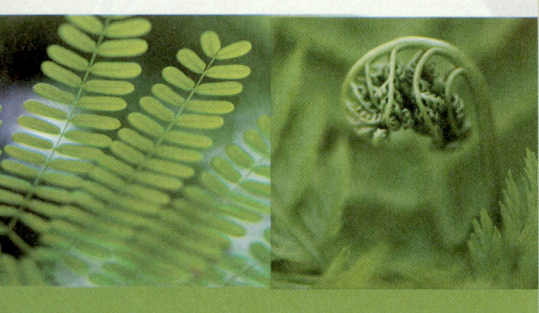

BRIEF Outline

LEARNING Outcomes

After completing this chapter, you will be able to:

- Discuss the anatomy and physiology of the pediatric cardiovascular system.
- Describe cardiovascular disorders to include both congenital and acquired disorders.
- Discuss clinical manifestations, diagnostic procedures, medical management, and nursing interventions related to cardiovascular disorders.
- Explain appropriate nursing interventions for children with cardiovascular disorders.

Cardiovascular disorders in children can result from congenital heart anomalies or defects or acquired heart diseases. These disorders pose serious health threats. Connor (2002) estimates that one-third of children born with a congenital heart disease will die, with most of those deaths occurring in the first year of life. Due to the serious nature of cardiovascular disorders, the health care of these children may require frequent hospitalizations, including admissions to the intensive care unit. Nursing care for these children can be challenging. The LPN/LVN assists the physician and RN in providing safe, effective care to these children. Check the nurse practice act for your state and facility policy to determine whether specific interventions are within the scope of practice.

Anatomy and Physiology

To understand the pathology of heart defects, it is important to review the normal structure of the fetal heart (Figure 19-1A ■). Because fetal blood is oxygenated in the placenta, the lungs in the fetus only need enough blood to perfuse lung tissue. In the fetal heart, there are two structures to decrease the flow of blood to the fetal lungs. They are the foramen ovale

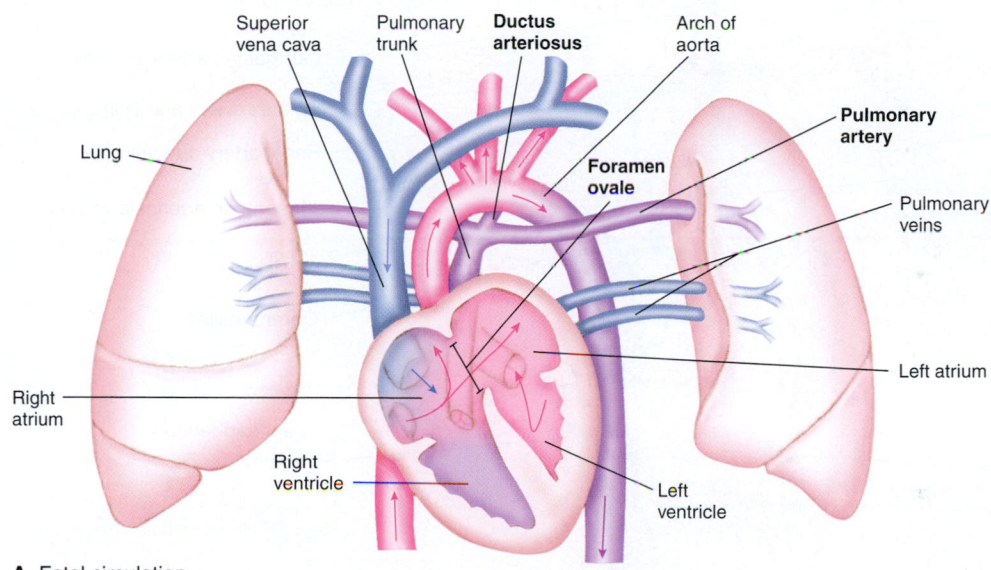

A Fetal circulation

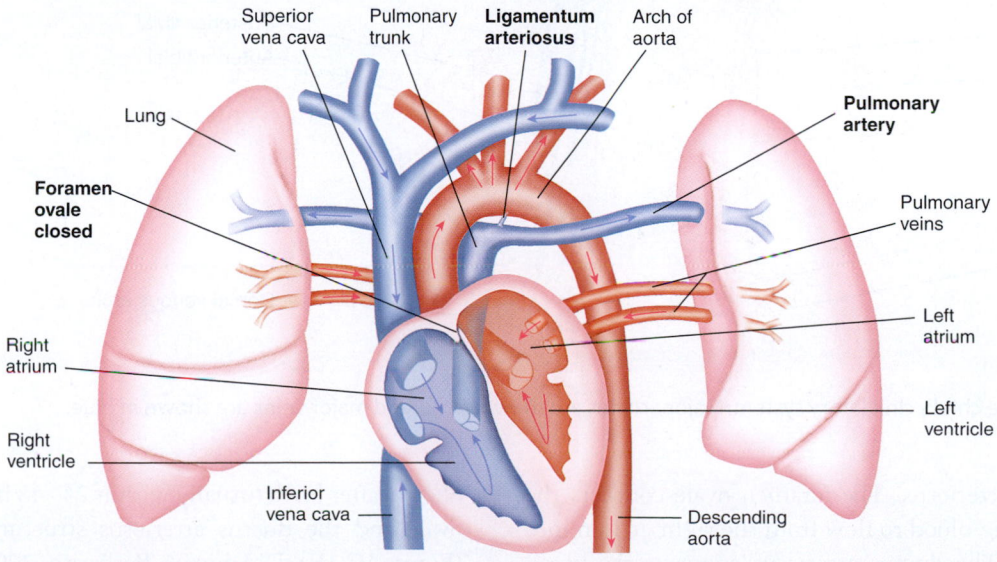

B Newborn circulation

Figure 19-1. ■ **(A)** Fetal circulation. Notice the open ductus arteriosus above the heart and the flow of blood through the foramen ovale in the center of the heart. **(B)** Newborn circulation. Note that the ductus arteriosus has closed showing two separate structures: the pulmonary arteries and the aortic arch.

MAJOR ARTERIES

MAJOR VEINS

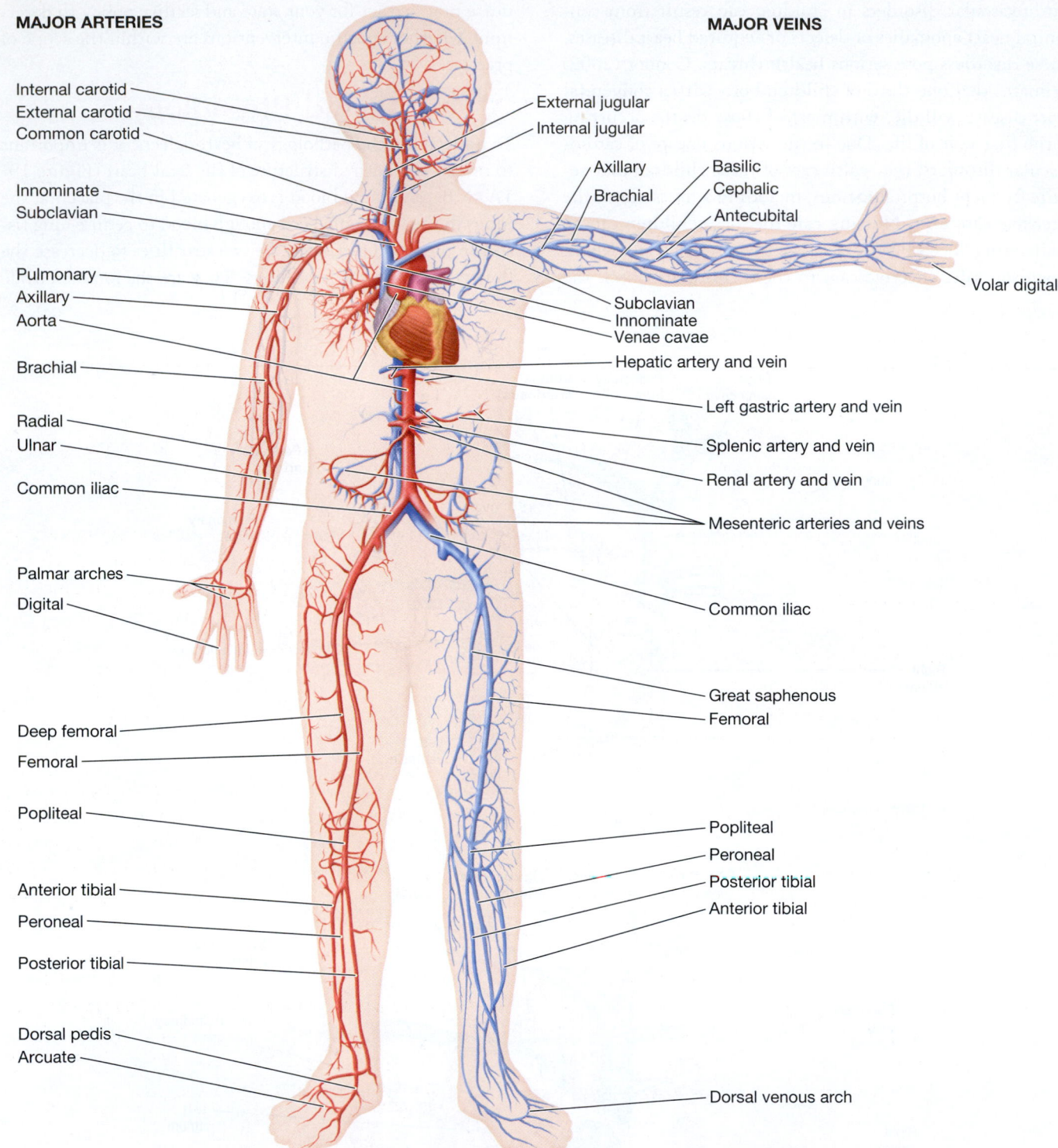

Internal carotid
External carotid
Common carotid

Innominate
Subclavian

Pulmonary
Axillary
Aorta

Brachial

Radial
Ulnar

Common iliac

Palmar arches
Digital

Deep femoral

Femoral

Popliteal

Anterior tibial

Peroneal

Posterior tibial

Dorsal pedis
Arcuate

External jugular
Internal jugular

Axillary   Basilic
Brachial   Cephalic
              Antecubital

Volar digital

Subclavian
Innominate
Venae cavae

Hepatic artery and vein

Left gastric artery and vein

Splenic artery and vein

Renal artery and vein

Mesenteric arteries and veins

Common iliac

Great saphenous
Femoral

Popliteal
Peroneal
Posterior tibial
Anterior tibial

Dorsal venous arch

Figure 19-2. ■ The child's circulatory system. Major arteries are shown in red, and major veins are shown in blue.

and the ductus arteriosus. The foramen ovale connects the two atria, allowing blood to flow from the right atrium into the left atrium. The ductus arteriosus connects the blood flow from the pulmonary artery into the aortic arch.

At birth, with the infant's first breath, blood flow to the lungs must increase dramatically to allow full oxygenation.

Shortly after birth (usually within 24–48 hours), the foramen ovale and the ductus arteriosus structures normally close (Figure 19-1B) (D'Amico & Barbarito, 2007). Now the right side of the heart pumps blood to the lungs for oxygenation, and the left side of the heart pumps oxygenated blood throughout the body. Figure 19-2 ■ illustrates the arteries and veins in the body. The pressure in the left side of the heart becomes higher than the pressure in the right side. An infant's heart muscle fibers are not developed fully, and the ventricles are not as compliant to **stroke volume** (the amount of blood forced out by the ventricles during a heart contraction). Therefore, the infant is very sensitive to volume and pressure overloads. **Cardiac output** is the total volume of blood forced out of the ventricles in 1 minute. Cardiac output is calculated by multiplying stroke volume by heart rate. Three things affect cardiac output. First is the **preload,** which is the volume of blood in the ventricles at the end of diastole. Second is the **afterload** or the resistance against which the ventricles pump. Finally, the **contractility,** or the ability of the ventricles to stretch, affects cardiac output.

Variations from these normal findings affect the health of the newborn and are discussed in this chapter. See Chapters 6 and 9 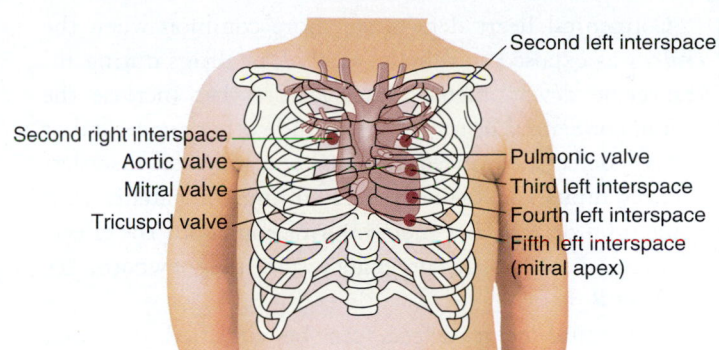 for a review of fetal and newborn cardiovascular function.

Figure 19-3. ■ Points for auscultating the heart.

Brief Assessment Overview

HISTORY

To obtain client history for an assessment of a client's cardiovascular system, several questions need to be asked. Inquire about a family history of cardiac disease. Ask the child or parent if there is any weakness or fatigue that develops upon physical exertion. Inquire about symptoms of cyanosis, edema, dizziness, or poor weight gain.

PHYSICAL

To perform a brief focused assessment of the cardiovascular system, the nurse would:

- Observe the child's body posture (e.g., squatting is often seen in a child with tetralogy of Fallot, hyperextension of the neck is seen with hypoxia).
- Observe for respiratory difficulty.
- Observe for edema, abdominal distention, or signs of dehydration.
- Inspect nail beds, sclera, and skin tone (Box 19-1 ■).
- Monitor body temperature, respiratory rate, and blood pressure (see Procedures 13-1, 13-3, and 13-4).

- Palpate the peripheral pulse, and auscultate the apical pulse (see Procedure 13-2).
- Palpate for pitting edema if present.
- Auscultate heart and breath sounds (see Procedures 13-2 and 13-3). Figure 19-3 ■ illustrates areas for auscultating the heart.

Arterial oxygen saturation is a key indicator of cardiac health. The normal amount of oxygen saturation in a child's blood is 95% to 98%. Table 19-1 ■ provides lab values for arterial oxygen saturation. Also see Procedure 13-27 , Monitoring Oxygen Status.

Congenital Heart Anomalies and Defects

Many congenital anomalies (e.g., patent ductus arteriosus, atrial septal defect, ventricular septal defect, coarctation of the aorta, tetralogy of Fallot, transposition of the great vessels) are identified at birth or within the first few weeks of life. It is important for the nurse to have an understanding of the pathology, symptoms, and related nursing care for these conditions. If the anomaly is life threatening, surgery is usually performed immediately to correct the defect. Other anomalies are not repaired until the child is stronger and better able to withstand the surgical procedure. Sometimes repair is performed in stages, and complete reconstruction may take months or years.

BOX 19-1	CULTURAL PULSE POINTS

Cyanosis in Dark Skinned Children

When assessing cyanosis and decreased hemoglobin levels in dark-skinned children, such as those of Mediterranean descent or African heritage, look for an ashen tone instead of a blue hue. Look closely at the conjunctiva, sclera, soles of the feet, palms of the hands, tongue, lips, or nail beds to assist in the assessment.

TABLE 19-1	
Pediatric Lab Values for Oxygen Saturation	
Normal	95–98%
Mild hypoxemia	90–95%
Moderate hypoxemia	85–90%
Severe hypoxemia	85% or lower

Congenital heart defects are more common when the child was exposed to rubella, alcohol, or drugs during intrauterine development. Other factors that increase the risk of congenital heart defects include other congenital or genetic defects, advanced maternal age, maternal disorders such as lupus and diabetes, and siblings or parents with congenital defects. For more information about the effects of these disorders on pregnancy and the newborn, see Chapter 8 ⚭.

Congenital heart defects can be classified into four groups according to the way the defect affects circulation: defects with increased pulmonary blood flow, defects with decreased pulmonary blood flow, defects that obstruct systemic blood flow, and mixed defects.

DEFECTS WITH INCREASED PULMONARY BLOOD FLOW

Three heart defects that increase the blood flow to the pulmonary system are an atrial septal defect (ASD; Figure 19-4 ■), a patent (open) ductus arteriosus (PDA; Figure 19-5 ■), and a ventricular septal defect (VSD).

Atrial Septal Defect

ASD describes the opening in the **septum** (wall) between the left and right atria that remains when the foramen ovale fails to close within a few hours after birth. Blood

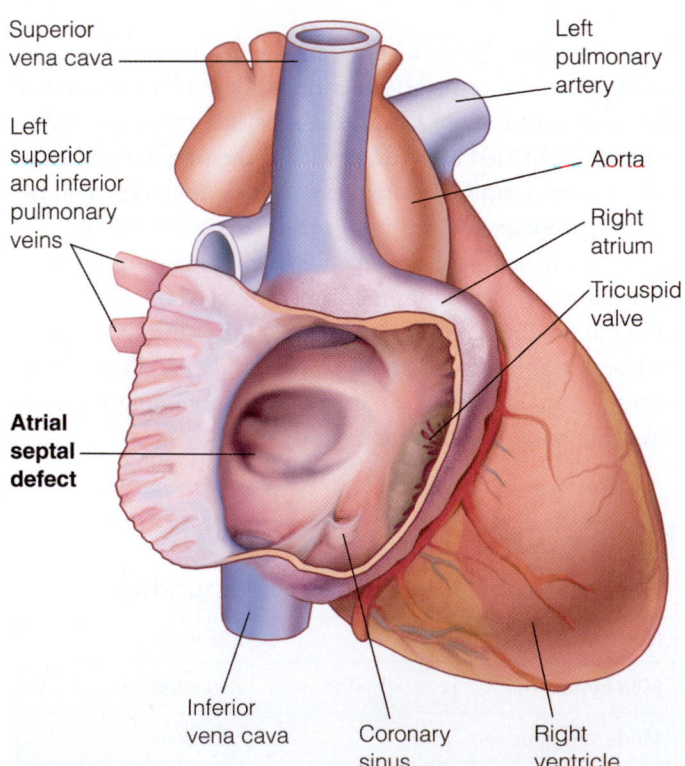

Figure 19-4. ■ Atrial septal defect. Note that the defect is an opening between the right and the left sides of the heart.

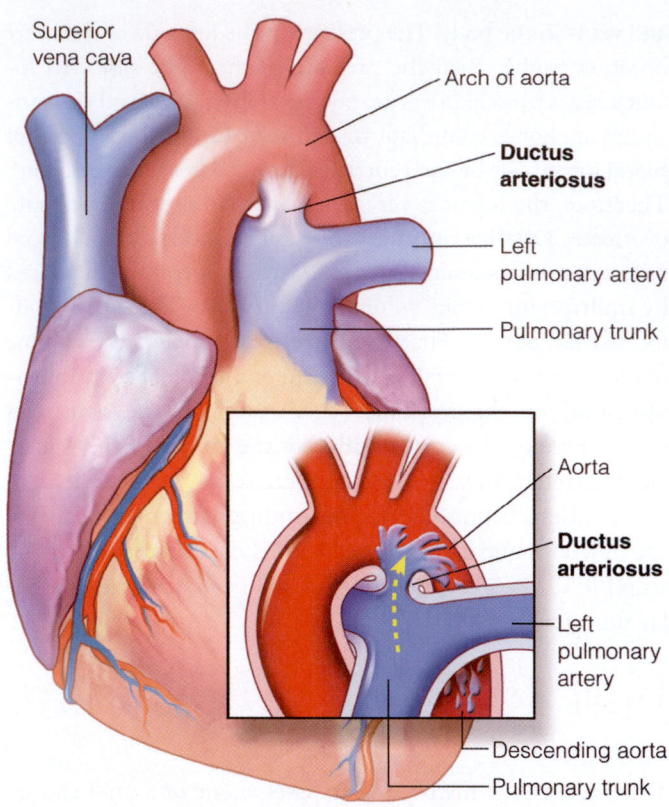

Figure 19-5. ■ Patent ductus arteriosus. Note that the connecting duct between the pulmonary artery and the aortic arch is still open.

flows directly from the left atrium into the right atrium, increasing the amount of blood in the right side of the heart. Increased pressure on the right side of the head results in ventricular hypertrophy and increased pulmonary artery blood flow.

MANIFESTATIONS/DIAGNOSIS. The young child with ASD may be asymptomatic. Diagnosis may not occur until the preschool years, when symptoms of fatigue, delayed growth, and congestive heart failure occur. A soft systolic heart murmur may also be auscultated due to increased pulmonary artery blood flow. An echocardiogram and chest x-rays are used to identify the defect.

TREATMENT. The ASD can be closed or patched through a surgical process or by cardiac catheterization using a septal occluder (Figure 19-6A ■).

Patent Ductus Arteriosus (PDA)

A PDA (see Figure 19-5) occurs when the ductus arteriosus fails to close. Closure is initiated with the first breath, and it normally occurs within 15 hours after birth but can take up to 3 months. In this defect, blood is pushed from the aorta to the pulmonary artery, resulting in an increase in blood flowing to the lungs. The increase in blood flowing to the lungs causes right ventricle hypertrophy and increased pressure in the pulmonary circulation.

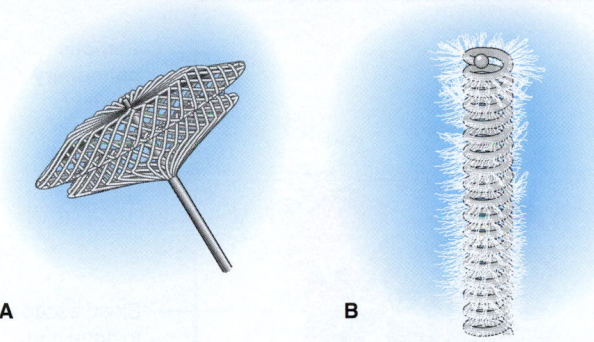

Figure 19-6. ■ **(A)** Septal occluder is used to close an atrial septal defect and less commonly to close a ventricular septal defect. **(B)** Coil used to close a patent ductus arteriosus. The coil of wire covered with tiny fibers occludes the ductus arteriosus when a thrombus forms in the mass of fabric and wire.

MANIFESTATIONS.   Clinical manifestations of a PDA include a full, bounding pulse; dyspnea; tachypnea; and delayed growth patterns. Figure 19-7 ■ illustrates selected heart patterns. The infant with a PDA is at risk for respiratory infections and endocarditis due to increased pulmonary blood flow. The child is also at risk for congestive heart failure (CHF), hepatomegaly, and intercostal retractions. A continuous systolic murmur can be auscultated, and a pulmonic thrill may be palpated at the left sternal border second to fourth intercostals space on a child with a PDA.

DIAGNOSIS.   A PDA can be diagnosed by chest x-ray, electrocardiogram (ECG), or echocardiogram.

TREATMENT.   The symptomatic infant with a PDA is given indomethacin, or a nonsteroidal anti-inflammatory that is

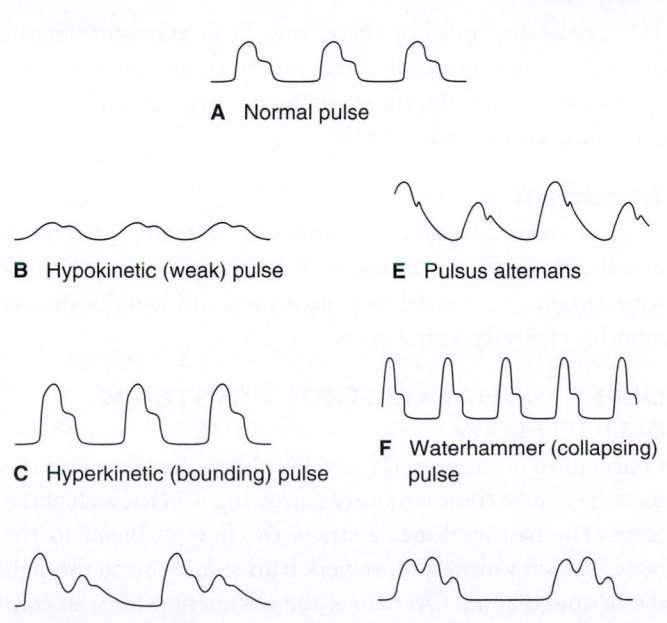

Figure 19-7. ■ Types of pulse patterns.

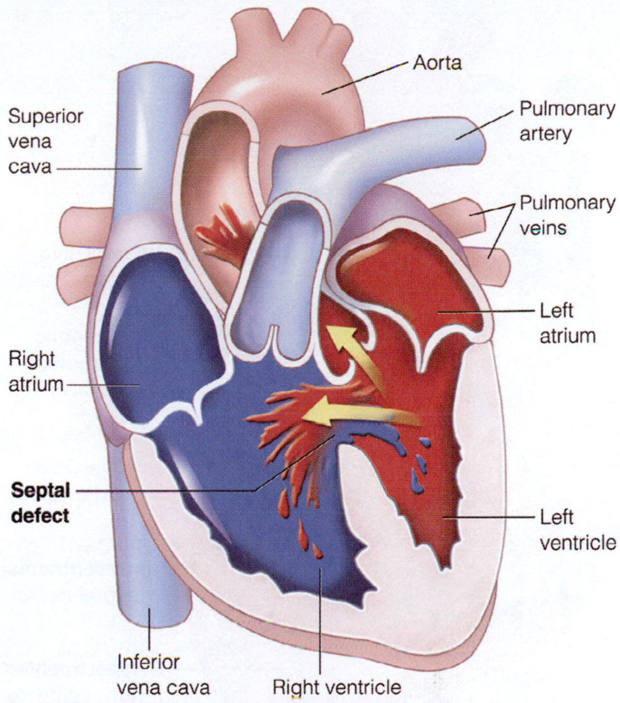

A Normal pulse

B Hypokinetic (weak) pulse

C Hyperkinetic (bounding) pulse

D Bigeminal pulse

E Pulsus alternans

F Waterhammer (collapsing) pulse

G Pulsus bisferiens

Figure 19-8. ■ Ventricular septal defect. Note the opening between the right and left ventricles.

also a prostaglandin inhibitor, intravenously to stimulate the closure of the ductus arteriosus. If unsuccessful, a surgical **ligation** (obstructing a vessel or duct using suture or wire ligature; see Figure 19-6B) of the PDA may be necessary. In some children, closure may be accomplished via a transcatheter, obstructive device.

Ventricular Septal Defect

A ventricular septal defect or VSD (Figure 19-8 ■) results from an abnormal opening in the septum between the ventricles. This allows blood to flow directly from the left ventricle to the right ventricle. The size of the VSD determines the degree of problems the child will have.

MANIFESTATIONS.   Most children with a VSD are asymptomatic. If symptoms are present, the child may have dyspnea, tachypnea, delayed growth patterns, reduced fluid intake, or congestive heart failure (CHF). The child may have symptoms of pulmonary disease, such as pulmonary hypertension. A systolic murmur can be auscultated.

DIAGNOSIS.   A VSD can be diagnosed with a chest x-ray, ECG, or echocardiogram. Small VSDs may close spontaneously and not require medical intervention.

TREATMENT.   If surgical closure is required, it is done prior to age 2 years to prevent pulmonary artery hypertension. Pulmonary artery hypertension can lead to infectious endocarditis and cardiac failure. A **Rashkind procedure (balloon atrial septostomy)** may be performed to relieve

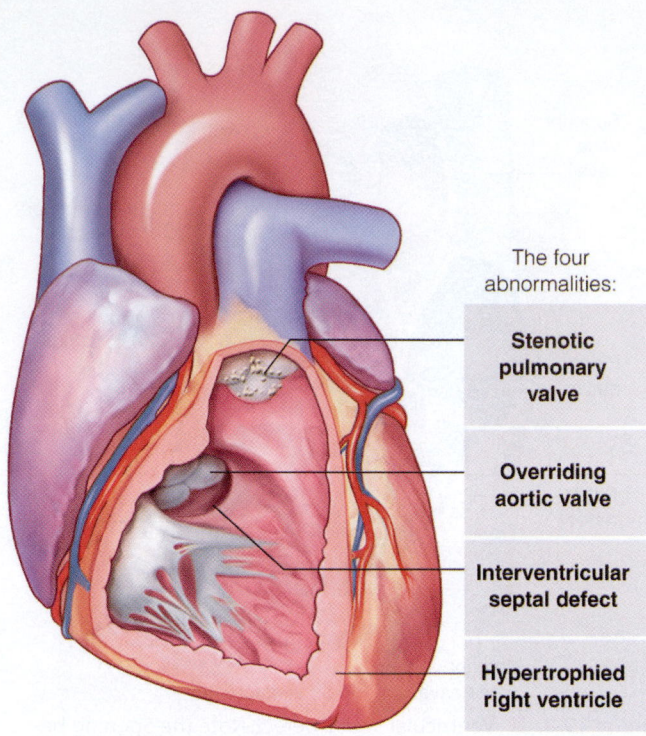

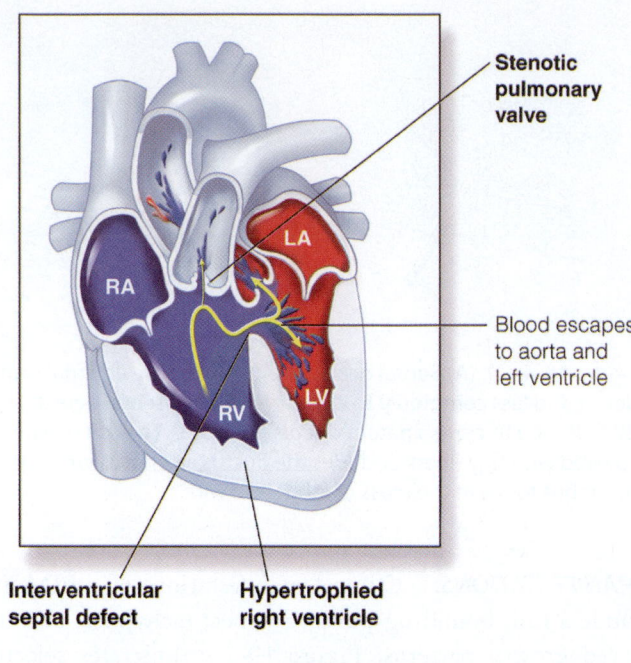

The four abnormalities:

Stenotic pulmonary valve

Overriding aortic valve

Interventricular septal defect

Hypertrophied right ventricle

Stenotic pulmonary valve

Blood escapes to aorta and left ventricle

Interventricular septal defect

Hypertrophied right ventricle

Figure 19-9. ■ Tetralogy of Fallot involves four distinct problems: pulmonary stenosis, ventricular septal defect, right ventricular hypertrophy, and an overriding aorta.

CHF until a more permanent surgical treatment can be accomplished. During the Rashkind procedure, an enlargement of the existing opening in the cardiac septum is made, allowing better mixing of oxygenated blood from the lungs with the systemic blood. Because the child will be at risk for endocarditis, prophylactic antibiotic administration prior to these procedures will be necessary.

DEFECTS WITH DECREASED PULMONARY BLOOD FLOW

When blood flow is decreased to the lungs, the amount of oxygen to all tissues decreases. Only one congenital heart defect that decreases blood flow to the lungs will be discussed here. Tetralogy of Fallot (TOF) is a combination of four defects: pulmonary stenosis, VSD, right ventricular hypertrophy, and an overriding aorta (Figure 19-9 ■). **Pulmonary stenosis** is a narrowing of the pulmonary valve. As the right ventricle tries to push blood through the tight pulmonary valve, the ventricular muscle enlarges (right ventricular *hypertrophy*). As pressure in the right ventricle rises, blood is pushed through the VSD into the aorta, where it mixes with oxygenated blood from the left ventricle and is pumped throughout the body. The mixing of oxygenated and unoxygenated blood results in the common symptom of cyanosis.

Manifestations

Clinical manifestations of TOF are determined by the severity of pulmonary stenosis. The infant may become cyanotic and hypoxic (Figure 19-10 ■). Other symptoms include delayed growth, polycythemia, metabolic acidosis, exercise intolerance, and clubbing of the fingers. **Clubbing** is an enlargement of the end of the fingers associated with disorders causing cyanosis. A systolic murmur may be heard in the pulmonic area.

Diagnosis

TOF can be diagnosed by chest x-ray, ECG, echocardiogram, or cardiac catheterization. The combined presence of pulmonary stenosis, VSD, right ventricular hypertrophy, and an overriding aorta denotes TOF.

Treatment

Surgical correction of the disorder is necessary prior to 6 months of age for the infant with severe symptoms. Otherwise, surgery can be delayed until the child is older than 6 months, typically 1 to 2 years.

DEFECTS THAT OBSTRUCT SYSTEMIC BLOOD FLOW

Coarctation of the aorta (Figure 19-11 ■) is a *narrowing* of the aorta. The most common site of narrowing is in the arch of the aorta. The narrowed area restricts the flow of blood to the body. The left ventricle must work hard to force blood through the narrowed aorta. Over time, the obstruction leads to congestive heart failure. With coarctation of the aorta, blood pressure will usually be higher in the arms than in the legs.

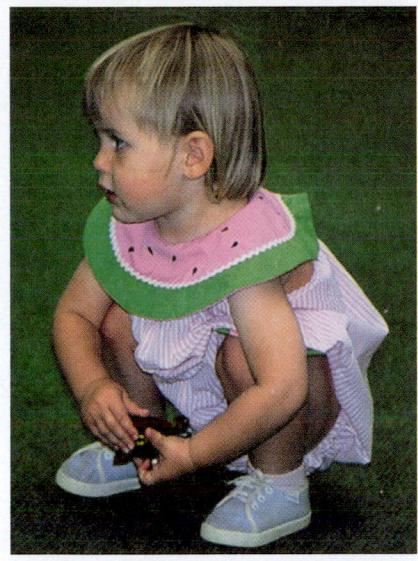

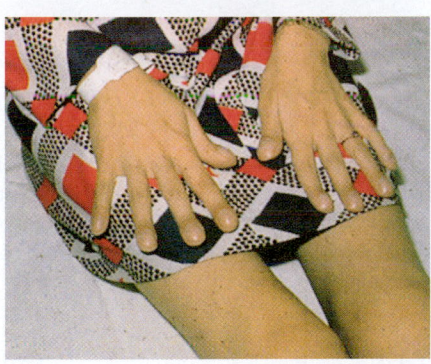

Figure 19-10. ■ (**A**) A child with cyanotic heart defect squats (assumes a knee-chest position) to relieve cyanotic spells. (**B**) Clubbing of the fingers is one manifestation of a cyanotic defect in an older child.

Manifestations

The degree of constriction dictates the severity of symptoms. Children with coarctation of the aorta may be asymptomatic, and their growth patterns may be unaffected. Or they may have CHF and altered blood pressure, with lower blood pressure and weak pulses in the legs due to reduced blood flow through the descending aorta; higher blood pressure; and strong, bounding pulses in the arms, neck, and head. Femoral pulses are weak or absent, and the older child may have weakness and pain in the legs following exercise.

Diagnosis

Diagnosis of coarctation of the aorta can be made by ECG, chest x-ray, or MRI.

Treatment

Repair of the disorder is ideally performed in the first year of life. Balloon dilation, anastomosis, or surgical resection relieves the symptoms. However, the coarctation may recur.

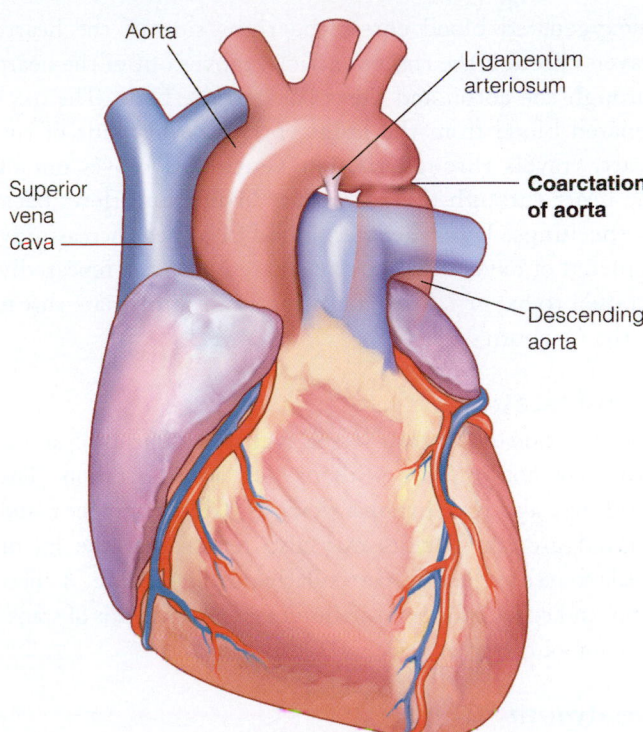

Figure 19-11. ■ Coarctation of the aorta. In most instances, the narrowing occurs in the aortic arch.

The nurse must teach parents to observe closely for the return of signs and symptoms of coarctation of the aorta.

MIXED DEFECTS

Mixed defects are those that affect both systemic and pulmonary circulation. When the positions of aorta and pulmonary artery are reversed (Figure 19-12 ■), the result is **transposition of the great arteries.** In this condition,

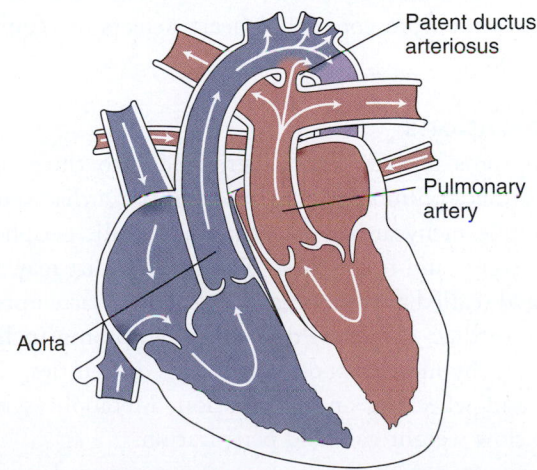

Figure 19-12. ■ Transposition of the great arteries. Note that the pulmonary artery and aorta are switched. Survival initially depends on the patent ductus arteriosus and foramen ovale. About 5% of children with congenital heart disease have this condition (Grifka, 1999).

unoxygenated blood enters the right side of the heart, travels through the right ventricle, moves out of the heart through the aorta, and flows back to the body. The oxygenated blood from the lungs enters the left side of the heart, travels through the left ventricles, moves out of the heart through the pulmonary artery, and flows back to the lungs. Unoxygenated blood becomes increasingly depleted of oxygen, while oxygenated blood is repeatedly exposed to oxygen. This condition is an immediate threat to the newborn's life.

Manifestations

Transposition of the great vessels is characterized by cyanosis that may not improve with oxygen administration. The child may also have hypoxia, acidosis, CHF, tachypnea, and delayed growth. Parents may also report that the infant needs to rest frequently, particularly during feeding. A chest x-ray and echocardiogram are used for the diagnosis of transposition of the great vessels (TOG).

Treatment

Prompt treatment is necessary. Prostaglandin E_1 is given to the newborn intravenously to maintain patency of the ductus arteriosus prior to surgical intervention. Surgical intervention, an arterial switch, can be performed before 1 week of life. Balloon atrial septostomy (Rashkind procedure described previously) may also be performed at 1 week to 3 months of age.

Acquired Heart Diseases

CONGESTIVE HEART FAILURE

In CHF, a child has circulatory deficits that decrease cardiac output and can lead to cardiogenic shock (Figure 19-13 ■). CHF can result from congenital heart defects or acquired heart defects.

Manifestations

The symptoms of CHF can be grouped into three categories: cardiac, pulmonary, and metabolic. Cardiac symptoms include tachycardia, poor capillary refill, peripheral edema, fatigue, and restlessness. The child's heart may also be enlarged (called **cardiomegaly**) as the body attempts to maintain cardiac output. Pulmonary symptoms include dyspnea, tachypnea, cyanosis, feeding difficulties, and crackles and wheezing on auscultation. Metabolic symptoms are slow weight gain and perspiration.

Diagnosis

A diagnosis of CHF is based on the previous symptoms. An x-ray of the heart can detect cardiomegaly or pulmonary edema.

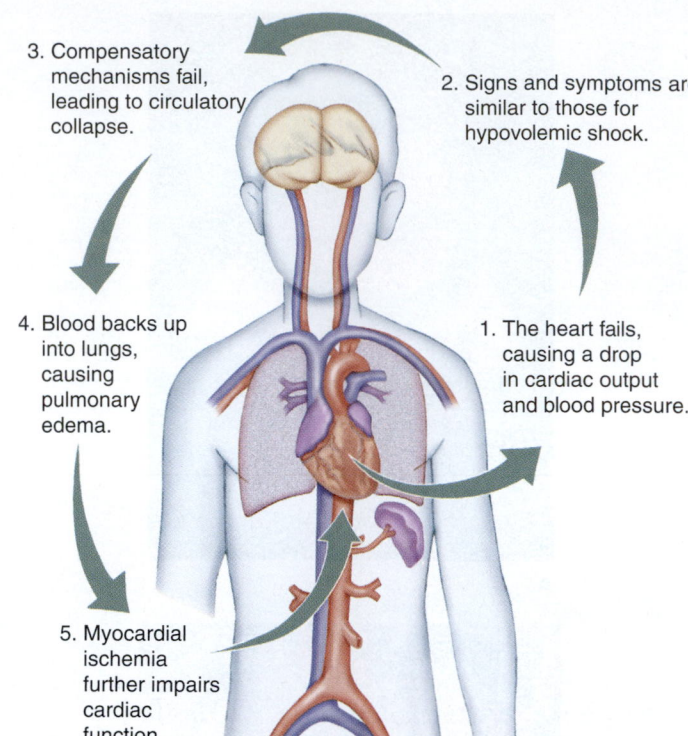

3. Compensatory mechanisms fail, leading to circulatory collapse.

2. Signs and symptoms are similar to those for hypovolemic shock.

4. Blood backs up into lungs, causing pulmonary edema.

1. The heart fails, causing a drop in cardiac output and blood pressure.

5. Myocardial ischemia further impairs cardiac function.

Figure 19-13. ■ Cardiogenic shock. When the heart fails, cardiac output and blood pressure decrease. Blood backs up into the lungs, causing pulmonary edema. Inadequate amounts of oxygen reach the myocardium, impairing the heart's pumping action. The result is cardiogenic shock.

Treatment

Children with CHF are treated with diuretics, potassium supplements, and **inotropic** (increases myocardial contractility) medications to increase the effectiveness of the heart. Heart transplantation may be required for children with end-stage cardiomyopathy. The nursing care for children with CHF is similar to that for children with other cardiac disorders. Priorities include a thorough assessment of the child's condition, promoting oxygenation, administering prescribed medications effectively, facilitating growth and development, and providing necessary teaching and support to the family.

SYSTEMIC HYPERTENSION

Elevated blood pressure in children is often secondary to kidney disease, coarctation of the aorta, hyperthyroidism, increased intracranial pressure (ICP), and side effects of certain medications. Hypertension may also be genetic or the result of family history and is called primary or essential hypertension.

Severe hypertension can cause headaches, dizziness, and visual disturbances in children. A diagnosis of hypertension is made following three separate measurements of elevated blood pressure. Laboratory tests such as blood urea nitrogen (BUN), creatinine, blood glucose, electrolytes, complete

TABLE 19-2

Pharmacology: Antihypertensives

DRUG (COMMON BRAND NAME AND GENERIC)	USUAL ROUTE/DOSE	CLASSIFICATION AND PURPOSE	SELECTED SIDE EFFECTS	DON'T GIVE IF
Inderal (propranolol hydrochloride)	Child: PO 1 mg/kg/day in two divided doses Neonate: PO 0.25 mg/kg every 6–8 hours	Beta-adrenergic antagonist for hypertension	Confusion, fatigue, drowsiness, bradycardia, paresthesia of the hands	Pulse is less than 60 bpm or systolic blood pressure is less than 90 mm Hg
Aldomet (methyldopa)	Child: PO 10–65 mg/kg/day in two to four divided doses IV 20–65 mg/kg/day in four divided doses	Central-acting hypertensive	Sedation, drowsiness, decreased mental acuity, sodium and water retention, nasal stuffiness	Child is receiving other drugs that decrease consciousness or if the child has decreased level of consciousness

blood count, urinalysis, and a lipid panel are also done. An echocardiogram is used to assess the degree of cardiac involvement.

Clinical management of hypertension in children includes weight reduction for children who are overweight; a high-fiber diet low in calories, sodium, and fat; and regular exercise. Adolescents should be taught about the hazards of smoking and alcohol consumption. Antihypertensive medications are given to children with severe hypertension. Table 19-2 ■ describes drugs used to correct hypertension in children.

Nursing Considerations

Obtaining an accurate blood pressure measure is important. The appropriate size blood pressure cuff is essential. The child and family should be taught to take the blood pressure accurately. The blood pressure should be taken at different times during the day and after the child is at rest for at least 5 minutes (see Procedure 13-4 ⦾).

The nurse can assist the child and family in making nutritional food choices that will help maintain a healthy blood pressure. The nurse should discuss specific foods appropriate for keeping the blood pressure low. The teaching plan should also include food choices at restaurants and fast-food restaurants. Box 19-2 ■ describes herbs and vitamins that can be used as aids for the heart. However, herbs and vitamin supplements should be used with caution in children. Teach parents to review these with their care provider.

HYPERLIPIDEMIA

Hyperlipidemia is a condition characterized by increased total cholesterol, low-density lipoproteins, and triglycerides accompanied by decreased high-density lipoproteins. Children rarely exhibit symptoms of hyperlipidemia. Diagnosis is made by blood screening. See Table 19-3 ■ for expected laboratory values for cholesterol.

BOX 19-2 COMPLEMENTARY THERAPIES

Herbs and Vitamins for the Heart

In adults, several natural products have been said to promote heart health. These products are vitamin E supplementation, garlic, and the herb hawthorn. It is inappropriate to automatically assume that these same products are useful for children.

Herbal products are basically untested on children, and their production is unregulated in the United States. Parents who choose to give herbal products to their children should be advised to use products produced in developed countries to avoid contamination of lead, mercury, and steroids.

The National Institutes of Health (NIH) does report an apparent link between heart health and vitamin E supplementation. Parents of children should be taught about sources of vitamin E in foods. Foods containing vitamin E are almonds, sunflower seeds, peanut butter, spinach, broccoli, and kiwi. Physicians may recommend vitamin E supplementation for children with specific cardiac disorders. The following dosages of vitamin E are recommended by the NIH:

- Ages 1–3: 9 IU/day
- Ages 4–8: 10.5 IU/day
- Ages 9–13: 16.5 IU/day
- Ages 14 and older: 22.5 IU/day

Children with hyperlipidemia should be encouraged to maintain a low-fat, low-cholesterol diet. They should implement a regular exercise plan. If these measures do not lower the lipid levels, cholesterol-lowering medication may be prescribed. See Health Promotion Issue on pages 610 and 611.

Nursing Considerations

The nurse should assist the child and family in making appropriate food choices (see Nutrition sections of Chapter 12 ⦾). Referral to a nutritionist may be necessary. Appropriate food

(Text continues on p. 612.)

MediaLink Calculating BMI

HEALTH PROMOTION ISSUE

PROMOTING A HEALTHY HEART IN CHILDREN

Maria, the parent of a 7-year-old boy, Jason, asks the pediatrician's nurse what she can do to help her son avoid heart disease. Maria has been told by her family physician that there are many risk factors for heart disease in her family's history. Her son is 4 feet 2 inches tall and weighs 120 pounds. He enjoys reading, drawing, and playing educational video games. Maria and her husband smoke one pack of cigarettes per day. Their diet consists of mostly convenience foods.

DISCUSSION

Heart disease has been linked to being overweight or having a body mass index (BMI) over the 95th percentile, high blood pressure, high cholesterol, diabetes, or cardiovascular disease before age 55 for men or 65 for women. When a family member smokes, it also increases the child's risk.

The BMI is determined by assessing gender, height, and weight. A score is

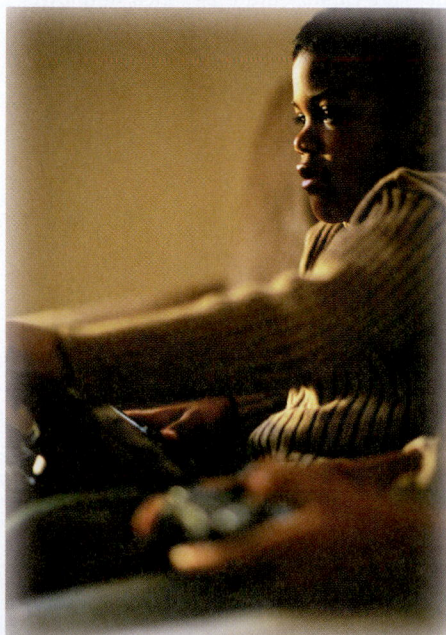

Gerard Launet\Getty Images-PhotoAlto Royalty Free)

then derived. If this score is less than or equal to the 5th percentile, the child is considered underweight. A BMI of 85th percentile to 95th percentile puts the child at risk for being overweight.

Hypertension can be defined as an average systolic and/or diastolic blood pressure that is more than 95th percentile for gender, age, and height on more than two occasions. To measure a child's blood pressure appropriately, the nurse uses auscultation and ensures that an appropriate size blood pressure cuff is used.

The American Heart Association suggests that children with a family history of high cholesterol or early heart disease have fasting lipids tested after age 2. Total cholesterol higher than 170 mg/dL is considered to be borderline. A level greater than 200 mg/dL is considered to be elevated. A low-density lipoprotein higher than 110 mg/dL is considered to be borderline, and a level more than 130 is considered to be elevated. A high-density lipoprotein of less than 35 mg/dL should be evaluated further, as should triglycerides that are higher than 150 mg/dL.

Prevention of cardiac disorders should include maintaining a healthy weight, remaining normotensive, keeping cholesterol levels within normal limits, preventing the development of diabetes, and avoiding smoking. There are many lifestyle considerations to assist in the prevention of heart disease. The nurse can be instrumental in assisting children and parents to develop ways to implement preventative measures.

PLANNING AND IMPLEMENTATION

Following a thorough assessment of Maria and her son's medical and social

history, the nurse must develop a plan to address their needs. The LPN/LVN consults with the RN and the pediatrician. Together, their plan will provide health maintenance and factors to help Maria's son prevent heart disease. Elements of the plan will also provide Maria and her husband with health benefits.

The nurse calculates Jason's BMI using a standardized chart. With a weight of 120 lb and height of 4 ft, 2 in., Jason's BMI is 33.8, which is above the 95th percentile. His ideal weight should be 61 lb. The nurse, dietician, and pediatrician develop a plan for diet and exercise to help Jason manage his weight.

Jason, as a 7-year-old, needs about 2,000 cal/day. To lower his weight, fewer calories and increased energy expenditure are needed. The nurse and the dietician decide to assess Jason's current diet by having him keep a 24-hour food and beverage journal with the assistance of his mother. Later, they will use this journal to help him maintain healthy habits.

The diet that the nurse and the dietician design is low in sugar, fat content, and calories. They teach Jason the importance of healthy food choices and of eating three modest-size meals and two snacks daily. Beverages can constitute a high percentage of calories in a child's diet. Sodas and fruit juices should be avoided. Low-fat milk and water are better choices.

Jason needs to understand portion sizes to help him avoid overeating. He should be taught how to choose foods that fit into the food pyramid. Eating protein-rich foods at each meal and for each snack will keep Jason from being hungry.

The nurse spends time talking with Maria about food preparation. They discuss cooking methods such as baking, broiling, and grilling that can lower fat content and calories. They discuss buying fresh fruits and vegetables and preparing them for easy access. They discuss the fat and calorie content of favorite fast foods. Maria agrees that Jason will need to avoid fast-food meals in order to control his weight.

Jason does not have a regular pattern of exercise. Maria states that he enjoys sedentary activities such as reading, drawing, and video games. The nurse discusses a variety of activities with Jason to determine what type of activities he might enjoy. They discuss walking to the park or riding his bike several times a week. He also said he could take over the chore of walking the dog for his mother. They discuss rewarding himself with reading or drawing only after he has exercised. The nurse encourages Jason to do sit-ups and push-ups when watching television.

The nurse discusses with Maria and her husband about providing a good fitness example for Jason. The nurse suggests exercising together as a family. They could take the stairs in public places instead of riding the elevator. They could park the car some distance from the store and walk briskly to their shopping destination. They could encourage Jason to get involved in a team sport such as soccer, which would give him the opportunity to exercise and build relationships with other active children.

The nurse also discusses with Maria and her husband about keeping a positive attitude during the time they are changing their current habits of diet and exercise. They should not react heavy handedly or punish Jason if he eats something unhealthy or does not exercise every day. Instead, if they remain complimentary and encouraging, Jason will be more likely to stick with the plan for diet and exercise.

The nurse explains to Maria and her husband that living in a smoking environment puts Jason in a higher risk category for heart disease. She also tells them that growing up in a household where smoking is the norm increases the chance that he will smoke as an adult. The nurse encourages Maria and her husband to join a smoking cessation class offered by a local hospital.

The nurse assists the pediatrician in assessing Jason's blood pressure, cholesterol, and blood glucose. At this time all values are normal, but the pediatrician and the nurse plan to monitor this physical data on a regular basis. They also plan to schedule regular office visits to monitor Jason's weight. They will encourage Jason and his family to use the journal to record daily diet and beverage intake, as well as the type of exercise he does and the length of time spent in the activity. They will also encourage them to use the journal to record fears, struggles, thoughts, and feelings related to the weight management plan. Maria and her husband could also use the journal to record their successes and struggles with smoking cessation.

SELF-REFLECTION

Use the previous guidelines for heart disease risk factors to determine your personal risk. Do you know your cholesterol levels? What is your blood pressure? What is your blood glucose? Calculate your BMI. Are there changes that you need to make in order to decrease your own risk for heart disease? Develop a personal plan for improvement and discuss the plan with a trusted friend who will provide you with accountability.

SUGGESTED RESOURCES

For the Nurse

- Kavey, R. E., Daniels, S. R., Lauer, R. M., Atkins, D. L., Hayman, L. L., & Taubert, K. (2003). American Heart Association guidelines for primary prevention of atherosclerotic cardiovascular disease beginning in childhood. *Circulation, 107*(11), 1562–1566.
- National High Blood Pressure Working Group on High Blood Pressure in Children and Adolescents. (2004). The fourth report on the diagnosis, evaluation, and treatment of high blood pressure in children and adolescents. *Pediatrics, 114*(2), 555–576.

For the Client

- http://pediatrics.aappublications.org This website shows how hypertension can be determined in boys.
- Bernardini, R. (2003). The truth about children's health: The comprehensive guide to understanding, preventing, and reversing disease. New York: PRI.
- Sothern, M., & Almen, T. (2003). Trim kids: The proven 12-week plan that has helped thousands of children achieve a healthier weight. London: Harper Collins.
- www.keepkidshealthy.com This website can be used to calculate an individual's BMI and find additional information on preventing heart disease.

TABLE 19-3

Laboratory Values for Cholesterol

TEST	NORMAL	BORDERLINE LEVELS	HIGH LEVELS
Total cholesterol	Less than 170 mg/dL	170–199 mg/dL	More than 200 mg/dL
Low-density lipoproteins	Less than 110 mg/dL	110–129 mg/dL	More than 130 mg/dL
Triglycerides	100 mg/dL	100–150 mg/dL	More than 150 mg/dL
High-density lipoproteins	More than 35 mg/dL	Less than 35 mg/dL	—

choices for a low-fat, low-cholesterol diet include egg substitutes, chicken instead of red meats, and low-fat margarines and salad dressings.

Children with sedentary lifestyles are at greater risk for hyperlipidemia. The nurse can be instrumental in assisting the child and family with healthy lifestyle changes. Thirty minutes of aerobic activity, three to four times a week is necessary to lower the child's lipid levels. The child should choose activities that are enjoyable.

KAWASAKI SYNDROME

Kawasaki syndrome, an acute systemic inflammatory illness, is also known as mucocutaneous lymph node syndrome. Kawasaki syndrome is more common in Asian children and male children (Taubert, 1994) but does affect other children as well. It is the most common cause of acquired heart disease in children, and it is increasing in incidence.

Manifestations

Three distinct phases of Kawasaki syndrome can be identified. In the acute phase, the child is admitted to the hospital with fever, **conjunctival hyperemia** (an increased amount of blood in the conjunctiva), red throat, swollen hands and feet, rash, and enlarged cervical lymph nodes. The acute phase lasts for several weeks. As the child progresses from the acute to the subacute phase, the skin on the lips, hands, and feet slough off or develop **fissures** (cracks or lines present on skin tissue) (Figure 19-14 ■). The child experiences joint pain. The heart is affected by thrombosis, large aneurysms of the coronary arteries, and myocardial infarction. The child gradually progresses through convalescence with a decrease of inflammation. Most children fully recover, but damage to the heart is permanent and can lead to later complications.

Diagnosis

A diagnosis of Kawasaki syndrome is made by evaluating the child's symptoms, and blood work such as erythrocyte sedimentation rate, platelet count, C-reactive protein level, and white blood cell count, all of which will be elevated. The child

may have mild anemia, thrombocytosis, and hypoalbuminemia. An echocardiogram may also show vascular changes.

Treatment

Children with Kawasaki syndrome will most likely be hospitalized during treatment. The child is given IV immunoglobulin and oral aspirin. High doses of these medications are given to prevent cardiac damage.

Nursing Considerations

In the acute phase, take the child's temperature every 4 hours and administer large doses (80–100 mg/kg/day) of aspirin as ordered. Due to the antiplatelet action of aspirin, it is important to assess for bleeding. Monitor the conjunctiva, oral mucosa, and skin every 8 hours for increasing edema, spreading of the red rash, and peeling of the skin. Assess the child for signs of dehydration and malnutrition. Auscultate the heart every 4 hours for abnormal sounds and rhythm.

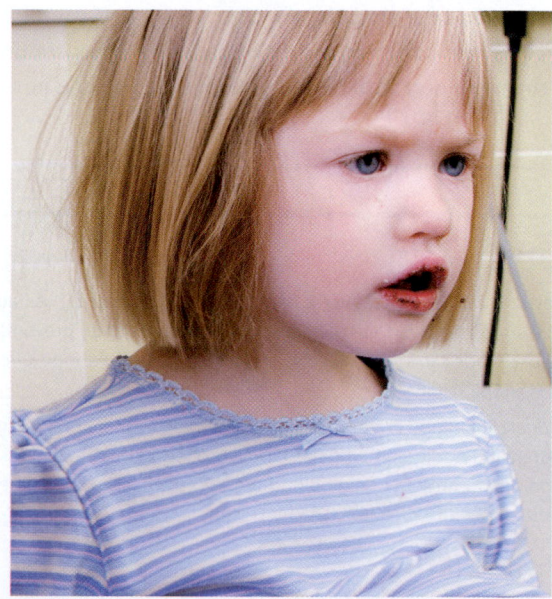

Figure 19-14. ■ This child has returned for one of her frequent follow-up visits to assess her cardiac status after treatment for Kawasaki syndrome. Notice the lips that show the inflammation and cracking.

Because Kawasaki syndrome is very uncomfortable, all care should be provided as gently as possible. It is important to keep linens clean, dry, and free of wrinkles. Provide oral care using foam applicators to decrease trauma and bleeding of the gums. Bathe the child with cool water to decrease fever. A bed cradle may be needed to keep linens off the sensitive skin.

Fluid balance can be maintained by administering IV fluids. It may be difficult for the child to eat due to irritation of the oral mucosa. Soft foods of moderate temperature should be offered.

Activity is important to prevent complications of bed rest. However, periods of rest are also important to prevent cardiac complications. The child may be reluctant to move due to swollen, painful joints. Turn the child every 2 hours and provide passive and active range-of-motion (ROM) exercises to prevent skin breakdown and respiratory complications. Administer analgesics before activity to help keep the child comfortable.

All procedures should be explained to the child and family. Encourage parents to hold and rock the child to provide a sense of security. Teach them to provide care at home, as well as the administration and possible side effects of medications.

ACUTE RHEUMATIC FEVER

Acute rheumatic fever (ARF) is an inflammatory disorder that can follow a group A beta-hemolytic *Streptococcus* infection of the throat (pharyngitis, tonsillitis). Rheumatic fever is more common in children between 6 and 15 years old. There has been a decrease in the number of cases of rheumatic fever due to the use of antibiotics in the treatment of beta-hemolytic strep infections. Although the exact pathology is unknown, it is believed that the group A beta-hemolytic *Streptococcus* triggers an autoimmune response that damages the heart, joints, central nervous system (CNS), and skin. ARF tends to recur, and with each recurrence, there is a threat of further damage to the heart.

Manifestations

Rheumatic fever most often occurs following a strep throat infection. The child could have had a mild sore throat that was relatively asymptomatic or a more severe respiratory illness. Within a few days to 6 weeks, the child presents with enlarged, painful, inflamed joints; a red rash; and a temperature of 100.4°F (38°C) or higher. The most commonly affected joints are the knees, elbows, and wrists. There may be increased heart rate, irregular rhythm, and abnormal sounds. Tachycardia, atrial fibrillation, murmurs, and friction rub may be caused by inflammation of the heart. Most commonly, the mitral and aortic valves are permanently damaged by rheumatic fever. If the heart is involved, the child should be hospitalized during the acute phase of the illness.

Erythema marginatum, a red skin rash, rarely occurs with rheumatic fever. This transient rash is characterized by nonpruritic, red, macular lesions that blanch in the center. Frequently, the rash may be found on the chest, abdomen, buttocks, and proximal limbs. Although erythema marginatum is unpleasant, it does not cause permanent skin damage.

If the CNS is involved, the condition is known as *Sydenham chorea* (**St. Vitus's dance**). Changes in the CNS rarely occur until late in the disease process, possibly after other symptoms have subsided. The child experiences involuntary facial and upper extremity movements. There may be abnormal electroencephalogram (EEG) findings that gradually return to normal. **Chorea** (involuntary, spasmodic movements of the limbs and face) can last for a few weeks or as long as 2 years. Eventually the child returns to normal functioning.

Diagnosis

Diagnosis of ARF is based on clinical manifestations. Diagnostic laboratory findings will include presence of antistreptolysin O (ASO) titer, the antistreptococcal antibody.

Treatment

The treatment of ARF includes the administration of antibiotics, anti-inflammatories, and steroids for severe **carditis** (inflammation of the heart).

> ### clinical ALERT
>
> Polyarthritis of ARF responds better to the anti-inflammatory effects of aspirin than to acetaminophen or ibuprofen. Parents should be instructed to follow the physician's orders about medication administration and to recognize and report symptoms of Reye's syndrome. For more information on Reye's syndrome, see Chapter 26 ⚭ .

Nursing Considerations

The assessment of the child must include a detailed assessment of these body systems. In the acute phase of rheumatic fever, the child is assessed every 4 hours for elevated temperature and heart function. Tepid baths or cool compresses may be provided to decrease temperature and provide comfort. IV fluids are monitored carefully because fluid overload could lead to CHF. Antibiotics and aspirin are prescribed. The nurse provides quiet activities to prevent the child from overtaxing the heart.

During the recovery phase, the child will be cared for at home. Parents need to be reassured that the rash, chorea, and arthritis will subside. The child will need to have limited activities but should be able to return to school and function normally. The child may remain on long-term antibiotic therapy.

BOX 19-3   CLIENT TEACHING

Topics for Discharge After Acute Rheumatic Fever

- **Activity limited to prevent heart damage:** Plan quiet activities such as computer and board games and reading. As activities increase and the child returns to school, arrange periods of rest.
- **Medication:** Long-term antibiotic therapy is necessary. It is important to take medication as prescribed to prevent heart damage.
- **Future health care:** Tell future health care providers, including dentists and surgeons, of history of rheumatic fever. Prophylactic antibiotics may need to be given before procedures. Do not ignore future sore throats; the child may need increased antibiotics.

clinical ALERT

It is important to tell future health care providers, including dentists and surgeons, of the history of rheumatic fever. Prophylactic antibiotics may be prescribed prior to invasive procedures.

Client teaching is important for long-term care after discharge (Box 19-3 ■). The child and parents should understand the need to prevent infection, treat sore throats, and monitor heart function.

Evaluation of heart function during and following ARF is a crucial part of care. The child and parents should be able to verbalize the need for follow-up evaluation. They should also be able to state the type and dosage of medications, the signs of infection, and the guidelines for seeking medical attention.

NURSING CARE

PRIORITIES IN NURSING CARE

When caring for children with cardiac disorders, priority should be given to several aspects of care. It is important to assess oxygen status and to promote oxygenation in these children (Figure 19-15 ■). Positioning the child to facilitate breathing and correctly administering oxygen therapy will be the focus of care. Nursing care should also promote energy conservation in these children because they tire easily and have compromised circulation. Assessment of the child's respiratory and cardiac status, as well as fluid and electrolyte balance, is essential.

ASSESSING

Children with congenital and acquired heart defects exhibit signs and symptoms of CHF. These include, but

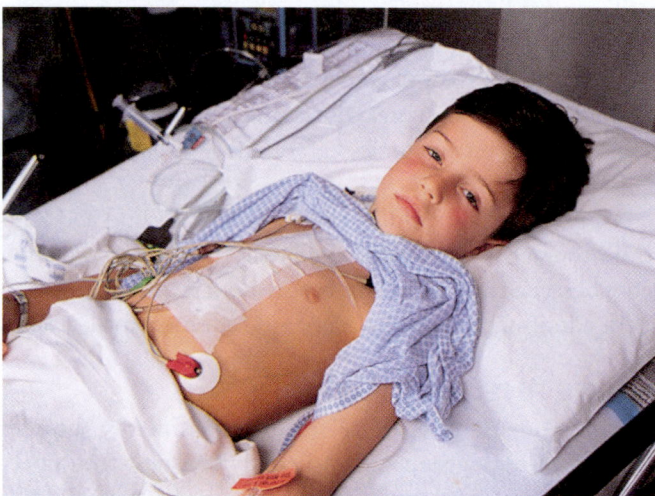

A

B

Figure 19-15. ■ (A) This child is continuously monitored for congestive heart failure. (B) This child with atrial septal defect repair is placed in a position that assists breathing.

are not limited to, altered vital signs, heart murmurs, cyanosis, respiratory distress, fluid retention, and activity intolerance. It is important for the nurse to monitor vital signs correctly, document them, and monitor for changes. See Procedures 13-1 to 13-4 ◗◗. Some heart murmurs are loud and easily heard. Others are soft and can only be detected by a trained practitioner. Murmurs are graded according to the intensity of the sound from grade 1 to grade 6. A grade 1 murmur can barely be heard, while a grade 6 murmur is heard without a stethoscope. Cyanosis can be either constant, generalized cyanosis or cyanosis around the mouth **(circumoral)**, seen only when the child is active, nursing, or crying. Signs of respiratory distress include tachypnea, orthopnea, grunting, flaring nostrils, and chest retractions (see Figure 9-18 or 18-3 ◗◗). Fluid retention may be evidenced by bulging fontanels, fewer than six wet diapers per day, moist lung sounds, and generalized tissue edema. Restlessness, crying, and lethargy can be signs of intracranial edema. Young children may display activity intolerance by increased respiratory effort, resting frequently, or squatting while at play.

DIAGNOSING, PLANNING, AND IMPLEMENTING

Prior to surgical intervention, the following diagnoses may be applicable:

- Activity Intolerance, related to impaired circulation
- Risk for Infection, related to inadequate defense mechanisms
- Imbalanced Nutrition: More than Body Requirements, related to excess intake of sodium- and/or fat-containing foods
- Impaired Skin Integrity, related to hyperthermia or peripheral edema
- Risk for Imbalanced Fluid Volume, related to impaired circulation.

Nursing diagnoses for children who have had surgery for heart defects might include:

- Ineffective Breathing Pattern, related to pulmonary edema, increased work of breathing, or poor respiratory effort
- Decreased Cardiac Output, related to mechanical defects
- Acute Pain, related to operative site.

Goals for the child are as follows:

- To tolerate activity by balancing rest and activity
- To be free of signs and symptoms of infection
- To demonstrate an improved diet based on prescribed regimen
- To have lesion-free skin
- To maintain fluid and electrolyte balance
- To improve breathing and reduce need for oxygen
- To appear more comfortable, as observed by parents
- To take food orally.

Nursing interventions are supportive measures for the child and family.

- Group activities and alternate them with periods of rest to promote energy conservation. *It is important to conserve the child's energy, balancing rest and activity.*
- Encourage a balanced diet with adequate iron, protein, and vitamins. Diet should be low in sodium and fat. Supplements may be needed. *Adequate nutrients are needed to produce red blood cells, maintain tissue integrity, and maintain fluid balance.*
- Establish a routine of skin care to include assessing on a daily basis, changing positions frequently, keeping diaper area clean, changing bed linens frequently, and providing mouth care prn. *These measures will prevent skin breakdown and improve tissue perfusion that is currently compromised.*

- Instruct child and parents in the importance of hand hygiene, especially after toileting, before meals, and after interacting with other children. *Prevention of transfer of harmful bacteria is essential to preventing infection.*
- Encourage maintenance of all immunizations. *Immunizations will prevent a majority of serious childhood diseases.*
- Closely monitor the child's intake and output. See Procedure 15-1. *Intake and output is an essential measure of the child's fluid and electrolyte status.*
- Weigh the child daily. See Procedure 13-7. *Subtle changes in weight can assist in the diagnosis of fluid and electrolyte imbalances.*
- Monitor lab values such as urine-specific gravity, BUN, and electrolytes. Report abnormal findings. *Slight changes in these values indicate fluid and electrolyte imbalances. These imbalances may not be tolerated by the child with a cardiovascular disorder and must be addressed promptly.*
- Position the child to assist respiration. *Upright positions allow for adequate inspiration and expiration.*
- Encourage the use of slow, deep abdominal breathing during times of respiratory distress. *Slow, deep abdominal breathing can ensure adequate oxygen exchange and reduce anxiety.*
- Monitor oxygen saturation. Report abnormal findings. See Table 19-1. Also see Procedure 13-27, Monitoring Oxygen Status. *Oxygen saturation provides data about the child's ability to use available oxygen.*
- Older children and adolescents need to be taught that smoking increasingly compromises respiratory health. *The nurse explains the risks of smoking in an effort to deter this behavior.*
- Explain oxygen therapy and the necessity of it to the child and parents. See Procedure 13-26. *This teaching should assist compliance.*
- Administer prescribed medications and treatments in a timely manner. Monitor continually until the child is stable. Observe closely for side effects. See Procedures 13-29 through 13-38. *This may be the primary role of the RN. LPNs/LVNs assist or administer medications as state regulations and facility policy allow.*
- Provide emotional support to the family. *Parents and family will be anxious and concerned about the child's health. This may interfere with learning about the condition.*
- Reinforce teaching about the child's condition. For example, if an infant becomes cyanotic, the parent can place the infant supine and bend the knees to bring the child to a knee-chest position. *Reinforcement of teaching can be useful. The knee-chest position increases vascular resistance in the lower extremities.*
- Help the child hospitalized with a cardiac condition to feel some sense of control. *Examples of measures that can increase a child's sense of control are allowing the child to have input regarding the day's schedule (i.e., when to bathe), or giving the child a choice of acceptable food items.*

EVALUATING

Children with cardiac defects should be evaluated frequently for fluid balance, signs of infection, and side effects of medication. The nurse will monitor to be sure the child stabilizes over a few hours to days postoperatively. Oxygen will gradually be reduced. The child will be comfortable and able to take oral nutrients. Parents should be able to verbalize and demonstrate needed home care prior to discharge. Encourage follow-up appointments to evaluate health status, including normal growth and development patterns. Because many cardiac defects can be long term and life threatening, therapeutic communication is valuable in evaluating the infant's and family's emotional status.

NURSING PROCESS CARE PLAN
Child with Hypertension

Branson, age 13, has been recently diagnosed with hypertension. Branson's mother asks the pediatric nurse how to help Branson lower his blood pressure. She knows he needs to lose weight and reduce the stress in his life. She is also concerned about the antihistamines that Branson takes daily for his environmental allergies. She states, "The physician said that his allergy medicine might make his blood pressure worse."

Assessment. The client has a height of 5 ft, 4 in., and weighs 175 lb. Vital signs are T 97.8, P 100, R 18, BP 140/90. Branson states, "I'm always concerned about my grades. It's very important to me to make all As. I want to be able to get into an Ivy League college." Client says he does not have many friends, and other students only make fun of him anyway. Denies any hobbies, sports activities, or other interests.

Nursing Diagnosis. The following important nursing diagnoses (among others) are established for this client:

- Anxiety, related to threat to role status
- Imbalanced Nutrition: More than Body Requirements, related to lack of basic nutritional knowledge and lack of physical exercise.

Expected Outcomes. The expected outcomes for the plan of care might include the following:

- Demonstrates anxiety-relieving strategies
- Lists foods to assist in maintaining appropriate intake of calories, fats, and other nutrients
- Participates in a regular exercise program.

Planning and Implementation. The following interventions are planned and implemented for Branson:

- Encourage verbalization of anxious thoughts related to academic success.
- Provide teaching on creating a calm environment.
- Discourage the use of caffeine or other stimulants.
- Teach anxiety-reducing techniques such as breathing patterns, relaxation methods, meditation, massage, etc.
- Design, along with Branson, a regular schedule for assessing body weight.
- Obtain an accurate record of food intake.
- Obtain an accurate record of daily physical activity.
- Provide teaching on appropriate daily intake of calories and nutrients.
- Suggest appropriate food choices.
- Assist Branson in developing an exercise regimen.

Evaluation. At the follow-up visit, the nurse inquires as to whether Branson is experiencing less stress. He states that he is really enjoying his regular physical activity at the gym. This time gives him an opportunity to get his mind off his studies. He is walking on the track and lifting weights with his trainer four times a week after school. He has also made a new friend at the gym who has similar interests. He and his new friend sometimes spend time at the book store together.

The nurse asks Branson about his diet. He states that he is learning to like fruits and vegetables. He has replaced meals of pizza and soda with sandwiches of meat, cheese, and lettuce and bottles of water. He also states that his desire for sweets is diminishing, and he is excited to have lost 5 pounds already.

Critical Thinking in the Nursing Process

1. Excessive sodium in the diet may contribute to hypertension. Provide suggestions for Branson to reduce the sodium in his diet.
2. Design a plan for teaching Branson to monitor his blood pressure.
3. How can Branson manage his allergies and reduce his intake of antihistamines?

Note: Discussion of Critical Thinking questions appears in Appendix I.

Note: The references and resources for this and all chapters have been compiled at the back of the book.

MediaLink Hypertension

Chapter Review

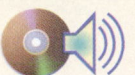 **KEY TERMS** by Topic

Use the audio glossary feature of either the CD-ROM or the Companion Website to hear the correct pronunciation of the following key terms.

Anatomy and Physiology
stroke volume, cardiac output, preload, afterload, contractility

Congenital Heart Anomalies and Defects
septum, ligation, Rashkind procedure (balloon atrial septostomy), pulmonary stenosis, clubbing, coarctation, transposition of the great arteries

Acquired Heart Diseases
cardiomegaly, inotropic, hyperlipidemia, conjunctival hyperemia, fissures, erythema marginatum, St. Vitus's dance, chorea, carditis, circumoral

KEY Points

- An infant's heart muscle fibers are not developed fully, and the ventricles are not as compliant to stroke volume. Therefore, the infant is very sensitive to volume and pressure overloads.

- Volume and pressure overloads cause CHF in infants.

- CHF is characterized in children according to the type of heart defect. Symptoms of left-sided heart defects are cyanosis, dyspnea, respiratory rales, orthopnea, tachycardia, fatigue, and restlessness. Right-sided heart defects are characterized by distended neck veins, tachycardia, liver enlargement, weight gain, and edema.

- Congenital heart defects may arise when the fetus is exposed to infections, such as rubella, alcohol, or drugs *in utero*.

- Congenital heart defects can be classified into four groups according to the way the defect affects circulation: defects with increased pulmonary blood flow, defects with decreased pulmonary blood flow, defects that obstruct systemic blood flow, and mixed defects.

- Elevated blood pressure in children is often secondary to kidney disease, coarctation of the aorta, hyperthyroidism, increased ICP, and side effects of certain medications.

- Obtaining an accurate blood pressure measure in children with cardiovascular disorders is important. The appropriate size blood pressure cuff is essential.

- Nursing care for children with cardiac disorders should include assessing oxygen status and promoting oxygenation and energy conservation. Assessment should also include fluid and electrolyte balance.

- Because rheumatic fever most often occurs following a strep throat infection, the nurse must educate parents on the symptoms and encourage them to report these symptoms.

- Polyarthritis of ARF responds better to the anti-inflammatory effects of aspirin than to acetaminophen or ibuprofen. Therefore, parents should administer aspirin only under the supervision of the physician and be instructed to report symptoms of Reye's syndrome.

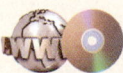 **EXPLORE Media**Link

Additional interactive resources for this chapter can be found on the Companion Website at www.prenhall.com/towle.

Click on Chapter 19 and "Begin" to select the activities for this chapter.

For chapter-related NCLEX-style questions and an audio glossary, access the accompanying CD-ROM in this book.

Animations

Heart

Heart sounds

Chambers of the human heart

Dysrhythmia

Congenital heart defects

Capillary pressure

FOR FURTHER Study

Chapter 6 discusses fetal circulation.

For more information about the effects of maternal disorders on pregnancy and the newborn, see Chapter 8.

Chapter 9 discusses care of the newborn; Figure 9-2 illustrates newborn circulation; Figure 9-18 illustrates areas and levels of retraction in an infant.

Nutrition is discussed by age group in Chapter 12.

See Procedures 13-1 through 13-4 for additional information on taking a child's vital signs.

For more information on Reye's syndrome, see Chapter 26.

Figure 18-3 illustrates the child's respiratory tract and areas where retractions may be seen.

Critical Thinking Care Map

Caring for a Client with Acute Rheumatic Fever

NCLEX-PN® Focus Area: Physiologic Integrity

Case Study: Mrs. Ness called the pediatrician's office and reported her 10-year-old daughter, Emma, has symptoms of a red rash; a temperature of 101°F; and sore, painful wrists and elbows. Upon reviewing the client's chart, the LPN notes that Emma had a positive strep culture 3 weeks ago and received a prescription for penicillin.

Nursing Diagnosis: Acute Pain related to joint inflammation

COLLECT DATA

Subjective	Objective
_____	_____
_____	_____
_____	_____
_____	_____
_____	_____
_____	_____
_____	_____

Would you report this? Yes/No

If yes, to: _____

Nursing Care

_____
_____
_____
_____
_____
_____
_____
_____
_____
_____
_____
_____
_____
_____

How would you document this? _____
_____
_____
_____

Compare your documentation to the sample provided in Appendix I.

Data Collected
(use those that apply)

- "I'm just not hungry. Nothing tastes good."
- "The medication caused diarrhea, so we didn't finish the prescription."
- Reports joint pain to be a 6 on a scale of 10
- Takes Tylenol every 4 to 6 hours for joint pain
- "Rash doesn't itch".
- Denies sore throat
- Reports resolution of diarrhea since discontinuing medication
- Right wrist enlarged
- Winces when wrist and elbow are moved
- Vital signs: T 101.1, P 110, R 12, BP 110/60
- Diffuse macular lesions noted on chest and abdomen
- Throat without erythema

Nursing Interventions
(use those that apply; list in priority order)

- Teach the child and parent to properly clean skin and prevent moisture.
- Develop a plan to re-evaluate the child's pain.
- Monitor the child's hydration level and encourage additional oral intake.
- Note the size, color, and any exudate related to the child's rash.
- Teach the child and parent the proper administration of prescribed pharmacologic agents to include route, dosage, side effects, reportable symptoms, and drug interactions.
- Use cooling measures to lower body temperature.
- Teach the child and parent nonpharmacologic methods of pain relief such as gentle joint massage, ROM exercises, application of heat, control of environmental factors (lighting, noise, room temperature), and relaxation techniques.
- Thoroughly assess the child's pain. Include location, characteristics, onset/duration, frequency, quality, intensity, precipitating factors, and relief methods.

NCLEX-PN® Exam Preparation

1 The nurse is caring for a child with congestive heart failure and has just finished teaching the parents about diuretics and why they are given. The nurse realizes more teaching is needed when the father states:

1. "The diuretic should be given at the same time each day.
2. "The diuretic helps take away the fluid."
3. "If my child throws up the diuretic, I can give him another right away."
4. "I realize my child has to be monitored closely while on the diuretics."

2 A child has been diagnosed with Kawasaki disease. The father is asking about the disease, and the nurse explains that Kawasaki disease is:

1. a circulatory deficit with decreased cardiac output.
2. a mixed cardiac defect that affects both the systemic and the pulmonic circulations.
3. an inflammatory disorder caused by group A beta-hemolytic *Streptococcus* infection.
4. a systemic, acute inflammatory disease also known as mucocutaneous lymph node syndrome.

3 The nurse is caring for a child with Kawasaki disease. The child is in the subacute phase of the disease, which would explain which manifestation?

1. swollen hands and feet
2. sloughing off of the skin on the lips, hands, and feet
3. no outward signs and symptoms
4. enlarged cervical lymph nodes

4 The nurse has assumed care of a child with suspected rheumatic fever. The lab reports have just come back. The nurse reviews them and knows that which lab report would be helpful in confirmation of this diagnosis?

1. antistreptolysin O titer
2. erythrocyte sedimentation rate
3. glucose tolerance test
4. red blood count

5 The nurse is monitoring the intake and output of an infant with congestive heart failure. Which of the following indicators alerts the nurse that the child is accumulating fluid?

1. sunken fontanel
2. bradycardia
3. crackles heard on auscultation
4. capillary refill of 2 seconds

6 A nurse is caring for an infant with a diagnosis of tetralogy of Fallot (TOF). The nurse knows that there are four defects associated with TOF. They are:

1. left ventricular hypertrophy, arterial septal defect, aortic stenosis, and overriding aorta.
2. right ventricular hypertrophy, pulmonary stenosis, arterial septal defect, and overriding pulmonary artery.
3. right ventricular hypertrophy, pulmonary stenosis, ventricular septal defect, and overriding aorta.
4. left ventricular hypertrophy, pulmonary stenosis, arterial septal defect, and overriding aorta.

7 The nurse is caring for a child with a diagnosis of coarctation of the aorta who has congestive heart failure. The nurse is also alert to the other following possible conditions for this diagnosis, which are:

1. weak, thready pulses in the right arm and bounding pulses in the lower extremities.
2. strong, bounding pulse in the left arm and thready pulses in the lower extremities.
3. strong, bounding pulses in the arms and thready, weak pulse in the right femoral artery.
4. strong, bounding pulse in both arms and thready, weak pulses in the legs.

8 The mother of a child with a diagnosis of transposition of the great arteries asks what kind of medication the nurse is giving the child. The nurse tells the mother that the child is receiving prostaglandin E_1. The mother asks why this medication is necessary. The nurse replies that the medication:

1. maintains adequate cardiac output and oxygen saturation.
2. prevents endocarditis.
3. is given prophalactically to prevent infection before surgery.
4. prevents the progression of central nervous system involvement.

9 The nurse is caring for a child with Kawasaki disease and reviews the medication orders expecting to find orders for:

1. aspirin and immune globulin.
2. cephalosporin and furosemide.
3. glucagon and phenobarbital.
4. digoxin and cisplatin.

10 A nurse is caring for a 15-year-old child with hyperlipidemia and is implementing a teaching plan for this child. Select the interventions the nurse anticipates for this client.

1. low-fat, low-cholesterol diet
2. pain medication
3. regular exercise plan
4. consultation with a dietitian
5. anticoagulants
6. cholesterol-lowering medications

Answers for Review Questions, as well as discussion of Care Plan and Critical Thinking Care Map questions, appear in Appendix I.

Chapter 20

Care of the Child with Hematologic or Lymphatic Disorders

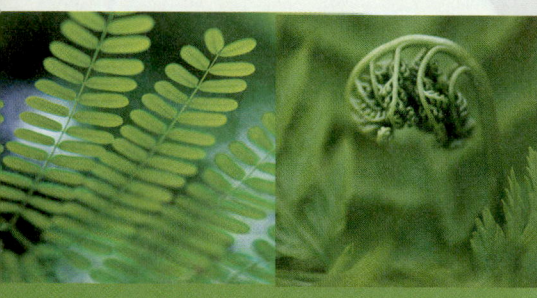

HEALTH PROMOTION ISSUE:
Dealing with Side Effects of Chemotherapy

NURSING PROCESS CARE PLAN:
Client with Sickle Cell Anemia

CRITICAL THINKING CARE MAP:
Client with Hodgkin's Lymphoma

BRIEF Outline

Anatomy and Physiology
Brief Assessment Overview
Bleeding Disorders
Anemias

Thalassemia
Hodgkin's Lymphoma
Leukemia
Nursing Care

LEARNING Outcomes

After completing this chapter, you will be able to:

- Describe the anatomy and physiology associated with the hematologic system.
- Describe the anatomy and physiology associated with the lymphatic system.
- Discuss the clinical manifestation of disorders of the hematologic and lymphatic systems.
- Discuss the medical management of disorders of the hematologic and lymphatic systems.
- Discuss nursing considerations related to disorders of the hematologic and lymphatic systems.

Disorders of blood and lymph in children range from life altering (causing fatigue) to life threatening (leukemia). They may be inherited (e.g., sickle cell disease) or not (e.g., leukemia). Because blood and lymph support all body organs and systems, these disorders can have profound effects. Care of children with blood and lymph disorders will entail emotional support and teaching, as well as physical care.

Anatomy and Physiology

Hematology is the study of blood and blood-forming tissues. It includes the study of the bone marrow, blood, spleen, and lymph system. Knowledge of hematology is important to client care because it assists the nurse in determining the body's ability to deliver oxygen and other important nutrients to the body.

Blood cells are produced in the bone marrow by a process called **hematopoiesis.** The function of blood includes transportation of oxygen and other nutrients to the body; regulation of fluids, electrolytes, and acid-bases; and protection of the body through clotting and infection control.

Blood is composed of plasma and a variety of blood cells (Figure 20-1 ■). **Plasma** is mainly water. It also includes proteins such as albumin, globulin, and fibrinogen. Plasma contain small amounts of waste products, ions, gases, and nutrients. The three types of blood cells are erythrocytes, leukocytes, and thrombocytes. **Erythrocytes** are also called red blood cells (RBCs). RBCs carry oxygen and carbon dioxide to the body's tissues and regulate the body's acid-base balance. These RBCs are pliable and able to change their shape so they can be transported in the narrow passages of the capillary. RBCs are produced by a process called **erythropoiesis** and destroyed by a process called **hemolysis.**

Leukocytes are also called white blood cells (WBCs). WBCs are involved in infection control for the child. There are two types of WBCs: the *granulocyte* and the *agranulocyte.* When a harmful bacteria, virus, or atypical cell is noted by the WBC, the granulocyte can destroy it. The agranulocyte provides the body's immune response by assisting in the development of antibodies. A common agranulocyte is the *lymphocyte.* (Disorders of the immune system are discussed in Chapter 21 ⬭.)

The **thrombocytes,** also called platelets, assist the body's clotting mechanism. These cells are important in minimizing blood loss when a child is involved in an injury. Following an injury, vasoconstriction occurs to decrease bleeding from the site. After vasoconstriction, platelets begin the process of clumping or **agglutination.** Platelets also activate clotting factors so coagulation can occur. Examples of clotting factors are fibrin and thrombin.

The body has a mechanism in place so excessive clotting does not occur, compromising circulation. Anticoagulants

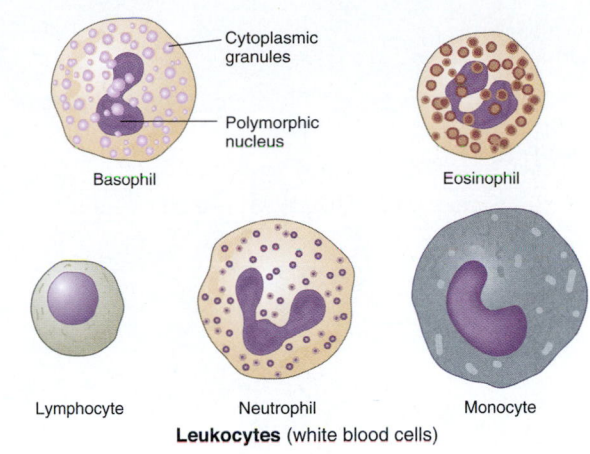

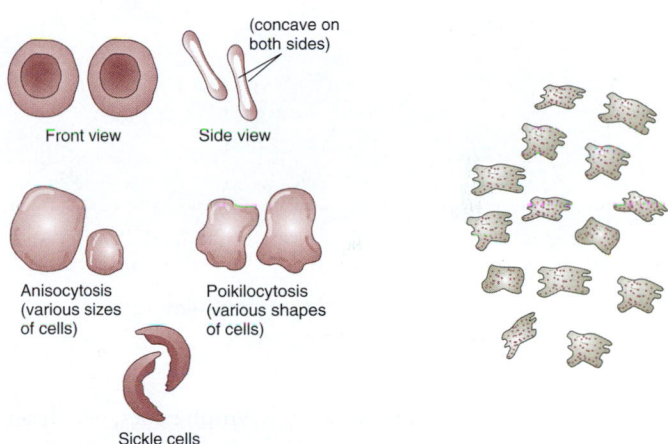

Figure 20-1. ■ Types of blood cells: *leukocytes* (white blood cells) at top, *erythrocytes* (red blood cells) at bottom left, *platelets* (also called *thrombocytes*) at bottom right.

are agents that keep blood from clotting or dissolve fibrin when it forms.

The liver, spleen, and lymphatic system are also parts of the hematologic system. The liver produces the coagulants. The spleen produces RBCs during fetal development; filters RBCs and their by-products; and stores lymphocytes, monocytes, and platelets.

The lymphatic system (Figure 20-2 ■) transports fluid and filters the fluid between the interstitial spaces and the intravascular system. The lymphatic system is also important in the body's immune response. When the body is fighting infection, more granulocytes are produced. Debris from destruction of bacteria or viruses is carried away by lymph. An acute infection causes swelling of the lymph nodes as the body works rapidly to destroy and remove infection. For this reason, lymph nodes are important in physical assessment. This system consists of lymph, lymphatic capillaries, ducts, and lymph nodes.

Lymph capillaries and ducts form a circulation system that drains lymph and fluid from tissues. Lymph contains

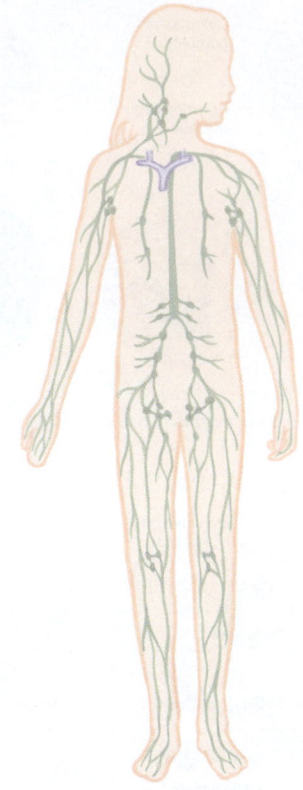

Figure 20-2. ■ Lymph system in the child. (DK Images)

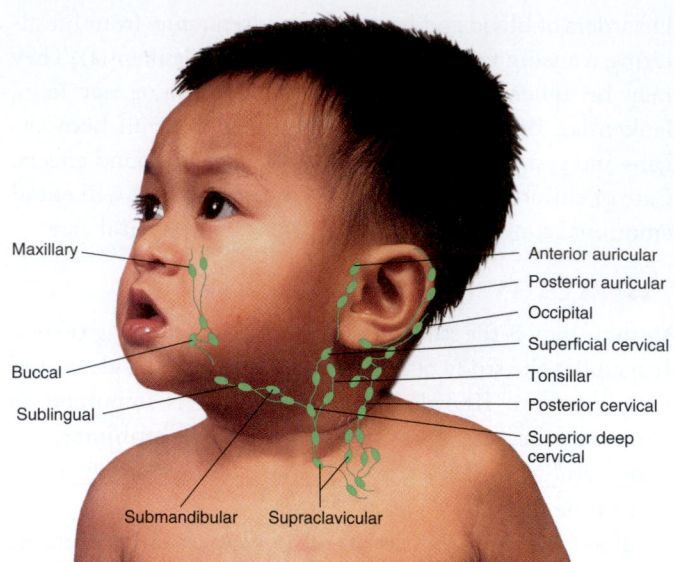

Maxillary
Buccal
Sublingual

Anterior auricular
Posterior auricular
Occipital
Superficial cervical
Tonsillar
Posterior cervical
Superior deep cervical

Submandibular   Supraclavicular

A

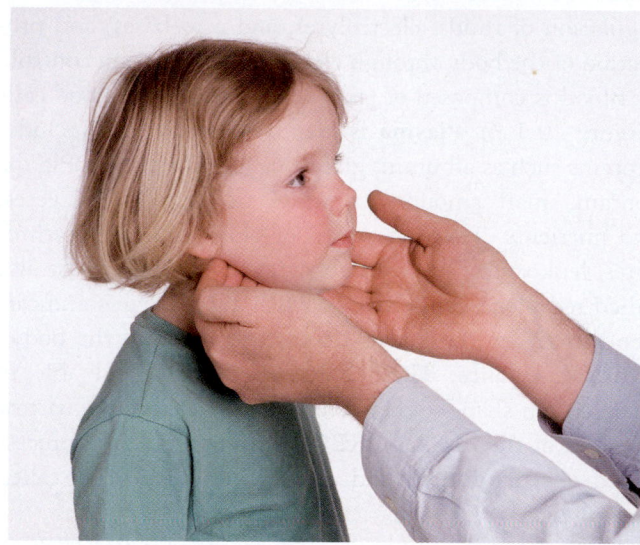

B

Figure 20-3. ■ (**A**) The lymph nodes in the neck are often palpated to determine the presence of infection. (**B**) Care provider assessing the lymph nodes in a young client. (**B**: © Dorling Kindersley)

leukocytes. The lymph flows through lymph nodes, which act as filters. The body has both deep (impalpable) and superficial (palpable) lymph nodes. The body has two collecting ducts for lymph fluid. The right lymphatic duct drains the upper body, and the thoracic duct drains the lower body. Eventually, all lymph is returned to the intravascular system. (Disorders of the cardiovascular system are discussed in Chapter 19 ⬭.)

Brief Assessment Overview

HISTORY

- Inquire about the child's activity level. Has the child had weakness or fatigue?
- Has there been a recent illness or infection? Any fever? Any weight loss?
- Has the child been in contact with anyone with an illness or infection?
- Does the child bruise easily? Any bleeding?
- Inquire about the family history related to cancer, anemia, and other blood and lymph disorders.
- Any weight loss or gain?

PHYSICAL ASSESSMENT

- Observe for bruising, noting location, size, and color.
- Palpate for lymph nodes (Figure 20-3 ■), noting size, mobility, consistency, tenderness, and temperature.

Bleeding Disorders

Bleeding disorders are the result of a decreased amount of blood clotting factors or a decreased number of platelets. Often there are few symptoms until after 6 months of age, due to the limited mobility of the child. Once the infant becomes more mobile, excessive bruising may be evident. It is important to evaluate the infant to differentiate bleeding disorders from child abuse. More information on recognizing child abuse can be found in Box 17-7 and in Chapter 27 ⬭.

HEMOPHILIA

Hemophilia is a rare hereditary X-linked recessive disorder causing a deficiency in a specific blood clotting factor. The disorder almost exclusively affects males.

Manifestations

The hallmark symptom is bleeding into soft tissue and joints or prolonged bleeding during invasive procedures such as dental procedures, surgery, or trauma. Parents may first notice symptoms of joint pain, tenderness, and edema caused by bleeding into the joint. Bruising, nosebleeds, and hematuria may also be noted.

Diagnosis and Treatment

Diagnosis of hemophilia is made based on history, physical examination, and laboratory tests. Laboratory tests reveal decreased factor VIII or IX and prolonged activated partial thromboplastin time. Usually, prothrombin time, thrombin time, fibrinogen, and platelet counts are within normal limits. Treatment of hemophilia includes transfusion of the missing clotting factor. In mild cases, desmopressin acetate or DDAVP (a synthetic drug that increases factor VIII activity) is effective. Aminocaproic acid has an unlabeled use of stopping bleeding related to dental procedures (Bindler, 2006).

Nursing Considerations

Parents and children should be taught safety measures to prevent injury, and they should be taught to avoid medications that alter blood clotting, such as those containing aspirin. Bracelets identifying the child as a hemophiliac may help medical personnel to provide necessary care in case of bleeding.

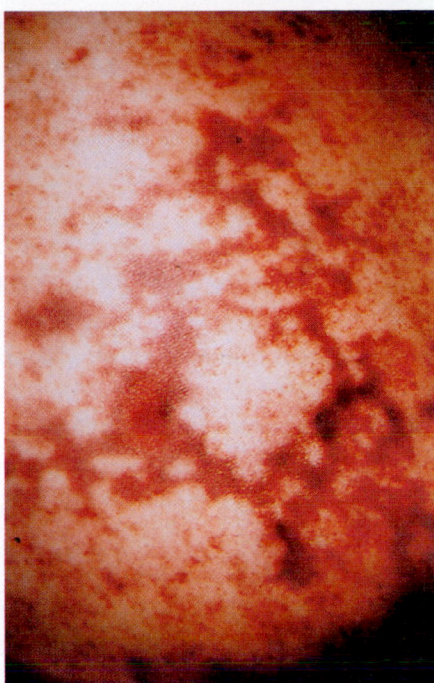

Figure 20-4. ■ Nonpalpable purpura with bleeding into the tissue below the skin. (Courtesy of the Department of Hematology/Oncology, Children's Medical Center, Washington, DC.)

---

clinical ALERT

To prevent excessive bleeding in children with hemophilia, avoid:

- Rectal temperatures
- Rectal suppositories
- Frequent blood pressure monitoring
- Unnecessary invasive procedures such as intramuscular or subcutaneous injections and venipunctures
- Medications containing aspirin
- Contact sports.

IDIOPATHIC THROMBOCYTOPENIA

Idiopathic thrombocytopenic purpura (ITP) is a bleeding disorder of unknown cause that leads to a decrease in the number of platelets. Thrombocytopenia is more common in children between the ages of 2 and 5 years. Frequently, the child has had a recent viral infection such as chickenpox or rubella.

Manifestations

Symptoms include **purpura** (a rash in which blood cells leak into the skin, as shown in Figure 20-4 ■), **petechiae** (pinpoint microhemorrhages under the skin), hematuria, blood in the stool, nosebleeds, and **ecchymosis** (larger hemorrhage into the skin). The disorder may spontaneously go into permanent remission. **Remission** is defined as lack of evidence of any clinical symptoms of a disorder.

Diagnosis and Treatment

Diagnosis of ITP is made through reviewing the child's history and physical findings. Laboratory data include a decreased platelet count, decreased antiplatelet antibodies, presence of antinuclear antibodies, and positive direct Coombs' test. Corticosteroid therapy is indicated for platelet counts less than 50,000 mm^3/dL. For platelet counts less than 20,000 mm^3/dL, IV immune globulin is administered. Platelet replacement may be required if the child is experiencing hemorrhage. If the disorder continues long term, a splenectomy may be performed with some success in controlling the disorder.

Nursing Considerations

Nursing care would include controlling bleeding (Box 20-1 ■) and teaching the child and family measures to decrease risk of bleeding. Parents should also be aware of the signs and symptoms of occult (hidden) bleeding, such as tarry stool (*melena*). Occult blood may be present with tumors of the GI tract, ulcers, or inflammatory bowel disease.

Anemias

Anemia is a decrease in the number of RBCs, a decrease in hemoglobin, or both. Anemia can be caused by blood loss, a destruction of RBCs, or a decrease in production of RBCs.

BOX 20-1 NURSING CARE CHECKLIST

First Aid for Bleeding

- ☑ Obtain assistance from another health care worker.
- ☑ Apply personal protective equipment.
- ☑ Apply direct pressure with sterile gauze to the site of bleeding for at least 15 minutes.
- ☑ If gauze becomes soaked, do not remove. Add additional gauze.
- ☑ Raise the site of bleeding above the heart while applying pressure.
- ☑ Apply ice packs to promote vasoconstriction.
- ☑ If bleeding has not slowed after 15 minutes of these measures, apply additional pressure to the pulse site above the wound.
- ☑ Monitor vital signs closely.
- ☑ If the child does not have venous access, initiate access to administer IV fluid or blood replacement as ordered.
- ☑ Offer emotional support to the child and his or her family.

Three types of anemia—iron-deficiency anemia, sickle cell anemia, and thalassemia—all of which affect children, are discussed.

IRON-DEFICIENCY ANEMIA

Iron-deficiency anemia is a condition that results when the demand for stored iron is greater than what the body can supply. The number of RBCs may be normal, but the hemoglobin level is low, resulting in decreased oxygen-carrying capacity. The cause of iron-deficiency anemia in infants can be blood loss, but more commonly it is due to poor intake of iron and iron-rich foods after 6 months of age. Infants have adequate iron stores from birth to 4 to 6 months. In children and adolescents, iron-deficiency anemia may develop during periods of rapid physical growth.

Manifestations

The child with iron-deficiency anemia will appear pale, tired, and irritable (Figure 20-5 ■). If undiagnosed or untreated for a long period of time, the child can display tachycardia, muscle weakness, systolic heart murmur, and growth retardation, as well as be mentally delayed. Over time, the nail beds become deformed.

clinical ALERT

Anemia may be associated with *pica*, a craving to eat substances that are not food. A child who is seen eating dirt, clay, chalk, glue, ice, starch, or hair should be assessed to determine whether anemia is the cause. Teach parents to recognize and report these symptoms promptly.

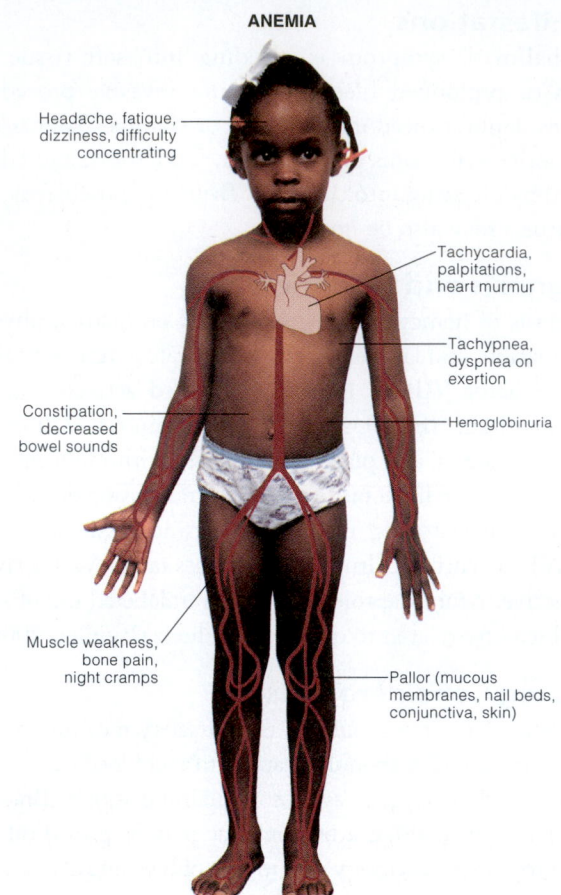

ANEMIA

Headache, fatigue, dizziness, difficulty concentrating

Tachycardia, palpitations, heart murmur

Tachypnea, dyspnea on exertion

Constipation, decreased bowel sounds

Hemoglobinuria

Muscle weakness, bone pain, night cramps

Pallor (mucous membranes, nail beds, conjunctiva, skin)

Figure 20-5. ■ Multisystem effects of anemia.

Diagnosis

Diagnosis of iron-deficiency anemia is made by history, physical examination, and laboratory tests. Hemoglobin, hematocrit, reticulocyte counts, serum ferritin, and serum iron concentration will be decreased while RBC count and total iron-binding capacity are increased. See Table 20-1 for classifications of iron-deficiency anemia.

Treatment

Treatment for iron-deficiency anemia includes administration of oral supplemental iron preparations (Table 20-2 ■). Dietary counseling is also important to ensure adequate dietary intake of iron. For instance, children are more apt to eat raisins and

TABLE 20-1

Hemoglobin Levels in Anemia

ANEMIA CLASSIFICATION	HEMOGLOBIN LEVEL
Mild	9.5–11 g/dL
Moderate	8–9.4 g/dL
Severe	Less than 8 g/dL

TABLE 20-2

Pharmacology: Drugs for Iron Deficiencies

DRUG (COMMON BRAND NAME AND GENERIC)	USUAL ROUTE/DOSE	CLASSIFICATION AND PURPOSE	SELECTED SIDE EFFECTS	DON'T GIVE IF
Feosol (ferrous sulfate)	For deficiency: under 6 years old, 75–225 mg/day PO; 6–12 years old, 600 mg/day PO	Iron preparation	Nausea; heartburn; constipation; black, tarry stools	Crushed; within 1 hour of bedtime; undiluted
Feostat (ferrous fumarate)	For deficiency: 3 mg/kg tid PO For supplementation: 3 mg/day once daily PO For the infant: 1–15 mg/kg/day PO	Iron preparation	As above	As above
Fergon (ferrous gluconate)	For deficiency: 100–300 mg/day PO For supplementation: 100–300 mg/day PO	Iron preparation	As above	As above

enriched cereals or breads than green, leafy vegetables. Re-evaluation of laboratory findings is necessary after 2 months of treatment. If findings are satisfactory, iron supplementation is decreased and laboratory tests are repeated in 6 months to determine if dietary intake is sufficient.

Nursing Considerations

Parents should be taught to provide a diet high in iron, such as dark green and deep yellow fruits and vegetables, dried fruits such as raisins, red meats, fish, poultry, and whole grains. Box 20-2 ■ lists foods that can help in absorption of iron. Infants who are formula fed should be given formulas containing iron. When solid food is introduced, iron-fortified cereals are encouraged.

Because young children have difficulty swallowing pills, liquid iron preparation may be ordered. Liquid preparations should be diluted and given through a straw or placed on the back of the tongue to prevent staining of the teeth. Liquid iron preparation may not be compatible with milk or juice. Iron preparations may turn the stool black, cause constipation, and create an unpleasant aftertaste. Adequate fluids, a high-fiber diet, and exercise will help the child avoid constipation.

clinical ALERT

Iron overdose is possible, and parents should be taught to recognize the symptoms. These symptoms include abdominal pain, vomiting, blood diarrhea, shortness of breath, and shock. Immediate recognition and prompt reporting of these symptoms are essential. The child will need immediate treatment.

BOX 20-2   COMPLEMENTARY THERAPIES

Foods to Increase Absorption of Iron

Vitamin C–containing foods can increase the absorption of iron when ingested at the same time. The nurse can give the child and parent several examples of meals that will facilitate absorption of iron:

- hamburger with tomato slice
- chicken and broccoli casserole
- spinach salad with orange slices
- whole-grain cereal (dry) sprinkled over fresh strawberries
- baked fish with a glass of pure fruit juice fortified with vitamin C

SICKLE CELL ANEMIA

Sickle cell anemia is a hereditary disorder affecting the formation of hemoglobin. Normal hemoglobin (Hgb) is replaced by hemoglobin S (Hgb S) that causes the RBC to form an "S" or "C" shape (Figure 20-6 ■). The abnormally shaped RBCs cannot travel normally through the capillaries, resulting in decreased blood flow and decreased oxygen-carrying capacity.

Sickle cell anemia is a recessive trait affecting primarily African Americans, but it has been found in other races as well. Approximately 1 in 12 African Americans carries the recessive gene, but most do not exhibit symptoms of sickle

Hemoglobin S and Red Blood Cell Sickling

Sickle cell anemia is caused by an inherited autosomal recessive defect in Hb synthesis. Sickle cell hemoglobin (HbS) differs from normal hemoglobin only in the substitution of the amino acid valine for glutamine in both beta chains of the hemoglobin molecule.

When HbS is oxygenated, it has the same globular shape as normal hemoglobin. However, when HbS off-loads oxygen, it becomes insoluble in intracellular fluid and crystallizes into rodlike structures. Clusters of rods form polymers (long chains) that bend the erythrocyte into the characteristic crescent shape of the sickle cell.

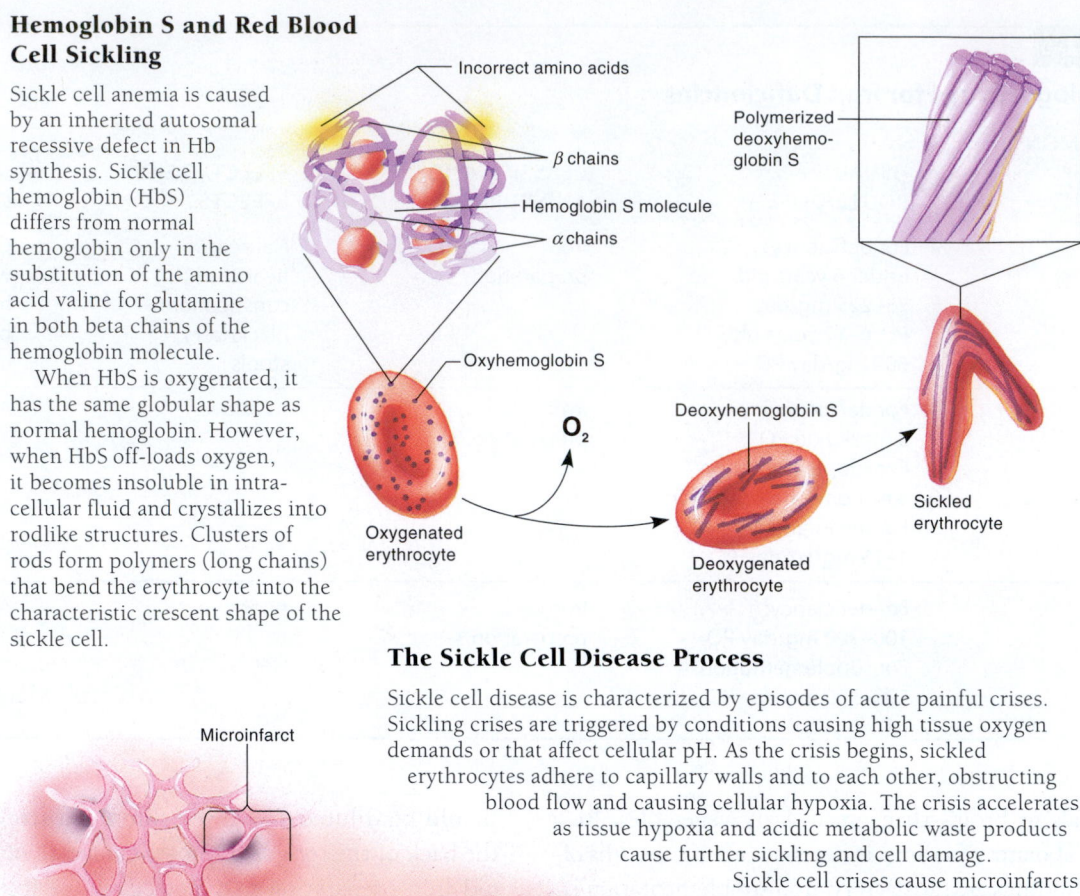

The Sickle Cell Disease Process

Sickle cell disease is characterized by episodes of acute painful crises. Sickling crises are triggered by conditions causing high tissue oxygen demands or that affect cellular pH. As the crisis begins, sickled erythrocytes adhere to capillary walls and to each other, obstructing blood flow and causing cellular hypoxia. The crisis accelerates as tissue hypoxia and acidic metabolic waste products cause further sickling and cell damage.

Sickle cell crises cause microinfarcts in joints and organs, and repeated crises slowly destroy organs and tissues. The spleen and kidneys are especially prone to sickling damage.

Figure 20-6. ■ Pathophysiology of sickle cell anemia. Obstruction of capillaries causes acute pain.

cell anemia. If both parents carry the recessive gene, there is a 25% chance that each child will have sickle cell anemia. Such parents should be counseled about the possibility of having a child with sickle cell anemia.

Manifestations

The infant with sickle cell anemia will be asymptomatic until approximately 4 to 6 months of age because sickling is inhibited by fetal hemoglobin. Not all RBCs will be misshapen,

and the infant will be healthy much of the time. During periods of stress, such as rapid growth or illness, more sickle-shaped cells will be released into the circulation. Sickle cells have a short life span, living 10 to 20 days instead of the usual 120 days of normal RBCs. The difficulties associated with sickle cell anemia are a combination of sickle cells obstructing circulation (**vaso-occlusion**) and anemia from not enough normal RBCs and hemoglobin. They result in pathologic changes to body systems and structures (Table 20-3 ■).

TABLE 20-3

Effects of Sickle Cell Anemia on Body Structures and Systems

ORGAN AFFECTED	PATHOLOGIC CHANGES
Brain	Stroke (cerebrovascular accident), headache, aphasia, convulsions, visual disturbances
Bones	Infections and bone degeneration resulting from chronic ischemia (osteoporosis, osteomyelitis, spinal deformities, aseptic necrosis of the femoral head)
Eyes	Diminished vision from retinal detachment, retinopathy
Extremities	Vaso-occlusion and chronic ischemia leading to peripheral neuropathy, weakness, arthralgia
Kidneys	Ischemia leading to enuresis, hematuria, inability to concentrate urine
Liver	Impaired blood flow leads to enlargement and scarring (hepatomegaly, cirrhosis)
Penis	Obstruction of microcirculation and engorgement of penis (priapism)
Skin	Decreased peripheral circulation (leg ulcers)
Spleen	Infarct in spleen leads to fibrosis (nonfunctioning spleen, increased number of infections); crisis involving spleen can be life threatening within hours

Source: Data from Ball, J., & Bindler, R. (2003). *Pediatric nursing care for children,* 3rd ed. Upper Saddler River, NJ: Prentice Hall.

Children with sickle cell anemia experience symptoms characterized as a sickle cell crisis (see Figure 20-6). The **sickle cell crisis** is an acute episode of severe symptoms. The crisis may be brought on by fever, dehydration, altitude, vomiting, emotional distress, fatigue, alcohol consumption, pregnancy, or excessive physical activity.

During a sickle cell crisis, the child will experience severe pain, localized to the area of the vaso-occlusion. For example, an obstruction in the spleen would cause severe left upper quadrant pain. If occlusions occur close to the dermis, discoloration, pallor, and coolness would be present. Nausea, fever, swelling and pain in the joints, vomiting, anorexia, and diarrhea may also be present.

The three most common types of sickle cell crisis (Box 20-3 ■) are:

BOX 20-3

Types of Sickle Cell Crisis
Vaso-occlusive (Thombotic) Crisis
- Most common type of crisis; painful
- Caused by stasis of blood with clumping of cells in the microcirculation, ischemia, and infarction
- Signs include fever, pain, and tissue engorgement

Splenic Sequestration
- Life-threatening crisis; death can occur within hours
- Caused by pooling of blood in the spleen
- Signs include profound anemia, hypovolemia, and shock

Aplastic Crisis
- Diminished production and increased destruction of red blood cells
- Triggered by viral infection or depletion of folic acid
- Signs include profound anemia and pallor

Source: London, M., Ladewig, P., Ball, J., & Bindler, R. (2007). *Maternal and child nursing care,* 2nd ed. Upper Saddle River, NJ: Pearson Education.

- Vaso-occlusive (or thrombotic)—most common
- Splenic sequestration
- Aplastic.

Diagnosis

Diagnosis of sickle cell anemia can be made for infants through hemoglobin electrophoresis. For children older than 6 months, a Sickledex test is used for screening purposes. If the Sickledex is positive, a hemoglobin electrophoresis can verify the diagnosis. The Hgb will be decreased, and the reticulocyte count will be increased.

Treatment

If given early in crisis, a blood transfusion can relieve the anemia and make the sickled blood less thick or viscous. Whole blood, packed RBCs, fresh frozen plasma, cryoprecipitate, clotting factors, or albumin may be prescribed. Parenteral analgesics are administered routinely to control pain. Continuous IV infusion of fluid is common during crisis to correct dehydration. Oxygen therapy may also be implemented. Because the child with sickle cell anemia has a decreased ability to fight infection, prophylactic antibiotic administration is given.

clinical ALERT

The child who requires frequent blood transfusions is at risk for **hemosiderosis** (iron overload, the buildup of iron in tissues and organs). Therefore, an iron-chelating agent such as deferoxamine is also given, which binds to iron so it can be excreted by the kidneys. Vitamin C may also be used to promote iron excretion.

Nursing Considerations

The child should be observed closely for signs of anemia, including pallor, fatigue, lethargy, and irritability. If the child is under physical stress, mild cyanosis may be present. The nurse should encourage a diet high in calories and protein, with adequate fluid intake. Because children who are chronically ill are at greater risk for infection, and infection can stimulate crisis, it is essential to prevent infection. Immunizations, including the pneumococcal vaccine, should be kept up to date. The child should avoid contact with infected persons. Frequent hand washing is a must. Prophylactic antibiotic administration may be prescribed.

Administration of blood products is often the role of the registered nurse, who starts the infusion and documents that the blood to be infused matches the child's blood type. The LPN/LVN should follow state regulations and facility policies regarding administration of blood. In many states, LPNs/LVNs may administer blood products once they are IV certified. LPNs/LVNs may monitor the infusion and the client and obtain vital signs frequently. The LPN/LVN should also be aware of the clinical manifestations of blood transfusion reaction (Box 20-4 ■). These include urticaria, respiratory distress, fever, chills, headache, chest or back pain, hypotension, nausea, productive cough, and distended neck veins.

Assisting the child with sickle cell anemia in pain management is a priority nursing task. A combination of nonpharmacologic and pharmacologic techniques should be used. Nonpharmacologic techniques include positioning, breathing and relaxation techniques, distraction, massage, and warm baths. The nurse should ensure the routine administration of pharmacologic pain relief methods in addition to the nonpharmacologic methods.

Knowledge about the disease helps ensure compliance with preventative measures and treatment. Family members should be encouraged to share their feelings. Because sickle cell anemia is a chronic, life-threatening, genetic disease, a lot of additional stress will be placed on the family unit. Family members need help coping with guilt, fear, and depression. Support groups may be available to assist and support families of sickle cell children.

Thalassemia

Thalassemia is an inherited disorder caused by abnormal hemoglobin synthesis. Thalassemias are classified as either *beta* or *alpha*. Children of Mediterranean descent and those from the Middle East, Asia, or Africa are more likely to have these conditions (Box 20-5 ■). Beta thalassemia is an autosomal recessive disorder, so if both parents are carriers, each child has a 25% chance of having the condition.

Both beta and alpha thalassemias are defects in the production of hemoglobin. In beta thalassemia, the RBCs are fragile and can be easily destroyed.

Manifestations

The by-product of hemolysis is *hemosiderin*, which can be deposited in the skin of the child, creating a tanned appearance. As anemia progresses, the child can have pathologic fractures and skeletal deformities. Pallor, lethargy, activity intolerance, headache, and bone pain are also clinical manifestations. The liver and spleen may also become enlarged.

The symptoms of alpha thalassemia are similar to beta thalassemia. They are, however, typically milder in nature unless the child's genes are affected. When this occurs, the fetus may develop hydrops fetalis and congestive heart failure.

Diagnosis and Treatment

Thalassemia can be detected by genetic testing in pregnancy. History, symptoms, and physical examination assist in the formation of a diagnosis in the infant or child. Laboratory tests include hemoglobin electrophoresis, complete blood count (CBC), chest x-ray, and magnetic resonance imaging (MRI) of the liver.

BOX 20-4	ASSESSMENT

Clinical Manifestations of Blood Transfusion Reaction

- Urticaria
- Respiratory distress
- Fever
- Chills
- Headache
- Chest or back pain
- Hypotension
- Nausea
- Productive cough
- Distended neck veins

Note: In many states, LPNs/LVNs may administer blood products once they are IV certified.

BOX 20-5	CULTURAL PULSE POINTS

Genetic Risk for Thalassemia

Health officials in Greece have developed extensive public service campaigns to advise citizens of their potential genetic risk for thalassemia. Prenatal screening programs have been successful in reducing the incidence of the disease. Therapeutic abortion rates are also high among women who discover the trait in the fetus they are carrying. Thalassemia is a risk for all women of Mediterranean descent.

Medical management of thalassemia is supportive and not curative. The child may be given blood transfusions every 2 to 4 weeks. An iron-chelating agent (e.g., deferoxamide) is given to prevent iron overload (*hemosiderosis*). If the spleen is enlarged, a splenectomy may be considered.

Nursing care for the child with thalassemia is similar to other forms of anemia and includes strategies to minimize infection, help the child conserve energy, and teach the parent and child about the disease and treatment.

Hodgkin's Lymphoma

Hodgkin's lymphoma (Figure 20-7 ■) is a rare, malignant disorder of the lymphoid system. In children younger than 14 years, Hodgkin's disease is rare. The incidence of the disease increases with age and is especially high in 15-year-old males. With early diagnosis and treatment of Hodgkin's lymphoma, the long-term prognosis is favorable (80–90% survival rate).

Manifestations

The symptoms of Hodgkin's disease include nontender, firm, enlarged lymph nodes usually in the cervical and supraclavicular area. Occasionally, the mediastinal lymph nodes are involved, resulting in respiratory distress from pressure against the trachea. Some adolescents experience fever, night sweats, and weight loss.

The erythrocyte sedimentation rate and leukocyte counts may be elevated. Research indicates a relationship between herpes virus, cytomegalovirus, and Epstein–Barr virus and Hodgkin's disease. Hodgkin's disease has been reported in families, suggesting a genetic factor as well.

Diagnosis

Diagnosis is made by lymph node biopsy. Once the diagnosis is made, further tests must be made to determine the

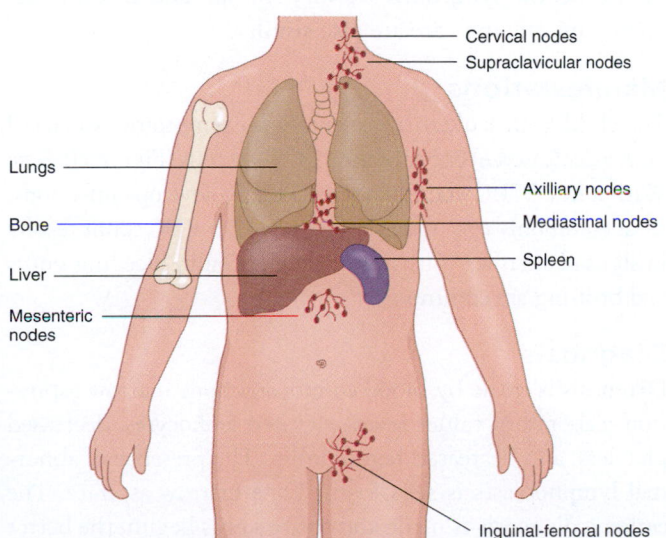

Figure 20-7. ■ Hodgkin's disease. Lymph nodes and organs affected in Hodgkin's disease in children.

Cervical nodes
Supraclavicular nodes
Lungs
Bone
Liver
Mesenteric nodes
Axilliary nodes
Mediastinal nodes
Spleen
Inguinal-femoral nodes

BOX 20-6

Staging of Hodgkin's Lymphoma

- Stage I: The disease is confined to a single lymph node area.
- Stage IE: The disease progresses from the single lymph node area to adjacent regions.
- Stage II: The disease is in two or more lymph node areas on one side of the diaphragm.
- Stage IIE: The disease extends to adjacent regions of at least one of the affected nodes.
- Stage III: The disease is in lymph node areas on both sides of the diaphragm.
- Stage IIIE: The disease extends into adjacent areas or organs.
- Stage IIISE: The disease extends into adjacent areas or organs and/or into the spleen.
- Stage IV: The disease has spread from the lymphatic system to one or more other organs, such as the bone marrow or liver. Lymph nodes associated with these organs may or may not be affected.

---

extent to which the disease has spread throughout the body. This process, called **staging**, is a process of naming the extent of the spread of cancer. It is necessary to help the physician plan the specific treatment. The tests usually consist of computed tomography (CT) or MRI scans, lymphangiogram, blood counts, bone marrow biopsy, and staging laparotomy. Box 20-6 ■ shows the staging system for Hodgkin's lymphoma.

Treatment

Treatment usually consists of a combination of four or five antineoplastic agents. Table 20-4 ■ lists the antineoplastic agents commonly used to treat Hodgkin's lymphoma. There are several reasons for using a combination of antineoplastic agents. First, there is less chance that the cancer cells can develop a resistance to one of the drugs. Second, drug combinations allow the health care provider to select drugs with different patterns of toxicity; therefore, damage is prevented to other body organs. Third, selecting drugs that affect cells

TABLE 20-4

Combination Antineoplastic Agents Used to Treat Hodgkin's Lymphoma

COMBINATION	DRUGS INCLUDED
ABVD	Adriamycin, bleomycin, vinblastine, dacarbazine
MOPP	Mechlorethamine, vincristine(oncovin) procarbazine, prednisone
BCVPP	Carmustine (BiCNU), cyclophosphamide, vinblastine, procarbazine, prednisone

at different stages of their growth cycle allows higher numbers of malignant cells to be destroyed. Side effects of antineoplastic drugs include bone marrow depression, nausea, vomiting, stomatitis, and hair loss. Many are excreted unchanged in the urine. Low-dose radiation may be added to the treatment plan.

Nursing Considerations

The side effects of antineoplastic drugs, coupled with the disease process and radiation treatments, may make the child feel tired, sick, and embarrassed by the change in appearance. The adolescent, who felt invincible prior to developing Hodgkin's disease, may suddenly be confronted with his or her own mortality. Because exposure to infection must be avoided when WBCs are low, the child may need to decrease contact with his or her friends, remain home from school, and limit social interaction. The child's lack of contact with the peer group could lead to feelings of isolation, depression, and anger.

Because many antineoplastic agents are given intravenously, in most cases, these drugs are administered by an RN with preparation beyond his or her original degree. This training is usually offered by the clinical facility. The LPN/LVN caring for the client would need to work closely with the RN. Clients must be assessed for signs of infection, open lesions, and bleeding. Their mental health status should be evaluated and emotional support provided. Precautions must be taken to prevent the care provider from being contaminated by body fluids containing the antineoplastic drugs.

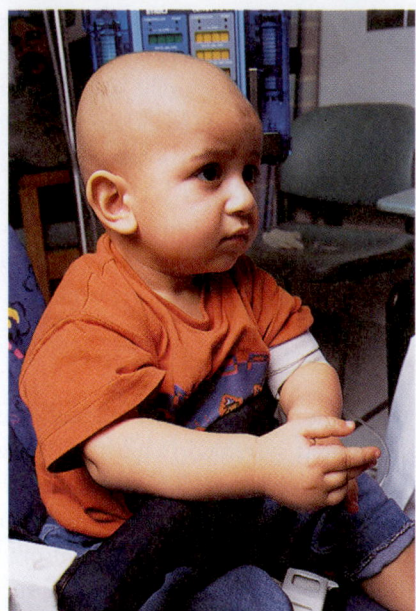

Figure 20-8. ■ Acute lymphoblastic leukemia is the most common type of leukemia in children and the most common cancer affecting children younger than 5 years.

Leukemia

Leukemia is cancer of the blood-forming organs. It is characterized by an increase of abnormal WBCs. Several different types of leukemia are differentiated by the rate of disease progression and the specific cells affected. Chronic leukemia, although common in adults, is rare in children. The exact cause of leukemia is unknown, yet some researchers theorize that exposure to viruses before or after birth can predispose a child to leukemia. Two types of acute leukemia, acute lymphoblastic leukemia and acute myeloid leukemia, are common in children and are discussed here.

ACUTE LYMPHOBLASTIC LEUKEMIA

Acute lymphoblastic leukemia (ALL) is the overproduction of immature lymphocytes. ALL, the most common leukemia of childhood, has the highest incidence in Caucasian boys who are 3 to 4 years of age (Figure 20-8 ■).

Normally, lymphocytes are formed from stem cells in the bone marrow and migrate to lymphatic tissue where they become mature functioning cells. In ALL, the lymphocytes divide rapidly but fail to mature. Lymphoblasts (immature lymph cells) have no normal function. As lymphoblast numbers rise, fewer and fewer normal lymph cells are made,

and the high numbers of lymphoblasts crowd out normal WBCs, RBCs, and platelets.

ACUTE MYELOGENOUS LEUKEMIA

Acute myelogenous leukemia (AML) occurs when cancer cells develop in the bone marrow (*myeloid tissue*). AML is a less common form of leukemia in children. In AML, cancer cells replace normal bone marrow. Immature WBCs, RBCs, and platelets are found circulating throughout the body. Because in both ALL and AML bone marrow is replaced by blast cells, the symptoms are very similar. Diagnosis, treatment, and nursing care are also similar.

Manifestations

The child with leukemia presents with symptoms associated with a decreased number of normal blood cells (Figure 20-9 ■). With a low WBC count, the child easily develops infections, most commonly respiratory infections. Low RBC count results in signs of anemia. With a low platelet count, bleeding gums and bruising are common.

Diagnosis

Diagnosis is made by blood counts and bone marrow aspiration. Laboratory values reveal elevated leukocytes, decreased platelets, and decreased hemoglobin. The presence of abnormal lymphoblasts is seen in the bone marrow aspirate. The earlier a diagnosis is made and treatment is begun, the better the prognosis. Left untreated, the life expectancy of a child with AML is several weeks to 6 months.

LEUKEMIA

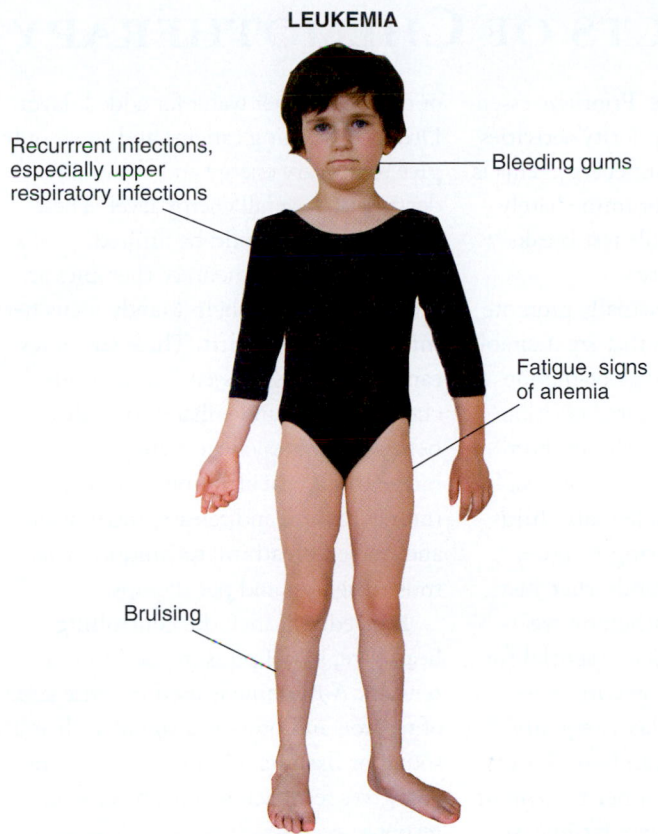

Recurrrent infections, especially upper respiratory infections

Bleeding gums

Fatigue, signs of anemia

Bruising

Figure 20-9. ■ Multisystem effects of leukemia (M. C. Schlachter Photography)

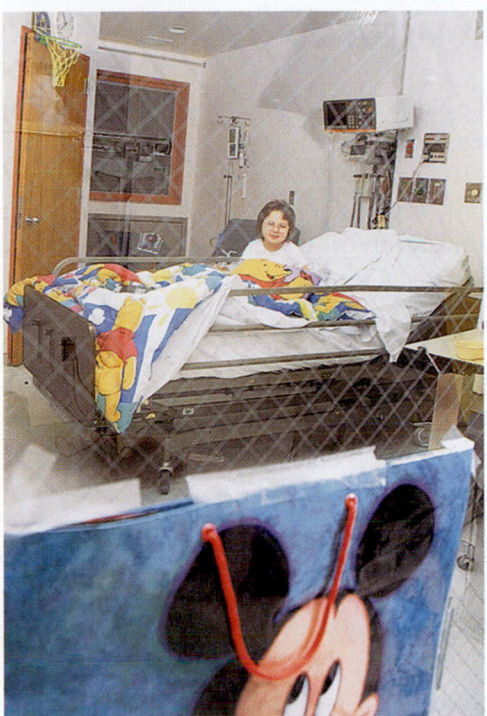

Figure 20-10. ■ Protective isolation. The child undergoing bone marrow transplantation is hospitalized in a special sterile unit while receiving chemotherapy before the transfusion. The child will remain in the unit for several weeks afterward until the new marrow produces enough cells to maintain health.

Treatment

Treatment might include antibiotics, blood replacement, chemotherapy, and radiation. After remission is achieved, bone marrow transplant can be beneficial if a suitable donor is available. During treatment or after bone marrow transplantation, the child must be protected in as sterile an environment as possible, while the body rebuilds its defenses (Figure 20-10 ■). (See Health Promotion Issue on pages 632 and 633.)

Nursing Considerations

Assessment of bruising, bleeding, fever, and symptoms of infection during treatment should be done frequently. Chemotherapy is very damaging to the kidneys, so renal function must be monitored with specific gravity, intake and output, and daily weight. Chemotherapy and radiation can be harmful to the rapidly growing mucous membranes of the gastrointestinal system, resulting in nausea, vomiting, constipation, and sores in the mouth. Nutritional status and fluid balance should be assessed closely.

The child with leukemia needs periods of rest coupled with safe activities. During the acute phase of the illness, the child may not have enough energy for a lot of physical activity, but quiet play can help maintain mobility as well as provide the child with a diversion from thoughts of cancer.

Having an acute life-threatening illness causes a lot of fear for the child and for the parents and family. Because of the rapid onset of symptoms of leukemia, the child appears well one day and extremely ill the next. Hospitalization, numerous invasive diagnostic procedures, and administration of toxic chemotherapy contribute to the fear and anxiety. The nurse is instrumental in providing support and teaching. The nurse also helps organize interdisciplinary resources to assist the client and family. Referral to family support groups may be made on request.

NURSING CARE

PRIORITIES IN NURSING CARE

When caring for children with hematologic and lymphatic system disorders, priority nursing care includes improving tissue perfusion, infection prevention, injury prevention, improving nutritional status, adequate pain management, and improving activity intolerance. Administer iron replacement therapy as ordered. Encourage dietary intake of foods containing iron. Provide a safe environment for the child. Implement

(Text continues on p. 634.)

DEALING WITH SIDE EFFECTS OF CHEMOTHERAPY

Nine-year-old Mandy recently completed her second chemotherapy treatment for leukemia. Her mother reports that Mandy had no side effects with the first treatment but has recently been fatigued to the point of not having enough energy to eat. Mandy and her mom have also noticed that Mandy's hair seems to be falling out. Mandy is crying frequently and refusing to go out in public, including school.

Mandy's mom wonders if these side effects are normal. She asks the nurse for advice on dealing with these issues. She is interested in anything that will make Mandy feel more comfortable, increase her energy, and cause her to feel better about herself so she can continue her normal activities.

DISCUSSION

Fatigue is the most frequent symptom reported by cancer patients. This fatigue can feel quite different from general fatigue. It may also appear suddenly and may not be relieved by rest. The child may only see resolution of fatigue once her condition stabilizes.

Hair loss or *alopecia* is a common occurrence following chemotherapy. Alopecia can be thinning of the hair, loss of clumps of hair, or a complete loss of all hair, including hair on the head, face, arms and legs, underarms, and pubic area. The remaining hair may become dull and dry. The hair usually grows back. The new hair, however, may be a different color and texture.

PLANNING AND IMPLEMENTATION

Fatigue

Encouraging rest for a child with fatigue due to chemotherapy is the most important nursing action. The nurse should make specific suggestions to assist Mandy and her mother in achieving an adequate amount of rest for Mandy. Carefully review Mandy's schedule. Prioritize essential activities. Do these priority activities when Mandy has the most energy. This is usually in the morning or immediately following a meal. Schedule rest breaks and naps between activities.

Physical activity can actually promote energy. Discuss activities that are desirable to Mandy. Begin with range-of-motion exercises performed in a seated position and progress to leisurely walks of short distance or exercise in a swimming pool.

A healthy diet and adequate fluids are essential for combating fatigue. The nurse can teach Mandy that just like getting her chemotherapy treatment on a regular basis is essential for fighting the leukemia, getting adequate nutrition every day is equally important. The nurse can help Mandy view nutrition as part of her treatment.

Large meals can increase fatigue, so several small meals are more effective. Healthy snacks such as fruit juice, fruits, vegetables, soups, cheese, peanut butter, and nuts should be readily available.

The nurse should explain to Mandy that the fluids she drinks can also increase or decrease her fatigue. The best fluid to consume is water. Most clients enjoy water that is very chilled. Mandy can be encouraged to squeeze a slice of lemon, lime, or orange into her water for added flavor. Drinks containing caffeine and sugar only give temporary energy and eventually decrease the overall energy level. These types of drinks should be limited.

Several complementary therapies are available that may help Mandy focus her mind, body, and spirit. These therapies can reduce stress, lessen fatigue from chemotherapy, and enhance overall well-being. Examples of these therapies are biofeedback, visualization, massage, muscle tension and release, meditation and prayer, breathing techniques, yoga, music therapy, and pet therapy.

Biofeedback includes controlling heart rate, blood pressure, and muscle tension. A machine is used to sense signs of tension and provide a signal such as a sound or flashing a light. The machine also gives feedback when a relaxation response occurs.

Visualization creates a mind picture. Visualization can reduce fear, promote positive thinking, and increase relaxation. Mandy can create mind pictures of herself as an energetic child or of her leukemia being rid from her body by the chemotherapy.

Many health care practitioners believe in the power of healing touch. Massage therapy involves touch and different

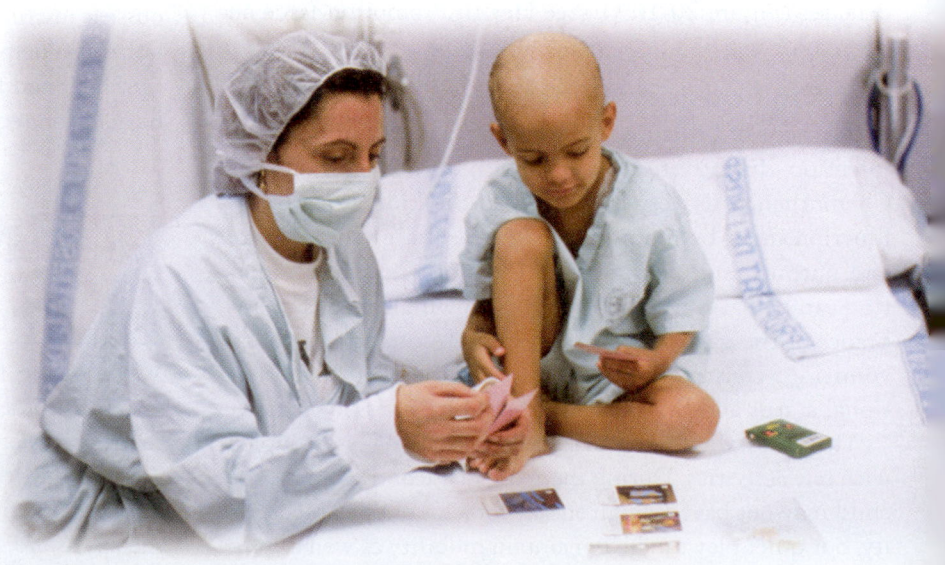

(Geoff Tompkinson\Photo Researchers, Inc.)

methods of stroking and kneading the muscles of the body. The nurse can refer Mandy to a licensed massage therapist for massage therapy.

Mandy can learn several techniques for relieving tension at home between visits to the massage therapist. The nurse can teach these simple techniques. Mandy should find a comfortable, quiet environment. Taking slow, deep breaths will promote relaxation. Instructions for muscle tension and release are as follows: Breathe in through the nose, tensing the toes. Then breathe out through the mouth, releasing the tension and relaxing completely. Take several deep breaths, enjoying the relaxed state. Continue the process with all muscle groups, progressing from toe to head.

Meditation is a relaxation technique and state of mind allowing the client to focus his or her energy and thoughts. In meditation, the client can repeat a positive word or short phrase. For example, Mandy could repeat, "I have energy. My body is healing." The nurse should assess the family's spiritual beliefs. If prayer is a familiar practice, it should be encouraged. Prayer can provide strength, comfort, and inspiration throughout the cancer experience. The nurse may also want to refer Mandy to a pastor or priest.

The nurse can assist Mandy in becoming aware of her breathing. Paying attention to rate and depth of breathing can assist Mandy in recognizing stress and promoting states of relaxation. Teach breathing awareness as follows: Ask the client to sit up straight, placing one hand, palm down, over the abdomen with the other hand on top; ask the client to breathe in and out normally, paying attention to how the abdomen rises and falls; and encourage the client to imagine a balloon in the abdomen, expanding during inspiration and collapsing during expiration. Mandy should be encouraged to slow her rate and rhythm of breathing when she detects stress in her life.

Yoga is described as a science of the inner world of the body and mind consciousness. It involves stretching, muscle tone, and relaxation. Yoga can be learned by taking a class, reading a book, or watching a videotape. The nurse can refer Mandy to available resources.

Music therapy can enhance physical comfort and reduce fatigue. Music is effective by activating the right brain and stimulating the autonomic nervous system. The nurse should encourage Mandy to decrease unpleasant noises by using earphones and turning off the television and radio, which can increase anxiety. The nurse can assist Mandy in attaining resources for relaxing music.

Pet therapy has been shown to improve the life span of clients, decrease blood pressure, and increase relaxation. Caring for a pet or just having a pet present is a source of comfort and provides a distraction or focus for clients. Interactions with pets allow clients to exercise their nurturing instinct and to feel safe and accepted unconditionally. Any pet—a dog, a cat, a bird, or a fish—could be beneficial for Mandy.

Mandy should keep a journal of her diet, activity, and fatigue level. Mandy and her mom should review this daily and make adjustments as needed. Mandy should also bring this journal to her health care visits for review.

Alopecia

The nurse can help Mandy learn to care correctly for her hair and scalp during chemotherapy treatments. A mild shampoo, soft hair brush, and low heat during drying of the hair can help minimize hair loss. Using chemicals such as hair color, perms, or relaxing agents can irritate the scalp and increase the risk of hair loss. The nurse might suggest a shorter hairstyle. This would make hair loss easier to accept. Suggestions for preventing sun damage to the scalp include regular use of sunscreen and wearing a head covering such as a hat, cap, or scarf when outdoors.

When hair loss occurs, Mandy will need information about covering her head if she so chooses. Some children decide to purchase a wig prior to complete hair loss to obtain a more correct color and style match. The nurse can help Mandy's mom file for health insurance reimbursement because the cost of a wig is typically covered when the client is receiving chemotherapy.

Anger and depression are common emotions expressed by clients who lose their hair. The nurse can assist Mandy and her mom in dealing with these emotions. The complementary therapies described here might be effective. Talking or journaling about the emotions may also prove to be helpful. The nurse may be able to put Mandy in contact with another young girl who has experienced hair loss during chemotherapy.

SELF-REFLECTION

What is your reaction when you see a child with alopecia? Shock? Horror? Pity? Sorrow? What unspoken messages are given to children when we compliment their hair? What messages are conveyed when we express approval only when their hair is well groomed and neat?

SUGGESTED RESOURCES

For the Nurse

- www.cancer.gov The National Cancer Institute website provides information to health care professionals and the public on various types of cancer.
- www.leukemia.org The Leukemia and Lymphoma Society website provides information to health care professionals and the public on leukemia and lymphoma.

For the Client

- www.bio-medical.com This website provides more information on biofeedback and provides resources for the necessary equipment.
- www.holistic-online.com This website offers information on complementary therapies that may be implemented to decrease stress and fatigue.
- www.alopeciaareata.com This website offers information on the causes of hair loss in children and provides suggestions for dealing with hair loss.

measures to prevent the spread of harmful bacteria. Provide pharmacologic and nonpharmacologic pain methods. Assist the child with activities of daily living (ADLs) and encourage periods of rest.

ASSESSING

To assess clients with these disorders adequately, the nurse should obtain a complete history, including past medical history and family history. Baseline physical data includes weight, height, vital signs, inspection of the skin, and palpation of the lymph nodes.

DIAGNOSIS, PLANNING, AND IMPLEMENTING

Some common nursing diagnoses for children with these disorders include:

- Ineffective Tissue Perfusion, related to reduced hemoglobin content of the blood
- Risk for Infection, related to excessive white blood cell production
- Risk for Injury, related to hematologic alterations
- Imbalanced Nutrition: Less Than Body Requirements, related to inadequate dietary intake of iron
- Acute Pain, related to hematologic alterations
- Activity Intolerance, related to decreased oxygen supply.

Outcomes for these children include:

- Tissue perfusion improves as evidenced by sensation, temperature, and color within normal limits.
- Child will be free of symptoms of infection.
- Child will avoid physical injury.
- Laboratory values will be within normal limits.
- Child will state that pain level is improved.
- Child will participate in ADLs without symptoms of fatigue.

For children with hematologic and lymphatic system disorders, the following interventions apply:

- Monitor fluid, electrolyte, and laboratory status. *Slight changes in these values could further compromise tissue perfusion.*
- Evaluate capillary refill, peripheral pulses, and edema. *Alteration in these findings may indicate compromised tissue perfusion.*
- Instruct the child and parents on the importance of hand washing. *Hand washing minimizes exposure to harmful bacteria.*
- Encourage the child and parents to avoid contact with individuals who are known to be ill. *This minimizes the child's exposure to harmful bacteria and viruses.*
- Assist the child with ambulation, prn. *Assistance with ambulation can prevent falls.*
- Remove environmental hazards. *Poor lighting, walkway obstructions, and stairways are examples of environmental hazards that may contribute to the risk for injury.*

- Assess diet for nutritional content. *Accurate evaluation of the child's diet gives the nurse data for developing a teaching plan specific to his or her client.*
- Develop a meal plan to increase the dietary intake of iron. *A specific plan will take into consideration a child's likes and dislikes and improve compliance.*
- Teach the use of nonpharmacologic methods of pain relief. *Nonpharmacologic methods of pain relief can supplement pharmacologic methods and assist in the reduction of pain.*
- Correctly administer pharmacologic pain relief methods. *The correct administration of pharmacologic agents for pain relief will be most effective.*
- Prioritize daily activities. *The child will have energy for important activities and not be tired by activities that are unnecessary.*
- Encourage frequent periods of rest. *Rest can restore the child's energy levels.*

EVALUATING

The nurse collects data for frequent assessment of the child with these disorders to determine effectiveness of treatment. The goal of treatment for children with hematologic disorders is a return to normal blood count levels. The child's energy level will return to normal, and he or she will be free of infection and hemorrhage. The child with lymphatic disorders will be free of infection and edema.

NURSING PROCESS CARE PLAN
Client with Sickle Cell Anemia

An 8-year-old girl was admitted yesterday to the facility in sickle cell crisis. Her family was vacationing when the crisis began, and they drove several hours back by car in order to admit their daughter to her "home" hospital. A blood transfusion and fluids have been administered. She is receiving oxygen at 2 liters per minute. The parents state that their son has a cold, but that they "were sure Yolanda did not have it" when they started their trip. When you enter the room, Yolanda is moaning. She cries when you say it is time to reposition her in bed. She states she does not want to have a position change because "it hurts too much to move."

Assessment. When caring for Yolanda, the following data should be collected:

- Status of pain: location, intensity, duration, alleviating factors
- Vital signs
- Intake and output
- Skin (pallor, cyanosis, tenting)
- Review of lab work.

Nursing Diagnosis. The following important nursing diagnosis (among others) is established for this client:

■ Acute Pain, related to sickle cell crisis resulting from vaso-occlusion in lower extremities

Expected Outcome. Client will state pain relief sufficient to allow movement, position changes, and range of motion exercises.

Planning and Implementation

■ Administer pain medication promptly. *Pain of sickle cell is difficult for the child to manage and should be addressed before it becomes too severe.*

■ Position the child carefully. *Careful positioning can prevent undue pain in joints and extremities.*

■ Encourage the child and the family to notify the nurse if pain-relieving measures are not successful. *Management of the child's pain must include using alternative measures if the currently prescribed methods are not effective.*

■ Ask the child and the family about nonpharmacologic pain relief measures that have been helpful in the past.

Use these nonpharmacologic measures when providing care. *Nonpharmacologic measures complement pain medications.*

Evaluation. Yolanda reports warm compresses prior to position changes reduce the discomfort and make movement easier.

Critical Thinking in the Nursing Process

1. What conditions may have led to the sickle cell crisis?
2. When performing physical interventions with this client, what concern will be most important?
3. What nonpharmacologic interventions can be used in this situation?

Note: Discussion of Critical Thinking questions appears in Appendix I.

Note: The references and resources for this and all chapters have been compiled at the back of the book.

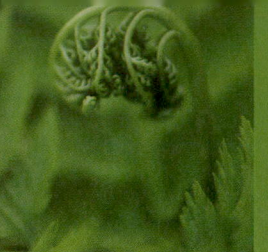

Chapter Review

 **KEY TERMS** by Topic

Use the audio glossary feature of either the CD-ROM or the Companion Website to hear the correct pronunciation of the following key terms.

Anatomy and Physiology
hematology, hematopoiesis, plasma, erythrocytes, erythropoiesis, hemolysis, leukocytes, thrombocytes, agglutination

Bleeding Disorders
hemophilia, idiopathic thrombocytopenic purpura (ITP), purpura, petechiae, ecchymosis, remission

Anemias
anemia, iron-deficiency anemia, sickle cell anemia, vaso-occlusion, sickle cell crisis, hemosiderosis

Hodgkin's Lymphoma
staging

Leukemia
leukemia, acute lymphoblastic leukemia (ALL), acute myelogenous leukemia (AML)

KEY Points

- The primary oxygen-carrying cell in the body is the erythrocyte or red blood cell.

- The primary cell in the body that helps prevent infections is the leukocyte or white blood cell.

- The primary cell in the body that assists with clotting is the thrombocyte or platelet.

- The priority nursing intervention when caring for a child with hemophilia is to prevent bleeding.

- Emergency measures are necessary to control bleeding of the child with hemophilia. These include applying pressure, elevating the site, applying ice, monitoring vital signs, and obtaining venous access.

- When caring for the child with iron-deficiency anemia, the nurse must teach the child and family about adequate dietary sources of iron.

- Liquid iron preparation causes staining of the teeth. The nurse can administer these preparations through a straw to prevent this complication.

- A common complication of iron supplementation is constipation. Fluids, exercise, and fiber are appropriate preventative measures for this complication.

- Children who have sickle cell crises experience pain. The nurse must be vigilant in assisting the child to properly manage his or her pain.

- Common types of leukemia in children include acute lymphoblastic leukemia (ALL) and acute myelogenous leukemia (AML).

- Preventing infection in children with leukemia is a priority nursing intervention.

- Children, especially adolescents, must be assisted by the nurse in dealing with the side effects of antineoplastic drugs, which include bone marrow depression, nausea, vomiting, stomatitis, and hair loss.

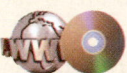 **EXPLORE MediaLink**

Additional interactive resources for this chapter can be found on the Companion Website at www.prenhall.com/towle.

Click on Chapter 20 and "Begin" to select the activities for this chapter.

For chapter-related NCLEX-style questions and an audio glossary, access the accompanying CD-ROM in this book.

Animations

Sickle cell anemia

Leukemia

Interactivities: Match the lymphatic system

Hemodynamics

FOR FURTHER Study

Musculoskeletal signs of child abuse are described in Box 17-7.

Disorders of the cardiovascular system are discussed in Chapter 19.

Disorders of the immune system are discussed in Chapter 21.

More information on child abuse can be found in Chapter 27.

Client with Hodgkin's Lymphoma
NCLEX-PN® Focus Area: Physiologic Integrity: Reduction of Risk Potential

Case Study: Yolanda is a 15-year-old Black female recently diagnosed with Hodgkin's lymphoma. She has completed her first cycle of chemotherapy. She and her mother ask what they should expect over the next few weeks.

Nursing Diagnosis: Risk for Infection, related to immunocompromised status following chemotherapy

COLLECT DATA

Subjective	Objective
_____	_____
_____	_____
_____	_____
_____	_____
_____	_____
_____	_____
_____	_____

Would you report this? Yes/No

If yes, to: _____

Nursing Care

_____
_____
_____
_____
_____
_____
_____
_____
_____
_____
_____
_____
_____
_____

How would you document this? _____
_____
_____
_____

Data Collected
(use those that apply)

- States that she wants to see her friends as soon as possible and go to the movies
- Current weight 110 lb
- Height 5 ft, 4 in.
- Vital signs: T 99.0, P 59, R 12, BP 120/80
- WBC count 5,000 mm^3
- "The doctor said I could go about my normal life."
- Family history of breast cancer
- Mother reports that Mandy's best friend has the flu

Nursing Interventions
(use those that apply; list in priority order)

- Monitor white blood cell count.
- Encourage frequent mouth care regimen.
- Teach client to monitor for symptoms of infection such as fever, redness, cold symptoms, etc.
- Teach good hand washing habits.
- Assess client's spiritual beliefs.
- Screen visitors for those who may be ill.
- Facilitate communication between client and his or her family.
- Avoid large crowds.
- Encourage well-balanced diet high in protein.

Compare your documentation to the sample provided in Appendix I.

NCLEX-PN® Exam Preparation

TEST-TAKING TIP The words *more instruction is needed* (as in question 2) indicate that the answer that will properly complete the sentence is NOT a true statement.

1 The nurse is caring for a pediatric client with sickle cell anemia. The parents ask the nurse about the causes of the disease. Which response by the nurse best describes the cause of this disease?

   1. "It is caused by a recessive trait that primarily affects African Americans."
   2. "It is caused by a demand for iron in the bloodstream."
   3. "It is an inherited disorder caused by abnormal hemoglobin synthesis."
   4. "It is a rare, malignant disorder of the lymphatic system."

2 The nurse is instructing the father of a child with sickle cell anemia about sickle cell crisis and causes. The father verbalizes understanding, but the nurse realizes more instruction is needed when he identifies which of the following as a major contributor in a sickle cell crisis?

   1. iron deficiency
   2. fever
   3. stress
   4. vomiting

3 The nursing instructor is conducting a lecture about hematologic disorders in children and leads the discussion about the causes of thalassemia. The nurse tells the students that children who are at greatest risk for this blood disorder are those who are:

   1. of German American heritage.
   2. of Australian descent.
   3. of Swedish descent.
   4. of Mediterranean descent.

4 The nurse knows that which of the following blood values indicate sickle cell disease?

   1. high Hgb and low reticulocyte count
   2. low Hgb and low reticulocyte count
   3. high Hgb and high reticulocyte count
   4. low Hgb and high reticulocyte count

5 A nurse is reading the health record of her client with Hodgkin's disease. Which of the following symptoms would the nurse expect to see in the record considering the diagnosis?

   1. tender, soft lymph nodes in the femoral area
   2. nontender, soft tumors in the abdominal area
   3. nontender, hard lymph nodes in the cervical area
   4. tender, soft tumors in the popliteal area

6 The nurse has just completed teaching the parents of a child who has just been started on chemotherapy. The mother has been instructed about infection control during therapy. The nurse realizes the mother understands the teaching when she says:

   1. "I will make sure to keep my child away from public places to prevent infection."
   2. "It is all right for my child to go skiing as long as I give him vitamin C to prevent infection."
   3. "The chemotherapy won't affect my son as long as he eats well."
   4. "My son doesn't have to have blood tests until the chemotherapy has ended."

7 The nursing instructor asks a nursing student in the class to describe acute lymphoblastic leukemia (ALL). The instructor realizes the nursing student does not need further instruction in the disease when the student states:

   1. "ALL occurs when cancer cells develop in the bone marrow."
   2. "ALL is the overproduction of immature lymphocytes."
   3. "ALL is a rare hereditary sex-linked disorder."
   4. "ALL is a malignant disorder of the lymphatic system."

8 The nurse is reviewing the physician's orders for a child with hemophilia. Indicate the orders that the nurse might expect to see written in the child's chart. Choose all that apply.

   1. Avoid rectal temperatures.
   2. Avoid unnecessary invasive procedures.
   3. Avoid salicylates.
   4. Avoid carbonated beverages.
   5. Avoid rectal suppositories.

9 A 5-year-old child is hospitalized with a suspected diagnosis of idiopathic thrombocytopenic purpura. The laboratory technician has just drawn the child's blood. Because of the suspected diagnosis, the nurse expects to see the following results on the child's lab report:

   1. increased platelet count, positive Coombs' test
   2. decreased platelet count, increased antiplatelet antibodies
   3. positive direct Coombs' test, absence of antinuclear antibodies
   4. decreased platelet count and antiplatelet antibodies

10 The nurse is discussing iron-deficiency anemia and knows the child with this disorder may crave substances that are not food, a condition called pica. Select the following substances that children with this disorder may crave and eat:

   1. dirt
   2. hair
   3. glass
   4. starch
   5. anchovies
   6. chalk
   7. glue

Answers for Review Questions, as well as discussion of Care Plan and Critical Thinking Care Map questions, appear in Appendix I.

Chapter 21

Care of the Child with Immune Disorders

BRIEF Outline

Anatomy and Physiology
Brief Assessment Overview
Congenital Immune Disorders
HIV and AIDS
Juvenile Rheumatoid Arthritis
Systemic Lupus Erythematosus

Organ Transplantation
Allergies
Immunotherapy
Nursing Care

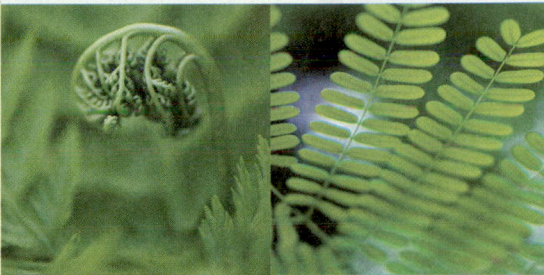

HEALTH PROMOTION ISSUE:
Disclosing HIV Status: A Difficult
Task for Teens

NURSING PROCESS CARE PLAN:
Child with an Organ Transplant

CRITICAL THINKING CARE MAP:
Caring for a Client with AIDS

LEARNING Outcomes

After completing this chapter, you will be able to:

- Discuss the anatomy and physiology of the pediatric immunologic system.
- Describe immunologic disorders to include HIV, AIDS, juvenile rheumatoid arthritis, and allergies.
- Discuss clinical manifestations, diagnostic procedures, medical management, and nursing interventions related to immunologic disorders.
- Describe the care of children requiring organ transplants.

The immune system provides the child vital protection against many illnesses and diseases. A functioning immune system allows the child to coexist with other children and adults and to avoid or minimize illness or disease. However, when the immune system does not function properly, diseases and conditions such as allergies, juvenile arthritis, or possibly AIDS could affect the child. This chapter reviews the anatomy and physiology of the immune system and discusses a variety of disorders related to the immune system.

Anatomy and Physiology

The primary role of the immune system is to recognize and eliminate foreign substances. The foreign substances are called **antigens.** When the immune system recognizes these antigens, **antibodies** or proteins are produced. The antibodies will now be available to attack the antigen should it invade the body in the future. This process is called the **immune response.**

NATURAL IMMUNITY AND ACQUIRED IMMUNITY

There are two types of immunity: natural and acquired. **Natural immunity** is present at birth and lasts about 3 to 6 months. It includes:

- Intact skin, which prevents foreign substances from entering the body
- Body pH, which maintains an environment that is hostile to antigens
- Antibodies against certain antigens, which were passed to the child during pregnancy and breastfeeding
- Body processes of inflammation and phagocytosis, which fight antigens.

Acquired immunity is developed over a period of time after birth by exposure to foreign substances. Acquired immunity is developed through humoral immunity and cell-mediated immunity.

Humoral Immunity

Humoral immunity destroys bacteria, viruses, parasites, allergens, and other foreign substances by producing antibodies called **immunoglobulins.** The types of immunoglobulins and their basic functions are described in Table 21-1 ■. The production of immunoglobulins begins in early infancy but is not complete until age 6 or 7. The body's first response to antigens is called the **primary immune response.** Figure 21-1 ■ illustrates the events in the body's primary immune response. This first response produces antibodies within 3 days. It is important to note that the individual does not show symptoms when this first exposure and response occur. However, the primary

TABLE 21-1	
Types of Immunoglobulin (Ig) and Functions	
IMMUNOGLOBULIN	**ACTION**
IgM	First antibody produced with primary immune response
	Mediates *cytotoxic* (cell-killing) response
	Activates *complement* (serum protein complex that is activated by the antigen-antibody complex in an immune reaction)
IgG	Only immunoglobulin to cross placenta
	Active against bacteria, bacterial toxins, and viruses
	Activates complements
IgA	Prevents binding of viruses to cells of respiratory and GI tracts
IgD	Function not fully understood
IgE	Primarily responsible for allergic reactions

Source: Adapted from Ball, J., & Bindler, R. (2006). *Child health nursing: Partnering with children & families.* Upper Saddle River, NJ: Prentice Hall, Table 27-2, p. 959.

response prepares the body to respond quickly to second or repeated exposure.

The **secondary immune response** occurs when the child is exposed to the antigen in the future. Within 24 hours, the previously produced antibodies provide protection for the child.

Cell-Mediated Immunity

Cell-mediated immunity provides the child with protection against bacteria, viruses, fungi, and tumors. This process develops early in the child's life. Cell-mediated immunity is also the process that causes rejection of organs that have been transplanted. The thymus produces lymphocytes, which directly attack the foreign substances. Figure 21-2 ■ (lower left) illustrates the actions of the thymus. T lymphocytes, B lymphocytes, and natural kill (NK) cells play an important role in cell-mediated immunity.

Immunizations provide **active immunity.** In active immunity, an antigen is given, and antibodies are produced (see Figure 21-1) to provide immunity if the body is exposed in the future. Active immunity is the mechanism by which immunizations provide protection against childhood diseases that used to claim thousands of infants' lives. **Passive immunity** is provided by administering immunoglobulins to protect children against diseases to which they may have been exposed already. For example, a child with Kawasaki syndrome (see Chapter 19 ⬭) is given large doses of

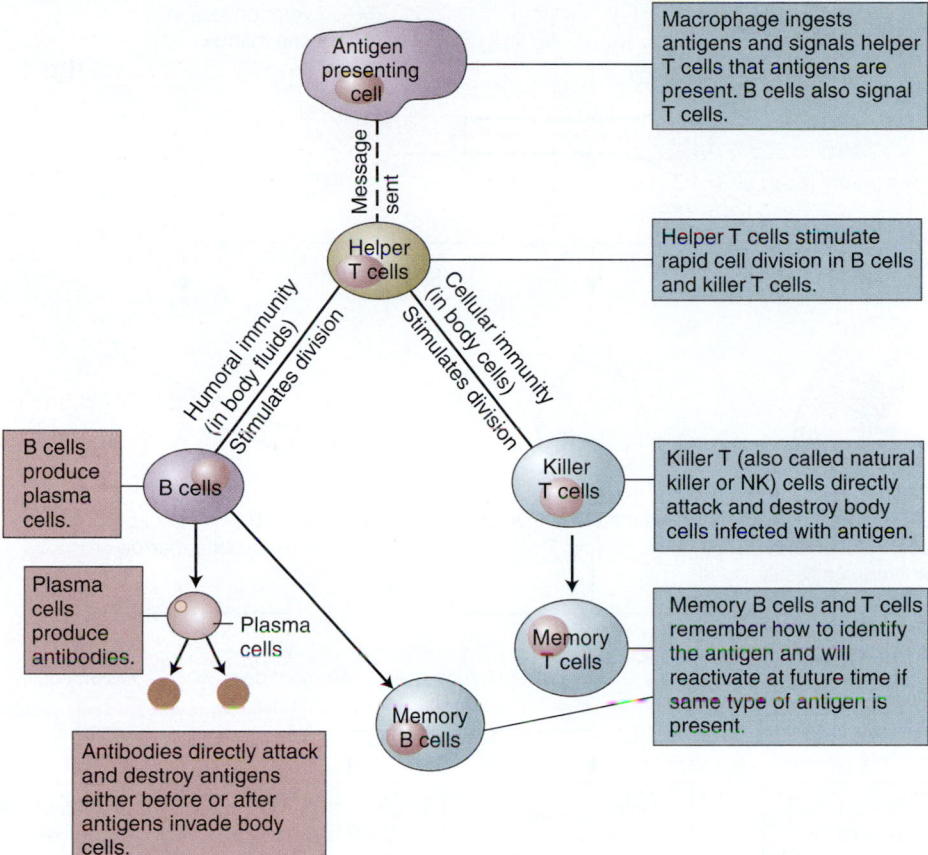

Figure 21-1. ■ Primary immune response.

immunoglobulins for a period of time to counter the effects of the disease. For more information about immunizations, see Chapter 26 ⬭ and the childhood immunization schedule in Appendix II ⬭.

Brief Assessment Overview

HISTORY

- Inquire about recent illnesses and infections. Ask especially about unexplained fevers.
- Does the child suffer from allergy symptoms?
- Inquire about stiffness or pain in the joints.
- Inquire about the child's appetite.
- Review immunization record.

PHYSICAL

- Obtain height and weight.
- Obtain vital signs.
- Inspect the oral cavity. (With immunosuppression, there may be thrush.)
- Inspect the skin for lesions.
- Assess range of motion (ROM) in joints.
- Palpate the lymph nodes (see Figures 20-2 and 20-3 ⬭).

Congenital Immune Disorders

SEVERE COMBINED IMMUNODEFICIENCY DISEASE

In severe combined immunodeficiency disorder (SCID), both humoral and cellular immunity is absent. There is a lack of functioning T and B cells. In infants with SCID, genetic mutations lead to impaired lymphoid development. B lymphocytes may appear in normal numbers but do not function effectively. NK cells are few. Infants often become symptomatic (highly susceptible to infection) by 3 months of age because maternal antibodies are lost. Resistant oral candidiasis may be the first infection noted. Treatment involves IV immunoglobulin, hematopoietic stem cell transplant with a histocompatible donor, and prophylactic antibiotics. Enzyme replacement therapy is helpful in certain cases.

clinical ALERT

Children with T-cell deficiencies may experience graft-versus-host reaction with normal blood transfusions. They must be given irradiated blood products that are negative for cytomegalovirus in order to avoid this risk.

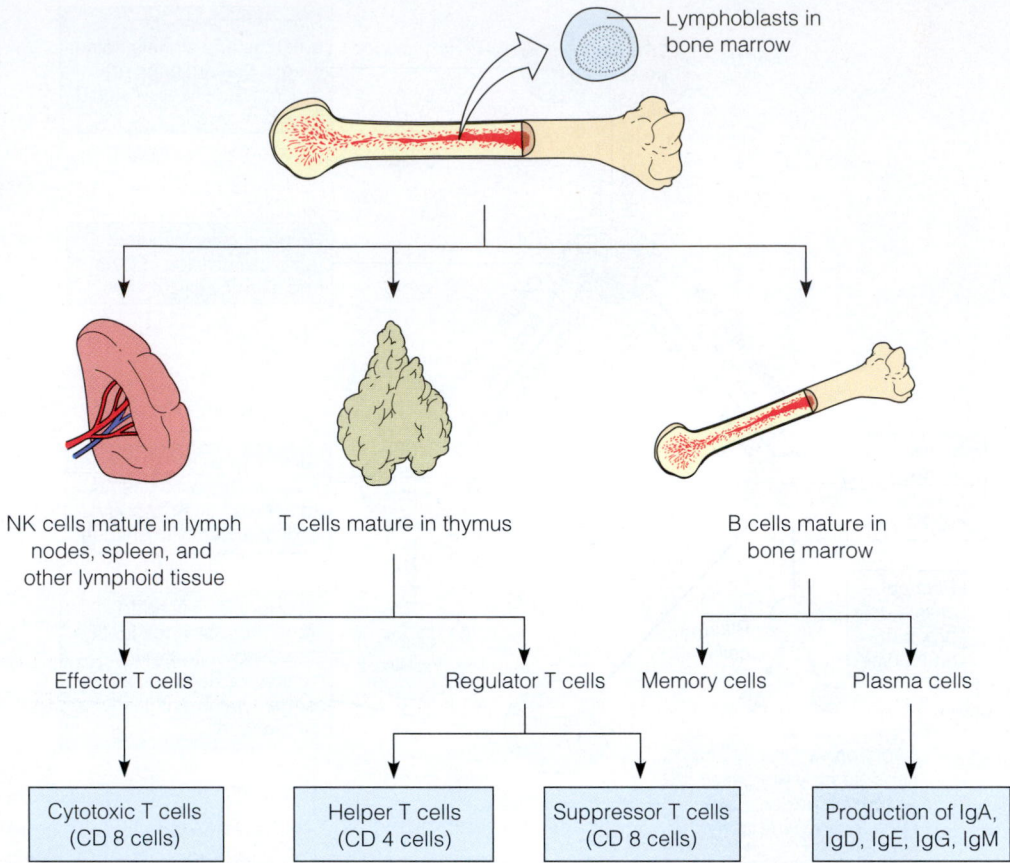

Figure 21-2. ■ The development and differentiation of lymphocytes shows how cell-mediated immunity works.

COMMON VARIABLE IMMUNODEFICIENCY

In common variable immunodeficiency (also called *acquired hypogammaglobulinemia*), there is a low level of circulating immunoglobulins of all classes. This disorder appears equally in male and female adolescents and young adults. Clients present with susceptibility to infection. Treatment is by regular administration of immunoglobulins and antibiotics to protect against infection.

HIV and AIDS

HIV is a retrovirus that causes the end-stage condition AIDS. AIDS is characterized by a defect in cell-mediated immunity that makes it difficult or sometimes impossible for the affected child to fight infection. In 2004, approximately 9,443 children under the age of 13 in the United States were living with AIDS.

HIV is transmitted to children primarily through perinatal transmission (see Chapter 8 ⬭). During pregnancy, the virus can cross the placenta and infect the fetus (see Chapter 7 ⬭). During birth, the newborn can be infected by exposure to maternal blood, amniotic fluid, or genital tract secretions. In the postpartum period, the newborn can contract the disease by exposure to breast milk of the HIV-positive mother. Adolescents typically contract HIV through unprotected sexual activity and IV drug use. See the Health Promotion Issue on pages 644 and 645.

Because of the risk of perinatal transmission, the Centers for Disease Control and Prevention (CDC) has recommended HIV screening as a routine part of prenatal care. Women who refuse to be tested should be questioned about the reasons for refusal, and counseling should be provided. The screening test should be offered again later in the pregnancy. The woman may be reluctant to find out the diagnosis. However, the nurse should teach the client that risk for perinatal transmission is significantly reduced if the mother receives zidovudine (AZT) therapy during pregnancy and if the infant is delivered by cesarean section.

Infection with the virus during the perinatal period shortens the time frame between seroconversion to the condition of AIDS. The time frame between exposure, seroconversion, and disease development can be within 2 years of birth.

Manifestations

Clinical manifestations include chronic otitis media, fever, skin irritation, failure to thrive, lack of weight gain, chronic diarrhea, hepatosplenomegaly, lymphadenopathy, and oral

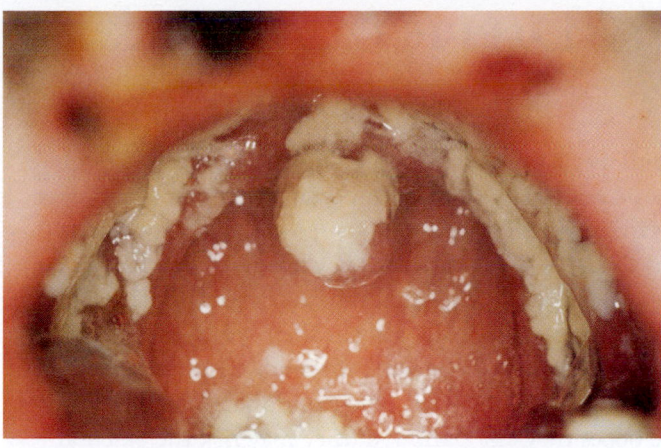

Figure 21-3. ■ Oral thrush is a common finding in clients with HIV. (Biophoto Associates/Photo Researchers, Inc.)

candidiasis. Although rare, Kaposi's sarcoma can develop. It is manifested as purple papules that begin on the feet and spread across the skin.

Oral candidiasis, or **thrush,** is a chronic condition caused most commonly by the fungus *Candida albicans.* Thrush is seen as white patches on the oral and pharyngeal mucosa (Figure 21-3 ■) that may easily bleed. The fungal infection can also be found in the diaper region, under the arms, or on the neck. (Fluconazole or itraconazole is the treatment of choice for oral candidiasis. These medications are applied directly to the affected tissue.) Candidiasis is also discussed further in Chapter 24. ◑◔

Diagnosis

The presence of HIV is determined with the polymerase chain reaction test or the enzyme-linked immunoabsorbent assay (ELISA). This blood test (ELISA) may initially be negative, especially in the newborn. Testing is repeated as necessary, and HIV is confirmed following two positive tests. A newer test, called the OraQuick Advance HIV1/2 Antibody Test, uses oral fluids obtained by swabbing the upper and lower gums. Results are available in 20 minutes, and positive results have been found to be 99% accurate.

Treatment

During pregnancy, HIV-positive mothers are treated with the antiretroviral agent AZT to prevent transmission to the fetus. Most obstetricians will perform a cesarean section to further reduce the fetus's risk of exposure to the virus. After birth, the newborn is also treated with AZT to reduce the risk of transmission. Newborns can be treated prophylactically with antibiotics and immune globulin to prevent bacterial infections. In children in whom HIV is confirmed, antiretroviral therapy is used, usually combining several drugs (Table 21-2 ■).

Nursing Considerations

The nursing care of children with HIV/AIDS primarily involves reducing infection and transmission and promoting adequate growth and development. To reduce infection, the nurse must use proper sterile technique when performing invasive procedures, as is appropriate for all clients. Invasive procedures should be avoided if possible.

(Text continues on p. 646.)

TABLE 21-2

Pharmacology: Antiretroviral Agents Used to Treat HIV

DRUG (COMMON BRAND NAME AND GENERIC)	USUAL ROUTE/DOSE	CLASSIFICATION AND PURPOSE	SELECTED SIDE EFFECTS	DON'T GIVE IF
Retrovir (zidovudine)	100–180 mg/m^2 every 6 hours PO for children 3 months–13 years	Nucleoside reverse transcriptase inhibitors used to suppress viral load	Fever, malaise, myalgia, headache, nausea, vomiting, anorexia, cough, rash	Client is anemic or has a granulocyte count above 750/mm^3
Norvir (ritonavir)	400–600 mg/m^2 PO bid for children 2–16 years	Protease inhibitors used in combination with other antiretroviral agents to suppress viral load	Weakness, nausea, diarrhea, vomiting	Client has suppressed liver function
Rescriptor (delavirdine mesylate)	400 mg PO tid for children greater than 16 years	Nonnucleoside reverse transcriptase inhibitors used in combination with other antiretroviral agents to suppress viral load	Rash, headache, dizziness, chest pain	At the same time as an antacid In the presence of fever, blistering rash, oral lesions, conjunctivitis, muscle or joint pain

MediaLink

HIV/AIDS

DISCLOSING HIV STATUS: A DIFFICULT TASK FOR TEENS

Marilyn, age 16, came to the family practice office because she was constantly feeling tired and had been losing weight over the past few months. The nurse took a careful health history that included a past sexual history. Marilyn had a prescription for birth control pills and stated that she was faithful in taking her pills daily. She further stated that she was sexually active, with three to four encounters monthly. She knew each of the guys with whom she had sex, but they rarely used a condom.

Marilyn's mother accompanied her this morning and is aware of her sexual activity. After discussing the health history with the nurse practitioner, the nurse drew an ELISA screen to test for HIV, and the nurse practitioner performed a pelvic exam and Pap smear. A follow-up appointment is scheduled for Marilyn. The nurse teaches Marilyn the importance of avoiding sexual contact until the lab results can be interpreted.

At the follow-up visit, the nurse practitioner tells Marilyn that the ELISA test is positive and that her Pap smear was negative. The nurse tells Marilyn that another ELISA test is necessary and gains consent to draw the specimen. The nurse explains that two separate specimens must be drawn to confirm a diagnosis of HIV infection.

When the second ELISA results are obtained, Marilyn is told that she is infected with HIV. She immediately states that there is no way that she could have the virus. She states that she used her birth control pills faithfully and knew all of her partners well enough to know that they are not HIV positive.

The nurse patiently listens to Marilyn, while her mother cries. The nurse understands that Marilyn and her mother are not ready to receive information about her diagnosis. She makes an appointment with them in 2 days. She does discuss with Marilyn the importance of abstaining from sexual contact until they have had a chance to discuss the issue further.

At the return visit, Marilyn states that she does not want anybody to know about her diagnosis other than her mother. When the nurse explains the necessity of disclosing her diagnosis to her past partners, Marilyn becomes angry and states that she hopes they all have the virus and become gravely ill.

Marilyn had been told by a friend that there was medicine that prevented you from passing the virus on to others. This was the medicine Marilyn wanted to take. Marilyn stated she did not plan to curtail her sexual activity and knew that her partners would not agree to wear a condom. In fact, if she asked them to, they would know that something was wrong. She did not plan to tell anybody that she was HIV positive.

The nurse and nurse practitioner work on a plan to inform Marilyn and her mother about the disease, its treatment, and the lifestyle changes that are necessary.

DISCUSSION

Adolescents are physically developing into adulthood. The hormones of adolescence increase the sex drive and cause teens to be preoccupied with the opposite gender. Physically, they are capable of having sexual intercourse but emotionally and cognitively they often demonstrate risky behaviors related to sexuality.

Acceptance among peers is of utmost importance to teens. They want to be accepted and not stand out as different. They fear rejection. Fear of rejection can cause teens to make decisions about their behavior that may not be wise. If friends want them to go somewhere or do something that is not allowed, they may risk the parental consequences instead of risking their peers' rejection.

Because their cognitive development allows them to think abstractly, teens begin to feel that they are invincible, possibly immortal. They can easily believe that they are wise and do not need the advice and direction offered by authority figures. This is a hazard of adolescence, that teens seek independence but are not yet mature enough to know the ramifications of their decisions.

Teens who have been diagnosed with HIV fear rejection if they disclose their diagnosis. They do not want to be labeled as sick or unclean. They fear that people will shun them.

Some teens may initially deny their diagnosis, hoping that it will go away. Some can even create a magical thinking scenario where they never deal with the disease process. However, teens who try to pretend to others are rarely able to pretend to themselves. Often, feelings of despair, anxiety, and depression overwhelm teens who attempt to ignore their diagnosis.

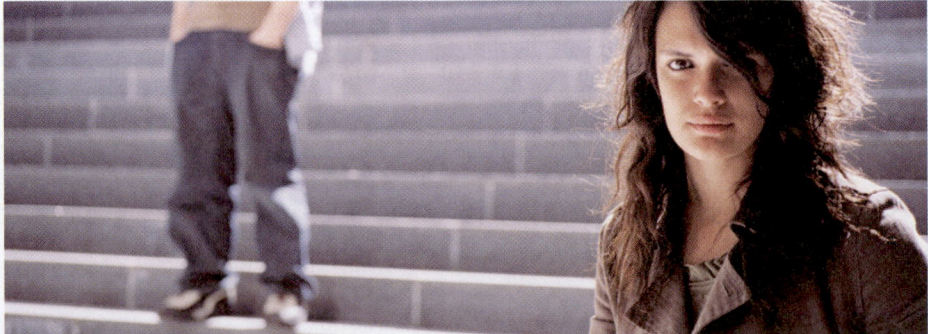

(Spohn Matthieu\Getty Images Royalty Free /PhotoAlto)

Teens who are struggling with the diagnosis and the decision to disclose need support from a caring health care professional who can guide them into correct thinking and decision making. The nurse can play an important role in listening to the teen's concerns and giving appropriate information. The nurse can also help the teen prepare him- or herself to disclose the diagnosis (when ready) by assisting with the right words to use and by helping decide on the right timing for disclosure.

The nurse can discuss the benefits of nondisclosure with the teen. By disclosing the diagnosis to only a few trusted individuals, the teen can ensure that the condition will not be discussed by those the teen does not want to tell. Nondisclosure prevents acquaintances from making judgments.

Nondisclosure also has risks. Teens who do not admit to their diagnosis are less likely to follow the medical regime. Lack of proper medical treatment can further complicate the condition. Teens who choose to keep their diagnosis from friends and family lose the advantage of social support.

Besides this risk to the infected teen, nondisclosure also allows further spread of the virus. Past partners have the right to know about their exposure and the necessity of seeking testing for themselves. Future partners have the right to be informed about their probable exposure, if they have sex without adequate protection.

Many websites and AIDS hotlines can provide teens a safe place to disclose their diagnosis. These sites allow teens to practice how they will tell others about their condition and to receive feedback from teens who have struggled with the same decisions.

PLANNING AND IMPLEMENTATION

The nurse develops an extensive teaching plan for Marilyn that includes classroom learning, written materials, videos, peer counseling, and regular follow-up visits to the family practice clinic. The following content outline was developed:

- General knowledge about HIV/AIDS
- Transmission of HIV/AIDS
- Medical treatment of the disease
- The importance of social support
- How to discuss her condition with others.

Marilyn needs to understand that there is no current cure for HIV/AIDS but that early intervention and continued treatment can increase the quality of life. Transmission of the virus can occur through contact with body fluids. This can occur during oral-penile contact, oral-vaginal contact, vaginal-penile contact, penile-rectal contact, substance abuse with needles and syringes, contact with blood such as sharing razors or toothbrushes, handling used feminine hygiene products, and so on. Marilyn should be encouraged to use condoms with each sexual encounter. She should understand that this will be necessary for the remainder of her life.

Marilyn needs to understand her prescribed medical regime. She needs to know about each drug, its side effects, and specific information about taking these drugs correctly. She needs to understand when to report symptoms of complications. She should have phone numbers to reach the health care provider any time of the day or night.

Marilyn will need emotional support to help her avoid feelings of rejection and isolation. The nurse can help Marilyn identify those people in her life who can lend her positive support and those who might give negative feedback. The nurse can assist Marilyn with role-playing. The nurse can allow Marilyn to practice telling people about her diagnosis. The nurse may refer Marilyn to support groups with teens her age who can assist Marilyn in developing ways to tell her trusted friends and family.

As Marilyn becomes confident in managing her disease, she may want to help others who are HIV positive. The nurse should assess for this readiness and encourage Marilyn to use the things she learns to help others. The nurse can refer Marilyn to agencies that provide services to teens with a diagnosis of HIV.

SELF-REFLECTION

What medical secret have you kept for yourself or possibly for a family member or friend? Why was it important to keep that secret? What were the benefits of keeping this secret? What were the risks of keeping this secret?

SUGGESTED RESOURCES

For the Nurse

- www.aids-alliance.org The AIDS Alliance for Children, Youth and Families creates and shares information about programs that work for women, youth, children, and families affected by HIV/AIDS. They provide a forum for consumers and health care providers to advocate for public policies related to HIV/AIDS.

- www.thebodypro.com An online source for health care professionals caring for clients with HIV/AIDS.

For the Client

- www.advocatesforyouth.org This website provides information about adolescent sex and issues related to HIV/AIDS. Public policy and political issues are also summarized, and teens are encouraged to speak out related to these issues.

- www.thebody.com An online resource for individuals living with HIV/AIDS.

BOX 21-1   **CLIENT TEACHING**

Care of the HIV Child at Home

- Remind parents and caregivers that HIV virus cannot be spread by sneezing, coughing, hugging, or touching the child.
- Exposure to body fluids and blood creates the greatest risk of exposure. Situations in which this may occur includes trauma, accidents, or fights with another child where the skin integrity is compromised.
- Gloves should be used when diapering a child, cleaning wounds, and wiping up urine, feces, or vomit.
- Use disposable towels for wiping spills. Use disposable diaper wipes.

- To clean a surface exposed to body fluids, mix 1 tablespoon liquid chlorine bleach in 1 quart of water.
- Dispose of diapers, diaper wipes, gloves, and towels exposed to body fluids in a leak-proof container such as a plastic bag.
- Encourage parents and caregivers to wash their hands with soap and water for at least 10 seconds after removing gloves.
- Linens exposed to body fluids can be washed separately, adding 1/2 cup liquid chlorine bleach to the washing detergent.
- Encourage parents and caregivers to prevent the sharing of eating utensils. Children should be prevented from putting toys in their mouth and sharing them. Toys and eating utensils can be washed normally in the dishwasher or with hot soap and water.

Mothers who are HIV positive must avoid breastfeeding. The family should be taught proper hand washing techniques to prevent the spread of infection. The family must also understand the importance of avoiding other children and individuals with infections of all types because the child with HIV is more susceptible to any infection (Box 21-1 ■). Diseases such as tuberculosis can be devastating. The importance of immunizations should be emphasized to the family. See Appendix II ⚭ for the immunization schedule.

Promoting adequate respiration and nutrition will also be important in assisting the child with HIV/AIDS to avoid infection. The nurse can encourage the child to perform deep breathing exercises. The diet of these children should be assessed carefully for adequate nutritional content, including calories, protein, vitamins, and antioxidants. See Chapter 22 ⚭ for a nutritional assessment. Referral to a registered dietician may be necessary.

Due to the medical regime and frequent hospitalizations, children with HIV/AIDS are at risk for developmental delays. The nurse should assess physical and mental functioning, as well as provide assistance to parents regarding activities to promote growth and development.

Juvenile Rheumatoid Arthritis

Juvenile rheumatoid arthritis (JRA) is a chronic disorder causing joint inflammation. It is **autoimmune** in nature, meaning that in this disorder, the body attacks itself, perceiving its own cells as foreign substances. In JRA, tissues surrounding joints may also be affected. Periods of remission are common in children. In fact, 70% of children will have permanent remission by the time they become adults.

Manifestations

Symptoms include both systemic and musculoskeletal changes. The child presents with fever, rash, **lymph-** **adenopathy** (enlarged lymph nodes), **splenomegaly** (enlarged spleen), and **hepatomegaly** (enlarged liver), indicating a systemic inflammatory process. The child may have a limp or favor one extremity over the other. Pain, stiffness, swelling, and loss of movement may be seen in one or more large joints such as the knees.

Diagnosis

JRA is usually diagnosed by presentation of clinical symptoms. Laboratory findings include positive rheumatoid factor, human leukocyte antigen B27, and antinuclear antibody.

Treatment

The medical management of JRA includes medication and physical therapy. The priorities of care are to relieve pain and prevent joint contractures. On occasion, surgery is performed to reduce pain and improve joint function. Salicylates (aspirin) or nonsteroidal anti-inflammatory drugs (NSAIDs) are used to reduce inflammation. These drugs can cause gastrointestinal (GI) upset, and the child should be monitored closely for this and other side effects.

Physical therapy is essential in the treatment plan. ROM exercises, hydrotherapy, and muscle strengthening exercise help prevent contractures (Figure 21-4 ■). Warm compresses are used to relieve discomfort and swelling. The child should be provided with adequate nutrition to promote healing (Box 21-2 ■).

Nursing Considerations

The care of the child with JRA usually occurs in the community. The family must be taught the importance of medication management, side effects, and need for physical therapy. The child should remain in school and have contact with peers as much as possible. Activities should be planned to enable the child to develop a positive self-image.

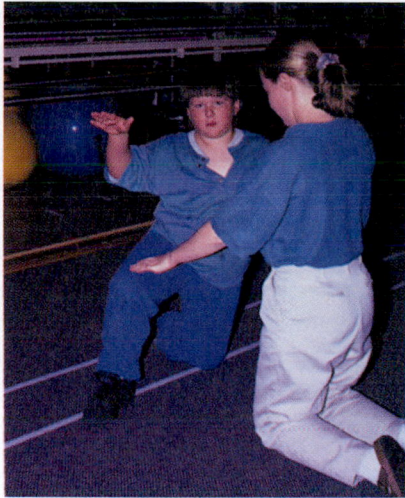

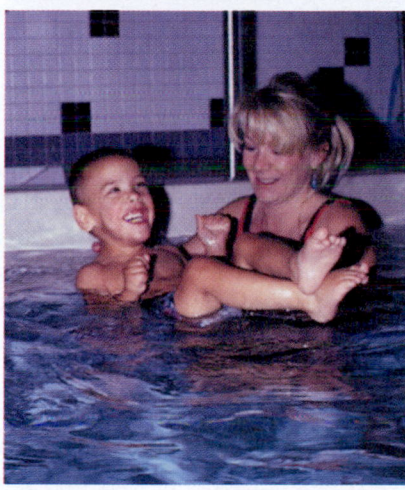

Figure 21-4. ■ (A) Stretching exercises are an important part of physical therapy for a child who has juvenile rheumatoid arthritis. (B) Swimming is very helpful for maintaining joint function in children with JRA.

BOX 21-2	NUTRITION THERAPY

Foods for Children with Juvenile Rheumatoid Arthritis

Inflammation caused by juvenile rheumatoid arthritis can be quite painful for children. Certain foods may have natural anti-inflammatory properties and promote joint health in those with this disorder. Pineapple contains the enzyme bromelain, which is associated with reducing inflammation. Flavonoids such as blueberries, tomatoes, broccoli, and apples decrease inflammation and strengthen connective tissues. Salmon, trout, and tuna contain omega-3 fatty acids, which relieve stiffness and pain in the joints. Ginger contains shogoals and gingerols, which are antioxidants and anti-inflammatories. Ginger can be added to foods and found in beverages in many health food stores.

Certain foods can also increase inflammation in the joints. Children with rheumatoid arthritis should limit or avoid dairy products, eggs, hydrogenated oils, refined sugars, white flour, soy, corn and wheat products, caffeine, potatoes, green pepper, and eggplant.

Referral should be made for home care. The American Juvenile Rheumatoid Arthritis Association can be a valuable resource for families.

The child should be routinely evaluated for decreased pain and swelling in joints, increased mobility, and side effects of medication. With adequate treatment, the prognosis is favorable for complete recovery.

Systemic Lupus Erythematosus

Systemic lupus erythematosus (SLE) is an autoimmune disease of the connective tissue and blood vessels that causes inflammation in any organ of the body. According to the Arthritis Foundation, 25,000 children and adolescents in the United States have SLE. It occurs more frequently than leukemia, cystic fibrosis, or muscular dystrophy. There is a higher incidence of SLE in African American, Asian, and Hispanic children in the United States.

Manifestations

The child with SLE may have an erythematous butterfly rash across the nose, cheeks, and cheekbones (called a *malar rash*). Figure 21-5 ■ shows this characteristic rash. Many SLE clients are photosensitive. Exposure to sun causes a diffuse maculopapular rash (see Figure 24-3. ⬭ for skin lesions). The disease is characterized in most children by swollen and painful joints. They may experience alopecia, *Raynaud's phenomenon* (pallor, numbness, and pain in the extremities, usually caused by exposure to cold), mouth ulcers,

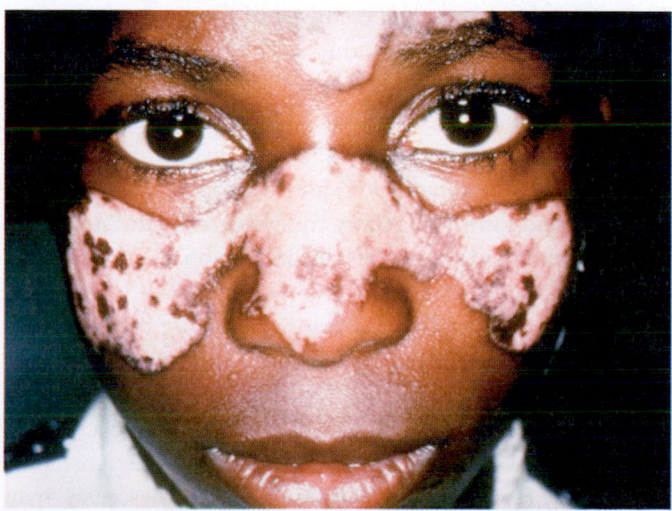

Figure 21-5. ■ Butterfly rash of systemic lupus erythematosus.

anemia, headache, memory loss, weight loss, fatigue, and low-grade fever. If the kidneys become inflamed, the child may develop nephritis. When the brain is inflamed, seizures and mood changes can occur. An inflamed heart may manifest as pericarditis or myocardial infarction. Inflammation of the lungs results in pleuritis. The disease is characterized by periods of exacerbation (brought on by sun exposure, stress, or infection) and remission.

Diagnosis

Diagnosis of SLE is made by observing for the physical findings and the presence of positive antinuclear antibodies (ANA), anti–double-stranded DNA antibodies (anti-DNA), and antiphospholipid antibodies. The complete blood count (CBC) will show decreased red blood cells (RBCs), platelets, and white blood cells (WBCs). The urinalysis may show the presence of blood, protein, and cast cells. A kidney biopsy may be necessary. To determine the extent of involvement of other organs, x-rays, electrocardiogram (ECG), echogram, electroencephalogram (EEG), magnetic resonance imaging (MRI) scans, or computed tomography (CT) scans may be necessary.

Treatment

Medications used to treat SLE include NSAIDs such as Naprosyn, Advil, or Tolectin, which help control the discomfort associated with inflammation. Antimalarials such as Plaquenil (hydroxychloroquine) are prescribed to help control the skin rash of SLE. The most commonly used medications for SLE are corticosteroids. Immunosuppressants such as Imuran and Cytoxan may also be prescribed. Long-term prognosis depends on how severely internal organs are involved. The 5-year survival rate for children is 78% to 92% (Stichweh et al., 2004).

Nursing Considerations

The nurse should teach the child and family to take corticosteroids properly. Be sure the child understands the possible side effects, including hunger leading to weight gain, mood changes, worsening acne, jitteriness, and insomnia. Corticosteroids may also cause hypertension, immunosuppression, growth retardation, and hyperglycemia. Caution the child and family to report these side effects. Emphasize that stopping corticosteroid administration abruptly can be dangerous.

Infection prevention is a priority nursing intervention. Children with SLE should understand the signs and symptoms of infections and be instructed to report them promptly to their health care provider. These children should also be diligent about keeping immunizations up to date. Children with SLE, particularly adolescents, may struggle with disturbed body image. This is primarily due to symptoms such as rash and alopecia. The nurse can help the child explore his or her feelings and develop ways to manage them.

The child must be taught the importance of protecting the skin from sun exposure. The nurse can help the child understand the importance of using sunscreen daily; wearing appropriate clothing, including a hat; and decreasing time spent outdoors. The nurse must help the child with SLE and family to assess the child's diet in order to help combat growth retardation or the side effects of steroid use (including weight gain). The child's diet should include fruits and vegetables and be low in salt and sugar.

Organ Transplantation

Transplanting organs and tissues dates back to the fourth century BC when a Chinese surgeon is said to have successfully switched the hearts of two clients. The first blood transfusion in 1667 is said to have occurred when a physician transfused the blood of a lamb into a 15-year-old boy with a malignant fever. The first human-to-human blood transfusion occurred in 1818, when a husband donated blood for his wife who was dying of blood loss following childbirth. The first bone transplant took place in 1668, when Russian scientists replaced a man's skull with that of a dog. Today, surgeons are able to transplant most major organs and tissues with human organs and tissue, animal organs and tissue, and manufactured organs. However, it is important to recognize that some religious groups oppose organ donation (Box 21-3 ■), so parents may refuse consideration of such surgery for their children.

ORGAN DONATION

Donors for organs and tissues can come from both living and deceased individuals or animals. Blood, skin, marrow, and kidneys can be donated from a living human or (in the case of skin) from the needy recipient. An **autogenous graft** is a skin graft in which skin is transplanted from one site to another site in the same recipient. A **xenograft** is an organ or tissue obtained from an animal for transplantation into a human. Major organs necessary for life, such as the heart, lung, liver, kidneys, corneas, bone, and pancreas, are harvested from individuals who are classified as brain dead and incapable of sustaining life on their own or from recently deceased individuals. Declaration of brain death in the client is confirmed by clinical signs and medical testing. Clinical signs of brain death include diagnosis of an irreversible condition, apnea with an arterial $PaCO_2$ of at least 60 mm Hg, lack of response to deep stimuli, no spontaneous movement, lack of gag or corneal reflex, lack of oculocephalic reflex or doll's eye maneuver, and absence of toxic or metabolic disorders. Medical testing used to confirm brain death includes

BOX 21-3   CULTURAL PULSE POINTS

Religious Beliefs Related to Organ Donation

- The **Amish** will consent to organ transplant but believe that it is God who ultimately heals.
- **Baptists** have adopted resolutions to encourage physicians to use organ transplantation to save lives and to encourage the public to donate their organs and tissues.
- **Buddhists** call organ transplantation a matter of individual conscience and an act of compassion.
- **Christian Scientists** rely on spiritual rather than medical healing. They do not have any specific statements regarding organ transplantation and consider this issue a matter of personal choice.
- **Episcopalians** promote organ and tissue transplantation and donation. The church relates this act of kindness to the life of Jesus Christ, who gave his life so that others may live.
- **Hindus** believe that organ transplantation is an individual decision and that it is ethical to use body parts to alleviate the suffering of other humans.
- **Jehovah's Witnesses** allow organ transplantation as long as all blood is drained from the organ or tissues prior to transplantation and any blood transfused is autologous blood, taken from the organ recipient prior to surgery.

- **Judaism** encourages organ transplantation. In 1992, the Rabbinical Council of America (Orthodox) stated that the *pikuach nefest,* an ancient requirement to save lives if possible, promotes organ donation despite Jewish laws that forbid mutilation of the body.
- **Lutheran** doctrine states that organ donation is a humanitarian act and an expression of sacrificial love for one's neighbor.
- **Roman Catholics** consider organ transplantation an act of charity. In 1990, Pope John Paul II made a statement in favor of organ donation in the form of living tissues or from those who are deceased.
- **Seventh-Day Adventists** strongly promote organ transplantation and the religion runs transplant hospitals. One example is Loma Linda University Medical Center in Southern California, which specializes in pediatric heart transplantation.
- **United Methodists** encourage organ donation and transplantation. Their 1992 resolution further states that prior to harvesting the organs, death must be determined by a reliable source and there should be no measure to hasten death. The religious organization encourages their pastors to discuss organ donation as a routine part of their hospice care.

cerebral blood flow studies and EEG. Common causes for organ transplantation are shown in Table 21-3 ∎.

Donor Screening and Donor Consent

Donors must be screened for compatibility. Individuals who abuse intravenous drugs; have severe hypertension; have pre-existing infections of HIV, hepatitis B or C, syphilis, tuberculosis, or septicemia; have a malignancy; and some with diabetes mellitus are not candidates for organ donation. It is best to obtain the client's consent for organ donation. However, if this is not possible due to the nature of the illness or injury, a family member can give consent for organ donation. This is emotionally easier for the family if they know what the child wants. A donor card, which can be obtained at a hospital or on the Internet, can communicate the child's preferences about organ donation.

Living donors, those donating organs such as kidneys, need psychological care to determine if they are emotionally stable enough to donate the organ. It must be documented that they understand the associated risks. Follow-up care is also important to assist the donor in coping with feelings of fear and isolation during physical recovery.

Nursing Considerations

The recipient of organ donation requires careful preoperative and postoperative care. Preoperatively, the child will need to be evaluated physically and emotionally to determine his or her level of readiness for surgery. Children are often very direct in their questions. Table 21-4 ∎ provides possible nursing responses to common questions that children might ask. Most of these families have been waiting a long time for an organ to become available. They may be so excited that an organ has been found that they fail to consider that the organ may not function properly. Immunosuppressive drugs may be required to suppress the immune response and prevent rejection of the organ. Immunosuppressive agents are usually used in combination, and the regime varies according to the agency and the type of organ to be transplanted. The child's physical condition is documented through a variety of medical and laboratory tests. The nurse also helps maintain the carefully controlled environment that is used to protect the organ recipient from exposure to micro-organisms.

Postoperative care also includes both emotional and physical care. Some research studies have linked organ transplantation with posttraumatic stress syndrome for both the parents and recipients of organ donation. Fear of rejection of the organ is a common concern among organ recipients. Following surgery, the nurse will be responsible for evaluating the return and maintenance of the function of the organ that was transplanted. For instance, the child who was a recipient of a kidney should be evaluated for urinary function and fluid and electrolyte balance. The child who was a recipient of a heart should be evaluated for cardiac status.

MediaLink   Organ donor

TABLE 21-3

Common Causes for Organ Transplantation

ORGAN TRANSPLANTED	COMMON CAUSES
Heart and heart valves	Coronary artery disease, cardiomyopathy, valvular disease, congenital defects, viral infections
Intestine	Short bowel syndrome, Crohn's disease, inflammatory bowel disease, congenital defects, trauma
Kidney	Diabetes, hypertension, renal failure
Liver	Hepatitis C, alcoholism
Lung	Cystic fibrosis, primary pulmonary hypertension, idiopathic pulmonary fibrosis, chronic obstructive pulmonary disease (COPD)
Pancreas	Type 1 diabetes
Blood	Surgery, trauma, burns, incompatibility such as Rh factor
Bone, tendons, marrow, stem cells	Cancer, arthritis, trauma; marrow is used for sickle cell anemia, aplastic anemia, leukemia, Hodgkin's disease, lymphoma
Cornea	Corneal damage, keratoconus
Skin	Burns, trauma, cancer, foot ulcers due to diabetes
Arteries and veins	Atherosclerosis, trauma, aneurysms

Rejection of the transplanted organ is a major issue in the postoperative period. The rejection can occur immediately, within minutes or hours, or within days or months. The nurse must constantly monitor for signs of rejection.

clinical ALERT

Signs of rejection include laboratory values outside the normal range and lack of improvement of clinical symptoms related to the disease process prior to surgery.

Rejection may require removal of the transplanted organ or additional immunosuppressive therapy. Infection is also a particular hazard following organ transplantation therapy. The nurse must be diligent in observing for clinical symptoms of infection and reporting them promptly.

Allergies

An **allergy** is an altered reaction to an antigen or allergen. Common allergens include pet fur, cockroaches, cow's milk, dust, egg whites, medications, mites, mold, pollen, peanuts, seafood, shellfish, soy, tree nuts, and wheat. Reactions to an allergen do not occur until a repeated exposure takes place.

Manifestations

Clinical manifestations of allergies can be mild (Figure 21-6 ■), severe, or life threatening. Table 21-5 ■ outlines the various types of reactions.

Diagnosis and Treatment

Careful history taking is required to assist in diagnosing allergies. Intradermal skin testing (Figure 21-7 ■) can be done to identify specific antigens. Food allergens can be

TABLE 21-4

Questions a Child Might Ask About Organ Transplantation

QUESTION	NURSING RESPONSE
What is a transplant?	A transplant is a surgery to take out your old, diseased organ and replace it with a healthy one.
Why do I need a new organ?	Your (heart, lung, kidney, etc.) is not working right. To keep you from getting sicker, you need a new organ.
Where do these organs come from?	Some organs that are transplanted come from a friend or family member or even a stranger. These organs are ones that the person can live without. Some organs come from people who have died and have asked that their organs be used to help others.
Will I live at the hospital while I'm waiting for my organ?	No, you can live at home while you wait for the right organ to help you. You may have to get to the hospital quickly, though, when there is an organ found for you.
Will my life be better after the transplant?	Most children who have a transplant will get better soon. Right after the surgery you will need to take medicine and rest. Soon you should be able to go back to school. Your family and your doctor will keep a close watch over you.

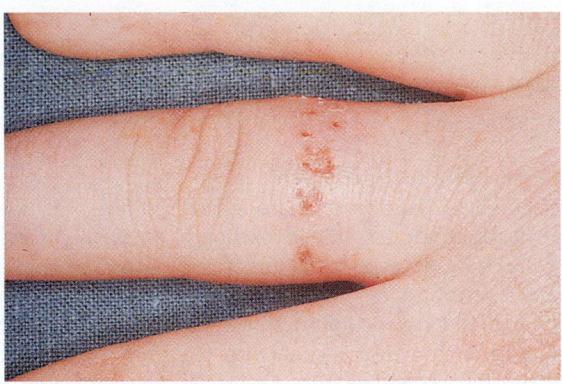

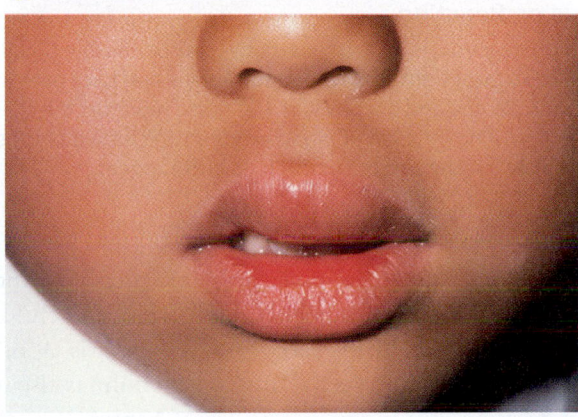

Figure 21-6. ■ (**A**) Inflammation of the skin caused by the metal salts in jewelry. (**B**) Inflammation of the lip caused by allergic reaction to peanuts. (**A.** Biophoto Associates/Photo Researchers, Inc., **B:** Photo Researchers, Inc.)

identified by removing foods one at a time and observing for the allergic reaction. Once the allergen or allergens are identified, the allergen must be avoided.

Oral antihistamines can be administered to decrease the symptoms of allergic reactions. If the child is allergic

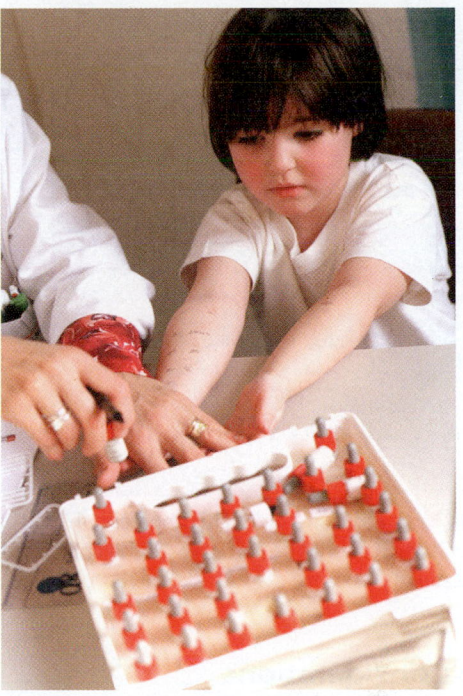

Figure 21-7. ■ Skin testing to determine the source of allergic reaction. (PHANIE/Photo Researchers, Inc.)

to medications, desensitization may allow the child to take medications that may be necessary for treatment of diseases. **Desensitization** is the process of administering doses of medication in increasing increments in an effort to avoid the allergic reaction. For example, penicillin is a medication that causes frequent allergic reactions in children. However, it is necessary for treatment of several infections. Desensitization may allow the child to be treated with penicillin when he or she encounters certain infections.

TABLE 21-5

Types of Allergic Reactions

TYPES	EXAMPLES	OCCURS	CLINICAL MANIFESTATIONS
Type I—localized or systemic	Hay fever, pet fur, insect bite	Within seconds or minutes of exposure	Rhinitis, sneezing, hives, urticaria, wheezing, vomiting, diarrhea, anaphylaxis
Type II—tissue specific	Reaction to blood transfusion, hemolytic disease of the newborn	Within 15–30 minutes of exposure	Symptoms vary but include fever and dyspnea
Type III—immune complex	Serum sickness, acute glomerulonephritis	Within 6 hours of exposure	Urticaria, fever, joint pain
Type IV—delayed	Tuberculin skin test, contact dermatitis, allograft tissue rejection	Within several hours after exposure	Symptoms vary but include fever, erythema, and pruritus

MediaLink Allergic rhinitis

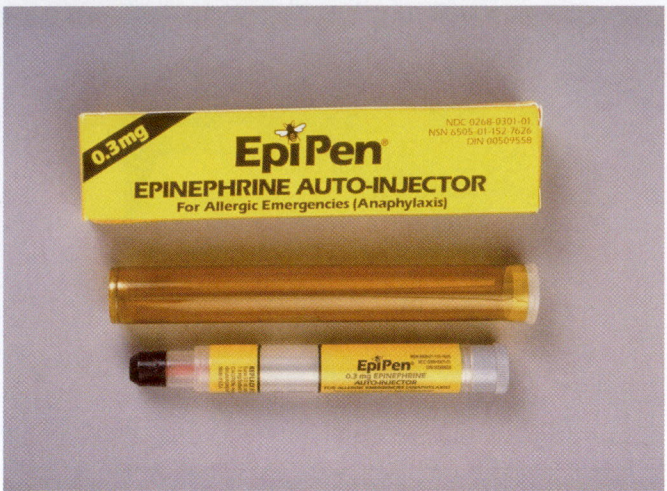

Figure 21-8. ■ Parents and older children need instruction in use of the EpiPen, which should be carried with the child at all times. (Pearson Education/PH College)

Nursing Considerations

The nurse can be instrumental in providing the child and family with assistance in how to avoid allergens. This may require removing pets from the home, controlling dust, placing plastic covers on beds and pillows, removing carpet, using high-efficiency air filters, and controlling and removing mold. The child who is allergic to bee or wasp stings must understand the use of premeasured, single-dose epinephrine or the EpiPen (Figure 21-8 ■). A prescription is required, and the EpiPen should be available at the school, day care center, and home. The nurse can teach the child to use the EpiPen properly. The child should also understand the care of the EpiPen. Care of the EpiPen includes storing it out of direct sunlight or extreme temperatures and checking the expiration date often.

LATEX ALLERGY

Latex allergy is an IgE-mediated response to repeated exposure to latex. (IgE is a type of immunoglobulin that is primarily responsible for allergic reactions.) Reactions to latex can be type I (local or systemic) or type IV (delayed hypersensitivity). Clients who have sensitivities/allergies to bananas, avocados, potatoes, chestnuts, and tropical fruits can also be at risk for developing an allergy to latex. Latex can be found in several health care products such as gloves, drains, adhesives, and catheters. Fortunately, nonlatex products are available. Latex substitutes must be used when the allergy is identified.

Immunotherapy

Immunotherapy is the prevention and treatment of disease using the administration of allergens, immunostimulants, immunosuppressants, interferon, and immune globulin.

Immune globulin can be given intramuscularly or intravenously. Both routes can be useful when treating children following exposure to diseases such as hepatitis A or B, rubella, rubeola, and varicella. Immune globulin is also useful in treating Kawasaki disease (see Chapter 19 ⦾), AIDS, and idiopathic thrombocytopenic purpura (see Chapter 20 ⦾).

Children should be assessed carefully for hypersensitivity reaction or infusion reaction. Manifestations of hypersensitivity reaction and infusion reaction are listed in Box 21-4 ■.

NURSING CARE

PRIORITIES IN NURSING CARE

When caring for children with immune disorders, nursing care should be focused on gathering a thorough history of the child's condition. This is especially important when determining what allergen is causing the allergic reaction. Preventing infection through the use of aseptic and sterile technique and reverse isolation is important for the child with HIV/AIDS and organ transplantation. Children with JRA are often in pain and therefore intolerant to activity. The nurse should provide comfort measures and assistance with activities of daily living. Long-term illnesses such as HIV/AIDS, conditions requiring organ transplant, and JRA are emotionally taxing on both the children and their families. The nurse must encourage the expression of feelings and concerns related to the disease process and the health care required.

ASSESSING

In children with immune disorders, the nurse collects data about signs and symptoms of infection, including fever, decreased breath sounds, fatigue, and skin irritation or lesions. Nutritional status, height, and weight (see Procedures 13-6 to 13-8 ⬯; see also Chapter 14 ⬯) will give the nurse an indication of the child's general condition. Following organ transplantation, the nurse observes for signs and symptoms of organ rejection. For the child with JRA, joint mobility and joint pain are checked and recorded. The nurse must also assess the caregiver for signs and symptoms of role strain. Manifestations of role strain include physical symptoms of GI upset, headaches, and insomnia; emotional symptoms of stress, anger, and anxiety; and socioeconomic symptoms of withdrawal from social activities and diminished work productivity.

DIAGNOSING, PLANNING, AND IMPLEMENTING

Possible nursing diagnoses for children with immune disorders include:

- Imbalanced Nutrition: Less Than Body Requirements, related to chronic immune disorders
- Impaired Skin Integrity, related to altered immune status
- Delayed Growth and Development, related to physical disability and chronic immune disorder
- Activity Intolerance, related to chronic pain
- Risk for Infection, related to suppressed immune system
- Risk for Caregiver Role Strain, related to stress concerning child's immune disorder.

Outcomes for children with immune disorders include that the child will:

- Maintain weight and body mass within normal limits (WNL).
- Demonstrate intact skin and mucous membranes.
- Achieve milestones related to physical, cognitive, and psychosocial development as expected.
- Participate in physical activity within symptoms of intolerance.
- Be free of symptoms of infection.

The caregiver will:

- Demonstrate balance in providing care to the child.

Nursing interventions for children who have immune disorders include the following actions:

- Provide small frequent meals with items that are pleasing to the child. *Smaller meals are better tolerated. The child will be more likely to eat if he or she has a choice of foods.*

- Create a pleasant environment for mealtime. *The environment is essential for the child to enjoy his or her food and maintain adequate intake.*
- Protect the skin from injury by frequent position changes; pressure-reducing mattress; and clean, wrinkle-free linens. *These measures reduce pressure and friction and therefore protect skin integrity.*
- Encourage ambulation as tolerated, including passive and active ROM exercises. *These measures will increase circulation and muscle tone and also strengthen muscles and joints.*
- Offer age-appropriate toys. *The correct toys will stimulate appropriate development.*
- Conduct and document frequent assessment of the child's developmental level. *This strategy will allow caregivers to intervene quickly if developmental delays are noted.*
- Refer to and support the use of physical therapy. *This service will assist the child in maintaining joint function and will help prevent contractures.*
- Assist with activities of daily living, being careful to encourage the child's continued participation. *Assistance will help the child avoid fatigue. Continued participation will aid in building muscle strength and activity tolerance.*
- Provide protection from individuals who have current infections. *Children with immune disorders need protection from infections.*
- Follow universal precautions and proper hand washing techniques. *Using these measures provides protection from nosocomial infections.*
- Encourage family members to express feelings and concerns. *Expression of feelings will assist with decreasing anxiety.*
- Refer family members to community resources. *Additional support services can relieve some of the caregiver's burden.*

EVALUATING

The child with immune disorders should be evaluated for adequate nutritional status, skin integrity, appropriate growth and development, tolerance to activity, and risk for infection. Caregivers who manage the care of children with immune disorders should be evaluated for excessive stress and ineffective coping.

NURSING PROCESS CARE PLAN
Child with an Organ Transplant

Riley, age 4, is diagnosed with cardiomyopathy. She is awaiting transplantation of a heart. Her mother is concerned because her sister's son, who is also 4, speaks using short sentences and loves to skip and hop. Riley uses short phrases to communicate and can walk well but does not skip or hop. Riley's mother wants to know if she should be worried.

Assessment. The following data should be collected as soon as possible:

- Perform a developmental screening to determine Riley's developmental level in each of the following areas: physical, gross motor, fine motor, language, socialization, cognition, and family relationship.
- Determine Riley's mother's knowledge related to developmental levels.
- Determine Riley's mother's expectations for Riley's future.

Nursing Diagnosis. The following important nursing diagnosis (among others) is established for this client:

- Risk for Altered Development related to chronic illness (cardiomyopathy).

Expected Outcome

- Riley will achieve developmental milestones in each of the following areas: physical, gross motor, fine motor, language, socialization, cognition, and family relationship.

Planning and Implementation

- Instruct Riley's parents about normal development of the 4-year-old child.
- Teach them activities to promote normal development.
- Suggest age-appropriate toys.
- Encourage Riley's parents to promote normal development despite her illness.

- Assist Riley's parents in establishing a method for positive rewards and feedback when Riley accomplishes developmental milestones.
- Suggest a follow-up plan to monitor Riley's developmental progress.

Evaluation. Riley and her parents implement a plan to monitor and promote her developmental progress. They have implemented activities to encourage Riley in motor skills, language, socialization, and cognition. Spending specific time together also promotes family relationships. They are keeping monthly pediatric visits to monitor their success.

Critical Thinking in the Nursing Process

1. Develop a plan for promoting Riley's motor skills.
2. Develop a plan for promoting Riley's language skills.
3. List at least five toys that will aid in promoting Riley's developmental progress.

Note: Dicussion of Critical Thinking questions appears in Appendix I.

Note: The references and resources for this and all chapters have been compiled at the back of the book.

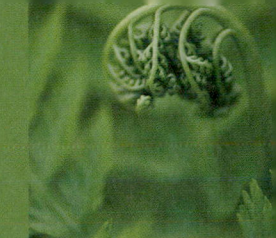

Chapter Review

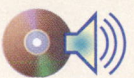

KEY TERMS by Topic

Use the audio glossary feature of either the CD-ROM or the Companion Website to hear the correct pronunciation of the following key terms.

Anatomy and Physiology
antigens, antibodies, immune response, natural immunity, acquired immunity, humoral immunity, immunoglobulins, primary immune response, secondary immune response, cell-mediated immunity, active immunity, passive immunity

HIV and AIDS
oral candidiasis, thrush

Juvenile Rheumatoid Arthritis
autoimmune, lymphadenopathy, splenomegaly, hepatomegaly

Organ Transplantation
autogenous graft, xenograft

Allergies
allergy, desensitization

Immunotherapy
anaphylactic shock

KEY Points

- The primary role of the immune system is to recognize and eliminate foreign substances.

- There are two types of immunity: natural and acquired.

- The child can contract HIV via the placenta during pregnancy, by exposure at birth, or through breast milk. The adolescent can be exposed to the virus by sexual contact.

- The child who develops AIDS is immunocompromised. The nurse must be diligent in assisting the child and family in preventing infections.

- Both JRA and SLE cause inflammation and therefore discomfort and pain in affected children. The nurse must assist the child in maintaining mobility and preventing pain.

- Corticosteroid therapy is commonly prescribed for treatment of SLE. The side effects of these medications include hunger leading to weight gain, mood changes, worsening acne, jitteriness, insomnia, hypertension, immunosuppression, growth retardation, and hyperglycemia.

- Kidneys, hearts, bone marrow, tissues, corneas, and other organs can be transplanted in children. The nurse can assist in preparing the child for organ transplantation and providing postoperative care to prevent rejection of the organ.

- Common allergies in children include pet fur, cockroaches, cow's milk, dust, egg whites, medications, mites, mold, pollen, peanuts, seafood, shellfish, soy, tree nuts, and wheat.

- Careful history taking is required to assist in the diagnosis of allergies.

- Anaphylactic shock is a systemic reaction to an allergen that occurs within minutes or up to 2 hours after exposure. Anaphylaxis is characterized by itching, hives, soft tissue edema, cough, dyspnea, pallor, perspiration, and tachycardia. These symptoms, if not treated promptly, can lead to respiratory distress and death.

EXPLORE MediaLink

Additional interactive resources for this chapter can be found on the Companion Website at www.prenhall.com/towle.

Click on Chapter 21 and "Begin" to select the activities for this chapter.

For chapter-related NCLEX-style questions and an audio glossary, access the accompanying CD-ROM in this book.

Animations

HIV/AIDs

Cell division

Allergic rhinitis

FOR FURTHER Study

For information on how the HIV virus can cross the placenta and infect the fetus during pregnancy, see Chapter 7.

See Chapter 8 for additional information on HIV.

Nutritional status, height assessment, and weight assessment are provided in Procedures 13-6 to 13-8.

See Chapter 14 for additional information on the child's general condition.

Kawasaki syndrome is discussed in Chapter 19.

For further discussion on idiopathic thrombocytopenic purpura, see Chapter 20.

For a nutritional assessment, see Chapter 22.

Skin lesions and candidiasis are discussed further in Chapter 24.

See Chapter 26 for information on infectious diseases.

See Appendix II for the childhood immunization schedule.

Critical Thinking Care Map

Caring for a Client with AIDS

NCLEX-PN® Focus Area: Safety and Infection

Case Study: Joe, age 15, recently had two positive polymerase chain reaction tests and was told that he was HIV positive. The condition and its implications were explained to Joe by the nurse. The nurse's teaching focused on preventing infection, promoting nutritional health, and providing knowledge about the disease process and the prescribed treatment. Immediately following the nurse's discussion, Joe said he wanted to continue going to high school and was sure that his friends were not at risk for contracting the virus.

Nursing Diagnosis: Risk for Infection

COLLECT DATA

Subjective	Objective
_____	_____
_____	_____
_____	_____
_____	_____
_____	_____
_____	_____

Would you report this? Yes/No

If yes, to: _____

Nursing Care

_____

_____

_____

_____

_____

_____

_____

_____

_____

_____

How would you document this? _____

_____

_____

Compare your documentation to the sample provided in Appendix I.

Data Collected
(use those that apply)

- Note anxious behaviors such as wringing hands and pacing.
- "I feel really tired."
- "I'm very strict about my diet. It is low fat and low calorie."
- Intake and output
- Weight
- "I really don't like to take medicine. Can't I just take it when I think about it?"
- Skin turgor
- Vital signs
- "My best friend has the flu."
- Lab results to include CBC, blood or wound cultures, serum protein, and albumin
- "I'd feel like a nerd if I wore that mask to school."
- Skin assessment for wounds and wound drainage

Nursing Interventions
(use those that apply; list in priority order)

- Refer Joe to a nutritionist to plan an alternative diet.
- Instruct Joe in hand washing and other techniques to avoid contamination with harmful bacteria or viruses.
- Review immunization schedule and recommend required immunizations as appropriate.
- Monitor intake and output by encouraging Joe to keep a food and fluid diary.
- Monitor Joe's weight at follow-up visits to determine nutritional status.
- Teach Joe and his parents to recognize symptoms of infections, colds, and flu in themselves, family members, friends, or others with whom they may come in contact.
- Teach Joe about the long-term effects of life as an HIV-positive client.
- Use a pre- and posttest to determine Joe's level of understanding of his diagnosis and treatment regime.
- Make sure Joe and his parents understand the proper handling, storage, and preparation of food.
- Make frequent follow-up appointments with Joe to monitor lab values.

NCLEX-PN® Exam Preparation

1 A nurse is assigned to care for an adolescent with a latex allergy diagnosis. The nurse is taking the client's history and, in order to determine the client's risk factors associated with latex allergies, asks about an allergy to which foods? Choose all that apply.

1. cheese
2. potatoes
3. milk
4. avocados
5. yogurt
6. bananas

2 The nurse is working at a health care clinic and is scheduled to give immunizations today. The nurse knows that the immunizations provide:

1. protection from all communicable diseases.
2. natural immunity from diseases.
3. nonhumoral immunity from diseases.
4. acquired immunity from diseases.

3 A young mother who is HIV positive has followed all recommended prenatal precautions and has just delivered a female child by cesarean section. After the infant is examined, the physician states that the infant has no outward symptoms of HIV. The nurse realizes that the mother needs more education about the possibility of HIV transmission to her infant when she states:

1. "I know there is still the potential my child will have HIV."
2. "I will be breastfeeding my infant since she does not appear to have HIV."
3. "I realize we all must learn to wash our hands before and after caring for the baby."
4. "I understand my baby will be treated with AZT to reduce the risk of HIV transmission."

4 A 10-year-old child has been diagnosed with juvenile rheumatoid arthritis. The nurse realizes this is a chronic autoimmune disorder that causes joint inflammation. What symptom is not associated with this disease?

1. fever
2. rash
3. lymphadenopathy
4. rhinitis

5 The nurse is aware of a child who is being evaluated for brain death following a traumatic injury to the head. The child has been on a respirator for 2 weeks. The nurse knows the following two medical tests will be used in the evaluation of brain death:

1. cardiac enzymes and electroencephalogram.
2. cerebral blood flow studies and electrocardiogram.
3. electroencephalogram and cerebral blood flow studies.
4. electroencephalogram and serum glucose testing.

6 The nurse is caring for a pediatric client after a kidney transplant. The nurse knows this client has the potential for organ rejection and monitors the following closely:

1. urinary function, fluid and electrolyte balance.
2. cardiac function, range of motion, and edema.
3. $Paco_2$ 60 mmHg, respirations over 30.
4. thrombophlebitis and periorbital edema.

7 In a pediatric clinic, the mother of a 3-month-old child tells the nurse the child does not gain weight, and has constant ear infections, fever, mouth infection (oral candidiasis), and diarrhea. Upon examination, the physician confirms the child also has hepatosplenomegaly. The nurse suspects the child has a diagnosis of:

1. juvenile rheumatoid arthritis.
2. latex allergies.
3. HIV.
4. chronic otitis media.

8 The nurse realizes the following nursing interventions should be instituted for a child with a suspected diagnosis of HIV:

1. avoidance of infection and proper nutrition.
2. antibiotic therapy and careful skin care.
3. exercise regime and range of motion.
4. administration of oral antihistamines and penicillin.

9 The nurse is attempting to explain humoral immunity to a child's mother who has inquired about her child's ability to fight off illness during a well-baby visit to the clinic. The nurse tells the mother the following about humoral immunity so the mother will understand:

1. "Humoral immunity is present at birth and protects the child from everything."
2. "Humoral immunity occurs after the age of 10."
3. "Humoral immunity destroys bacteria, viruses, and allergens."
4. "Humoral immunity takes place at the same time as puberty."

10 You are caring for an adolescent with a known sensitivity to latex. In preparing for his or her care, you select nursing interventions to care for this client to prevent an allergic response to latex. Choose all that apply.

1. Use only nonlatex gloves.
2. Remove all latex materials from the room.
3. Use medications that are stored in glass.
4. Use special blood pressure cuffs.
5. Noninvasive latex products can be kept in the room.
6. A latex-free cart should be kept in or near the client's room.

Answers for Review Questions, as well as discussion of Care Plan and Critical Thinking Care Map questions, appear in Appendix I.

Chapter 22

Care of the Child with Gastrointestinal Disorders

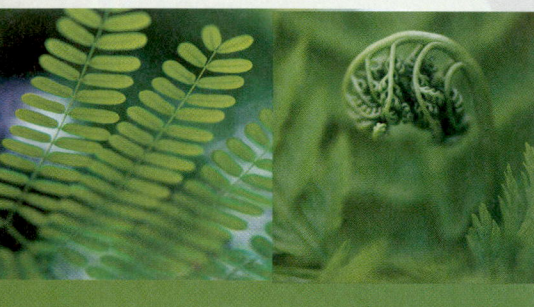

HEALTH PROMOTION ISSUE:
Childhood Obesity and Fast Foods

NURSING PROCESS CARE PLAN:
Care of a Child with Bilateral Cleft Lip

CRITICAL THINKING CARE MAP:
Caring for a Client with Gastroenteritis

BRIEF Outline

Anatomy and Physiology
Brief Assessment Overview
Congenital Gastrointestinal Defects
Gastrointestinal Inflammation
Intestinal Parasites

Malabsorption Disorders
Nutrition Disorders
Hepatic Disorders
Motility Disorders
Poisonings
Nursing Care

LEARNING Outcomes

After completing this chapter, you will be able to:

- Describe the basic structures and functioning of the gastrointestinal tract and accessory structures.
- Describe major gastrointestinal disorders in clear, simple terms.
- Discuss clinical manifestations, diagnostic procedures, and medical management related to gastrointestinal disorders.
- Explain appropriate nursing interventions for children with gastrointestinal disorders.

Gastrointestinal disorders in children include congenital malformation, malabsorption conditions, and problems with motility. The role of the LPN/LVN in caring for these children is one of assisting with data collection and monitoring the effectiveness of treatments. Most therapeutic interventions ordered for gastrointestinal disorders can be administered by the LPN/LVN.

Anatomy and Physiology

PRIMARY ORGANS

The primary organs of the gastrointestinal system consist of a series of hollow tubelike structures through which food is digested and solid waste is eliminated (Figure 22-1 ■). The entire system is lined with a mucous membrane. Food is propelled through the system by wavelike contractions of the smooth muscle (**peristalsis**) that lies underneath the mucous membrane.

The oral cavity is formed by the hard and soft palate, the cheeks, and the tongue. Extending from the center of the soft palate is a cone-shaped process, the uvula. The soft palate and uvula prevent food and fluid from entering the nasal cavity during swallowing. The tongue is made of skeletal muscle attached to the mandible and hyoid bone in the neck. A thin membrane or **lingual frenulum** attaches

the tongue to the floor of the mouth. The tongue is covered with small raised bumps called **papillae.** The sensory receptors for salt, sour, sweet, and bitter are located on the sides of the papillae. The mucous membrane covering the front of the mouth and the inside of the lips is called the **gingiva.** The teeth formed in the mandible and maxilla erupt through the gingiva beginning at around 6 months of age and continue until all 20 deciduous teeth are in place by 2 years of age. Around 6 years of age, the deciduous teeth are replaced by permanent teeth. The 32 permanent teeth are generally in place between 17 and 24 years of age. Three pairs of salivary glands empty their secretions into the oral cavity. The largest of the salivary glands, the **parotid gland,** is located below and in front of the ears at the angle of the jaw. The parotid ducts open into the **buccal space** (area inside the cheek by the second molars). The **submandibular glands** lie behind the mandible and secrete saliva into the submandibular (Wharton's) ducts opening on each side of the lingual frenulum. The **sublingual glands** (glands under the tongue) open into the floor of the mouth. These structures are illustrated in Figure 22-2 ■.

The esophagus attaches the oral pharynx to the stomach. At the lower end of the esophagus, the **cardiac sphincter** acts to prevent food and gastric acid from being pushed from the stomach into the esophagus.

The stomach is a muscular backward C-shaped pouch located just under the diaphragm. Regions of the stomach are identified by their shape or underlying tissue. The rounded top of the stomach is the **fundus.** The area around the cardiac sphincter is the **cardiac region.** The inner curved area of the stomach is the **lesser curvature,** and the outer area is the **greater curvature.** At the bottom of the stomach, surrounding the **pyloric sphincter** is the **pylorus** (the muscular tissue surrounding and controlling the stomach outlet). When the stomach is empty, its lining lies in folds called **rugae.** When food enters the stomach, hydrochloric acid and digestive enzymes are released from the gastric glands inside the mucous membrane. Mucus is also produced to prevent damage to the mucous membrane from the potent gastric juices. Three layers of muscles contract to mix food with digestive acid and enzymes and form a semiliquid substance called **chyme.** The chyme stays in the stomach several hours before it is propelled through the pyloric sphincter into the small intestine.

The small intestine is divided into three sections. The first section is the duodenum. The common bile duct and pancreatic duct empty into the duodenum. The mucous membrane contains small glands that release intestinal juice (digestive enzymes). The main processes of chemical digestion take place in the duodenum. The second section of the small intestine is the jejunum, and the third section

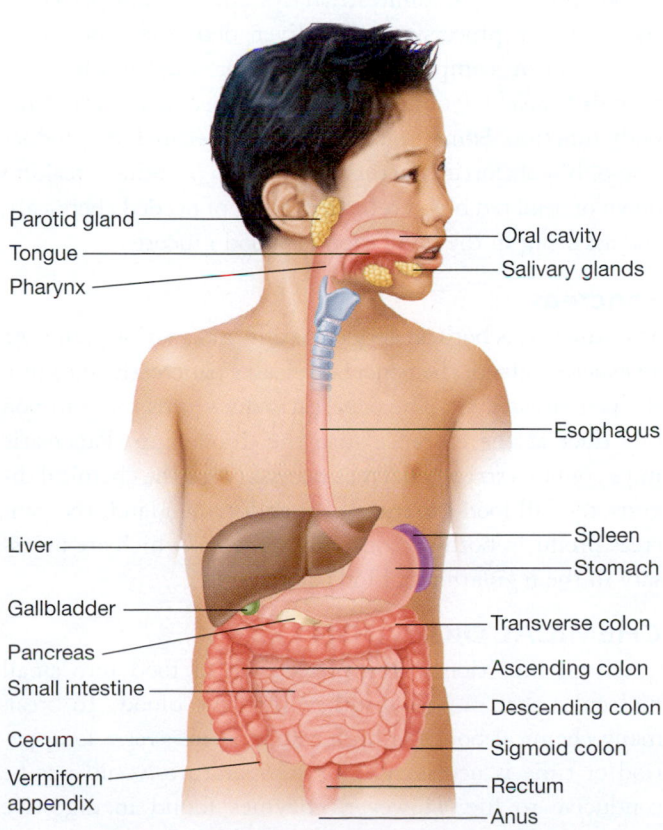

Parotid gland
Tongue
Pharynx

Oral cavity
Salivary glands

Esophagus

Liver
Gallbladder
Pancreas
Small intestine
Cecum
Vermiform appendix

Spleen
Stomach
Transverse colon
Ascending colon
Descending colon
Sigmoid colon
Rectum
Anus

Figure 22-1. ■ Organs of the alimentary canal and related accessory organs.

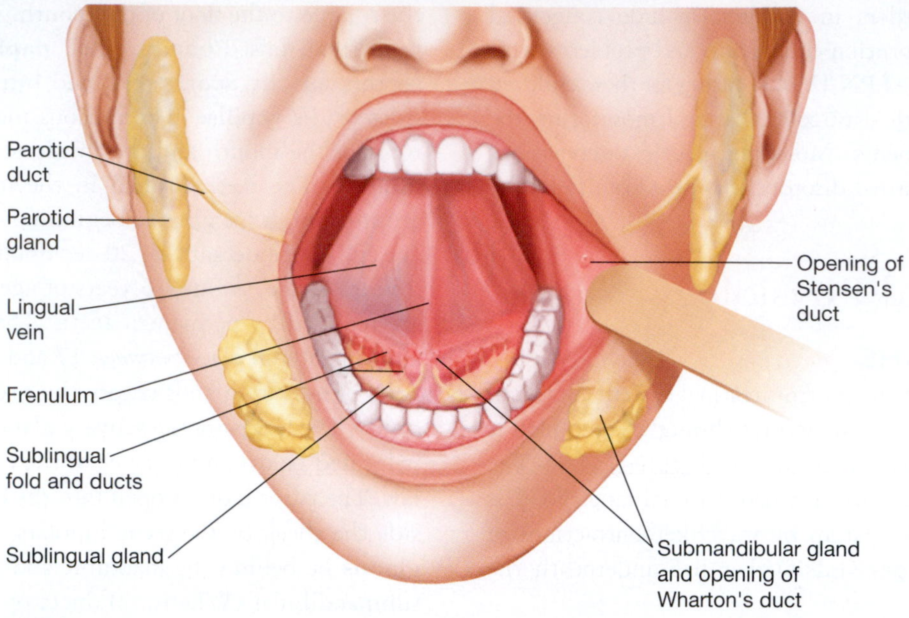

Figure 22-2. ■ Salivary glands.

is the ileum. Absorption of nutrients occurs mainly in the jejunum and ileum. The ileocecal valve connects the ileum of the small intestine and cecum of the large intestine. The inner lining of the small intestine lies in folds called *plica*. Covering each plica are small, finger-like structures called *villi* (singular, *villus*). Inside each villus is a capillary network and lymph vessel into which nutrients are absorbed. The cells along the outer side of the villi have a brush border or microvilli. These folds and projections greatly increase the surface area inside the intestines and thereby increase the absorption of nutrients.

The large intestine or colon is divided into several sections. First, the *cecum* is located in the lower right quadrant of the abdomen. Hanging from the lower end of the cecum is the appendix. Chyme, entering the cecum, is propelled by peristalsis upward through the ascending colon, through the transverse colon, the descending colon, and into the sigmoid colon. As the chyme moves through the large intestine, water is removed, leaving the solid waste or feces in a compacted mass. Feces remains in the rectum and sigmoid colon until it is expelled through the anus.

ACCESSORY ORGANS

The two accessory organs of the digestive system are the liver and pancreas (see Figure 22-1).

Liver

The liver, located in the upper right quadrant of the abdomen, just below the diaphragm, is the largest gland in the body. One function of the liver is to produce and excrete bile. Bile flows from the liver into the hepatic duct and cystic duct and then into the gall bladder, where it is stored

and concentrated. When food enters the duodenum, the gall bladder contracts, forcing the bile out the cystic duct and the common bile duct and into the duodenum. Bile acts as an *emulsifier*, breaking large molecules of fat into smaller molecules of fat. All chemicals that are absorbed into the blood from the gastrointestinal system are transported to the liver for processing. The liver detoxifies chemicals, breaks down compounds (*catabolism*), and builds compounds (*anabolism*) of many substances necessary for normal body function. Some functions of the liver include production of blood clotting factors and plasma proteins, breaking down of dead red blood cells, recycling of needed chemicals, and assisting in the regulation of blood glucose.

Pancreas

The pancreas is both an endocrine and an exocrine gland. As an exocrine gland, the pancreas releases pancreatic juice into the pancreatic duct. The pancreatic duct joins the common bile duct at the entrance into the duodenum. Pancreatic juice contains strong enzymes necessary for the chemical digestion of all food groups. As an endocrine gland, the pancreas produces both glycogen and insulin, which are necessary in the regulation of blood sugar.

CHEMICAL DIGESTION

Chemical digestion is the breakdown of food into small molecules that can be absorbed into the blood. To break many chemical bonds, a high temperature over a long period of time is necessary. This temperature would not be conducive to life. However, enzymes found in digestive juices speed up chemical reactions and allow them to occur within the normal body temperature.

Chemical digestion begins in the mouth. *Amylase* found in saliva changes starch (a polysaccharide) into maltose (a disaccharide). If swallowing occurs too rapidly, this reaction will not take place. When food enters the stomach, hydrochloric acid and *protease* (pepsin) found in gastric juice break large molecules of protein into smaller molecules. Many chemical reactions occur in the duodenum. Chyme leaving the stomach is highly acidic. The fluids in the duodenum are alkaline, changing the pH of the chyme. Bile is excreted over the chyme. As stated previously, bile breaks large molecules of fat into smaller molecules. Pancreatic juice contains three enzymes. Lipase changes small molecules of fat into fatty acids, monoglycerides, and glycerol. Protease (trypsin) changes proteins into amino acids and peptides. Amylase changes starch into maltose. Intestinal juice contains several enzymes. Peptidase changes peptides into amino acids. Maltase changes maltose into glucose. Lactase changes lactose into galactose and glucose. Sucrase changes sucrose into glucose. At the end of chemical digestion, glucose, galactose, amino acids, fatty acids, and glycerol are absorbed into the blood.

Brief Assessment Overview

HISTORY

The symptoms of many gastrointestinal disorders appear over time. The family should be questioned about the child's symptoms, including appetite, vomiting, diarrhea, constipation, and abdominal pain. The specific foods the child has eaten in the past 24 hours may be important when allergies or foodborne infections are being considered. If anyone else in the family has similar symptoms, they should be reported.

PHYSICAL

A general inspection is performed at the start of a health assessment. A child who appears far above average in weight may be one of the growing numbers of children for whom obesity will be a lifelong issue. The nurse can plan to provide client information about healthful diets and the importance of proper nutrition. The Health Promotion Issue on pages 662 and 663 discusses one aspect of this concern. Obesity is discussed in Chapter 27 under Psychological Disorders and Associated Manifestations.

The physical assessment of the gastrointestinal system of children begins with inspection of the abdomen. The abdomen should appear symmetric, round, or flat when the child is supine. There should not be indentation or bulging of the abdominal muscles at the midline or around the umbilicus.

The abdomen should be auscultated using the diaphragm of the stethoscope. Bowel sounds occur every 10 to 30 seconds and have a high-pitched quality. Auscultate for at least 5 minutes before reporting that bowel sounds are absent. Absent bowel sounds may indicate peritonitis or paralytic ileus.

Hyperactive bowel sounds indicate gastroenteritis or a partial obstruction.

Palpation should be done last because it can alter bowel sounds if done prior to auscultation. Light palpation is used to assess the softness or firmness of the abdominal muscles and the presence of any tenderness. Deep palpation is used to assess the size and consistency of the liver and other organs, except in certain instances such as Wilms' tumor (discussed in Chapter 23). Deep palpation is not a responsibility of the LPN/LVN, although it is important to understand. Palpation is best accomplished when the child is supine, with the knees bent. To help the child relax, ask the child, "How soft can you make your tummy?" If the child is ticklish, firm pressure should be used. Do not pretend to tickle because the child will tighten the abdominal muscles, making it difficult to feel the underlying tissue.

At times, the anal area must be visualized and assessed. Children have a sense that their privacy has been invaded when the perineum is examined. Having a parent hold a child or be present by the child's head can give a sense of security. The anus should be inspected for redness, swelling, fissures, and drainage. A rectal examination should only be performed by a trained examiner.

Gastrointestinal system disorders include congenital anomalies, as well as inflammation, malabsorption, and motility problems. The liver is an accessory organ to the gastrointestinal system, so hepatic disorders are also covered in this chapter. The focus of nursing care is to maintain nutrition and fluid balance and to promote elimination of solid waste.

Congenital Gastrointestinal Defects

Congenital defects of the gastrointestinal system, the most common of the congenital defects, require surgical correction but are not usually immediately life threatening. If detection and correction are not made in a timely manner, however, aspiration, malnutrition, and obstruction could result.

CLEFT LIP AND CLEFT PALATE

Cleft lip and cleft palate commonly occur together but can be found separately (Figure 22-3 ■). When the medial nasal and maxillary processes fail to join, the result is a **cleft palate.** There is an opening between the roof of the mouth and the floor of the nasal passage. If the upper lip fails to join medially, a **cleft lip** is the result. Cleft lip can be unilateral or bilateral. Cleft palate could be complete (through bone and tissue) or partial (involving the bone structure but not the overlying mucous membrane). So, when assessing every newborn, it is important not only to visualize the palate, but also to feel the palate with the little finger to be sure the bones are intact.

(*Text continues on p. 664.*)

HEALTH PROMOTION ISSUE

CHILDHOOD OBESITY AND FAST FOODS

An overweight single mother brings her two young children in for wellness checks. The 2-year-old is at the 50th percentile for height, the 98th for weight. The 5-year-old is at the 65th percentile for height, the 96th for weight. The mother insists that she does not have a lot of snack food around the house. "We usually just eat out when I pick them up on the way home from work."

DISCUSSION

Childhood obesity has increased since the mid-1980s and may be approaching epidemic status (Shulman, 2004). The National Health and Nutrition Examination Survey data indicate that 15% of children and teens between 6 and 19 years are overweight (Binns & Ariza, 2004). It is estimated that 25% to 30% are obese (Moran, 1999). What are some implications of obesity? What is causing this increase in childhood obesity?

Few problems in childhood have such an impact on the life of the individual as obesity. Obesity is associated with many physical complications, including type II diabetes mellitus, coronary artery disease, pulmonary dysfunction, stroke, and arthritis. Obesity can also disable the individual emotionally, including poor body image, low self-esteem, social isolation, and feelings of depression and rejection.

Obesity is not only an individual's problem, but it also causes social concern. For example, the cost of treatment of the complications of obesity will put additional strain on the national health care budget. The obese individual may need to take more sick days off work and therefore be less productive.

What is the difference between being overweight and being obese? Both overweight and obesity are an unhealthy accumulation of body fat. The body mass index (BMI) is the standard for determining if an individual is overweight or obese. The BMI is determined by dividing the individual's weight in kilograms by their height in meters squared. For example, a child weighs 45 lb (20.45 kg) and is 42 in. tall. The height in meters squared would be 1.1 m^2 (42 in. = 105 cm = 1.05 m). The BMI would be 18%. Children with a BMI between the 85th and 95th percentile are considered to be overweight. Children over the 95th percentile are considered to be obese. (*Note:* See Appendix II ∞ for growth charts to determine percentile.)

PLANNING AND IMPLEMENTATION

There are many causes of the increase in obesity in children. Heredity is one factor that cannot be changed. Other factors can be changed with positive results. In many households, children spend most of their personal time sitting in front of a computer or television. With little activity, children do not burn the calories they consume. By limiting a child's sedentary activities and encouraging participation in physical, motion-oriented activities, parents can help children slow or prevent the deposition of body fat.

Diet is the second factor that can be adjusted. Fast food has become a prominent feature in the diet of families. Consumption of fast food by children increased fivefold between 1970 and 1995, while the number of fast-food restaurants doubled. Several dietary factors may cause excessive weight gain from fast-food consumption. They include massive portion size; high energy-density foods; an appeal to taste preference for fats, sugar, and salt; high content of saturated and trans fat; high glycemic load; and low fiber.

Little research has been conducted on the effects of fast food on body weight. Without sufficient data, many support the claim that fast food can be

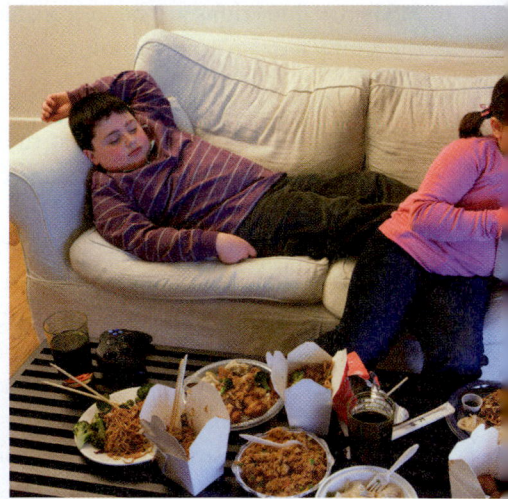

(Getty Images/Digital Vision)

part of a healthy diet. One study by Bowman, Gortmaker, Ebbeling et al. (2004) included 6,212 children and adolescents from 4 to 19 years. On a typical day, more than 30% of the children ate fast food. These children consumed more total calories; more fat; more carbohydrates, including sugar and sweetened beverages; less fiber; less milk; and fewer fruits and vegetables. These same children made poorer food choices on days when they did not consume fast food. The study concluded that fast-food consumption has an adverse effect on dietary quality that could increase risk for obesity.

In response to political pressure, many fast-food restaurants are providing information about the nutrition content of their menu items. Many fast-food restaurants are giving nutritious choices, including salads, fruit, and milk. Advertisements for meat sandwiches complimented with vegetables are becoming more common. It will be up to parents to ensure that children select the healthier foods.

NURSING CONCERNS

When assessing a child's nutritional status, the nurse should ask about the frequency and content of fast-food meals. The child should be weighed and measured, and the BMI calculated. Children over the 85% percentile should be evaluated for complications such as hypertension, diabetes, and hyperlipidemia. The child's activities should be assessed in relation to calories burned. It is important to assess the child's emotional status and the impact the child's weight has on quality of life.

Parents and children should be taught the impact that being overweight or obese has on their general health. Although it is necessary to discuss complications of being overweight, it is important to stress how well the child will feel when he or she has more energy following weight loss. Point out the benefits of weight loss, instead of dwelling on the risks and complications.

The family may need a referral to a nutritionist. It should be suggested that meals at a fast-food restaurant be reserved for a special occasion instead of being a daily event. Suggest that when fast food must be consumed, the restaurant selected should offer nutritious meals, and the food choices should reflect a balanced meal, with as low a fat content as possible.

Parents should encourage their children to become physically active. Limiting computer or television time may be necessary. Scheduling activities daily that require active participation will help burn calories and establish lifelong habits of physical exercise.

Obesity in children is becoming a major health concern. The problem results, in part, from the rapid pace at which parents live. The rush-rush of today's lifestyle necessitates rapid meal production and encourages parents to purchase fast foods for their families. These high-calorie, high-fat meals, coupled with sedentary activities of children, result in obesity. The nurse should provide teaching and support as families try to break the cycle and improve their health.

SELF-REFLECTION

Do you find time each day to take a break for some enjoyable physical activity? Do you give yourself several portions of fruits and vegetables daily? If you are in a hurry, do you seek out healthful food options?

SUGGESTED RESOURCES

- Bowman, S., Gortmaker, S., Ebbeling, C., Pereira, M., & Ludwig, D. (2004). Effects of fast-food consumption on energy intake and diet quality among children in a national household survey. *Pediatrics 113*(1), 112–118.

- Nestle, M. (2002). Food politics: How the food industry influences nutrition and health. Berkeley: University of California Press.

- Freeland-Graves, J., & Nitzke, S. (2002). Position of the American Dietetic Association; Total diet approach to communicating food and nutrition information. *Journal of the American Dietetic Association 102*, 100–108.

- Taveras, E., Berkey, C., Rifas-Shiman, S., Ludwing, D., et al. (2005). Association of consumption of fried food away from home with body mass index and diet quality in older children and adolescents. *Pediatrics 116*(4), e518–e524.

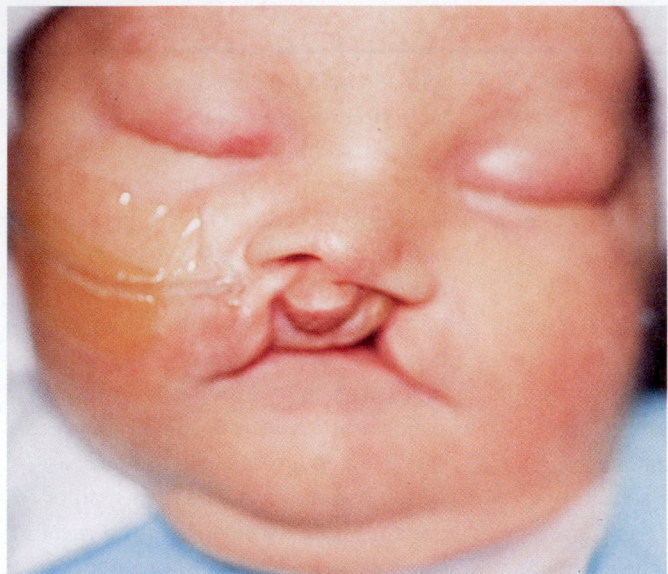

A

B

Figure 22-3. ■ **(A)** Bilateral cleft lip. **(B)** Repaired bilateral cleft lip. (Courtesy of Dr. Elizabeth Peterson, Spokane, WA.)

The cause of clefts is a combination of genetic and environmental influences. There is an increased incidence in families with a history of clefts. In the United States, cleft lip and cleft palate are more common in Native Americans and Asians than in Whites and Blacks. Since 1996, when cereal was fortified with folate in an attempt to decrease neural tube defects, the incidence of cleft lip and palate has decreased. The data suggest a correlation between folate and facial formation (Wong, Eskes, Kuihpers, et al., 1999).

Cultural Considerations

Infants in many developing countries do not have access to surgical treatment for cleft lip and palate. Medical teams from the United States and Canada may travel to these countries to perform surgery and teach surgical techniques to local doctors. Children from other countries may also be brought to this country for surgery.

Preoperative Nursing Considerations

The most immediate concern when a baby is born with a cleft lip or cleft palate is providing nutrition. The newborn with a cleft lip cannot make a seal around the nipple. Air leading between the cleft in the lip and the nipple prevents suction to draw the milk into the mouth. The small amounts of milk that do enter the mouth may leak out instead of being swallowed.

The newborn with a cleft palate will be unable to compress the nipple between the tongue and the palate. Milk that enters the mouth can enter the nasal cavity, and then drain from the nose or down the back of the throat. When milk drains down the throat without coordinated swallowing, the child is at risk for choking. Milk that pools in the nasal passages increases the risk for sinus and middle ear infections. Repeated middle ear infections can damage the tympanic membrane, resulting in hearing loss.

Prior to surgical repair, the baby must be fed. Special feeding equipment such as a long nipple with enlarged holes or a *Breck feeder* (syringe with a rubber tube) may be used. Parents will need instruction on the use of special equipment. Parents will also need encouragement and emotional support to handle this additional responsibility in the care of their child.

Sucking increases the strength of the muscles of the mouth that are needed for speech. When the lip and palate are not formed correctly, teeth may not erupt or may erupt out of alignment. A space may be present between the front teeth. The teeth, lips, and palate are used in forming sounds. When these structures are not formed properly, speech therapy is often required.

Surgical Correction

The surgical correction of cleft lip is usually accomplished in the first 3 months of life. To achieve the best cosmetic effect, the priority of care is to protect the suture line from trauma and infection. A **Logan clamp** (a metal bow taped to both sides of the suture line) or a butterfly bandage is frequently used to decrease tension on the suture line. Depending on the extent of the defect, the absence of infection, and the amount of suture line trauma, complete closure may be accomplished in one surgery. Cosmetic revision may need to be done at a later date.

Postoperative Nursing Considerations

Postoperatively, fluids are given through a dropper or syringe. The infant cannot suck until the suture line has healed. The infant should be placed supine or in a side-lying position to avoid rubbing the suture line on the bed. Soft restraints over the elbows may be used to keep the child from rubbing the suture line or sucking on the thumb or fingers. Antibiotic ointment is generally placed on the suture line to prevent infection. The infant should be medicated for pain as necessary to prevent crying and stress on the suture line.

Surgical closure of a cleft palate may need to be accomplished in stages, depending on the extent of the cleft. Closure of a cleft palate is usually begun at 4 to 6 months of age, with complete closure accomplished by age 2. As with cleft lip repair, preventing trauma and infection of the suture line is important. To prevent trauma, the nurse should teach the family to avoid putting hard or sharp objects into the child's mouth, including suction catheters, tongue blades, straws, forks, and toothbrushes. Once healing is complete, the child will need to be referred to a speech therapist.

Parents anticipate the birth of their "pretty" baby. When the child is born with an obvious facial defect, the family experiences the loss of their "perfect" child. Although in most cases corrective surgery can provide closure of the defect, a permanent scar remains. Nursing care is needed to allow families to express their grief or disappointment and to model a positive response to the newborn.

ESOPHAGEAL ATRESIA AND TRACHEOESOPHAGEAL FISTULA

Esophageal atresia and tracheoesophageal fistula may be found separately but are most commonly found together. When the esophagus ends in a blind pouch before entering the stomach, the anomaly is called **esophageal atresia.** The proximal end of the lower segment of the esophagus is also a closed pouch. **Tracheoesophageal fistula** is a connection between the trachea and the esophagus. The most common type of anomaly, illustrated in Figure 22-4 ■, occurs when the upper segment of the esophagus ends in a blind pouch connected to the trachea. The lower segment of the esophagus is connected to the trachea by a fistula. This formation is described as an esophageal atresia with proximal and distal tracheoesophageal fistula. Oral intake will be unable to enter the stomach (resulting in vomiting); instead, it will enter the trachea through the fistula, causing aspiration.

Esophageal atresia and tracheoesophageal fistula are potentially life threatening.

Manifestations

The infant with esophageal atresia and tracheoesophageal fistula presents with copious amounts of thin mucus shortly after birth. The secretions clear with suctioning, but they soon reappear. If a tracheoesophageal fistula is present, the stomach may become distended with trapped air. If the defects are not identified prior to feeding, the infant will regurgitate the feeding, or the feeding will be aspirated into the lungs. Severe respiratory distress will occur, and aspiration pneumonia may develop.

Diagnosis and Treatment

To diagnose this disorder, an attempt is made to pass a 5 or 8 French nasogastric tube into the stomach. The tube meets resistance and can be advanced only a short distance. X-ray, ultrasound, and echocardiogram are performed to confirm diagnosis.

Treatment is aimed at preventing respiratory complications until the defect can be surgically repaired. In the absence of other anomalies, surgical repair is usually completed in the first few days of life to separate the trachea from the esophagus and join the esophageal segments. If other anomalies are present, gastrostomy feedings may be necessary until the infant is stabilized (Figure 22-5 ■). (See also Procedure 13-21 ⊙⊙.)

Postoperatively, the infant should not be fed orally for 7 to 14 days to allow for healing. Once oral feedings begin, they are usually tolerated.

IMPERFORATE ANUS

Imperforate anus occurs when the membrane between the anal pit and the colon fails to break down.

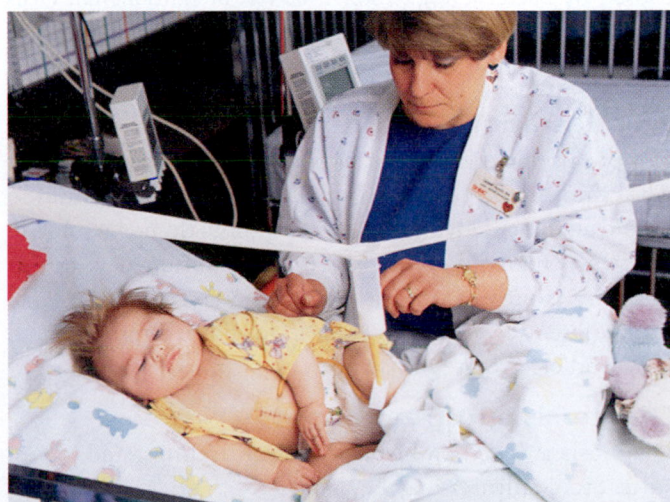

Figure 22-5. ■ Gastrostomy tube feeding into stomach. This type of feeding may be given to a child with tracheoesophageal fistula prior to surgery.

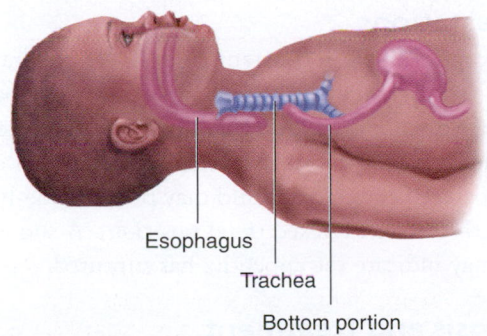

Esophagus

Trachea

Bottom portion of esophagus

Figure 22-4. ■ Esophageal atresia and tracheoesophageal fistula. Most commonly, the upper segment of the esophagus ends in a blind pouch connected to the trachea; a fistula connects the lower segment to the trachea.

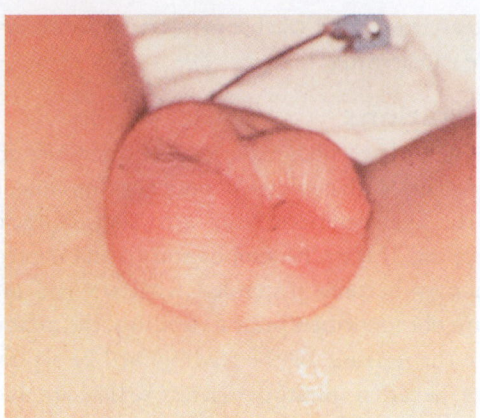

Figure 22-6. ■ Imperforate anus.

Manifestations

On inspection of the perineum, a thin membrane may be seen covering the anus or an obvious malformation can be seen, including a flat anus or deep dimple. If meconium is not passed within 24 hours of birth, an imperforate anus should be suspected. Anomalies of the urinary and reproductive systems should be suspected, especially if meconium is present in the urine. Figure 22-6 ■ illustrates this anorectal anomaly.

Treatment

Surgical correction, occurring shortly after birth, is a relatively simple procedure if no other anomaly is present. The baby should not receive oral intake until the anus is opened surgically. Feeding the infant would stimulate peristalsis and could cause rupture of the colon. If surgery is delayed, IV fluid and nutrition will be necessary.

Gastrointestinal Inflammation

GASTROENTERITIS

Gastroenteritis, or inflammation of the stomach, may be caused by bacteria (e.g., *Escherichia coli* or salmonella), virus (e.g., rotavirus), toxins, and allergies. The illness may resolve without complications or cause mild to severe dehydration.

Manifestations

Symptoms include nausea, vomiting, diarrhea, and fever. The child should be offered small amounts of clear fluid to help overcome dehydration. If symptoms do not resolve in 24 to 48 hours, signs of severe dehydration develop, or bleeding is present, the parents should consult a physician immediately. See Chapter 15 ⚭ for more information on fluid and electrolyte imbalances.

Diagnosis and Treatment

Diagnosis is based on history, clinical findings, and lab results. Stool cultures may be done.

If the child is hospitalized, the treatment would include IV fluids, electrolytes, and antibiotics. The child would be

MediaLink Probiotics

BOX 22-1	COMPLEMENTARY THERAPIES

Probiotics

When children are given a long course of broad-spectrum antibiotics, the normal intestinal flora can be destroyed. In such situations, the use of **probiotics** (foods or supplements containing live beneficial organisms) may be helpful to restore the normal flora. Many dairy manufacturers are enhancing foods with probiotics. Fermented foods such as miso, tempeh, soy sauce, and yogurt contain active probiotic cultures.

Individuals who have been on long-term antibiotic therapy may need large quantities of these foods to re-establish the normal flora in the gastrointestinal tract. In these cases, probiotic supplements in the form of powder or capsule may be better. These supplements, which contain *Lactobacillus, Acidophilus,* and bifidobacteria, should be kept refrigerated. Symptoms of diarrhea, bloating, and flatus should resolve within a few weeks.

Some practitioners believe that the Western diet, which is high in sugar and animal fat, prevents the normal flora from flourishing. They recommend a diet high in fiber and probiotic supplements for everyone (Pick, 2006).

Probiotics may have helpful effects beyond the gastrointestinal tract. They have also been studied in relation to prevention of atopic dermatitis in children (Kalliomäki, Salminen, Poussa, et al., 2003).

placed on enteric precautions, and a gown and gloves would be required when caring for the child.

Once vomiting and diarrhea subside, the child's diet should be progressed to full liquids and soft foods for a few days. Box 22-1 ■ provides information that might assist digestion.

APPENDICITIS

Appendicitis is inflammation of the vermiform appendix, a small sac at the end of the cecum. Appendicitis is most common in boys between 10 and 16, and rarely occurs before 2 years of age. Initially, there is a blockage of the lumen of the appendix followed by infection and inflammation. If the infection is not relieved or the appendix removed, the risk of rupture and subsequent peritonitis is great (Figure 22-7 ■).

Manifestations

The child presents with constant right lower quadrant pain. There is usually **rebound tenderness** following palpation (increase in discomfort when abdominal pressure is released). The child usually exhibits a fever, nausea, and an elevated white blood cell count. The child may prefer a side-lying position with the knees flexed (fetal position). A sudden relief of pain may indicate the appendix has ruptured.

Diagnosis and Treatment

Diagnosis may be more difficult in a child than in an adult because a child's symptoms and pain perception may be more generalized. Computed tomography (CT)

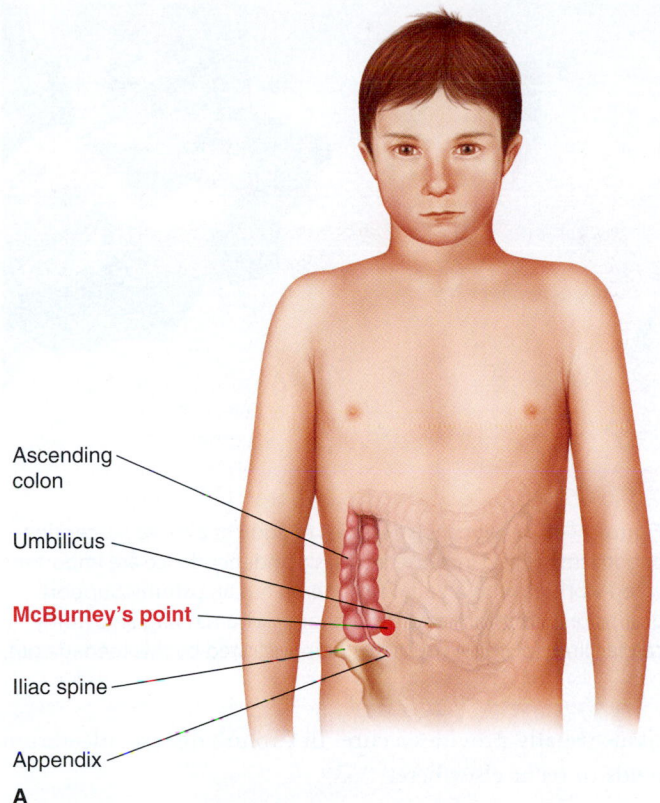

Ascending colon

Umbilicus

McBurney's point

Iliac spine

Appendix

A

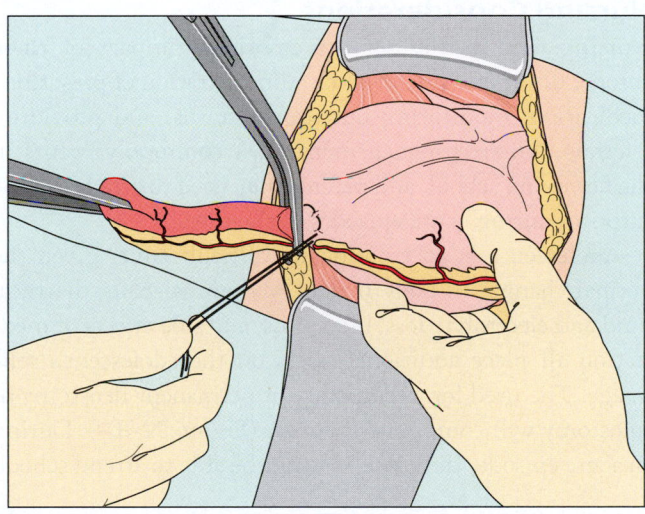

B

Figure 22-7. ■ (**A**) McBurney's point is the common location of pain in children and adolescents with appendicitis. (**B**) Appendectomy. The appendix and cecum are brought through the incision to the surface of the abdomen. The base of the appendix is clamped and ligated. The appendix is then removed.

with contrast is increasingly used. X-rays may or may not show a *fecalith* (a hard mass of feces) in the right lower quadrant. Tests may be performed to rule out a variety of possible disorders, such as urinary tract infection, inguinal hernia, sickle cell crisis, testicular torsion, pelvic inflammatory disease, and gastroenteritis.

The medical treatment of appendicitis is surgical intervention as soon as possible (see Figure 22-7B). Routine preoperative care should be provided, including surgical consent, an IV infusion, and sedation. With an uneventful surgical procedure, the child may be discharged within 12 to 24 hours. Routine discharge teaching should be given to the child and parents.

If the appendix ruptures prior to surgery, peritonitis spreads rapidly. If untreated, small bowel obstruction, electrolyte imbalance, and septic shock result. In this case, the nurse should anticipate a longer, more complex course of nursing care.

Nursing Considerations

Following surgery, the child should be monitored frequently for signs of infection and small bowel obstruction. Intravenous antibiotics will be administered, and IV fluids will be given until bowel function returns. Once bowel sounds are heard, small amounts of clear fluid are offered, and the diet is gradually progressed as tolerated. A small bowel obstruction would be treated with nasogastric decompression.

The child will be hospitalized approximately 1 to 5 days postoperatively. Prior to discharge, the child and parents should be instructed in use of pain medication, antibiotic administration, incision care, and the need for follow-up visits to the surgeon.

Evaluation of progress is based on a return of bowel function, a return of white blood cell count to normal, and a decrease in discomfort. The child and parents should verbalize an understanding of discharge instructions. The child should be able to return to normal activities within a few days. Vigorous activities such as contact sports should be avoided until approved by the physician.

INFLAMMATORY BOWEL DISEASE

Inflammatory bowel disease is two separate chronic disorders of the intestine:

- **Crohn's disease** (random inflammation of the entire gastrointestinal tract that involves all layers of the bowel wall)
- **Ulcerative colitis** (inflammation with sloughing of the mucosa of the large intestine).

These two disorders have similar symptoms and treatment but different pathology. It was once believed that these were diseases of young adults. However, the incidence of both disorders has increased in adolescence. The etiology is uncertain, but there is a strong support for a genetic association (Box 22-2 ■).

Manifestations

Crohn's disease begins as a small, localized ulcer, and then grows in size and depth. The onset of symptoms is gradual, with abdominal cramps followed by diarrhea. These symptoms subside in a few days and then recur, becoming more severe each time. Over time, the child develops anorexia, weight loss, and general malaise.

Ulcerative colitis also begins with abdominal cramps and diarrhea. Lower abdominal pain occurs before and during a bowel movement and stops with the passage of stool and flatus. The stool is mixed with mucus and blood. Weight loss and delayed growth occur over time.

Diagnosis and Treatment

Diagnosis is based on determining the location and extent of involvement. Stool specimens are used to rule out an infectious process. Biopsy is taken during a colonoscopy. Laboratory studies are useful in identifying secondary conditions such as anemia, electrolyte imbalance, and malnutrition.

Medical treatment for both disorders involves the administration of corticosteroids, antibiotics, and antidiarrheal medication (Table 22-1 ■). For moderate to severe Crohn's disease, including fistula-forming disease, immunosuppressants such as Remicade (infliximab) are administered. The goal of nutritional therapy is to provide adequate calories and nutrients for growth without aggravating the inflammation and diarrhea. Total parenteral nutrition (TPN) is often given during an acute episode when the bowel must be rested. TPN can be used to improve nutrition by increasing the amount of protein, carbohydrates, vitamins, and minerals to aid in healing. At times, surgery is needed. A temporary colostomy or ileostomy is performed to allow the lower small intestine or colon to rest and heal. In ulcerative colitis, the removal of the affected

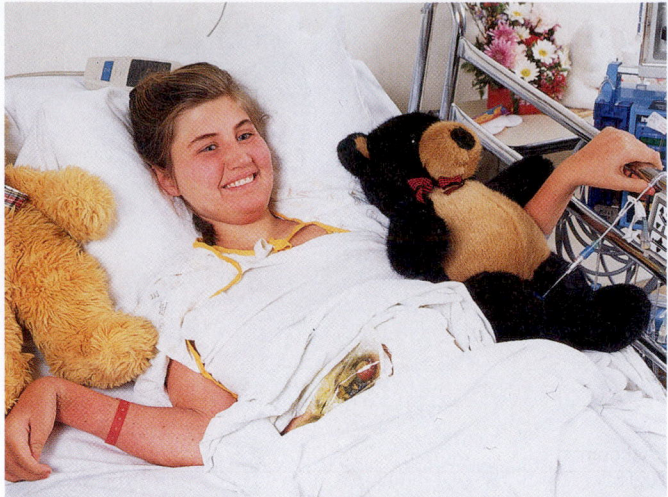

Figure 22-8. ■ Nursing strategies to address altered perception of body image and increase feelings of independence are important when working with an adolescent who has an ostomy. Support groups or a visit from another teenager who has had an ostomy can facilitate positive coping, as demonstrated by this teenage girl.

tissue usually provides a cure. In Crohn's disease, ulceration tends to recur elsewhere.

Nursing Considerations

Nursing care focuses on the emotional impact of these chronic disorders, teaching the administration of prescribed medication, monitoring nutritional status, and providing referrals. Nursing management most commonly occurs in the home and school, and parents may need to arrange home tutoring during acute episodes of the disease.

Adolescence is an emotionally difficult time, given the normal changes in body image. Abdominal pain, diarrhea, fluid and electrolyte loss, blood loss, and side effects of medication all place additional stress on the adolescent's self-image. The need for a temporary or permanent ileostomy or colostomy will compound the issue (Figure 22-8 ■). During an acute episode, the client may not be able to attend school,

TABLE 22-1

Pharmacology: Drugs Used for Inflammatory Bowel Disease

DRUG (COMMON BRAND NAME AND GENERIC)	USUAL ROUTE/DOSE	CLASSIFICATION	SELECTED SIDE EFFECTS	DON'T GIVE IF
Kaopectate, Imodium (loperamide)	1–2 mg bid-tid follow with 0.1 mg/kg/dose after each loose stool	Antidiarrheal	Constipation, toxic megacolon in clients with ulcerative colitis	Child has severe diarrhea (consult care provider)
Remicade (infliximab)	Child over 6 years 5 mg/kg IV over 2 hours; may repeat ×2 at 4-week intervals	Immunosuppressant	Fatigue, fever, pain, headache, dizziness, infections	Suspected or identified infection is present

which may limit support from friends. Encourage the adolescent to maintain contact with friends by telephone, e-mail, cards, and visits. Referral to visiting nurses and support groups for children with ostomies and the Crohn's Colitis Foundation may be useful.

Because adolescents can provide a lot of their own care, instructions should be given to both the client and the parents. Demonstration and return demonstration in care of central venous catheters and administration of TPN, including maintaining sterile technique, operating infusion pumps, and obtaining blood glucose levels, are important aspects of teaching. Teaching should also include the importance of adhering to the prescribed medication regimen, with an emphasis on continuing the medications even when the client is asymptomatic. If an ostomy is required, teaching must include the care of the site, bag change, and odor management. Procedure 22-1 ■ describes the steps in ostomy care.

Intestinal Parasites

Intestinal parasites occur most frequently in tropical regions but can occur in any area of the United States. Typically, outbreaks occur in areas where water is not treated,

---

PROCEDURE 22-1   Ostomy Care

Purpose
- To assess and care for the skin around the stoma
- To collect stool
- To maintain odors for client comfort and self-esteem

Equipment
- Disposable gloves
- Bedpan
- Solvent (presaturated sponges or liquid)
- Moisture-proof bag for disposal of pouches
- Cleaning materials, including toilet tissue, warm water, mild soap, washclothes, towel
- Skin barrier (paste, powder, water, or liquid skin sealant)
- Stoma measuring guide
- Pen or pencil, scissors
- Clean ostomy appliance (pouch) with belt (optional)
- Tail closure clamp
- Deodorant (liquid or tablet)

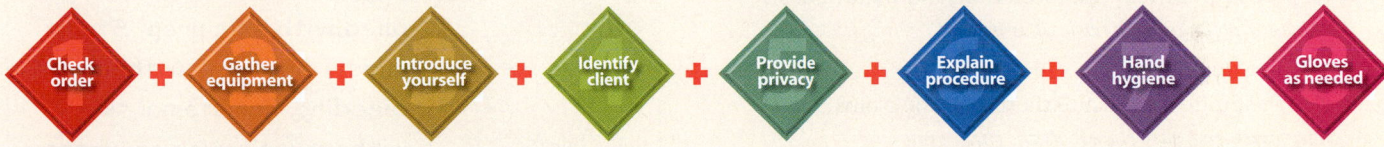

Check order + Gather equipment + Introduce yourself + Identify client + Provide privacy + Explain procedure + Hand hygiene + Gloves as needed

Interventions

1. Determine the need for appliance change.
   - Assess the used appliance for fluid leakage. *Fluid leakage can irritate and damage skin.*
   - Ask client about discomfort at or around the stoma. *Discomfort around stoma could indicate skin irritation and breakdown.*
   - Assess fullness of pouch. *Pouch should be emptied or changed when one-third to one-half full. The weight of an overfilled pouch can cause it to detach from the skin, causing spillage and skin irritation.*

2. Select appropriate time.
   - Avoid changing pouch close to meals or visiting hours. *Odor may reduce the appetite, offend visitors, or embarrass the client.*
   - Avoid times when increased peristalsis would increase drainage. *Food intake and certain medications will increase peristalsis. It is better to avoid these times so stool does not leak out of the stoma and onto the skin or linen.*

3. Prepare the client.
   - Explain the procedure to the client and parents. *Parents will need to provide care at home. Older children may learn self-care. Changing the pouch should not be painful, but it might be distasteful. Generally, it is not much different than changing a dirty diaper.*
   - Position the client in a supine position or sitting in the bathroom. *If the client is unable to get out of bed, the supine position is used. Sitting or standing in the bathroom may be the position used in the home and should also be used in the hospital.*

4. Empty the pouch.
   - Don gloves, unfasten the belt (if one is present). *Gloves are recommended to prevent contaminating hands.*
   - Empty the pouch through the bottom tail by opening the clamp and squeezing the stool into the bedpan or toilet. *Emptying the pouch before removal prevents spillage onto the client's skin.*

- Assess the amount, color, and consistency of stool. *Assessment is necessary to determine if bowel is functioning properly.*
- If the pouch is attached to the skin and no leaks are apparent, the bag can be rinsed with warm water, drained into the bedpan or toilet, and the clamp reapplied. *As long as the appliance is attached to the skin and no skin irritation is apparent, the appliance can be reused. It should be changed every 48 to 72 hours.*

5. Remove the appliance.
   - Peel the pouch off slowly while supporting the client's skin. *Keeping the skin taut lessens discomfort and prevents skin abrasions.*
   - Dispose of the pouch in a moisture-proof bag.

6. Clean the stoma and surrounding skin.
   - Gently wipe any excess stool from the stoma with toilet tissue and dispose of it in moisture-proof bag or toilet.
   - Wash stoma and surrounding skin with warm water (and soap) using washcloth. Rinse and dry the skin with towel. *Soap may dry the skin and so may not be used. The stoma has no sensory neurons, so cleaning will not cause discomfort but may stimulate peristalsis.*
   - Use special cleanser to remove hard, dry stool, or remnants of old stoma adhesive. *Special cleansers emulsify to prevent damage to the skin.*
   - Rinse and pat dry. *Skin must be dry before new pouch is applied.*

7. Assess the stoma (Figure 22-9 ■).
   - Inspect stoma for redness, swelling, size, and bleeding.
   - Inspect skin for redness, ulceration, and irritation. *Slight redness after appliance removal is normal.*

8. Apply new appliance.
   - Use the guide to measure the size of the stoma. *Stoma size varies and may change as the child grows.*
   - Be sure opening in the pouch adhesive is the correct size. Cut to fit if needed. *Some pouches come with standard size openings, whereas others need to be cut to fit. The entire stoma should fit through the opening.*
   - Apply skin barrier (powder, paste, or liquid). Follow manufacture's directions. *A variety of products are available.*

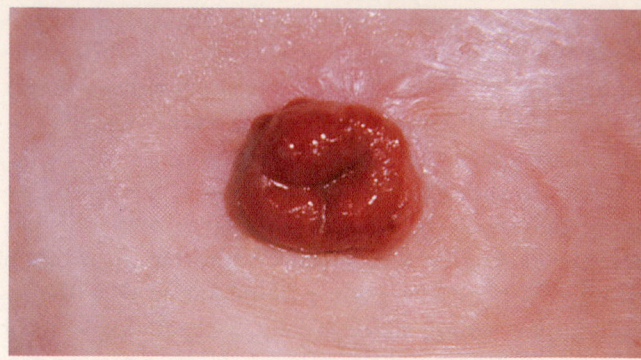

Figure 22-9. ■ Healthy-appearing stoma (Courtesy of Carol Williams, RN, BS, University of California Davis Medical Center.)

Parents should be taught to use the product(s) they will be using at home. Skin barrier protects the tissue from stool and moisture.
- Center the pouch over the stoma. *The adhesive from the pouch should not touch the stoma. Adhesive can irritate and damage the stomal tissue.*
- Gently press against the skin.
- Place deodorant in the pouch. Close the tail of the pouch with the clamp. *Deodorant is optional.*
- Dispose of supplies. Air freshener may be needed.

SAMPLE DOCUMENTATION

(date and time)   Ostomy appliance removed, skin and stoma cleansed with warm water. Fresh pouch applied with skin prep. Stoma moist, dark red, without bleeding. Peristomal skin without irritation or ulceration. Client denies discomfort. _____

J. House, LPN

---

poor sanitation exists, or food is not properly cooked. However, children are also exposed to larva or eggs from playing in contaminated dirt at playgrounds and in sandboxes. Infected children playing in wet or dirty diapers can transfer eggs or larva to the soil, where others can become infected. The most common intestinal parasites are included in Table 22-2 ■.

Manifestations

Symptoms of intestinal parasites include abdominal cramps, diarrhea, and weight loss. Some parasites lay eggs at the anal opening, resulting in anal irritation and itching. Severe infections may result in intestinal obstruction and liver and lung involvement.

Diagnosis and Treatment

The organism is identified by laboratory examination of stool specimen. Treatment involves administration of prescribed medication. Generally, all family members and others in direct contact with the infected child should be treated. Follow-up stool examination is necessary to ensure cure. Repeat medication regimen may be required. Preven-

TABLE 22-2

Common Intestinal Parasites

PARASITE	TRANSMISSION	SYMPTOMS	TREATMENT
Giardiasis Organism: protozoan *Guardia lamblia*	Person to person, unfiltered water, infected food, animals. Organisms enter through mouth, feed in the duodenum and jejunum, and are excreted in stool.	Abdominal cramps; foul-smelling, loose, or watery stool containing gelatinous material.	Medication: furazolidone (has fewer side effects but is more expensive), quinacrine
Pinworms Organism: nematode *Enterobius vermicularis*	Discharged eggs inhaled or hand to mouth. Eggs hatch in intestine in 15–28 days; larvae migrate to cecum After mating, mature female leaves out the anus. Can move to vagina and urethra.	Worm movement causes intense itching, especially at night when female leaves anus.	Medication: mebendazole, pyrantel, pamoate, piperazine citrate Repeat treatment in 2–3 weeks. All family members should be treated.
Roundworms (Ascariasis) Organism: nematode *Ascaris lumbricoides*	Eggs carried hand to mouth. Eggs hatch in small intestine. Larva can penetrate intestinal villi, enter portal circulation and liver. Some ascend to upper respiratory tract, are swallowed, move to small intestine, and cycle repeats. Some eggs are excreted in stool.	Severe infection results in intestinal obstruction, peritonitis, jaundice and lung involvement.	Medication: mebendazole, pyrantel, pamoate, piperazine citrate Check stools in 2 weeks and monthly for 3 months. Intestinal obstruction may require surgery. All family members should be treated.
Hookworms Organism: nematode *Necator americanus*	Direct contact with infected soil. Larvae attach to and penetrate skin. Travel in blood to lungs, move in sputum to throat and are swallowed. Worms live in small intestine, feed on villi causing bleeding. Eggs excreted in stool, hatch in damp shaded soil.	Severe infection results in anemia and malnutrition. Larvae on skin may cause irritation, burning, and itching.	Medication: mebendazole, pyrantel pamoate Examine stool in 2 weeks and monthly for 3 months. All family members should be treated.
Visceral larva migrans (Toxocariasis) Organism: nematode *Toxocara canis* or *Toxocara catis* (commonly found in dogs and cats)	Ingestion of eggs from soil. Hatch in intestine. Mobile larva migrate to liver and eventually all organs, including brain. They encapsulate in dense fibrous tissue.	Low-grade fever, recurrent upper airway disease, hepatomegaly, pulmonary infiltration, neurologic problems. Hypereosinophilia in blood.	None specific Infection usually resolves spontaneously. Deworm household pets. Keep away from animal droppings.

tion includes frequent hand washing, covering sandboxes when not in use, and frequent diaper changes with perineal care for infected children.

Malabsorption Disorders

Malabsorption disorders result from lack of nutrients in the diet, an inability of the small intestine to absorb nutrients, or liver disorders that can result in lack of bile for digestion and alter metabolism of nutrients.

CELIAC DISEASE

Celiac disease (*gluten-sensitive enteropathy* or *sprue*) is a chronic malabsorption syndrome in which the child is unable to digest gluten, a protein found in wheat, barley, rye, and oats. The inability to digest gluten results in an increase in the amino acid glutamine, which is toxic to the mucous membrane in the small intestine. Over time, the intestinal villi are damaged. Initially, fat absorption is affected, resulting in **steatorrhea** (fat in the stool). Eventually, absorption of protein, carbohydrates, calcium, iron, and fat-soluble vitamins is affected. Research is being conducted to determine the existence of a genetic influence in the child developing celiac disease.

Manifestations

Symptoms do not begin until the child has ingested solid foods containing gluten, usually in the first 2 years of life. When gluten is introduced into the diet, the child experiences chronic diarrhea, vomiting, and failure to grow. The stools are large, foul-smelling, greasy, and frothy.

Diagnosis and Treatment

Diagnosis is based on symptoms, fat content in the stool, and intestinal biopsy.

The child improves rapidly when gluten is eliminated from the diet. Vitamin supplements may be prescribed if the child is malnourished. Growth patterns usually return to normal within a year.

Nursing Considerations

The family of a child with celiac disease must establish a plan for lifelong avoidance of gluten-containing foods. When any such serious disorder is identified, parents will need time to adjust to the diagnosis and to incorporate new information and lifestyle requirements. The nurse provides emotional support for this transition, as well as information and referrals. A nutritionist or celiac support group can assist the family in developing a variety of recipes focusing on viable foods (e.g., fruits, vegetables, meat, rice).

Teach parents that the child with celiac disease will need to avoid gluten (wheat, rye, barley) completely and for life. Parents must not reintroduce these foods once symptoms disappear. Reintroduction of gluten puts the child at risk for growth retardation and development of gastrointestinal cancer as an adult. Also teach parents to read labels carefully for "hidden" sources of gluten. Some examples of unexpected gluten-containing foods are:

- Mayonnaise
- Many types of vinegar
- Catsup
- Canned soup

Diet will need to be reviewed and reinforced as the child grows. This is especially true for adolescence, when peer group pressure may cause the child to want to abandon the required diet in order to "fit in."

LACTOSE INTOLERANCE

Lactose intolerance is a congenital or acquired disorder in which the child fails to produce lactase, an enzyme needed in the digestion of lactose. Lactose or milk sugar is found in milk and milk products. The child rapidly develops diarrhea as soon as milk is consumed.

Implementing a lactose-free diet relieves the symptoms. In the newborn, soy formulas are used instead of breastfeeding or milk-based formula. In the older child, eliminating milk and milk products from the diet is necessary. (Many soy substitutes are now available.) In some children, adding enzyme tablets such as LactAid to the milk or sprinkling it on food corrects the problem.

Nutrition Disorders

KWASHIORKOR

Kwashiorkor is a deficiency in protein in the diet that results in muscle wasting. It is most common in underdeveloped countries, where malnutrition is common. Frequently, the protein deficiency occurs even when the diet is nearly adequate in calories.

Manifestations

Symptoms may develop after the child has been weaned from the breast due to the birth of a sibling. Because of the lack of protein in the diet, the child fails to grow, muscles waste, and there is edema in the abdomen. Anorexia, diarrhea, and vomiting may occur. The hair becomes thin, brittle, and lightens in color due to the lack of melanin. Skin breaks down and becomes infected. The child is irritable at first and then becomes mentally dull. Figure 22-10 ■ shows the multisystem effects of malnutrition.

Treatment

Treatment is mainly preventive. Although kwashiorkor may never be totally eradicated worldwide, many organizations are working to supply sufficient quantities of protein in the diet to prevent starvation. Powdered protein, sprinkled on the culturally prepared food, can relieve the problem. In established cases of kwashiorkor, the addition of protein to the diet may prevent more serious growth retardation but may not correct the existing damage.

RICKETS

Rickets is a condition caused by a vitamin D deficiency. Vitamin D is necessary for the proper absorption and utilization of calcium and phosphorus. When deficiency exists, the result is failure of the bones to develop. The child may manifest bowlegs, knock-knees, beading along the ribs (*rachitic rosary*), and improper formation of teeth.

The widespread use of vitamins and fortified foods has nearly eliminated rickets in North America. However, parents should be encouraged to provide well-balanced meals and exercise in the sunlight (because the skin synthesizes vitamin D when exposed to the sun).

SCURVY

Scurvy is caused by a lack of vitamin C in the diet. Vitamin C is a water-soluble vitamin that is destroyed by heat. Because vitamin C is not stored in the body, daily intake is required. The main sources of vitamin C in the diet are citrus fruits and raw leafy vegetables. Vegetables should be cooked in small amounts of water at low heat to prevent destruction of vitamin C. Vitamin C tablets may be used to supplement the diet.

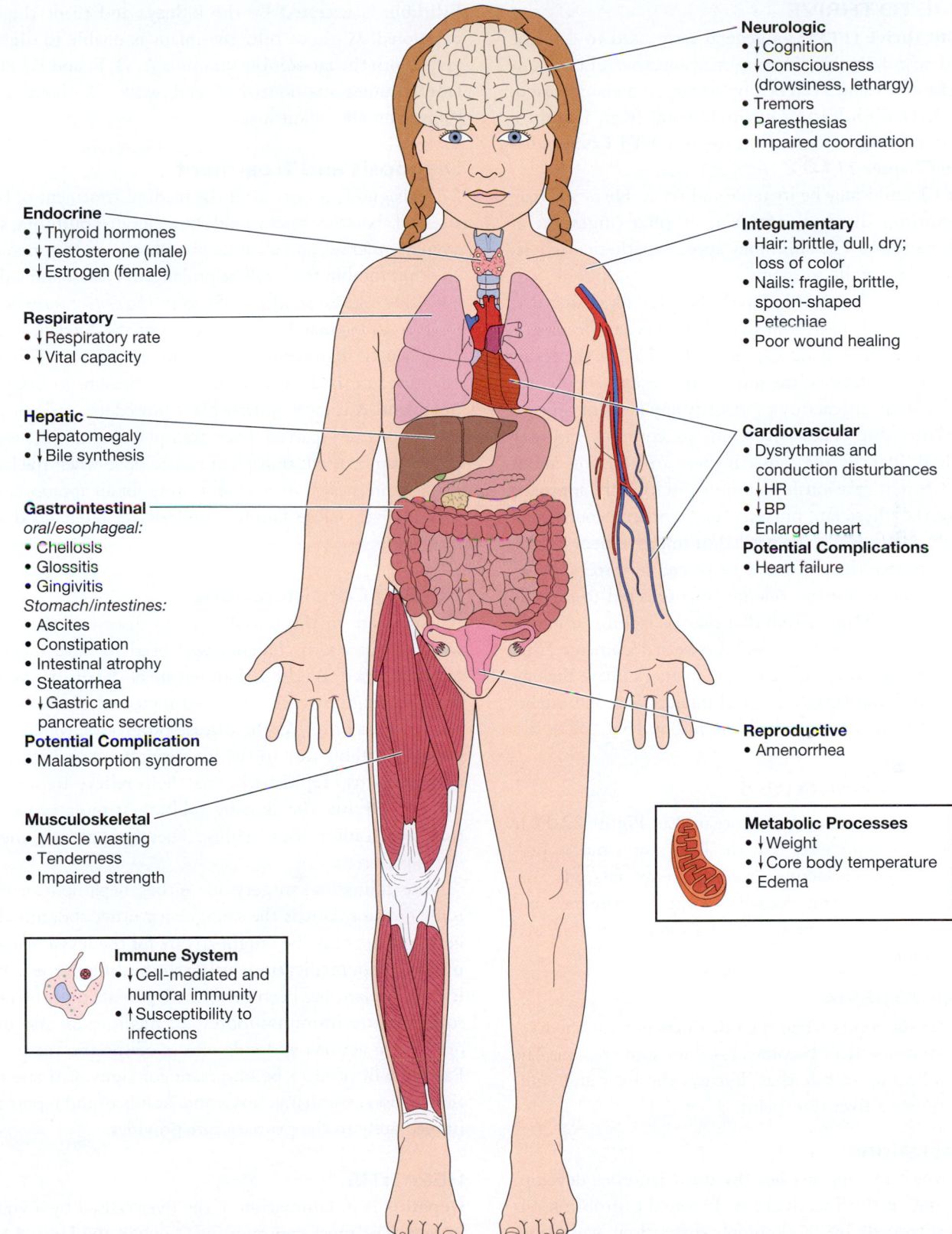

Neurologic
- ↓Cognition
- ↓Consciousness (drowsiness, lethargy)
- Tremors
- Paresthesias
- Impaired coordination

Endocrine
- ↓Thyroid hormones
- ↓Testosterone (male)
- ↓Estrogen (female)

Integumentary
- Hair: brittle, dull, dry; loss of color
- Nails: fragile, brittle, spoon-shaped
- Petechiae
- Poor wound healing

Respiratory
- ↓Respiratory rate
- ↓Vital capacity

Hepatic
- Hepatomegaly
- ↓Bile synthesis

Cardiovascular
- Dysrythmias and conduction disturbances
- ↓HR
- ↓BP
- Enlarged heart

Potential Complications
- Heart failure

Gastrointestinal
oral/esophageal:
- Chellosis
- Glossitis
- Gingivitis

Stomach/intestines:
- Ascites
- Constipation
- Intestinal atrophy
- Steatorrhea
- ↓Gastric and pancreatic secretions

Potential Complication
- Malabsorption syndrome

Reproductive
- Amenorrhea

Metabolic Processes
- ↓Weight
- ↓Core body temperature
- Edema

Musculoskeletal
- Muscle wasting
- Tenderness
- Impaired strength

Immune System
- ↓Cell-mediated and humoral immunity
- ↑Susceptibility to infections

Figure 22-10. ■ Multisystem effects of malnutrition.

FAILURE TO THRIVE

Failure to thrive (FTT) is a general term used to describe the child who fails to gain weight or loses weight for unknown reasons. Causes can be physical (e.g., malabsorption, heart or liver disorders) or environmental (e.g., failure to bond with parents or neglect by caregivers). FTT is also discussed in Chapter 27 ⚭.

The FTT child may be irritable and weak. He or she may have vomiting, diarrhea, anorexia, or **pica** (ingestion of nonfood material). The child may appear apathetic, listless, and exhibit "rag doll" limpness.

The child may be admitted to the hospital for evaluation. Malabsorption and heart and liver disorders can be identified and treated with good success. When FTT is the result of environmental factors, the nurse must be alert in observing child-parent interaction to identify any areas of concern in the relationship. These situations are complex and may take time to identify the cause. If there are concerns about the child-parent relationship, a multidisciplinary approach involving the physician, nurses, social workers, counselors, and family agencies may be needed. If improvement cannot be demonstrated, the child may be placed in foster care. In the hospital environment, one nurse is selected to provide the nurturing and interaction that may be lacking at home.

The prognosis is questionable. It has been documented that children who have been starved emotionally can have lifelong problems involving language, social interactions, and intelligence (see the importance of bonding in Box 16-1 ⚭).

Hepatic Disorders

The liver is one of the most vital organs (see Figure 22-1). It is important to remember that the liver stores blood; produces blood clotting factors; stores proteins, fats, glucose, iron, and vitamins; and detoxifies drugs, hormones, and other substances. Two common liver disorders are addressed in this chapter.

BILIARY ATRESIA

Biliary atresia occurs when the bile ducts outside the liver fail to form properly or become closed for some reason. The result is a backup of bile that destroys the liver and commonly requires a liver transplant.

Manifestations

Initially, the baby appears healthy until jaundice develops in the second or third week of life. Elevated bilirubin levels are accompanied by abdominal distention and **hepatomegaly** (enlarged liver). The infant is easily bruised, has prolonged bleeding time, and experiences **pruritis** (itching). Within a short time, **splenomegaly** (enlarged spleen) develops. Because of the absence of bile, the stools become off-white or clay colored and are the consistency of putty.

Bilirubin is excreted by the kidneys and turns the urine teacolored. Without bile, the infant is unable to digest fat and absorb the fat-soluble vitamins A, D, E, and K. The infant becomes malnourished and weak. Without a liver transplant, the infant dies.

Diagnosis and Treatment

Early diagnosis is critical in the medical treatment of biliary atresia. Laboratory tests would show elevated bilirubin, serum aminotransferase, and alkaline phosphatase and ammonia levels. Prothrombin time will be prolonged. Ultrasound will rule out other causes of illness. Surgery (*hepatoportoenterostomy* or *Kasai procedure*) may be done to connect the duodenum to the porta hepatis segment of bile duct inside the liver. This surgical procedure is done as a palliative measure to delay liver transplant. Advances in transplant procedures make it possible to perform partial liver transplantation. Because live donors can be used, transplant can be done when the baby is in optimum health instead of waiting for an appropriate-size cadaver liver. Close family members are often good tissue matches.

Nursing Considerations

Nursing care in the initial stage of disease is the same as with any newborn. Parents will need to have diagnostic tests explained. As the serious nature of the disease becomes more evident, parents will need increased emotional support and teaching. As the disease progresses, the baby will become irritable due to the intense itching and accumulation of toxins. Tepid baths may help relieve itching temporarily. Drying the skin by rubbing stimulates vasodilation, which intensifies itching. Therefore, patting the skin dry is preferred.

Care following surgery for either hepatoportoenterostomy or transplant is the same as any other abdominal surgery. Parents must be taught to care for the incision and administer pain medication during the healing process. When liver transplant has been performed, parents must be taught to administer immunosuppressant medication, and to recognize the actions and side effects of specific medication. Parents will need to be observant for signs of tissue rejection (nausea, vomiting, fever, and jaundice) and report them immediately to the primary care provider.

HEPATITIS

Hepatitis is inflammation of the liver caused by a viral infection. The most common infections in the United States are from hepatitis A virus (HAV), hepatitis B virus (HBV), hepatitis C virus (HCV), and hepatitis D virus (HDV). Hepatitis E virus (HEV) is more common in unclean water in developing countries. Table 22-3 ■ compares the common causes of hepatitis.

TABLE 22-3

Common Causes of Hepatitis

ORGANISM	MODE OF TRANSMISSION	INCUBATION	CLINICAL MANIFESTATION	IMMUNIZATION AVAILABLE
Hepatitis A virus	Fecal-oral route, person to person, contaminated water or food (shellfish)	4 weeks (10–50 days)	Acute onset (may be less acute in young children). Children usually do not become jaundiced. Flulike symptoms.	Immune serum globulin Hepatitis A vaccine
Hepatitis B virus	Blood and body fluids	1–6 months	Nausea, vomiting, anorexia, fatigue, upper right quadrant pain, hepatomegaly.	Hepatitis B immune globulin Hepatitis B vaccine
Hepatitis C virus	Blood and blood products	6–7 weeks	Frequent episodes of flulike symptoms without jaundice. Risk of liver cancer.	None
Hepatitis D virus	Blood and blood products Found with HBV infection	2–8 weeks	Same as HBV. Causes fulminating hepatitis.	Hepatitis B vaccine
Hepatitis E virus	Fecal-oral route from water in developing countries	2–9 weeks	Severe flulike symptoms. High mortality in pregnancy and fetal loss.	None

clinical ALERT

Nurses and other health care workers could come in contact with the blood or body fluids containing hepatitis virus. Standard precautions should be used at all times. It is recommended that health care workers receive three doses of hepatitis B immunization.

Hepatitis A, commonly called *infectious hepatitis*, is highly contagious. Because it is transmitted primarily by the fecal-oral route during the early stages of the illness, large numbers of people can become exposed. The HAV lives on surfaces for up to 1 month, so diaper changing tables should be cleansed frequently. Children often become infected from day care workers who change diapers and then prepare food. Although HAV is mild in most people, in those individuals with pre-existing liver disease, HAV infection could cause liver failure and death.

Hepatitis B, commonly called *serum hepatitis*, is a serious illness. Transmission of HBV occurs through blood and body fluids exchange, including sexual contact, sharing IV needles, and from mother to fetus. Those individuals testing positive for HBV should also be tested for HDV.

Hepatitis C is transmitted through blood and blood products. Children requiring repeat blood transfusion for treatment of sickle cell disease or hemophilia are at risk for developing HCV. IV drug use, body piercing, and multiple sexual partners increase the risk.

Hepatitis D is found in conjunction with HBV. When signs of liver failure are more acute than would be expected in an individual with HBV, HDV infection should be suspected. Children with HBV coupled with HDV are at extreme risk for developing **fulminating hepatitis** (progressive, total destruction of the liver). These children die within 2 weeks unless a liver transplant is completed.

Hepatitis E is transmitted in contaminated water in developing countries. Most commonly, outbreaks of HEV occur shortly after a heavy rain when groundwater becomes contaminated with runoff from outdoor septic systems.

The body's response to the hepatitis virus is the same. At first, the virus attacks the **parenchymal** cells (functional part of an organ), resulting in local degeneration and necrosis of

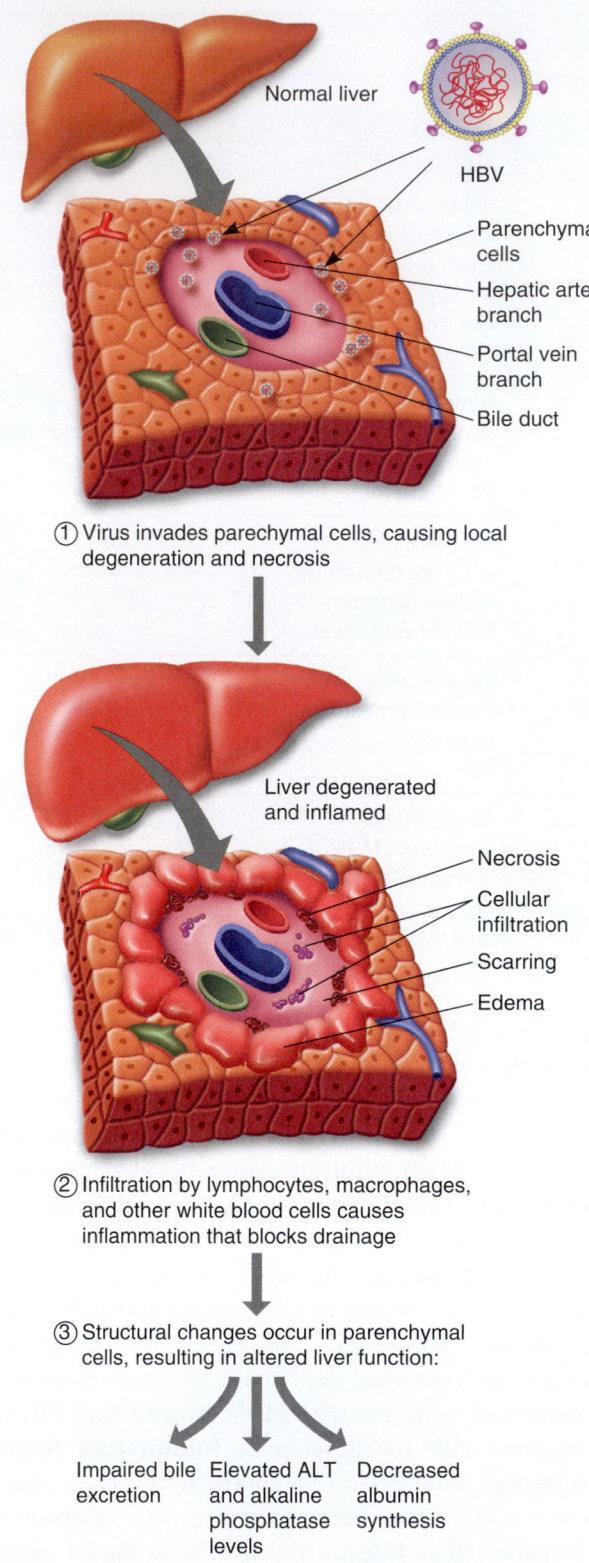

① Virus invades parechymal cells, causing local degeneration and necrosis

Normal liver

HBV

Parenchymal cells

Hepatic artery branch

Portal vein branch

Bile duct

Liver degenerated and inflamed

Necrosis

Cellular infiltration

Scarring

Edema

② Infiltration by lymphocytes, macrophages, and other white blood cells causes inflammation that blocks drainage

③ Structural changes occur in parenchymal cells, resulting in altered liver function:

Impaired bile excretion	Elevated ALT and alkaline phosphatase levels	Decreased albumin synthesis

Figure 22-11. ■ Pathophysiology of hepatitis. The hepatitis virus causes degeneration and necrosis of the liver, which results in abnormal liver function and illness.

the tissue (Figure 22-11 ■). This stimulates the inflammatory process. Swelling and an accumulation of white blood cells blocks the drainage of bile. The backup of bile further damages the liver tissue, resulting in an elevation in bilirubin,

and ALT and alkaline phosphatase in the blood. The liver fails to produce enough albumins, resulting in generalized edema. In most cases, the body's immune system is able to destroy the hepatitis virus, stopping the liver destruction. Regeneration of liver tissue occurs in approximately 3 months. Serology studies would show positive for antibodies to one or more of the hepatitis viruses. For children with a pre-existing liver disorder or an impaired immune system, continued liver destruction could result in death.

clinical ALERT

When hepatitis is present, the liver is unable to detoxify and metabolize drugs at the usual rate. Medications should be administered carefully and the child monitored closely for both side effects and toxic effects.

PHENYLKETONURIA

Phenylketonuria (PKU) is an autosomal recessive inherited disorder that affects the body's ability to use protein. Normally, a liver enzyme, phenylalanine hydroxylase, breaks down the amino acid phenylaline into tyrosine. Children with PKU have a deficiency in this enzyme.

Manifestations

As phenylalanine builds up in the blood, it causes a musty odor of the body and urine, as well as vomiting, irritability, seizures, hyperactivity, and rash. Over time, elevated levels of phenylalanine result in mental retardation.

Diagnosis

State laws require all infants to be screened for PKU. To ensure accurate results, the infant must receive either breast milk or formula for several days. Tests performed on the infant who leaves the birthing center 24 hours after delivery should be repeated. PKU is also discussed under newborn care in Chapter 9 ◎◎. Figure 9-27 ◎◎ shows the heel stick performed on newborns to test for PKU.

Treatment

Special formulas, such as albumaid XP, lofenalac, and minafen, are used in treatment until the child is ready for solid food. Then a diet low in phenylalanine is maintained for life. The diet must also meet the child's requirements for growth. The phenylalanine diet would be low in meat, milk products, and aspartame. Modified protein in which phenylalanine has been removed can be used. If diet modifications are not followed for at least the first 6 years, there is a significant impact on the child's IQ. The modified diet must be followed for life. If adults fail to follow the diet, their IQ will remain the same, but they will have difficulty focusing on tasks and processing rapidly (Box 22-3 ■). Because this is a disorder that requires lifelong changes in diet, nursing considerations are similar to those for celiac disease.

Phenylketonuria

PKU is more common in communities with numerous intermarriages over several generations. It is rare in African, Jewish, and Japanese populations.

Motility Disorders

Motility disorders prevent gastrointestinal contents from moving through the system in a normal manner.

GASTROESOPHAGEAL REFLUX

Gastroesophageal reflux disease (GERD) is a condition caused by a relaxation of the cardiac sphincter. The relaxation of the cardiac sphincter allows gastric contents to return to the esophagus. Some "spitting up" is considered normal in infants, but continued regurgitation can lead to aspiration, pneumonia, or apnea. The infant will appear hungry, irritable, and have a history of vomiting. He or she will eat but still lose weight.

Gastroesophageal reflux is more common in premature infants and children with neurologic impairment. Treatment of gastroesophageal reflex depends on the severity of the disorder. Mild cases may be treated by adding rice cereal to thicken the feedings, positioning the child upright 30 degrees after feeding, and avoiding acidic juices. Medications may be prescribed to reduce stomach acid.

Severe cases of gastroesophageal reflux may require surgery such as a *Nissen fundoplication* (which anchors the lower esophageal sphincter below the diaphragm and reinforces the high-pressure area). A gastrostomy tube will be left in place for approximately 6 weeks. Parents will need to be taught to administer gastrostomy feedings and to care for the insertion site.

PYLORIC STENOSIS

Pyloric stenosis is an obstruction of the pyloric canal caused by a thickening of the pyloric sphincter and narrowing of the passageway between the stomach and the duodenum (Figure 22-12 ■). As the stomach tries to push food through the narrowed lumen, the mucous membrane becomes inflamed and swollen, narrowing the lumen further and eventually causing total obstruction.

Manifestations

The disorder occurs most commonly in 5-week-old firstborn boys. The infant with pyloric stenosis is usually asymptomatic until 2 to 4 weeks after birth, appearing healthy but possibly regurgitating a small amount of milk after feeding. Parents report the child to be a "good eater." As the pylorus narrows, the child begins to vomit after every feeding.

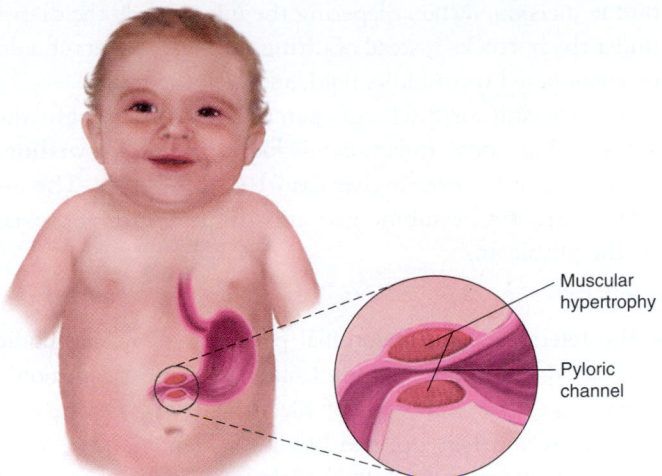

Figure 22-12. ■ Pyloric stenosis results in symptoms of projectile vomiting and visible peristalsis.

Within a few weeks, the vomiting becomes projectile, and the emesis may be ejected up to 3 feet from the infant. The infant becomes dehydrated, loses weight, and passes fewer and smaller stools.

A small round mass may be felt in the right upper quadrant, and peristaltic waves may be seen across the abdomen. The infant may appear irritable and uncomfortable, or, if severe dehydration is present, he or she may be lethargic. The infant with pyloric stenosis becomes very ill with dehydration in just a few days. It is important for the parents to obtain medical attention immediately.

Diagnosis and Treatment

An abdominal ultrasound is most commonly used to diagnose this disorder; x-ray may also be performed. As soon as the diagnosis is made, plans for urgent surgery are developed. Surgical correction by **pyloroplasty** (procedure in which the pyloric canal is widened) is the treatment of choice. The infant usually recovers rapidly after surgery, with a very positive prognosis, and is usually discharged in a few days.

Nursing Considerations

Nursing care focuses on meeting the infant's needs for fluids and nutrition, promoting comfort, preventing infection, and supporting the parents. Because projectile vomiting will continue until surgery, the infant should be kept NPO. IV therapy will be used to establish fluid and electrolyte balance. By monitoring the infant's intake and output, including emesis and urine specific gravity, the nurse can evaluate the effectiveness of therapy.

Postoperatively, the infant is given small amounts of clear liquid. If clear liquids are tolerated, the infant will be advanced to formula or breastfeedings. To provide for the infant's comfort, acetaminophen or other analgesics are given as prescribed. Parents should be instructed to avoid pressure on the incision. When diapering the infant, slide the diaper under the buttocks instead of lifting the legs. Parents should be encouraged to swaddle, hold, and rock the infant.

In planning for discharge, parents should be taught the signs of incisional infection, including redness, swelling, discharge, and a fever higher than 101°F (38.5°C). The infant should not be submerged in bathwater until approved by the physician.

COLIC

Colic refers to acute abdominal pain caused by spasmodic contractions of the intestines. Colic occurs most commonly during the first 3 months of life. Infants cry loudly, pull their arms and legs up, and become red in the face. They may expel flatus or belch frequently, spitting up mucus and undigested milk or formula. The exact cause of colic is unknown, but contributing factors include swallowing air during feeding, eating too rapidly, overeating, overexcitement, and an anxious mother. Colic may be relieved by picking the infant up, burping (bubbling) gently, and giving some warm water to drink. Rocking and soothing the infant in a calm manner provides reassurance. Colic is not serious, and most infants are healthy and continue to gain weight.

INTUSSUSCEPTION

Intussusception is one of several causes of mechanical obstruction of the small bowel (Figure 22-13 ■) seen in children. It occurs when one portion of the intestine telescopes into another portion. The most common site for intussusception is the ileocecal valve. As telescoping occurs, the walls of the intestine rub together, producing inflammation, swelling, and obstruction. Swelling causes a decrease

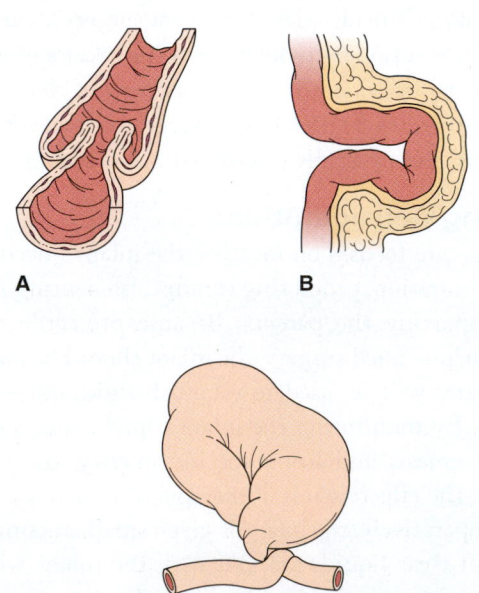

Figure 22-13. ■ Selective causes of mechanical obstruction. **(A)** Intussusception. **(B)** Incarcerated hernia. **(C)** Volvulus.

in blood flow to the intestine, resulting in ischemia, necrosis, perforation, and hemorrhage. Intussusception is one of the most common causes of intestinal obstruction in children. It occurs more frequently in boys between the ages of 2 months and 5 years than in other groups.

Manifestations

The child with intussusception presents with sudden severe abdominal pain, vomiting, and passage of brown stool. Periods of comfort may be followed by a recurrence of pain. As the condition worsens, the stool resembles currant jelly. A palpable abdominal mass may be felt.

Diagnosis and Treatment

Diagnosis is made from the history and barium enema studies. In some cases, the installation of barium moves the intestine back into place. If this does not occur, surgery will be required to reduce the telescoping bowel and remove damaged tissue.

Nursing Considerations

Nursing care focuses on pain management, maintaining fluid balance and nutrition, and supporting parents. The child will be kept NPO and may have a nasogastric tube to suction until the bowel is returned to its normal location. Postoperative care is routine, including administration of IV fluids, analgesics, and assessments. After normal bowel function returns, the child is offered clear liquids and is advanced to full feedings as tolerated.

Parents should be taught to care for the child at home, including watching for infection and administering prescribed medication. Surgery is usually successful in correcting the problem, but parents should be encouraged to seek medical attention if symptoms recur, if the child develops a fever, or if appetite decreases.

HERNIA

Hernia is a protrusion of the stomach or intestine through a malformation or enlarged opening in the normal musculature. In the infant, three locations are common:

- Umbilical hernia
- Inguinal hernia.
- Diaphragmatic hernia, rare but the most life threatening, is corrected shortly after birth (see Chapter 9 ∞).

Umbilical hernia (see Figure 9-42 ∞) results from protrusion of abdominal contents through a weakened umbilical ring and is most common in African American girls. *Inguinal hernia*, a protrusion of abdominal contents through a weakened inguinal ring, is more common in boys. The hernia appears as a soft swelling below the umbilicus or in the groin. The hernia grows larger with coughing, crying, or straining.

Parents should be instructed not to push on the hernia or apply tape, straps, or coins. These actions can cause the intestine to strangulate (see Figure 22-13B). Some defects resolve spontaneously by 3 to 4 years of age. Others are surgically repaired, requiring a short hospital stay.

MECKEL'S DIVERTICULUM

Meckel's diverticulum occurs when the connection between the yolk sac and the intestine in the embryo fails to atrophy. The result is a **diverticulum** (an outpouching) in the ileum, usually near the ileocecal valve. The pouch contains gastric or pancreatic tissue that secretes acid and enzymes, causing irritation and ulceration.

Manifestations

Symptoms appear by 2 years of age. Painless bleeding (either dark stools or bright red bleeding) occurs as a result of ulceration and obstruction. Abdominal pain is unusual, but when it occurs, it may resemble appendicitis, **volvulus** (twisted bowel; see Figure 22-13C), or intussusception.

Diagnosis and Treatment

Diagnosis is usually based on history because the diverticulum is usually small and does not fill with contrast medium. If untreated, perforation and peritonitis could result. Treatment involves surgical removal of the diverticulum and any damaged tissue. Once healing occurs, prognosis is good.

HIRSCHSPRUNG'S DISEASE (MEGACOLON)

Hirschsprung's disease (also called **megacolon**) is a condition in which the autonomic parasympathetic ganglia that normally cause peristalsis in the intestine are absent. The result of inadequate motility causes mechanical bowel obstruction of the large intestine. Hirschsprung's disease is more common in boys and often occurs with congenital heart defects, Down syndrome, and other neurologic syndromes.

Manifestations

Symptoms vary depending on the extent of the defect and the age of the child. In newborns, the first symptom may be failure to pass meconium, refusal to suck, abdominal distention, and meconium emesis. Older children may have a history of abdominal distention and constipation alternating with diarrhea.

clinical ALERT

Because newborns are frequently discharged from the hospital within 24 hours of birth, parents must be instructed to observe for meconium passage, abdominal distention, and vomiting. If the newborn fails to pass stool or the abdomen becomes distended, parents should contact the primary care provider.

Diagnosis and Treatment

Diagnosis is made by history, radiographic contrast studies, and biopsy. In mild cases, treatment includes high-fiber diet, adequate fluids, stool softeners, and isotonic enemas. More severe cases require surgery to remove the affected bowel. At times, a colostomy is performed. If a small portion of the bowel is affected, the colostomy may be reversed, and **reanastomosis** (reconnection) may be performed at a later date. If large areas of the bowel are affected, the colostomy may be permanent.

Nursing Considerations

Nursing care includes careful observation of the newborn for the passage of meconium. When the diagnosis is made later in infancy or childhood, a careful history of growth patterns, nutritional intake, and bowel habits must be obtained. Parents will need instruction on administering medication, giving saline enemas, and managing a colostomy, including proper drainage, skin care, and bag changing. Parents must be taught to watch for malabsorption of nutrients, including poor growth and malnutrition. Referral to an enterostomal nurse specialist and ostomy support groups may be helpful.

Poisonings

Poisoning, the ingestion of a toxic substance, is a common cause of injury or death in children between 1 and 4 years of age. Recall from Chapter 11 ⊘ that the developmental task of children in this age group is to explore their environment. Young children frequently put objects and fluid into their mouth, potentially resulting in poisoning (Table 22-4 ■). The Poison Prevention Packaging Act of 1970 mandates child protective devices for all potentially toxic substances such as household cleansers and medication. However, some adults find these protective lids difficult to remove and will not tighten them or will leave the lid off. Other substances found in the home are potentially hazardous and are not regulated by law. For example, many household plants, including Boston ivy, poinsettia, philodendron, lily-of-the-valley, daffodil, azalea, and rhododendron, are toxic if ingested. Cosmetics; nail care products; weed, bug, and rodent killers; paints; and furniture polish are also highly toxic.

Most poisonings occur in the home. Parents who suspect a child has ingested a poisonous substance should call the local poison control center (PCC) immediately. The PCC can ask the parents questions about the substance, advise the parents about treatment to begin at home, and direct the parents on the need for emergency treatment. The possibility of intentional ingestion should be considered with older children. If the child vomits, the emesis should be brought to the emergency department.

Emergency treatment for poisoning is based on the goal of preventing further absorption of the poison and reversing its effects.

TABLE 22-4

Poisons

TYPE OF POISON	SOURCES	CLINICAL MANIFESTATION	TREATMENT	PREVENTION
Corrosives: acids and alkaline	Cleansers: toilet cleaner, drain cleaners, bleach Batteries	Burns around mouth, throat, and stomach; respiratory obstruction; drooling; pain	Do NOT induce vomiting Dilute with water Give activated charcoal	Keep cleansers and batteries out of reach of children. Keep lids tightly closed.
Hydrocarbons: distillates of petroleum	Gasoline, kerosene, furniture polish, paint thinners, oils	Coughing, vomiting, respiratory distress, lethargy	Do NOT induce vomiting/gastric lavage Provide supportive care Decontaminate skin	Keep gasoline products out of reach of children. Do NOT store in other containers. Keep lids tightly closed.
Salicylates: aspirin	Products containing aspirin	Nausea/vomiting, tinnitus, bleeding, convulsions, death	If alert, induce vomiting IV sodium bicarbonate Vitamin K	Keep in locked medicine cabinet. Keep lid tightly closed.
Acetaminophen	Many over-the-counter products, in combination with narcotics	Nausea/vomiting, pallor, hepatic involvement	Induce vomiting/gastric lavage Give charcoal or Mucomyst	Keep in locked medicine cabinet. Tell children drug is NOT candy.
Heavy metals: mercury, lead	Paints, pesticides, water from lead pipes, broken thermometers	Tremors, memory loss, cognitive defects	Remove causative agent Provide chelation therapy (see text)	Remove potential causes from environment. Use digital thermometers.

clinical ALERT

The priorities of treatment for a child with poisoning can be recalled with the mnemonic SIRES:

- **S**tabilize the child's condition.
- **I**dentify the toxic substance.
- **R**everse its effects.
- **E**liminate the substance from the child's body.
- **S**upport the child (and parents) physically and psychologically.

When the child arrives in the emergency department, the airway, breathing, and circulation must be monitored continuously and cardiopulmonary resuscitation (CPR) performed if needed. An IV line should be established and blood drawn for toxicology. Parents, family, and child (if applicable) should be questioned about the events leading up to the poisoning. The type of poison, the amount of chemical, the amount of time the child was unsupervised, allergies, and pre-existing disorders should be determined.

The process of reversal or elimination of the substance from the child's body depends on the specific agent ingested. See Table 22-5 ■ for methods commonly used to reverse the effect of poisons. Syrup of ipecac is no longer recommended because it can be harmful in some situations and may not remove all poison (West, 1997). Activated charcoal binds with poisonous chemicals to slow or prevent absorption.

Once the emergency phase of treatment is over, the child and parents will need continued physical and emotional support. Depending on the degree of damage from the toxic agent, the child may recover without deficit, or he or she may have life-changing deficits of gastrointestinal, neurologic, cardiovascular, hepatic, and renal functions. The age and development of the child will guide the amount of emotional support that will be needed. Parents, however, will need emotional support to deal with feelings of guilt, blame, and

TABLE 22-5

Methods to Treat Poisoning

TYPE OF TREATMENT	PROCESS OR AGENT
Gastric lavage	■ Insert largest gastric tube possible through mouth. ■ Instill and aspirate normal saline until returns clear. ■ Less effective than vomiting, used for neurologically depressed, diminished gag reflex, or uncooperative children. ■ Use in acid ingestion to prevent continued damage. ■ Contraindicated in alkaline ingestion due to possible damage to esophagus.
Activated charcoal	■ Assess level of consciousness before giving orally. ■ Can be given by gastric tube. ■ Give in opaque cup with a lid and straw so child cannot see black liquid. ■ Give after vomiting stops; aspiration of charcoal can damage lung.
Cathartics	■ Increases elimination of toxic substance and minimizes absorption.
Antidote and antagonist	■ There are only a few agents. ■ Narcan is common for opiate ingestion.
Other (depending on child's condition)	■ Diuretics. ■ Fluids. ■ Anticonvulsants. ■ Hemodialysis. ■ Antiarrhythmics. ■ Exchange transfusion.

shame. Conflict between parents might occur. If a babysitter or other care provider is involved, additional emotional stress will be placed on the family. In some instances, child protection services may be called and the child placed in protective custody while the situation is under investigation.

LEAD POISONING

Lead poisoning (toxic levels of lead in the blood) is decreasing in the United States but remains a concern in many poor families living in older housing in inner cities or rural areas. The main sources are from lead-based paint, drinking water flowing through lead pipes, lead holding tanks or pipes and tanks soldered with lead, food grown in lead-contaminated dirt, and airborne lead from smelters and battery manufacturing plants.

Children are at greater risk for toxic levels because they absorb and retain more lead in proportion to body weight than adults. Children younger than 7 years are particularly at risk. Young children often chew on crib rails, pencils, or other

BOX 22-4   **CULTURAL PULSE POINTS**

Use of Lead in Traditional Medicines

Some traditional medicines contain large amounts of lead. Mexican Americans use azarcon and greta to treat empacho (a colic-like illness). Asian communities use chifong, tokuwan, pay-loo-ah, ghasard, bali goli, and kandu. Middle Eastern communities use alkohl, kohl, surma, saoot, and cebagin.

painted surfaces when teething. They ingest small quantities of paint that over time can build to toxic levels. Lead interferes with normal cell function, particularly nervous system, blood cells, kidneys, and vitamin D and calcium metabolism. Once in the body, lead is deposited in bones and teeth. It is slowly released from the bones. Even when the source is removed, toxic levels can take time to be resolved.

Manifestations

Symptoms include cognitive deficit, learning disabilities, hearing impairment, and growth delays. Lead ingestion by pregnant women can cause fetal malformation, low birth weight, and premature birth.

Diagnosis and Treatment

A blood test (Pb-B) is the most useful tool in the screening, diagnosis, and monitoring of lead poisoning. Treatment is with **chelation therapy,** the administration of a chemical that will bind to the lead and increase the rate of excretion. Calcium disodium ethylenediamine tetraacetate (CaNa$_2$EDTA), dimercaprol (BAL), d-penicillamine, or succimer (DMSA) may be used alone or in combination for several days followed by a rest period and then repeated. Before the child is discharged, a lead-free environment must be assured.

Nursing Considerations

Nursing implications include community teaching regarding lead poison risks, environmental assessment, and screening individuals at risk. The school nurse should suspect lead poisoning in children with learning disabilities and children with growth delays. Nurses must teach the parents about individual risk, administration of chelation therapy, and the need to avoid all sources of lead. This teaching may find resistance in some cultures (Box 22-4 ■).

NURSING CARE

PRIORITIES IN NURSING CARE

Priorities for the nurse in caring for children with gastrointestinal disorders include the following:

- Early detection and treatment of gastrointestinal conditions
- Prevention of fluid and electrolyte imbalance due to vomiting and diarrhea
- Maintaining adequate nutrition for growth requirements
- Promoting elimination of solid waste.

ASSESSING

Children with gastrointestinal disorders should be assessed for the presence of active bowel sounds, abdominal tenderness, vomiting, diarrhea, and constipation. Parents of young children or the older client should be questioned about the frequency, color, amount, and odor of the stool. Questions should be asked about usual feeding habits and recent changes in those habits. When a child presents with flulike symptoms, it is important to ask if the child has been around anyone testing positive for hepatitis or if there has been possible exposure from contaminated blood, blood products, or contaminated water.

DIAGNOSING, PLANNING, AND IMPLEMENTING

The following nursing diagnoses may be pertinent to the care of young children with gastrointestinal disorders:

- Deficient Fluid Volume
- Altered Nutrition: Less than Body Requirements
- Risk for Infection
- Risk for Body Image Disturbance, related to jaundice (older child)
- Pain, related to disorder or surgery.

Expected outcomes for children with gastrointestinal disorders would include the following, among others:

- Maintain adequate hydration.
- Obtain necessary nutrients to provide for healing and growth.
- Remain free of infection.
- Express an understanding of the condition and how it is expected to resolve.
- State pain is within acceptable limits.

Nursing interventions might include:

- Administer fluids (either intravenously or orally) as ordered. *Maintaining fluid balance is a high priority when the gastrointestinal system is not functioning properly. Refer to Chapter 15 ⚭ for more information.*
- Advance diet from clear liquid to full liquid to soft as ordered and tolerated. *Often, the child will be NPO for diagnostic tests, surgery, or to rest the gastrointestinal system and allow for healing. Once a diet can be resumed, it is best to advance the diet slowly.*
- Administer medication, including antiemetics, antibiotics,

antidiarrheals, and laxatives as ordered. *Medications are frequently ordered to stop vomiting and diarrhea and stimulate defecation if the child is constipated. Antibiotics may be ordered to treat gastrointestinal infections or prior to bowel surgery.*

- Teach parents and child (if appropriate) the care of medical appliances in use at home. *Medical appliances such as intestinal tubes, tube feeding pumps, and colostomy drainage bags may be used in the treatment of gastrointestinal disorders. Parents (and older children) must be taught to care for insertion sites, skin around appliances, and any other equipment.*
- Teach parents regarding follow-up care. *Many gastrointestinal disorders are chronic in nature and require continued medical supervision.*

EVALUATING

Signs of dehydration will subside, a normal elimination pattern will return, vomiting will stop, and the child will gain weight. Postoperatively, the child will be evaluated for return of normal gastrointestinal function. Parents should be able to verbalize understanding of home care.

NURSING PROCESS CARE PLAN
Care of a Child with Bilateral Cleft Lip

John was born with a bilateral cleft lip. He has been cared for at home and is strong enough for surgical correction. John has been admitted to the pediatric unit from surgery.

Assessment. VS: T 99.2 (R), P 90, R 36, Wt 12.5 lb (5.7 kg). John is awake and crying. An IV of lactated Ringer's solution is infusing in his left hand. Logan clamp is present across the surgical site. His diaper is wet.

Nursing Diagnosis. The following important nursing diagnoses (among others) are established for this client:

- Pain related to surgical procedure
- Risk for Trauma of the surgical site.

Expected Outcomes. The following expected outcomes have been identified:

- Infant is resting comfortably.
- Operative site is undamaged.

Planning and Implementation

- Medicate for pain as ordered. *Keeping the infant comfortable will decrease crying and trauma to the suture line.*
- Apply elbow restraints. Restrain on back. *Jacket restraint prevents bending the elbows and rubbing the face or sucking the*

thumb. Restraining on back prevents rubbing face on the bed. Restraint will also protect the IV site.

- Clean suture line as ordered. *Cleaning the suture line prevents infection and aids in healing.*
- Teach parents use of restraints and suture line care at home. *Continued care will be needed after discharge until healing is complete in several weeks.*
- Do not put anything in the mouth. *This prevents trauma to the suture line.*

Evaluation. John will rest comfortably with minimal crying. The suture line will remain intact without signs of infection. Parents can verbalize home care.

Critical Thinking in the Nursing Process

1. Should John be medicated for pain before or after feeding?
2. If John cannot have anything put in his mouth, how will he be fed?
3. How will the nurse know that John is getting enough nutrition?

Note: Discussion of Critical Thinking questions appears in Appendix 1.

Note: The references and resources for this and all chapters have been compiled at the back of the book.

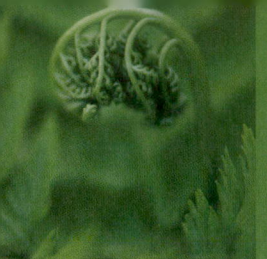

 ## KEY TERMS by Topic

Use the audio glossary feature of either the CD-ROM or the Companion Website to hear the correct pronunciation of the following key terms.

Anatomy and Physiology

peristalsis, lingual frenulum, papillae, gingiva, parotid gland, buccal space, submandibular glands, sublingual glands, cardiac sphincter, fundus, cardiac region, lesser curvature, greater curvature, pyloric sphincter, pylorus, rugae, chyme

Congenital Gastrointestinal Defects

cleft palate, cleft lip, Logan clamp, esophageal atresia, tracheoesophageal fistula

Gastrointestinal Inflammation

gastroenteritis, probiotics, appendicitis, rebound tenderness, Crohn's disease, ulcerative colitis

Malabsorption Disorders

celiac disease, steatorrhea, lactose intolerance

Nutrition Disorders

kwashiorkor, rickets, scurvy, failure to thrive (FTT), pica

Hepatic Disorders

biliary atresia, hepatomegaly, pruritis, splenomegaly, hepatitis, fulminating hepatitis, parenchymal, phenylketonuria (PKU)

Motility Disorders

motility disorders, gastroesophageal reflux disease (GERD), pyloric stenosis, pyloroplasty, colic, intussusception, hernia, diverticulum, volvulus, Hirschsprung's disease, megacolon, reanastomosis

Poisoning

poisoning, chelation therapy

KEY Points

- Gastrointestinal disorders are potentially life threatening due to fluid and electrolyte imbalance and malnutrition.

- Vomiting and diarrhea must be treated rapidly in children to prevent dehydration.

- Congenital malformation of the gastrointestinal system may require multiple surgeries to correct; therefore, nutrition is provided by IV administration of TPN.

- Most metabolic disorders require lifelong treatment.

- Families may need to be taught to administer nutrition by tube feeding or IV when long-term treatment is required.

- Health promotion activities include a low-fat, high-fiber diet and exercise to prevent or treat obesity.

FOR FURTHER Study

Phenylketonuria (PKU) is also discussed under Newborn Care in Chapter 9. Figure 9-27 shows the heel stick performed on newborns to test for PKU.

Children who have been starved emotionally can have lifelong problems involving language, social interactions, and intelligence; see Box 16-1.

Failure to thrive and obesity are also discussed in Chapter 27.

See Appendix II for growth charts to determine percentile.

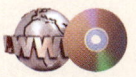 ## EXPLORE MediaLink

Additional interactive resources for this chapter can be found on the Companion Website at www.prenhall.com/towle.

Click on Chapter 22 and "Begin" to select the activities for this chapter.

For chapter-related NCLEX-style questions and an audio glossary, access the accompanying CD-ROM in this book.

Animations

Digestive system

Gavage tube

Critical Thinking Care Map

Caring for a Client with Gastroenteritis
NCLEX-PN® Focus Area: Physiologic Integrity: Basic Care and Comfort

Case Study: Jonathan's mother calls the pediatrician's office and reports that Jonathan has been vomiting and having diarrhea for the past 2 days. He is lethargic and not drinking his bottle. The infant is 7 months old.

Nursing Diagnosis: Imbalanced Nutrition: Less than Body Requirements

COLLECT DATA

Subjective	Objective
_____	_____
_____	_____
_____	_____
_____	_____
_____	_____

Would you report this? Yes/No

If yes, to: _____

Nursing Care

_____
_____
_____
_____
_____
_____
_____
_____
_____
_____
_____
_____
_____
_____

How would you document this? _____
_____
_____
_____

Compare your documentation to the sample provided in Appendix I.

Data Collected
(use those that apply)

- Current weight: 12 lb
- Previous weight: 16 lb
- Diffuse red area across buttocks
- Mother reports no fluid or solid intake in the past 48 hours
- Mother states infant enjoys playing with trucks
- Mucous membranes pale
- Vomiting x6/day
- Diarrhea x10/day
- Immunizations up to date
- Hyperactive bowels sounds in all four quandrants
- Mother reports infant is lethargic

Nursing Interventions
(use those that apply; list in priority order)

- Obtain a thorough nutrition history.
- Apply topical agents as ordered for rash.
- Assess for signs and symptoms of dehydration.
- Weigh daily.
- Administer next series of immunizations.
- Develop a plan with the parents for nutritional and fluid replacement.
- Administer antiemetics as ordered.
- Provide age-appropriate toys for play.
- Assess for possible causes of vomiting and diarrhea.
- Monitor lab values carefully.

NCLEX-PN® Exam Preparation

TEST-TAKING TIP It is often possible to eliminate words that are meant to distract, such as "always" and "never," especially when discussing client outcomes.

1 A 2-week-old infant is recovering from surgery for pyloric stenosis. The mother comments, "Now that the surgery is over, Timmy should not have intestinal obstruction ever again." An appropriate nursing response would be:

1. "You need to talk with the doctor about your son's future."
2. "You are correct, Timmy will never again experience intestinal obstruction."
3. "Recurrence of obstruction is unlikely, but we will review symptoms you should watch for."
4. "Timmy will not have obstruction as a child but will have digestive problems as an adult."

2 A pediatric client has been diagnosed with rickets. The nurse knows the child's mother understands the treatment when she states that she will give the child additional amounts of:

1. milk, cheese, and yogurt.
2. ice cream, jello, and pudding.
3. whole grain cereal and bread.
4. citrus fruit.

3 The symptom that the nurse must monitor most closely when pyloric stenosis is suspected is:

1. anorexia.
2. infrequent bowel movements.
3. projectile vomiting.
4. colicky abdominal cramps.

4. To prevent trauma to the surgical site after a cleft palate repair, the nurse should avoid placing _____ _____ inside the infant's mouth.

5 The nurse is providing teaching to parents of an infant with Hirschsprung's disease. Which of the following statements best describes Hirshprung's disease?

1. It results in frequent evacuation of solids, liquids, and gas.
2. There is passage of excessive amounts of meconium.
3. It results in excessive peristaltic movements within the gastrointestinal tract.
4. The colon has a segment with limited nerve supply that prevents normal movement.

6 A 4-month-old has gastroesophageal reflux but is thriving without other complications. Which of the following should the nurse suggest to minimize reflux?

1. Discontinue breastfeeding.
2. Position the baby with his head up after feeding.
3. Give continuous nasogastric tube feeding.
4. Decrease frequency of feedings as much as possible.

7 The nurse is caring for a baby with probable intussusception. He had diarrhea before admission, but while waiting for a barium enema, he passes a normal brown stool. Which of the following is the most appropriate nursing action?

1. Notify the physician.
2. Measure abdominal girth.
3. Continue with preparation for barium enema.
4. Take vital signs, including blood pressure.

8 The nurse would consider which of the following a positive outcome in evaluating an infant with failure to thrive?

1. The family depends on nursing staff for care.
2. The family demonstrates nurturing behaviors toward the infant.
3. The infant maintains admission weight.
4. The infant makes slow progress on developmental milestones.

9 Which of the following is most important when assessing a child with poisoning?

1. Determine what was taken and the treatment provided by parents.
2. Determine medication allergies.
3. Give ipecac before activated charcoal.
4. Induce vomiting.

10 A 12-year-old client has a fever and complains of abdominal pain. The school nurse:

1. calls the physician.
2. checks for rebound tenderness.
3. recommends a laxative.
4. applies a heating pad.

Answers for Review Questions, as well as discussion of Care Plan and Critical Thinking Care Map questions, appear in Appendix I.

Chapter 23

Care of the Child with Genitourinary Disorders

BRIEF Outline

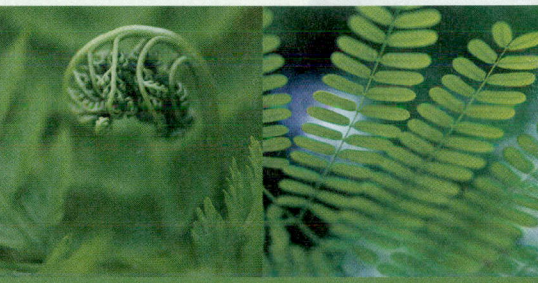

NURSING PROCESS CARE PLAN:
Child with Nephrotic Syndrome

HEALTH PROMOTION ISSUE :
Assisting the Young Teen with
Her First Pap Smear

CRITICAL THINKING CARE MAP:
Caring for a Client with Vaginitis

LEARNING Outcomes

After completing this chapter, you will be able to:

- Discuss the anatomy and physiology of the pediatric urinary and reproductive systems.
- Describe urinary and reproductive disorders to include urinary tract infections, acute and chronic renal failure, Wilms' tumor, hypospadias, phimosis, cryptorchidism, ambiguous genitalia, and menstrual disorders.
- Discuss clinical manifestations, diagnostic procedures, medical management, and nursing interventions related to urinary and reproductive disorders.
- Explain appropriate nursing interventions for children with urinary and reproductive disorders.

The **genitourinary system** consists of structures of the urinary system and the reproductive system. In this chapter, the anatomy and physiology of both systems are reviewed.

Disorders of the urinary system and the reproductive system are also discussed.

URINARY (RENAL) SYSTEM

Anatomy and Physiology

The structures of the urinary system include the kidneys, ureters, bladder, urethra, and renal arteries and veins (Figure 23-1 ■). The primary functions of the urinary system include waste excretion; homeostasis, fluid, electrolyte, and acid-base balance; regulation of blood pressure; regulation of calcium metabolism; and stimulation of erythrocyte development.

Early in pregnancy, the kidneys develop and begin to assist in the maintenance of amniotic fluid levels. Urine production begins during the third month of gestation. The placenta filters the fetus's blood and maintains homeostasis. At birth, the newborn's kidneys take over these functions.

Growth of the kidney continues until adolescence. The process of filtration becomes refined by age 2. Urine output also increases as the child ages. Urinary output is as follows:

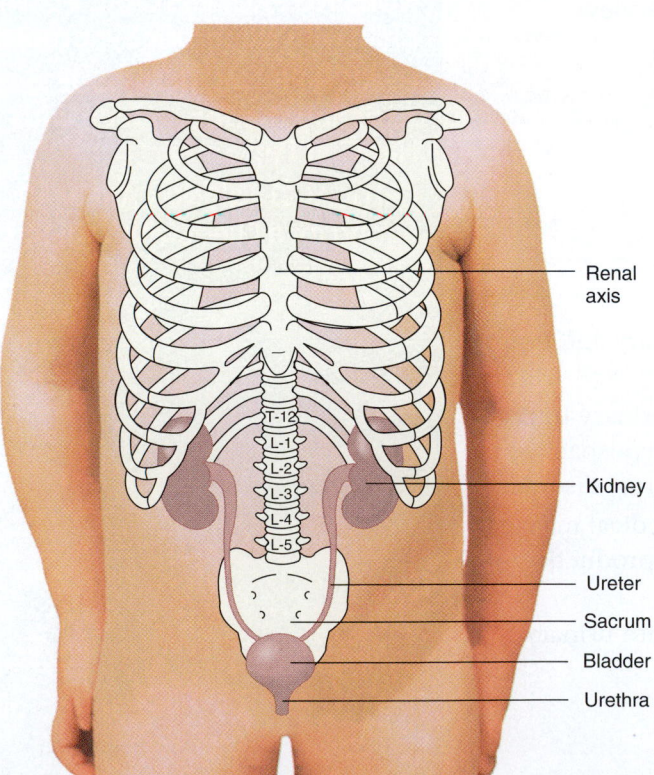

Figure 23-1. ■ The kidneys are located between the twelfth thoracic (T12) and the third lumbar (L3) vertebrae. (Kidneys do not concentrate urine until about 2 years of age.)

- For an infant, 2 mL/kg/hr
- For a child, 0.5–1 mL/kg/hr
- For an adolescent, 40–80 mL/hr.

An estimate of a child's bladder capacity in ounces can be made by adding 2 to the child's age in years. The sum approximates the ounces of bladder capacity in the child (London, Ladewig, Ball, Bindler [2007], p. 1630). For example, the normal amount of urine a 1-year-old child's bladder can hold is 3 oz (90 mL).

Brief Assessment Overview

HISTORY

- Ask about patterns of urination. Include amount, color, and number of times per day (for an infant, number of diapers per day).
- Ask if the child complains of pain, burning, frequency, or urgency when voiding. Any of these symptoms could indicate the presence of a urinary tract infection (UTI).
- Ask about toilet training.
- Ask about involuntary urination. Ask when and how often it occurs. In an older child (school age), ask if there are situations that are associated with involuntary urination (e.g., sleeping overnight in a strange place).
- Inquire about recent weight gain. It is especially important to note sudden increases in weight that seem unusual to the parents because this may indicate kidney malfunction.
- Inquire about past urinary disorders. Some people are prone to UTIs.
- Require family history as it relates to urinary disorders.

PHYSICAL

- Weigh the child.
- Inspect for adequate hydration. Perform test for skin turgor.
- Inspect extremities for edema.
- Observe for bladder distension. Improper functioning of the urinary system may result in bladder distension.

Disorders of the urinary system that affect the child include congenital anomalies, infections, and tumors. Because one of the functions of the urinary system is to eliminate waste, disorders affecting the urinary system pose a significant risk to the health of the child.

Congenital Urinary Defects

Defects of the urinary system are commonly found with defects of the lower gastrointestinal tract and reproductive system. The first concern is to determine that the infant is able to urinate. Most commonly, the newborn voids in the first 24 hours of birth. If this does not occur, intervention is more immediate. The newborn who does not void within 24 hours may be assessed for urethral stenosis or absent kidneys or ureters. Only common disorders of the urinary tract are discussed in this chapter.

URETHRAL MALPOSITION

Typically in the male child, the urethra opens at the tip of the penis. **Hypospadias** occurs when the urethra opens on the *ventral* (lower) surface of the penis. **Epispadias** occurs when the urethra opens on the *dorsal* (upper) surface of the penis (Figure 23-2 ■). Epispadias may occur in females, but it is quite rare. In females with epispadias, the urethra opens by a separation of the labia minora and a fissure of the clitoris.

Both hypospadias and epispadias are congenital anomalies that occur when the urethral folds fail to fuse over the urethral groove during fetal development. Hypospadias commonly occurs in combination with congenital inguinal hernias, undescended testes, and **chordee** (a congenital anomaly that causes a ventral curvature of the penis, which is caused by fibrous tissues along the corpus spongiosum). Epispadias can be associated with **bladder exstrophy** (Figure 23-3 ■), a defect usually corrected in the first 48 hours of life, in which there is an absence of part of the abdominal wall and anterior wall of the bladder, causing the posterior wall of the bladder to protrude through the defect.

Manifestations

The opening, in hypospadias or epispadias of the male, can be found anywhere along the shaft of the penis. A dimple or pit may be seen along the ventral or dorsal side of the penile shaft (see Figure 23-2).

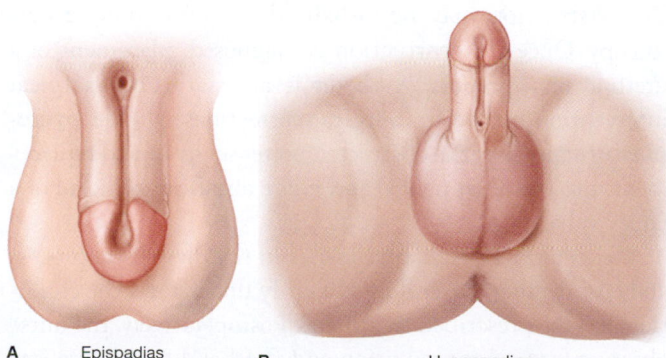

A   Epispadias   **B**   Hypospadias

Figure 23-2. ■ (A) Epispadias; the urethra is on the dorsal surface of the penis. (B) Hypospadias; the urethra is on the ventral surface of the penis.

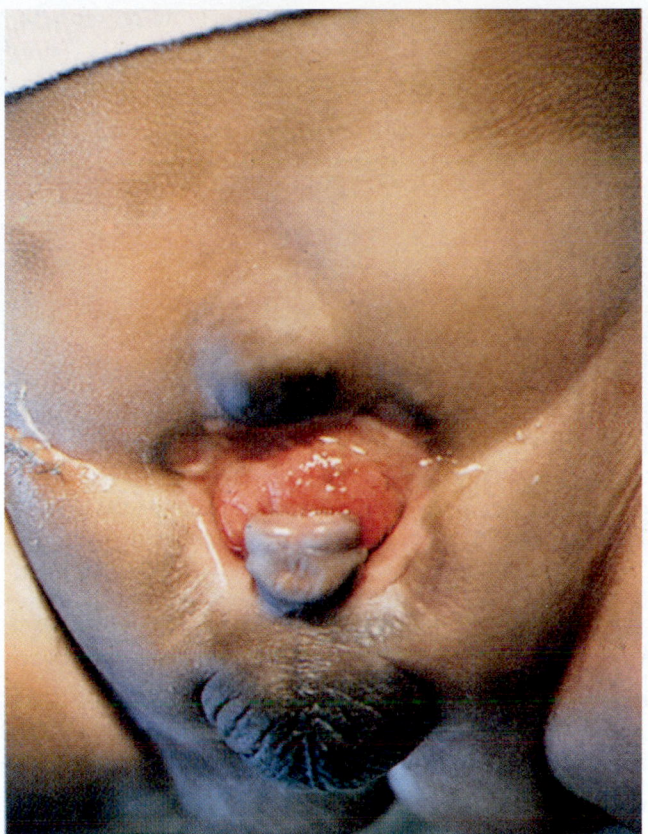

Figure 23-3. ■ This child has bladder exstrophy, noted by extrusion of the posterior bladder wall through the lower abdominal wall. Until surgery can be performed, the bladder mucosa must be protected from trauma and irritation. A sterile, saline-soaked dressing maintains moisture; it is covered with a sterile plastic wrap. The surrounding area must be cleaned daily. Skin sealant is applied to protect surrounding skin from leaking urine.

Diagnosis and Treatment

Diagnosis is made by documenting physical findings. Prenatally, the defect may be seen on ultrasound. Genetic testing may also be done.

Surgical correction is needed for hypospadias and epispadias, usually during the first year of life. Infants are not circumcised in an effort to preserve the foreskin for use in the cosmetic repair. The surgery moves the position of the urethra to correct urinary function. Following surgery, the infant will have a urethral stent to keep the urethra open.

Nursing Considerations

The nurse observes the infant postoperatively for edema, dysuria, bleeding, infection, and pain. Because of the urinary stent, the infant needs to be double diapered (Figure 23-4 ■). Maintaining hydration will assist adequate urinary output. The nurse needs to document the child's intake and output carefully, noting any lack of urinary drainage for 1 hour. (See Procedure 15-1 ⬤⬤.) Be aware that the urine will be blood tinged for a few days.

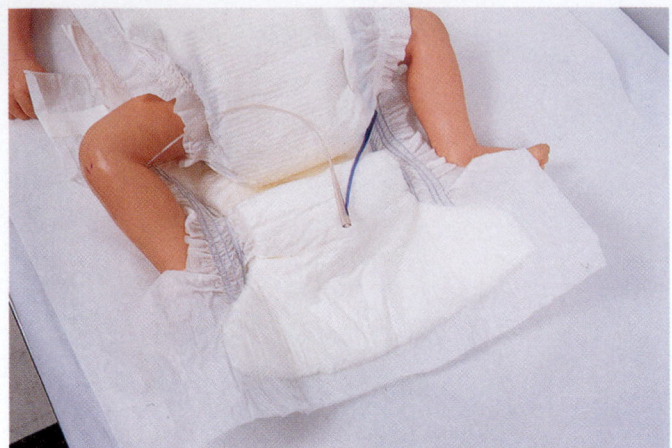

Figure 23-4. ■ The double-diapering technique protects the urinary stent after surgery for hypospadias or epispadias repair. The inner diaper collects stools; the outer diaper, urine.

Following surgery, the infant may have bladder spasms. Anticholinergics and analgesics are administered by the nurse. Antibiotics are administered prophylactically to prevent infection. Box 23-1 ■ provides steps for the nurse to take to prevent and/or recognize symptoms of postoperative infection.

Obstructive Uropathy

Obstructive uropathy is a condition in which the structure or function of the urinary system is altered, resulting in obstruction of urine flow (Figure 23-5 ■). Obstructions can be congenital or acquired. A congenital cause for urinary obstruction is **polycystic kidney.** In this condition, one or both

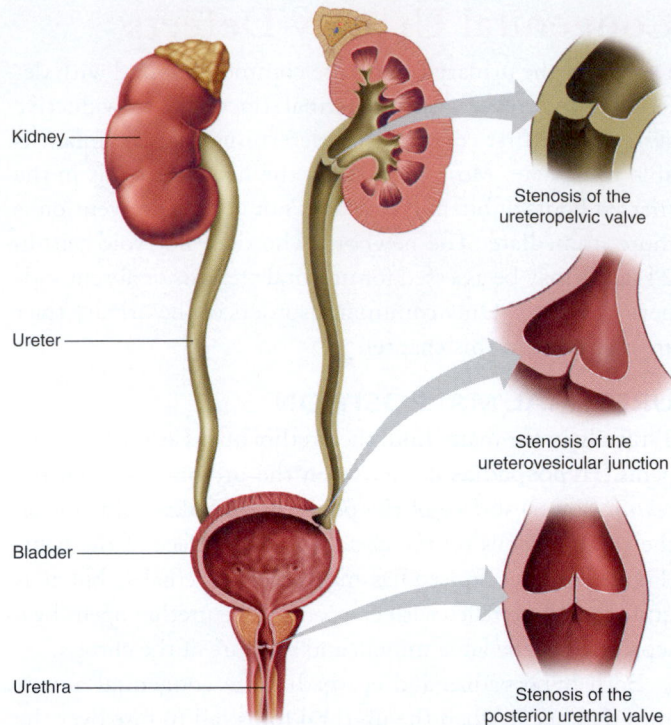

Figure 23-5. ■ The common sites of obstruction in the upper and lower urinary tract. Upper urinary tract infections are often unilateral. Renal failure is most likely to occur when both kidneys are affected by hydronephrosis.

kidneys are enlarged and contain fluid-filled cysts. Acquired causes include tumors, kidney stones (**nephrolithiasis**), and crystal formations caused by medications.

Manifestations

As urine flow from the kidney to the bladder is blocked, urine will back up causing **stasis** (pooling of urine or other body fluids). Stasis can lead to UTIs, loss of renal function, and hydronephrosis. **Hydronephrosis** is the distension of the renal pelvis caused by increased pressure due to urine backup.

Diagnosis and Treatment

The obstruction may be visualized by ultrasound or cystoscopy. Once the obstruction is diagnosed, placement of a urethral or suprapubic catheter is necessary until surgical intervention can occur. Surgical corrections include **pyeloplasty** (removal of the obstructed ureter segment and replacement into the renal pelvis) and **valve ablation** (removal of a faulty valve).

Preoperatively, the nurse assists in the diagnostic process and ensures that the child and family understand the condition and the prescribed treatment. Postoperatively, the nurse observes for urinary retention and fluid and electrolyte imbalances.

Upon discharge, many children will have a stent, catheter, or urinary diversion device. Parents need specific instructions

---

BOX 23-1 | **NURSING CARE CHECKLIST**

Preventing Postoperative Infection

☑ Change all dressings with sterile technique.

☑ Keep drains and stents free of obstruction.

☑ Observe closely for signs of infection, including:
- Change in vital signs: increased temperature, increased pulse
- White, puslike drainage from the wound
- Foul odor from the wound
- Edema and redness around the wound
- Increasing report of pain
- Increasing irritability
- Decreasing appetite.

☑ Report symptoms of infection promptly to physician.

☑ Administer antibiotics properly.

☑ Teach caregiver, upon discharge, to administer the entire course of prescribed antibiotics and report symptoms of infection promptly.

on how to care for these devices, how to maintain hygiene (see Figure 23-4), and when to report complications.

Urinary Tract Infections

Urinary tract infections (UTIs) are a group of bacterial infections that include **cystitis** (bladder infection) and **pyelonephritis** (kidney infection). UTIs can be a single acute episode or a chronic recurrent or persistent infection. In the infant, UTIs are more common in males, primarily due to structural defects. In the young child, UTIs are more common in females, usually caused by *Escherichia coli* entering the urethra and progressing to the bladder. Younger children also have shorter bladders, which increase their risk for UTIs.

UTIs can also be caused by **vesicoureteral reflux,** a defect of the vesicoureteral valve. Normally, when urine enters the bladder, pressure builds and closes the vesicoureteral valve. If there is a defect in this valve, closure does not occur and urine refluxes into the ureter. Urinary stasis leads to UTIs. Vesicoureteral reflux may resolve spontaneously. If dilation of the kidneys occurs, surgical intervention may be necessary.

Manifestations

Signs of UTI in the infant are less specific than in older children. Whenever an infant presents with unexplained illness, the possibility of UTI should be suspected. Symptoms of UTI include fever, nausea and vomiting, anorexia, strong-smelling urine, abdominal pain, **dysuria** (painful urination), and **hematuria** (blood in the urine). In the infant and young child who is nonverbal, dysuria may be displayed as crying during urination. The continent child may suddenly develop incontinence or hesitancy, due to fear of pain.

Diagnosis

Urinalysis can detect hematuria and the presence of white blood cells and nitrites (Table 23-1 ■). However, to determine the exact causative agent, a urine culture is necessary. A sterile urine specimen is collected by the nurse (see description of this in Procedure 13-14 ⚭). Proper collection of the sample is essential to the accuracy of the findings. A clean-catch specimen may be obtained if the child is cooperative. A sterile single-use, self-adhering urinary bag or catheterization may be used to collect a sample in the incontinent child. (Urinary catheterization in a child is described in Procedure 13-24. ⚭)

TABLE 23-1		
Lab Values for Urinalysis		
CHARACTERISTIC	**NORMAL VALUE**	**NURSING CONSIDERATIONS**
Bacteria	None to few organisms present	Normally residing bacteria from the perineum may contaminate the specimen.
pH	4.50–8.0	Normal urine is slightly acidic. Urinary tract infections may cause the urine to become alkaline.
Color	Clear, straw colored, amber	Bacteria or vaginal discharge may cause the urine to be cloudy. Concentrated urine will be dark. Urine that contains blood will be red in color.
Odor	Slight, nonoffensive odor	Urine containing bacteria may smell foul.
Glucose	Negative	Presence of glucose in the urine may indicate high blood glucose levels.
Protein	Negative	Presence of protein in the urine may indicate glomerular kidney disease.
Red blood cells	Negative on gross examination; 0–5 per high-powered field	Blood in the urine may indicate UTI or other kidney diseases.
White blood cells	Negative; less than 2 per high-powered field	Presence may indicate UTI.
Specific gravity	Newborn: 1.001–1.020; Child: 1.005–1.030	Increased values may indicate renal disease.
Ketones	Negative	Present in diabetes mellitus, starvation, or in children who have ingested an excessive amount of aspirin.

MediaLink UTI

Treatment

The primary treatment for UTI is administration of antibiotics. Parenteral antibiotics are required for children with pyelonephritis. Oral or IV fluids can assist in maintaining urinary function.

Prophylactic antibiotic administration is indicated for children with structural defects such as vesicoureteral reflux.

Nursing Considerations

In most circumstances, a UTI can be prevented. The parents should be taught to clean the perineum thoroughly with each diaper change. The young child who is being toilet trained should be taught to wipe from front to back. The perineum should be washed daily. Discourage the use of bubble baths and hot tubs that can irritate the urethra and increase the chance of infection. Box 23-2 ■ provides information about preventing UTIs.

Acute Postinfectious Glomerulonephritis

Acute postinfectious **glomerulonephritis** (APIGN; inflammation of the glomeruli) usually results from the body's immune response following an infection (Figure 23-6 ■). This condition is also called *acute poststreptococcal glomerulonephritis* if caused by *Streptococcus*. Infecting organisms related to glomerulonephritis are group A beta-hemolytic *Streptococcus*, *Staphylococcus*, *Pneumococcus*, and coxsackievirus. It is the most common type of kidney inflammation. It is most often seen in children between the ages of 2 and 12 years, and it is twice as common in boys as in girls. Antibiotic therapy to kill the infecting agent does not prevent this disorder from occurring. APIGN results when immune complexes, deposited in glomeruli, obstruct capillary blood flow. The condition can lead to acute or chronic renal failure.

Manifestations

Children with glomerulonephritis may be asymptomatic. Others have a sudden onset of flank pain, irritability, malaise, and fever. Other symptoms include gross or microscopic hematuria, dysuria, edema, hypertension, and oliguria.

Diagnosis and Treatment

Urinalysis and serum studies are performed. An electrocardiogram may also be done to look for changes caused by circulatory overload. Treatment for children with glomerulonephritis is supportive, including bed rest in some cases, antihypertensive medication, and fluid restriction. The nurse should monitor the child's fluid status by planning fluid restriction and documenting intake and output. See

| BOX 23-2 | COMPLEMENTARY THERAPIES |

Preventing Urinary Tract Infections

There are several nonpharmacologic measures parents can use to help prevent UTIs in their children.

- Risk of bacterial contamination can be reduced by:
  - In female children, wiping the perineum from front to back after urination, defecation, and during regular hygiene to keep harmful bacteria found in the stool away from the urethra.
  - Avoiding the use of bubble bath, which is a skin irritant that provides a medium for growth of harmful bacteria.
  - Decreasing the use of harsh soaps, shampoos, and detergents, which can be skin irritants.
  - Limiting bath times to 15 minutes. Children should urinate immediately following the bath to remove harmful bacteria.
  - In the infant, changing diapers frequently.
  - Supplying children with white cotton underwear. Synthetic fibers and fabric dyes can be skin irritants.
  - Providing loose-fitting pants, shorts, tights and underwear to avoid skin irritation.
  - Quickly removing wet clothing such as dance or exercise wear and bathing suits to avoid skin irritation.
- A diet with plenty of fiber helps prevent constipation. Constipation distends the rectum and distorts the bladder, which hinders complete emptying of the bladder.
- Drinking clear liquids routinely flushes harmful bacteria from the urinary tract. Cranberry juice may change the acidity of the urine and cause it to be less likely to become infected.
- Emptying the bladder every 4 hours during the day and once before bedtime helps remove harmful bacteria regularly.
- For males, retracting the foreskin and cleaning the head of the penis daily keeps an uncircumcised child clean.

Source: Data from the American Academy of Family Physicians and Lynn Cates, MD, FAAP, The Dr. Spock Company; National Women's Health Information Center. (2003). A lifetime of good health: Your guide to staying healthy. Washington, DC: US Department of Health and Human Services; National Kidney and Urologic Diseases Information Clearinghouse. How can urinary tract infections be prevented? Bethesda, MD: Author.

Procedures 15-1 and 15-3 ⚭. If tests are positive for streptococcal infection, antibiotics are administered, and the family may be tested and treated for strep as well (Ball & Bindler, 2006). Further infection should be prevented by reducing exposure to pathogens.

Nursing Considerations

The child's skin integrity is compromised by bed rest. The nurse can reposition the child frequently and keep linens wrinkle free. Maintaining adequate nutritional intake may be a challenge for the nurse. The child with glomerulonephritis has a decreased appetite, so the nurse will have to encourage the child to eat.

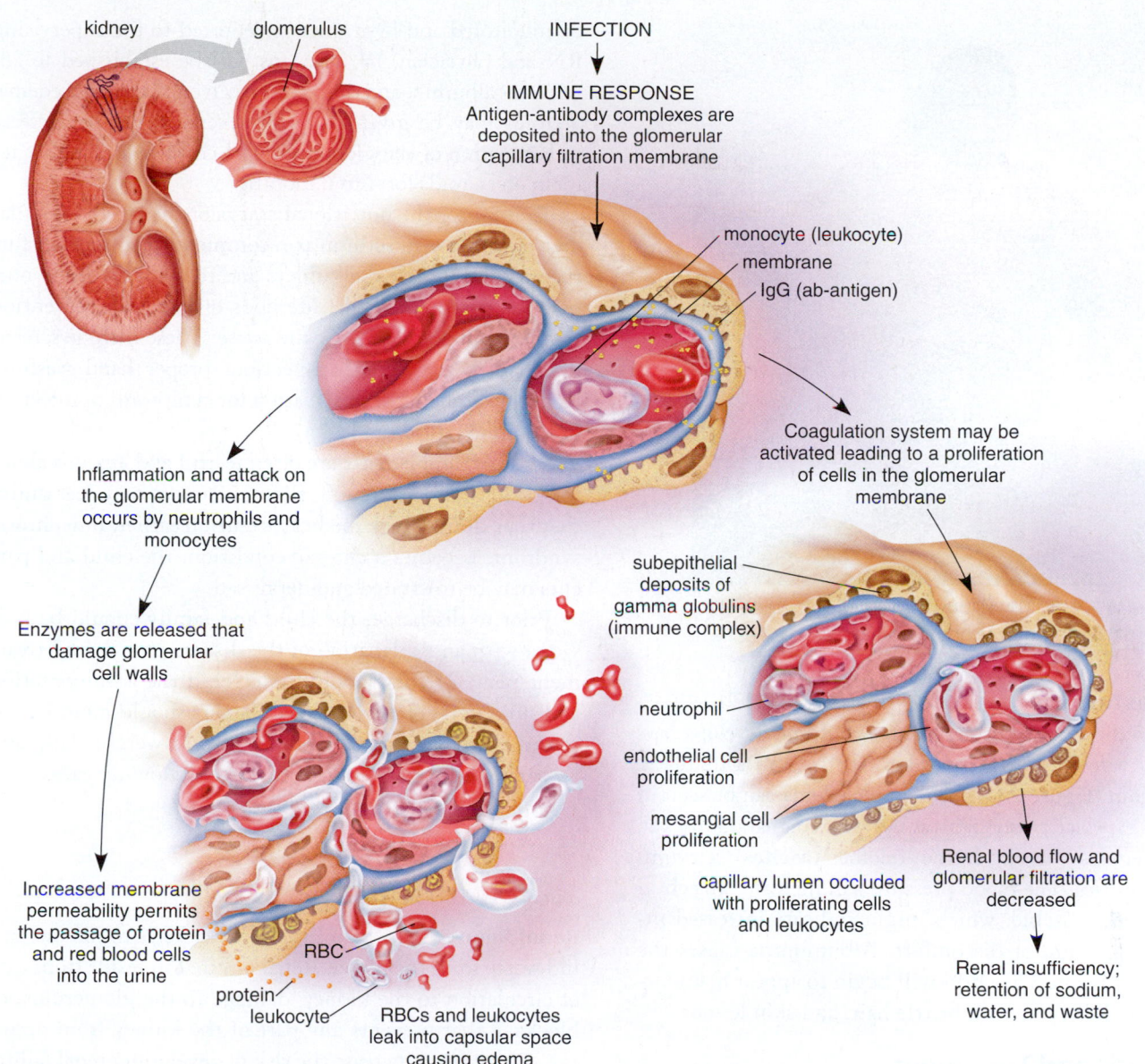

kidney   glomerulus

INFECTION

IMMUNE RESPONSE
Antigen-antibody complexes are
deposited into the glomerular
capillary filtration membrane

monocyte (leukocyte)
membrane
IgG (ab-antigen)

Coagulation system may be
activated leading to a proliferation
of cells in the glomerular
membrane

Inflammation and attack on
the glomerular membrane
occurs by neutrophils and
monocytes

subepithelial
deposits of
gamma globulins
(immune complex)

Enzymes are released that
damage glomerular
cell walls

neutrophil

endothelial cell
proliferation

mesangial cell
proliferation

Increased membrane
permeability permits
the passage of protein
and red blood cells
into the urine

RBC

capillary lumen occluded
with proliferating cells
and leukocytes

Renal blood flow and
glomerular filtration are
decreased

protein
leukocyte

RBCs and leukocytes
leak into capsular space
causing edema

Renal insufficiency;
retention of sodium,
water, and waste

Figure 23-6. ■ In acute postinfectious glomerulonephritis, an immune response to group A beta-hemolytic *Streptococcus* causes inflammation and damage to the glomerular membrane. Protein and red blood cells can pass through glomerular cell walls into the urine. Damaged cells block blood flow to the glomeruli. Renal insufficiency results, leading to retention of sodium, water, and waste.

Most cases of APIGN resolve completely. Gross signs generally resolve in a few weeks. Lab values for microscopic hematuria may take up to 2 years to return to normal, while lab values for proteinuria may be abnormal for up to 12 months. Parents should be forewarned about these findings.

Nephrotic Syndrome

Nephrotic syndrome is a clinical state characterized by edema, **proteinuria** (protein in the urine), **hypoalbuminemia** (low blood albumin levels), **hyperlipidemia** (high blood lipids), and altered immunity. *Primary nephrotic syndrome*, also called minimal-change nephrotic syndrome (MCNS) affects only the kidneys and frequently follows an infection such as *pyelonephritis* (inflammation of the kidney pelvis). Primary nephrotic syndrome is most often seen in children. *Secondary nephrotic syndrome* results from a multisystem disorder such as diabetes, systemic lupus, or sickle cell anemia. Nephrotic syndrome affects more male children between the ages of 2 and 7 than any other group.

In nephrotic syndrome, the glomerular permeability is altered, allowing albumin to move from the blood to the urine. This results in hypoalbuminemia and proteinuria. The shift in albumin changes the osmotic pressure of the blood. The kidney reabsorbs sodium and water, resulting in edema. A low osmotic pressure stimulates the liver to make lipoproteins (*cholesterol*), leading to hyperlipidemia. As immunoglobulins are excreted, the child's immunity is decreased.

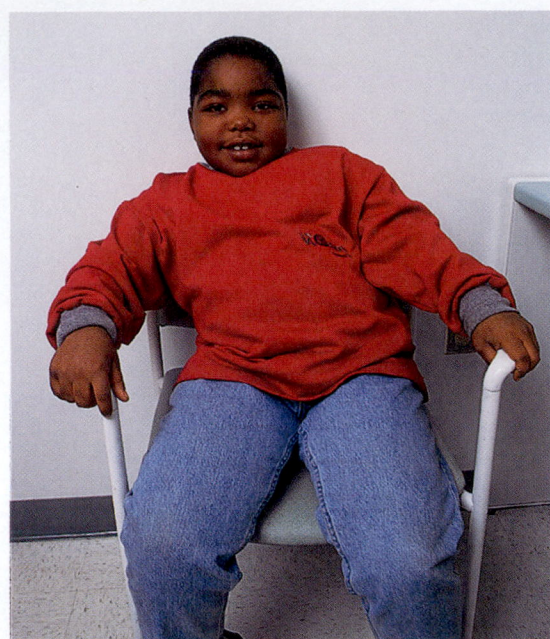

Figure 23-7. ■ Young boy with edema characteristic of nephrotic syndrome or renal failure.

Manifestations

Edema in the child with nephrotic syndrome develops rapidly over a few days to 2 weeks, resulting in a dramatic weight gain (Figure 23-7 ■). Notable edema can be seen in the face, especially **periorbital edema** (edema around the eyes). Edema is also seen in the abdomen (**ascites**), scrotum, and extremities. The blood pressure will increase. The child may become irritable, which might indicate increased intracranial pressure or discomfort. Albuminuria causes the urine to be foamy. The child will begin to appear malnourished with dull eyes; dull, brittle hair; and skin lesions.

Diagnosis and Treatment

When nephrotic syndrome is suspected, a urinalysis is performed to determine the presence of protein in the urine. Typical findings are 3+ to 4+ protein. A 24-hour urine specimen may reveal as much as 15 g of protein. Hematuria may also be detected.

Treatment of nephrotic syndrome is focused on reducing proteinuria and edema and on preventing infection while the child is immunocompromised. Oral corticosteroids are given initially to reduce proteinuria and edema. Diuretic therapy may be necessary to further reduce the edema. Potassium supplementation may be necessary if hypokalemia develops in children taking diuretics. Cyclophosphamide (Cytoxan) can be given to improve symptoms, but this further compromises the child's immunologic status.

Nursing Considerations

The child with nephrotic syndrome should be weighed daily to determine resolution of edema. The blood pressure should

be monitored and hypertension reported to the supervising RN and physician. IV infusions will be established to administer albumin, and diuretics are given to decrease edema. Steroids may be given daily for several weeks to decrease inflammation of the glomeruli. The child will probably remain on steroids for 4 to 6 months.

To improve the nutritional status of the child, a regular diet that is low in sodium is recommended to prevent further protein loss by the kidneys and to allow return of normal blood protein levels. Methods of infection prevention should be implemented by the nurse. These include screening visitors for signs of infection, proper hand washing techniques, and close observation for symptoms of infection in the child.

Children and parents are often fearful and anxious about the child's life-threatening illness. Parents may feel guilty that they did not seek medical attention earlier. If nephrotic syndrome becomes a chronic condition, the child and parents may be frustrated and depressed.

Prior to discharge, the child and family should be provided with an explanation of the disease process and treatment plan. Parents should understand the administration and side effects of medications. Parents should monitor and record the urine protein and the child's weight daily and verbalize the need for routine medical follow-up care.

Acute and Chronic Renal Failure

Renal failure is the inability of the kidneys to remove liquid waste from the blood. Renal failure can result from lack of circulation to the kidney, damage to the glomerulus, or blockage that prevents any part of the kidney from draining. Factors that increase the risk of developing renal failure include severe dehydration, hypotension, accidental poisoning, repeated infection, and trauma.

Acute renal failure (ARF) is the sudden onset of diminished kidney function resulting in the imbalance of fluids and electrolytes. **Chronic renal failure (CRF)** is a progressive, irreversible loss of kidney function. CRF can progress to **end-stage renal disease (ESRD)**, a condition in which kidney function is less than 10% and the child requires dialysis or kidney transplantation to survive.

Manifestations

Specific symptoms of ARF may not appear in the child until the disease is advanced. However, oliguria is usually one of the first symptoms noticed. Nonspecific symptoms include pale skin, headache, nausea, and fatigue. The child may have difficulty concentrating. As the disease progresses, edema (see Figure 23-7), tachycardia, and hypertension become evident. In addition to the previous symptoms, children with

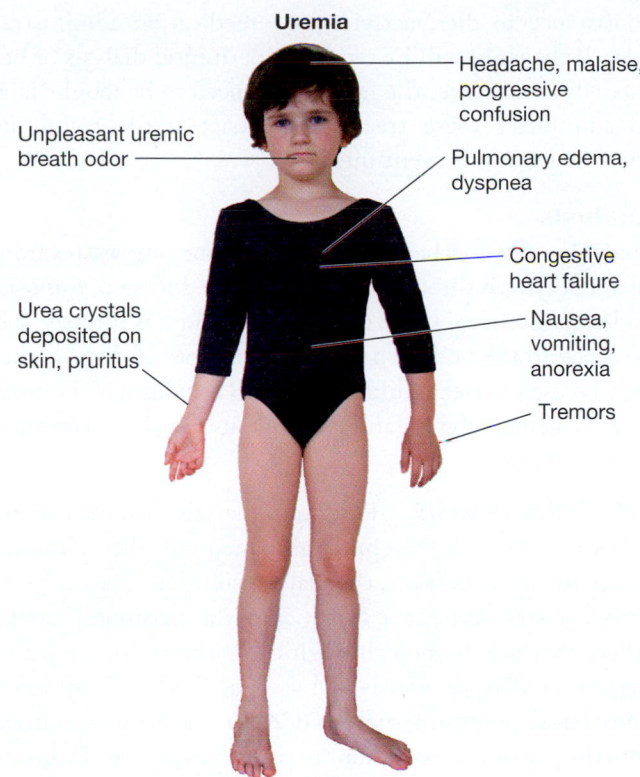

Uremia

Headache, malaise, progressive confusion

Unpleasant uremic breath odor

Pulmonary edema, dyspnea

Congestive heart failure

Urea crystals deposited on skin, pruritus

Nausea, vomiting, anorexia

Tremors

Figure 23-8. ■ Multisystem effects of uremia.
(M. C. Schlachter Photography)

TABLE 23-2

Lab Values for Children with Renal Failure

LAB	NORMAL	FINDING
Blood urea nitrogen (BUN)	Infant: 5–15 mg/dL	Increased
	Child: 5–20 mg/dL	Increased
Serum creatinine	Newborn: 0.8–1.4 mg/dL	Increased
	Infant: 0.7–1.7 mg/dL	Increased
	2–6 years old: 0.3–0.6 mg/dL	Increased
	Over 6 years old: 0.4–1.2 mg/dL	Increased
Serum potassium	Infant: 3.6–5.8 mEq/L	Increased
	Child: 3.5–5.5 mEq/L	Increased
Serum sodium	Infant: 134–150 mEq/L	Increased or decreased
	Child: 135–145 mEq/L	Increased or decreased
Bicarbonate (HCO_3)	24–28 mEq/L	Decreased

CRF have decreased mental alertness, anemia, and growth retardation caused by demineralization of bone. In ESRD, all body systems become affected when waste is not eliminated. **Uremic syndrome** develops in ESRD (Figure 23-8 ■). Uremic syndrome is characterized by nausea, vomiting, anorexia, uremic breath odor, anemia, **uremic frost** (urea crystals deposited on the skin), pruritus, malaise, headache, confusion, tremors, pulmonary edema, dyspnea, and congestive heart failure.

Diagnosis

Urinary output is measured carefully, usually by indwelling catheter (see Procedure 13-14 ⚭). Oliguria in renal failure in children is defined as urine output less than 1mL/kg/hr. For example, a child weighing 8 kg would have a urine output of less than 8 mL/hr. Increased laboratory values include serum creatinine, blood urea nitrogen (BUN), and serum potassium. Arterial bicarbonate may be decreased. Serum sodium may be increased or decreased, depending on the child's fluid status. Table 23-2 ■ shows lab values in children with renal failure. Kidney function tests such as an intravenous pyelography may be ordered to determine size, structure, and function of the kidneys, ureters, and bladder.

Glomerular filtration rate is used to determine the extent of CRF in children. The glomerular filtration rate depicts the kidney's ability to filter plasma properly. In CRF, this

rate is decreased. Table 23-3 ■ reviews normal glomerular filtration rates for the pediatric client.

Treatment

Children in ARF who have fluid volume deficit are typically admitted to pediatric intensive care units for IV fluid replacement. Solutions used are normal saline or lactated Ringer's. If blood loss is the cause of fluid volume deficit, albumin is given.

Children in ARF with fluid overload require diuretic therapy and oral fluid restriction. Hyperkalemia is treated

TABLE 23-3

Normal Glomerular Filtration Rates

AGE OF CHILD	NORMAL GFR
Infants, 1 week	40.6 ± 14.8 mean GFR
Infants, 2–8 weeks	65.8 ± 24.8 mean GFR
Infants, 8 weeks–2 years	95.7 ± 21.7 mean GFR
Children, 2–12 years	133.0 ± 27.0 mean GFR
Males, 13–21 years	140.0 ± 30.0 mean GFR
Females, 13–21 years	126.0 ± 22.0 mean GFR

with Kayexalate (see Table 15-4). This medication can be given orally or by enema.

CRF requires strict dietary management in order to provide the child with adequate calories for growth needs while restricting foods that might complicate fluid and electrolyte imbalances. Pharmacologic agents for children with CRF include vitamin and mineral supplementation, phosphate-binding agents to prevent bone demineralization, growth hormones to stimulate growth, hematopoietic growth factors and iron supplementation to treat anemia, and antihypertensive agents to treat hypertension.

Some children can be managed with a combination of medication and diet therapy, while other children progress rapidly to ESRD that requires dialysis or kidney transplant. See the next section for more information on dialysis. For more information about organ transplantation, see Chapters 21 and 28 ⊙⊙.

Nursing Considerations

The child with renal failure should be assessed for signs of fluid overload, including weight gain, pitting edema, pulmonary edema, and ascites. A priority nursing task is strictly monitoring intake and output. See Chapter 15 ⊙⊙ for more information on this procedure. Urinary output should be monitored, including the color and odor of the urine. Blood values (including serum electrolytes, BUN, creatinine, and bicarbonate levels) should be monitored closely. Abnormal levels should be reported to the supervising RN and physician.

Medications must be administered as directed in order to achieve the desired effect. The child must be monitored for side effects of medication, signs of electrolyte imbalance, and alterations in blood pressure. The child will need small frequent feedings in order to meet additional nutrition demands.

In a child with renal failure, infection places additional burden on the kidneys and can speed the progression of the disease. Sites for infection include respiratory, urinary, and gastrointestinal tracts and dialysis sites. The nurse must be an effective role model for the child and family in preventing infection.

The child and family should be assessed for signs of undue stress brought on by life-threatening chronic illness. The need for ongoing dialysis is expensive, and the limited number of dialysis facilities dictates the family's place of residence. The child and family need emotional support in dealing with a chronic life-threatening illness. Both the National Kidney Foundation and local support groups can be valuable resources for the nurse and the family.

In planning home care, the needs of the child and family should be identified well before discharge. Help the family plan medication administration times that work around dialysis and that fit their routine. Stress the importance of

consistency in diet, activity, and medication administration. If the child will be receiving peritoneal dialysis or hemodialysis at home, the family will need to be taught how to administer these treatments. Strict sterile technique must be used to prevent infection.

Dialysis

Dialysis is the mechanical process of removing wastes from blood or lymph through the processes of diffusion, osmosis, and ultrafiltration. Once the blood or lymph is filtered, it is returned to the body. There are three types of dialysis that may be used to treat children with CRF and/or ESRD: peritoneal, hemodialysis, and continuous renal replacement therapy (CRRT).

PERITONEAL DIALYSIS. Peritoneal dialysis involves placing a catheter through the child's abdomen into the peritoneal cavity to infuse *dialysate*, the dialysis solution. The dialysate draws wastes and extra fluids into the peritoneal cavity, where they are drained through the catheter. Two types of peritoneal dialysis are available. The first is continuous ambulatory peritoneal dialysis (CAPD). Dialysate is infused into the peritoneal cavity four to five times per day. Drainage of the fluid occurs when the collection chamber is lowered below the pelvis. The second method of peritoneal dialysis is called automated peritoneal dialysis. The process of infusing dialysate and removing it is automated and occurs approximately five times over a 10-hour period.

clinical ALERT

The nurse must carefully assess the child undergoing peritoneal dialysis for peritonitis and abdominal hernia. The child with peritonitis may have cloudy dialysate following dialysis, as well as fever, vomiting, diarrhea, and abdominal tenderness or pain.

HEMODIALYSIS. In hemodialysis, the child's blood is removed from the body and flows through a *dialyzer* (a machine that removes wastes and extra fluid), and then is returned to the body (Figure 23-9 ■). The child will have an external shunt or an arteriovenous fistula. Children with CRF and/or ESRD need hemodialysis three times weekly. Each dialysis session lasts 3 to 4 hours.

clinical ALERT

The nurse must be vigilant to observe for complications related to hemodialysis. These complications include hypotension, thrombosis, infection, fluid and electrolyte imbalances, and shock. **Disequilibrium syndrome** is a complication caused by cerebral edema. Symptoms of disequilibrium syndrome include fatigue; nausea; vomiting; tremors, which can progress to delirium; seizures; and coma.

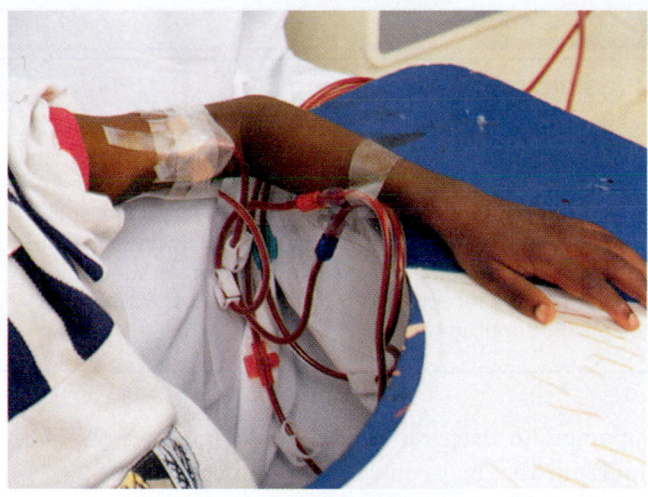

A

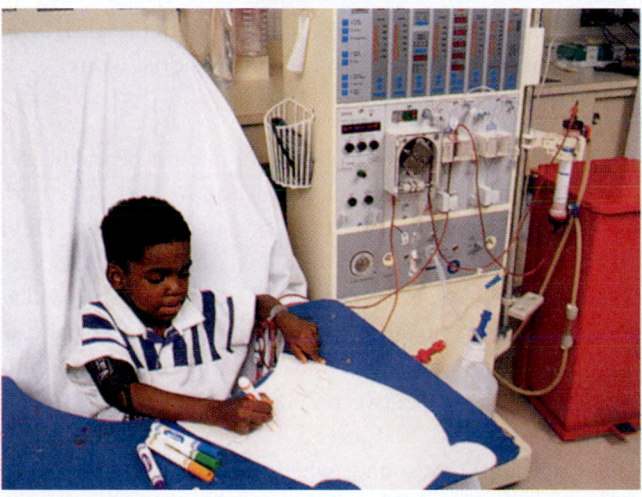

B

Figure 23-9. ■ This child is undergoing hemodialysis. (**A**) A surgically implanted vascular graft is being used here. One needle is placed in the arterialized end of the graft (red tubing), and one needle is placed in the venous end (blue tubing) for blood return. (**B**) The child is able to draw or perform other quiet activities during dialysis treatment. Note that the child's blood pressure is monitored carefully throughout treatment.

CONTINUOUS RENAL REPLACEMENT THERAPY.   Continuous renal replacement therapy (CRRT) provides the child with continuous hemodialysis, 24 hours per day. CRRT is an inpatient procedure often requiring that the child be admitted to the pediatric intensive care unit.

Wilms' Tumor or Nephroblastoma

Wilms' tumor or **nephroblastoma** is a highly metastatic, cancerous tumor of the kidney. It is most common in children between 2 and 5 years of age. Even in the absence of other anomalies, a genetic link is suggested. A gene that promotes normal kidney function is missing in a child with Wilms' tumor.

Manifestations

A child with Wilms' tumor may be asymptomatic. Commonly, parents palpate an abdominal mass while bathing the child. The mass may be unilateral or bilateral; it is usually firm and contains several lobes. Hematuria, hypertension, and abdominal pain may be present.

Diagnosis

Diagnosis is made on the basis of ultrasound. Magnetic resonance imaging (MRI) of the lungs, liver, spleen, and brain are necessary to determine metastasis. These procedures are frightening to the child and parents, and thorough explanation is important. Parents are usually allowed to stay with the child during diagnostic tests. The diagnosis will provide the staging of the tumor (Table 23-4 ■).

Treatment

Surgery to remove the kidney and affected lymph nodes is usually scheduled as soon as possible. Follow-up chemotherapy and/or radiation may be necessary to ensure destruction

TABLE 23-4	
Staging of Wilms' Tumor	
STAGE OF WILMS' TUMOR	**CANCER LOCATION**
Stage I	Cancer is found only in the kidney and can be completely removed by surgery.
Stage II	Cancer has spread beyond the kidney to fat or soft tissue or blood vessels. The cancer can be completely removed by surgery.
Stage III	Cancer has spread within the abdomen and cannot be completely removed by surgery. The cancer may have spread to the lymph nodes (small bean-shaped structures found throughout the body that produce and store infection-fighting cells) near the kidney, blood vessels, or the peritoneum (tissue that lines the abdomen and covers most organs in the abdomen).
Stage IV	Cancer has spread to the lungs, liver, bone, or brain, or to lymph nodes outside the abdomen and pelvis.
Stage V	Cancer cells are found in both kidneys when the disease is first diagnosed.

of the tumor. If the tumor has metastasized to the other kidney or to other organs, prognosis is poor.

Nursing Considerations

Due to the highly metastatic nature of Wilms' tumor, signs should be placed on the chart and in the head of the bed warning all health care providers to avoid palpating the child's abdomen. Preoperative and postoperative care follows routine protocols.

clinical ALERT

Do *not* palpate the abdomen of a child with potential Wilms' tumor. These tumors are fragile. Palpation could cause the tumor to rupture, dispersing cancerous cells throughout the abdomen.

The postoperative nursing care focuses on pain management and fluid balance. A large incision is needed to remove the kidney, and the shift in the internal organs can cause discomfort for the child. Gentle handling is important, but the child will need to be encouraged to turn, cough, and deep breathe to prevent complications.

Fluid balance should be monitored by daily weight, intake and output, and urine specific gravity. The blood pressure should be monitored to assess shock and the function of the remaining kidney.

During chemotherapy, the child should be monitored for side effects, infection, and function of the remaining kidney. Parents should be taught home care and the need for continued follow-up visits prior to discharge. The remaining kidney needs to be protected from infection and injury. Parents may want to overprotect the child, but it will help the positive development of the child to maintain as normal a lifestyle as possible.

Enuresis

Enuresis is urinary incontinence occurring in a child who is capable of obtaining bladder control. (Box 23-3 ■ describes physiologic factors that relate to toilet training.) *Nocturnal enuresis* occurs during the night, and *diurnal enuresis* occurs during the day. Enuresis can be a result of familial tendencies, difficulty in arousing, decreased bladder capacity, abnormal circadian rhythms, abnormalities of the urethra, developmental delays, or sleep apnea.

Diagnosis

To diagnose enuresis in children, historical data must be gathered. It is important to determine a family history of enuresis. There should be a discussion of how the family is currently managing the problem. It should also be determined how the child was toilet trained, if applicable. It is

BOX 23-3

Physiology of Toilet Training

At birth, a child's bladder capacity is 20 to 50 mL. This capacity increases gradually until reaching 700 mL in adulthood. When "stretch receptors" found in the bladder wall are stimulated, urination is initiated. Children younger than 2 years are incapable of maintaining bladder control because they do not have sufficient nerve development to be able to detect the stimulation of these stretch receptors. Complete bladder control may not be possible until age 4 or 5.

important to determine if there are any stressors in the child's life that may contribute to enuresis.

Other laboratory tests that can assist in the diagnosis are urinalysis and urine culture. Diagnostic studies may include bladder capacity, uroflow measurement, and ultrasound scans of the bladder to measure residual urine.

Treatment

Treatment for enuresis can be a combination of medication and behavioral modifications. Medications used are antidiuretics, anticholinergics, or tricyclic antidepressants (Table 23-5 ■). The child's behavior related to fluid intake and voiding is modified in an effort to develop new habits that will assist the child in controlling the bladder at night. Total fluid intake for the day is divided into portions that are administered as follows: 40% between 7 A.M. and noon, 40% between noon and 5 P.M., and 20% after 5 P.M. For children older than 7 years, an alarm that sounds when the child begins to void at night can assist the child in waking and voiding in the bathroom (Box 23-4 ■). Positive reinforcement and rewards can be implemented when the child is able to remain dry. These reinforcements should be specifically motivating for the child. If the child has diurnal enuresis, a 2-hour voiding schedule can be used to teach the child to empty the bladder completely.

NURSING CARE

PRIORITIES IN NURSING CARE

When caring for children with urinary disorders other than renal failure, the nurse should seek to maintain renal function and fluid balance. Children with infections should be monitored for changes in body temperature, elevated white blood cells (WBCs), and poor urine output. Monitor closely for signs and symptoms of fluid deficit or fluid overload. See Chapter 15 ◯◯ for more information on fluid and electrolyte imbalances. Oral and IV intake must be carefully assessed to avoid excess intake. The nurse carefully collects data and records daily intake and output.

TABLE 23-5

Pharmacology: Medications Used for Treatment of Enuresis

DRUG (COMMON BRAND NAME AND GENERIC)	USUAL ROUTE/DOSE	CLASSIFICATION AND PURPOSE	SELECTED SIDE EFFECTS	DON'T GIVE IF
Tofranil (imipramine hydrochloride)	25–50 mg PO 1 hour before bedtime	Tricyclic antidepressant for nocturnal enuresis	Sedation, drowsiness, orthostatic hypotension, arrhythmias, blurred vision, dry mouth, urinary retention	Child has respiratory disorder, cardiovascular disorder, blood disorder, or hepatic disorder
Levsin or Levsinex Timecaps (hyoscyamine sulfate)	0.0625–0.125 mg PO prn, maximum dosage for child 2–12 is 0.75 mg/day	Anticholinergic (parasympatholytic) relaxes smooth muscle of the bladder, increasing bladder capacity	Drowsiness, blurred vision, dry mouth, constipation, urinary retention	Child has diabetes mellitus or cardiac disease
DDAVP or Stimate (desmopressin acetate)	5–40 mcg intranasal spray at bedtime or 0.2–0.6 mg PO at bedtime for children greater than 6 years	Vasopressin to relieve polyuria	Transient headache, nasal congestion, heartburn, shortness of breath	Child has cardiac disease, marked edema
Ditropan (oxybutynin chloride)	0.2 mg/kg PO 2–4 times/day for child 1–5 years; 5 mg PO 2 times/day for child greater than 5 years	Anticholinergic (parasympatholytic) relaxes smooth muscle of the bladder, increasing bladder capacity	Drowsiness, blurred vision, dry mouth, constipation	Child has GI obstruction, myasthenia gravis, glaucoma, severe colitis, urinary retention, severe cardiac disease

BOX 23-4   **CLIENT TEACHING**

Use of Enuresis Alarm

Parents and children must understand how the enuresis alarm functions and how it is to be used (Mercer, 2003). Teach parents the following:

- The average child will need to use the enuresis alarm for 10 to 12 weeks to achieve success in staying dry.
- Attach the alarm to close-fitting cloth underwear. Do not attach it to loose clothing such as boxer shorts or pajamas. Do not attach it to disposable diapers.
- When the alarm sounds, go to the child's room and observe the child's response. Tell the child to put his or her feet on the floor and walk to the bathroom. Help the child if necessary. Turn off the alarm only after the child puts his or her feet on the floor.
- Recognize that in the beginning, the child will have voided by the time he or she wakes up or the parents arrive. The measures of progress include:
  - Reduced number of episodes of wetting per night
  - Increased length of sleep time before wetting

- Decreased amount of urination (spotting) before the child puts his or her feet on the floor.
- After a wetting episode, reattach the alarm to clean dry underpants.
- Keep a chart to track events, and praise the child for progress.
- Consider giving prizes for cooperation and improved performance. Prizes may include stickers for each time the child goes without assistance to the bathroom or a larger prize, such as a meal out or some form of entertainment, for the first completely dry night.
- Remind parents that the greatest reward for the child is their praise.
- Once the child is able to stay dry through the night, continue use of the alarm until there have been 2 continuous weeks without an episode of enuresis. Then use the alarm every other night for 2 or more weeks of consecutive dryness.
- If the child has a wetting episode during this time, begin the 2-week "weaning period" again. Do not be hasty about this phase of the training. Relapse is common when training is cut off prematurely.

ASSESSING

Children with urinary disorders should be assessed for intake and output. Urine should be monitored for amount, color, clarity, odor, and specific gravity. (Normal specific gravity of urine is 1.010 to 1.025.) Assess the abdomen using light palpation to prevent damage to internal organs. Assess the child for signs of dehydration or fluid excess, including the presence of edema and monitoring daily weights.

DIAGNOSING, PLANNING, AND IMPLEMENTING

Numerous nursing diagnoses could apply to the child with urinary disorders and their families. Nursing diagnoses might include:

- Risk for Infection, related to urinary stasis
- Excess Fluid Volume, related to impaired kidney function
- Risk for Deficient Fluid Volume, related to impaired kidney function
- Impaired Urinary Elimination, related to structural or functional impairment of the urinary system.

Nursing interventions follow the general health guidelines presented in previous chapters of this book. Adaptation of interventions with the child is addressed as follows:

- Encourage children to drink water and a variety of juices daily. Frozen pops and frozen juice can be used to increase fluid intake. *Adequate fluid intake is essential to proper kidney function. Additional fluids may be needed during times of illness, infection, and fever.*
- Follow doctor's orders for fluid restriction in children with urinary disorders. See Procedure 15-3 ⚭ for more information on managing fluid restrictions. *When sodium and water retention are present, fluids should be limited.*
- Administer medications as ordered, such as analgesics and steroids. *Dysuria may make the child reluctant to void. If surgery is needed, the child must be medicated for comfort. Steroids reduce the immune response.*
- Provide instruction to the child and parents about care. Be aware of family strain, and refer to RN and social worker as necessary. *The life-threatening nature of urinary disorders contributes to family strain. The long-term effects and treatment contribute to caregiver strain.*
- Provide client teaching concerning signs of infection after surgery (Box 23-5 ■).

EVALUATING

The child's condition is evaluated by blood and urine analysis, weight loss, and a return of general health. Monitor closely for side effects of medications. The function of the kidneys (or a remaining kidney) must be evaluated frequently. Report any signs of urinary infection or renal failure

---

| BOX 23-5 | CLIENT TEACHING |

Signs of Infection After Surgery

Teach parents to understand the following signs and symptoms of infection and to report them promptly to the primary care provider. Signs of infection include:

- Increased temperature
- Cloudy urine
- Foul odor from the surgical site
- Purulent drainage
- Decreased feeding
- Increased fussiness.

---

to the physician immediately. Repeat urine samples may be done after treatment with antibiotics to determine complete eradication of the causative organism.

Due to the strain of acute life-threatening illness on the child and family, frequent evaluation of family functioning is important. Referral to support groups and agencies may be necessary.

NURSING PROCESS CARE PLAN
Child With Nephrotic Syndrome

James, a 22-month-old child, has been admitted to the pediatric unit with a diagnosis of possible nephrotic syndrome. James has gained 2 lb in the last week and a half. His mother states, "His face is so swollen, I can hardly recognize my own child." Laboratory reports indicate a low blood albumin and high proteinuria. James is irritable and whines most of the time.

Assessment
- 2+ edema
- Crackling lung sounds
- Vital signs: P 150, R 48

Nursing Diagnosis. The following important nursing diagnosis (among others) is established for this client:

- Excess Fluid Volume, related to altered urinary function.

Expected Outcomes. Intake and output will be within 100 mL by third hospital day.

Planning and Implementation
- Measure and record intake and output every 8 hours.
- Check output hourly. If no urinary catheter, weigh diapers.
- Monitor specific gravity.
- Take daily weights.
- Reposition every half-hour.

- Anticipate respiratory distress by monitoring breath sounds, respiratory effort, and level of consciousness.
- Administer IV fluids via appropriate equipment.
- Administer medications with attention to dosage and potential effect on electrolytes and blood protein levels.

Evaluation

- Review intake and output record to determine balance.
- Edema in body will be less than on admission.
- Lung sounds will be clear.
- Weight will be the same as 2 weeks ago.

Critical Thinking in the Nursing Process

1. Explain the importance of repositioning James every half-hour.
2. What information would you obtain from weighing diapers, and why is it important?
3. What actions might you take to support James's family during his hospitalization?

Note: Discussion of Critical Thinking questions appears in Appendix I.

REPRODUCTIVE SYSTEM

Anatomy and Physiology

The reproductive system consists of internal and external organs that will, when mature, assist the individual in achieving conception and assist the female in maintaining pregnancy and achieving childbirth. The organs of the male are the penis, scrotum, testes, prostate, and epididymis. These organs function to produce, protect, and transport sperm; regulate hormone production; and provide sexual pleasure later in life.

Female reproductive organs include the ovaries, fallopian tubes, uterus, cervix, vagina, and vulva. These organs function to produce, protect, and transport ova; regulate hormone production; and provide sexual pleasure later in life (see Figure 4-13). The phases of sexual maturation (called *Tanner's stages*) are described in Table 11-12 .

Puberty is the maturation process of the reproductive system. At the end of this process, the individual is capable of reproduction. In males, the onset of puberty occurs between ages 10 and 15. During puberty, the penis, testes, and scrotum enlarge. New hair develops on the face, in the pubic area, and in the axillae. Mature sperm are able to be produced.

In females, the onset of puberty occurs between ages 8 and 13. During puberty, breasts enlarge, menstruation begins, and new hair develops in the pubic area and in the axillae. For more information about the changes of puberty, see Chapter 4 .

Brief Assessment Overview

HISTORY

- Ask about family history of reproductive disorders.
- Inquire about redness, swelling, or discharge from the genitalia.
- Ask about burning or itching of the genitalia.
- Inquire about lumps or masses on the child's genitalia.

- For the older child and adolescent, ask about sexual abuse. See Chapter 27 for a more detailed description of this assessment.

PHYSICAL

- Inspect external genitalia for color, size, hair distribution, lumps or masses, drainage, and symmetry of the organs.
- In males, note placement of the urinary meatus and determine whether the child is circumcised.

Although the reproductive system is immature until puberty, many congenital anomalies of the urinary system also affect the reproductive system.

Ambiguous Genitalia

Ambiguous genitalia (**pseudohermaphroditism**) is a rare condition in which it is difficult to determine the gender of the child. In this circumstance, chromosomal analysis may be necessary. Not only is the reproductive system affected, but also, in many cases, the urinary and intestinal systems are affected. Surgical reconstruction is usually done in stages, with the primary goal being normal functioning of the urinary and intestinal systems. Depending on the degree of defect, reproductive function may be lost. See Chapter 9 for information about care of the child with ambiguous genitalia.

Male Disorders

HYDROCELE

Hydrocele (Figure 23-10) is the accumulation of fluid in the scrotum. During fetal development, fluid becomes trapped in the tunica vaginalis. When the scrotum is palpated, a round, smooth, and nontender mass is noted. The scrotal sac can also be *transilluminated* (have a light shown through it) to detect the presence of fluid. Most hydroceles resolve spontaneously in the first 2 years of life. The

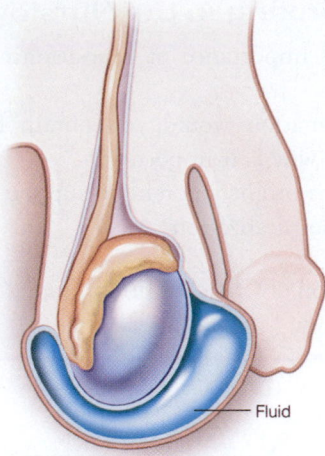

Figure 23-10. ■ Hydrocele is a nontender, fluid-filled mass within the tunica vaginalis.

nurse should assist the family in understanding this disorder. Parents may also be concerned that the enlargement of the scrotum is permanent. The nurse should provide teaching about the probable spontaneous resolution of the condition.

PHIMOSIS

Phimosis is the inability to retract the foreskin of the penis due to a tightened prepuce. At birth, the infant's foreskin is not retractable due to adhesions. As the child grows, retraction of the foreskin should occur. Complications of phimosis include **balanoposthitis** (inflammation or infection of the glans penis) and **paraphimosis** (the inability to return the foreskin over the glans, causing constriction of the penis).

Phimosis is treated surgically by *circumcision* (the removal of the foreskin). Circumcision in the older child can be traumatic and painful. The nurse can assist with anxiety-reducing techniques in the preoperative period. Chapter 9 ⊙ has more information about circumcision.

CRYPTORCHIDISM

Cryptorchidism (undescended testicle) is a condition in which one or both testicles fail to descend into the scrotum. Descent of the testes may occur *in utero* or may take place by the time the infant is 3 months old. Cryptorchidism can occur due to lower testosterone levels or due to a structural defect, such as a shortened spermatic cord.

Diagnosis of cryptorchidism is made by physical examination and confirmed by ultrasound, computed tomography (CT) scan, or MRI. At birth, the infant is screened for cryptorchidism by using the Ballard Gestational Assessment Scale. See Chapter 9, Figure 9-9 ⊙, for more information on using this assessment tool. Findings of undescended testicles at birth require follow-up examinations.

BOX 23-6

Testicular Self-Examination

Testicular self-examination is important for all males ages 15 to 35, but especially for the young man with a history of cryptorchidism. Young men should choose a day of the week, perhaps their birthday, and examine the testicles in the following manner every month:

- Examination can be done in front of a mirror or in the shower.
- Lubrication makes the skin around the testicle move easier. In the shower, soap is appropriate. Outside the shower, lotion can be used.
- Place the index and middle fingers under the testicle with thumbs on top. Roll the testicle gently between the thumbs and fingers. Feel for any lumps or masses. This should not be painful.
- Differentiate between the epididymis and any lumps. The epididymis lies above and behind the testicle. It is soft and smooth and may be slightly tender.
- Contact your physician promptly if any masses, lumps, or unexpected pain or tenderness are noted.

Medical treatment of cryptorchidism includes administration of human chorionic gonadotrophin, although this treatment is not widely accepted in the United States. Prior to age 2, a surgical procedure called an *orchiopexy* may be performed to reposition the testicle into the scrotal sac. Children with cryptorchidism have a 35 to 50 times greater risk of testicular cancer. These children should be taught the technique of testicular self-examination (Box 23-6 ■). See Chapter 5 ⊙ for more information on testicular cancer.

TESTICULAR TORSION

If the spermatic cord becomes twisted, a condition called testicular torsion occurs (Figure 23-11 ■). This condition

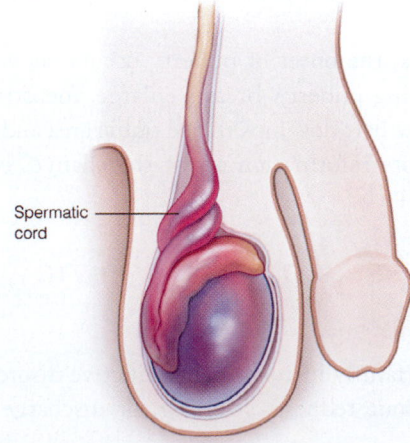

Figure 23-11. ■ Testicular torsion occurs most frequently in adolescents. It requires immediate surgical intervention.

may occur in newborns, but more commonly occurs in early adolescence. The young male experiences intense scrotal pain accompanied by nausea and vomiting. Because ischemia develops quickly, surgical correction is necessary within 4 hours of the onset of symptoms.

Female Disorders

As is true for other body systems, primary care of the reproductive system is best. For females, regular gynecologic examinations often begin during the late teenage years or when they become sexually active. Nursing care involves sensitivity to the embarrassment or fear the client might experience when approaching a gynecologic exam. The Health Promotion Issue on pages 704 and 705 addresses this topic.

IMPERFORATE HYMEN

The **hymen** is the mucous membrane, skin, and fibrous tissue that covers the introitus of the vagina at birth. An *imperforate hymen* is a hymen that does not allow passage of vaginal secretions or menses. The female child may have no symptoms until the onset of puberty. Obstruction of menses increases uterine pressure and results in abdominal discomfort and distension.

The hymen may be removed surgically. Young girls will need information related to their anatomy. They will also need reassurance that this condition will not affect their future sexuality or ability to bear children.

FEMALE CIRCUMCISION

Female circumcision is a type of surgical procedure performed on young girls for cultural purposes rather than medical ones. In some cultures, this procedure may be performed on infants as young as 1 day old, while in other settings it may be performed on the adolescent or young adult woman. Three types of female circumcision are typically seen:

- *Sunna* is the excision of part or all of the clitoris.
- The second type is the excision of the entire clitoris and the labia minora. Following this type of circumcision, the edges of the labia minora are sewn together, leaving a small opening for urination and menstruation.
- *Infibulation* is the third type of female circumcision. In this procedure, the entire clitoris and labia minora are excised and the labia majora is scraped. The edges are then sewn together leaving only a small opening for urination and menstruation.

This cultural norm in some African, Asian, and Middle Eastern societies is said to be done in order to control a woman's sexuality, to ensure her virginity until marriage, to reduce her to her expected cultural role, to protect her from rape, to enhance feminine hygiene, and as a religious ritual (Reichert, 1998).

Girls who are exposed to this surgical procedure are at risk for hemorrhage, pain, and infection. Psychological complications include anxiety, depression, and frigidity. Intercourse is painful, if possible at all. Childbirth may also not be possible.

Nurses should learn about the practice of female circumcision, especially among the population they serve. Children who present with symptoms of complications from female circumcision should be treated with dignity and respect. Encourage the child to talk about her feelings about her body. The child needs to be able to trust the nurse. The child and her family need to be educated about the possible complications of this practice.

MENSTRUAL DISORDERS

As puberty begins, adolescent girls may develop menstrual disorders. Menstruation may be painful (*dysmennorhea*), or menstrual cycles may be irregular. Dysmenorrhea is due to the release of prostaglandins during the menstrual cycle, and it accompanies ovulatory cycles. Prostaglandin inhibitors such as ibuprofen are an effective treatment for dysmenorrhea. Nonpharmacologic pain relief methods for dysmenorrhea include a low sodium diet to reduce bloating, heat application to the lower abdomen and back, rest, and exercise. For more information on dysmenorrhea, see Chapter 5 🔗.

Adolescents can experience *metrorrhagia* or bleeding between menstrual cycles. Some young girls may spot during ovulation or experience breakthrough bleeding if they are on oral contraceptives. Vaginal irritation such as vaginitis may also cause bleeding. Any bleeding between periods that is not associated with the previous explanations should be reported to the physician because it may be a sign of uterine cancer or ovarian cysts.

Amenorrhea (the absence of menses) can occur in the adolescent who is under severe stress, has a chronic illness, is dieting extremely, or is exercising strenuously. Amenorrhea is also a sign of pregnancy. For more information about amenorrhea, see Chapter 5 🔗.

Premenstrual syndrome (PMS) is also a menstrual disorder that often affects teens. PMS is caused by hormonal imbalance and is characterized by irritability, depression, edema, and breast tenderness that occurs prior to the start of the menstrual cycle each month. For more information on PMS, see Chapter 5 🔗.

VAGINITIS

Vaginitis is the inflammation of the vagina. Vaginal irritation may be caused by the insertion of foreign objects, infection with *Streptococcus* or *E. coli*, infestation of pinworms, or chemical irritation from hygiene products such as douches, soaps, and perfumes. It may also be caused by *Candida albicans* (often appearing when a girl becomes

(*Text continues on p. 706.*)

ASSISTING THE YOUNG TEEN WITH HER FIRST PAP SMEAR

Seventeen-year-old Dana presents to the family planning clinic requesting birth control pills. She had a baby 18 months ago and states that she does not want to be pregnant again. She is accompanied by her mother and her toddler son, Gray.

The LPN takes Dana's history. Dana has been sexually active since she was 14 years old. She has never used any form of birth control, including condoms, and has had at least five sexual partners. Dana states that she has never had a Pap smear and confesses that she does not really know what one is. She says that her friend told her that it was painful and that she should never have one.

Dana says that she is afraid of having a Pap smear. She just wants the nurse practitioner to give her a prescription for birth control pills because she needs to go to work.

The LPN and nurse practitioner review Dana's history and discuss her situation. It is determined that a Pap smear is indicated based on her past medical history. Together, they devise a teaching plan to help Dana understand the importance of this procedure.

DISCUSSION

The Papanicolaou test, commonly called the Pap smear, is a screen for cervical cancer. A physician, nurse practitioner, nurse midwife, or physician's assistant will take a small sample of cervical cells, which are sent to the laboratory for examination. Prior to becoming cancer, cervical cells go through cellular changes. The Pap smear is designed to detect these cervical cellular changes prior to their becoming cancerous.

According to the American Cancer Society and the American College of Obstetricians and Gynecologists, a woman should have her first Pap smear at age 21 or within 3 years of becoming sexually active, whichever comes first. These recommendations were made based on the risk of cervical cancer to this age group. The most common cause of cervical cancer is infection with the human papillomavirus (HPV). This virus is most often transmitted sexually. The Pap smear can detect infection with HPV. Other risk factors for developing cervical cancer include smoking, having multiple partners (more than two), having sexual intercourse before age 18, having sexual intercourse with males who have multiple partners, and infection with sexually transmitted infections, including HIV.

The Pap smear is part of a complete gynecologic examination. The comprehensive examination can include, but is not limited to, personal and family medical history, weight measurement, urinalysis, hematocrit and hemoglobin check, blood pressure check, auscultation of heart and lungs, an abdominal exam, a breast exam, teaching about breast self-exam, a pelvic exam, and evaluation for contraception or conception readiness.

Prior to the Pap smear, the client must completely disrobe below the waist. The LPN will supply a disposable gown and drape. The client is placed in a private room and a chaperone, usually the nurse, is provided for the client's comfort and to assist the practitioner.

Most examination tables are covered with disposable paper. Tables are padded and have stirrups to support the woman's feet. Stirrups are metal and can be cold. The woman can wear socks to be more comfortable.

The practitioner uses a vaginal speculum to separate the vaginal walls and visualize the cervix. The nurse can position an examination light toward the perineum and apply water-soluble lubricant to ease insertion of the speculum. The speculum can be made of plastic or metal.

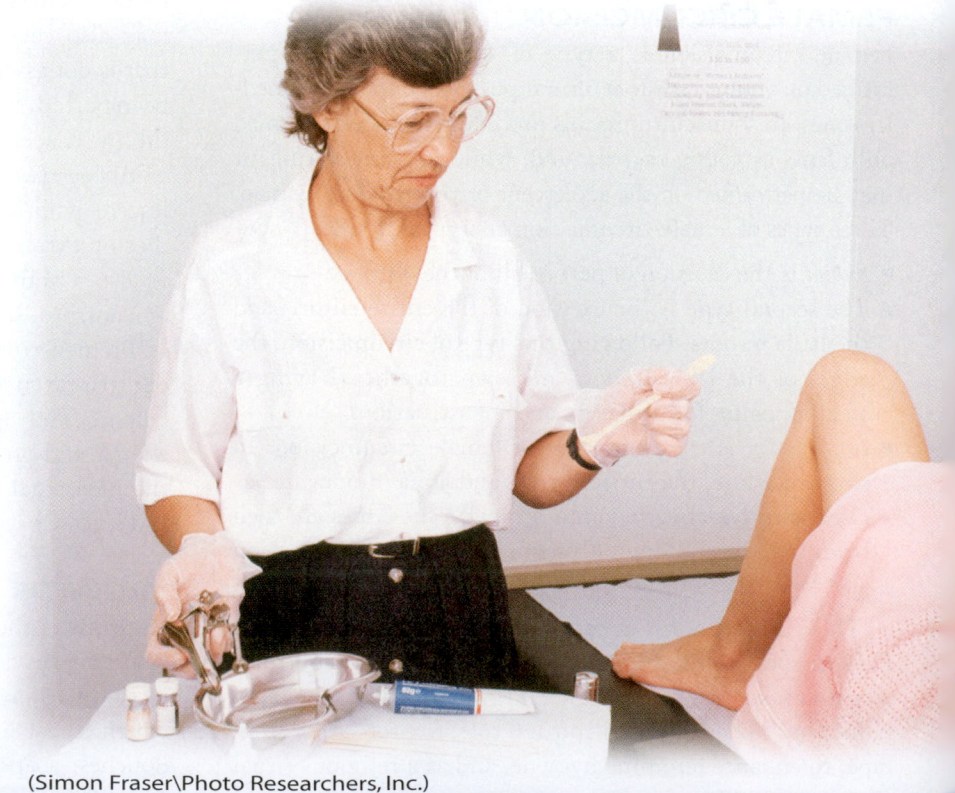

(Simon Fraser\Photo Researchers, Inc.)

Both the speculum and the lubricant can be prewarmed to promote comfort.

A small wooden spatula, plastic scraper, cotton swab, or brush is used by the practitioner to obtain cervical cells. The cells are then placed on a glass slide and may be sprayed or mixed with a fixative agent. The nurse is usually responsible for properly preparing, labeling, and processing the specimen and then sending it to the lab.

Most results from the Pap smear are available within 1 to 2 weeks. The clinic may send postcards through the mail for negative results. Clients are usually called when positive results are determined, meaning that abnormal cervical cells were identified. This positive result is classified as cervical inflammation or irritation. It may be caused by an infection; dysplasia; or early signs of cancers, carcinoma *in situ* (cancer cells detected only in the top layer of the cervix), or advanced cervical cancer.

PLANNING AND IMPLEMENTATION

The LPN and nurse practitioner understand that a woman's first experience with a Pap smear will affect her approach to this vital health screening for the rest of her life. Dana has expressed fear of the procedure and a lack of knowledge about its importance. Typical emotions that accompany the first Pap smear are anxiety, fear of finding cancer or other health issues, fear of pain, and embarrassment.

The LPN decides to discuss Dana's concerns with her first. She asks Dana to tell her about her fears regarding the Pap smear. Dana states that she is embarrassed and afraid that the nurse practitioner will think she has not kept herself clean enough. Dana asks if she can come back when she has recently used a vaginal douche. The LPN tells Dana that using douches or other feminine hygiene products can actually make the test invalid.

The nurse asks Dana the date of her last menstrual period. Dana does not understand why that matters. The nurse explains that having her period during the Pap smear also interferes with the test results. Dana states that her last menstrual period was 2 weeks ago.

Dana is still concerned about the discomfort she may experience during the Pap smear. The nurse explains the procedure step by step and answers Dana's questions carefully and patiently. The nurse is careful not to tell Dana that there will be no discomfort, but she does give her some suggestions for making the procedure less uncomfortable. She teaches Dana simple deep abdominal breathing. She also shows Dana which muscles are most likely to become tense and gives her some suggestions for releasing the tension in these muscles.

Dana is also concerned about bleeding after the procedure. Her friend reported that she bled heavily for several days. The nurse explains to Dana that a small amount of vaginal spotting is common for several hours after the Pap smear. There may be a need to wear a panty liner to protect her clothes, but the spotting should go away by the next morning. The nurse tells Dana that if she is still spotting the next morning or if there is bleeding heavier than spotting, she should call the clinic and report these symptoms.

The nurse has also assessed that Dana needs some further teaching. After the nurse validates that Dana has an understanding of the indications and results, she discusses with Dana the risks of her unprotected sexual activity.

Because the LPN and the nurse practitioner accurately assessed Dana's emotional and physical needs, Dana consented to the Pap smear. The procedure was performed easily by the nurse practitioner with the assistance of the LPN. Dana's need for birth control and protection from sexually transmitted infections was discussed, and she left the clinic after receiving an injection of Depo and several samples of condoms. The LPN made a follow-up appointment for Dana in 1 month.

SELF-REFLECTION

At what age did you have your first Pap smear? What was the indication for this procedure? Try to remember your feelings before, during, and after the Pap smear. Do you remember the nurse assisting with this procedure? Did he or she assess your emotional response to the procedure?

SUGGESTED RESOURCES

For the Nurse

- Condon, M. (2004). *Women's health: Body, mind, spirit: An integrated approach to wellness and illness.* Upper Saddle River, NJ: Prentice Hall.
- Lichtman, R. (2005). *Gynecology: Well-woman care* (2nd ed.). Upper Saddle River, NJ: Prentice Hall.
- Varney Burst, H. (2004). *Varney's midwifery* (4th ed.). Sudbury, MA: Jones and Bartlett.
- Youngkin, E., & Davis, M. (2004). *Women's health: A primary care clinical guide* (3rd ed.). Upper Saddle River, NJ: Prentice Hall.

For the Client

- Greydanus, D. (2003). *American Academy of Pediatrics: Caring for your teenager.* New York, NY: Bantam.
- Lopez, R. I. (2003). *The teen health book: A parent's guide to adolescent health and well-being.* New York, NY: W. W. Norton & Company.
- Reisser, P. (2002). Teen health guide. Colorado Springs, CO: Focus on the Family.

sexually active) or trichomoniasis (the most frequently diagnosed STD). Sexual abuse must also be ruled out when a child or adolescent presents with vaginitis. For more information on caring for the child who has experienced sexual abuse, see Chapters 5 ⊙⊙ and 27 ⊙⊙.

Manifestations

The client with vaginitis may complain of pruritus, pain, and vaginal discharge or bleeding. Discharge may have a foul odor.

Diagnosis and Treatment

An examination of the child's external genitalia and collection of a specimen of the vaginal discharge is necessary. The drug of choice for *C. albicans* is nystatin ointment. Miconazole (Monistat) may also be ordered and administered as a vaginal suppository. For trichomoniasis, metronidazole (Flagyl) is often ordered.

Nursing Considerations

The nurse can help the young girl avoid contact vaginitis by teaching her to wipe her perineum from front to back, therefore avoiding infestation of the vagina with harmful bacteria from the rectum. The nurse can also discourage the use of bubble baths and feminine hygiene products such as douches or sprays. The nurse can encourage daily cleansing of the perineum with warm water and mild soap, as well as frequent changes of tampons and sanitary pads during menstruation. Caution young girls that wet clothes can cause vaginal irritation. Wet swimsuits and exercise clothing should be removed promptly. Teach girls that cotton underwear absorbs moisture more effectively than synthetic materials.

NURSING CARE

PRIORITIES IN NURSING CARE

Disorders related to the reproductive system can cause anxiety and embarrassment for children and their families. The nurse must be sensitive to these emotions and take care to communicate (verbally and nonverbally) in a professional manner. The use of humor is *not* appropriate in these situations. Listen carefully to expressed concerns, and assess carefully and respectfully for any unexpressed concerns. It is also important for the nurse not to assume that all families share Western values and viewpoints about sex and sexuality (Box 23-7 ■).

ASSESSING

Nursing assessments for children with reproductive disorders includes monitoring for signs and symptoms of infection. The nurse should carefully assess lab values, per-

| BOX 23-7 | CULTURAL PULSE POINTS |

Conflict with "American" Values

Young women of Egyptian heritage face many conflicts related to their sexuality. Egyptians and others from Middle Eastern or Eastern cultures have traditional religious beliefs that forbid sexual activity outside marriage. It is expected that women will be virgins when they get married. Parents may be hesitant to discuss issues of birth control, sexually transmitted diseases, and teenage pregnancy with their daughters because they fear it would promote premarital sexual activity. Parents may evoke strict policies on their daughter's activities away from home. Some parents may consider returning to their native country with their daughter, rather than risk having them influenced by American values.

sonal hygiene practices, and other factors that might increase the child's risk for infection. Assess for the child's verbal and nonverbal reactions to his or her physical characteristics. Pay close attention to statements that reflect self-criticism.

Acute pain is often associated with disorders of the reproductive system. The nurse should assess for verbal and nonverbal symptoms of pain using age-appropriate pain scales. Myths are prevalent related to disorders of the reproductive system. The nurse must be careful to determine the child's and the family's level of knowledge related to the condition and the prescribed treatment.

DIAGNOSING, PLANNING, AND IMPLEMENTING

Nursing diagnoses for children with reproductive disorders include:

- Risk for Infection, related to surgical procedure
- Risk for Disturbed Body Image, related to anatomic alterations
- Acute Pain, related to menstrual irregularities
- Deficient Knowledge, related to changes of puberty.

Some outcomes for children with reproductive disorders might include:

- Child will remain free of signs and symptoms of infection.
- Child and family will accept current body structure and function.
- Child will remain free of pain.
- Child and family will accurately state information regarding the condition and prescribed treatment.

The nurse's role in providing support to these clients would include the following:

- Teach the child and family the importance of preventing infections of the reproductive system, especially in the postoperative period. *Knowledge of the risks of infection will motivate the child and family to use preventive measures.*

- Use hand washing between contacts with other clients and procedures with this child. *Harmful bacteria can be effectively removed by friction and running water.*

- Teach parents the importance of their responses to the child's physical characteristics. *Children often take their cue about their body image from their parents.*

- Parents of children with physical alterations in the reproductive system need clear information about the nature of the alteration and the future consequences. *Accurate information allows the family to form an accurate mind-set about the child's condition.*

- Provide pharmacologic and nonpharmacologic pain relief measures as necessary. *Pharmacologic pain relief measures provide physiologic relief of pain, while nonpharmacologic pain relief measures reduce tension and therefore relieve psychological aspects of pain.*

- Select age-appropriate teaching methods to instruct the child and family about the condition and prescribed treatment. *Cognitive development must be considered in order to convey information accurately.*

EVALUATING

The nurse reviews stated outcomes to determine if goals were met. Follow-up pain assessments are important when administering pharmacologic pain medications. Signs and symptoms of infection should be reported promptly. The nurse confirms the child's and family's understanding of the condition and the prescribed treatment by having them verbalize information.

Note: The references and resources for this and all chapters have been compiled at the back of the book.

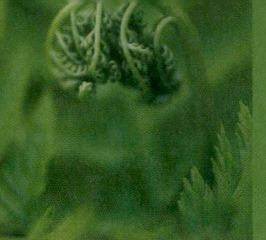

Chapter Review

KEY TERMS by Topic

Use the audio glossary feature of either the CD-ROM or the Companion Website to hear the correct pronunciation of the following key terms.

Introduction
genitourinary system

Congenital Urinary Defects
hypospadias, epispadias, chordee, bladder exstrophy

Obstructive Uropathy
obstructive uropathy, polycystic kidney, nephrolithiasis, stasis, hydronephrosis, pyeloplasty, valve ablation

Urinary Tract Infections
cystitis, pyelonephritis, vesicoureteral reflux, dysuria, hematuria

Acute Postinfectious Glomerulonephritis
glomerulonephritis

Nephrotic Syndrome
nephrotic syndrome, proteinuria , hypoalbuminemia, hyperlipidemia, periorbital edema, ascites

Acute and Chronic Renal Failure
renal failure, acute renal failure (ARF), chronic renal failure (CRF), end-stage renal

disease (ESRD), uremic syndrome, uremic frost, dialysis, disequilibrium syndrome

Wilms' Tumor or Nephroblastoma
Wilms' tumor, nephroblastoma

Enuresis
enuresis

Ambiguous Genitalia
pseudohermaphroditism

Male Disorders
phimosis, balanoposthitis, paraphimosis, cryptorchidism

Female Disorders
hymen, vaginitis

KEY Points

- The primary functions of the urinary system include waste excretion; homeostasis; fluid, electrolyte, and acid-base balance; regulation of blood pressure; regulation of calcium metabolism; and stimulation of erythrocyte development.

- It is important for the nurse to know the normal bladder capacity for the child according to age group. Urinary output needs to be measured carefully.

- Most commonly, the newborn voids in the first 24 hours of birth. The newborn who does not void within 24 hours may be assessed for urethral stenosis or absent kidneys or ureters.

- In the male infant, UTIs are more common due to structural defects. In the young female child, UTIs are more common due to *E. coli* entering the urethra and progressing to the bladder. Shorter urethras also increase their risk for UTIs.

- Symptoms of UTI include fever, nausea and vomiting, anorexia, strong-smelling urine, abdominal pain, dysuria, and hematuria. The infant and young child may cry during urination. The continent child may suddenly develop incontinence or hesitancy due to fear of pain.

- Renal failure is the inability of the kidneys to remove liquid waste from the blood. Renal failure can be acute or chronic.

- The child with renal failure should be assessed for signs of fluid overload, including weight gain, pitting edema, pulmonary edema, and ascites.

- The nurse can help the young girl avoid contact vaginitis by teaching her to wipe her perineum from front to back, therefore avoiding infestation of the vagina with harmful bacteria from the rectum.

- Disorders related to the reproductive system can cause anxiety and embarrassment for children and their families. The nurse must be sensitive to these emotions and take care to communicate in a professional manner.

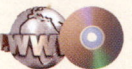

EXPLORE MediaLink

Additional interactive resources for this chapter can be found on the Companion Website at www.prenhall.com/towle.

Click on Chapter 23 and "Begin" to select the activities for this chapter.

For chapter-related NCLEX-style questions and an audio glossary, access the accompanying CD-ROM in this book.

Animations

Renal corpuscle

Erectile dysfunction

FOR FURTHER Study

For reproductive anatomy, see Figures 4-9 and 4-13; for more information about changes of puberty, see Chapter 4 and Figure 4-22.

See Chapter 5 for more information on male and female reproductive disorders.

For additional information on newborn issues, see Chapter 9.

Phases of sexual maturation are described in Table 11-12.

Collection of urine specimens is described in Procedure 13-14. Urinary catheterization in a child is described in Procedure 13-24.

For fluid and electrolyte imbalances and monitoring I & O, see Chapter 15; Table 15-4 discusses potassium regulation.

See Chapter 27 for sexual abuse assessment.

For more about organ transplantation, see Chapters 21 and 28.

Critical Thinking Care Map

Caring for a Client with Vaginitis
NCLEX-PN® Focus Area: Physiologic Integrity

Case Study: Mrs. Freidman has made an appointment with the pediatrician for her 14-year-old daughter, Casey. Casey reported to her mother yesterday that her vulva was swollen and painful and that she was experiencing intense itching. Mrs. Freidman has accused Casey of having sexual intercourse because she believes that is the only way a woman can have the symptoms Casey is describing. Casey denies having sexual intercourse.

Nursing Diagnosis: Deficient Knowledge (parent)

COLLECT DATA

Subjective

_____
_____
_____
_____
_____
_____

Objective

_____
_____
_____
_____
_____
_____

Would you report this? Yes/No

If yes, to: _____

Nursing Care

_____
_____
_____
_____
_____
_____
_____
_____
_____
_____
_____

How would you document this? _____
_____
_____
_____

Compare your documentation to the sample provided in Appendix I.

Data Collected
(use those that apply)

- Report of swollen vulva
- Intact hymen
- Report of vulvar pain
- Vulva edematous
- Vital signs: T 98.6, P 60, R 12, B/P 110/70
- Report of vulvar itching
- Mrs. Freidman is waving arms and pacing in examination room
- "Casey has had sex and that's why she has these symptoms."
- "I have not ever had sex with anyone."
- Vulva red
- Small amount of white vaginal discharge noted.

Nursing Interventions
(use those that apply; list in priority order)

- Assist physician to obtain vaginal specimen.
- Describe methods of preventing vaginitis.
- Explain the physiology and causes of vaginitis.
- Obtain urine specimen for pregnancy test.
- Describe the signs and symptoms of vaginitis.
- Assess Mrs. Freidman's knowledge level regarding vaginitis.
- Explain medical treatment of vaginitis.
- Counsel Casey on the hazards of sexual activity.
- Present teaching in a nonjudgmental manner.

NCLEX-PN® Exam Preparation

1 A nurse is caring for a child who has just returned from surgery where he underwent repair for epispadias. The parents are concerned when they see a slight amount of blood in the urinary collection bag. The nurse tells the parents:

1. "I will call the surgeon right away."
2. "Your child will probably need a blood transfusion."
3. "A slight amount of blood in the urine is normal following this surgery."
4. "The catheter will be taken out soon."

2 The nurse is discussing the discharge plans for a newborn with hypospadias. What statement by the parents indicates their understanding of the plan?

1. "Our child will have to have frequent blood tests."
2. "Our child will have to be catheterized frequently."
3. "A special support will have to be worn by our child until surgery."
4. "Our child won't be circumcised right away in order to save tissue for repair."

3 In a child with a diagnosis of urinary tract infection, the nurse knows the child may experience the following symptoms:

1. hematuria, dysuria, nausea, and vomiting
2. oliguria, hematuria, and seizures
3. proteinuria, oliguria, and hypoalbuminemia
4. hyperlipidemia, hypoalbuminemia, and hyperproteinuria

4 The nurse reviews the laboratory report of a child with possible glomerulonephritis. The nurse knows which finding is associated with such a diagnosis?

1. hematuria
2. decreased pH
3. *Streptococcus*
4. glucosuria

5 A nurse is caring for a child with symptoms of uremic frost, nausea, vomiting, anorexia, uremic breath odor, anemia, pruritis, and pulmonary edema. The nurse knows these symptoms are most likely caused by:

1. hypospadius.
2. bladder exstrophy.
3. epispadius.
4. uremic syndrome.

6 The nurse is conducting an assessment of a child with a potential Wilms' tumor. In the course of the assessment, the nurse avoids which method of gathering data?

1. obtaining a urine sample
2. taking the child's temperature
3. obtaining a radial pulse
4. palpating the abdomen

7 The nurse is reviewing the plan of care for an infant with the diagnosis of bladder exstrophy and targets which of the following priority diagnoses?

1. potential for infection
2. excess fluid volume
3. impaired tissue integrity
4. deficient knowledge of parents

8 The parents of an infant with bladder exstrophy ask the nurse about the condition. The nurse explains this condition is caused by:

1. a congenital disorder inherited from the father.
2. an intrusion of the bladder, which is abnormally located in the renal pelvis.
3. an extrusion of the bladder through a lower abdominal wall defect.
4. a condition due to low folic acid intake by the mother during pregnancy.

9 The nurse is caring for a child admitted to the medical center with a diagnosis of nephrotic syndrome and selects the following data that can be found on assessment (choose all that apply):

1. hypoalbuminemia
2. protein in the urine
3. edema
4. uremic frost
5. hyperlipidemia
6. decreased immunity

10 The nurse selects the following teaching items for the parents of a 2-year-old, partially toilet trained, female child with a diagnosis of urinary tract infection (choose all that apply):

1. Clean the perineum after each diaper change.
2. Wipe the child from front to back.
3. Avoid bubble baths.
4. Avoid putting the child in a commercial hot tub.
5. Do not use disposable diapers.

Answers for Review Questions, as well as discussion of Care Plan and Critical Thinking Care Map questions, appear in Appendix I.

Chapter 24

Care of the Child with Integumentary Disorders

BRIEF Outline

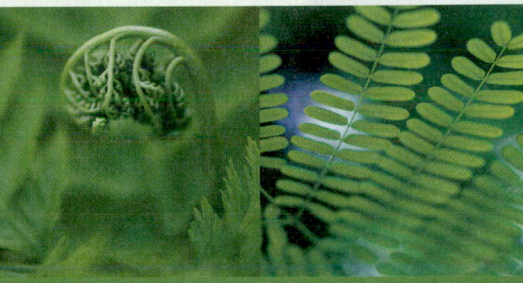

NURSING PROCESS CARE PLAN:
Client with Cellulitis

HEALTH PROMOTION ISSUE:
Teens and Tanning

CRITICAL THINKING CARE MAP:
Caring for a Child with Eczema

LEARNING Outcomes

After completing this chapter, you will be able to:

- Review the basic structure and function of skin, and describe differences between the skin of a child and an adult.
- Discuss common congenital disorders of skin, their treatment, and nursing care.
- Discuss common infections and infestations of skin in children, as well as treatment and nursing care.
- Discuss various types of skin trauma in children, as well as treatment and nursing care.

Many changes occur in the skin from the time of birth to adolescence. Skin disorders are common among pediatric clients. The LPN/LVN plays an important role in assisting the client and family as they cope with common skin disorders. Important priorities for the LPN/LVN are promoting healthy skin care to the pediatric client and providing methods to prevent skin infections while decreasing pain and discomfort. Psychological and social development may be altered if skin disorders lead to disfigurement.

Skin serves several functions. The main function of the skin is to protect the body from pathogens that may cause infections. Temperature regulation can also be influenced by the skin when the blood vessels dilate (allowing heat to dissipate from the body) and through perspiration (allowing evaporation of fluids). Production of serum creates an oily barrier that helps prevent fluid loss. Sensory receptors provide information about pain, touch, pressure, and temperature. Sensory input is delivered to the brain so the body can adapt to the outside environment. The outer layer of the skin participates in the production of vitamin D.

Anatomy and Physiology

The integumentary system is the largest organ system in the body. It includes the skin and its associated structures: hair, nails, sebaceous and sweat glands, blood vessels, nerve endings, and sensory organs (Figure 24-1 ■). The skin is the first line of defense against infection. Injury to the skin may pose multiple health risks to the pediatric client.

The **epidermis** is the outer thin layer of the skin. It consists of two layers.

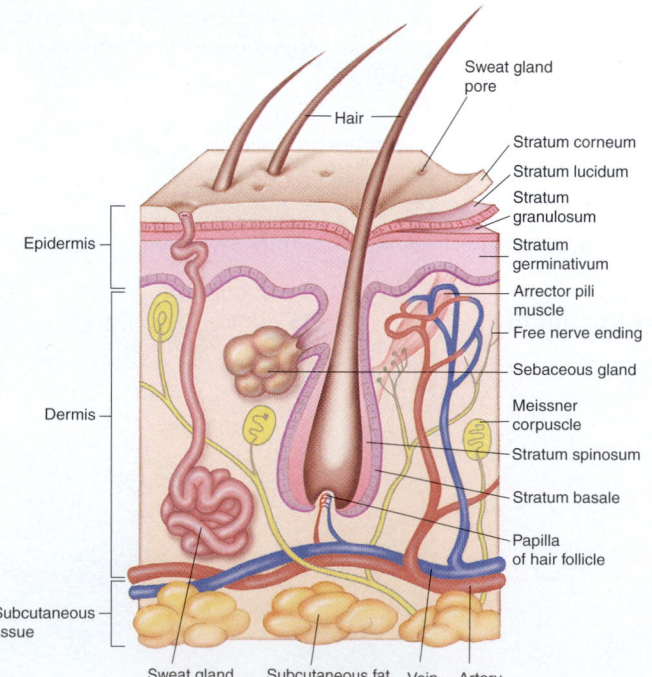

Epidermis

Dermis

Subcutaneous tissue

Hair

Sweat gland pore
Stratum corneum
Stratum lucidum
Stratum granulosum
Stratum germinativum
Arrector pili muscle
Free nerve ending
Sebaceous gland
Meissner corpuscle
Stratum spinosum
Stratum basale
Papilla of hair follicle

Sweat gland   Subcutaneous fat   Vein   Artery

Figure 24-1. ■ Anatomic view of skin and accessory structures.

- *Stratum corneum* (horny cell layer), which consists of flattened dead, keratinized cells.
- *Stratum germinativum* (basal cell layer), where cells multiply, grow, and move toward the skin's surface, causing the surface layer to be replaced about every 4 weeks. The stratum germinativum also contains melanocytes that secrete **melanin,** a pigment that adds color to the skin.

The **dermis** is the inner, thicker layer of the skin, which contains most of the associated structures (e.g., hair, nails, sebaceous and sweat glands, blood vessels, nerve endings, sensory organs). The dermal layer is highly vascular and provides nourishment to the epidermis. Fibrous connective and collagen tissue within the dermis provides strength and allows the skin to stretch with body movements. Collagen is produced by *fibroblast cells* (the primary cell type in the dermis). Nerve endings within the dermis provide sensations of pain, pressure, temperature, and touch.

ASSOCIATED STRUCTURES

Hair

Hair covers the majority of the body except the lips, palms of the hands, and soles of the feet. Hair consists of the shaft (the visible part of the hair) located in the epidermis and the root located deep within the dermal layer of the skin, all of which make up the hair follicle. The **arrector pili,** an involuntary muscle, surrounds the hair follicle and pulls the hair upright when it contracts. This response is due to cold external temperatures or fear. Hair located on the scalp, eyelids, eyebrows, and ear canals aids in keeping dust and insects from entering the body. Hair that is shiny, lustrous, and not easily plucked reflects good nutritional status in the client. Hair that is dry, brittle, thinning, and easily plucked indicates poor nutritional status. The color of the hair is provided by melanocytes (found in the hair shaft). A decrease in the number of functioning melanocytes causes color changes in the hair.

Nails

Nails consist of keratinized epidermal cells. The body of the nail is visible and pink in color because of the vascular nail bed underneath. Nail growth occurs at the nail root, which lies under the cuticle. Healthy nails are firm and transparent but may appear pink over the body of the nail. Nails that are brittle may often indicate poor nutritional status.

Sebaceous Glands

Sebaceous glands are located in the dermis and secrete sebum. Sebum has a lubricating effect on the skin. It helps keep the skin soft and the hair supple. It also aids in preventing the growth of bacteria. Secretion of sebum from the sebaceous glands is stimulated by sex hormones that increase during puberty. Sebaceous glands are located over the entire body, except on the palms of the hand and soles of the feet.

The face, scalp, upper chest, and back contain more sebaceous glands than other parts of the body.

Sweat Glands (Sudoriferous Glands)

Sweat glands (sudoriferous glands) are *exocrine* glands (i.e., they have ducts). Eccrine glands and apocrine glands are two types of sweat glands that secrete fluids to the surface of the skin.

- *Eccrine glands* are small but distributed throughout the body. They play a role in maintaining body temperature by allowing body heat to dissipate as sweat when it is brought to the top of the skin for evaporation.
- *Apocrine glands* are deeper in the dermis and open into the hair follicles. These sweat glands are larger, are found in the axillae and genital areas, and begin functioning at the onset of puberty. Once the sweat produced by the apocrine glands comes in contact with bacteria on the skin, it produces a distinct body odor.

Subcutaneous Layer

The subcutaneous layer, also referred to as the *superficial fascia*, is directly under the dermis. (The word *subcutaneous* means "under the skin.") The subcutaneous layer includes elastic, fibrous, and adipose tissue. The main functions of this layer are to cushion internal organs, store fat for energy, insulate the body, and connect the skin to the surface of the muscles.

GROWTH AND DEVELOPMENT

The skin of the newborn is high in water content and very thin (Figure 24-2 ■). It can absorb harmful chemicals more readily than older skin. Because the epidermis is not strongly attached to the underlying dermis, friction may cause blistering. Care must be taken to handle the newborn gently. Newborns have little subcutaneous fat, so heat loss is rapid. (See Figure 9-4 ⚭ for an illustration of brown fatty tissue in newborns.) The newborn's body regulates temperature through the eccrine sweat glands (see also Figure 9-3 ⚭); the apocrine glands do not yet function. Skin contains little melanin at birth, so skin tones are lighter.

As children grow, the skin thickens, and the epidermis and dermis become more tightly bound. Eccrine glands increase their function, and apocrine glands begin functioning at puberty. Increased melanin creates a full skin tone and protects the body against the harmful rays of the sun.

Pediatric clients are more prone to skin infections than adults. If a skin infection develops, it is more likely to produce systemic symptoms in children. Subcutaneous fat is decreased in preterm and term newborns, making them more sensitive to environmental changes. The epidermis of the newborn is thinner, which makes it more susceptible to blisters from friction if careful handling is not practiced. The pH level of the newborn's skin is more alkaline than that of the older child; because of this, it is more prone to infections. The eccrine glands mature around 2 to 3 years of age, allowing the child to regulate body temperature more easily. The skin of the young child is drier and chaps easily because sebum is not excreted by the sebaceous glands until 8 to 10 years of age. The hormonal surge during adolescence increases sebum production, leading to increased incidence of acne vulgaris (discussed later in the chapter).

Brief Assessment Overview

Assessment of the skin can be a window into systemic problems involving oxygenation, circulation, nutrition, and hydration. All equipment should be gathered prior to the

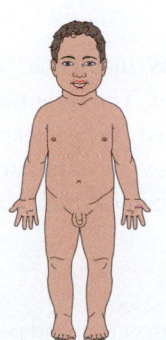
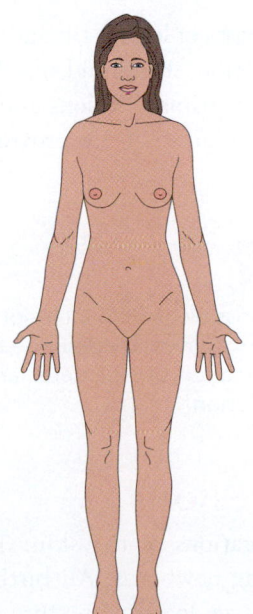

Body surface area of adult much greater in relation to internal organs

Sebaceous glands increase production in adolescence

Sweat glands have greater production in adolescents and young adults

Epidermis thicker in adult with more fat and subcutaneous tissue

Figure 24-2. ■ Adult versus child integumentary system.

examination. Equipment includes a clear flexible metric ruler, marking pen, penlight, and disposable gloves. The LPN/LVN would use a clear, flexible, metric ruler to measure the size of lesions, patches of skin discolorations, and wound size. A marking pen may be used to define borders so the provider can inspect for the increasing or decreasing size of lesions, skin discolorations, and wounds. A penlight provides focused lighting for the LPN/LVN during the assessment. A Wood's lamp and glass slides for special procedures would be available for the provider to use during the examination. To ensure standard precautions are followed, disposable gloves should be available to the LPN/LVN and the provider. The LPN/LVN should prepare the environment, ensuring proper lighting, temperature, and privacy.

HISTORY

Review past health history and family history for any skin health issues such as eczema, pruritus, lesions, lice, scabies, changes in hair or hair loss, changes in nails, or any other infections or infestations. For present health status, inquire about allergies (food, medication, fabrics, metals, or pollens), current medications (topical or systemic), and skin care habits (bathing, use of skin care products, and use of sunscreen).

PHYSICAL

Inspection and palpation are the two main techniques used during assessment of the skin. Inspect the skin for color pigment changes (pallor, jaundice, cyanosis, or erythema) and for location of birthmarks such as port-wine stains or strawberry hemangiomas (discussed later). (For mongolian spots, see Figure 9-15 ⬭.) Palpate the skin to assess moisture, texture, turgor, and temperature. The dorsal side of the examiner's hand is used because it is more sensitive to temperatures changes.

Identify the major types of lesions (including tattoos and piercings) and note location, shape, and size. It is important to differentiate between primary lesions and secondary lesions. (Box 24-1 ■ and Figure 24-3 ■ provide descriptions and pictures.)

> **clinical ALERT**
>
> Inspect suspicious or possible malignant lesions by using the acronym ABCDE: **A** = asymmetry of shape, **B** = border irregularity, **C** = color variation, **D** = diameter larger than 6 mm, **E** = elevation of lesion.

Congenital Lesions

Birthmarks are discolorations of the skin. They can be a common finding among newborns. All birthmarks should be examined for color, size, location, texture, and elevation. Some birthmarks may be an indicator of disease and may require further investigation. Appearance of birthmarks may be upsetting to parents. The LPN/LVN provides support and education to the family about birthmarks.

CAPILLARY (STRAWBERRY) HEMANGIOMA

Strawberry (or capillary) hemangioma is a benign cutaneous tumor that involves the capillaries in the dermis. Strawberry hemangioma (Figure 24-4A ■) may appear a few weeks after birth and is more common in girls and premature infants. During the first year, capillary hemangiomas may enlarge. By 2 to 3 years of age, the hemangiomas will begin to decrease.

Manifestations

Clinical manifestations include a bright red area of skin that is flat in the beginning but will elevate with growth. The surface is rough and has a rubbery feel to it. The margins are well defined. Most hemangiomas are found on the face and head.

Diagnosis

Diagnosis is made by inspection and palpation of the hemangioma, documenting location, color, and size. Monitoring the growth of the vascular tumor is also helpful for diagnostic purposes.

Treatment

Medical treatment may not be indicated once the hemangioma begins to resolve spontaneously. Oral prednisone may be given once a day for 7 to 10 days, then tapered to the lowest most effective dose for 4 to 6 weeks to help slow the growth of the hemangioma. A rest period of 2 to 4 weeks may be needed between prednisone treatments. For some children, hemangioma treatment may include laser therapy to reduce the size. If the hemangioma is extensive and causing a problem to the airway, eyes, or ear canal, or if feeding is compromised, subcutaneous injections of alfa-2a or interferon alfa-2b may be needed.

PORT-WINE STAINS

Port-wine stains are permanent vascular stains that involve the vascular bed in the dermis. They are most commonly found on the face and head (see Figure 24-4B). As the child grows, the color may darken and the birthmark thickens.

Manifestations

Clinical manifestations include a pink to reddish-purple stain on the face or head. The color may depend on the depth of dermal tissue involved. When deeper vessels of the dermis are involved, the port-wine stain darkens. If located on the face, the birthmark becomes thick with a *verrucose* (wartlike) nodular surface.

Diagnosis

Diagnosis is made by inspection and palpation of the port-wine stain in relation to the location, color, and size. Port-wine stains

BOX 24-1 ASSESSMENT

Common Skin Lesions

Primary Lesions (see Figure 24-3)

Cyst—a fluid-filled or semisolid sac originating in the subcutaneous tissue or dermis
Examples: epidermoid (skin) cyst or sebaceous cyst seen in acne

Macule, Patch—a discolored spot that is even with the skin's surface; macules are less 1 cm, patches are greater than 1 cm
Examples: (of macule) freckles, petechiae; (of patch) port-wine stains, mongolian spots

Papule, Plaque—a circumscribed, solid elevation of the skin
Examples: (of papule) elevated mole, warts; (of plaques) psoriasis, actinic keratosis

Nodule, Tumor—a circumscribed, elevated mass of tissue extending deeper into the dermis than a papule; nodules are 0.5–2 cm; tumors are greater than 2 cm and may have irregular borders
Examples: (of nodule) squamous cell carcinoma or small lipoma (fatty growth); (of tumor) hemangioma, carcinoma

Pustule—a small, circumscribed elevation of the skin containing purulent matter
Examples: infected pimple

Vesicle, Bulla—a small, circumscribed elevation of the skin containing fluid; vesicles are less then 0.5 cm; bullae are greater than 0.5 cm
Examples: (of vesicle) herpes simplex or cold sore; (of bulla) contact dermatitis or large burn blisters

Wheal—a circumscribed, slightly reddened papule or irregular plaque of edema of the skin, usually accompanied by intense itching
Examples: insect bites, hives

Secondary Lesions (see Figure 24-3)

Atrophy—a semitransparent, paperlike, sometimes wrinkled skin surface; a wasting of the skin
Examples: aged or sun-damaged skin, striae ("stretch marks")

Crust—blood, pus, or serum that has dried on the surface of the skin after injury
Examples: scab (after abrasion injury), eczema

Erosion—a wearing away of the superficial epidermis by friction or pressure
Examples: scratches, ruptured vesicles

Fissure—a deep furrow or slit extending into the dermis
Examples: athlete's foot lesions, cracks at the sides of the mouth with dehydration

Keloid—excess scar tissue; hyperplastic scar tissue with irregular bands of collagen, usually formed after trauma, surgery, burn, or severe skin disease
Examples: enlarged scars from ear piercing

Lichenification—leathery hardening and thickening of the skin, caused by scratching or rubbing
Examples: chronic dermatitis

Scales—a small thin plate of epidermis that is shed from skin tissue
Examples: dandruff, eczema, dry skin

Scar—fibrous tissue that replaces normal tissue after injury
Examples: healed surgical wound, healed acne

Ulcer—superficial loss of tissue, usually with inflammation, on the surface of the skin or mucous membrane
Examples: decubitus ulcers (pressure sores), chancres

Vascular Lesions

Ecchymosis—purplish patch caused by extravasation (leaking) of blood into the skin; like petechiae but >3 mm diameter

Hematoma—localized mass of extravasated blood that is confined within an organ or tissue

Petechiae—tiny hemorrhagic spots, from pinpoint to pinhead size

Port-wine stain—a large, congenital vascular nevus with a purplish color; usually found on the head and neck (see Figure 24-4B)

Purpura—condition characterized by hemorrhaging into the skin

Spider angioma—dilated arteriole in the skin with radiating capillary branches that look like the legs of a spider

Strawberry mark—a small capillary hemangioma that resembles a strawberry in size, shape, and color; usually disappears in early childhood

Source: Ramont, R., & Niedringhaus, D. (2006). *Comprehensive nursing care.* Upper Saddle River, NJ: Prentice Hall.

do not blanch. Examination should rule out any structural malformations that are sometimes associated with port-wine stains, such as glaucoma or tumors of the blood or lymph vessels in the pia-arachnoid (refers to the pia mater and arachnoid layers of the meninges protecting the brain and spinal cord).

Treatment

Medical treatment may depend on the location and size of the port-wine stain. If the birthmark is small, cosmetics may be used to cover the stain. If large, a series of laser treatments may be necessary.

Nursing Considerations

Support and encouragement are vital to families of infants with congenital lesions. For children with strawberry hemangiomas, a series of photographs may be taken over time. This visual record of progressive involution of the hemangioma will offer encouragement. If laser treatments are used to correct strawberry hemangiomas or port-wine stains, care should be given to prevent any trauma such as picking at the scab. Only water is used to clean these areas and to blot them dry. Sometimes a topical antibiotic ointment is applied to the area. Sunlight should be avoided for a few weeks, and then sunscreen (at least SPF 15 or higher) should be applied for continual protection.

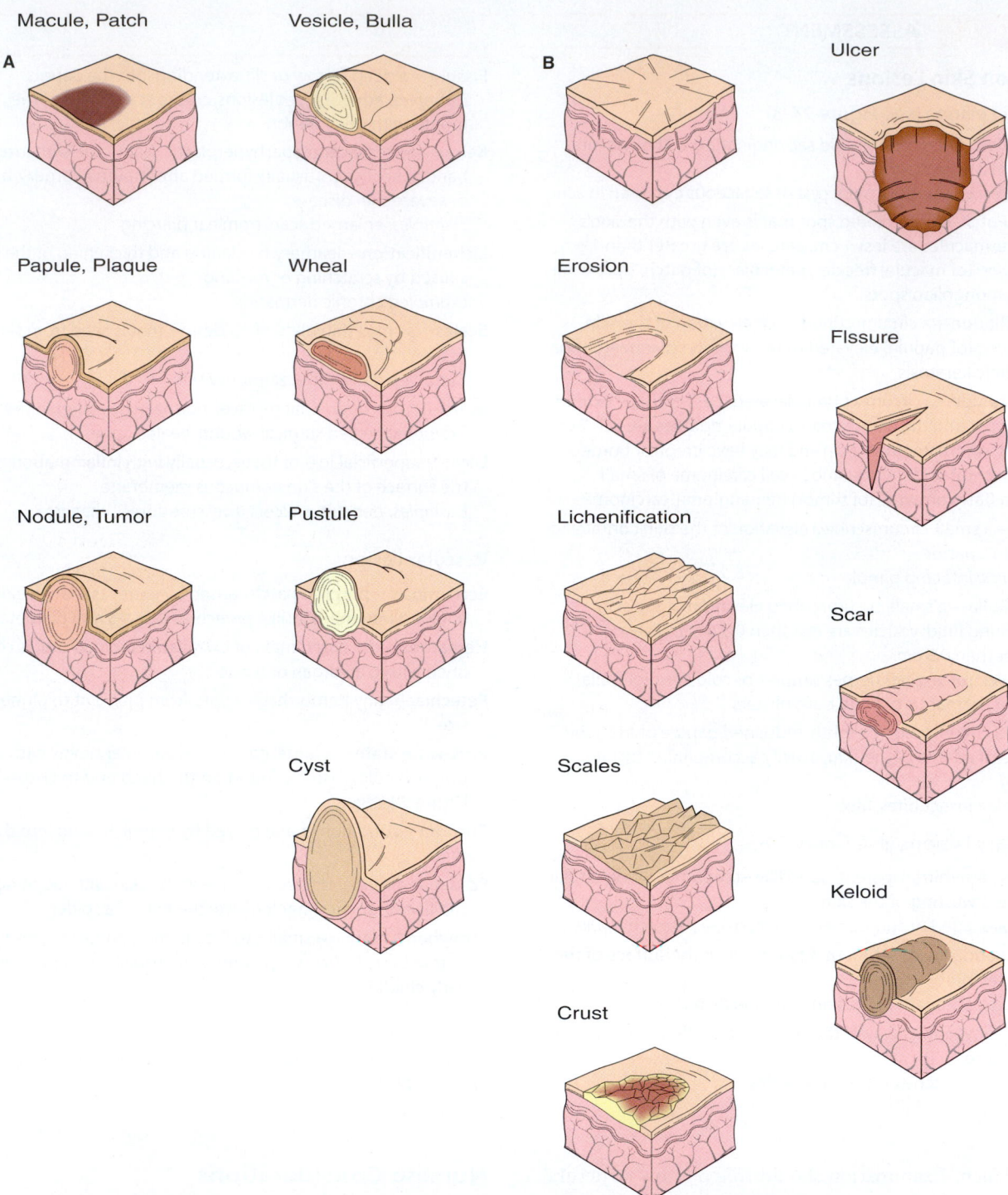

Figure 24-3. ■ Vascular skin lesions. (**A**) Primary skin lesions. (**B**) Secondary skin lesions.

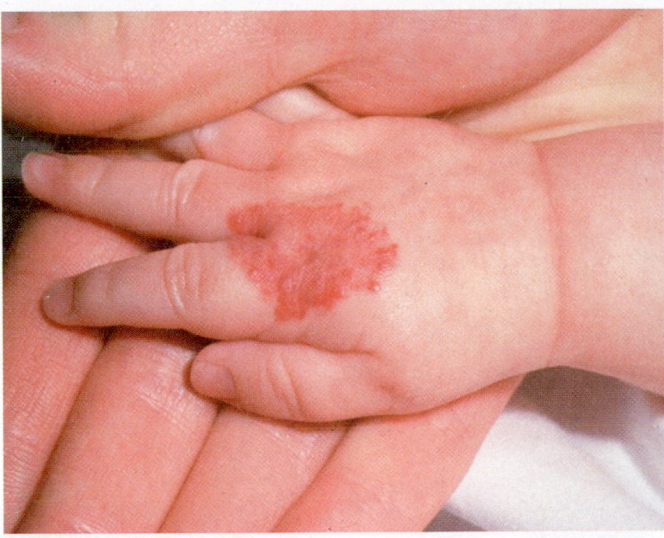

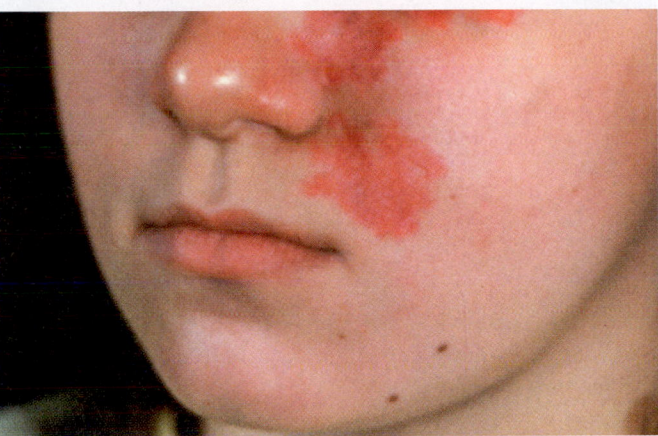

Figure 24-4. ■ **(A)** Capillary (strawberry) hemangioma. **(B)** Port-wine stain. (**A.** H. C. Robinson/Science Photo Library/Photo Researchers, Inc. **B.** Custom Medical Stock Photo, Inc.)

Skin Disorders

MILIARIA

Miliaria is also known as *prickly heat*. Eccrine (sweat) glands become blocked when the child is exposed to high environmental temperatures and increased humidity. This reaction may cause backup pressure of sweat, which escapes to surrounding tissue and causes the skin to itch and feel prickly.

Manifestations

Clinical manifestations include minute vesicles with papules. Erythema surrounds the vesicles and papules (see Figure 24-3). Itching is present.

Diagnosis

Diagnosis is made by inspection and palpation of the skin.

Treatment

Medical management involves providing a cool environment and allowing for good ventilation. Cool baths and dusting powders may decrease itching.

Nursing Considerations

Nursing care includes advising parents to monitor the room temperature and to avoid being outside if the temperature is too humid.

INTERTRIGO

Intertrigo is skin irritation caused when opposing skin creates friction. Excessive heat and moisture may cause sweat to be retained between skin folds or in areas where skin rubs together. Areas commonly irritated include the neck, axillae, groin, and intergluteal folds. Obese children are more prone to intertrigo.

Manifestations

Clinical manifestations include inflammation and erythema of the skin, especially in areas where skin has rubbed together. Skin may appear warm and moist. *Candida* infection (discussed later) may also be present.

Diagnosis

Diagnosis is made by inspection and palpation of the skin and skin folds for inflammation, moisture, and redness.

Treatment

Medical treatment involves applying nonmedicated powder to affected areas. Treatment using 1% hydrocortisone cream may also be needed if a candidal infection is present. Weight loss may help prevent rubbing of skin folds.

Nursing Considerations

Nursing care is directed at keeping the affected area clean and dry. Encourage parents to expose the child's skin to air and light for short periods of time to help dry the skin. Instruct parents that clothing should be appropriate for environmental temperature and should not be tight or binding.

Inflammatory Disorders

DERMATITIS

Dermatitis is a general term meaning inflammation of the dermis or skin. When a foreign substance, known as an **irritant**, irritates the skin, the cells release histamine. Histamine causes blood vessels to dilate, resulting in redness, heat, and swelling. Itching and pain are also common. At times, vesicles or blisters form, open, drain, and develop a crust. Dermatitis is classified by the location and cause of the irritation, which may stem from an allergen or an irritant. Contact dermatitis, diaper dermatitis, and seborrheic dermatitis are common inflammatory conditions of the skin and are prevalent in infants and children.

CONTACT DERMATITIS

Contact dermatitis can stem from allergens (poison ivy, poison oak, latex, or nickel) or from repeated exposure to irritants (detergents, bleaches, soaps, lotions, urine, and stool). Inflammation is usually limited to the area of contact. Latex may cause both an allergic and an irritant reaction in some infants and children.

Manifestations

Clinical manifestations of allergic contact dermatitis include reddened papules that ooze, crust, itch, and are edematous (see Figure 21-6 ⬭). Reactions to allergens may develop within 12 to 72 hours after exposure and last up to 3 to 4 weeks. Contact dermatitis caused by irritants manifests itself by localized redness, edema, and scaling of the skin. Reactions appear shortly after exposure to the irritant. They disappear quickly once the irritant is removed.

Diagnosis

Diagnosis is made by obtaining a thorough history of any repeated or prolonged use of common substances known to cause contact dermatitis. Physical examination is done by inspection and palpation of the lesions. Skin testing may be ordered to identify specific allergens and/or irritants that affect the skin.

Treatment

Medical treatment includes proper cleansing of the affected area with mild soap and thorough rinsing of the skin. Hydrocortisone topical ointment may be prescribed to relieve the inflammation. Medication may be prescribed to relieve pruritis. Advise the family to avoid irritants known to affect the skin.

Nursing Considerations

Nursing care begins by collecting data to identify any irritants that have come in contact with the skin. The nurse educates the family on methods to avoid common household products known to cause contact dermatitis.

   If the contact dermatitis covers a large area of the body, fails to resolve, or gets worse in a short time, or if signs of infection are present, the infant should be seen by a physician or health care provider. Instruct the family on how to recognize signs of infection.

DIAPER DERMATITIS

Diaper dermatitis (Figure 24-5 ■) is caused by irritation from urine and/or stool and is more common in infants. Breastfed infants have a lower pH and therefore are not as prone to diaper dermatitis as bottle-fed infants. Introduction of formula or solids foods changes the pH level, leaving the infant more prone to diaper dermatitis. At times, the diaper area can become infected with *Candida albicans*.

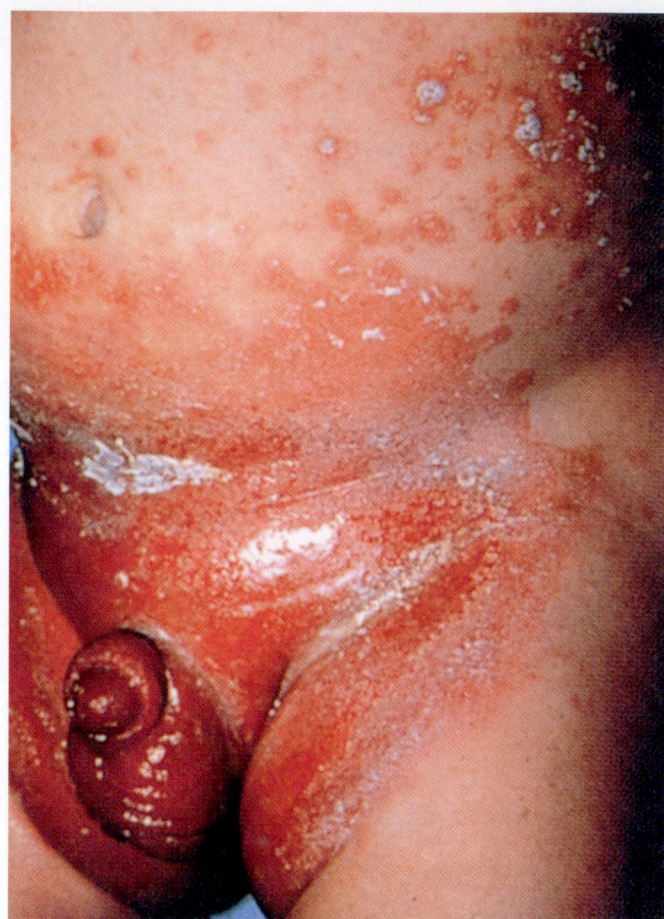

Figure 24-5. ■ Diaper dermatitis. (Courtesy of the Centers for Disease Control and Prevention, Atlanta, GA.)

Manifestations

Clinical manifestation includes red, edematous, and blistered skin in the diaper region. Skin folds may be free of irritation because they do not come in contact with the soiled diaper.

Diagnosis

Diagnosis is made by inspection and palpation of the lesions located in the diaper area.

Treatment

Medical management may include treating the area with a 0.25% to 1% hydrocortisone cream with each diaper change and then applying a sealant to help protect against moisture. The area should be cleansed with mild soap and water at each diaper change, and the diaper area should be allowed to air-dry. Application of 1% hydrocortisone cream and antifungal creams may be used to treat *Candida albicans*.

Nursing Considerations

Nursing care begins by educating the parents on prevention methods that decrease the risk of diaper dermatitis. Encourage parents to use superabsorbent diapers. Instruct parents to change soiled diapers immediately and thoroughly cleanse the area with mild soap and water. Tell parents to avoid using diaper wipes because the solution may further irritate the skin. Barrier creams or sealants (Balmex, Destin, or zinc oxide) may be used to protect the skin from moisture. With a doctor's order, a 0.25% to 1% hydrocortisone ointment may be applied before any ointment to seal out moisture.

SEBORRHEIC DERMATITIS

Seborrheic dermatitis, known as *"cradle cap"* in babies, may be the result of changes in sebaceous glands. Adolescents may also present with seborrheic dermatitis, commonly known as "dandruff," which may begin with the onset of puberty.

Manifestations

Clinical manifestations include oily, yellow, scaly patches on the scalp and forehead with mildly erythematous skin underneath.

Diagnosis

Diagnosis is made by inspection and palpation of lesions on the scalp and forehead.

Treatment

Medical treatment for infants includes daily shampooing with a mild nonmedicated shampoo. Emollients can be left in place for a few minutes to loosen and lift the crusts, and then removed with a soft bristle hairbrush or fingertips. Adolescents may use a medicated dandruff shampoo.

Nursing Considerations

Nursing care includes educating parents on proper cleansing of the scalp and forehead. Demonstrate proper holding during the shampoo to avoid getting it in the child's eyes. The cheeks and eyelids can be washed with baby shampoo. Encourage parents to apply an emollient on the scalp for 20 minutes prior to cleansing. Vigorous brushing with a soft baby hairbrush is helpful in removing the scales. Instruct adolescents to adapt a regular hygiene regime for shampooing and to switch to a medicated shampoo product. Encourage adolescents to seek treatment as soon as symptoms begin.

ECZEMA

Eczema (Figure 24-6 ■) is a chronic inflammatory skin disorder. The cause of eczema is unknown but has been associated with an immune dysfunction of the skin. A combination of external factors (allergens/irritants) and a family history of allergies, asthma, or hay fever has been linked to eczema. If the eczema is severe in the infant or appears before age 2 years, the cause is likely to be related to food allergies. Common food allergies include eggs, milk, peanuts, wheat, soy, and fish. Common irritants include wool, soaps and detergents, some perfumes and cosmetics, chlorine, dust, sand, and even cigarette smoke. If eczema persists during childhood and into adolescence, it is less acute.

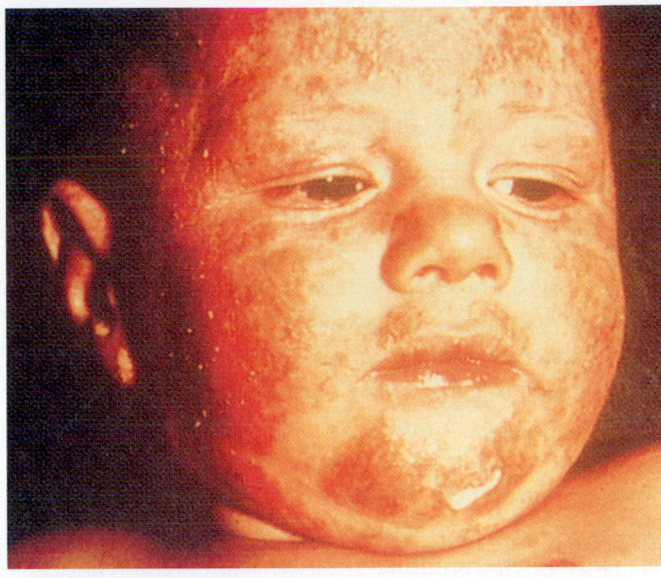

Figure 24-6. ■ Chronic eczema.

Self-esteem is an issue with children and adolescents because of changes in appearance of skin during flare-ups. Eczema flare-ups are more common during the winter months when the air is dry.

Manifestations

INFANTS. Clinical manifestations for infants with eczema include erythematous areas of skin with papulovesicular lesions that rupture and crust. Areas that are affected in infants include cheeks, scalp, forehead, neck, trunk, and extensor surfaces of extremities. The infant is irritable and restless due to intense pruritis.

CHILDREN. For children older than 2 years to puberty, the skin appears erythematous, dry, and scaly, and may include papules that rupture and *weep* (drip serous fluid). Pruritis is also present. Skin behind the knees, around the wrist, the sides of the neck, and around the mouth is most commonly affected. Adolescents may also develop lesions on the eyelids, earlobes, fingertips, toes, and nipple area.

Diagnosis

Diagnosis begins by collecting a comprehensive health history. Data relating to age of onset, presence of asthma or hay fever in parents, location of flare-ups on the body, flare-ups occurring prior to age 4, skin rash occurring prior to age 2, and episodes of dry skin in the past year are helpful for diagnosis. Physical exam includes inspection and palpation of papules and vesicles that have ruptured and formed a yellow, crusty exudate. Skin testing may be done to isolate food allergies.

Treatment

Medical treatment involves hydrating and lubricating the skin to minimize pruritis, while determining triggers that lead to flare-ups. Emollients (Eucerin), oral antihistamines (Benadryl), and topical (1% to 2.5% hydrocortisone) and oral corticosteroids are used to treat eczema. If lesions become infected, topical or oral antibiotics may be prescribed.

Nursing Considerations

The LPN/LVN works closely with children and their families to identify and remove allergens or irritants that cause flare-ups. Encourage regular use of moisturizing lotions and creams to keep skin lubricated to prevent drying and cracking of skin. Apply wet compresses soaked in aluminum acetate solution to help remove crusts and decrease inflammation. Encourage children and adolescents to shower after swimming in pools with chlorine water and after excessive sweating. Encourage children to apply a lubricant after bathing to help seal in moisture. Loose-fitting clothing and soft fabrics help minimize skin irritation. Wash clothes in mild detergents and rinse well. During winter months, keep the environment cool with constant humidity levels. Fingernails should be cut short in infants and children to prevent excessive skin irritation from scratching. Antihistamines may be used at night to decrease itching so the child can rest well. Educate parents to recognize signs of infections and to report them immediately. Encourage children and adolescents to express feelings about their appearance. Low self-esteem is common in children with eczema.

ACNE VULGARIS

Acne vulgaris (acne) is a common skin condition that mostly affects adolescents (Figure 24-7 ■). During puberty, sebum (oil) production from the sebaceous glands increases (under the influence of androgens), and epithelial cells shed at a faster rate. Hair follicles in the skin become blocked, trapping sebum under the skin and causing **comedones** (whiteheads and blackheads) to develop. These blocked follicles provide a rich environment for *Propionibacterium* acnes to grow, causing inflammation. Papules, pustules, and nodules develop in the skin. Acne lesions are commonly found on the face, chest, shoulders, and back.

Manifestations

Clinical manifestations include formation of comedones (whiteheads and blackheads), pustules, and papules over the surface of the skin.

Diagnosis

Identification of comedones, pustules, and papules are used to diagnosis acne vulgaris. Physical exam includes inspection and palpation of the lesion.

Treatment

Topical medications such as tretinoin (Retin-A) or adapalene (Differin) are used to treat mild acne. Medical treatment also includes the use of systemic antibiotics, such as doxycycline, erythromycin, or tetracycline, for 3 months. For more severe acne, isotretinoin (Accutane) may be prescribed.

Nursing Considerations

Nursing management includes supporting and educating the adolescent on proper care of acne lesions. Educate the adolescent to care for skin properly and avoid oil-based cosmetics or lotions. Encourage the client to maintain prescribed medical treatments, and explain that improvement of skin lesions may take up to 3 months. Some acne medications make the skin more sensitive to sunlight, so use of sunscreen should be encouraged. Advise the client to avoid picking or squeezing the lesions, which may push the infected material deeper into the follicle, prolonging inflammation and infection.

> **clinical ALERT**
>
> If Accutane is prescribed, explain that pregnancy should be avoided. Accutane has a teratogenic effect on the developing fetus. Girls who are sexually active should be informed about adopting two forms of contraception to prevent pregnancy (London, Ladewig, Ball, and Bindler, 2007, p. 1869).

NURSING CARE

PRIORITIES IN NURSING CARE

The priority for nursing care of children with inflammatory skin conditions focuses on identification of the lesions so appropriate medical treatments may begin as soon as possible. The LPN/LVN assists the family and child in identifying any irritants that may have come in contact with the skin. It is important to assist the adolescent with acne vulgaris to

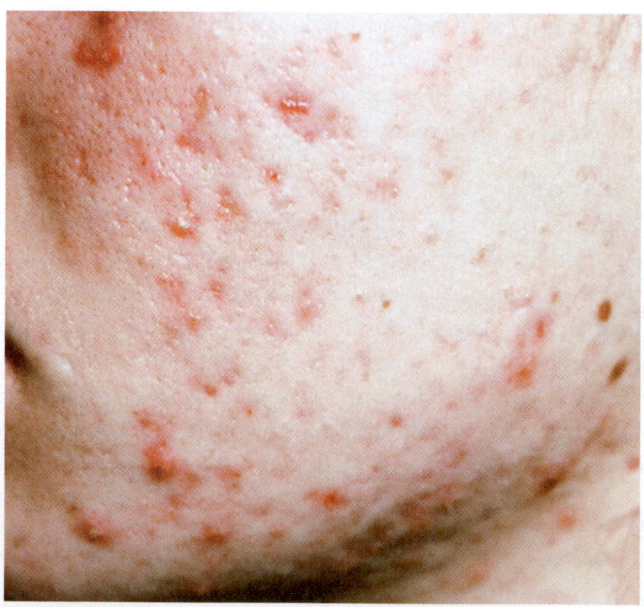

Figure 24-7. ■ Acne lesion. (Medical-On-Line Ltd.)

identify any triggers that may have precipitated the outbreak. The LPN/LVN educates families on proper hygiene methods for bathing and shampooing.

ASSESSING

Children with inflammatory skin conditions should be assessed for any change in color, texture, temperature, and moisture of the skin. Document the location of the lesions, and assess whether the lesions are spreading to other areas of the body. Collect data concerning any irritants that may have been in contact with the skin. Assess for the presence of pruritis, which may lead to secondary infections if the child scratches the lesions. Assess effectiveness of treatments for the lesions with lotions and ointments. Collect data about the child's ability to cope with changes in body image, especially in clients with eczema and acne vulgaris.

DIAGNOSING, PLANNING, AND IMPLEMENTING

The following nursing diagnoses may be used in planning nursing care for the child with an inflammatory disorder:

- Impaired Skin Integrity, related to allergies or irritants
- Acute Pain, related to itching and scratching
- Risk for Infection, related to open lesions
- Disturbed Body Image, related to prolonged treatments for healing.

Typical outcomes for a child with an inflammatory skin disorder might include:

- Skin lesions identified and healed
- Irritants removed
- Pain level decreased
- No signs of secondary infection
- Verbalizes understanding of the healing process.

Nursing interventions related to children with inflammatory disorders include:

For Diaper Rash and Infant's Skin

- Encourage frequent diaper changes. *Removes irritants (urine and stool) away from skin to promote healing.*
- Expose diaper area to open air. *Moisture increases skin irritation. Exposing skin to open air allows skin to dry.*
- Assist families to identify irritants that cause skin to become inflamed. *Eliminating exposure to common irritants will decrease flare-ups and allow skin to heal.*

For Infections, Infestations, Bites, and Contact Dermatitis

- Encourage child to avoid picking and scratching lesions. *Scratching skin lesions increases the chance of infection entering the skin tissue.*
- Educate parents to recognize signs of infection. *Secondary infections may occur if the lesions are exposed to bacteria.*

- Instruct parents on how to cleanse the affected area. *Proper cleansing and drying are vital to reducing risk for infection and promoting the healing process.*
- Administer medicated creams and lotions as scheduled. *Adhering to the prescribed medication schedule will promote healing.*

For Acne and Other Conditions of Adolescents

- Encourage the adolescent to express concerns about appearance of skin associated with acne. *This allows the adolescent to convey feelings about altered skin condition. The nurse is able to dispel any misconceptions about causes and treatments with acne.*

EVALUATING

The LPN/LVN documents whether redness or swelling have increased or decreased over a period of time and whether the client perceives that the itching has increased or decreased. Improvement of skin texture is also documented. Medicated lotions and creams are evaluated for effectiveness. Determine the family's ability to adopt good hygiene practices. Determine whether the child understands the healing process and the time involved. The family and child verbalize common allergens and irritants that affect outbreaks of eczema or contact dermatitis.

Parasitic Infestations

Parasites are living organisms that get their food source from another living host. *Pediculosis* and *scabies* are infestations by lice and *Sarcoptes* mites, respectively. Lice and mites are arthropods that get their food supply by sucking blood from a human host. These infestations are transmitted by direct skin-to-skin contact or by sharing of personal items that have come into contact with the infestation.

PEDICULOSIS

Pediculosis is an infestation with parasites (lice) that live on the outside of a human host. *Pediculus capitis* (head lice) is found most commonly in children from 3 to 10 years of age (Figure 24-8 ■). Preschools and elementary schools have occasional outbreaks of head lice among children in the same classroom. Lice are often found behind the ears on the back of the scalp where the female louse lays eggs (viable **nits**) that hatch within 8 to 10 days. *Pediculus corporis* (body lice) and *Phthirus pubis* (pubic lice or **crabs**) are two other forms of lice infestations.

Manifestations

Clinical manifestations include intense itching over the scalp area and viable nits (eggs) located on one side of the hair shaft.

Diagnosis

Diagnosis is made by inspection, using a bright light and magnifying glass over the affected area. Detection of head

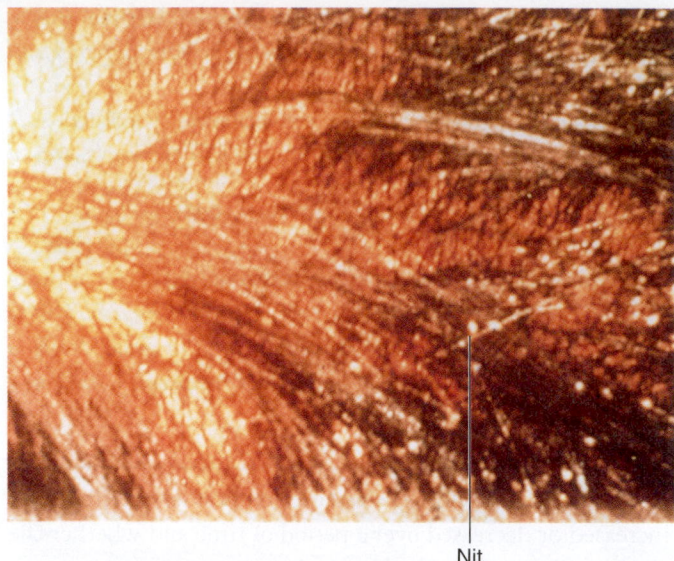

Nit

Figure 24-8. ■ Head lice nits in the hair.

lice is aided by examining sections of hair and the back of the scalp (over the occipital area and behind the ears) for tiny viable nits attached to the base of hair shafts. In severe cases, lice are visible to the naked eye.

Treatment

Medical treatment involves using a *pediculicide* (lice-killing) shampoo, such as permethrin (Nix). The hair is combed with a fine-tooth comb dipped in vinegar to help remove stubborn nits and nit shells. A second treatment is applied in 7 days to ensure that all nits are killed.

Nursing Considerations

Nursing care focuses on teaching parents and/or children how to kill the parasite and alleviate itching. Demonstrate how to inspect for lice by checking the scalp over the occipital area of the head and by separating small amounts of hair to look for any nits. Instruct parents to remove any nits before they hatch. All family members should be examined for the presence of lice so treatment may be initiated immediately. Instruct parents to inform the child's school so precautions may be taken in the classroom to prevent spread of the infestation. Advise parents to follow directions carefully on the prescribed shampoo. Some providers then suggest drying the hair and combing it with a fine-tooth comb dipped in vinegar to remove stubborn nits. This process may need to be repeated again in 7 days to kill any eggs that may have hatched after shampooing.

It must be stressed that parents will need to wash all bedding, towels, and hair accessories in hot water and dry them in a hot dryer. Upholstered furniture should be vacuumed, and the vacuum bag should be discarded. Personal items that cannot be washed, such as pillows, toys, and stuffed animals, should be sealed in a plastic bag for

2 weeks. This breaks the cycle of infestation by preventing any lice that hatch from finding a new host.

SCABIES

Scabies is an infestation caused by the mite *Sarcoptes scabiei*. The lesions are mainly found on the hands and feet and in the folds of the skin. Once the scabies mite finds a human host, it burrows into the epidermis and lays eggs. In 2 to 4 days, the eggs hatch and the immature mites travel toward the surface of the skin, where they mature and grow. If left untreated, scabies mites continue this cycle every 14 to 17 days. Ova and feces from the scabies mites come in contact with the skin and cause irritation and pruritus (Figure 24-9 ■). This usually appears about 1 month after infestation.

Manifestations

Clinical manifestations include erythematous papules, vesicles, and even pustules. Pruritus is present and is more severe at night. Lesions may appear on the face, head, neck, chest, abdomen, waist, axillae, web of fingers, buttocks, intergluteal folds, palms of the hands, and soles of the feet. Lesions may appear as a thin gray burrow that ends with a *vesicle* (blister).

Diagnosis

Diagnosis is made by obtaining a complete history and general physical examination. Skin scrapings are inspected under the microscope for the presence of mites, eggs, or feces.

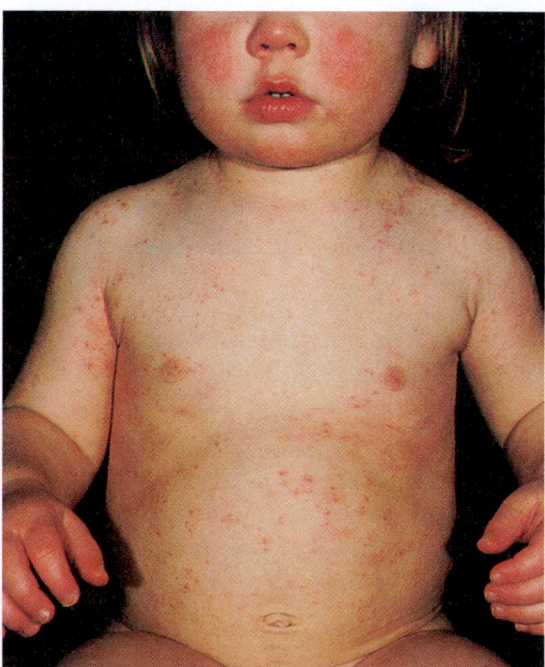

Figure 24-9. ■ Diffuse scabies in an infant. The lesions are most numerous around the axillae, chest, and abdomen. (From Habif, T. P. [1990]. *Clinical dermatology: A color guide to diagnosis and therapy* [2nd ed.]. St. Louis, MO: Mosby-Year Book, p. 298. With permission from Elsevier.)

Treatment

Medical treatment may include treatment with premethrin cream (Elimite) and good hygiene practices to prevent recurrent infestations. Recommend washing all clothing, linens, and towels in hot (140°F) water and drying them at high heat to kill any remaining mites.

Nursing Considerations

Once diagnosis is made, the child needs to shower, dry thoroughly, and apply 5% permethrin lotion. All household members should be treated at the same time, regardless of whether they have symptoms. Instruct the child to leave the cream or lotion on for 8 to 12 hours before showering again. Much of the care for scabies resembles the care for pediculosis. The nurse teaches good hygiene practices and instructs parents to wash clothes, bed linens, and towels on a regular basis. Items that cannot be washed or dry-cleaned should be sealed in a plastic bag for 5 days. Nonjudgmental nursing care will increase the family's compliance with treatment regimens and will lessen embarrassment about the situation.

Skin Infections

Any break in skin integrity provides an opportunity for infection to take hold (see chain of infection in Figure 26-1).

Introduced lesions, such as piercings and tattoos, increase the risk of infection. Box 24-2 ■ discusses some of the issues involved in these forms of ornamentation.

WARTS (PAPILLOMAVIRUS)

Warts are benign tumors in the epithelial cells of the skin that are caused by the human papillomavirus (HPV). Common warts are found on the skin surface, and plantar warts are found on the feet. Warts can be transmitted from person to person, or the infection may transfer from one site to another on the same person (referred to as *autoinoculation*). Plantar warts may develop from contact on surfaces such as locker room floors. A compromised immune system in children may increase the risk for developing HPV, therefore leaving children more susceptible to warts.

Manifestations

Warts (Figure 24-10 ■) appear on the surface of the skin as rough, scaly papules and nodules that are the same color of the skin. They are painless and are most commonly found on the dorsal surface of the hand and around the nails of the fingertips. Plantar warts are more common in adolescents; they appear as papules and plaques on the bottom of the feet. Due to the pressure and irritation of walking, they can be quite painful.

BOX 24-2	CULTURAL PULSE POINTS

Tattoos and Piercings

Among some cultures and subcultures, tattoos and body piercings are considered to be important adornments. Parents may have piercings performed on their children while they are still infants, or tattoos and piercings may be a way of celebrating the onset of puberty or the approach of adulthood. Nurses should be informed about the care involved when having these procedures so they can provide teaching.

Youth who want tattoos or piercings must follow state regulations. Parental consent may be required. Because piercings and tattoos both compromise skin integrity, these procedures carry certain risks of infection. In all cases, proper care of the skin as it heals is essential to prevent local infection. More important, safety guidelines need to be followed by those performing the piercings or tattooing to prevent systemic infections, including life-threatening ones such as hepatitis, tetanus, or HIV.

According to La Leche League (2005), proper tattooing procedures include:

- Sterilization of equipment with an autoclave
- Bagging of equipment after use
- Single-use needles, gloves, ink, cups, and posts
- Thorough hand washing with disinfectant soap.

Likewise, piercings should only be done with new needles, and universal precautions should be followed during the procedure.

Care of the skin while it heals after tattooing includes:

- Daily washing with a mild soap and water
- No picking of scabs
- No sun exposure.

Care of the skin after piercing is done one to five times per day until healing is complete (Children's Hospital Boston, 2006). Healing time ranges from about 4 weeks (for the tongue) to a year (for ear cartilage or the navel). Care includes:

- Washing the hands before touching the pierced area
- Removing crusty skin from the site and jewelry with warm water
- Washing the skin and jewelry with antibacterial soap, rinsing well, and patting the area dry with a paper towel (*Note:* Cloth towels are not used because they may harbor bacteria.)
- Allowing air to the site to promote healing (Antibacterial ointment is not used.)
- Preventing sweat, dirt, body fluids, alcohol or hydrogen peroxide, or tight clothing from coming into contact with the site until healing is complete; these may cause irritation or infection
- Avoiding hot tubs and swimming pools until skin has completely healed.

There is no evidence to suggest that tattooing, or tattoo removal, affects breastfeeding (La Leche League, 2005). However, most professionals will not tattoo a woman who is pregnant, and it is recommended that a woman wait a year after childbirth before getting a new tattoo.

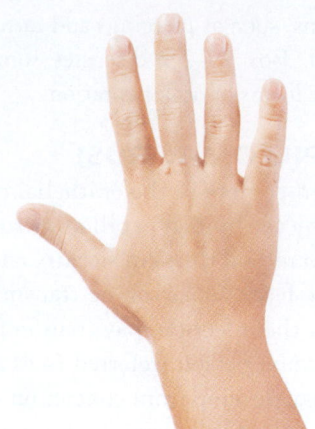

Figure 24-10. ■ Warts on a child's hand. (Maksym Bondarchuk/ Shutterstock)

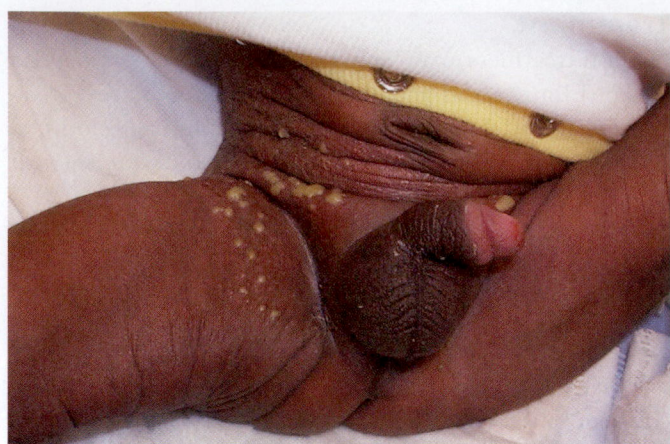

Figure 24-11. ■ Bullous impetigo. (Courtesy of Dr. William H. Sorey, University of Mississippi Medical Center.)

Diagnosis

Diagnosis is made by inspection of papules and nodules that appear rough and scaly.

Treatment

Medical treatment is individualized, ranging from no treatment to destroying the wart by physical or chemical methods. Removal of the wart may require the use of chemical substances or peeling agents, **cryotherapy** (freezing with liquid nitrogen), laser therapy, or applying duct tape over the wart.

Nursing Considerations

The nurse explains that treatments involving the applications of peeling agents may take up to several months to see improvement. If pain is associated with treatment, encourage parents to reduce the frequency. Once the pain decreases, instruct them to continue therapy as directed. Encourage the child to avoid picking the wart. This will reduce the risk of autoinoculation.

IMPETIGO

Impetigo is a superficial skin infection that appears on the face, hands, neck, or extremities and is caused by streptococci or staphylococci. Insect bites, burns, scratches, and lacerations provide a portal of entry for the bacteria. It is highly contagious and can be transferred between children and adults, especially if towels, linens, and clothing are shared with the infected person. Poor sanitation and close living conditions place children at risk for contracting impetigo. This infection is primarily seen during the summer months when the temperature is hot and humid and children are more prone to insect bites, scratches, and lacerations.

Manifestations

Clinical manifestations include vesicles or pustules, edema, and redness surrounding the lesion (Figure 24-11 ■). Once the vesicle ruptures, the lesion is covered with a loosely adherent, honey-yellow crust. If the crust is removed, a new honey-yellow crust will form.

Diagnosis

Diagnosis is made by inspecting and palpating the lesions for a honey-yellow–colored crust and exudate. Disposable gloves should be worn by the LPN/LVN during assessment. Bacterial cultures may be obtained for diagnosis.

Treatment

Medical treatment involves soaking the crusted lesion in warm water, scrubbing with medicated soap to remove the crust, and applying a topical bactericidal ointment (e.g., mupirocin or bacitracin) to the lesion for 1 week. A systemic antibiotic may be used if no improvement is seen with topical ointments.

Nursing Considerations

The nurse educates the family that even minor cuts and scratches to the skin pose a threat for invasion of bacteria. Remind the family that impetigo is highly contagious and that towels, bed linens, and clothes must not be shared with a family member who is infected with impetigo. Instruct parents to wash and remove the crust several times a day and to follow orders for applying topical bactericidal ointment. Tell them to return to the clinic if the lesions do not improve because a systemic antibiotic may be necessary.

CELLULITIS

Cellulitis is a bacterial infection of the dermis and subcutaneous tissue. Recent upper respiratory infections, sinusitis, otitis media, or an abscessed tooth may result in cellulitis affecting the face and neck region. Injury that compromises the skin barrier such as trauma, scratches, or bug bites may cause cellulitis in the extremities. Cellulitis may also occur at an IV insertion site if standard precautions are not followed by the LPN/LVN. *Staphylococcus aureus, Streptococcus pneumoniae, Hemophilus influenza*, and beta-hemolytic and group A *Streptococcus* are common causative organisms. Onset is usually rapid.

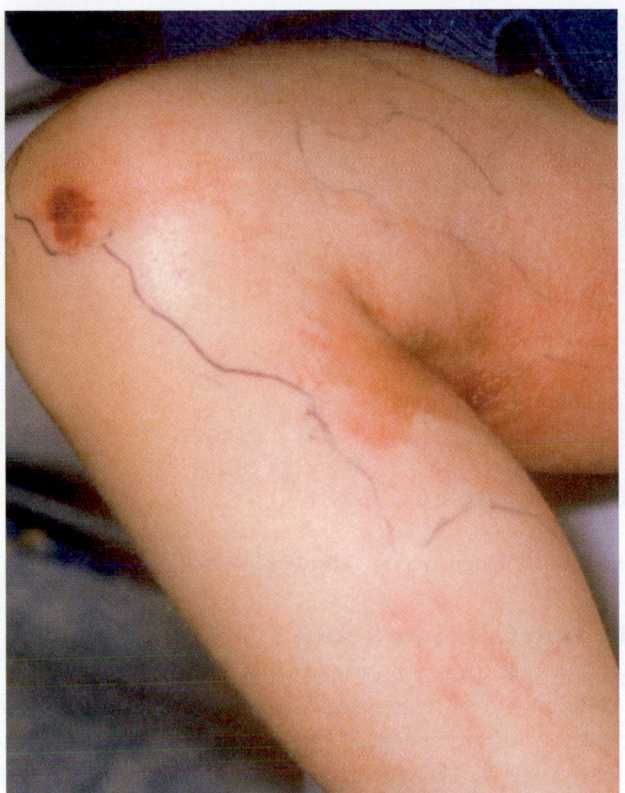

Figure 24-12. ■ Cellulitis. Markings on leg show fullest extent of infection. (Medical-On-Line Ltd.)

Manifestations

Clinical manifestations of local symptoms around the infected site include edematous skin that is red, tender, and warm to touch (Figure 24-12 ■). There may be red streaks extending out from the infected area. Systemic symptoms indicating septicemia include fever, headache, pain, chills, malaise, and lymphangitis.

Diagnosis

Diagnosis is made by evaluating lab results for a complete blood cell count (including a differential) and by analyzing results from cultures drawn from the infected site. Blood cultures may be taken if the child appears toxic.

Treatment

Children with cellulitis of the trunk, extremities, or perianal area may be treated with oral antibiotics on an outpatient basis. When the case is severe or the face and larger areas of the body are affected, the child may be hospitalized and treated with IV antibiotics.

Nursing Considerations

Nursing considerations include strict adherence to antibiotics administration to achieve therapeutic blood levels and prevent sepsis. The nurse ensures that the child has an opportunity to rest and elevate the affected area. Warm compresses are applied to improve circulation and promote healing of the skin tissues. To avoid spread of infection, parents and child are taught to wash hands frequently, especially when caring for the infected area. Instruct the parents to return to the pediatrician's office immediately if they notice any signs of sepsis or spread of infection.

HERPES SIMPLEX TYPE I

Herpes simplex type I ("fever blister," "cold sore," or "canker sore") is a viral infection caused by herpes simplex virus type I (HSV-I). The virus is passed from the infected person to others by direct contact. The virus remains latent, possibly from childhood, until individual triggers activate a response. Fever, emotional upset, menses, cold, or sun exposure are triggers that initiate an outbreak of the virus. HSV-I poses a serious threat to newborns. (See Chapter 5 and Table 8-4 ⚭ for more information about herpes.)

Manifestations

Clinical manifestations include a tingling or burning sensation at the affected site. A single vesicle or a cluster of vesicles appears over red inflamed skin. Lesions are found near the mouth, and some are found on the buccal mucosa. Usually, the vesicles dry and heal in 8 to 10 days.

Diagnosis

Medical diagnosis is made by inspection of the lesion, with attention to the presence of vesicles that appear reddened and crusted. A culture may be obtained for analysis.

Treatment

Medical treatment with acyclovir (Zovirax) is initiated at the first indication of symptoms.

Nursing Considerations

The nurse encourages the child to report symptoms of a herpes outbreak early so medication can begin as soon as possible to decrease the length of the outbreak. Instruct the child on methods to prevent spreading of the lesions by using good hand washing techniques. Help the child identify what triggers the outbreak of the lesions and develop a plan to minimize the triggers.

Fungal Infections

DERMATOPHYTES (RINGWORM)

Dermatophytes are fungi that mainly affect the surface of the skin, hair, and nails. Tinea (sometimes called **ringworm**) is a term used to describe a group of fungal infections of the

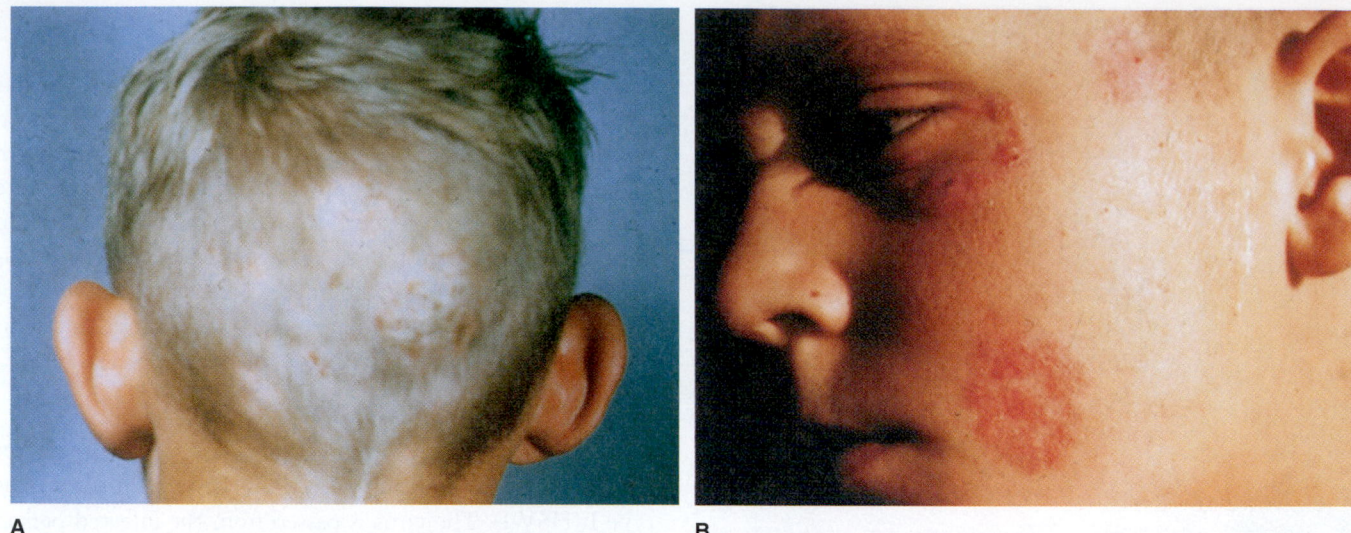

Figure 24-13. ■ **(A)** Tinea capitis. **(B)** Tinea corporis. (Courtesy of the Centers for Disease Control and Prevention, Atlanta, GA.)

skin that are transmitted from human to human or from animals to human. The different types of fungal (tinea) infections are named after the location of the fungal infection on the body: tinea capitis (of the head), tinea corporis (of the body), tinea pedis (of the foot), and tinea cruris (of the groin).

Manifestations

- **Tinea capitis** is a scalp fungus. It most commonly affects children between the ages of 3 and 10 years. When the fungus invades the scalp, the hair becomes brittle and breaks off, leaving circular patches of scalp showing the hair loss. Papules form around the edges of the ring and become scaly and red in color (Figure 24-13A ■).
- **Tinea corporis** has a circular reddened patch on the skin with raised borders. The lesions can become scaly (see Figure 24-13B).
- **Tinea pedis** is referred to as "athlete's foot." The skin between the toes and on the soles of the feet becomes red, with deep scaly fissures that are painful and itchy.
- **Tinea cruris,** referred to as "jock itch," causes the skin in the groin area to become red and scaly, with raised papules or vesicles forming a circular rash.

Diagnosis

Diagnosis is made by obtaining a skin scraping of the lesion and viewing it under a microscope to detect fungal growth.

Treatment

Medical treatment involves the use of antifungal topical ointments, powders, or sprays. Superficial fungal infections may be treated with over-the-counter medications such as Tinactin, Micatin, Lotrimin, and Lamisil. If the fungal infection is deep into the skin, Diflucan or Sporonax may be prescribed.

Nursing Considerations

Nursing care focuses on preventing the spread of infection, encouraging good hygiene practices, and promoting comfort. To prevent spread of tinea capitis and tinea corporis, instruct children not to share hairbrushes, combs, pillows, towels, clothes, or hats. Advise children with tinea cruris and tinea pedis to keep the infected area clean and dry. Recommend loose-fitting clothing that will keep moisture out and decrease friction from fabric that can cause skin irritation. Teach children that, to prevent tinea pedis, they must wear shoes at all times in public lockers rooms and showers. Encourage parents to administer medication for the entire prescribed period, even up to 7 days after the infection has resided. Fungal infections may need to be treated for 6 months to a year.

ORAL CANDIDIASIS (THRUSH)

Oral candidiasis (**thrush**) is a yeastlike fungal infection that is caused by *Candida albicans* (see Figure 21-3 ⬤⬤). It generally affects newborns born vaginally from an infected mother. It may also be a chronic condition in young children receiving antibiotics or corticosteroids, or in those who have an immune disorder.

Manifestations

Oral candidiasis (thrush) appears as white plaques on the tongue, palate, or buccal mucosa that bleed easily. Nutritional intake may be decreased due to pain and discomfort with breastfeeding or feeding. Candida lesions may also be present in the diaper area of an infant who has diaper dermatitis.

Diagnosis

Oral candidiasis is diagnosed by inspection of the oral mucosa or by fungal culture. Microscopic examination from skin scrapings of the lesion is also used for diagnosis.

Treatment

Medical treatment for thrush includes the use of oral and topical antifungal medications such as nystatin oral suspension or clotrimazole. Fluconazole or itraconazole may be prescribed if the infection is severe or if immunocompromised children have oropharyngeal candidiasis. Systemic *Candida* infections are treated with IV amphotericin B.

Nursing Considerations

Nursing care involves teaching the parents to use a swab when applying nystatin oral suspension to the tongue surface and buccal mucosa, and then allowing the infant to swallow the remaining suspension. This procedure is done after feedings. Older children can be taught to swish the suspension in the mouth before swallowing. Nursing care also focuses on decreasing the risk of reinfection by instructing the parents to sterilize bottle nipples and pacifiers for 20 minutes in boiling water. Instruct parents to follow directions on antiseptic sprays when disinfecting toys that cannot be autoclaved. The child who uses a corticosteroid inhaler should be taught to rinse the mouth well with water after use. Spacers should also be rinsed in water after use. Instruct breastfeeding mothers to apply nystatin oral suspension to the nipple area to prevent reinfection.

NURSING CARE

PRIORITIES IN NURSING CARE

When caring for children with skin infections or infestations, the priority of care revolves around diagnosing the organism. Focus care on preventing the spread of infection and eradicating the infestation (head lice or mites). Explain to families how skin infections such as impetigo and HSV-1 are spread from person to person. Instruct families on how to eliminate parasites by teaching them to establish good hygiene practices and protect the home environment. Provide nursing care in a nonjudgmental way to decrease embarrassment about fungal and parasitic infections. Promote compliance with prescribed medication procedures.

ASSESSING

Children with skin infections should be assessed for signs of erythema, vesicles or pustules, edema, fever, malaise, and texture of skin lesions. Collect data on drainage from lesions, documenting color, order, and crusting. Assess oral mucosa for white plaques. Assess presence of pruritis. Inspect hair shafts at base of head for presence of female louse eggs (viable nits). Assess the family's compliance with medication routines.

DIAGNOSING, PLANNING, AND IMPLEMENTING

The following nursing diagnoses may be used in planning nursing care for the child with skin infections and infestations:

- Risk-Prone Health Behavior, related to poor hygiene practices
- Impaired Skin Integrity, related to ruptured vesicles and crusting of lesions
- Impaired Body Image, related to visible parasites on hair and skin
- Interrupted Breastfeeding, related to pain and discomfort from infected oral mucosa
- Risk for Infection, related to spread of organisms from person to person
- Self-Care Deficit: Bathing/Hygiene, related to lack of knowledge on bathing and shampooing.

Typical outcomes for a child with a skin infection or infestation might include:

- Regular hygiene practices followed
- Skin remains intact and free of drainage from lesions
- Body image improved
- Breastfeeding resumed
- No signs of infection noted among family members
- Verbalizes importance of good hygiene practices.

Nursing interventions for some of the nursing diagnoses have been discussed previously in this chapter and are not repeated here. Additional nursing interventions are as follows:

- Instruct parents on how to soak and remove crusts from impetigo lesions several times a day. *Promotes healing.*
- Educate parents to recognize signs of infection. *Prompt medical attention is needed to prevent spread of infection.*
- Apply warm compresses over skin infected with cellulitis. *Improves circulation and promotes healing.*
- Monitor antibiotic therapy. *Helps achieve a therapeutic blood level to decrease infection.*
- Encourage frequent hand washing. *Prevents spread of infection.*
- Educate parents on how to apply medicated lotions or creams to lesions. *Protects skin and improves healing.*
- Inform parents to wash all towels, bed linens, and clothes when lice and scabies are detected. *Prevents spread of lice to other family members. Washing in hot water and heated drying will eradicate lice and scabies.*
- Demonstrate proper application of antifungal medication to the oral mucosa in infants. *Swabbing nystatin oral suspension to the tongue and oral mucosa to infants following feedings will help promote healing of thrush and continued breastfeeding. Older children should be taught how to swish and swallow.*

EVALUATING

The LPN/LVN documents no signs of infection. Infections are not spread to other members of the family. The LPN/LVN verifies that the parents are following recommendations for washing towels, linens, and clothing to eradicate parasites. The LPN/LVN observes the parent as he or she applies medicated lotion and creams to infected skin tissue. Listen to determine if parents can recall signs of infection and verbalize when to return to the pediatrician's office.

NURSING PROCESS CARE PLAN
Client with Cellulitis

Mrs. B calls the pediatrician's office to report that her daughter Lucy, age 12, woke up this morning complaining of headache, chills, and pain in her right calf. Last week at camp, Lucy injured her leg on a piece of old wood in the lake while canoeing. The camp nurse accompanied Lucy to the emergency room where she received stitches in her right calf. The mother states the leg is swollen, with red streaks spreading out from the wound.

Assessment. The LPN/LVN should gather the following information over the telephone:

- Onset of symptoms
- Complaints of chills, fever, or malaise
- Color of skin around the wound
- Swelling in the leg
- Drainage from the wound
- Pain associated with walking
- Pain level.

When the child is seen in the pediatrician's office, gather the following data:

- Vital signs
- Condition of skin around the wound
- Lab work
- Inspect stitches and approximation of wound
- Assess for lymphangitis.

Nursing Diagnosis. The following important nursing diagnosis (among others) is established for this client:

- Risk for Infection related to tissue trauma from a foreign object.

Expected Outcomes
- Will be free of infection
- Will remain pain free with weight bearing

Planning and Implementation
- Review lab work and report abnormalities immediately. *To identify infection and type of bacteria.*

- Instruct child to rest and elevate leg. *To reduce swelling and promote comfort.*
- Explain the importance of following the advised medical regimen for antibiotic therapy. *To prevent complications associated with systemic infections and to achieve therapeutic blood levels of antibiotics.*
- Explain the importance of hand washing while caring for the wound. *To prevent spread of infection.*
- Demonstrate proper technique for dressing changes. *To ensure proper care of wound.*
- Apply warm compresses over the infected area. *To enhance circulation to the area and promote healing.*
- Instruct parents to recognize signs of infection. *Cellulitis may lead to septicemia.*
- Explain to parents the need to return to the pediatrician's office if infection worsens. *Spread of infection could cause the child to become seriously ill and require hospitalization.*

Evaluation. Inflammation of the skin tissue should begin to subside within 48 hours after initiating antibiotic therapy. Temperature will return to normal range. The child should be able to bear weight on the leg once inflammation and pain decrease. Skin tissue will be free of redness, drainage, and edema. Complications leading to septicemia are prevented.

Critical Thinking Questions

1. Lucy notices that the redness in her right calf has traveled above her knee and appears to have red streaks that lead to the wound. What is causing changes in the skin tissue?
2. Lucy has been admitted to the hospital and is placed on IV antibiotics. How do you explain to Lucy why she now has IV medication?
3. Mrs. B. asks what she can do to help Lucy be more comfortable at home. How do you respond?

Note: Discussion of Critical Thinking questions appears in Appendix I.

Burns

Burns can occur at any age; however, in the young child, burns are more common in boys between 1 and 4 years of age. At this age, children are exploring their environment. They can reach hot pans on the stove, pull and chew on electrical cords, ingest cleaning agents and chemicals, grab a hot curling iron, and explore the fire in the fireplace. School-age children and adolescents venture outside to explore. They may come in contact with matches, fireworks, and electrical wires (when climbing trees and voltage towers). They may experiment with mixing chemicals. Most burns can be prevented, and parents must be alert to hazards in and around

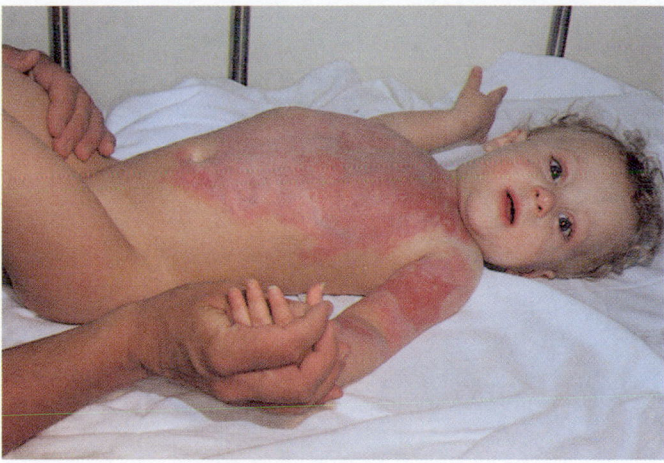

A

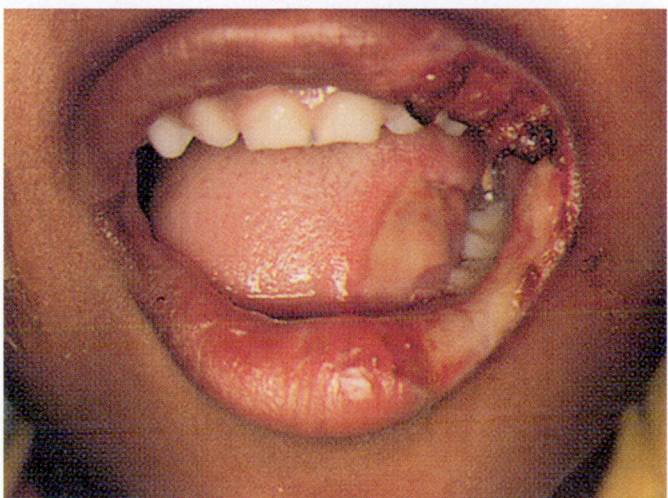

B

C

Figure 24-14. ■ **(A)** Thermal (scald) burns are the most common burn injury in infancy. **(B)** Burns of the hands or feet that are distributed like gloves or stockings are associated with child abuse. **(C)** Electrical burn caused by biting an electric cord. **(B:** Roy Alson, PhD, MD FACEP, FAAEM.)

the child's environment. There are four types of burns (Figure 24-14 ■):

- **Thermal burns** are caused by flame and hot objects such as coffee, grease, or stoves (Figure 24-14A and B).
- **Chemical burns** are caused by strong acids or alkaline, such as the chemical found in cleansers containing lye, toilet cleaners, or preparations used to open clogged drains.
- **Electrical burns** (Figure 24-14C) are caused by contact with exposed electric wires. As the electricity travels through the body, it burns the tissue at point of entrance and at point of exit.
- **Radiation burns** are caused by exposure to radiation, the most common type being sunburn.

Burns may also be evidence of child abuse. Any unusual burn occurring in a pattern could suggest deliberately induced burns. Examples are the circles of cigarette burns or a burn that covers the area like a glove or a stocking.

Manifestations

Burns are assessed for burn depth (thickness) and burn area (percentage of body surface area [BSA]). Burn depth is described as partial thickness or full thickness. Partial-thickness burns (sometimes called first- and second-degree burns) may be superficial or deep. Skin appears red, may blister, blanches with pressure, and is painful and sensitive to cold air. The skin may regenerate, but some scarring may result. Full-thickness burns include third-degree burns. Skin will appear brown, may form **eschar** (dead matter sloughed off the skin surface), and may be white to gray in color. Decreased sensation to pain is associated with full-thickness burns. These burns require skin grafting because the skin cannot regenerate.

Burn area is an estimate of the amount of body surface area (BSA) damaged (Figure 24-15 ■). The process for estimating the amount of body surface damage is the same as for an adult. However, the percent of body surface is different for a child than for an adult because of the different body proportions. For example, if a 1-year-old were burned on the back of the head (8.5%) and upper back (6.5%), the burn area would be 15%. (For an adult, it would be 13.5%.)

Diagnosis

Diagnosis for burns is based on assessment of the thickness of the burn and use of the Lund and Browder chart (see Figure 24-15) to determine the percentage of body surface area (BSA) burned.

Treatment

The initial treatment of a burn is to stop the burning process by removing the cause. Because the child's status may change rapidly due to smoke inhalation and swelling of the airway, monitoring of **a**irway, **b**reathing, and **c**irculation (the ABCs)

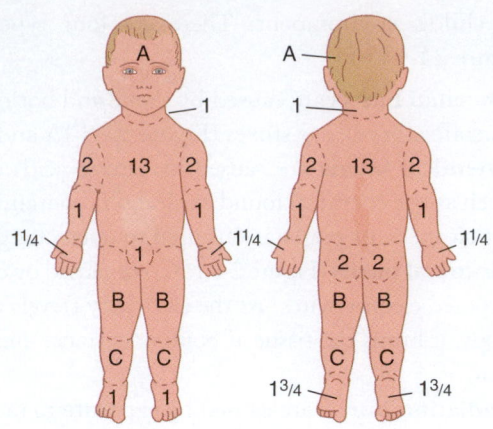

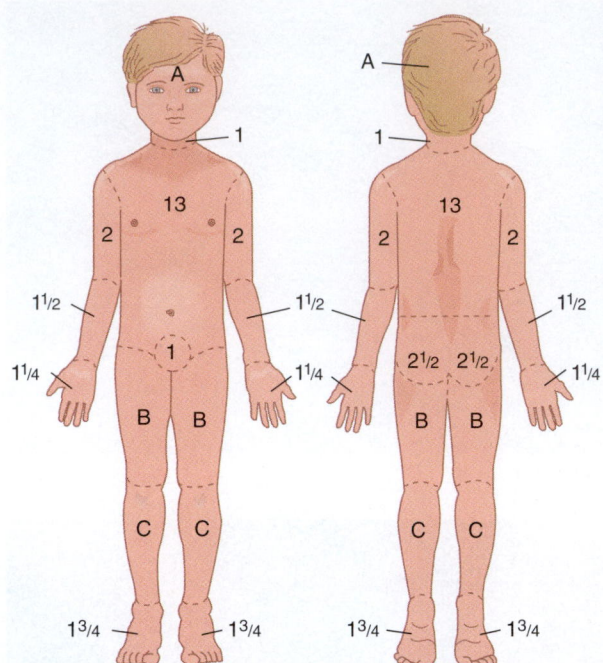

Relative Percentages of Areas Affected by Growth

Area	Age in years					
	0	1	5	10	11	Adult
A = $1/2$ of head	$9^{1}/_2$	$8^{1}/_2$	$6^{1}/_2$	$5^{1}/_2$	$4^{1}/_2$	$3^{1}/_2$
B = $1/2$ of one thigh	$2^{3}/_4$	$3^{1}/_4$	4	$4^{1}/_2$	$4^{1}/_2$	$4^{3}/_4$
C = $1/2$ of one lower leg	$2^{1}/_2$	$2^{1}/_2$	$2^{3}/_4$	3	$3^{1}/_4$	$3^{1}/_2$

Figure 24-15. ■ Classifications of burns in children. These charts determine percentage of skin surface area involved in pediatric burn injuries. (Adapted from Artz, C. P. & Moncrief, J. A. [1969]. *The treatment of burns* [2nd ed.]. Philadelphia: Saunders. With the permission from Elsevier.)

is essential. Medical treatment also focuses on replacing fluid loss, managing pain control, preventing infection, promoting nutrition to improve tissue healing, and salvaging viable burned tissue. Box 24-3 ■ describes a common remedy for mild superficial burns.

Nursing Considerations

A serious burn is an emergency. Continued monitoring of the ABCs is a priority. Shortly after a burn, fluid shifts from the blood vessels to the interstitial space (see Figure 15-2 ⚭), resulting in low blood volume. With severe burn injuries, fluid volume must be replaced to prevent hypovolemic shock.

BOX 24-3 **COMPLEMENTARY THERAPIES**

Herbal Therapy with Aloe Vera Gel

Aloe vera gel is found in many lotions, sunscreens, and cosmetics. Aloe vera has antibacterial, anti-inflammatory, and antiviral actions. Clinical trials have shown that aloe vera accelerates healing of burns, abrasions, frostbite, and canker sores. Itching can also be decreased with the use of aloe vera. Parents often keep aloe vera in the home to treat mild injuries in children. Contact dermatitis is a rare side effect associated with aloe vera. Aloe vera gel is difficult to stabilize in lotions or other commercial products. The best source of aloe vera gel is directly from the broken leaf of a plant.

Source: Data from Kemper, K., Gardiner, P., & Coles, D. (2001). The skinny on herbal remedies for dermatologic disorders. *Contemporary Pediatrics, 7*, 103; Atherton, P. (1997). Aloe vera: Myth or medicine? *Positive Health* 20 June/July. The International Aloe Science Council. (2002). The complete story of aloe vera.

IV hydration should be initiated with lactated Ringer's or normal saline. Nutritional requirements for calories and protein are increased to promote healing of skin tissue. Enteral feedings may begin within 6 hours of the burn injury. The LPN/LVN assesses the level of pain associated with procedures and administers pain medication according to the prescribed schedule to decrease pain during procedures. Continually evaluate effectiveness of pain medication. Comfort measures such as relaxation techniques, diversional activities, and therapeutic touch can be used in addition to pain medication. Demonstrate proper wound care and methods to prevent infection prior to discharge. Provide psychological support to the child and family. Allow the child to talk about his or her feelings, concerns, and fears. Provide referrals for social support, and encourage families to join community support groups.

NURSING CARE

PRIORITIES IN NURSING CARE

When caring for a child with a burn injury, priority of care may be determined by the classification of the burn itself. Moderate burns require dressing changes and teaching prior to discharge. Severe burns require hospitalization and extensive treatments. In general, the nurse assists with immediate care of the burn injury to maintain the ABCs. Care focuses on fluid replacement, pain control, and prevention of infection. Psychological support for the child and family is paramount during the recovery process.

ASSESSING

The role of the LPN/LVN in burn care is one of continued data collection and monitoring of the child for complications.

DIAGNOSING, PLANNING, AND IMPLEMENTING

The following nursing diagnoses can be used to plan and implement care of the burned child:

- Impaired Physical Mobility, related to joint stiffness and bed rest
- Acute Pain related to tissue damage
- Deficient Fluid Volume, related to fluid shift and loss from damaged tissue
- Risk for Infection, related to loss of protective layers of the skin
- Imbalanced Nutrition: Less than Body Requirements, related to increased need for calories and protein
- Disturbed Body Image, related to body disfigurement
- Anxiety (parent and child), related to burn injury and lengthy hospitalization.

Possible outcomes for children with burn injuries may include:

- Child will remain free of secondary infections.
- Pain will be controlled.
- Nutrition will be adequate for weight gain and tissue repair.
- Child will verbalize feelings about the burn injury and identify sources of support.

The following nursing interventions should be implemented in caring for the child and family:

- Administer narcotics or other analgesics as needed prior to dressing changes. Keep the wound covered to decrease discomfort and prevent infection. A bed cradle may be used to keep linen off the wound. *Burns can be very painful, so the child must be adequately medicated. Covering the wound decreases pain stimulation from contact with air and linen.*
- For minor burns, teach parents how to care for the wound and change the dressing (Figure 24-16 ■). *Minor burns are treated on an outpatient basis. Parents must understand how to protect the wound, how to frequently provide dressing changes, and how to recognize signs of infection should they occur.*
- Follow doctor's orders and facility guidelines in changing dressings, whirlpool baths, debridement, and ointment application. *To promote healing, the eschar must be removed. Check facility policy to determine if this is an LPN/LVN function.*
- Strictly follow doctor's orders regarding care of skin graft and donor site. *A skin graft must remain fixed to underlying tissue until circulation is re-established. Care must be taken to prevent injury to the graft site. The donor site should be kept clean and dry to promote healing.*
- Keep room temperature warm to prevent hypothermia. Avoid heat lamps. *When there is large destruction of skin, the*

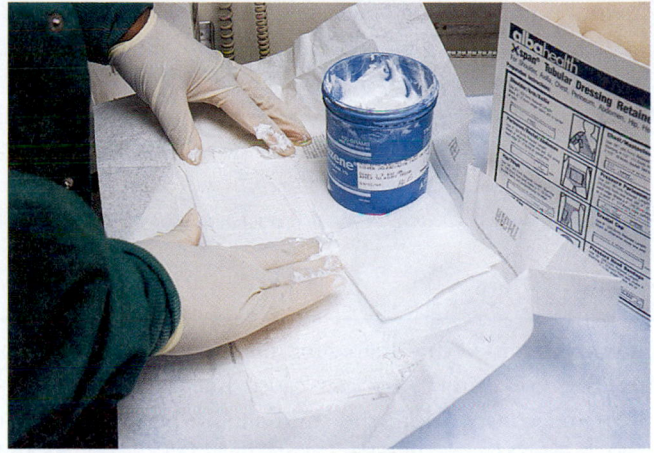

A

B

Figure 24-16. ■ Serious burns are most often treated in the ICU or in a specialized burn center. (**A**) Care of burns must done with sterile technique to prevent introduction of infection to the compromised area. (**B**) The treated wound is covered with a sterile gauze.

body's thermoregulation mechanism is altered and the child develops hypothermia. Heat lamps should be avoided to prevent further burns.

- Administer oral and IV fluids as ordered. Monitor intake and output and hematocrit. *Fluid shifts from vascular to interstitial space and leaks from damaged skin. Fluid balance must be monitored and maintained.*
- Administer high-protein nutrition, either oral or total parenteral nutrition (TPN) as ordered. *Proteins are needed for tissue repair.*
- Encourage activity within limitations of wound healing process. Books, games, and movies may be used for the child confined to bed. Physical therapy may be used to maintain and regain strength and movement. *Physical activity is necessary for muscle strength, growth, and positive mental outlook.*
- Use therapeutic communication techniques to help child and family cope with disfigurement. Refer family to RN and social worker as necessary. *The child may need support in dealing*

with altered body image. Parents may need support in dealing with guilt and change in child's appearance. Burn treatment is expensive, so the family may need support with financial obligations.

■ Teach the family how to care for the wound, skin graft, and donor site at home. *The healing of a burn generally takes several weeks or months to complete. The child may be discharged from the hospital and readmitted for surgery for follow-up treatment.*

EVALUATING

The child should be evaluated for infection and wound healing. Because immobility can cause pneumonia, contractures, and constipation, the child should be evaluated for these complications. Parents should be able to verbalize and demonstrate an understanding of home care.

Trauma. to Skin from the Environment

SUNBURN

Overexposure to the sun's ultraviolet rays can damage the outer surface of the skin, resulting in a burn injury. A combination of low levels of melanin in children, a thin epidermal layer, and long periods of time spent in the sun places children at higher risk for sunburns. Children and adolescents who have had repeated sunburns or severe blistering from the sun are more likely to develop melanoma and basal cell carcinoma than those who have protected themselves from the sun's harmful rays.

In a relatively short time (30 minutes to 4 hours), sun exposure can cause the skin to become red and tender. If exposure is prolonged, edema, vesiculation, bullae, or blistering may result. Other symptoms of sunburn may include headache, fatigue, chills, and malaise.

Treatment includes symptomatic care. Increase oral fluids, cool compresses, and topical corticosteroid (only to intact skin) over the burned area to relieve pain and discomfort.

Prevention is the best medicine. Teach children and parents to apply sunscreen (SPF 15 or greater), to wear protective clothing, and to avoid sun exposure between 10 A.M. and 4 P.M. when the sun's rays are the strongest. These simple methods will greatly decrease the risk of developing melanoma later in life.

MELANOMA

Malignant melanoma is the most serious of all skin cancers. Although rare in children younger than 14 years, it is increasing among adolescents. There is an increased risk of developing melanoma in children with dysplastic nevus syndrome, congenital nevi, or an immunodeficiency state. Melanoma arises from **melanocytes** (pigment-producing

cells) in the dermis and epidermis. Damage to the pigment-producing cells is most often caused by a cumulative effect from the sun's ultraviolet rays. The use of tanning beds and excessive exposure to the sun has been associated with malignant melanoma.

Manifestations

Clinical manifestations include lesions (or moles) with color variations of brown, tan, or black; an irregular border; and a diameter greater than 6 mm (Figure 24-16 ■). The lesion may become ulcerated or may bleed.

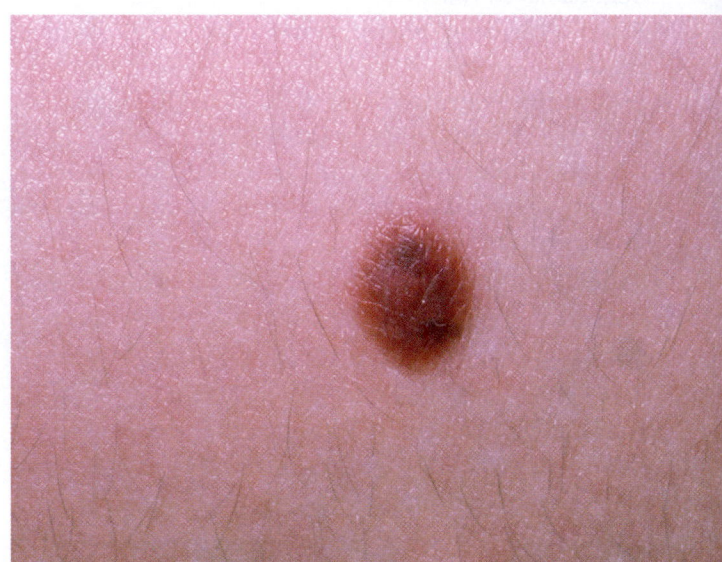

A

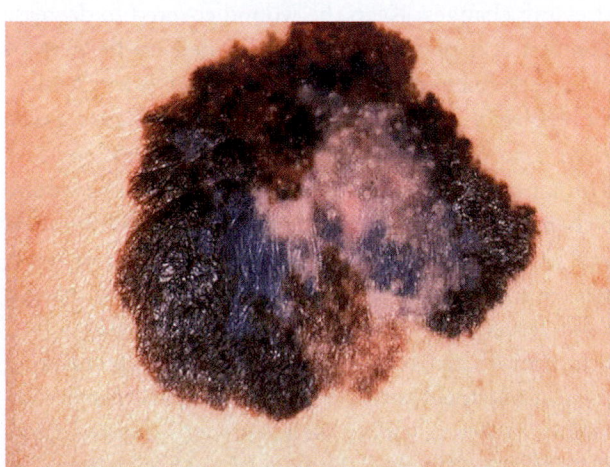

B

Figure 24-16. ■ (A) Benign juvenile melanoma on the nose of a child; this is a superficial skin tumor that is most common in children. Note symmetric shape and even brown tone. (Dr. P. Marazzi/Photo Researchers, Inc.) (B) Malignant melanoma. Note the asymmetric shape and black areas of the melanoma. (CDC/ Carl Washington, M.D., Emory Univ. School of Medicine; Mona Saraiya, MD, MPH)

Diagnosis

Diagnosis is made by inspection and palpation of the lesion. A biopsy of the lesion is done to determine malignancy. History assessment is collected to determine skin care practices related to sun exposure.

Treatment

Medical treatment includes surgical removal of the lesion. Melanoma may spread to other parts of the body, so surrounding tissue is also removed.

clinical ALERT

It is important to teach children and parents to pay attention to moles and other markings. Teach the warning signs of melanoma, and stress that early attention is essential for a successful cure.

Nursing Considerations

Nursing care focuses on prevention, educating parents and children about the harmful effects of the sun's ultraviolet rays, and teaching parents to seek medical attention if suspicious skin lesions or moles are noticed. Instruct the parents to apply sunscreen with SPF 15 or higher year round when the child is outside and to avoid the sun during peak hours (10 A.M. and 4 P.M.). Teach that it is wise to cover up with long-sleeved shirts, long pants, and hats that protect the face when outside. Discourage use of tanning beds. Encourage parents and teach older children to inspect the skin for any suspicious lesions or moles and to report any changes in color, shape, or size to their pediatrician. The Health Promotion Issue on pages 734 and 735 discusses teens and tanning.

FROSTBITE

Overexposure to low environmental temperatures may cause skin and tissue damage known as **frostbite.** A combination of high concentration of water in skin cells and exposure to extremely low temperatures (below $-2°C$) causes ice crystals to form in the tissue. Areas most commonly affected include the hands and feet (especially fingers and toes), as well as the cheeks, nose, and ears.

Manifestations

Skin may appear pale and white and have decreased sensation. If deeper tissues such as the dermis and subcutaneous tissue are involved, the skin first appears cyanotic with mottling and then becomes red and edematous. Blisters or bullae may appear after rewarming. If frostbite is severe, the skin tissue may become *necrotic* (dead). The client may lose tissue such as fingers, toes, tip of the nose, or earlobes.

Diagnosis

Diagnosis is made by inspection and palpation of the skin tissue that has been exposed to extremely low temperatures.

Treatment

Immediate medical treatment requires placing the child in a warmer environment and removing wet clothes. Rewarm the affected area slowly by submerging in warm water between 100.4 to 104.0°F (38–40°C) for 10 to 15 minutes. Analgesics are given to decrease pain that is associated with the rewarming process. Cleanse the area with saline and cover with a sterile dressing.

Nursing Considerations

Nursing care focuses on rewarming the affected area while protecting the skin tissues from further injury. Monitor the affected area for increase in circulation and return of sensation. Assess the need for pain medication as sensation returns. If hospitalization is required, maintain sterile technique during dressing changes, follow prescribed antibiotic therapy regimens, and encourage proper nutrition to promote healing of skin tissue. Educate children to layer clothing and to wear hats, gloves, and an extra pair of warm socks when outside in cold temperatures. Instruct children to come inside when hands and feet feel numb or sting.

BITES

Children of all ages learn by playing and by exploring the environment around them. Sometimes the environment can pose a health threat when children come into contact with animals, insects, or even snakes. Toddlers and young children sometimes experience human bites. Often the bites may be harmless, but every bite warrants assessing, especially if the skin barrier has been damaged. Severe systemic problems may develop if the child encounters a severe reaction to the bite, which could progress to anaphylaxis (see Chapter 21 ⌘).

Manifestations

Clinical manifestations for animal bites include redness, edema, and lacerations at the site of injury. The wound may drain, and cellulitis may develop. Symptoms related to insect bites may depend on the insect itself and may cause either a local reaction or a systemic reaction. Some local reactions from insect bites include redness, itching, pain, hives, papules, and edema at the point of entry. Some systemic reactions include wheezing, urticaria, laryngeal or angioedema, and possibly anaphylaxis. Clinical manifestations for snake bites include burning at the puncture site, redness, ecchymosis, edema, dizziness, hypotension, tachycardia, sweating, and nausea and vomiting.

Diagnosis

Diagnosis is made by inspection and palpation of the skin tissue at the site of the animal or insect bite. Identification of the source of the bite (i.e., animal, insect, or snake) is helpful in diagnosis. Lab work is done for snake bites to determine whether the snake was venomous.

(*Text continues on p. 736.*)

HEALTH PROMOTION ISSUE

TEENS AND TANNING

Jesse, a 15-year-old, female comes to the pediatrician's office with her mom for a wellness visit. She has no history of health problems and is currently well. Jesse and her mom are experiencing some communication difficulties. Jesse challenges her mom's authority frequently. Jesse wants a membership to the tanning salon for her 16th birthday. Jesse states that she is unhappy with her pale skin and wants to be tanned. The nurse notes that Jesse is pale, freckled, and has auburn hair and blue eyes. Jesse thinks tanning will make her more beautiful and is especially hopeful that she can get a tan before the prom. Her mom asks the nurse if there are any health risks related to the tanning salon.

DISCUSSION

The tanning salon industry is a $5 billion a year business with more than 28 million customers annually. The U.S. Food and Drug Administration (FDA) has set forth guidelines related to the proper use of tanning beds. These guidelines regulate the amount of exposure in the first week of tanning and then gradually increase to a maximum exposure weekly. Studies have shown that more than 95% of tanning salon users do not follow the FDA guidelines but use the tanning beds without discretion.

Lights used by tanning salons emit mainly ultraviolet A radiation which has been linked with more rapid changes in pigmentation. Overexposure to ultraviolet A radiation has been linked to skin damage involving loss of elasticity and premature aging. An adolescent is particularly at risk be-

cause the effects of ultraviolet damage are cumulative. So more exposure, over a long period of time, places the teenager at greater risk.

Tanning in salons has been linked to burns of the skin and the cornea. Suggested use of tanning salons includes covering sensitive areas of the skin and wearing eye protection. Exposure to the light emitted from a tanning bed may cause photosensitivity. Not all skin types respond in the desired manner to this light. Rashes and urticaria may occur. Tanning salons are linked with both melanoma and nonmelanoma skin cancers. It appears that excessive tanning damages the skin's DNA, which in turn blocks the immunosuppressant characteristics of the skin. Tanning, whether in the natural sunlight or from artificial lamps, accelerates aging of the skin. This effect includes wrinkling of exposed skin and loss of moisture.

Psychologically, tanning in salons can be addictive. A report by the *Journal of the American Academy of Dermatology* found that people felt more relaxed and less tense following exposure to ultraviolent lamps. They compared the emotions of these people to

others who were exposed to a tanning bed where the lamp contained a placebo lamp rather than an ultraviolent lamp. It is believed that tanning may stimulate secretion of endorphins and produce feelings of well-being.

PLANNING AND IMPLEMENTATION

The nurse should use this opportunity to thoroughly assess Jesse's skin health. What is the texture of her skin? What is her coloring? Fair-skinned, freckled individuals are at greater risk for skin cancer. Does she have any unusual moles, lumps, or discolored areas? This assessment could also be an opportunity for the nurse to teach Jesse how to conduct a skin self-assessment. Encourage Jesse to see a dermatologist for a baseline assessment. She should perform the skin self-assessment monthly. Teach Jesse to examine all of her skin, including those hard-to-visualize places. It may be necessary to perform the examination with a mirror and a light source to increase visibility. Moles need to be assessed for changes related to symmetry, border, color, and diameter. Moles

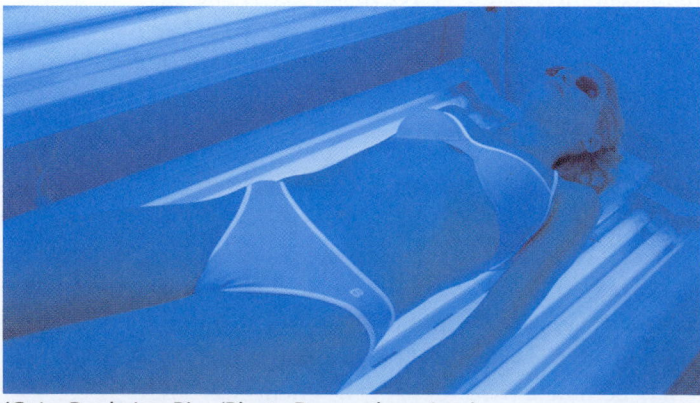

(Ct La Baule Les Pins/Photo Researchers, Inc.)

that are asymmetric or have irregular borders should be considered suspicious. Moles that have more than one shade of brown, black, or tan need to be assessed by a dermatologist. Moles that are one-fourth of an inch in diameter or larger are also suspicious for melanoma. Jesse should also be aware of any mole that suddenly gets larger or becomes elevated. A mole that is crusty, oozes, or bleeds needs to be reported promptly to the physician. Itching, pain, and tenderness in the area of a mole are also reportable symptoms.

The nurse has the opportunity to teach Jesse about the risks of tanning salons. Each risk should be explained in a clear, concise manner. Because adolescents have a tendency to not believe bad things will happen to them, color pictures of the skin effects caused by exposure to ultraviolet light can help Jesse clearly understand the hazards. Teenagers may be particularly affected by accelerated aging caused by exposure to tanning salons.

This situation provides the perfect opportunity for the nurse to teach Jesse about protection from the harmful effects of the sun. The sun is most powerful during the hours of 10:00 to 16:00. Jesse should limit her exposure to the sun during these hours and always liberally apply a sunscreen with a sun protection factor of at least 15. Liberal application of sunscreen is equal to 1 oz of sunscreen per application. Read the labels of sunscreens and choose one that blocks both UVA and UVB rays. The sunscreen should contain avobenzone, titanium dioxide, and transparent or microdispersed zinc oxide in the ingredient list. Sunscreen should be reapplied every few hours or more often when swimming or perspiring heavily. Jesse should avoid the use of tan accelerating products as they will increase her risk of health hazards from exposure to ultraviolent light.

Certain medications could also accelerate the hazardous effects of ultraviolent light. Some of these medications are tetracycline, sulfa drugs, anti-inflammatory medications, and diuretics. The nurse should teach Jesse that she should avoid exposure to the sun or tanning beds when she is taking any of these medications.

General teaching about skin health should be provided to Jesse so she can develop healthy habits early in life. The skin, especially that on the face, should be washed two times a day with a mild, nonabrasive soap and warm water. Rinsing with cool water helps to close the pores. Immediately following bathing, a quality moisturizer should be applied. Even if Jesse's skin is oily, a mild moisturizer will be of benefit. To nourish her skin, Jesse's diet should contain a variety of fruits, vegetables, protein, and whole grains. She should also drink 8 to 10 glasses of water daily. Jesse should understand that regular exercise improves circulation, skin tone, and color. Adequate rest nightly provides a healthy glow to the skin. The nurse should also relate to Jesse that smoking increases the aging process of the skin and should be avoided.

The nurse could suggest Jesse use self-tanning lotions or creams to achieve a bronze appearance without the risks of UVA exposure. Self-tanning products contain dihydroxyacetone (DHA). This substance is a sugar that interacts with dead surface cells in the epidermis, adding temporary color to the skin and making it somewhat darker. As the dead cells slough off, the color will fade, usually within 1 week. The nurse should remind Jesse that these products do not offer any protection from the harmful rays of the sun and that SPF protection still needs to be applied with exposure to the sun.

SELF-REFLECTION

Look at the models in a variety of fashion magazines. Do they appear to have a tan? What about actresses in television shows or movies? Are they tanned? If so, what message does this give to impressionable youth? Are you comfortable with your skin color, or do you try to artificially change it? List the ways you have compromised your skin health. What changes could you make in skin care regimen that could protect your skin from sun damage?

SUGGESTED RESOURCES

For the Nurse

- **www.fda.gov** This website contains the U.S. Food and Drug Administration's suggestions about tanning salons.

For the Client

- **www.skincancer.org** This website is the official site of the Skin Cancer Foundation. It offers much information about the risks of skin cancer and preventive measures.

Treatment

Medical treatment involves irrigation of the wound and possible removal of dead tissue. Surgical repair or closure of the wound may be necessary. Antibiotics are prescribed to treat infection. If rabies cannot be ruled out from the animal, the child may need to receive human rabies immune globulin (HRIG) or human diploid cell rabies (HDCV) vaccine.

Nursing Considerations

Nursing care is focused on assessing local and systemic reactions to bites and stings. The source of the bite must be identified in order to determine whether the source is venomous or if the animal has rabies. Demonstrate to parents how to clean and dress wounds. Discuss ways to prevent insect bites and stings with the parents and child. Prevention methods include:

- Applying insect repellents containing DEET (diethyl-toluamide)

clinical ALERT

Because of the thinness of the epidermis in children, DEET must be used with caution. Many manufacturers recommend applying DEET to a child's clothing, shoes, and hat rather than to the child's skin. Avoid repellents containing more than 10% DEET. If DEET is used on the skin, teach parents to have children wash with soap and water to remove DEET once they are inside.

- Wearing protective clothing when outdoors
- Covering the head with a hat
- Avoiding sweet-smelling lotions, creams, or perfumes that would attract insects
- Inspecting household pets for fleas and ticks; paying attention to proper use of pet products and product warnings labels
- Teaching parents to observe for signs of infection and treat with antibiotics
- Encouraging children to avoid touching or handling strange animals, insects, or snakes.

NURSING CARE

PRIORITIES IN NURSING CARE

Caring for a children who has experienced a trauma from outside sources requires an understanding of how the children interacts with their environment. Nursing care begins by identifying the source of the trauma whether it stems from extreme environmental temperatures (sunburn or frostbite) or from animals, insects, or snakes. Children are curious about their surroundings. Nurses play an important role in promoting safety during play while educating children about hazards outside their home.

ASSESSING

Identify the source of the injury: a fire or electrical source, a bite from animals or insects, overexposure to sun, or a cold injury due to low environmental temperatures. Assess for allergic reactions, either local or systemic. Note color, texture, and turgor of skin tissue. Assess for presence of lesions, lacerations, scrapes, puncture wounds, or blistering resulting from injury. Document the location of injury on the skin's surface, and note the amount of BSA involved. Assess the child's psychological response to the trauma, and note coping mechanisms.

DIAGNOSING, PLANNING, AND IMPLEMENTING

The following nursing diagnoses may be used in planning nursing care for the child with skin conditions related to environment or trauma. (Some previously mentioned nursing diagnoses for burn clients are not repeated here.)

- Hyperthermia, related to ultraviolet rays from the sun
- Hypothermia, related to overexposure to low environmental temperature
- Risk for Infection, related to interruption of skin barrier due to animal bites, burns, or frostbite
- Acute Pain, related to rewarming of skin from frostbite or from uncomfortable procedures for burn injuries
- Impaired Skin Integrity, related to environmental trauma
- Disturbed Body Image, related to altered skin structures due to trauma.

Typical outcomes for a child with conditions related to environment or trauma.

- Expresses understanding for decreased exposure to harmful environmental conditions
- Skin remains intact and free of infection
- Decreased pain level reported
- Improved self-image and self-esteem as evidenced by returning to normal social activities.

Nursing interventions related to children with conditions related to environment or trauma follow. (Some nursing interventions related to children with a burn injury have been discussed and are not repeated here.)

- Assess for signs of infection resulting from injury. *Prompt treatment is necessary to prevent spread of infection.*
- Demonstrate proper procedures to clean and dress wounds. *Prevents spread of infection and promotes healing.*
- Administer analgesics for pain. *Procedures for burn injuries and the rewarming process for frostbite can be very*

painful. Analgesics promote comfort during procedures and allow the child to rest.

- Monitor for signs of local or systemic allergic reactions related to insect or snake bites. *Systemic reactions include wheezing, urticaria, tachycardia, nausea and vomiting, laryngeal or angioedema, hypotension, dizziness, or anaphylactic shock.*
- Educate child to protect skin from harmful ultraviolet rays. *Decreased exposure to the sun will protect the skin from sunburn, which could be severe and could compromise skin integrity. Severe burns that blister may increase risk of developing melanoma.*
- Educate parents to dress their child appropriately when playing outside in cold weather. *Overexposure to environmental temperatures for a prolonged period of time may cause damage to skin tissue.*
- Provide a safe environment for the child to express feelings about disfigurement due to skin trauma. *Positive communication and acceptance will allow the child to feel secure and to express emotions related to disfigurement.*

EVALUATING

The LPN/LVN evaluates skin tissue for signs of infection. Pain medication is evaluated for effectiveness. Watch for local or systemic allergic reactions to insect or snake bites. Monitor the family's ability to support and care for injuries related to trauma. Evaluate the child's ability to cope with altered appearance due to trauma. Evaluate the family's ability to dress the child appropriately during cold winter months.

Note: The references and resources for this and all chapters have been compiled at the back of the book.

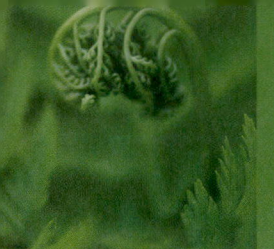

Chapter Review

 **KEY TERMS** by Topic

Use the audio glossary feature of either the CD-ROM or the Companion Website to hear the correct pronunciation of the following key terms.

Anatomy and Physiology
epidermis, melanin, dermis, arrector pili

Inflammatory Disorders
dermatitis, irritant, contact dermatitis, diaper dermatitis, *seborrheic dermatitis*, comedones

Parasitic Infestations
pediculosis, nits, crabs, scabies

Skin Infections
cryotherapy, impetigo, cellulitis

Fungal Infections
ringworm, tinea capitis, tinea corporis, tinea pedis, tinea cruris, thrush

Burns
thermal burns, chemical burns, electrical burns, radiation burns, eschar

Trauma to the Skin from the Environment
melanocytes, frostbite

KEY Points

- Functions of skin include protecting the body from pathogens; regulating temperature; preventing dehydration; providing sensory receptors for pain, touch, pressure, and temperature; and aiding production of vitamin D.

- Contact dermatitis can stem from allergens (poison ivy, latex, nickel) or repeated exposure to irritants (detergents, lotions, urine, stool).

- Breastfed infants are not as prone to diaper dermatitis.

- Eczema has been associated with an immune dysfunction of the skin. Eczema flare-ups are more common during winter. Eczema is not contagious.

- Acne affects many adolescents. Treatment may be topical or systemic. Nursing care involves emotional and physical effects of the disorder.

- Impetigo is highly contagious. Poor sanitation and close living conditions place children at risk for contracting impetigo.

- Cellulitis is a bacterial infection of the dermis and subcutaneous tissue. Onset is usually rapid. Cellulitis requires medical attention; if not treated, septicemia may result.

- Dermatophytes are fungi that mainly affect the surface of the skin, hair, and nails. Tinea (ringworm) describes fungal infections of the skin that are transmitted from human to human or from animals to human.

- Oral candidiasis appears as white plaques on the tongue, palate, and/or buccal mucosa that bleed easily.

- Pediculosis is infestation with lice, a parasite that lives on the outside of a human host. Nursing care for head lice focuses on methods to kill the parasite and alleviate itching.

- Burns are assessed for burn depth and burn area. Major burns require hospitalization and possible grafting.

- Melanoma usually arises from cells damaged by overexposure to the sun's ultraviolet rays.

- Nursing care for frostbite focuses on rewarming the area while protecting skin tissues from further injury.

- Nursing care for bites focuses on local and systemic reactions, and teaching about how to prevent future instances of trauma.

 **EXPLORE Media**Link

Additional interactive resources for this chapter can be found on the Companion Website at www.prenhall.com/towle.

Click on Chapter 24 and "Begin" to select the activities for this chapter.

For chapter-related NCLEX-style questions and an audio glossary, access the accompanying CD-ROM in this book.

Animations

Eczema

FOR FURTHER Study

See Chapter 5 and Table 8-4 for more information about herpes.

See Figure 9-4 for an illustration of brown fatty tissue in newborns. Mongolian spots are shown in Figure 9-15.

For an illustration of interstitial space, see Figure 15-2.

Anaphylaxis, oral candidiasis, and contact dermatitis are discussed in Chapter 21.

The chain of infection is illustrated in Figure 26-1.

Caring for a Child with Eczema

NCLEX-PN® Focus Area: Physiologic Integrity: Basic Care and Comfort

Case Study: Sarah's mother calls the pediatrician's office and reports that her 12-year-old daughter has been scratching the skin around her neck and behind her knees for the past 3 days and is unable to rest at night due to constant itching. The area now looks very red and scaly with yellow, crusted sores.

Nursing Diagnosis Risk for Impaired Skin Integrity

COLLECT DATA

Subjective	Objective
_____	_____
_____	_____
_____	_____
_____	_____
_____	_____
_____	_____

Would you report this? Yes/No

If yes, to: _____

Nursing Care

_____
_____
_____
_____
_____
_____
_____
_____
_____
_____
_____
_____

How would you document this? _____
_____
_____
_____

Compare your documentation to the sample provided in Appendix I.

Data Collected
(use those that apply)

- T 98.8
- Lesions on neck are dry and scaly
- Ruptured papules with yellow crust behind knees
- Enjoys playing with her baby brother
- Mother states that they have had a lot of fish over the last week
- Stopped attending youth group with friends
- Menses began 2 months ago
- Mother states child is now wearing a small amount of makeup
- Child reports her skin itches and the sores leak fluid more during winter
- Child states she likes milk and cookies
- Mother states the child does not shower after swimming
- Child states she sleeps late on weekends

Nursing Interventions
(use those that apply; list in priority order)

- Administer antipyretics.
- Obtain a thorough nutrition history.
- Hydrate skin with lotions and creams.
- Encourage wool clothing during winter months.
- Encourage showering after swimming.
- Administer oral antihistamines.
- Instruct to keep fingernails short.
- Encourage child to wear loose-fitting clothing.
- Keep environmental temperatures cool.
- Apply wet compresses to lesions that are crusted.
- Encourage a regular exercise program.

NCLEX-PN® Exam Preparation

1 The nurse is reviewing a list of instructions with a parent for an infant with oral candidiasis. Select all instructions that should be included on the list.
1. Swab oral mucosa with oral nystatin.
2. Clean bottle nipples in cool water.
3. Disinfect all toys.
4. Place stuffed animals in a plastic bag for 5 days.
5. Report rash in the diaper area.

2 A 12-year-old is receiving oral antibiotics due to a deep cut behind his left knee after falling off his bicycle. The child has returned for a follow-up visit. Which of the following assessment findings should be reported immediately to the nursing supervisor?
1. lymphangitis
2. last tetanus shot 6 months ago
3. limps when walking
4. pedal pulse of 76

3 Which of the following assessment findings is characteristic of port-wine stains?
1. color is deep yellow to orange in appearance
2. does not blanch
3. located on the folds of the neck
4. laser treatments may be needed

4 The environmental temperature should be kept cool and _____ for children with eczema.

5 When taking a family history, the nurse discovers that both parents have a history of asthma. Which of the following skin disorders has been associated with asthma?
1. eczema
2. intertrigo
3. diaper dermatitis
4. tinea infections

6 The nurse is caring for an infant with seborrheic dermatitis. Which of the following symptoms would the nurse expect?
1. red blisters on the buttocks
2. yellow scaly patches on scalp
3. erythematous papules on back of neck
4. erythema in the folds of the skin

7 The nurse is discussing treatments for a 16-year-old with acne. Which of the following statements is correct about acne treatments?
1. "Oil-based skin products are best."
2. "Avoid using sunscreen while taking acne medication."
3. "It may take up to 3 months to see improvement in the skin."
4. "Tetracycline is contraindicated for adolescents with acne."

8 Which of the following nursing interventions is recommended for a child with impetigo?
1. Apply nystatin to open lesions.
2. Elevate extremities that have lesions.
3. Place toys in a plastic bag for 2 weeks.
4. Soak and remove crust on lesions several times a day.

9 Which of the following prevention methods should be followed to decrease the risk of melanoma? Use all that apply.
1. Avoid late afternoon sun between 4 P.M. and 6 P.M.
2. Apply sunscreen of SPF 15 or greater.
3. Use a tanning bed instead of the sun for tanning.
4. Report moles that are black with irregular borders.
5. Wear long-sleeved cotton clothing when outside.

10 A teenager is complaining that between his toes are red, scaly areas with deep fissures that itch and are painful. What should the nurse recommend the teenager do to avoid this skin condition in the future?
1. Wear flip-flops at all times in the locker room.
2. Apply Elimite cream on toes for 2 weeks.
3. Nothing; this is common among teenagers.
4. Wear tight-fitting wool socks.

Answers for Review Questions, as well as discussion of Care Plan and Critical Thinking Care Map questions, appear in Appendix I.

Chapter 25

Care of the Child with Endocrine Disorders

BRIEF Outline

Anatomy and Physiology
Inborn Errors of Metabolism
Pituitary Disorders
Thyroid Disorders

Adrenal Disorders
Pancreatic Islet Disorders
Nursing Care

LEARNING Outcomes

After completing this chapter, you will be able to:

- Identify the location of each endocrine gland, the hormones produced, and the function of each.
- Discuss the interrelationship of the normally functioning endocrine system.
- Discuss disorders of each endocrine gland, including pathology, diagnostic procedures, and medical treatment.
- Explain appropriate nursing interventions for children with endocrine disorders.
- Discuss teaching topics for children with diabetes and their parents.

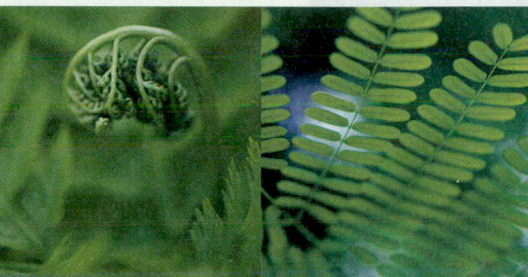

NURSING PROCESS CARE PLAN:
Care of a Client with Growth Hormone Deficiency

HEALTH PROMOTION ISSUE:
Metabolic Syndrome (Metabolic X Syndrome)

CRITICAL THINKING CARE MAP:
Caring for a Client with Type I Diabetes Mellitus

Endocrine disorders are some of the most difficult disorders to diagnose, but they can have some of the farthest-reaching effects. Many endocrine disorders are identified only over time and as other diagnoses are ruled out. Furthermore, once a disorder is identified, it can still take a lot of time and effort before treatment is adjusted to an appropriate level. Although endocrine disorders are generally treated by specialists, it is important for the LPN/LVN to be aware of their manifestations. By recognizing and reporting symptoms, the LPN/LVN may assist in identification of an endocrine disorder.

Anatomy and Physiology

The endocrine system performs the function of communication and slow, long-lasting control of various other body systems (Figure 25-1 ■). **Hormones,** proteins produced by endocrine glands, are secreted into the blood, where they are transported to the target organs. Hormones are the main regulators of growth and development, metabolism, and reproduction.

The blood level of most hormones is regulated by a negative feedback mechanism. Negative feedback involves two

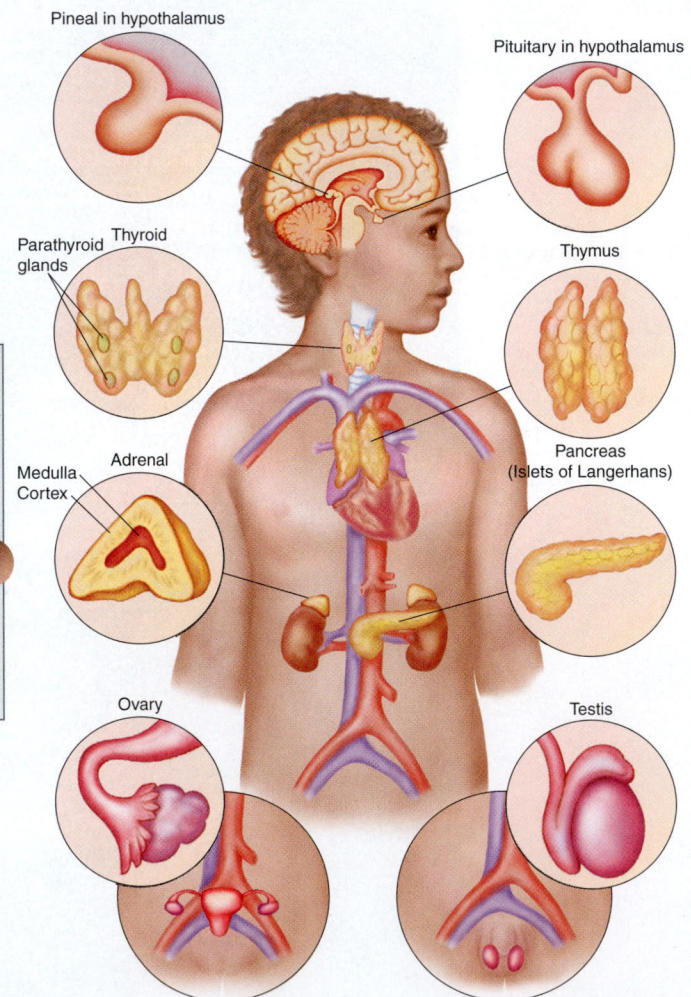

Figure 25-1. ■ Major organs and glands of the endocrine system.

Pineal in hypothalamus

Pituitary in hypothalamus

Parathyroid glands

Thyroid

Thymus

Medulla
Cortex

Adrenal

Pancreas
(Islets of Langerhans)

Ovary

Testis

Negative Feedback Loop

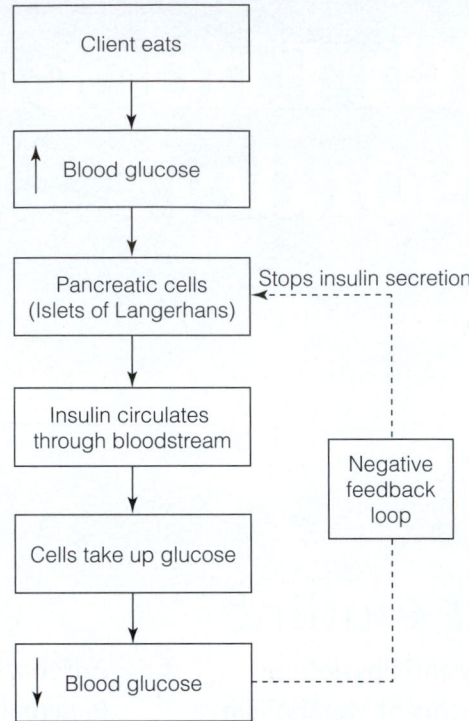

Client eats

↑ Blood glucose

Pancreatic cells
(Islets of Langerhans)   Stops insulin secretion

Insulin circulates
through bloodstream   Negative
feedback
loop

Cells take up glucose

↓ Blood glucose

Figure 25-2. ■ Negative feedback mechanism with blood glucose and insulin.

or more substances working in opposition to each other. An increase in one causes a decrease in the other. In **negative feedback** mechanisms, high levels of a hormone in the blood inhibit (switch off) hormone production. Low levels trigger (switch on) hormone production, much the way a thermostat would turn heat off or on in a house. Negative feedback can be illustrated using the regulation of blood glucose as an example (Figure 25-2 ■). Following a meal, the blood glucose level increases. The islet cells in the pancreas register the high glucose level and cause the pancreas to secrete the hormone insulin. Insulin aids transport of glucose out of the blood and into body cells. When glucose moves out of the blood into cells, the blood glucose levels decrease, and the cells in the pancreas register reduced levels of glucose and "switch off" insulin production. This is a *negative feedback* mechanism because production of a chemical (in this case, insulin) slows or stops when glandular tissue receives feedback that no more of the chemical is needed.

In **positive feedback,** an increase in one substance causes an increased response until some major event occurs that causes a decrease in the substance. The hormone oxytocin is regulated by a positive feedback mechanism. Oxytocin is responsible for stimulating contractions of the uterus during labor. Once started, secretion of oxytocin continues until delivery (the major event) has occurred. Then oxytocin secretion slows.

Although most hormones are produced and excreted by endocrine glands, one group, **prostaglandins,** are produced by various tissues in the body. Researchers are discovering that prostaglandins have an effect on respiration, blood pressure, gastrointestinal secretions, and reproduction. Through continued study of these complex hormones, causes of diseases and new treatments may be found.

Before studying specific pediatric endocrine disorders, a review of each endocrine gland and its specific hormones is warranted. Table 25-1 ■ provides an overview for review of the endocrine system.

TABLE 25-1

Review of Endocrine Glands and Effects

GLANDS	LOCATION	SECRETIONS	TARGET TISSUE	EFFECTS
Pineal	Buried deep in the brain	Melatonin	Gonads, pigment cells	Regulates body cycles
Pituitary Anterior (adenohypophysis)	Located at the base of the skull behind the base of the nose in the sella turcica A strip of tissue (pars intermedia) separates the anterior and posterior	Growth hormone (GH)	Many organs	Stimulates growth; essential for proper metabolic regulation
		Thyroid-stimulating hormone (TSH)	Thyroid gland	Stimulates thyroid secretions
		Adrenocorticotropic hormone (ACTH)	Adrenal cortex	Stimulates the adrenal cortex to release cortisol and aldosterone, regulates glucose homeostasis
		Follicle-stimulating hormone (FSH)	Gonads	Stimulates spermatogenesis in males, stimulates ovarian follicles in females
		Luteinizing hormone (LH)	Gonads	Stimulates ovulation and corpus luteum formation, stimulates secretion of testosterone in males
		Prolactin (PRL)	Mammary gland	Stimulates breast milk production
Posterior (neurohypophysis)		Antidiuretic hormone (ADH)	Kidneys	Stimulates reabsorption of water by the kidneys
		Oxytocin	Uterus	Stimulates contractions
			Mammary gland	Stimulates milk ejection
Thyroid gland	Located over the trachea	Thyroxine (T4), triiodothyronine (T3)	Most cells	Regulates the rate of metabolism
		Calcitonin	Bone	Maintains proper levels of calcium in the blood
Parathyroid glands	Bean-shaped structures embedded in the posterior surface of the thyroid gland	Parathormone (PTH)	Bone, kidneys, digestive tract	Maintains calcium and phosphate balance in the body, activates vitamin D
Thymus gland	Consists of two lobes located in the mediastinum beneath the sternum	Thymosin Thymin		Development of the immune system blocks the transmission of neuromuscular nerve impulses
Adrenal glands (suprarenals)	Located on top of the kidneys *Outer portion is the *adrenal cortex,* and the inner core is the *adrenal medulla*	**Cortex** Glucocorticoids (cortisol)	Kidney tubules, many organs	Involved in carbohydrate, protein, and fat metabolism and the body's stress reaction

(continued)

TABLE 25-1

Review of Endocrine Glands and Effects (continued)

GLANDS	LOCATION	SECRETIONS	TARGET TISSUE	EFFECTS
		Mineralocorticoids (mainly aldosterone)		Regulates electrolyte and water balance
		Gonadocorticoids		Secretes sex hormones in small amounts
		Medulla Epinephrine (adrenalin) Norepinephrine (noradrenalin)	Smooth muscle, cardiac muscle, blood vessels	Increases body metabolism, released during the "flight-or-fight" reaction Contracts the blood vessels, increases the blood pressure, slows the GI tract, and dilates the pupils
		Dopamine		Dilates systemic arteries, increases cardiac and urinary output
Pancreas (islets of Langerhans)	Located adjacent to the stomach and is connected to the duodenum of the small intestines by the pancreatic duct	Glucagon	Liver, adipose tissue	Targets the liver to release glycogen, causing an increase in the blood sugar
		Insulin	Liver, skeletal muscles, adipose tissue	Moves glucose out of the blood and into the cells
		Somatostatin		Interferes with release of the growth hormone and glucagons
Ovaries		Estrogens	Female reproductive structures	Promote the growth and development of the female characteristics
		Progesterone	Uterus	Responsible for the secretion of the corpus luteum, maintenance of the lining of the uterus in pregnancy
			Mammary glands	Stimulates development
Testes		Testosterone	Many organs	Stimulates development of the male characteristics and growth spurt at puberty
			Male reproductive systems	Stimulates development of sex organs and spermatogenesis

PINEAL GLAND

The pineal gland, a pinecone-shaped mass of tissue, is located in the roof of the third ventricle, deep inside the brain. The principle hormone produced by the pineal gland is **melatonin.** Melatonin is produced in darkness, and its production is interrupted when light enters the eyes. Melatonin regulates body cycles such as the sleep/wake cycle and inhibits *gonadotropic* (sex-organ promoting) hormones.

PITUITARY GLANDS (HYPOPHYSIS)

The pituitary gland is a small, pea-size gland suspended from the hypothalamus of the brain by a small stalk of tissue. Because the pituitary gland exerts control over other glands,

it is commonly called the "master gland." The pituitary gland is divided into the anterior and posterior lobes. Only the posterior lobe is connected by nerves to the hypothalamus. The anterior lobe is connected to the hypothalamus by blood vessels.

Anterior Pituitary Gland

The anterior lobe of the pituitary gland (adenohypophysis) secretes growth hormone, prolactin, and **trophic hormones** (hormones that stimulate other endocrine glands). The trophic hormones are:

- Thyroid-stimulating hormone
- Adrenocorticotropic hormone

- Follicle-stimulating hormone
- Luteinizing hormone.

Growth hormone (GH) promotes normal growth by speeding the movement of amino acids from the blood into cells. The cells use amino acids for growth. GH also speeds fat breakdown and slows glucose breakdown. Adequate glucose is needed for metabolism during periods of increased growth. By slowing glucose breakdown, the blood glucose remains high. As mentioned previously, high blood glucose stimulates the release of insulin from the pancreas. This is an example of the interrelationship of the endocrine glands.

Prolactin (lactogenic hormone), secreted during pregnancy, stimulates breast development and milk production (lactation). Shortly after delivery, prolactin allows the breast tissue to release milk when the nipple is stimulated.

Thyroid-stimulating hormone (TSH), as the name implies, stimulates the thyroid gland to increase secretion of thyroid hormones. Thyroid hormones are discussed later in this section.

Adrenocorticotropic hormone (ACTH) stimulates the adrenal cortex to increase in size and to secrete larger amounts of its hormones, especially cortisol (hydrocortisone). These hormones are also discussed later in this section.

Follicle-stimulating hormone (FSH) and **luteinizing hormone (LH)** stimulate the ovary to ripen and release ova. These hormones are sometimes called *sex steroids*. FSH also stimulates the ovarian follicle to secrete estrogen. In males, FSH and LH stimulate the production of sperm. LH also stimulates the interstitial cells in the testes to secrete testosterone. These hormones are discussed in Chapter 4 ⚭.

Posterior Pituitary Gland

The posterior pituitary gland (neurohypophysis) secretes two hormones: antidiuretic hormone and oxytocin. The hypothalamus produces these hormones. They are then transported to the posterior pituitary gland through neurons. The posterior pituitary gland releases these hormones when needed.

Antidiuretic hormone (ADH) accelerates the reabsorption of water from the urine back into the blood in the renal tubules. The result is a decrease in urinary output. ADH, therefore, is important in preventing dehydration.

Oxytocin is secreted at the beginning of labor to cause uterine contractions. This hormone is discussed in Chapter 7 ⚭.

THYROID GLAND

The thyroid gland is located in the neck just below the larynx. Following intervention by TSH, the thyroid gland secretes two thyroid hormones, thyroxine and triiodothyronine.

After the thyroid gland produces **thyroxine (T_4)** and **triiodothyronine (T_3)**, it stores these hormones until they are needed. Both T_4 and T_3 contain iodine. To produce ad-

equate amounts of thyroid hormones, iodine is needed in the diet. Thyroid hormones stimulate cellular metabolism by speeding up the release of energy from food. Every cell in the body is influenced by thyroid hormones.

The thyroid gland also secretes calcitonin. **Calcitonin** decreases the concentration of blood calcium by inhibiting the release of calcium from the bone. Any increase in blood calcium stimulates the secretion of calcitonin. This is important to prevent a harmful excess of blood calcium.

PARATHYROID GLANDS

The parathyroid glands, usually four, are located behind the thyroid gland. They secrete **parathyroid hormone (PTH)**. PTH increases the concentration of blood calcium by stimulating the breakdown of hard bone matrix, thus releasing the calcium into the blood. A low blood calcium level stimulates the secretion of PTH. Calcitonin and PTH work together to maintain a normal blood calcium level.

THYMUS

The thymus gland is located in the *mediastinum* (the underside of the sternum). In children, it extends upward to the lower edge of the thyroid. The thymus atrophies in puberty. The thymus secretes **thymosin**, a group of hormones that together play an important role in the development and function of the body's immune system. The thymus is more active in childhood, which may explain the shrinking of the gland once the immune system is mature.

ADRENAL GLANDS

The adrenal glands are located on top of each kidney. On the surface, each adrenal gland appears to be only one organ, but in reality it is two separate endocrine glands. The outer layer is the *adrenal cortex*, and the inner layer is the *adrenal medulla*. Each layer secretes different hormones with quite different actions:

- The adrenal cortex secretes corticoids. The outer zone of the adrenal cortex secretes the mineralocorticoids, mainly aldosterone. The middle zone of the adrenal cortex secretes the glucocorticoids, mainly cortisol or hydrocortisone. The inner zone secretes weak sex hormones or androgens.
- The adrenal medulla secretes epinephrine and norepinephrine.

Mineralocorticoids control the blood levels of minerals, mainly sodium chloride. **Aldosterone** increases blood sodium and decreases potassium by influencing the renal tubule. The renal tubule, under the influence of aldosterone, speeds up the reabsorption of sodium back into the blood so less will be lost in the urine. This also increases the reabsorption of water and decreases urine volume. At the same time, the renal tubules decrease the reabsorption of potassium so more will be lost in the urine.

Glucocorticoids have several functions:

1. They help maintain the blood glucose levels by increasing **gluconeogenesis**, the conversion of amino acids and fatty acids to glucose in the liver. Glucorticoids promote the breakdown of tissue proteins, mainly muscle tissue, into amino acids. The amino acids then enter the blood and are transported to the liver, where gluconeogenesis takes place.
2. Glucocorticoids help maintain blood pressure by working with other adrenal hormones to partially constrict blood vessels.
3. Glococorticoids have an anti-inflammatory effect.
4. Glucocorticoid secretion is one of the first responses to stress.

Androgens are secreted in small amounts by both males and females. In males, so much testosterone is secreted by the testes that androgens are insignificant. In females, androgens stimulate the female sex drive.

Nerve impulses conducted by the sympathetic nervous system stimulate the adrenal medulla. During times of stress, the adrenal medulla rapidly releases **epinephrine (adrenalin)** and **norepinephrine (noradrenalin)**. These hormones cause the body to be geared for strenuous activity ("fight-or-flight" reaction). Under the influence of epinephrine, the pulse and blood pressure increase, the bronchi dilate, peristalsis slows, the urinary sphincter tightens, and the pupils dilate. (See the section on sympathetic and parasympathetic response in Chapter 16 .)

PANCREAS (PANCREATIC ISLETS, ISLETS OF LANGERHANS)

The pancreas, a large gland located in the left quadrant of the abdomen just below the stomach, is the only organ that is both an exocrine and an endocrine gland. As an exocrine gland, the pancreas produces digestive enzymes. This function is discussed in Chapter 22 . The pancreatic islets or islets of Langerhans are microscopic groups of cells located throughout the pancreas. There are two kinds of islet cells: alpha and beta cells. Alpha cells secrete glucagon. Beta cells secrete insulin.

Glucagon increases the blood glucose by stimulating glycogenolysis in the liver. **Glycogenolysis** is the chemical process of changing stored glycogen into glucose. An increase in blood glucose stimulates the secretion of **insulin**, the only hormone that decreases blood glucose. Insulin accelerates the movement of glucose out of the blood, through the cell membrane, and into the cell. As blood glucose falls, glucagon is once again stimulated. Insulin and glucagon, therefore, work together to maintain the blood glucose level in a normal range of 80 to 120 mg/100 mL of blood.

Endocrine system disorders result from an overproduction or an underproduction of hormones or from not enough target cells responding to hormones. Because the endocrine system regulates metabolism, some metabolic disorders affecting children are discussed here, even though they may not be directly related to a specific hormone.

Endocrine disorders, with the exception of diabetes, are rare in children. All endocrine disorders will cause the child and family to make lifestyle adjustments. For example, most endocrine disorders in children require lifelong treatment and monitoring. Some require adjustment in dietary intake and daily (or several times daily) blood monitoring. Hormone replacement therapy may be expensive.

Inborn Errors of Metabolism

Phenylketonuria (PKU) was discussed in Chapter 22 .

GALACTOSEMIA

Galactosemia is an autosomal recessive disorder of carbohydrate metabolism. Galactosemia results from a deficiency in galactose-1-phosphate uridyltransferase (GALT), one of the three enzymes necessary for the conversion of sugar galactose into glucose. High levels of galactose in the blood result in damage to the kidneys, liver, brain, and eyes. Many children develop gram-negative infections.

Manifestations

Within a few days after birth, the baby develops vomiting and diarrhea, does not eat well, becomes hypoglycemic, and develops an enlarged liver. If not diagnosed and treated, the child will become mentally retarded and develop jaundice, ascites, cataracts, seizures, lethargy, and coma. Death usually occurs within 1 month.

Diagnosis

Routine screening of the newborn is done in all but six states. In these six states, diagnosis is made in symptomatic babies from history and laboratory tests.

Treatment

Infants with galactosemia are placed on lactose-free or galactose-free formulas. The child will be on a galactose-free diet (no milk or milk products) for life. Many children who follow a strict diet still develop complications of galactosemia, including learning disabilities, speech defects, visual disturbances, and ovarian failure.

Nursing Considerations

Nursing responsibilities focus on teaching the parents and child about the prescribed diet and referring the family to a nutritionist for counseling. Parents must learn to screen foods and medication for hidden lactose that has been used as filler. The parents should be referred for genetic counseling.

MAPLE SYRUP URINE DISEASE

Maple syrup urine disease (MSUD) is an autosomal recessive disease that affects amino acid metabolism. A missing or defective enzyme prevents the breakdown of three essential amino acids: leucine, isolucine, and valine (Box 25-1 ■). The result is alpha ketoacidosis. All three amino acids are necessary for normal hair, skin, and muscle formation. Leucine accumulates in the brain, causing cerebral edema, neurologic damage, and death.

Manifestations

Within days of birth, the infant becomes lethargic, has variable muscle tone, becomes irritable with a high-pitched cry, and the skin has a sweet smell.

Diagnosis and Treatment

Diagnosis is made by laboratory findings. Specially designed formulas with the three amino acids removed are prescribed. The diet should be rich in other amino acids, vitamins, minerals, and calories. The child needs special low-protein foods that are adequate for growth without causing a catabolic state (tissue breakdown). Daily urine testing for ketones is required to monitor the metabolic state.

Nursing Considerations

Nursing care includes teaching parents to maintain the prescribed diet. This includes mixing the special formula and developing a plan to prevent ketoacidosis on sick days. Referral to a nutritionist is helpful. Support groups can also help families by sharing tips for managing the child's condition.

TAY–SACHS DISEASE

Tay–Sachs disease is caused by an inherited abnormal gene. Because of this abnormal gene, the child does not have hexosaminidase A (HEXA), an enzyme that breaks down a fatty material called ganglioside GM2. Because the child lacks HEXA, the fatty material builds up in the brain, eventually causing nerve damage. Tay–Sachs is an autosomal recessive condition, which means that both parents must carry the abnormal gene for them to pass it on to the baby (Box 25-2 ■).

Manifestations

Infants with Tay–Sachs disease usually show symptoms between 3 and 6 months. Symptoms include muscle weakness

that progresses to paralysis. The child may become deaf and blind. Neurologic damage continues until death occurs at around age 5. Three related conditions have similar symptoms because they affect the same gene:

- A juvenile form appears between 2 and 5 years and progresses to death by age 15.
- A chronic form appears by age 5, with muscle weakness, slurred speech, tremors, and, sometimes, mental impairment.
- An adult form resembles the chronic form but appears between the teens and the 30s.

Diagnosis and Treatment

Diagnosis is through genetic testing. There is no effective treatment for Tay–Sachs disease. Medical management and nursing care are aimed at relieving symptoms, making the child comfortable, and preparing the child and family for death.

Those adults from high-risk groups should be encouraged to seek genetic counseling before becoming pregnant. If a woman is pregnant and both parents are carriers for Tay–Sachs disease, chorionic villus sampling can determine whether the fetus has the disease. Decisions can then be made about the status of the pregnancy.

Pituitary Disorders

Pituitary disorders in children may be caused by brain infections, infarction of the pituitary gland (associated with sickle cell disease), cranial injury, hypothalmic or pituitary tumors, or psychosocial deprivation. The following discussion concerns the most common pituitary disorders in children.

GROWTH HORMONE DEFICIENCY

Growth hormone deficiency (GHD) is a decrease in growth hormone that results from injury or disease of the hypothalamus or pituitary gland, inheritance, or genetic mutation. Because decreased function of the pituitary gland results in GHD, this disorder is often referred to as **hypopituitarism.**

Manifestations

Children with GHD have normal birth weights and lengths. Growing less than 2 in. (5 cm) a year, these children fall below the third percentile in growth by 1 year of age. Children with GHD tend to be overweight. Because growth hormone affects all cells, these children also develop hypoglycemic seizures, hyponatremia, jaundice, pale optic disc, and male genital problems (micropenis and undescended testicles). They maintain youthful facial features, higher-pitched voices, and delayed skeletal and sexual maturity.

Diagnosis and Treatment

Children below the third percentile for height should be referred to a pediatric endocrinologist. It is recommended that blood testing for growth hormone levels be done every 3 to 4 months. Treatment depends on the cause of the deficiency. Many children will receive subcutaneous injections of growth hormone three to seven times a week for at least 1 year or until normal height is achieved. Frequent monitoring will continue every 3 to 4 months, and injections will resume as needed. In some cases, the onset of puberty is delayed with medication to allow more time to achieve adult height.

Nursing Considerations

Nursing care consists of monitoring growth, teaching the family about the disorder and the treatment, and providing emotional support. Parents need to be taught to administer the injections. Growth hormone injections are expensive and may not be covered by insurance. Parents may need financial assistance and resources.

If hormone injections are not initiated at an early age, normal growth may not be achieved. People often treat short individuals differently based on their height, not their age. It is not uncommon for these social prejudices to affect the child's self-esteem. The emotional stress may be most notable during adolescence when the child is preoccupied by body image. Suggesting the child take part in sports that do not require a large physical stature (swimming, gymnastics, ice skating, etc.) and identifying positive role models who are successful despite their short stature may be helpful.

GROWTH HORMONE EXCESS

Growth hormone excess is rare in children. Most commonly, it results from a pituitary tumor. If growth hormone excess is coupled with precocious puberty, a hypothalmic tumor should be suspected. Because tall stature is valued in our society, a tall or rapidly growing child (especially a boy) may not be evaluated in a timely manner. Any child whose height is greater than predicted by parental height should be evaluated.

Diagnosis and Treatment

Diagnosis is made from history, laboratory findings, and radiologic studies. Treatment depends on the cause. If the epiphyseal plates remain open, high doses of sex hormones may be given to close the epiphyseal plates and stop growth.

Nursing Considerations

Nursing care involves teaching and emotional support. Like short stature, tall stature may be emotionally stressful for the child. Tall children may be treated as though they are older than their chronologic age.

PRECOCIOUS PUBERTY

Puberty normally begins between the ages of 8 and 13 years in girls and 9 and 14 years in boys. **Precocious puberty** is the presence of any secondary sex characteristics before the age of 8 in girls and before the age of 9 in boys.

Manifestations

Children with precocious puberty have both advanced bone age and reproductive changes. These children have a period of rapid growth followed by rapid closure of the epiphyseal plates. The end result is a short stature. Mood swings and emotional *lability* (changeability) may also be noted.

Diagnosis and Treatment

Diagnosis is made by monitoring the sex steroids, FSH and LH, as well as determining if other pituitary dysfunction exists. Occasionally, hormone treatment is necessary to suppress FSH and LH, but most commonly no medical treatment is required.

Nursing Considerations

The nurse should support parents and help them explain to the child that the changes in his or her body are normal, but just earlier than expected. It is important to remember that the child's emotional development will not match his or her physical development. The child may need support to deal with teasing by peers. Children with precocious puberty should be dressed for their chronologic age, not their physical development. Parents can encourage loose-fitting clothing to hide the body changes that are occurring. Parents need to be advised to talk with their child about sexuality and reproduction at an earlier age. The child and parents may need referral for counseling.

DIABETES INSIPIDUS

Diabetes insipidus is a rare disorder of the posterior pituitary gland. There are two types of diabetes insipidus that affect children:

1. Inadequate pituitary production of ADH. The first type of diabetes insipidus is failure of the pituitary gland to produce an adequate amount of ADH. Any trauma, inflammation, or pressure on the pituitary gland can cause the gland to slow or stop production of ADH.
2. Lack of response to ADH. The second, called *nephrogenic* (kidney-induced) diabetes insipidus, results from failure of the renal tubules to respond to ADH. Recall that ADH normally causes reabsorption of water from the renal

tubules. Without adequate ADH, or when the renal tubules fail to respond to ADH, water is not reabsorbed.

Manifestations

The end result of this disorder is excessive urine output (**polyuria**). When a large amount of water is lost, the child experiences **polydipsia** (excessive thirst). No matter how dehydrated the child becomes, the kidneys are unable to concentrate urine, as evidenced by a urine specific gravity of less than 1.010. Hypernatremia, increased serum sodium, is common. (See more on hypernatremia in Chapter 15 ∞.)

Diagnosis

Diagnostic tests include serum electrolytes, as well as serum and urine osmolality. Plasma arginine vasopressin (AVP) level before and during a fluid deprivation test confirms the diagnosis. During a fluid deprivation test, fluid is withheld from the child for up to 7 hours.

clinical ALERT

It is important to tell the parents that the child will become thirsty and irritable during the test. The test is stopped if the child loses 3% of body weight and develops a fever and hypotension.

Treatment

There are separate treatments for the two causes of diabetes insipidus. The treatment of ADH insufficiency is administration of desmopressin acetate (DDAVP). DDAVP is titrated so the urinary output is lowered and the child retains adequate caloric intake. DDAVP is not effective in controlling nephrogenic diabetes insipidus.

For nephrogenic diabetes insipidus, children are treated with diuretics, increased fluid intake, and salt- and protein-restricted diet. Box 25-3 ■ provides information about salt- and protein-restricted diets.

Nursing Considerations

Nursing responsibilities are to teach the parents how to manage their child's disease, to administer medication, and to recognize signs of complications such as dehydration and electrolyte imbalance. When the child becomes ill, it is important for the parents to seek medical attention right away and to communicate to health care providers the child's diagnosis of diabetes insipidus. Box 25-4 ■ provides client teaching about care of a child with diabetes insipidus.

Thyroid Disorders

Thyroid disorders are rare in children. However, when they do occur, they must be diagnosed and treated in a timely

---

BOX 25-3 | NUTRITION THERAPY

Foods for a Low-Salt, Low-Protein Diet

Low-Salt Diet

- The health care professional will order the amount of restriction (e.g., a 2-g Na diet). Most foods do contain some sodium, so foods that are lowest in sodium should be selected.
- The nurse reinforces the following guidelines to help the client (or parents) maintain a low-salt diet:
  - Check labels for Na (sodium).
  - Add no salt to foods.
  - Avoid salty snacks (chips, salty popcorn, pretzels with salt).
  - Avoid processed, prepared foods because they tend to contain higher levels of sodium.

Low-Protein Diet

- The health care professional will order the amount of restriction (e.g., a 40-g protein diet).
- The nurse reinforces the following guidelines to help the client (or parents) maintain a low-protein diet:
  - All meats and milk are high in protein (about 3 oz meat = 8 g protein).
  - Cereal/bread and vegetables are moderate to low in protein.
    - ½ cup cereal or 1 slice bread = 2 g protein
    - ½ cup vegetables = 1 g protein
  - Avoid seafood.
  - Limit meat to half of a serving.
  - Use bread and vegetables for food volume.

---

manner because thyroid hormones are necessary for cellular metabolism, mental functioning, and growth.

HYPOTHYROIDISM

Hypothyroidism is a disorder in which thyroid hormones are decreased. The cause can be congenital. It may also result from an autosomal recessive gene mutation, a deficiency in TSH, or inflammation of the thyroid gland.

Manifestations

Symptoms generally do not appear for a few months after birth (Figure 25-3 ■). The tongue and lips thicken, and the child has a dull expression. The child can also develop jaundice, hypotonia, bradycardia, lethargy, feeding problems, and cool extremities. Older children may develop precocious puberty, irregular menses, hair loss, slowing of growth, increased weight, and **goiter** (painless enlargement of thyroid gland).

Diagnosis and Treatment

In the newborn, diagnosis is made by mandatory screening of TSH and T_4. If TSH is elevated, the hypothyroidism is caused by the thyroid gland, not the pituitary gland.

BOX 25-4   CLIENT TEACHING

Child with Diabetes Insipidus

Teach parents that assisting the child with diabetes insipidus requires learning everyday maintenance, medicine administration, and warning signs of complications.

Medication Administration

■ Desmopressin acetate (DDAVP) is administered by intranasal drops or spray.
  • Put half of a dose in each nostril. (Review Procedure 13-29 ⮾ for steps on teaching parents about administering nasal medication.)
  • Solution should be kept in refrigerator.

Fluid Administration

■ Provide written signs of dehydration, and discuss warning signs with parents.
■ Instruct parents to measure intake and output. Fluid intake must equal fluid output.

■ Forewarn parents that the child who has compensated for high urine output may have difficulty decreasing intake when output has slowed with treatment. They should expect that the child will adjust in time.
■ Give fluids during the night as needed.
■ Acute illness increases metabolism and the risk of dehydration and electrolyte imbalance. Parents need to notify the physician immediately. They will also need to monitor intake and output more closely during times of acute illness.

Follow-up Care

■ Remind parents to schedule an appointment for blood work to monitor electrolytes.
■ Instruct parents that follow-up medical care is important to monitor the diagnosis.
■ Instruct parents to seek medical attention during times of illness.
■ Provide referral resources for home health nurse and respite care.

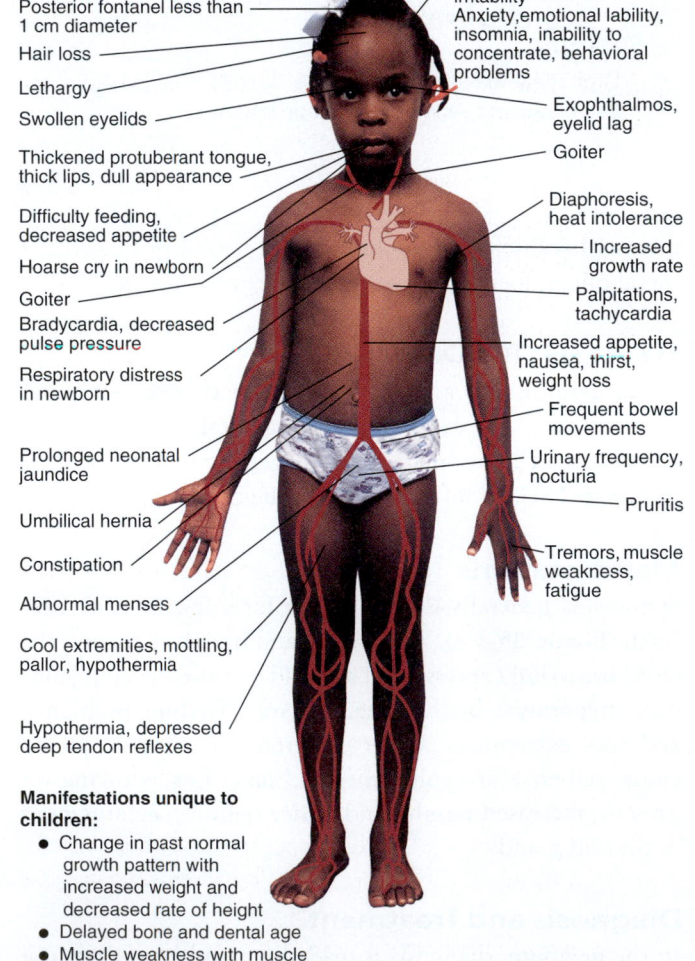

Hypothyroidism vs. Hyperthyroidism

Posterior fontanel less than 1 cm diameter
Hair loss
Lethargy
Swollen eyelids
Thickened protuberant tongue, thick lips, dull appearance
Difficulty feeding, decreased appetite
Hoarse cry in newborn
Goiter
Bradycardia, decreased pulse pressure
Respiratory distress in newborn
Prolonged neonatal jaundice
Umbilical hernia
Constipation
Abnormal menses
Cool extremities, mottling, pallor, hypothermia
Hypothermia, depressed deep tendon reflexes

Nervousness, restlessness, irritability
Anxiety, emotional lability, insomnia, inability to concentrate, behavioral problems
Exophthalmos, eyelid lag
Goiter
Diaphoresis, heat intolerance
Increased growth rate
Palpitations, tachycardia
Increased appetite, nausea, thirst, weight loss
Frequent bowel movements
Urinary frequency, nocturia
Pruritis
Tremors, muscle weakness, fatigue

Manifestations unique to children:
● Change in past normal growth pattern with increased weight and decreased rate of height
● Delayed bone and dental age
● Muscle weakness with muscle hypertrophy
● Delayed or very early puberty

Figure 25-3. ■ Multisystem effects of hypothyroidism and hyperthyroidism.

clinical ALERT

It is important to diagnose and treat hypothyroidism rapidly to prevent permanent mental retardation.

Levothyroxin (Synthroid) is often prescribed to treat hypothyroidism. As the child grows, the dose will need to be adjusted to maintain a normal hormone level. It is important for the child to be followed by a pediatric endocrinologist.

Nursing Considerations

As with other endocrine disorders, the nursing management involves parent teaching about the condition, the administration of medication, and the signs of inadequate hormone replacement. It is important to stress to parents the need for lifelong thyroid replacement therapy.

HYPERTHYROIDISM

Hyperthyroidism is extremely rare in children and adolescents. When it does occur, it is almost always associated with Grave's disease. **Grave's disease** is an autoimmune disorder in which antibodies attack the thyroid gland. When immunoglobulins attack the thyroid cells, the result is an overproduction of thyroid hormones. Congenital hyperthyroidism can occur in infants of mothers with Grave's disease when the immunoglobulins are transferred through the placenta. Other causes of hyperthyroidism are thyroid-secreting tumors of the thyroid, thyroiditis, and pituitary tumors that increase the production of TSH.

Manifestations

Symptoms of hyperthyroidism include an enlarged nontender thyroid gland (*goiter*), prominent or bulging eyes (**exophthalmos**), nervousness, restlessness, and irritability. Increased weight loss with increased appetite, heat intolerance, and muscle weakness occur when the condition remains untreated. Symptoms generally begin in the school-age child and may be present for several years before they are recognized and treated. The child's performance in school declines due to decreased ability to concentrate. They rapidly become fatigued and overheated in physical education class. They may have difficulty relaxing and sleeping.

Diagnosis and Treatment

Diagnosis is usually made with serum TSH, T_3, and T_4 autoantibodies specific for thyroid disorders, and thyroid scan. Antithyroid medications are usually the first choice of treatment. This treatment continues for approximately 2 years or until the thyroid decreases in size. Hyperthyroidism generally recurs every few years and requires repeated treatment.

The second choice of treatment is radiation with radioactive iodine to destroy the thyroid tissue. There is no evidence that this type of radiation increases the risk for cancer or birth defects in future children.

Thyroidectomy is the third option of treatment. Destruction or removal of the thyroid causes permanent hypothyroidism. After thyroidectomy, the client will require lifelong thyroid replacement therapy.

Nursing Considerations

Nursing care involves teaching the child and parents about the disorder and the chosen treatment. Because treatment is long term and relapse can occur, the child and family need emotional support and encouragement. The child with hyperthyroidism is easily fatigued and may need periods of rest, even at school. Children receiving radiation and their families need reassurance about the safety of radioactive iodine treatment.

Families anticipating thyroid surgery in their child will need routine preoperative teaching, as well as specific information about surgically induced hypothyroidism. Children may be very fearful of having their "throat cut" for thyroid surgery. They will need additional emotional support.

The priority for postoperative care is to maintain the airway and prevent blood loss. Swelling at the surgical site could obstruct the airway, and the physician would need to insert a tracheostomy tube to maintain respirations. Anticipating the child's return from the operating room, the nurse should have a tracheostomy tray at the bedside in preparation for emergency treatment should it be required.

Postoperatively, the nurse should observe closely for bleeding. The thyroid is a very vascular organ and bleeding could be excessive. When the child is lying flat, blood would drain onto the bed and pool under the child's head. The nurse should feel for wetness under the child neck with each assessment until the risk for bleeding has passed.

clinical ALERT

Swelling of the surgical site can cause airway obstruction. The child should be assessed closely for swelling, bleeding, hoarseness, and difficulty breathing. If the parathyroid glands were accidentally removed, the blood calcium level can drop to life-threateningly low levels. Signs of hypocalcemia include tingling and tetany. A syringe containing calcium should be kept at the bedside.

All cases of hyperthyroidism require regular follow-up appointments with a pediatric endocrinologist. Serum thyroid levels should be drawn on a regular basis. The child should also wear a medical alert bracelet identifying hyperthyroidism, or surgically induced hypothyroidism, and the specific medications.

Adrenal Disorders

Like other endocrine disorders, adrenal disorders are rare in children. However, when they do occur, prompt attention is needed.

CUSHING'S SYNDROME

Hyperfunction of the adrenal cortex is called **Cushing's syndrome.** Symptoms result from increased levels of glucocorticoids (especially cortisol). Cushing's syndrome can be caused by tumor of the adrenal cortex, an increased secretion of ACTH by the pituitary gland, or hyperplasia of the adrenal glands. In children, the most common cause of Cushing's symptoms (*cushingoid* or Cushing's-like features) is administration of corticosteroids for the treatment of other disorders. These children do not have actual Cushing's syndrome, only the symptoms.

Manifestations

Symptoms of Cushing's syndrome include a gradual, excessive weight gain and slow growth. It generally takes 5 years for the characteristics of **"moon face"** (round cheeks and double chin) and **"buffalo hump"** (fat deposits on the back between the shoulders) to develop. Other changes include delayed puberty and mental changes.

Diagnosis and Treatment

Diagnosis is based on clinical symptoms and abnormal laboratory findings of sodium, potassium, calcium, phosphorus, and glucose. Adrenal suppression tests reveal that adrenal cortisol output is not suppressed after administration of dexamethasone.

If cushingoid features are the result of hydrocortisone administration, treatment would be geared to the symptoms, to obtain and maintain normal electrolyte and glucose levels. If Cushing's syndrome is the result of tumor, surgical intervention is warranted. The prognosis for malignant tumors of the adrenal gland is poor.

Nursing Considerations

Nursing care includes monitoring of lab values, as well as client teaching about the pathology of the disorder and prescribed treatment.

> **clinical ALERT**
>
> Children receiving hydrocortisone must not be withdrawn from the medication rapidly. Rapid withdrawal could result in a life-threatening condition called *adrenal crisis*.

A child with Cushing's syndrome or drug-induced cushingoid features should wear a medical alert bracelet at all times. In an emergency, the primary care providers may look at lab values and misdiagnosis the child's condition. They may administer too high a dose of corticosteroids if they do not know the child is already taking these medications.

CONGENITAL ADRENAL HYPERPLASIA

Congenital adrenal hyperplasia (also called *adrenocortical hyperplasia*) is an autosomal recessive disorder that causes a deficiency in one of the enzymes needed for cortisol and aldosterone production. Congenital adrenal hyperplasia occurs more commonly in Native Alaskans (American Academy of Pediatrics Section on Endocrinology and Committee on Genetics, 2000). The most common form of congenital adrenal hyperplasia blocks the production of aldosterone, causing a loss of salt in the urine. A decrease in cortisol stimulates an increase in ACTH by the pituitary gland.

Manifestations

During fetal development, an increase in ACTH triggers an overproduction of androgens, resulting in ambiguous genitalia (**pseudohermaphroditism**); see Figure 9-44 🔗. In older children, precocious genitalia (transition to adult genitalia) may occur by 6 to 8 years of age. Epiphyseal plates close early, resulting in small stature.

Diagnosis and Treatment

Diagnosis is confirmed by elevated levels of serum 17-hydroxyprogesterone. Chromosome studies may be necessary to confirm the gender of the infant. These children may have life-threatening electrolyte imbalances. Because of this, lab tests must be performed often.

Treatment involves administration of glucocorticoid medication to suppress production of ACTH and androgens. Mineralocorticoids or additional salt intake may be necessary. Reconstructive surgery of the genitals may be necessary.

Nursing Considerations

Nursing care includes teaching and emotional support. Siblings, grandparents, other family members, and day care workers will also need instructions about the condition, as well as teaching about symptoms of electrolyte imbalance. Until gender is confirmed, the newborn should be referred to as "your infant" instead of "your son" or "your daughter." Genetic counseling and referral for counseling may be needed.

ADRENAL INSUFFICIENCY (ADDISON'S DISEASE)

Adrenal insufficiency (Addison's disease) is extremely rare in children. When it does occur, the child experiences a decrease in glucocorticoids and mineralocorticoids. The condition can be caused by trauma to the adrenal glands.

Symptoms progress slowly as the adrenal glands deteriorate. The child may present with weakness, fever, abdominal pain, hypoglycemia, dehydration, and shock. The client with Addison's disease may crave salt; the nurse can be aware of this while collecting data.

Addison's disease is diagnosed by low levels of serum cortisol and urinary 17-hydroxycorticoid. Serum values for sodium and glucose are low, and potassium is high. Treatment includes the administration of deficient hormones. Nursing care includes teaching and emotional support.

PHEOCHROMOCYTOMA

Pheochromocytoma is an adrenal tumor, most commonly benign and curable. The tumor occurs between the ages of 6 and 14. The adrenal tumor releases the catecholamines epinephrine and norepinephrine.

Manifestations

Symptoms include severe hypertension with a systolic blood pressure that may reach 250 mm Hg. The child may also experience blurred vision, headache, palpitations, weakness, polyuria, and polydipsia. Because the release of epinephrine and norepinephrine is intermittent, symptoms come and go. Attacks may occur weekly, monthly, or, in some cases, only during periods of stress.

Diagnosis and Treatment

Diagnosis is based on 24-hour urine studies to detect urinary catecholamines, vanillylmandelic acid (VMA) levels, and magnetic resonance imaging (MRI) to localize the tumor. Beta- and alpha-adrenergic blocking agents are given to control hypertension and catecholamine release. Surgical removal of the affected adrenal gland occurs approximately 14 days after medication has started. Following surgery, 24-hour urine studies are performed for several days to determine whether the entire tumor has been removed.

Nursing Considerations

Nursing care is mainly emotional support and pre- and postoperative teaching. Families should be taught how to monitor the child's blood pressure. Follow-up urine screening is done on a regular basis for the rest of the child's life.

Pancreatic Islet Disorders

DIABETES MELLITUS

The most common metabolic disorder in children is **diabetes mellitus,** a disorder of carbohydrate, protein, and fat metabolism. There are two types of diabetes mellitus. The majority of children have type I or insulin-dependent diabetes mellitus (IDDM). Non–insulin-dependent diabetes mellitus (NIDDM) or type II is usually contracted as an adult. However, the incidence of children and adolescents acquiring type II diabetes mellitus is increasing. Therefore, both types are discussed.

TYPE I DIABETES MELLITUS

The average age of onset of type I (insulin-dependent) diabetes mellitus (IDDM) is 10 to 14 years. Although there is a strong familial tendency to type I diabetes mellitus, there are no specific inheritance data (American Diabetes Association, 2000). Current research has identified a genetic marker that increases the child's susceptibility to the disease. Other environmental factors, such as viruses or chemicals in the diet, stimulate an autoimmune response that damages the islets of Langerhans (where insulin is produced). Antigens generate the production of antibodies that indicate the continued destruction of the islet cells.

As you recall, insulin is necessary for the transport of glucose into all body cells. When the beta cells are destroyed, the level of insulin falls and the level of blood glucose increases. Because cells need glucose for energy, there is a steep decrease in cell metabolism, and cells must convert protein and fat into glucose. When the level of blood glucose exceeds the renal threshold of 160 mg/dL, glucose is excreted in the urine (**glucosuria**). Glucose in the urine causes an increase in osmotic pressure that pulls additional water into the urine, resulting in increased urinary output (*polyuria*). With an excessive urinary output, the child will become thirsty (*polydipsia*). The cells become starved for glucose, triggering the appetite and resulting in **polyphagia** (excessive hunger).

To provide cells with needed energy, the liver metabolizes free fatty acids at an increased rate. Although this use of fatty acids increases the energy available to cells, it also results in an accumulation of acetyl coenzyme A (CoA) or *ketone bodies*. An increase in ketone bodies results in metabolic acidosis or **diabetic ketoacidosis** (DKA; discussed further in the next section).

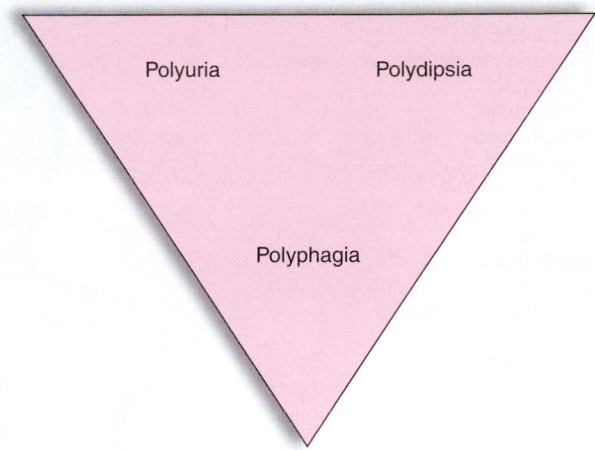

Figure 25-4. ■ Classic symptoms of diabetes mellitus.

Manifestations

The classic signs of type I diabetes mellitus include:

- The three Ps (Figure 25-4 ■):
  Polyuria
  Polydipsia
  Polyphagia
- Hyperglycemia
- Weight loss

Other symptoms include fatigue, headache, poor wound healing, and infection. Adolescent girls may have recurrent episodes of vaginitis caused by *Candida*, which thrives in a high-glucose environment. Symptoms generally develop over time, but most have been present for less than 1 month. The parents may bring their child to the health care provider with recognizable symptoms, or the child may present in the emergency room with DKA.

Figure 25-5 ■ shows early and late symptoms of type 1 and type 2 diabetes. It also illustrates the progressive and long-term complications of this complex disorder. Diabetic ketoacidosis is discussed in the next section.

Diagnosis and Treatment

Type I diabetes mellitus is diagnosed by nonfasting blood glucose (random glucose) levels over 200 mg/dL. A follow-up fasting blood glucose level would also be elevated over 126 mg/dL. The primary care provider may monitor an insulin test to detect the blood level of insulin. A C-peptide test, a byproduct of insulin production, may also be used in diagnosis.

The medical management of type I diabetes mellitus is to regain a normal blood glucose level with the administration of insulin. This may be either by repeated subcutaneous injections (Figure 25-6 ■) or by continuous subcutaneous insulin pump. The health care provider will prescribe a meal plan for the child to follow, in which approximately 50% to 60% of calories come from carbohydrates, 10% to 20% from protein, and 20% to 30% from

Diabetes

MediaLink

EARLY MANIFESTATIONS
- **Type 1 DM**
  - Polyuria (sometimes enuresis)
  - Polydipsia
  - Polyphagia
  - Weight loss
  - Glycosuria
  - Hyperglycemia
  - Fatigue
  - Vaginitis
- **Type 2 DM**
  - Obesity
  - Acanthosis nigricans
  - Polyuria
  - Polydipsia
  - Blurred vision
  - Glycosuria
  - Hyperglycemia

PROGRESSIVE COMPLICATIONS
- **Cardiovascular**
  - Lipid disorders
  - Hypertension

- **Metabolic**
  - Diabetic ketoacidosis
  - Hyperglycemic hyperosmolar nonketotic coma
  - Hypoglycemia
  - Androgen-mediated hirsutism, polycystic ovary syndrome, menstrual irregularities

- **Renal**
  - Albuminuria

- **Integumentary**
  - Impaired healing
  - Acne

LONG-TERM COMPLICATIONS
- **Eyes**
  - Diabetic retinopathy
  - Blurred vision

- **Cardiovascular**
  - Atherosclerotic heart disease
  - Peripheral vascular disease

- **Renal**
  - Proteinuria
  - Chronic renal failure

- **Neurologic**
  - Peripheral neuropathy
  - Paresthesias
  - Impotence in males

- **Impaired Immune System**
  - Recurrent infections

Immune System
- Impaired healing
- Chronic skin infections
- Periodontal disease
- Urinary tract infections
- Lung infections
- Vaginitis

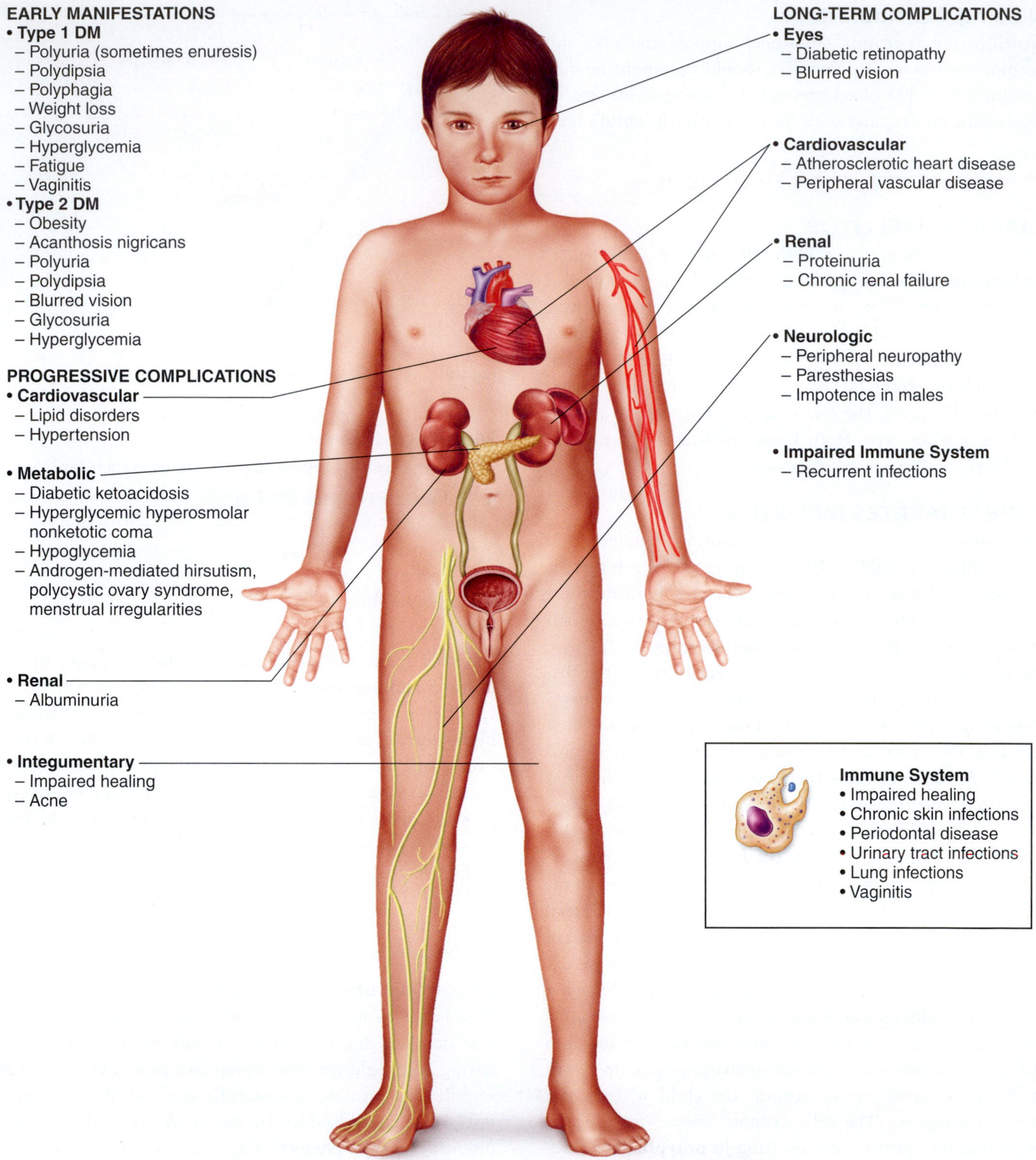

Figure 25-5. ■ Multisystem effects of diabetes mellitus.

fat. Exercise plays an important role in diabetes management by increasing the metabolism of glucose. Individuals who have high levels of activity may be able to have a higher caloric intake and lower doses of insulin. Exercise may result in decreased body weight, which decreases the need for insulin.

clinical ALERT

Blood glucose levels must be monitored during periods of exercise to prevent hypoglycemia. High carbohydrate juice or snacks should be available to treat hypoglycemia should it occur.

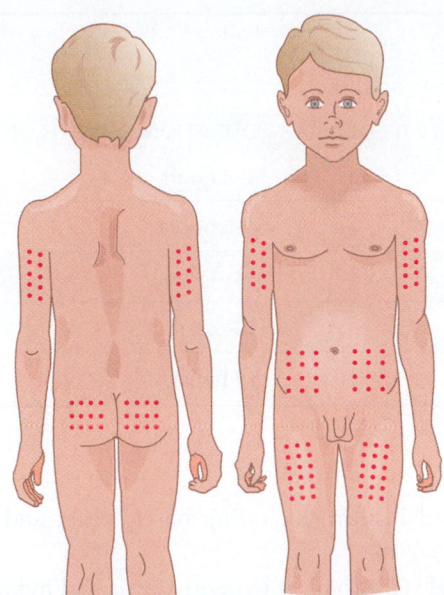

Figure 25-6. ■ Locations for rotating administration of insulin.

DIABETIC KETOACIDOSIS

DKA is the most common cause of death in diabetic children. The child may be seen initially in the emergency department and then transferred to a pediatric intensive care unit for continuous monitoring and treatment. The only cause of DKA is insufficient amount of insulin. Precipitating factors can be infection, other illnesses, or omission of insulin.

Manifestations

The classic signs of DKA include those of type I diabetes mellitus plus fruity or **acetone breath** (breath with odor of nail polish remover or rotting apples), deep labored breathing (**Kussmaul's respirations**), dehydration, decreased level of consciousness, and flushed dry skin. In late stages, DKA may present with electrolyte imbalances, arrhythmias, shock, and death. Manifestations of DKA are listed in Box 25-5 ■.

Diagnosis and Treatment

Values shown in Box 25-5 establish the diagnosis of DKA. DKA is a life-threatening emergency, and treatment must begin immediately to prevent further cell damage and death. If the child presents with DKA, immediate treatment involves IV infusion of isotonic fluids, most commonly, normal saline. The rate of infusion is geared to replace the deficit in 24 to 48 hours.

Blood glucose levels are decreased with the IV infusion of regular insulin. Insulin must be given IV because insulin cannot be absorbed from subcutaneous tissue when dehydration or acidosis is present. Because hypoglycemia could result if blood glucose levels are decreased rapidly, IV infusion of insulin is administered at a rate to decrease the blood glucose 100 to 150 mg/dL/hour. When the blood glucose level reaches 200 to 300 mg/dL, dextrose may be added to the IV fluids in order to prevent hypoglycemia.

clinical ALERT

Insulin will stick to plastic and glass tubing. Many hospitals are recommending that the pharmacy add albumin to the IV fluid to decrease this tendency. The tubing should be flushed to saturate the binding sites before the insulin is added to the solution.

BOX 25-5 ASSESSMENT

Diabetic Ketoacidosis

Lab Values
- Blood glucose greater than 300 mg/dL
- Serum ketones
- pH less than or equal to 7.3
- Bicarbonate less than 15 mEq/L
- Glycosuria
- Ketonuria
- Elevated blood urea nitrogen (BUN) and creatinine
- Possible electrolyte imbalances

Manifestations
- Weight loss
- Dehydration
- Flushed cheeks and ears
- Tachycardia
- Kussmaul respirations
- Acetone breath
- Altered level of consciousness
- Hypotension
- Abdominal or chest pain
- Nausea and vomiting

Late-Stage Manifestations
- Electrolyte imbalances
- Arrhythmias
- Altered consciousness
- Shock
- Death

Complication of DKA
- Cerebral edema (potentially life threatening; evidenced by headache, lethargy, very fast or very slow heartbeat, widening pulse pressure)

Source: Data from London, M. L., Ladewig, P. W., Ball, J. W., & Bindler, R. C. (2007). *Maternal & child nursing care* (2nd ed.). Upper Saddle River, NJ: Prentice Hall.

TABLE 25-2

Types of Insulin

TYPE OF INSULIN	ONSET (BEGIN EFFECT)	PEAK (MAXIMUM EFFECT)	DURATION (LENGTH OF EFFECT)
Lispro	15–25 minutes	30–90 minutes	3–4 hours
Regular	30–60 minutes	2–3 hours	4–6 hours
NPH	2–4 hours	4–10 hours	14–18 hours
Lente	3–4 hours	4–12 hours	16–20 hours
Insulin glargine (Lantus)	Not defined	Not defined	24 hours

DKA causes hydrogen ions to replace intracellular potassium. This initially causes serum potassium readings to be falsely elevated. In reality, the *total* body potassium is being depleted. Once urine output is established, IV potassium is administered. Other electrolytes must be closely monitored, and replacement may be necessary.

Nursing Considerations

The goals of nursing care are to stabilize the child's condition, to teach the child and family to manage the condition at home, and to prevent long-term complications. The first priority is to stabilize the child's condition. There is no protocol for the management of diabetes. Application of the entire nursing process on an ongoing basis is important. The nurse must be skilled in assessment, must understand the goals of treatment, and must be able to make rapid adjustments in the plan of care.

Nursing responsibilities in caring for the child with DKA are to administer the isotonic IV fluids; to monitor electrolytes, blood glucose, and acid-base balance; and to administer replacements as ordered. Once the child has stabilized, balanced nutrition will be given orally. Blood glucose will be monitored. Insulin will be administered subcutaneously to prevent further episodes of hyperglycemia.

Teaching the parents and the child is important for the long-term management of diabetes and the prevention of complications. Although the complete teaching plan is the responsibility of the RN, the LPN/LVN may be asked to provide instruction on the following topics:

- Blood glucose testing (see Chapter 13 ⊙⊙).
- Balanced nutrition with regular meals and snacks. (The American Diabetes Association offers help in adapting food needs, including an adapted food pyramid, and a food substitution list.
- Regular daily activity.
- Insulin administration (see Chapter 13 ⊙⊙).

- Prescribed insulin, including onset, peak, and duration (Table 25-2 ■).
- Signs and symptoms of hyperglycemia and hypoglycemia (Table 25-3 ■).
- Complications (see Figure 25-5).
- Health promotion activities to prevent injury:
  - Wearing shoes that fit the foot well
  - Filing nails straight across
  - Inspecting the feet daily for redness, swelling, or sores

TABLE 25-3

Signs and Symptoms of Hyperglycemia and Hypoglycemia

HYPERGLYCEMIA (BG OVER 120 mg/dl)	HYPOGLYCEMIA (BG LESS THAN 60 mg/dl)
Polyuria (excess urine)	Dizziness
Polydipsia (excess thirst)	Shakiness
Polyphagia (excess hunger)	Headache
Dry skin	Pallor
Flushed face	Visual disturbance
Blurred vision	Hunger
Muscle weakness	Fatigue
Weak, slow pulse	Tachycardia
Fruity or acetone breath	Disorientation (slow thought process)
Rapid respirations	Confusion
Confusion	Seizure
Coma	Coma
Death	Death

BOX 25-6	CLIENT TEACHING

Managing Diabetes During Sick Days

Maintain Normal Blood Glucose

- Monitor blood glucose every 2 hours.
- Take insulin as prescribed.
- Increase caloric intake with simple sugars in small amounts (sweetened gelatin, juice).

Prevent Dehydration

- Maintain fluid intake with small amounts of liquids frequently.
- Take antiemetics or antidiarrhea medication as recommended.

Decrease Activity

- Provide adequate rest periods.

Know Resources

- Contact primary care provider if normal blood glucose cannot be maintained.
- Contact primary care provider if unable to maintain fluid balance.

- Health promotion activities to prevent infection:
  - Bathing daily
  - Avoiding contact with infected individuals
  - Cleaning wounds, applying antibiotic ointment, and keeping wounds covered
- Management of type I diabetes mellitus during times of minor illness, such as cold and flu. Client teaching about this is discussed further under Nursing Care. Box 25-6 ■ provides guidelines for client teaching about care of a client with type I diabetes mellitus during illness.

Children should be encouraged to learn to manage their health needs. The young child can help assemble the equipment, can make choices about which finger to use for blood glucose testing, and can help in the selection of nutritious snacks. Older children can be taught to perform their own glucose testing, administer their insulin, and complete daily records.

The emotional support needed for the child depends on the age and stage of emotional development. Efforts should be made to enhance the child's feeling of autonomy and independence. The fewer changes the family has to make, the more supportive family members can be. Printed material should be provided to help the family learn and adjust to the changes. The child may need additional emotional support to handle the pressures of adolescence (e.g., what to do if friends want to get ice cream sundaes together). The family should be referred to home health or diabetes centers for continued in-depth teaching and support. The American Diabetes Association is

also an excellent source of information. Most schools do not allow children to have medication in their possession at school. Therefore, a plan for blood testing and insulin administration needs to be established. The school nurse should be informed of the child's diagnosis and plan of care. The school nurse may need to help the young child with blood testing or insulin administration at school. If other school personnel are to help the child, they must receive adequate instruction and supervision.

The child with newly diagnosed type I diabetes mellitus should be evaluated by the nurse and health care provider every few weeks until the condition has stabilized. The child and family should be able to verbalize an understanding of all teaching. The daily record of diet, blood glucose values, and amount of insulin administered should be reviewed and used as a basis for changes in insulin dosage.

TYPE II DIABETES MELLITUS

Type II diabetes mellitus occurs most commonly in adults older than age 40. However, the incidence of type II diabetes mellitus in individuals younger than 25 has increased since the mid-1990s. Type II diabetes accounts for 16% of childhood/adolescent diabetes. Many of these children have relatives with type II diabetes, are overweight, and are of African American, Hispanic, Asian, or Native American descent.

In type II diabetes, the body produces enough insulin, but for some reason the body is unable to use the insulin effectively. This condition is called **insulin resistance** and is a precursor to type II diabetes mellitus. Over several years, the production of insulin decreases, resulting in hyperglycemia.

Manifestations

Symptoms of type II diabetes develop slowly. Children may have polydipsia, polyuria, and polyphagia. They may be tired and develop frequent infections, but they do not have ketoacidosis.

Diagnosis and Treatment

Diagnosis is by fasting blood glucose test. Medical treatment of type II diabetes mellitus includes diet, exercise, blood glucose monitoring, and, in many cases, oral hypoglycemic agents or, less commonly, insulin (Table 25-4 ■). The diet should meet the nutritional needs of the growing child or adolescent but be low enough in calories to allow for weight loss. Exercise is intended not only to decrease the need for insulin, but also to burn calories for additional weight loss.

Oral hypoglycemic agents are not insulin. They stimulate the pancreas to produce insulin, and they make cell receptor sites more sensitive to insulin. Because type II diabetes mellitus has been unusual in children and adolescents, research is currently being conducted about the use of oral hypoglycemic agents in children and adolescents (Jacobson-Dickman & Levitsky, 2005).

TABLE 25-4

Pharmacology: Oral Hypoglycemics

DRUG (COMMON BRAND NAME AND GENERIC)	USUAL ROUTE/DOSE	CLASSIFICATION	SELECTED SIDE EFFECTS	DON'T GIVE IF
Glucophage (metaformin)	1 tablet 2–3 times a day	Oral antidiabetic drug	Dizziness, weakness, fatigue, shortness of breath, irregular pulse	Clients have abnormal renal function or when congestive heart failure is present
Glyburide (sulfonylurea)	2.5–5 mg every day	Oral antidiabetic drug	GI upset, weakness, fatigue	Client has low blood glucose levels

Nursing Considerations

Nursing responsibilities are similar to those for type I diabetes mellitus. Client and family teaching about the signs of hypoglycemia and hyperglycemia, the complications of diabetes, and treatment is consistent with all types of diabetes. Because oral hypoglycemic agents have not been used extensively in children and adolescents, it is important for the nurse to teach the family to monitor for side effects and report them to the health care provider in a timely manner.

METABOLIC SYNDROME (METABOLIC X SYNDROME)

In recent years, a set of conditions related to glucose metabolism has been identified and named metabolic (or metabolic X) syndrome. The Health Promotion Issue on pages 760 and 761 discusses this increasingly prevalent disorder.

NURSING CARE

PRIORITIES IN NURSING CARE

The priorities for nursing care of children with endocrine disorders include:
- Monitoring ordered lab values.
- Teaching the child/family to manage the condition at home.
- Providing information about specialists, support groups, and financial resources.

ASSESSING

The symptoms of many endocrine disorders are similar to symptoms of other disorders. Many affect the child's growth and development over time. The nurse should compare the client's data to the established standards of growth and development for the child's age.

DIAGNOSING, PLANNING, AND IMPLEMENTING

The specific endocrine disorder will determine the particular interventions needed. Diagnosis of disorders is usually made from serum levels of specific chemicals, as well as from symptoms and by eliminating other diagnoses.

Expected nursing diagnoses for children (and families) with endocrine disorders would include, but are not limited to, the following:

- Deficient Knowledge, related to the particular disorder
- Risk for Imbalanced Fluid Volume
- Caregiver Role Strain.

Outcomes for such nursing diagnoses would include:

- Expresses understanding of disorder, treatment, and ongoing management
- Maintains adequate hydration
- States plan to use personal network, support services, and referrals in long-term care of the child with an endocrine disorder.

Nursing interventions must be tailored to the specific needs of the client and family. Appropriate nursing actions include, but are not limited to, the following:

- Teach the child and family about the disorder and how to manage the day-to-day treatment. *Learning about a serious medical problem may be overwhelming. The family may need to hear information several times in order to retain learning.*
- Help the family plan alterations in diet, activity, and medication administration. Provide written materials for the parents' use later. *The parents can use the process of planning as a model. They may refer back to a sample plan when they are tired or overwhelmed.*
- Provide specific instructions and contact information concerning what to do when illness occurs in the child with an endocrine disorder. Stress the importance of Medic-Alert bracelets. *Acute illness may affect the endocrine disorder, and parents must keep the primary care provider informed of changes in*

the child's condition. Failure to notify medical personnel about the child's disorder may result in improper treatment and death.

- Provide referrals to home health nurses and school nurses if possible. *They may be beneficial resources in planning and implementing care.*

EVALUATING

Endocrine disorders in children affect their health for the rest of their lives. Periodic monitoring of serum levels is necessary to ensure stability of a child's condition. Dietary requirements change as a child grows. Diet restrictions should be reviewed and changes made to meet changing needs. Family dynamics and individual coping should be evaluated to ensure all needs are met.

NURSING PROCESS CARE PLAN
Care of a Client with Growth Hormone Deficiency

Juanita received a concussion at 9 months of age from a fall. At the time, she seemed to recover without incident. She is now 2 years old and is being seen in the pediatric endocrinologist office for failure to grow. She is in the 2nd percentile for growth for her age, but in the 20th percentile for weight. Except for failure to grow, Juanita's development is consistent with her age.

Assessment. Vital signs: T 97.2 (A), P 90, R 36, Wt. 24.5 lb (11 kg), Ht. 30.5 in. (77 cm). Juanita is alert and talkative. She is walking around the room holding a doll. Her speech is understandable, and she uses four- to five-word sentences. She has been referred from a health clinic due to slow growth.

Nursing Diagnosis. The following important nursing diagnosis (among others) is established for this client:

- Risk for Disproportionate Growth.

Expected Outcome. The following expected outcome was identified:

- Juanita will grow 2 in. in the next year.

Planning and Implementation

- Obtain serum growth hormone level as ordered by the primary care provider. *Serum growth hormone is needed for diagnosis and as a baseline for evaluation of treatment.*
- Discuss with parents the resources available to provide financial assistance to purchase prescribed growth hormone. *Growth hormone is expensive. Most parents will need financial assistance.*
- Teach parents the manifestations of GHD and the need for long-term follow-up assessments. *Parents need information in order to make informed choices. GHD requires treatment and follow-up assessment until the child reaches adult height.*
- Teach parents to administer the growth hormone injections as ordered. *Injections will be given three to seven times a week. It is less expensive and more convenient for parents to administer the medication.*
- Provide emotional support for parents and child. *The long-term effect of GHD can be frightening for parents. Children also need support because of the frequent injections. When the child gets older, support may be needed due to social pressure from peers.*
- Schedule follow-up appointments to monitor Juanita's growth, obtain serum growth hormone level, and assess side effects of medication.

Evaluation. Juanita will grow 0.5 in. in 3 months. Growth hormone level will be within normal range. No side effects of growth hormone replacement will be apparent.

Critical Thinking in the Nursing Process

1. What else can the nurse teach the parents that will help in Juanita's growth?
2. If Juanita does not receive growth hormone injections, will she grow more?
3. What suggestions may be offered to help Juanita accept a shot every day?

Note: Discussion of Critical Thinking questions appears in Appendix I.

Note: The references and resources for this and all chapters have been compiled at the back of the book.

HEALTH PROMOTION ISSUE

METABOLIC SYNDROME (METABOLIC X SYNDROME)

A young woman, unable to lose weight for more than a year, seeks assistance from her primary care provider. She states that she began putting on weight when she was 16 years old. She admits to a sedentary lifestyle but states that she does not have the energy to exercise. She is 62 lb over the expected weight for her height. The majority of the weight is around her abdomen. Her blood pressure is 142/88. Her laboratory tests determine that blood glucose level is high, triglycerides are elevated, and high-density lipoprotein (HDL) cholesterol is low. The primary care provider suspects she has a relatively newly identified disorder called metabolic syndrome.

DISCUSSION

Metabolic syndrome, also called metabolic X syndrome, is a group of related metabolic disorders, including obesity, insulin resistance, and complications of type II diabetes. Although these disorders have been known for years, the relationship and linking of these and other

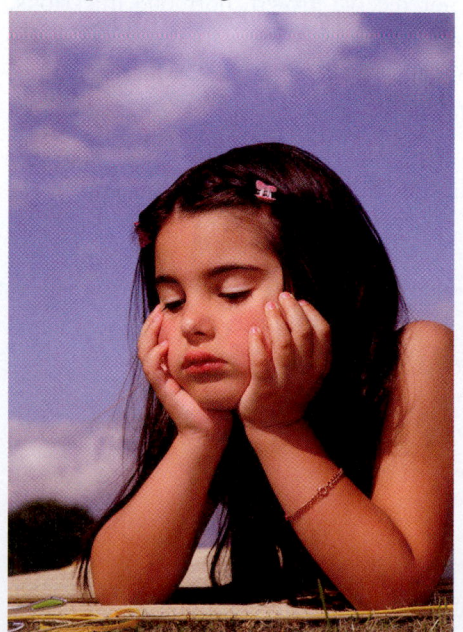

(marilyn barbone/Shutterstock)

disorders together is relatively new. Research is still underway to discover the cause of this life-altering syndrome and other disorders that may be linked to metabolic syndrome in the future.

One point is clear: Central obesity is a key factor in this syndrome. As noted in Chapter 22 ⚭, obesity is rapidly increasing in children. Many individuals, when seeking medical help to lose weight, state that their weight problem began during their teenage years. They admit to a high-calorie intake and a sedentary lifestyle. As overweight children grow, many may develop metabolic syndrome. However, not everyone who is overweight and inactive will develop this disorder. Researchers believe a genetic factor plays an important role as well. Further research is needed in this area. (See the Health Promotion Issue in Chapter 22 ⚭ for information on high-calorie diets and obesity in children.)

Metabolic syndrome places the individual at risk for other potentially life-threatening disorders. A buildup of plaque inside blood vessels, resulting from low HDL cholesterol levels, leads to coronary artery disease, cerebral vascular disease leading to stroke, and peripheral vascular disease. Insulin resistance or glucose intolerance is a precursor to type II diabetes. Metabolic syndrome is also being linked to fatty deposits in the liver, resulting in liver failure, renal failure, and cancer. Researchers in Australia have identified altered endocrine function related to metabolic syndrome. These include high estrogen levels in women, low testosterone levels in men, high cortisol levels, and low thyroid levels.

It is generally accepted that if clients exhibit three of the following criteria, they can be diagnosed with metabolic syndrome:

- Central obesity: fat deposits in and around the abdomen
- Atherogenic dyslipidemia: blood fat disorders (especially high triglycerides and low HDL cholesterol) leading to plaque buildup in blood vessels
- Insulin resistance or glucose intolerance
- Prothrombotic state: increased fibrinogen or plasminogen activator inhibitor (−1) in the blood leading to increased chance of thrombosis
- Elevated blood pressure of 130/85 mm Hg or higher
- Preinflammatory state: increased C-reactive protein in the blood, indicating an inflammatory process is in the early stage.

Diagnosis is based on clinical findings and abnormal laboratory values. Most of the tests must be repeated over time. Many individuals do not exhibit all the symptoms for years, so diagnosis takes time. However, when the individual has central edema and states that he or she has difficulty losing weight, the nurse should recommend laboratory testing be done to establish a baseline for future evaluation.

The waist measurement indicates central obesity. The waist measurement in women with central obesity is greater than 40 in. (102 cm); in men, it is greater than 35 in. (88 cm). The blood pressure may be elevated initially or gradually increase over time. The individual may have a history of polycystic ovarian disease. Depression, irritable bowel syndrome, chronic infections, and fatigue are all common complications seen with metabolic syndrome.

Laboratory findings show high blood glucose, low thyroid, and low HDL cholesterol. Estrogen levels will be elevated in women; testosterone levels will be lower in men. Estrogen results in calories being converted to fat. Liver function tests indicate a gradual decrease in liver function. Cortisol levels will be elevated.

PLANNING AND IMPLEMENTATION

There is no specific treatment for metabolic syndrome, nor is there a quick fix. Treatment is centered on weigh loss, maintaining blood glucose in normal ranges, and increasing activity. Diets must be altered to decrease calories while increasing protein and fiber. Activity should be increased to improve the efficiency of cell metabolism. Insulin resistance and increased blood glucose are often treated with oral hypoglycemics. Hypothyroidism is treated with synthetic hormone replacement. By increasing metabolism with increased thyroid, cell metabolism is increased, and more calories are burned. Anticholesterol and antitriglyceride medications may be given. Some herbal drugs such as pantethine, fish oil, and garlic can lower both cholesterol and triglycerides. Often these are enough to reduce weight, stabilize blood glucose, and increase the HDL cholesterol. Evaluation of these treatments is usually done at 3-month intervals.

Typically, the treatment for ovarian cysts is birth control pills that increase the estrogen and progesterone levels. Because of the high estrogen levels seen with metabolic syndrome, only low-level birth control pills can be used. An intrauterine device containing progesterone may be helpful in women who are unable to have additional estrogen.

Because of the multisystem effects of metabolic syndrome, it is important to prevent and treat central obesity in order to prevent the client from developing metabolic syndrome. Prevention begins in childhood by providing a diet that is adequate in fruits and vegetables, whole grain breads and cereals, meat, and milk products. The diet should be low in saturated fats. The nurse should teach children and parents to make healthy choices in their diet and to limit fast foods that are typically high in fats and calories.

Exercise is another key component in preventing obesity. Children should run, climb, or swim daily. Being involved in sports not only burns calories, but also improves social skills such as teamwork and fair play. Some children, however, do not enjoy sports, and it is hard to get them involved in physical activity. Encouraging them to walk or ride their bicycle to school, or to park away from the building so they will have to walk farther, will help them increase their activity. The nurse should help the family find other ways to increase activity in the child.

When assessing every child, the nurse should pay attention to the child's weight and fat distribution. If the child's weight is increasing faster than is expected, the nurse should discuss the child's diet and activity with the parents. By teaching parents about the potential for metabolic syndrome and the effect of obesity on the endocrine and other body systems, these disorders may be prevented.

When metabolic syndrome occurs, the nurse is responsible for teaching the individual about the syndrome, the prescribed treatment, and how to monitor the blood glucose level. The nurse assists in monitoring the effects and side effects of medication, the laboratory values, and the client's weight. Decreasing stress can help decrease the cortisol level and, therefore, decrease the effects on cell metabolism.

SELF-REFLECTION

Take notes for a day on your thoughts related to food and exercise. Do thoughts of food as a reward or a comfort pop into your mind? If you are planning to exercise, what are the thoughts that go through your mind? Do you recognize some thoughts that are self-defeating? Think of positive phrases that you can use as substitutes. For example, if you think, "I can't jog four blocks," you could substitute, "It doesn't matter if I jog or walk. What matters is that I am getting fresh air and exercise."

SUGGESTED RESOURCES

For the Nurse

■ Kidson, W. (1998). Polycystic ovary syndrome: A new direction in treatment. *Medical Journal of Australia, 169,* 537–540.

■ Largo, R. S., Gnatuk, C. L., Kunselman, A. R., & Dunaif, A. (2005). Change in glucose tolerance over time in women with polycystic ovarian syndrome: A controlled study. *Journal of Clinical Endocrinology and Metabolism, 90*(6), 3236–3242.

Chapter Review

KEY TERMS by Topic

Use the audio glossary feature of either the CD-ROM or the Companion Website to hear the correct pronunciation of the following key terms.

Anatomy and Physiology
hormones, negative feedback, positive feedback, prostaglandins, melatonin, trophic hormones, growth hormone (GH), prolactin (lactogenic hormone), thyroid-stimulating hormone (TSH), adrenocorticotropic hormone (ACTH), follicle-stimulating hormone (FSH), luteinizing hormone (LH), antidiuretic hormone (ADH), oxytocin, thyroxine (T_4), triiodthyronine (T_3), calcitonin, parathyroid hormone (PTH), thymosin, mineralocorticoids, aldosterone, glucocorticoids, gluconeogenesis, androgens, epinephrine (adrenalin), norepinephrine (noradrenalin), glucagon, glycogenolysis, insulin

Pituitary Disorders
growth hormone deficiency (GHD), hypopituitarism, precocious puberty, polyuria, polydipsia

Thyroid Disorders
goiter, Grave's disease, exophthalmos

Adrenal Disorders
Cushing's syndrome, "moon face," "buffalo hump," pseudohermaphroditism, pheochromocytoma

Pancreatic Islet Disorders
diabetes mellitus, glucosuria, polyphagia, diabetic ketoacidosis, acetone breath, Kussmaul's respirations, insulin resistance

KEY Points

- Endocrine disorders are potentially life threatening due to the lack of regulation of other body systems.

- Endocrine disorders display symptoms similar to those of other body systems, making diagnosis difficult at times.

- Endocrine disorders require long-term treatment.

- Some endocrine disorders are fatal.

- Families may need to be taught to monitor the child's condition and administer treatments, including medication.

- Many treatments of endocrine disorders are expensive and may not be covered by insurance. The nurse may need to provide resource information.

- Metabolic syndrome is an example of the complex nature of endocrine disorders.

EXPLORE MediaLink

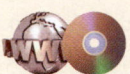

Additional interactive resources for this chapter can be found on the Companion Website at www.prenhall.com/towle.

Click on Chapter 25 and "Begin" to select the activities for this chapter.

For chapter-related NCLEX-style questions and an audio glossary, access the accompanying CD-ROM in this book.

Animations

Diabetes

Endocrine system

FOR FURTHER Study

Sexual steroid hormones are discussed in Chapter 4.

For further information on the hormone oxytocin, see Chapter 7.

Pseudohermaphroditism is illustrated in Figure 9-44.

See Procedures 13-13 and 13-35 for glucose blood tests and insulin administration.

For more on hypernatremia, see Chapter 15.

Sympathetic and parasympathetic responses are discussed in Chapter 16.

See Chapter 22 for a complete discussion on phenylketonuria and for additional information on the pancreas as an exocrine gland, high-calorie diets, and obesity.

Caring for a Client with Type I Diabetes Mellitus

NCLEX-PN® Focus Area: Physiologic Integrity

Case Study: Grey Wolf, an 11-year-old Native American boy, is admitted to the tribal clinic with a blood glucose of 48 mm/dL. He was diagnosed with type I diabetes mellitus 3 months ago. He has been having difficulty remembering to eat a snack before soccer practice.

Nursing Diagnosis: Risk for Injury, related to hypoglycemia

COLLECT DATA

Subjective	Objective
_____	_____
_____	_____
_____	_____
_____	_____
_____	_____
_____	_____

Would you report this? Yes/No

If yes, to: _____

Nursing Care

_____
_____
_____
_____
_____
_____
_____
_____
_____
_____
_____
_____
_____
_____

How would you document this? _____
_____
_____
_____

Compare your documentation to the sample provided in Appendix I.

Data Collected
(use those that apply)

- Irritable
- Thirsty
- Hungry
- Sweating
- Flushed
- Fruity/acetone breath
- Tremors
- P 102
- R 38

Nursing Interventions
(use those that apply; list in priority order)

- Obtain a thorough nutrition history.
- Administer regular insulin as ordered.
- Give orange juice with one packet sugar added.
- Start an IV of normal saline as ordered or as per facility policy.
- Give one ampule of sodium bicarbonate as ordered.
- Monitor blood glucose every 30 to 60 minutes.
- Review causes and signs of hypoglycemia.
- Review insulin administration techniques.

NCLEX-PN® Exam Preparation

1. Children are generally more physically active during the summer months. In caring for the child with type I diabetes mellitus, what changes in the plan of care should be expected?
   1. Decrease food intake.
   2. Increase food intake.
   3. Increase insulin dose.
   4. Decrease insulin dose.

2. The nurse is teaching an adolescent girl who has recently been diagnosed with type I diabetes mellitus. The nurse bases the teaching on the adolescent's:
   1. need to be unique, allowing her to select her diet without restriction.
   2. preoccupation with the future, allowing her to decline physical activity in favor of computer skills.
   3. need to feel in control, allowing her a larger share in decision making regarding the treatment plan.
   4. awareness of the severity of the disorder, motivating her to maintain a strict routine.

3. When a child develops diabetic ketoacidosis, the child's conditions is:
   1. an expected outcome of diabetes.
   2. best treated at home.
   3. extremely rare in children.
   4. a life-threatening situation.

4. An adolescent with a new diagnosis of diabetes is learning to give her own insulin injection. She correctly prepares the injection but cannot give herself the shot. The nurse should:
   1. give the shot and allow her to practice more.
   2. take her hand and make her give the shot.
   3. refer her to the doctor.
   4. tell her she can give the shot later.

5. A child with lupus has been placed on corticosteroids for an indefinite period of time. Which of the following are cushingoid symptoms associated with corticosteroid administration to children?
   1. weight gain and delayed puberty
   2. delayed growth and weight loss
   3. fat deposits and rapid growth
   4. moon face and precocious puberty

6. A diabetic adolescent has been admitted following an automobile accident. He is on bed rest, and his condition is stable. At 11:30 A.M., he develops a flushed face, increased urinary output, and fruity breath. Place the following interventions in priority order.
   1. Call the primary care provider.
   2. Administer regular insulin on sliding scale.
   3. Obtain a blood glucose level.
   4. Increase oral intake of water.
   5. Review the intake and output record.

7. The mother of an 8-year-old girl is concerned because her daughter is developing pubic hair and enlarged breast tissue. The nurse's best response would be:
   1. "Don't worry, girls don't get their period until age 12."
   2. "She is probably going to start her period soon, so you must get used to it."
   3. "At what age did you begin puberty?"
   4. "You had better tell her about menstruation soon."

8. After a thyroidectomy, a teenager is experiencing tingling and spasms of the hands. The nurse identifies this electrolyte imbalance as _____.

9. The nurse caring for a child with head trauma is ordered to monitor the urine-specific gravity. The doctor is concerned that the child will develop diabetes insipidus. Which of the following urine-specific gravity values should be reported immediately?
   1. 1.004
   2. 1.015
   3. 1.020
   4. 1.025

10. An overweight adolescent boy needs further instruction in type II diabetes mellitus when he states:
    1. "I have to walk at least 3 miles a day."
    2. "I should eat fruit for dessert instead of cake."
    3. "I can drink diet soda once a day."
    4. "If I take these pills, I will never need to take insulin shots."

Answers for Review Questions, as well as discussion of Care Plan and Critical Thinking Care Map questions, appear in Appendix I.

Chapter 26

Care of the Child with a Communicable Disease

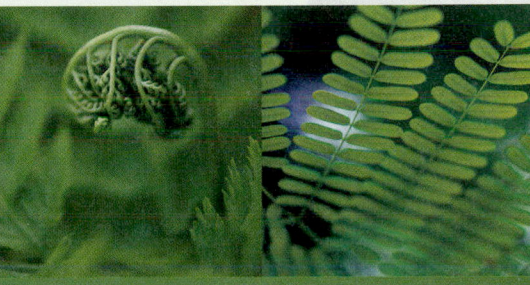

Brief Outline

Chain of Infection

Risk Factors for Communicable Diseases in Children

Immunizations

Client Teaching to Parents and Children

Common Infections

Infectious Diseases Transmitted by Insects or Animals

Sexually Transmitted Infections

Nursing Care

LEARNING Outcomes

After completing this chapter, you will be able to:

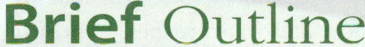

- Discuss the chain of infection.
- Explain the specific risk factors for communicable diseases in children.
- Describe methods of communicable disease prevention in children.
- Discuss clinical manifestations, diagnostic procedures, and medical management related to childhood communicable diseases.
- Explain appropriate nursing interventions for children with childhood communicable diseases.

HEALTH PROMOTION ISSUE: Avian Flu (Planning for the Management of Pandemic Influenza)

NURSING PROCESS CARE PLAN: Child with Chickenpox

CRITICAL THINKING CARE MAP: Caring for a Client Requiring Droplet Precautions

Diseases spread among children frequently and easily. **Communicable diseases** are diseases that are transmitted from one person to another by way of direct contact with body fluids (e.g., kissing) or indirectly through contact with contaminated objects (e.g., used tissues).

The nurse has an important role in recognizing these diseases and assisting the family in obtaining appropriate care. Communicable diseases can be prevented in many cases. Another important nursing role is client and family teaching regarding methods of disease prevention.

Chain of Infection

To transmit harmful organisms or **pathogens** from one child to another, there must be a reservoir, portal of exit, portal of entry, and susceptible host (Figure 26-1 ■). The **reservoir** is the site where harmful organisms grow and reproduce. Examples of reservoirs are humans, animals, insects, or soil. A **portal of exit** is the method in which the harmful organism leaves the reservoir. This could be through contact with infected body fluids such as blood or saliva. **Transmission** is the means by which the infectious agent travels from the portal of exit to the portal of entry. The **portal of entry** is the method in which the harmful organism enters a new host. This could be through the gastrointestinal tract, the integumentary system, or the respiratory system. The **susceptible host** is an individual who is at risk for contracting the disease caused by the harmful organism. Young children are more

susceptible to harmful organisms due to an immature immune system. The child who is ill, especially the child who is immunocompromised, will have a more difficult time fighting the harmful organism as well.

Harmful organisms are transmitted by direct and indirect methods. Direct methods of transmission of harmful organisms are methods in which there is direct contact with body fluids, skin, or mucous membranes. The indirect method of transmission of harmful organisms can also be called the **droplet method.** In this route of transmission, infected body fluids are released from the mouth or nose via sneezing, coughing, kissing, or just breathing and talking. Droplets can contact the susceptible host immediately, attach themselves to dust particles that are touched later by the host, or actually become suspended in the air. When harmful organisms become suspended in the air, the transmission is called **airborne transmission. Fomites** are inanimate objects that transmit harmful bacteria indirectly. Examples of these inanimate objects include personal hygiene items such as combs and hairbrushes, clothing, linens, eating utensils, food, water, and soil.

STAGES OF INFECTIOUS PROCESS

When children become ill with a communicable disease, there are four states of the infectious process: the incubation period, the prodromal period, illness, and the convalescent period.

The **incubation period** varies according to the specific disease. It is the time frame between the entry of the pathogen into the reservoir and the onset of clinical signs and symptoms. The pathogen multiplies in number during the incubation period.

The **prodromal period** occurs just prior to the onset of the clinical symptoms. During the prodromal period, the child may have nonspecific symptoms such as a low-grade temperature and lethargy. Children are contagious during this period, and because a specific disease is unrecognizable, they may come in contact with many individuals.

Illness is the stage in which clinical symptoms appear. Children are considered ill when they exhibit specific symptoms of the disease. The **convalescent period** is the time frame between the beginning of the resolution of symptoms and the restoration of wellness.

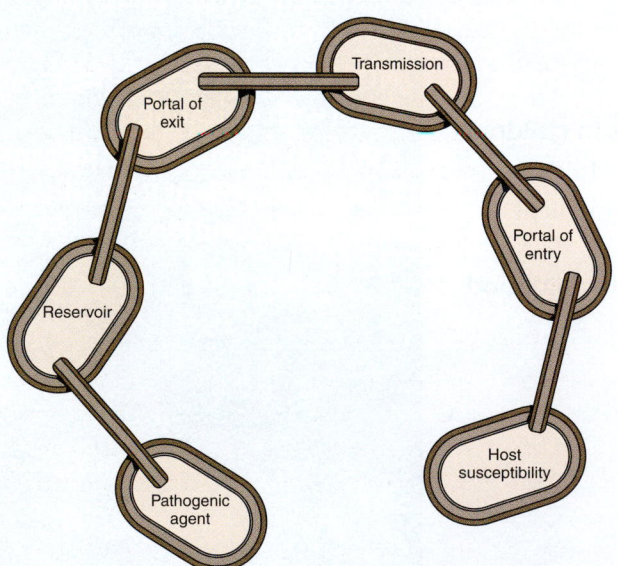

Figure 26-1. ■ Chain of infection. An effective chain of transmission for infection requires a suitable habitat, or reservoir, for the pathogen. A reservoir may be living or nonliving. Transmission may be direct or indirect. Direct transmission involves physical contact between the source of the infection and the new host. Indirect transmission occurs when pathogens survive outside humans before causing infection and disease. To achieve infection control, one of the links in the chain must be broken.

Risk Factors for Communicable Diseases in Children

A healthy person with a functioning immune system can fight many infections before he or she becomes acutely ill. When the organism enters the body, it becomes a foreign protein or antigen. With a healthy immune system, the body reacts rapidly by producing a specific antibody to stop or slow the growth of the antigen until white blood cells can destroy the organism. Once antibodies are produced, memory B cells and T cells remember how to identify the antigen and reactivate with the future exposure to the antigen. This process is called **active immunity.** Active immunity provides long-term protection. **Passive immunity** is the passing of antibodies from the person where the antibody was produced to another person. Passive immunity lasts only a short time. Antibodies are passed from mother to infant through the placenta, but in order for the infant to develop long-term immunity, he or she must actively produce the antibodies. As the child interacts with others in society, he or she will be exposed to various communicable diseases and develop antibodies to them.

The child is particularly susceptible to communicable diseases due to many factors. The child's immune system is immature. By age 1, the child will have adult levels of immunoglobulin M antibodies. The child has a lower number of neutrophils, the white blood cell that assists in the destruction of bacteria. See Chapter 21 ⚭ for more information on the child's immune system.

The child is also exposed to many varieties of harmful bacteria. Parents bring bacteria home from work, and siblings bring bacteria home from school. The developmental level of the child can also play a significant role in the child's risk of infection. A school-age child has the cognitive ability to understand the dangers of passing bacteria from the hand to the mouth. This child can therefore make a decision to wash his or her hands after toileting to avoid transmission of bacteria. The infant, toddler, and preschooler, however, do not have this cognitive ability.

Children in day care, mother's morning out programs, and church nurseries are exposed to a number of pathogens. They can also be exposed at family gatherings. The incidence of illness increases as children participate in these activities. Children share toys and food. They are exposed to infected droplets as other children sneeze on them and talk close to their face.

The child who is hospitalized is at risk for contracting a nosocomial or health care–associated infection. All children are susceptible, but those who are younger than 2 years and are immunocompromised or in a weakened state are at greater risk. The longer a child stays in the hospital, the greater the risk of contracting a nosocomial infection.

Children who travel with their parents to different parts of the world can be exposed to a variety of different diseases. For instance, malaria is prevalent in Southeast Asian countries, Central America, and South America, but not in North America. Children who travel to these areas must be protected from mosquito bites, the route of transmission of malaria. African sleeping sickness is prevalent in the tropical regions of Africa. It is transmitted through the bite of

the tsetse fly. The tsetse fly is not susceptible to insect repellent and can bite through lightweight clothing. It is important for parents to avoid taking children into areas inhabited by the tsetse fly. Mosquito netting placed over sleeping areas may help protect the child from these insects.

Children can also be exposed to infectious diseases that are carried into the geographic area in which they live. The Health Promotion Issue on page 768 and 769 discusses concerns about such a possibility: the transmission of avian flu.

Certain harmful organisms may be used as a weapon in an act of **bioterrorism** (release of deadly infectious agents for the purpose of causing chaos and fear). Common organisms that may be used include *Bacillia anthracis* (anthrax), *Clostridium botulinum* (botulism), *Yersinia pestis* (plague), variola major virus (smallpox), and *Francisella tularensis* (tularemia). These agents can be transmitted by breathing the aerosolized organism or by direct contact.

PRECAUTIONS AND SAFEGUARDS FOR CHILDREN

The most effective way to prevent the spread of communicable diseases is through consistent hand washing. Children may not always wash their hands after using the toilet, blowing their noses, sneezing, or before eating. Children put their hands and toys in their mouth, touch their nose and eyes, and thus spread infections. Teaching children how to wash their hands and insisting that they do so after using the toilet, before meals, and as often as feasible will help decrease the spread of communicable diseases. Making hand washing fun will often help children wash for the time required to destroy germs. For example, having children sing "Happy Birthday" two times while washing hands will ensure that they wash for at least 30 seconds. The nurse must insist parents wash their hands after using the bathroom or changing diapers and before preparing food. Often, a gentle reminder with information about the spread of infection is all that is necessary for parents.

In health care and hospital settings, procedures and precautions need to be implemented to control the spread of infection. Medical asepsis is a basic part of all procedures. The nurse uses health practices to reduce the number of harmful organisms (e.g., hand washing) and to prevent their spread (e.g., implementing precautions to isolate harmful bacteria to a specific area).

Universal precautions are defined by the Centers for Disease Control and Prevention (CDC) as a set of precautions designed to prevent transmission of HIV, hepatitis B virus (HBV), and other bloodborne pathogens when providing first aid or health care. Under universal precautions, blood and body fluids of *all* clients are considered to be *potentially* infectious for HIV, HBV, and other bloodborne pathogens.

(*Text continues on p. 770.*)

AVIAN FLU (PLANNING FOR THE MANAGEMENT OF PANDEMIC INFLUENZA)

Because of its geographic proximity, Honolulu is considered the gateway to the Americas by many Asian nations. Outside downtown Honolulu's Chinatown, the nurse works in a 24-hour free-standing medical clinic. On a daily basis, the clinic sees about 60 pediatric clients and 25 adult clients. More than 50% of these clients are tourists, and most of them are from Japan or China. The clinic is staffed by two family care physicians, a family nurse practitioner, two registered nurses, three LPNs, a laboratory technician, a receptionist, and a bookkeeper.

One glance at the clinic's population gives the staff concern that influenza will be brought to Americans from these Asian countries. Even the children who are now American citizens travel back to their homeland to visit relatives, or the relatives visit America on occasion. The Centers for Disease Control and Prevention (CDC) website shows that Cambodia, Vietnam, China, and Indonesia have the highest number of cases of avian flu and the highest number of deaths resulting from this strain of influenza in 2006.

Concerned about the avian flu and the impact it would have on this community, the staff at the medical clinic decide to be proactive and develop a plan before they have a real problem on their hands. Their initial step in developing the plan was to visit the CDC website for assistance.

DISCUSSION

Prior to discussing the situation, the team had to learn more about the avian flu. Following are some general definitions that will aid their work:

- The **seasonal flu,** also called the common flu, is a respiratory illness that can be transmitted from person to person. Generally, seasonal flu is caused by influenza A or B. Most people have some immunity to these strains. There is a vaccine available for the seasonal flu.

- The **avian flu,** also called the bird flu or H5N1, is caused by influenza viruses that occur naturally among wild birds. H5N1 is deadly to domestic birds. It can be transmitted from birds to humans. Currently, there is no human immunity and no vaccine available.

- **Pandemic flu** is a virulent human flu that causes a global outbreak of serious illness, or pandemic. Because there is little natural immunity, the disease can spread easily from person to person. Currently, there is no pandemic flu. However, there have been previous influenza pandemics such as the Spanish flu of 1918, the Asian flu of 1957, and the Hong Kong flu of 1968.

This H5N1 virus that now mainly affects birds can become dangerous to humans through two processes: the antigenic drift and the antigenic shift. The **antigenic drift** is the minor genetic change that occurs to the virus as it replicates within the host cells. The **antigenic shift** is an abrupt change or a major change in the virus. The antigenic shift makes the virus capable of infecting humans.

Allen (2006) describes the only known case of person-to-person transmission of the H5N1 virus. The transmission occurred in Thailand when an 11-year-child became ill after handling chickens that were dying. She was hospitalized with symptoms of the avian flu and was cared for by her mother, who did not have any contact with the chickens. The child died due to respiratory failure and shock. Her mother developed symptoms 3 days later and died of respiratory complications.

The incubation period of avian flu appears to be 2 to 10 days. Initial symptoms are flulike: chills, fever of 100°F to 103°F, persistent malaise, myalgia, headache, eye pain, photophobia, substernal burning sensation, nonproductive cough, sore throat, rhinitis, shortness of breath, and diarrhea (Sheff,

2006). Other possible symptoms include vomiting, abdominal pain, pleuritic pain, bleeding from the nose and gums, and conjunctivitis. Complications of the avian flu include pneumonia, acute respiratory distress, acute encephalitis, organ failure, and death.

Laboratory results include lymphocytopenia and decreased platelet counts. Radiologic findings include the presence of infiltrates and pneumonia. There are lab tests for the specific H5N1 virus. Respiratory specimens can be tested using virus culturing, antigen tests, or polymerase chain reaction assays.

Treatment for the avian flu is primarily supportive. Clinicians should attempt to prevent the worsening of symptoms. Most clients require admission to intensive care units to monitor fluid and electrolyte balance, oxygenation, circulatory status, and respiratory effort. Medication administration may include neuroaminidase inhibitors such as Tamiflu or Relenza, antibiotics to prevent secondary infections, and corticosteroids. Tamiflu can be given prophylactically to children who are 13 years of age or older. It can also be given to children 1 year of age or older with flu symptoms. Relenza can be given to

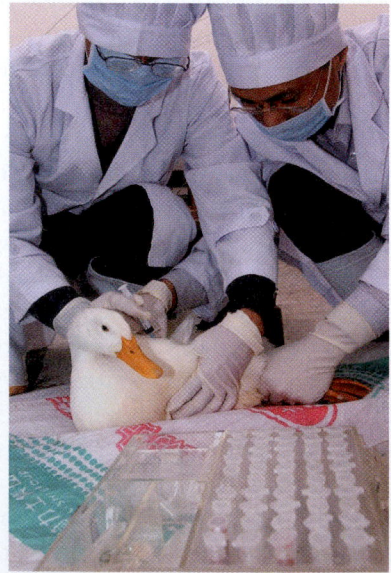

(Getty Images, Inc.)

children 7 years of age or older with flu symptoms. Both Tamiflu and Relenza need to be given within the first 48 hours following the onset of symptoms to have a positive effect. Oxygen administration, endotracheal intubation, and mechanical ventilation may be necessary.

Clients hospitalized with avian flu should be placed in a private room with standard and contact precautions. Staff members should have the proper equipment to protect themselves, including specially fitted respiratory masks, gloves, gown, and eye protection. Health care equipment such as stethoscope, thermometer, and sphygmomanometer should be dedicated to the client.

Currently, there is no vaccine available against the avian flu, but several companies are beginning efforts to produce sufficient antibodies to prevent infection.

PLANNING AND IMPLEMENTATION

Using the CDC's *Medical Offices and Clinics Pandemic Influenza Planning Checklist*, the staff of the medical clinic developed an action plan to ensure a proper response to an outbreak of the avian flu. Their first step was to develop a planning committee consisting of an administrator, a physician, a nurse, a receptionist, and a laboratory technician.

They assigned a committee member to monitor any health advisories regarding the avian flu both at the state level and at the federal level. Regular reports were given in the monthly committee meetings, and a mechanism was put in place to give urgent reports when necessary. For instance, this committee member would submit an urgent report when the influenza pandemic is in the United States, when it is in Hawaii, or when it is in Honolulu.

Data collection of influenza cases that present to their clinic was initiated. Analyzing these data allowed the committee to understand their needs for staffing and supplies if the number of cases greatly increased as they would with a pandemic situation. Reporting cases of pandemic influenza to local and state health departments will be essential. Therefore, one person from the committee was assigned to be the spokesperson for the clinic and manage this task. Contact information (including name, title, agency, telephone number, facsimile number, and e-mail) was obtained and placed in an easily identified location.

Education about the avian flu became the next task. The entire staff, full-time, part-time, and temporary, needed to be clear about the transmission of the virus, the recognizable symptoms, the treatment plan, and the prevention methods related to the avian flu. Their clients also needed to be educated regarding these same issues. A teaching curriculum was developed, including client handouts. Attention was given to the language and reading level of these materials. The CDC website provided many client education materials already translated into other languages including Spanish, Chinese, and Vietnamese.

It was also necessary to develop a plan for managing the barrage of telephone calls expected during a pandemic. A prioritization plan was developed for handling the clients who were most ill first. This included temporarily canceling physical exams and follow-up appointments to be able to handle the case load. The committee discussed designating separate days for influenza clients in order to decrease the risk of transmission to others. The waiting room situation had to be assessed because this could be a ready location for

transmission. Signs were made that directed clients with influenza symptoms to notify staff members immediately, sit in a designated area, use tissues to cover their cough, dispose of used tissues in designated receptacles, and use no-rinse hand sanitizer frequently.

Staffing was the next issue to be assessed. Priority was placed on administering influenza vaccine or antiviral prophylaxis, if necessary, to all personnel having client contact. The sick leave policy was also reviewed. What would happen if a staff member developed symptoms of the flu at work? What if staff members were needed to care for family members in their home who had symptoms of the flu? Were there enough temporary staff members available if they were needed?

Finally, the planning committee reviewed supplies that would be required during a pandemic outbreak. Supplies of masks, gloves, no-rinse hand sanitizer, syringes, alcohol swabs, and bandages were inventoried. A 2-week reserve inventory of these supplies was obtained. Suppliers of these items were contacted to determine how quickly the items could be acquired in an emergency situation.

This planning took time and energy. However, when the committee gave its final report to the entire staff, there was a sense of security that was experienced by all. With the proper education, supplies, personnel, implementation plan, and support persons identified, the medical clinic staff knew they were prepared to handle an avian flu outbreak in their community.

SELF-REFLECTION

What steps are you taking to personally protect yourself from the flu? Do you receive a flu shot annually? If you answered no, why not?

MediaLink

Avian flu

SUGGESTED RESOURCES

For the Nurse

- www.pandemicflu.gov

- Allen, P. (2006). Avian influenza pandemic: Not if, but when. *Pediatric Nursing, 32*(1), 76–81.

- Ray, M., & Walker-Jenkins, A. (2006). Confronting bird flu: Will pandemic avian flu be the next public health threat? *Lifelines, 10*(1), 21–29.

- Sheff, B. (2006). Avian influenza: Poised to launch a pandemic? *Nursing 2006, 36*(1), 51–53.

Standard precautions combine universal precautions and body substance isolation techniques, and apply to all clients in the hospital. Standard precautions include:

- Washing hands with plain soap and water before and after client contact.
- Wearing gloves when in contact with blood, body fluids, secretions, excretions, and other contaminated items. (Change gloves when they are contaminated, and wash hands before reapplying gloves.)
- Wearing a mask, eye protection, or a face shield when there is a possibility of contacting body fluids during certain procedures.
- Wearing a clean, nonsterile gown to protect skin and prevent soiling of the uniform by contact with body fluids. (Remove the gown promptly, and wash hands thoroughly.)
- Having designated client care equipment such as stethoscope, thermometer, and sphygmomanometer for clients with diseases that can be transmitted to others.
- Ensuring that employees who handle soiled equipment and linen are properly protected from exposure to infected body fluids.
- Handling sharp instruments properly to avoid exposure. (Do not recap used needles. Dispose of these items in proper receptacles.)
- Avoiding mouth-to-mouth resuscitation. Use mouthpieces, resuscitation bags, or other ventilation devices.
- Arranging for a private room for children who can transmit harmful bacteria via airborne or droplet transfer.

Transmission-based precautions include standard precautions *plus* airborne precautions, droplet precautions, or contact precautions. Airborne precautions protect others from diseases such as chickenpox and measles that can be transmitted by the airborne route. The child with these diseases needs to be in a private room that has negative air pressure. The door of the room should be kept closed. Everyone entering the room should wear a high-efficiency particulate air filter respirator mask. If the client leaves the room for any reason, he or she must wear the same type of protective mask.

Droplet precautions are implemented to prevent the spread of infection by the droplet route. A private room is necessary. The door may remain open. Individuals coming within 3 ft of the child must wear a surgical mask. If the client leaves the room for any reason, he or she must wear a surgical mask.

Contact precautions protect individuals from direct contact with the skin or indirect contact with inanimate objects that are infected with harmful organisms. Children requiring contact precautions should be in a private room. Gloves should be worn when entering the room and when providing care that would require contact with infected body fluids. Gowns must also be worn if there is a risk of contacting body fluids with the uniform and removed before leaving the client's room.

Reverse isolation can be used for the child who is immunocompromised. This form of precaution protects the child from harmful organisms that may be brought into the room by hospital personnel or family members. This form of precaution includes requiring every person who enters the child's room to wear gown, gloves, and a mask. Also, all equipment brought into the room needs to be carefully disinfected. Children who have recently had an organ transplant are often placed on reverse isolation. For more information about organ transplantation, see Chapter 21 ⌾. (See Appendix VIII ⌾ for a review of precautions.)

Immunizations

Immunization is the process of inducing resistance to communicable diseases. Immunization is accomplished by the use of **vaccine,** a product containing killed, live, recombinant, or conjugated micro-organisms administered parenterally to induce immunity. A *toxoid* is also considered a vaccine. The types of vaccines are listed in Table 26-1 ■. Refer to Chapter 13 and page 365 ⌾ for discussion about giving immunizations.

TABLE 26-1		
Types of Vaccine		
TYPE OF VACCINE	**DEFINITION**	**EXAMPLE**
Killed	Contains a micro-organism that is killed yet capable of causing the body to produce antibodies	Polio vaccine
Live	Contains a micro-organism that is live yet altered to be weakened, also called attenuated	Measles, mumps, rubella (MMR) vaccine
Recombinant	Contains a genetically altered micro-organism	Hepatitis B (HB) vaccine
Conjugated	Contains an altered organism that is paired with another substance	Haemophilus influenza type B (Hib)
Toxoid	A toxin that has been treated with heat or chemical to weaken the toxic effects while still retaining the ability to produce antibodies	Tetanus toxoid

The Advisory Committee on Immunization Practices of the CDC, the American Academy of Pediatrics (AAP), and the American Academy of Family Practitioners collaborate to develop the recommended immunization schedule for children.

See Appendix II ⚭ for the U.S. recommended immunization schedule from the CDC. Table 26-2 ■ lists nursing concerns for common pediatric immunizations. For additional information about immunizing, see page 365 ⚭.

TABLE 26-2

Nursing Considerations for Common Pediatric Immunizations

IMMUNIZATION TYPE	SIDE EFFECTS	NURSING CONSIDERATIONS
Diphtheria and pertussis vaccines and tetanus toxoid (DTaP) *Route:* Intramuscular *Dosage:* 0.5 mL May give at same time as all other vaccines in a separate site.	*Common:* Redness, pain, swelling, nodule at injection site; temperature up to 101°F (38.3°C); drowsiness, irritability, fussiness; anorexia within 2 days of injection. Increase in frequency and magnitude of local reactions with doses 4 and 5 (e.g., entire limb swelling). *Serious:* Allergic reaction, anaphylaxis; shock, fever above 102°F (38.8°C); febrile seizure; persistent inconsolable crying; coma or permanent brain damage.	Use same brand for all doses where feasible. Prior to immunization, ask about previous reaction to immunization. DTaP may coincide with or hasten the recognition of a seizure disorder. In children with a history of seizures with or without fever, give acetaminophen at the time of vaccine and then every 4 hours for 24 hours. Shake vaccine before withdrawing. Solution will be cloudy. If it contains clumps that cannot be resuspended, do not use. Inform parents of the chance of increased reaction to doses 4 and 5. Defer the vaccine if the child has a progressive neurologic problem until the child is stable. The series does not need to be restarted, regardless of when the previous dose was given.
Poliovirus vaccine (IPV) *Route:* Subcutaneous or intramuscular, depending on vaccine used *Dosage:* 0.5 mL May give at same time as all other vaccines in a separate site.	*Common:* Swelling and tenderness, irritability, tiredness. *Serious:* Allergic reaction or anaphylaxis.	Prior to immunization, ask if child has an allergy to neomycin, streptomycin, or polymyxin B (whichever of these antibiotics the specific vaccine to be used contains). Clear, colorless suspension. Do not use if it contains particulate matter, becomes cloudy, or changes color. All doses must be separated by at least 4 weeks. The series does not need to be restarted, regardless of when the previous dose was given.
Measles, mumps, rubella (MMR) vaccine *Route:* Subcutaneous *Dosage:* 0.5 mL May give at same time as all other vaccines in a separate site.	*Common:* Elevated temperature 1–2 weeks after immunization; redness or pain at injection site; noncontagious rash; joint pain. *Serious:* Allergic reaction, febrile seizure; meningitis (usually mild); encephalopathy; thrombocytopenia purpura; rare cases of coma and permanent brain damage.	Prior to immunization, ask if child has an allergy to neomycin or gelatin. Observe the child with an egg allergy for 90 minutes after injection. Inquire about immunosuppression. Instruct adolescent girls of childbearing age to avoid pregnancy for 3 months after immunization. Give tuberculosis test at same time as MMR or 4–6 weeks later. If MMR and Varivax are not given on the same day, space them at least 28 days apart. Reconstituted vaccine is a clear, yellow solution. Give entire contents of reconstituted vial even if more than 0.5 mL. As college students are at greater risk due to decreasing immunity, make sure they have received a second MMR dose.
Hepatitis B (HB) vaccine *Route:* Intramuscular *Dosage:* Engerix-B: 10 mcg or Recombivax HB: 5 mcg May give at same time as all other vaccines in a separate site.	*Common:* Pain or redness at injection site; headache; photophobia; altered liver enzymes. *Serious:* Allergic reaction or anaphylaxis; fever.	Prior to immunization, check status of mother's hepatitis B test and presence of other liver disease. *Note:* If mother has HbsAg+, vaccine must be given to infant within 12 hours of birth along with hepatitis B immune globulin at the same time in another site with a new needle and syringe. Shake vaccine before withdrawing. Solution will appear cloudy. Minimum spacing for children and teens is 4 weeks between doses 1 and 2, and 8 weeks between doses 2 and 3. The last dose in an infant series should not be given before 6 months of age. Vaccine brands can be interchanged for 3-dose series. The series does not need to be restarted, regardless of when the previous dose was given.

(continued)

TABLE 26-2

Nursing Considerations for Common Pediatric Immunizations (continued)

IMMUNIZATION TYPE	SIDE EFFECTS	NURSING CONSIDERATIONS
Haemophilus influenza type B (Hib) *Route:* Intramuscular *Dosage:* 0.5 mL May give at same time as all other vaccines in a separate site.	*Common:* Pain, redness, or swelling at site. *Serious:* Allergic reaction of anaphylaxis (extremely rare); fever.	Prior to immunizations, ask if child is immunosuppressed. Solution is clear and colorless. If the first dose is given between 7 and 11 months of age, 3 doses are needed. If the first dose is given at 12–14 months of age, give a booster dose in 8 weeks. If the first dose is given when the child is older than 15 months or younger than 5 years, only one dose is needed. Second and third doses can be given 4 and 8 weeks after the first. Use the same vaccine preparation for all doses of the primary series if possible. The series does not need to be restarted, regardless of when the previous dose was given.
Heptavalent pneumococcal conjugate vaccine (PCV) *Route:* Intramuscular *Dosage:* 0.5 mL	*Common:* Soreness, swelling, redness at injection site; mild to moderate fever; irritability, drowsiness, restless sleep, decreased appetite, vomiting and diarrhea, rash or hives. *Severe:* Allergic reaction or anaphylaxis.	Clear, colorless, or slightly opalescent liquid. In addition to infants, this vaccine is a priority for children ages 2–5 with sickle cell disease, asplenia, or HIV infection, or in those who are immunocompromised. The vaccine is also a priority for Native American and Native Alaskan children ages 2–5 because of their increased risk for pneumococcal disease. The series does not need to be restarted, regardless of when the previous dose was given.
Varicella virus vaccine *Route:* Subcutaneous *Dosage:* 0.5 mL	*Common:* Pain or redness at injection site; fever up to 102°F (38.8°C) in children. Less commonly, a mild vaccine-related rash may occur during first month after the injection. *Severe:* Allergic reaction or anaphylaxis; thrombocytopenia; febrile seizure; central nervous system manifestations.	Prior to immunization, ask if child is immunodeficient, on immunosuppression treatment, or has an allergy to neomycin or gelatin. Determine if a family member is immunocompromised. Clear, colorless to pale yellow liquid when reconstituted. Give the entire contents of the vial even if more than 0.5 mL. Instruct adolescent girls of childbearing age to avoid pregnancy for 3 months after immunization.
Hepatitis A *Route:* Intramuscular *Dosage:* 0.5 mL, 1 mL over 17 years for Vaqta, 1 mL over 18 years for Havrix May give at same time as all other vaccines in a separate site.	Rare reports of anaphylaxis reaction.	Shake well; slightly opaque white suspension. Can be given for postexposure prophylaxis against hepatitis A. Immune globulin and vaccine can be given at same time in different sites. Vaccine brands can be interchanged.
Influenza *Route:* Intramuscular (all ages), intranasal (5 years and older) *Dosage:* 0.25 mL in infants 6–35 months, 0.5 mL beginning at 3 years May give at same time as all other vaccines in a separate site.	*Common after injection:* May have soreness or swelling at injection site, fever, aches. Life-threatening allergic reactions are rare. *Common after intranasal vaccine:* Runny nose or nasal congestion, fever, headache or muscle aches, abdominal pain, and occasional vomiting.	Thawed intranasal vaccine is pale yellow, clear to slightly cloudy. Administered annually in autumn. Children with no history of influenza illness or vaccine need 2 doses 1 month apart. Intranasal dose is split (0.25 mL) with a dose divider clip. Administer in each nostril while child is sitting in an upright position. Insert the tip of the sprayer inside the nose and depress the plunger to spray. Children 8 years of age or younger who are receiving the influenza vaccine for the first time should get 2 doses separated by at least 4 weeks (injectable) and 6 weeks (intranasal). Must be reimmunized each year as immunity wanes.

Data from American Academy of Pediatrics. (2003). *Red Book: Report of the Committee on Infectious Disease* (26th ed.). Elk Grove Village, IL: Author; Immunization Action Coalition. (2004). *Mosby's drug consult 2004.* St. Louis: Mosby; Bindler, R.M., & L.B., Howry. (2005). *Pediatric drug with nursing implications.* Upper Saddle River, NJ: Prentice Hall.

BOX 26-1

New Vaccines on the Horizon

Otitis Media

Although still not approved by the U.S. Food and Drug Administration (FDA), a combination *Streptococcus pneumoniae* and *Haemophilus influenzae* vaccine studied in the Czech Republic and Slovakia was found to reduce the incidence of otitis media by 33% (Prymula, 2006).

Rotavirus

The FDA recently approved a vaccine against rotavirus, the most common cause of diarrhea in children. The CDC advises that children be given the three-dose series at 2 months, 4 months, and again at 6 months (Peck, 2006).

Meningitis

Recent outbreaks of meningitis on college campuses have led to the FDA's approval of a single-dose vaccine for adolescents age 11 or 12. If unvaccinated, children should receive the vaccine on entering high school or at age 15. Also, college students who will be living in dormitories and who have not been recently vaccinated should be immunized (Rosenfeld, 2006).

New vaccines are always in development. For example, each year vaccines are developed for the coming year to guard young children and individuals who are immunocompromised from the effects of influenza. Box 26-1 ■ provides information about some new pediatric vaccines that are in development.

Immunotherapy is the prevention and treatment of disease using the administration of allergens, immunostimulants, immunosuppressants, interferon, and immune globulin. Many communicable diseases can be treated by immune globulin to diminish the effects of the disease or prevent transmission of the disease. See further discussion of immune therapy in Chapter 21.

Client Teaching to Parents and Children

There are many ways in which families can reduce the transmission of communicable diseases among family members. Tissues used to blow the nose should be discarded in a trash receptacle immediately. All family members should wash their hands with soap and water or antibacterial gel after contact with body fluids and excrement. Hand washing should always follow toileting. If a child sneezes or coughs into the hands, the child should immediately wash them. However, recent thinking is that children should be taught to sneeze into the elbow instead of the hands to prevent disease transmission.

Toys can be a reservoir for harmful organisms. They should be washed with disinfectant regularly. During periods of communicability, children should not share toys because this increases the likelihood of transmission.

Some practices increase the risk of transmission of certain pathogens. These practices include nail biting, thumb sucking, sharing drinks and eating utensils, and putting items found on the floor or ground into the mouth. The older child can understand the hazards of these practices. However, the younger child's behavior will need to be monitored to prevent the transmission of harmful organisms in these ways.

REYE'S SYNDROME

Nurses must also teach parents about the risks that exist once children acquire a communicable disease. One serious possible result is Reye's syndrome. Reye's syndrome is an acute *encephalopathy* (a disorder characterized by inflammation of the brain). Untreated, the syndrome is often fatal. Symptoms of Reye's syndrome usually follow a viral illness and may be linked to the intake of aspirin. Because of this association, parents are taught to use acetaminophen or other fever reducers, not aspirin, to reduce fever in a child with a communicable disease.

Initial symptoms include nausea, vomiting, and lethargy but may progress quickly to marked changes in the level of consciousness. The child may become combative, use inappropriate language, have hyperreflexia, develop seizures, and become comatose.

Diagnosis of Reye's syndrome is based on history plus elevated liver enzymes and ammonia levels, decreased blood glucose levels, and prolonged prothrombin time. The ill child is admitted to the pediatric intensive care unit for supportive treatment and close observation. Respiratory ventilation may be necessary. Monitoring for increased intracranial pressure is essential. Intravenous fluids assist in treating hypoglycemia.

TEACHING EMERGENCY PREPAREDNESS

The nurse can assist families in preparing for emergencies such as bioterrorism. The AAP recommends that all families have a specified disaster plan. This organization suggests that children be involved in this planning. Children should also be encouraged to assist in creating a disaster kit. This kit should include several days' supply of food and water, pet supplies, warm clothing, rain gear, blankets, toiletries, battery-powered radio and flashlight with extra batteries, a credit card and supply of cash, a first aid kit, and copies of important documents. If a family member has a medical condition, extra medication and supplies need to be included in the kit. If there is an infant in the family and the mother is not breastfeeding, extra infant formula is a necessary element of the kit. The American Academy of Pediatrics offers a complete list of items for the disaster kit. Nursing care related to traumatic life events is discussed in Chapter 27 and Box 27-6, Effects of Disasters on Children.

Common Infections

Communicable diseases are considered to be acute illnesses. They typically have a limited duration and can be considered treatable in most cases. However, depending on the child's state of health, these diseases may prove to be complicated and severe.

It is important for the nurse to understand the route of transmission of these diseases and the incubation period.

Manifestations

Recognizing the clinical manifestations of these diseases can allow for prompt medical management. Many communicable diseases have a distinctive appearance. Figure 26-2 ■ shows clinical manifestations of several common communicable diseases.

Diagnosis and Treatment

Diagnosis is often by clinical manifestations. There may be a history of exposure to another child or children with the disease (particularly with school-age children). Treatment depends on the infectious agent but is generally supportive. Specific information about common pediatric communicable diseases, including transmission and incubation, manifestations, diagnostic tests, and nursing considerations, is provided in Table 26-3 ■. An important role for the nurse is teaching parents and the public how to prevent these childhood illnesses. The nurse must be prepared to assist the physician in providing medical treatment, with the goal of restoring health to the child.

(*Text continues on p. 783.*)

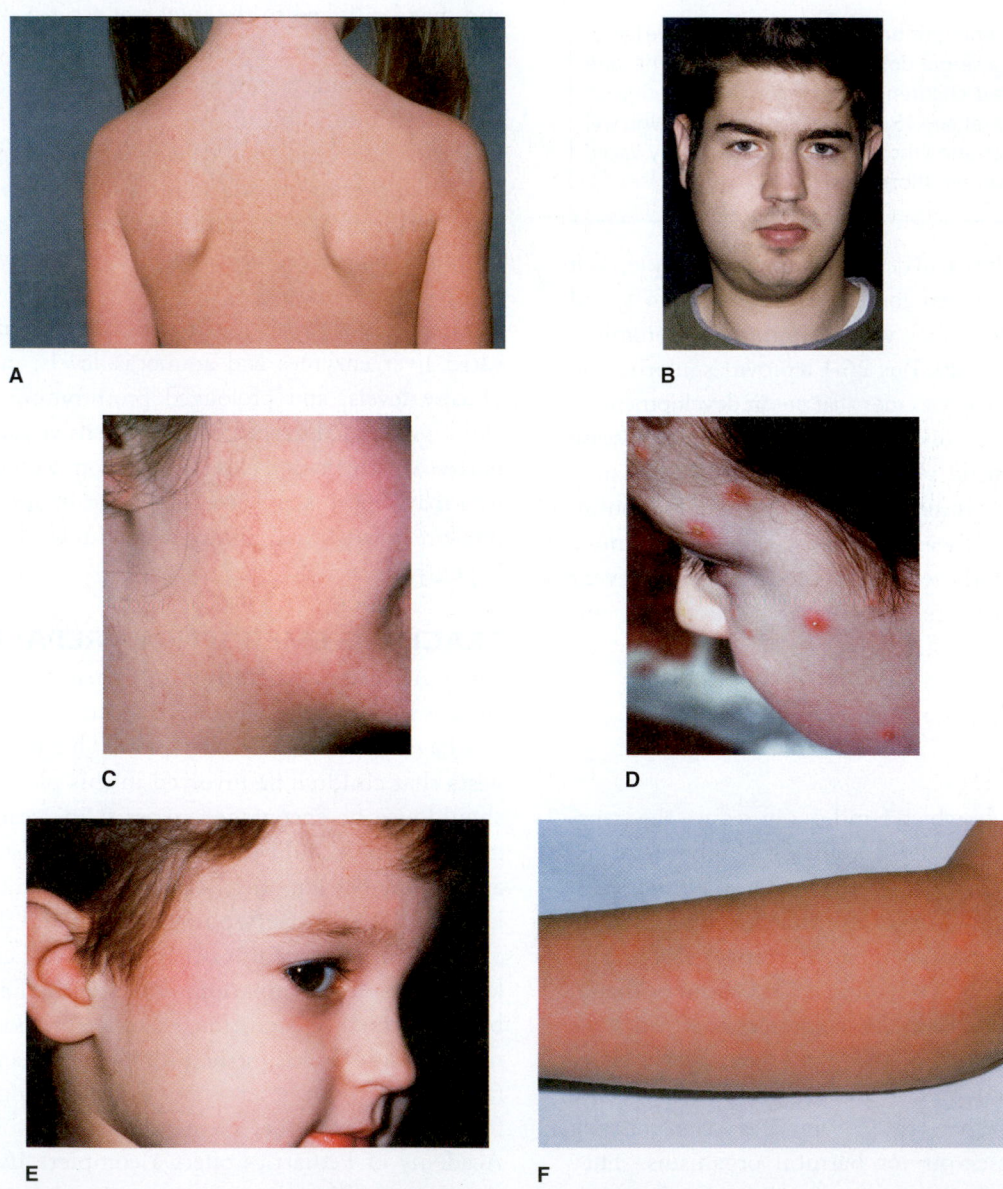

A

B

C

D

E

F

Figure 26-2. ■ Common infectious diseases of childhood. (**A**) Measles rash. (**B**) Mumps swelling. (**C**) Rubella or German measles. (**D**) Chickenpox lesions. (**E**) Fifth disease or erythema infectiosum. (**F**) Scarlet fever. (**A** and **C**. NMSB-Custom Medical Stock Photo, Inc. **D**. © Patrick J. Watson. **B**, **E** and **F**: Dr. P. Marazzi/Photo Researchers, Inc.)

TABLE 26-3

Common Communicable Diseases of Childhood

DISEASE AND CAUSATIVE ORGANISM	TRANSMISSION AND INCUBATION PERIOD	CLINICAL MANIFESTATIONS	DIAGNOSTIC TESTS AND MEDICAL TREATMENT	NURSING CONSIDERATIONS
Hepatitis B is caused by the hepatitis B virus (HBV).	*Transmission:* Exposure to body fluids, organ transplants, sexual contact, intravenous drug use and sharing of needles, transplacental, during birth or during breastfeeding. *Incubation period:* 1–6 months, with an average of 50 days. Children infected with HBV may become a carrier of the virus for life.	Fever, anorexia, nausea, vomiting, rash, arthralgia, pruritus, jaundice, right upper quadrant pain, darkening of the urine, clay-colored stools, hepatosplenomegaly	*Diagnostic:* Serologic testing to detect the presence of antigens and antibodies to HBV *Preventative measures:* Routine screening of pregnant women, 3-dose series of immunization against hepatitis B, hand washing *Medical treatment:* Bed rest, hydration, well-balanced diet, hepatitis B immune globulin (HBIG) for one-time exposure and infants born to infected mothers	■ Prevent the spread of the virus by good hand washing and other standard precautions. ■ Assist the child and family in planning a high-protein, high-carbohydrate, low-fat diet. ■ Assist the child with activities of daily living and quiet activities to promote rest. ■ Assess carefully for toxic effects of medications because drug metabolism can be altered with liver disorders.
Diphtheria is caused by *Corynebacterium diphtheriae.*	*Transmission:* Direct contact with mucous membranes, skin, or lesions of an infected period or a carrier. Transmission has also occurred indirectly by contact with contaminated surfaces. The bacteria may also reside in unpasteurized milk. *Incubation period:* 2–7 days or longer. Disease can be transmitted for a period of 2–4 weeks.	Low-grade fever, anorexia, malaise, foul-smelling rhinorrhea, sore throat with hoarseness, stridor or noisy breathing, cervical lymphadenitis. Children with diphtheria have a thick, bluish-white to grayish-black patchy, membranous lesion that can cover the tongue, soft or hard palate, and the pharynx.	*Diagnostic:* Cultures of the lesion *Preventative measures:* 5-dose series of immunization against diphtheria. The most common immunization against diphtheria is given in conjunction with tetanus and pertussis. *Medical treatment:* Administration of antibiotics and antitoxins after the child has been tested for sensitivity to horse serum. Observe carefully for airway obstruction.	■ Isolate the child to prevent transmission. ■ Observe carefully for airway obstruction. Keep oral airway and oxygen readily available at all times. ■ Suction prn. ■ Oral liquids may be a choking hazard. Give cautiously. ■ Provide oral hygiene frequently. ■ Assist the child with activities of daily living and quiet activities to promote rest.
Tetanus (lockjaw) is caused by *Clostridium tetani,* also called tetanus bacillus.	*Transmission:* Indirect contact with contaminated soil, manure, or tools through breaks in the skin or wound. The newborn can become infected if the umbilical cord is cut with a contaminated utensil. Not transmitted from person to person. *Incubation period:* 3 days to 3 weeks, with an average of 8 days.	Neck and jaw stiffness, difficulty chewing, difficulty swallowing, muscle spasms stimulated by noise or touch, spasms may progress to laryngospasm and compromise respiratory effort, abdominal rigidity progressing to **opisthotonos** or rigid hyperextension of the entire body. The newborn has difficulty sucking, irritability, and nuchal rigidity.	*Preventative measures:* 5-dose series of immunization against tetanus. The most common immunization against tetanus is given in conjunction with diphtheria and pertussis. A booster injection is necessary every 10 years for life. *Medical treatment:* Wound debridement, administration of antibiotics, muscle relaxants for spasms, tetanus immune globulin, nutritional support through enteral methods or total parenteral nutrition, mechanical ventilation is required.	■ Provide a quiet environment, reduce stimulation. ■ Provide wound care. ■ Provide skin care. ■ Observe closely for laryngospasm. Keep oral airway and oxygen readily available at all times. ■ Suction prn. ■ Maintain strict intake and output. ■ Monitor fluid and electrolyte balance.

(continued)

TABLE 26-3

Common Communicable Diseases of Childhood (continued)

DISEASE AND CAUSATIVE ORGANISM	TRANSMISSION AND INCUBATION PERIOD	CLINICAL MANIFESTATIONS	DIAGNOSTIC TESTS AND MEDICAL TREATMENT	NURSING CONSIDERATIONS
Pertussis (whooping cough) is caused by *Bordetella pertussis*.	*Transmission:* Direct and indirect contact with infected respiratory secretions. Risk for transmission is greatest in the catarrhal stage but may last 4 weeks into the paroxysmal stage. *Incubation period:* 5–21 days, with an average of 7–10 days	*Catarrhal stage:* Low-grade fever, rhinitis (coryza), sneezing, lacrimation (tearing), nonproductive cough. Symptoms may last 1–2 weeks. *Paroxysmal stage:* In children older than 6 months, the cough becomes worse at night. The child produces a "whooping" sound that is a high-pitched crowing sound. The loud cough is the child's effort to expel a thick mucous plug and is due to a narrowed glottis. The coughing episodes are very tiring for the child, and he or she may become cyanotic or red faced. Vomiting may even occur. The infant younger than 6 months will have periods of apnea instead of the characteristic cough. Symptoms may last 1–6 weeks. *Convalescent stage:* The cough resolves gradually and may return to the cough characteristic of the catarrhal stage.	*Diagnostic:* Culture and polymerase chain reaction testing. *Preventative measures:* 5-dose series of immunization against pertussis. The most common immunization against pertussis is given in conjunction with diphtheria and tetanus. *Medical treatment:* Administration of pertussis immune serum globulin, antibiotics, and corticosteroids; bed rest; removal of environmental factors that aggravate coughing; humidification of the environment, especially where the child sleeps; nutritional support; droplet precautions; oxygen administration	■ Assist the child with activities of daily living and quiet activities to promote rest. ■ Provide adequate ventilation and humidification of the child's room. ■ Suction gently prn. ■ Observe closely for airway obstruction. Keep oral airway and oxygen readily available at all times. ■ Monitor oxygen saturation levels, especially in the infant younger than 6 months. ■ Initiate droplet precautions. ■ Maintain strict intake and output. ■ Monitor fluid and electrolyte balance.
Haemophilus influenza type B+ (Hib) is caused by *Coccobacilli H. influenzae* type B. See Chapter 16 🔗 for more information on meningitis, a common manifestation of this bacterial infection.	*Transmission:* By direct contact or droplet inhalation. The child may transmit the bacteria during the 3 days following onset of symptoms. *Incubation period:* Unknown	Manifestations include: Meningitis—sudden onset of headache, stiff neck, irritability, nausea, vomiting, fever Epiglottitis—fever, sore throat, stridor, cough, swollen epiglottis Pneumonia—gradual onset of fever, chills, productive cough, pleuritic chest pain Septic arthritis—joint inflammation, stiffness, joint pain and tenderness	*Diagnostic:* Evaluation of cerebrospinal fluid (CSF) from a lumbar puncture *Preventative measures:* 4-dose series of immunization against Hib *Medical treatment:* Administration of antibiotics for infected child and other members of the household who have not been vaccinated	■ Initiate droplet precautions. ■ Monitor temperature closely and implement fever-reducing strategies. ■ Provide comfort measures specific to the condition.

		Cellulitis—localized heat, redness, pain and swelling, fever, chills, headache Sinusitis—swelling and drainage of the mucous membranes, sinus pressure, tenderness and pain, headache Otitis media—ear tenderness, pain and drainage, diminished hearing Bronchitis—productive cough, fever, back pain Pericarditis—fever, substernal chest pain, dyspnea, nonproductive cough		
Poliomyelitis is caused by poliovirus.	*Transmission:* Direct contact via the fecal-oral and respiratory route. Virus may be transmitted just before and just after onset of symptoms, although the virus may be shed in the feces and respiratory system for 1–6 weeks. *Incubation period:* 3–36 days, with an average of 7–10 days.	Fever, headache, nausea, vomiting, abdominal pain, neck and back pain. These symptoms, in some cases, progress to tremors of the extremities, positive Kernig's and Brudzinski's signs (see Chapter 16 for more information), hyperactive deep tendon reflexes (DTR), paralysis and respiratory distress. The child may develop progressive permanent paralysis, muscle atrophy, and/or severe arthritis.	*Diagnostic:* Stool or throat cell culture and evaluation of CSF from a lumbar puncture *Preventative measures:* 4-dose series of immunization against polio *Medical treatment:* Bed rest, pain management, respiratory support if necessary, physical therapy with the goal of restoring mobility	■ Initiate droplet precautions. ■ Observe closely for respiratory distress. Keep oral airway and oxygen readily available at all times. ■ Assist the child with activities of daily living and quiet activities to promote rest. ■ Administer pharmacologic and non-pharmacologic pain relief measures. ■ Implement measures to promote good body mechanics such as proper body alignment when in the bed and performing passive or active range-of-motion exercises.
Measles (*rubeola*) is caused by Mobillivirus.	*Transmission:* Direct or indirect with airborne droplets. *Incubation period:* 8–20 days. The child can transmit measles from the fourth day of the incubation period to 4 days after the rash appears.	High-grade fever, enlarged lymph nodes, malaise, coryza, cough, photophobia, conjunctivitis, **Koplik's spots** (small, irregular red spots with a bluish-white center appearing on the buccal mucosa). Two to 4 days after the onset of these symptoms, the child develops	*Diagnostic:* Serologic test for immunoglobulin (Ig) M measles antibody *Preventative measures:* 2-dose series of immunization against measles. The most common immunization against measles, MMR, is given in conjunction with mumps	■ Initiate droplet precautions. ■ Assist the child with activities of daily living and quiet activities to promote rest. ■ Assess lung sounds. ■ Suction prn. ■ With high fever, implement seizure precautions.

(continued)

TABLE 26-3

Common Communicable Diseases of Childhood (continued)

DISEASE AND CAUSATIVE ORGANISM	TRANSMISSION AND INCUBATION PERIOD	CLINICAL MANIFESTATIONS	DIAGNOSTIC TESTS AND MEDICAL TREATMENT	NURSING CONSIDERATIONS
		a red maculopapular, pruritic rash that spreads from the face to the trunk and extremities. The rash changes to brown in color, and eventually sloughing (**desquamation**) occurs.	and rubella. A booster injection is now recommended for the adolescent. *Medical treatment:* Immune globulin may be given to susceptible person up to 6 days after exposure. Bed rest. Administration of antipyretics, anitpruritics, cough suppressants, and antibiotics for secondary infections.	■ Provide skin care, especially when sloughing occurs. ■ Provide frequent oral care. ■ Limit excessive environmental lighting. Some children are sensitive to television.
Mumps (*parotitis*) is caused by *Rubulavirus*.	*Transmission:* Direct or indirect spread of respiratory secretions. The child may transmit the virus several days before and after the onset of parotitis. Children should not return to school until 9 days after parotitis occurs. *Incubation period:* 12–25 days.	Low-grade fever, headache, malaise. An earache soon develops, accompanied by unilateral or bilateral swelling of the parotid gland. The male child may develop **orchitis** (unilateral or bilateral inflammation of the testes accompanied by pain).	*Diagnostic:* Viral culture; serum mumps immunoglobulin (Ig) G antibody titer *Preventative measures:* 2-dose series of immunization against mumps. The most common immunization against mumps, MMR, is given in conjunction with measles and rubella. A booster injection is now recommended for the adolescent. *Medical treatment:* Administration of analgesics and antipyretics. Corticosteroids may be used.	■ Initiate droplet precautions. ■ Administer pharmacologic and non-pharmacologic pain relief measures. ■ Assist child with nutritional intake. Foods should be liquid or soft. Avoid sour foods, which intensify pain. ■ Maintain intake and output. ■ Monitor fluid and electrolyte balance.
Rubella (German measles or 3-day measles) is caused by an RNA virus.	*Transmission:* Direct or indirect spread via exposure to respiratory secretions, feces, or urine. The child may transmit the virus 7 days before to 5 days after the onset of the rash. Children should not return to school or day care until 7 days after the onset of the rash. *Incubation period:* 14–21 days with an average of 16–18 days.	Low-grade fever, headache, malaise, coryza, enlarged lymph nodes. **Forschheimer spots** (erythematous pinpoint lesions of the soft palate) may also occur. After 1–5 days of these prodromal symptoms, a pink, maculopapular rash begins on the face and spreads down the trunk. It disappears in the same order. The fetus exposed to the rubella virus during pregnancy may be born with congenital rubella syndrome. This syndrome is charac-	*Diagnostic:* Nasal cell culture; serum immunoglobulin (Ig) G or M antibody titer *Preventative measures:* 2-dose series of immunization against rubella. The most common immunization against rubella, MMR, is given in conjunction with measles and mumps. A booster injection is now recommended for the adolescent. *Medical treatment:* Administration of antipyretics	■ Initiate droplet precautions for the hospitalized child. Prevent contact with rubella nonimmune pregnant women. ■ Implement comfort measures.

	Transmission / Incubation	Manifestations	Diagnostic / Treatment	Nursing Interventions
		...terized by intrauterine growth retardation (IUGR), hepatosplenomegaly, thrombocytopenia, and dark purplish skin lesions.		
Varicella (chickenpox) is caused by varicella-zoster virus.	*Transmission:* Direct or indirect contact with airborne respiratory secretions, eye secretions, or vesicles. The infected child may transmit the virus up to 5 days before the onset of vesicles and is considered contagious until 6 days following this outbreak, when all vesicles have crusted over. *Incubation period:* 10–21 days	Low-grade fever, malaise, headache, mild abdominal pain and irritability; 24 hours later the child experiences an outbreak of pruritic macules that progress from papules to fluid-filled vesicles. Lesions begin on the trunk, scalp, and face, spreading to the remainder of the body, including the mouth, eyes, and perineum. Scarring can develop. The fetus exposed to the varicella virus during pregnancy may be born with congenital varicella syndrome. This syndrome is characterized by IUGR, skin scarring, limb hypoplasia (underdevelopment), eye defects, brain defects, and death.	*Diagnostic:* Tissue culture of vesicle *Preventative measures:* Varicella immunization any time after 12 months of age *Medical treatment:* Administration of antipyretics, antihistamines, and acyclovir to reduce the number of lesions for immunocompromised children. Varicella-zoster immune globulin many also be given to immunocompromised children.	■ If the child is hospitalized, implement droplet and contact precautions. Prevent contact with varicella nonimmune pregnant women. ■ Provide skin care. Soothing baths of oatmeal can be suggested. ■ Keep the child's fingernails short to discourage secondary infections from scratching. ■ Avoid the use of products containing aspirin because Reye's syndrome has been associated with the use of aspirin during a varicella outbreak.
Pneumococcal infection is caused by *Streptococcus pneumoniae.*	*Transmission:* Direct and indirect spread of respiratory secretions *Incubation period:* 1–3 days	Manifestations include: Meningitis—sudden onset of headache, stiff neck, irritability, nausea, vomiting, fever. Pneumonia—gradual onset of fever, chills, productive cough, pleuritic chest pain. Otitis media—ear tenderness, pain and drainage, diminished hearing. Bacteremia—fever of unknown origin	*Preventative measures:* 4-dose series of immunization against pneumococcal infection *Medical treatment:* Administration of antibiotics, primarily penicillin and antipyretics.	■ Monitor intake and output. ■ Encourage fluid intake. ■ Monitor for signs and symptoms of respiratory distress.

(continued)

TABLE 26-3

Common Communicable Diseases of Childhood (continued)

DISEASE AND CAUSATIVE ORGANISM	TRANSMISSION AND INCUBATION PERIOD	CLINICAL MANIFESTATIONS	DIAGNOSTIC TESTS AND MEDICAL TREATMENT	NURSING CONSIDERATIONS
Influenza is caused by *Orthomyxoviridae.*	*Transmission:* Direct and indirect contact with respiratory secretions *Incubation period:* 1–4 days	Abrupt onset of fever, chills, cough, malaise, muscle aches, headache, anorexia, nausea, vomiting, diarrhea	*Diagnostic:* Rapid influenza test using a nasal or throat specimen; viral culture *Preventative measures:* Annual immunization against influenza *Medical treatment:* Administration of nonaspirin antipyretics and antivirals	■ Initiate droplet and contact precautions. ■ Encourage fluids to prevent dehydration. ■ Assist the child with activities of daily living and quiet activities to promote rest.
Hepatitis A is caused by the hepatitis A virus (HAV).	*Transmission:* Exposure to contaminated stool, typically the fecal-oral route *Incubation period:* 4 weeks with an average of 10–50 days	Fever, anorexia, nausea, vomiting, rash, arthralgia, pruritus, jaundice (in less than 5% of cases)	*Diagnostic:* Serologic testing to detect the presence of antigens and antibodies to HAV *Preventative measures:* 2-dose series of immunization against hepatitis A. The first dose can be given at 12 months and the second dose at least 6 months later. Good hand washing, especially following diaper changes. Proper cleaning of changing surfaces and disposal of soiled diapers. *Medical treatment:* Bed rest, hydration, well-balanced diet, hepatitis A immune globulin for one-time exposure	See previous measures for hepatitis B.
Erythema infectiosum (*fifth disease*) is caused by human parvovirus B-19.	*Transmission:* Direct and indirect contact with respiratory secretions and blood *Incubation period:* 6–14 days	Stage 1—fever, chills, headache, malaise, body aches Stage 2—1 week later, a rash appears on the child's face. It is bright red and looks as if the child has been slapped. Circumoral pallor is also present. One to 4 days later, a lacy, erythematous, maculopapular rash appears on the trunk and limbs, progressing proximal to distal. Stage 3—rash begins to fade but can reappear if the skin is irritated as by the sun.	*Diagnosis:* Serologic testing to detect the presence of parvovirus B-19-specific immunoglobulin (Ig) M antibodies *Preventative measures:* Avoid contact with infected children. *Medical treatment:* Administration of antipyretics and analgesics	■ Provide skin care. Soothing baths of oatmeal can be suggested. ■ Protect child from exposure to sunlight.

Exanthem subitum (sixth disease or roseola) is caused by herpesvirus type 6.	*Transmission:* Unknown, respiratory secretions suspected *Incubation period:* 5–20 days, with an average of 10 days	If the fetus is exposed to the virus during pregnancy, fetal death may occur. Sudden onset of high-grade fever. The child may play normally and have a good appetite during the 3–4 days of high fever. The fever disappears abruptly and a pale, pink, maculopapular rash appears on the trunk and spreads to the face, neck, and extremities. The rash lasts 1–2 days. Exanthem subitum occurs mainly in children ages 6–36 months. *Medical treatment:* Hospitalization is rarely necessary; administer antipyretics.	■ Observe closely for febrile seizures. ■ Teach signs and symptoms to parents. ■ Encourage oral intake of fluids.
Mononucleosis is caused by the Epstein–Barr virus (EBV). Also called *infectious mononucleosis,* glandular fever, or the kissing disease.	*Transmission:* Direct and indirect contact with respiratory and genital tract secretions, also blood transfusions. *Note:* The virus can be shed for up to 18 months following the clinical disease. *Incubation period:* 10–50 days	High-grade fever that can last 3–6 days, chills, headache, anorexia, malaise, abdominal pain, left shoulder pain, sore throat, lymphadenopathy, hepatosplenomegaly, weakness, and lethargy, which can last several months. *Diagnostic:* Serologic monospot test; testing EBV antibodies by immunofluorescence. *Preventative measures:* Avoid contact with those who are known to have the disease. *Medical treatment:* Bed rest, administer corticosteroids for tonsillar swelling, antipyretics for fever and analgesics for pain.	■ Assist the child with activities of daily living and quiet activities to promote rest. ■ Due to the risk of liver and spleen rupture, teach the child and parents the importance of avoiding contact sports or rough play for approximately 4 weeks or until hepatosplenomegaly has subsided. ■ Encourage the child to maintain adequate hydration. ■ Older adolescents should be told to avoid kissing until several days after the fever has subsided.
Streptococcus A (strep throat) is caused by group A streptococci (GAS). This organism also causes impetigo, scarlet fever, scarlatina, and rheumatic fever. For more information on impetigo, see Chapter 24 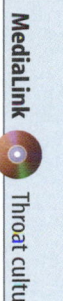.	*Transmission:* Direct contact *Incubation period:* 2–5 days	High-grade fever and chills with sudden onset, sore throat, dysphagia, malaise, headache, abdominal pain, anorexia, vomiting. Upon inspection, the pharynx appears bright red with white exudates. Cervical lymph nodes are tender. In toddlers, there may be a moderate temperature, rhinitis, *Diagnostic:* Secretions of the pharynx and tonsils are tested for the streptococcus, either by a rapid test or culture. *Preventative measures:* Avoid contact with those known to be infected. *Medical treatment:* Administer analgesics, antipyretics, antibiotics—penicillin is the drug of choice. If	■ If hospitalized, implement droplet precautions. ■ Provide a soft diet. ■ Offer saltwater gargles. ■ Encourage the child and the parents to take the entire prescribed antibiotic regime.

(continued)

MediaLink

Throat culture

TABLE 26-3

Common Communicable Diseases of Childhood (continued)

DISEASE AND CAUSATIVE ORGANISM	TRANSMISSION AND INCUBATION PERIOD	CLINICAL MANIFESTATIONS	DIAGNOSTIC TESTS AND MEDICAL TREATMENT	NURSING CONSIDERATIONS
For acute rheumatic fever, see Chapter 19 🔗.		irritability, and anorexia, not accompanied by sore throat. *Scarlet fever:* 12–48 hours following the onset of symptoms, a fine erythematous rash begins on the neck and spreads to the trunk and extremities. In 3–5 days, the rash begins to fade while the tips of the fingers and toes begins to peel. The tongue develops palatal petechiae. This is said to look like a strawberry and therefore is given the name "strawberry tongue."	the child is allergic to penicillin, erythromycin is given.	■ Encourage the child to replace toothbrush because the organism may be residing there.
Streptococcus B is caused by group B or beta streptococci (GBS).	*Transmission:* Direct contact with body fluids; intrauterine to the fetus *Incubation period:* less than 7 days	Newborn symptoms include: *Early onset:* Usually occurs within the first 24 hours of life. The newborn has respiratory distress, apnea, and signs of shock. Meconium-stained fluid may be seen at birth. *Late onset:* Between 1–4 weeks, the newborn may develop lethargy, fever, anorexia, and bulging fontanelles. Later effects include blindness, deafness, mental retardation, learning disabilities, and death.	*Diagnostic:* complete blood count, chest x-ray, culture of body fluids *Preventative measures:* Screening of pregnant women for GBS at 35–37 weeks. Intrapartum administration of ampicillin is indicated if the mother tests positive to reduce the risk of newborn infection. *Medical treatment:* Administration of antibiotics, particularly ampicillin and gentamycin.	■ Observe closely for symptoms of respiratory distress. ■ Keep the infant warm and free from drafts. Chilling increases the risk of respiratory distress. ■ Closely monitor intake and output.

Infectious Diseases Transmitted by Insects or Animals

Many infections are transmitted from human to human. However, some infections may be transmitted to humans from animals or from insects.

LYME DISEASE

Lyme disease is caused by *Borrelia burgdorferi*. It can be transmitted through a tick bite, with an incubation period of 3 to 32 days following the tick bite. Lyme disease is characterized by three stages. In stage 1, the child may have **erythema migrans** (Figure 26-3 ■; a red rash with a bull's eye appearance at the site of the bite). The rash will resolve spontaneously in 4 weeks. Other symptoms in stage 1 include malaise, headache, stiff neck, low-grade fever, and muscle or joint aches. Stage 2 is characterized by pain and swelling of the joints, facial palsy, meningitis, and atrioventricular (AV) block occurring 1 to 4 months after the bite. In stage 3, the child has advanced musculoskeletal pain, deafness, and encephalopathy.

Depending on geographic location, a client who presents with possible Lyme disease may need to be tested for babesiosis and possibly ehrlichiosis. Some emergency rooms routinely screen for these diseases. A client who is not improving with antibiotics should be suspected of having a second bloodborne parasite.

Diagnosis of Lyme disease is determined by enzyme-linked immunoabsorbent assay or the Western blot tests. Clinical management of the child with Lyme disease includes administering antibiotics, assisting the child in avoiding fatigue by encouraging rest and avoiding strenuous physical activity, and providing pharmacologic and nonpharmacologic pain relief measures.

Parents should be taught the proper method of removing a tick. The nurse can teach the parents to use tweezers to grasp the tick where it has attached to the child's body and to pull gently. Discourage them from squeezing the body of the tick. Teach them to inspect the tick to determine whether the entire tick was removed. (Disease transmission depends on the length of time the tick is attached [some say 24 hours]. If the body of the tick is removed but the head remains embedded in the skin, the disease can still be transmitted.)

ROCKY MOUNTAIN SPOTTED FEVER

Rocky Mountain spotted fever, also called *tickborne typhus fever* or *São Paulo typhus*, is caused by *Rickettsia rickettsii*. It is also transmitted through a tick bite. The incubation period is 2 to 12 days after a tick bite with an average of 7 days. The child with Rocky Mountain spotted fever may experience moderate to high fever, which lasts 2 to 3 weeks, malaise, abdominal and muscle pain, nausea and vomiting, a severe headache that is unrelieved, and conjunctival infection. A maculopapular rash that blanches begins on days 3 to 5 (Figure 26-4 ■). It is first found on the extremities and spreads to the trunk. It progresses from maculopapular in nature to petechial (see examples in Figure 24-3 ⬤⬤). There is also a risk of gastrointestinal bleeding, disseminated intravascular coagulation (DIC), pulmonary complications, encephalitis, neurologic dysfunction, and cardiac and renal complications.

Indirect immunofluorescent antibody assay, enzyme immunoassay, or indirect hemagglutination test may be used to diagnose Rocky Mountain spotted fever. Clinical management of children with Rocky Mountain spotted fever includes the administration of antibiotics. The drug of choice is doxycycline. Children should be observed carefully for abnormal bleeding. Emergency equipment should be available in case the child goes into shock. The nurse can help the child avoid fatigue by encouraging rest and discouraging strenuous physical activity. The nurse can also administer pharmacologic and nonpharmacologic pain relief measures.

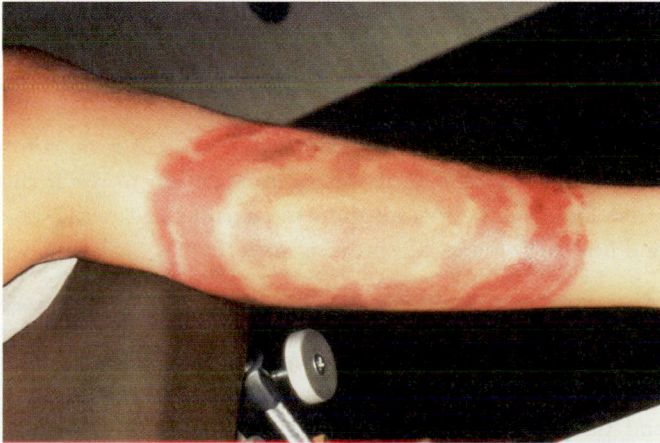

Figure 26-3. ■ Erythema migrans ("target" sign in Lyme disease). (Peter Arnold, Inc.)

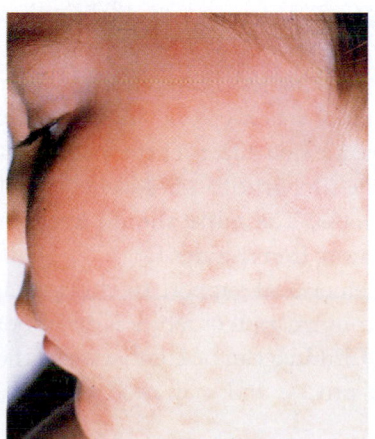

Figure 26-4. ■ Rocky Mountain spotted fever.

PROTECTION AGAINST TICK BITES

For children living in tick-prone areas, the nurse may assist the health care team in implementing preventative measures. These include a three-dose vaccination, LYMErix, to protect against *B. burgdorferi*. LYMErix is recommended for children ages 15 years and older. Children should learn to recognize and avoid tick-infested areas. When walking or playing in these areas, children should wear protective clothing. After being outdoors, the child and parents should routinely look for ticks carefully and remove them promptly. Inspect repellents containing DEET are effective in preventing tick bites. Parents should only apply this chemical when the child is in a high-risk area because there are associated side effects with this product. The insect repellent should not be used on the face, hands, or anywhere the child has a skin irritation. It should be washed off carefully with soap and water.

RABIES

Rabies is caused by *Rhabdoviridae*. Transmission of this harmful organism occurs due to a bite from an animal infected with rabies. The incubation period for *Rhabdoviridae* is 1 to 7 weeks, with an average of 6 weeks. The child is commonly asymptomatic during the incubation period. Initial symptoms include pain at the site of the bite, headache, fever, anorexia, and malaise. Half of the children develop **hydrophobia,** a reflex contraction at the sight of liquid accompanied by painful contractures in the muscles used for swallowing. Hallucinations, disorientations, manic episodes, seizures, stupor, coma, and death may occur. Diagnosis of rabies is confirmed by fluorescent antibody staining of the dead animal's brain tissue.

Clinical management of the child with rabies includes irrigating and washing the animal bite thoroughly as quickly as possible after the bite occurs. The wound may need suturing. It is important to administer human rabies immune globulin and human diploid cell rabies vaccine (HDCV) as soon as possible after the bite occurs. HDCV is given in five doses on days 0, 3, 7, 14, and 28. If the animal is found to be rabies free, the series may be stopped. For the child who is diagnosed with rabies, hospitalization is necessary, and contact precautions need to be implemented. The nurse should observe for side effects of the vaccine, which include irritation at the site, pruritus, headache, muscle aches, nausea, and dizziness. The nurse should keep the child with hydrophobia away from liquids.

Providing emotional support to children and their parents prior to confirmation of rabies is an important nursing intervention. Children can be combative in the latter stages of the disease process and may need sedation to avoid exhaustion.

Preventative measures related to rabies include vaccination of all domestic animals against rabies. Children should

---

BOX 26-2	CLIENT TEACHING

Recognizing a Rabid Animal

For an unvaccinated animal to become infected with rabies, it must suffer a bite from an infected animal. Early signs of rabies in an animal are behavioral changes, fever, slow eye reflexes, and chewing at the bite site. After several days, the animal will be irritable, restless, and aggressive; bark frequently; viciously attack inanimate objects; and appear disoriented. Finally, the animal will develop paralysis, starting with the limb that was bitten. As the throat and face become paralyzed, the bark changes, a foamy drool develops, and the jaw drops. Death usually occurs from respiratory paralysis.

---

be taught the dangers of interacting with stray or dead animals. Box 26-2 ■ provides information on how to recognize a rabid animal.

Sexually Transmitted Infections

Several sexually transmitted infections (STIs) may be acquired prenatally or at birth. These diseases include herpes, HIV, gonorrhea, and chlamydia. For more information about the newborn and these diseases, review Chapter 9 ⚭. HIV is discussed in Chapter 21 ⚭.

There are a variety of ways that children and adolescents can become infected with STIs. These include sexual experimentation, sexual play, molestation, and sexual abuse. Sexual abuse must be considered when a child presents to the health care provider with diseases such as syphilis and gonorrhea. See Chapter 5 ⚭ for discussion of these specific diseases. See Chapter 27 ⚭ for more discussion of sexual abuse.

NURSING CARE

PRIORITIES IN NURSING CARE

When caring for children with communicable diseases, the nursing care focus should be on determining symptoms and the degree of severity of the symptoms. Priority care of these children includes managing fever, preventing respiratory distress, promoting skin integrity, and ensuring comfort. The nurse uses skills in communication to teach the child and his or her parents how to manage the care at home and how to prevent the spread of infection.

ASSESSING

The nurse is responsible for assessing the child for symptoms of hyperthermia such as flushed skin, increased body and skin temperature, and increased heart and respiratory rates. Children with fevers should be observed for fluid loss and seizure activity. Observe the child for other signs of

Nontraditional Care of Communicable Disease

During periods of illness, alternative medical practices called *coining* and *cupping* may be practiced to relieve pruritus and symptoms of influenza such as muscle aches. This practice may be found among some people of Southeast Asian origin and also among Russian immigrants and Mexican American families.

In coining, a practitioner trained in the practice massages the client's chest, back, and shoulders with medicated ointment. A copper coin or silver spoon is then used to rub down the body parts in a linear fashion. Dark marks are left on the body for several days.

The practice of cupping is done by coating a small jar with alcohol. The jar is then held upside down, and a lighted match burns off the oxygen and creates a vacuum. The jar is then quickly placed on the skin. The vacuum draws the jar, creating a bruiselike mark. Such marks may appear at first glance to be physical child abuse. It is important to explore whether the child was treated with this culturally accepted practice. (See Figure 26-5.)

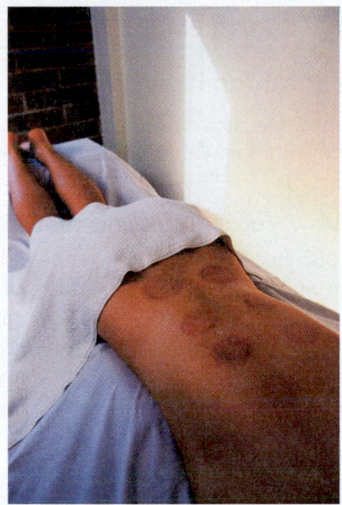

A

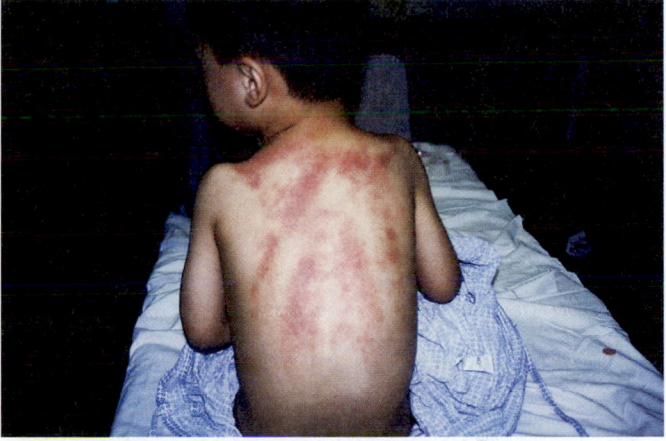

B

Figure 26-5. ■ Cupping (**A**) and coining (**B**) are non-Western healing practices of some cultural groups that must be distinguished from child abuse. (**A**: Getty Images, Inc.- Photodisc. **B**: Fran Nadel, MD.)

infections, including a change in activity level, a change in appetite, nausea and vomiting, and diarrhea.

Assessment of the child's respiratory status is important. Besides the respiratory rate, assess the depth and rhythm of respirations. Listen to breath sounds anteriorly and posteriorly. Characterize the child's cough. Evaluate the color and consistency of sputum. Look for restlessness, difficulty with speech, orthopnea, and cyanosis.

Ask the verbal child for a report of his or her discomfort and pain. Use pain scales appropriate to the child's age. Observe closely for nonverbal expressions of pain and discomfort such as grimacing, limited attention span, and withdrawal.

Assess the child's rashes and lesions for distribution, shape, color, size, and consistency. Determine the presence of prurititis and the degree of discomfort it is causing the child.

Note: Some Eastern cultures may practice traditional medicine that could raise suspicion of abuse. Box 26-3 ■ describes the practices of cupping and coining. Figure 26-5 ■ illustrates these practices.

DIAGNOSING, PLANNING, AND IMPLEMENTING

Nursing diagnoses for children with communicable diseases might include:

- Hyperthermia, related to the infectious process
- Ineffective Airway Clearance, related to airway spasm, excessive or retained secretions
- Acute Pain, related to skin lesions, pharyngitis, cough, chest congestion, etc.

- Impaired Skin Integrity, related to rash, pox, and swelling of the parotid gland.

Some outcomes for children with communicable diseases might include that the child will:

- Maintain body temperature within normal limits
- Have a patent airway
- Communicate lack of pain or reduced discomfort
- Be free of complications related to rash, lesions, and blisters (e.g., no purulent drainage, no bleeding of the lesions, no scarring).

The nurse's role in providing support to these children would include the following:

- Avoid the use of aspirin to relieve fever. Use acetaminophen or ibuprofen. *Aspirin increases the risk of Reye's syndrome.*
- Implement other methods of cooling the child, such as removing excess clothing, applying cool washcloths, using

BOX 26-4	COMPLEMENTARY THERAPIES

Methods for Soothing Itchy Skin

Chickenpox can cause extreme itching in children. Several natural remedies are available using common household products.

- Parents can mix ½ cup of vinegar into the bathwater.
- Oatmeal has also been found to relieve the discomfort caused by the virus. Parents can cook 2 cups of oatmeal according to manufacturer's directions. This mixture should be placed into a small cotton bag and secured at the top. The bag is then floated in a warm bath. As the water becomes milky, the solution should be splashed onto the lesions.
- A mixture of baking soda and water can be sponged onto the child's skin and allowed to dry thoroughly.

a circulating fan, or using a cooling blanket. *These methods supplement the use of antipyretics.*

- Encourage adequate intake of oral fluids. *This prevents dehydration.*
- Administer humidified oxygen as ordered.
- Encourage ambulation if there are no contraindications. If the child cannot ambulate, turn him or her from side to side every 2 hours. *This will promote movement of secretions.*
- Suction the nasopharynx or oropharynx. *This removes secretions blocking the airway.*
- Provide distractions and diversions such as board games, video games, movies, and puzzles. *This promotes comfort.*
- Manage environmental aspects such as soiled linens, bright lights, warm room temperature, and loud verbal conversations. *These aspects might contribute to the child's discomfort. For instance, a warm room increases the incidence of itching.*
- Provide antihistamines as ordered. Teach parents alternative forms of soothing itchy skin for use at home (Box 26-4 ■). *Antihistamines and alternative therapies assist in the control of itching.*
- Keep fingernails clean and short. *This decreases the risk of additional trauma to the skin and secondary infections.*
- If necessary, apply mittens. *This may prevent scratching.*
- Keep skin dry and clean. *Wet, dirty skin could aggravate itching.*

EVALUATING

Changes in vital signs, intake and output, and comfort levels need to be documented and reported to the supervising nurse. Changes in skin lesions need to be documented according to distribution, shape, color, size, and consistency. The effectiveness of analgesics, antipyretics, antibiotics, and antihistamines should be documented.

NURSING PROCESS CARE PLAN
Child with Chickenpox

Mrs. Word calls the family practice clinic because her 4-year-old daughter, Molly, has the chickenpox. Molly's sister had them last week. Mrs. Word is concerned because Molly is scratching her skin. Mrs. Word asks the nurse for suggestions to keep Molly from scratching. She is very concerned that scarring will occur, especially on Molly's face.

Assessment. The following data should be collected as soon as possible:

- History of present illness
- Risk factors that would contribute to impaired skin integrity such as bowel and bladder control, poor nutritional status, pre-existing skin conditions, impaired cognitive ability, and impaired circulation
- Other possible irritants such as restrictive clothing and harsh body soaps or laundry detergents
- Thorough skin assessment (see Chapter 24 ⦵)
- Current stage of the lesions, including color, distribution, skin temperature, moisture, erythema, and size of the lesions.

Nursing Diagnosis. The following important nursing diagnosis (among others) is established for this client:

- Risk for Impaired Skin Integrity, related to frequent scratching

Expected Outcomes

- Skin will show no evidence of scratching.
- There will be no complications related to scratching such as irritation, infection cellulitis, or scarring.

Planning and Implementation

- Encourage Mrs. Word to use a mild soap to keep Molly's skin clean and as free of bacteria as possible.
- If Molly still wears a diaper to bed, Mrs. Word needs to be taught that this can irritate her skin and increase irritation. Encourage Mrs. Word to awaken Molly and take her to the toilet once during the night.
- Cut Molly's fingernails short so they do not cut her skin. This could also provide a diversion activity if Mrs. Word chooses to give Molly a "manicure."
- Encourage Mrs. Word to keep Molly's hands busy during the day. She could color, paint, dress her dolls, play with modeling clay, or work puzzles.
- Suggest that Mrs. Word give Molly Benadryl (diphenhydramine hydrochloride) to prevent scratching when Molly is particularly uncomfortable.
- Suggest topical agents such as calamine lotion, oatmeal baths, or baking soda baths to make Molly more comfortable.

- Teach Mrs. Word how to recognize skin irritation, infection, and cellulitis.

Evaluation. Mrs. Word reports that Molly is enjoying her new easel and paints. She is administering Benadryl after lunch and giving her a nightly bath in baking soda. Many of the lesions are beginning to crust over.

Critical Thinking in the Nursing Process

1. Molly's Aunt Betty is 16 weeks pregnant. Aunt Betty is unsure whether she has had the chickenpox. What information would you give Mrs. Word concerning Aunt Betty's risk of contracting chickenpox?

2. What is the proper response to a parent who says he or she decided to tie the child's hands to the bed to keep them from scratching?
3. What information would the nurse give to parents to help them recognize symptoms of infection or cellulitis?

Note: Discussion of Critical Thinking questions appears in Appendix I.

Note: The references and resources for this and all chapters have been compiled at the back of the book.

Chapter Review

KEY TERMS by Topic

Use the audio glossary feature of either the CD-ROM or the Companion Website to hear the correct pronunciation of the following key terms.

Introduction
communicable diseases

Chain of Infection
pathogens, reservoir, portal of exit, transmission, portal of entry, susceptible host, droplet method, airborne transmission, fomites, incubation period, prodromal period, illness, convalescent period

Risk Factors for Communicable Diseases in Children
active immunity, passive immunity, bioterrorism, universal precautions, seasonal flu, avian flu, pandemic flu, antigenic drift, antigenic shift, standard precautions, transmission-based precautions, reverse isolation

Immunizations
immunization, vaccine

Common Infections
opisthotonos, Koplik's spots, desquamation, orchitis, Forschheimer spots

Infectious Diseases Transmitted by Insects or Animals
erythema migrans, hydrophobia

KEY Points

- The nurse has an important role in recognizing these diseases and assisting the family in obtaining appropriate care. Another important nursing role is client and family teaching regarding methods of disease prevention.

- For a disease to be transmitted from person to person, there must be a pathogen, reservoir, portal of exit, portal of entry, and susceptible host.

- Stages of the infectious process include the incubation period, the prodromal period, illness or the stage where clinical symptoms appear, and the convalescent period.

- The single most effective way to prevent the spread of communicable diseases is through hand washing.

- Nursing care for children with communicable diseases includes a variety of standards and precautions designed to prevent transmission of the disease or protect the child from additional harmful bacteria. The nurse must be able to implement the following precautions: universal, standard, airborne, droplet, contact, and reverse isolation.

- Immunizations are an essential tool to protect children against communicable diseases.

- Children living in tick-prone areas need added protection from tick bites, which may cause Lyme disease and Rocky Mountain spotted fever. This protection includes insect repellent, long-sleeved shirts, long pants, and a hat when in tick-prone areas and vaccination with LYMErix for older children.

- Comfort measures for children with communicable diseases include pain relief measures and measures to relieve pruritus.

EXPLORE Media Link

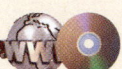

Additional interactive resources for this chapter can be found on the Companion Website at www.prenhall.com/towle.

Click on Chapter 26 and "Begin" to select the activities for this chapter.

For chapter-related NCLEX-style questions and an audio glossary, access the accompanying CD-ROM in this book.

Animations

Throat culture

FOR FURTHER Study

See Chapter 5 for more discussion about STIs.

For more information about the newborn, review Chapter 9.

Chapters 12 and 13 provide procedural steps for giving immunizations.

For more information on meningitis, see Chapter 16.

Acute rheumatic fever is discussed in Chapter 19.

For more information on HIV, the child's immune system, and organ transplantation, see Chapter 21.

For a review of skin assessment and disorders, see Chapter 24.

See Chapter 27 for more discussion about effects of disasters on children and sexual abuse.

See Appendix II for the U.S. recommended immunization schedule from the CDC.

See Appendix VIII for a brief review of precautions.

Caring for a Client Requiring Droplet Precautions

NCLEX-PN® Focus Area: Safety

Case Study: Wendy, a 2-year-old, is admitted to the pediatric unit with a diagnosis of diphtheria. She was recently adopted from an orphanage in Kiev, Russia. Due to her condition, she is placed on droplet precautions and is given a private room. Wendy's adoptive parents decide to stay overnight with her. However, the first time the nurse walks into the room with a mask on, Wendy begins to scream loudly and cry inconsolably.

Nursing Diagnosis Fear, related to unfamiliar environment and people

COLLECT DATA

Subjective	Objective

Would you report this? Yes/No

If yes, to: _____

Nursing Care

_____
_____
_____
_____
_____
_____
_____
_____
_____
_____
_____
_____

How would you document this? _____
_____
_____
_____

Data Collected
(use those that apply)

- Screaming loudly
- Crying inconsolably
- Harsh cough
- Clenched fists
- Resting with eyes closed in adoptive mother's arms
- Clutches toy stuffed frog while sobbing loudly
- T 99.6
- R 12 and labored
- Rhinorrhea
- Tightened jaw
- Immediately hides head in mother's lap when nurse with mask approaches

Nursing Interventions
(use those that apply; list in priority order)

- Monitor closely for signs of increasing respiratory distress.
- Keep oral airway, suction equipment, and Ambu bag close at hand.
- Provide Wendy with a mask to put on her frog.
- Stand further than 3 ft away from Wendy, remove the mask, and greet Wendy pleasantly each time the nurse enters the room. Replace mask. Repeat several times prior to moving close to Wendy.
- Administer oxygen as ordered.
- Suction prn.
- Avoid approaching Wendy or touching her unless she is being held by her adoptive mother or father.
- Administer antibiotics as ordered.
- Provide Wendy with age-appropriate diversional activities such as blocks.
- Give the child a surgical mask to try on.

Compare your documentation to the sample provided in Appendix I.

NCLEX-PN® Exam Preparation

1. The nurse has just completed instruction about active and passive immunity to a couple who is expecting their first child and realizes additional instruction is needed when the wife states:
   1. "My child will be protected for life from many diseases through passive immunity."
   2. "My child will develop active immunity by producing antibodies to specific organisms."
   3. "Through active immunity, my child will develop long-term protection against organisms."
   4. "Passive immunity is what my child gets from me and is short-term protection."

2. The mother of an 11-month-old is upset because her child seems to be frequently sick. From the knowledge the nurse has about communicable diseases and susceptibility of children that age, the nurse is able to share some educational points with the mother. The nurse tells the mother that:
   1. by age 1, the child will have adult levels of immunoglobulin M antibodies.
   2. the child has higher neutrophil levels so should be able to ward off disease.
   3. the child's immune system is fully mature at birth.
   4. the child must wear gloves when playing with others to prevent disease transmission.

3. The nurse is going to be caring for an infant who was exposed to the varicella virus before birth and has been diagnosed with congenital varicella syndrome. The nurse knows that this is characterized by certain symptoms, which are:
   1. asthma, rash, and otitis media.
   2. eye and brain defects and underdeveloped arms and legs.
   3. polydactyly, pneumocephalus, and rhinitis.
   4. urticaria, seborrhea, and psoriasis.

4. The nurse administers a DTaP immunization to a 6-month-old child at the physician's office. The mother calls the office the next day and tells the nurse that the area around the injection site is red and swollen. The nurse instructs the mother to:
   1. ignore the redness and swelling.
   2. rush the child to the nearest hospital.
   3. apply vinegar to the site.
   4. place a covered ice pack on the injection site.

5. The nurse is preparing an injection of measles, mumps, rubella vaccine and notices that the child is allergic to neomycin. The nurse plans to:
   1. administer the immunization.
   2. administer a smaller dose of the immunization.
   3. not give the immunization.
   4. give the immunization at a later date.

6. A child with roseola is brought into a clinic. While the nurse is providing instructions about care, the mother tells the nurse that she is worried that all of her children will contract roseola. The nurse tells the mother that:
   1. the disease is transmitted through uncooked foods.
   2. the disease is transmitted through contact with bodily fluids.
   3. the cause of the disease is unknown.
   4. the disease is transmitted through unpasteurized milk.

7. The nurse is providing home instructions to the parents of a child diagnosed with infectious mononucleosis. The nurse instructs the parents:
   1. to allow the child to return to school.
   2. to notify the physician if the child develops a fever of greater than 99.9°F.
   3. to keep the child supine for 1 week.
   4. to notify the physician if the child develops abdominal pain or left shoulder pain.

8. The nurse has listened to the news about the avian flu, its possibility of transmission, and its threat to humans. The parents of a child are in the clinic for a well-child visit and ask the nurse about the avian flu. The nurse responds:
   1. "The avian flu cannot be transmitted to humans."
   2. "There is a vaccine available for the avian-flu for children older than 3 years."
   3. "The avian flu is transmitted through eating the meat of infected pork."
   4. "There is no human immunity or vaccine available for the avian flu."

9. Select the statements about universal precautions that the nurse would use to explain this term. Choose all that apply.
   1. It is designed to prevent transmission of HIV.
   2. It is designed to prevent transmission of HBV.
   3. It is designed to prevent transmission of disease-producing micro-organisms transmitted by means of blood, tissue, and body fluids containing blood.
   4. It is a standard to follow when providing health care to clients.
   5. It is the same as transmission-based precautions.

10. Choose which statements describe standard precautions. Select all that apply.
    1. Use mouthpieces, resuscitation bags, or other ventilation devices for mouth-to-mouth resuscitation.
    2. Handle sharp instruments properly to avoid exposure.
    3. Wear a clean, nonsterile gown to protect skin and prevent soiling of the uniform by contact with body fluids.
    4. Immunize with the HBV vaccine.
    5. Wear masks, eye protection, or a face shield when there is a possibility of contacting body fluids during certain procedures.
    6. Hand wash with plain soap and water before and after client contact.

Answers for Review Questions, as well as discussion of Care Plan and Critical Thinking Care Map questions, appear in Appendix I.

Chapter 27

Care of the Child with Psychosocial Disorders

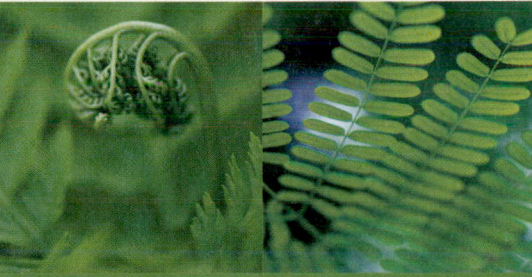

BRIEF Outline

Brief Assessment Overview

Psychological Disorders and Associated Manifestations

Nursing Care

Anorexia Nervosa and Bulimia

Nursing Care

Abuse and Family Violence

Nursing Care

Traumatic Events

Therapies to Assist the Child with Psychosocial Disorders

NURSING PROCESS CARE PLAN:
Client with Anorexia Nervosa

HEALTH PROMOTION ISSUE:
Preventing Infant Abduction

CRITICAL THINKING CARE MAP:
Caring for a Client with Attention-Deficit/Hyperactivity Disorder

LEARNING Outcomes

After completing this chapter, you will be able to:

- Describe an appropriate psychosocial assessment of the child.
- Describe psychosocial disorders to include autism, Asperger's syndrome, attention deficit disorder, Giles de la Tourette syndrome, anxiety, depression, anorexia nervosa and bulimia, child abuse (physical and emotional), and substance abuse.
- Describe associated manifestations of psychological disorders to include overeating and obesity and suicide.
- Discuss clinical manifestations, diagnostic procedures, medical management, and nursing interventions related to psychosocial disorders.
- Explain appropriate nursing interventions for children with psychosocial disorders.
- Discuss the impact of traumatic events and natural disasters on children.

Psychosocial health includes mental, emotional, social, and spiritual stability. Usually by age 8, children have developed the ability to think rationally and perceive situations realistically. The child who is emotionally healthy feels appropriately about life's circumstances. Stress is tolerated and coping skills are demonstrated. The child who is socially healthy has effective relationships, and his or her actions are appropriate in social situations. Spiritual health encompasses the child's belief system, his or her set of values, and how he or she makes choices; it includes the meaning given to life's circumstances (D'Amico & Barbarito, 2007). Psychosocial health is affected by many factors such as genetics, physical health, family, culture, geography, economic status, and self-concept. Alterations in a child's psychosocial health will affect about one-fourth of all children (Ball & Bindler, 2006). Some of these alterations will be short term, whereas others will have lifelong effects.

Brief Assessment Overview

To accurately assess the child, the nurse must review physical health, mental health, and spiritual health. **Holistic health** is a concept that approaches an individual's health as an integrated system rather than divided into physical, emotional, intellectual, and spiritual parts. Belief in this concept allows the nurse to understand that any alteration in the child's psychosocial health could have an effect on the physical health, while alterations in physical health could have psychosocial ramifications.

HISTORY

- Determine the child's past emotional or psychiatric problems.
- Determine the family history of emotional or psychiatric problems.
- Ask about the child's growth and development.
- Inquire about the child's performance in school and other organized activities.
- Inquire about the child's relationships with others.
- Determine the child's emotional response to illness and crises. Ask him or her to define the greatest source of comfort during these stressful times.
- Ask older children and teens to define their concept of hope and faith.
- Determine self-concept. Ask older children and teens how they would describe themselves to others.
- Ask specifically about the use of alcohol and street drugs.
- Ask older children and teens about eating disorders such as anorexia nervosa or bulimia.
- See the following sections for child abuse and sexual abuse screening.

PHYSICAL

- Observe the child's general appearance. Describe dress, hygiene, and grooming.
- If bulimia is suspected, inspect dental enamel of the teeth. Worn enamel can occur from gastric acid produced during purging.
- Describe the child's facial expression and affect.
- Observe the child's body posture and gait.
- Describe the child's speech patterns. Is the content of the child's speech appropriate? What is the tone, pace, and volume of the speech? Does the child talk to him- or herself? Is he or she aphasic or incoherent?

Psychological Disorders and Associated Manifestations

The ***Diagnostic and Statistical Manual of Mental Disorders, Fourth Edition*** (DSM-IV), which is published by the American Psychiatric Association, serves as the main diagnostic reference of mental health professionals in the United States. This resource includes diagnostic criteria for the most common mental disorders. It is also used for research purposes and by insurance companies to apply charges for services offered by mental health professionals. Appropriate use of the diagnostic criteria is said to require clinical training. Refer to a psychiatric nursing text for more information about this resource.

Psychological disorders include a wide range of disorders that may begin at birth or early childhood and may continue throughout life. These include psychological disorders such as autism, attention deficit disorders (ADDs), attention deficit hyperactivity disorders (ADHDs), anxiety, phobias, and depression. Also see Chapter 16 ⚭ for a further discussion of cognitive disorders.

Psychological disorders involve abnormalities in behavior, communication, and social interactions. Depending on the cause of the specific disorder, the child's development might progress to a point and then stop, progress to a point and then regress, or fail to develop beyond the infantile state.

Children with some psychological disorders engage in repetitive behaviors, including self-stimulating or self-destructive behaviors. The repetitive behaviors might include, but are not limited to, twirling in circles, head banging, and biting themselves. Some of these children may have difficulty sitting quietly for any length of time and focusing on a productive activity. They run around the room and "get into everything." Other children with psychological disorders focus on only one activity and seem to "block out" everything that is going on around them.

Difficulty with speech (both with talking and with understanding the spoken word) is common. Although some children may eventually learn to talk, abnormal patterns may develop. Cognitive abilities may correspond with intellectual deficits. Learning may be difficult, and the child may struggle in school. Other children may learn but have difficulty expressing what they know.

Children with psychological disorders demonstrate a wide range of social skills. They may have difficulty establishing relationships because of speech problems or lack of focus. Disrupted thought processes may cause the child to be anxious, develop phobias, overeat, or become depressed and even consider suicide. Some children and adults may be fearful of children with a psychological disorder and avoid interacting with them.

AUTISM AND ASPERGER'S SYNDROME

According to the Autism Society of America, **autism** is "a complex developmental disability that typically appears during the first three years of life and is the result of a neurological disorder that affects the normal functioning of the brain, impacting development in the areas of social interaction and communication skills." Children with autism have difficulty with verbal and nonverbal communication, social interactions, and leisure or play activities (Figure 27-1 ■)

Autism is found to affect boys more often than girls. There is no known cause for autism. It is believed to be genetically inherited. Autism is associated with congenital rubella syndrome, *fragile X syndrome* (a congenital disorder causing mental retardation), phenylketonuria, Down syndrome, and tuberous sclerosis.

Another disorder that is similar to autism is **Asperger's syndrome.** In this disorder, the child exhibits social isolation, communication difficulties, clumsiness, and a focused area of interest and attention. For instance, the child may be preoccupied with automobiles, knowing the names of all makes and models. Asperger's syndrome usually has a later onset than autism.

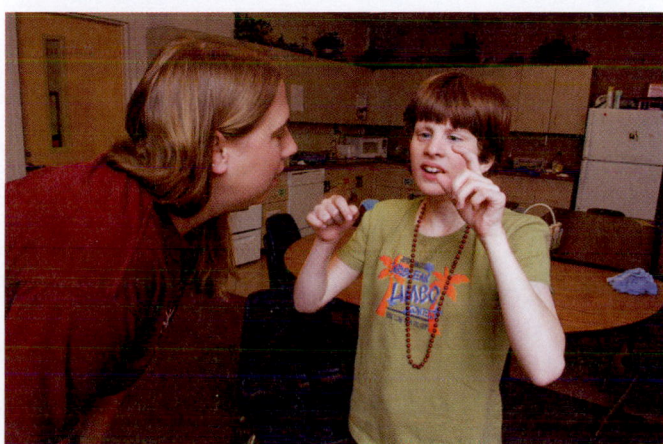

Figure 27-1. ■ Child with autistic disorder.
(Robin Nelson/PhotoEdit, Inc.)

Manifestations

Prior to diagnosis of autism, the infant may show a lack of response to sounds, have difficulty sleeping or sleep longer than expected, have difficulty feeding, avoid eye contact, or show little to no response to human interaction. The toddler who is autistic may suddenly be unable to communicate verbally. Words may be incessantly repeated. This is called **echolalia.** The toddler, who is expected to have stranger anxiety, demonstrates no fear in unfamiliar surroundings or around unfamiliar people. Toilet training may also be very difficult in the toddler with autism.

Autism is marked in the child by the presence of excessive repetitive behaviors such as hand movements or rocking. These rigid and obsessive behaviors are also called **stereotypy.** The child may appear stiff, unwilling to cuddle, and have an awkward gait. Repetitive sounds and loud responses to being touched are also noticed. The child is unable to interact with others socially and is often observed playing alone. Certain objects or toys have significance, and the child may not be able to eat, go to school, or go to sleep without them. They will also have either exaggerated responses to pain or a minimal response.

Diagnosis and Treatment

The diagnosis of autism is made by the presence of symptoms. Other conditions that may mimic symptoms of autism are ruled out by computed tomography (CT) scans, magnetic resonance imaging (MRI) scans, tests for lead poisoning, hearing tests, metabolic studies, and electroencephalograms. There are also several instruments available to use in screening for autism. For more information on these instruments, refer to a psychiatric nursing text.

Although there is no cure for autism, many researchers in the field agree that early, intensive interventions prior to age 5 can lead to behavior modification. A highly structured environment, with one-on-one interaction, is necessary for some children and therefore the parents and each caregiver need extensive training to promote success. Children may also be mainstreamed into public school systems. Eye contact, appropriate language, social skills, and proper methods of play are encouraged. Negative behaviors are discouraged by close supervision and consistency. Restraint may be necessary until the behavior is changed. Stimulants, selective serotonin reuptake inhibitors, and mood stabilizers may be prescribed to assist the interventions.

Nursing Considerations

It is important for the nurse caring for the child in either the outpatient or the inpatient setting to carefully determine the child's rituals and communication patterns. The setting for health care should be altered to accommodate the needs of the child. For instance, if the child has a specific toy that brings him or her comfort, he or she should be allowed to keep it with him or her. Parents should be encouraged to stay with the child to provide familiarity.

Children with autism may pose a safety risk due to repetitive behaviors such as head banging and the lack of fear of dangerous situations. The nurse can provide devices such as helmets and hand mittens to protect the child from injury. The environment should be carefully scrutinized, modified, and supervised to promote safety. Parents should receive referrals to agencies and support groups or long-term care facilities to assist them in managing care of the child with autism.

ATTENTION DEFICIT DISORDER AND ATTENTION DEFICIT/HYPERACTIVITY DISORDER

ADD and ADHD are most commonly identified as the older child enters school. ADD is a central nervous system (CNS) disorder characterized by inappropriate behaviors related to attention. ADHD involves inattention, hyperactivity, and impulsiveness. Worldwide, 6% to 8% of school-age children are diagnosed with ADHD (Faraone, 2003). In the United States, 3.8 million school-age children have the disorder (Vlam, 2006).

Manifestations

Children with ADD have difficulty finishing tasks. They are easily distracted and may move from topic to topic in their speech and activities. Some children with ADD are quietly distractible. They may have difficulty working with others.

Children with ADHD also have difficulty finishing tasks, but (unlike children with ADD) they fidget, may become loud, and disrupt others. Both ADD and ADHD children have difficulty maintaining social relationships, and they may be teased or shunned by other children.

Diagnosis

The child who is suspected of having ADD or ADHD should be evaluated by a mental health specialist, primary care physician, or advanced practice registered nurse. The health care professional reviews the medical and social history of the child. There are several tools available to assist in the diagnosis of ADHD. These include parent scales, teacher scales, and those that close relatives or caregivers complete. These scales assess achievement and performance in the classroom, self-esteem, interactions with others, impulsive behaviors, hyperactivity, ability to pay attention, and level of anxiety. The *Diagnostic and Statistical Manual of Mental Disorders* of the American Psychiatric Association's criteria for diagnosis include:

- At least six of nine inattentive symptoms and/or six of nine hyperactive or one impulsive symptom
- Duration of the symptoms longer than 6 months
- Symptoms evident in more than one setting (home, school, church, or community).

Treatment

If a diagnosis of ADD or ADHD is made, treatment may vary depending on the type and degree of disability. Treatment may include changing the environment, behavior modification, and medication.

Environmental changes include having the child use a separate desk in an area of the room where other students cannot distract him or her. However, ADD and ADHD children should also be made to feel important, valuable, and part of the class. Stimuli should be decreased. This can be accomplished by turning off the radio or television. However, some children benefit from listening to their head sets while working because it shuts out other external stimuli. Structure and routine need to be built into the child's day. Helping the child develop organizational skills is of great importance.

Professional counselors may be helpful in modifying the child's behavior and should be included in the care planning team. Establishing a system of rewards for appropriate behavior can help the child learn and foster a positive self-image. The expected behavior must be realistically achievable. If the child cannot receive frequent rewards, the behavior may not change. If consequences are necessary, they should follow quickly after the offense so the child can relate the consequence to the behavior.

The most commonly prescribed medications are stimulants. Common stimulants used in the treatment of ADD/ADHD are methylphenidate (Ritalin), dextroamphetamine sulfate (Dexedrine), and amphetamine sulfate (Adderal). Atomoxetine (Strattera), a specific noradrenergic reuptake inhibitor, is a more recent drug that is showing positive results. Other drugs such as antidepressants, antihypertensives, and arousal agents may also be used. The most recent medication approved by the U.S. Food and Drug Administration (FDA) is methylphenidate transdermal system (Daytrana). The patch is used once daily. It is designed to provide a sustained dosage and to stay on active children. Table 27-1 ■ lists some common medications used to treat ADD/ADHD and their usual side effects. Some medications may need to be taken at school. School personnel giving the medication should understand the safe administration of the drugs. "Drug holidays" may be implemented during vacation periods or during the summer months when academic performance is not required.

Nursing Considerations

The nurse should make sure parents understand the prescribed medication, including side effects. Insomnia can be prevented or corrected by taking the medication early in the day and by avoiding caffeine later in the day. It is also important to remove the computer, television, radio, and cell phone from the bedroom to eliminate activities that would

TABLE 27-1

Pharmacology: Medications Used to Treat ADD/ADHD

DRUG (COMMON BRAND NAME AND GENERIC)	USUAL ROUTE/DOSE	CLASSIFICATION AND PURPOSE	SELECTED SIDE EFFECTS	DON'T GIVE IF
Ritalin (methylphenidate hydrochloride)	5–10 mg before breakfast and lunch, increasing 5–10 mg/week prn. PO	Cerebral stimulant to provide mental focus	Dizziness, nervousness, insomnia, increase P&BP, blurred vision, dry mouth, loss of appetite if taken before meals (sometimes reported to slow growth)	After 6 P.M. to avoid insomnia
Adderall (amphetamine sulfate)	Child: 2.5–5 mg 1–2 times/day, increasing by 2.5–5 mg weekly PO Adolescent: 10 mg extended release once daily PO in morning; may increase by 5–10 mg at weekly intervals	Cerebral stimulant to provide alertness	Irritability, euphoria, palpitations, insomnia, restlessness	Within 6 hours of bedtime to avoid insomnia. Do not crush extended-release capsules.
Strattera (atomoxetine hydrochloride)	0.5–1.2 mg/kg/day PO	Psychotherapeutic agent to improve attentiveness and ability to follow through on tasks; diminishes hyperactivity	Anorexia, upset stomach, dizziness, tiredness, mood swings, insomnia, hypersomnia	The child reports hypotension or urinary retention
Wellbutrin (bupropion hydrochloride)	6 mg/kg/day PO	Antidepressant	Dizziness, agitation, insomnia, blurred vision, headache, tremor, nausea, vomiting, constipation, dry mouth	On an empty stomach
Provigil (modafinil)	100 mg/day PO	Cerebral stimulant, arousal agent	Headache, nausea	Child is less than 16 years old

prolong the initiation of sleep. The stimulant class of medications has a high potential for abuse. Discuss with the child and parents the need to secure medication at all times.

Families of children with ADD and ADHD require support. Parents may become frustrated with a child's behavior and inflict inappropriate punishments. A stable, routine environment will help the child focus. The parent needs to set boundaries and limits, and help the child learn to behave within them. Support groups may be beneficial to the parents.

The child with ADD or ADHD should be evaluated on a regular basis. Medications usually have an effect within the first 10 to 14 days of treatment. Behavior modification programs may take weeks or months to be effective. Small positive steps in behavioral change should be recognized.

ANXIETY

Anxiety is an emotion that everyone experiences at some time in life. However, in some people, the feeling is not related to actual past or upcoming events. When it exists consistently and out of proportion to reality, a diagnosis of anxiety may be made.

Manifestations

Subjective feelings of worry, helplessness, insecurity, and apprehension are characteristics of anxiety. Objective or physical symptoms often accompany these symptoms. These objectives symptoms include tachycardia, restlessness, diaphoresis, and trembling. Regressive behaviors may occur in some children. The child may experience enuresis and/or **encopresis** (a condition where the child delays defecation or experiences frequent soiling with feces). (For more information on enuresis, see Chapter 23 🔗.) Children with anxiety frequently learn to cope with it by withdrawing, avoiding situations, or becoming overly dependent on parents or other caregivers.

Generalized anxiety disorder (GAD) is also called overanxious disorder. The child is prone to excessive worry about the future. These worries are often imagined. Even if the worries never materialize, the child continues to demonstrate a pattern of worry. The child with **separation anxiety disorder (SAD)**, also called *anaclitic depression*, is fearful of separation from individuals or locations. Panic may set in as the child approaches the time and location of separation.

School phobia, also called school avoidance or school refusal, may be a type of SAD, although there may be other reasons the child refuses to go to school. Physical complaints usually accompany school phobia. These include stomachaches, headaches, and fever. School phobia may be associated with real stressors such as physical abuse or bullies. See the section on bullying later in this chapter for more information. School performance, sleep habits, and family and peer relationships are affected by school phobia. If the symptoms continue, the child's future education and employment may be affected. Children with school phobia have an increased risk of psychiatric disorders. Antidepressants may be effective in assisting the child to overcome the phobia.

Obsessive-compulsive disorder (OCD) is characterized by ritualistic thoughts or actions that interfere with activities of daily living. Children may have obsessions about germs, sexual activity, fears of traumatic events, or religious rituals. OCD may be associated with ADHD, tics, or hoarding behaviors. (*Note:* Tics may also occur in children as a result of high doses of medication.) Behavioral therapy can help the child learn to overcome fears and obsessions.

Treatment

All anxiety disorders should be recognized and dealt with promptly. Families and school personnel should be given proper information about the disorder and encouraged to assist in the relief measures. Real threats to the child's safety must be assessed and resolved if present. Children need to learn coping skills and relaxation techniques. Antidepressants and antianxiety medications may be used to assist the child with the initial relief of symptoms.

Nursing Considerations

The nurse can help the child develop coping methods. The child can be taught to replace negative thoughts with positive ones. For example, when the child feels anxious, he or she could repeat the phrase, "I am calm. I am in control." Physical activity decreases stress behaviors. Simply going on a 30-minute walk can help a child deal with symptoms of anxiety. Avoiding caffeine, tobacco, and other stimulants is essential to decreasing anxiety. The nurse should assess whether these habits are part of the child's life and, if so, encourage the child to replace these habits with healthy behaviors.

GILES DE LA TOURETTE SYNDROME

Giles de la Tourette syndrome is characterized by **tics** (sudden, rapid motor movements of the head, eyes, and upper body) and a variety of verbal noises. In Tourette syndrome, children may utter obscenities, profanities, or racial slurs (**coprolalia**) and may involuntarily gesture obscenely (**copropraxia**).

Tourette syndrome is believed to be genetically caused and occurs more commonly in boys than in girls. It is most often treated in children with pimozide (Orap), a dopamine receptor antagonist. The nurse must provide parental support and assist in helping the child achieve normal development. Because the tic behavior can occur more commonly during stressful periods, stress reduction techniques can be taught. If the child is unable to attend school while the tics are uncontrolled, the nurse can assist the parents in arranging for home tutoring.

DEPRESSION

Depression is a persistent feeling of sadness or hopelessness. It affects approximately 2% of children and 5% of adolescents with increased numbers in the older adolescent. Characteristics of depression include declining school performance, irritability, withdrawal from social activities, sleep disorders (either unable to sleep or sleeping all the time), appetite disturbance (either overeating or anorexia), headache, stomachache, difficulty concentrating, and difficulty making decisions. Box 27-1 ■ highlights signs of depression in the adolescent.

Depression can be a primary condition or secondary to learned behavior due to dysfunctional family traits. Depression can be seen with other psychiatric disorders, including ADHD, anxiety, bipolar disorder, or personality disorders. At times the depressed child maintains some degree of functioning until some crisis (e.g., a fight with parents, ending of a close relationship, or the loss of a friend) becomes the catalyst for extreme behavior. The child who is depressed may strike out at authority figures, as exhibited by violence at school, or direct the anger inward and hurt him- or herself.

BOX 27-1	ASSESSMENT

Manifestations of Depression

- Chronically depressed mood occurring for most of the day, more days than not
- Showing or describing mood as sad
- May be shown as irritability rather than depression
- Poor appetite or overeating
- Insomnia or hypersominia
- Low energy or fatigue
- Low self-esteem
- Poor concentration or difficulty making decisions
- Feelings of hopelessness
- Low interest
- Self-criticism; describing oneself as being uninteresting, incapable, or ineffective

Treatment

Treatment of depression in children is quite common because it is believed that depression can become worse with each episode (Eby, 2005). However, there have been some tragedies with children moving from depression to treatment to suicide.

clinical ALERT

Because of reports of increased suicidal thinking or aggressive behavior in children and adolescents taking antidepressant medications for psychiatric disorders, clear warnings now appear on FDA-approved antidepressant drugs. Parents must be cautioned to watch children carefully for these changes, especially during the first few weeks of treatment.

BIPOLAR DISORDER

Bipolar disorder is also called *manic depression*. In this disorder, children have mood swings that vary between mania and depression. Manic episodes are characterized by hyperactivity, irritability, aggression, and possibly hallucinations. Depressive episodes are marked by periods of sadness, sleep and eating disturbances, and social withdrawal. Ten to 20% of persons diagnosed with bipolar disorder commit suicide. Treatment is focused on stabilizing the child's mood by administering lithium, valproate (Depakote), or carbamazepine (Tegretol). Lamotrigine (Lamictal) is also used as a mood stabilizer (Eby, 2005).

SUICIDE

Suicide, the taking of one's own life, is the second leading cause of death for 15- to 19-year-olds. The rate of suicide has tripled since the mid-1950s. For every suicide that is completed, it is estimated that 100 to 200 attempts are made. Although females attempt suicide three to four times more often than males, males complete the act four times more often. Many suicides are reported as accidents because of family embarrassment or social stigma. Suicide can be an associated manifestation of psychological disorders.

Instability in the American family has increased. This lack of parental support, coupled with increased exposure to stressors at school, through peer groups, and at home, has left the adolescent unprepared. Tired of trying to handle the pressure alone, the teen becomes depressed and sees suicide as a way out. With easy access to firearms and drugs, it is not surprising that these become the usual method of suicide.

Early detection of depression (see Box 27-1) is key in preventing the tragedy of suicide or violence against others. When adolescents begin to contemplate suicide, their behavior may signal their thoughts and they need immediate help. It is important to seek help if the teen:

- Has behavior changes that last for a few weeks or longer
- Is showing four or more symptoms of depression
- Is doing poorly in school
- Is seriously withdrawn or isolated
- Is overly impulsive
- Is uninterested in activities that were once enjoyed
- Cries frequently
- Gives away treasured items
- Verbalizes suicidal thoughts such as "I don't want to live any longer."

If a child expresses suicidal thoughts, the nurse should not ignore the statement. The nurse should question the teen about depression and thoughts of suicide using therapeutic communication skills. If the teen admits suicidal thoughts (called *suicidal ideation*), the plan for suicide should be explored, including method and opportunity. The more lethal the method and the more realistic the opportunity, the higher the probability the teen will attempt suicide. The nurse should not leave the teen unattended until medical treatment is initiated.

The teen who is depressed should be referred immediately to a qualified professional for evaluation and treatment. Frequently, antidepressants are prescribed in conjunction with individual and family counseling.

In many cases, the risk for depression and suicide lessens with time and treatment. As the adolescent matures, he or she learns skills to cope with stress. In mild cases, an herbal remedy may be of use but should always be approved by the health care provider (Box 27-2 ■). For more details in working with the adolescent who has mental health conditions, refer to an adult mental health text.

OVEREATING AND OBESITY

Obesity may be an associated manifestation of psychological disorders. Obesity affects 11% to 16% of American children (*Healthy People 2010*) and is considered by some to have reached epidemic proportions. Non-Hispanics and Mexican Americans have higher rates of obesity than other ethnic

BOX 27-2	COMPLEMENTARY THERAPIES

St. John's Wort

A 2003 study at Case Western Reserve University of 33 children with a mean age of 10.5 years found that St. John's wort may be effective in treating children diagnosed with depressive disorders. St. John's wort, also called *Hypericum perforatum* or Klamathweed, occurs naturally as a shrub with yellow flowers. The plant can be processed into capsules, tablets, tinctures, teas, or lotions and has been associated with reduced symptoms of mild to moderate depression. Side effects are nausea, hives, fatigue, photosensitivity, restlessness, headache, dry mouth, dizziness, and confusion. Children must take St. John's wort only under the supervision of a physician. The following drugs have been found to interact negatively with St. John's wort: antidepressants, digoxin, immunosuppressants, antiretrovirals, loperamide, oral contraceptives, reserpine, theophylline, and warfarin.

groups. **Obesity** is defined as excessive weight and accumulation of body fat. Obesity is a body mass index (BMI) greater than or equal to the 95th percentile. Many children have learned a pattern of overeating from their families and appear well adjusted. Although the intake of "junk food" makes them feel good, the increased weight contributes to a poor body image, depression, and low self-esteem. Many children use overeating to compensate for insecurities, low self-esteem, poor body image, lack of parental attention, or feelings of stress, anxiety, and depression. The sedentary lifestyle of many children increases the risk of obesity. Watching television and playing video games instead of exercising greatly increases a child's risk of obesity.

A referral to a nutritionist may be appropriate to teach the child to make healthy food choices. If obesity is not corrected during adolescence, diabetes, orthopedic problems, and cardiovascular complications could develop in later years.

An extreme option for the adolescent who is severely obese is **bariatric surgery** (surgery to reduce stomach size). Strict criteria are required to even consider this life-altering option. The teen must have tried weight management techniques for longer than 6 months and failed. He or she must be physiologically mature and agree to psychological evaluations both before and after surgery. Psychiatric issues must be resolved or successfully managed prior to surgery. Female clients considering bariatric surgery must agree to avoid pregnancy for more than 1 year postoperatively. A supportive family is also required.

Nurses may not see the obese child until conditions related to obesity cause him or her to seek health care. Accurate weight and height are necessary. The nurse must carefully measure the child's blood pressure. Obtaining serum cholesterol, triglycerides, glucose, and hemoglobin A1 will assist in determining the presence of complications related to obesity. The nurse should focus on helping the family to meet the child's nutritional needs, managing related health conditions, and promoting self-esteem. The nurse can encourage exercise and activity programs that will not embarrass the child.

NURSING CARE

PRIORITIES IN NURSING CARE

When caring for children with psychological disorders, the nurse must assist the child and family to develop appropriate coping skills in order to effectively manage the disorder. The nurse can assist the family in helping the child achieve developmental milestones. Children with autism, Asperger's syndrome, ADD, ADHD, anxiety, and depression will benefit from nursing interventions aimed to assist the child to focus and communicate effectively. Preventing injury

and ensuring the child's safety are also priority nursing interventions. Finally, the nurse should assist the child and his or her family to seek healthy behaviors related to nutrition, rest, exercise, medication administration, and stress relief measures.

ASSESSING

When assessing the child suffering from psychological disorders, the nurse should take a thorough health history, including a birth history. Ask parents or caregivers to specifically describe the child's behavior. The nurse must also observe the child's behavior closely to validate these behaviors. Be sure to ask about these behaviors in a variety of settings. Determine if the child is behaving in a particular manner at school, at home, and in the community. A physical examination is also important, particularly for the child with depression and suicidal thoughts.

DIAGNOSING, PLANNING, AND IMPLEMENTING

Nursing diagnoses for children suffering from psychological disorders might include:

- Hopelessness, related to negative self-perception
- Chronic Low Self-Esteem, related to disturbance of thoughts
- Caregiver Role Strain, related to intensive care required to manage the child with a thought process disorder
- Impaired Verbal Communication, related to altered perceptions.

Some outcomes for children suffering from thought process disorders might include:

- The child will express hope for the future.
- The child will demonstrate behaviors associated with appropriate self-esteem.
- The caregiver will describe interventions for managing role strain.
- The child will verbalize thoughts and needs appropriately.

The nurse's role in providing support to these clients would include the following:

- Explore factors contributing to hopelessness with the child. *Verbalization of feelings allows the child to better understand and deal with emotions.*
- Positively reinforce behaviors that are desirable, such as making eye contact (in a child with autism) or putting things away (in a child with attention deficit). *Positive reinforcement yields encouragement for these behaviors.*
- Restrict negative comments about self, while allowing the child some opportunity to verbalize thoughts and feelings. *This decreases the chance of positively reinforcing negative behaviors.*
- Avoid any teasing or joking with the child who has low self-esteem. *These children are highly sensitive to negative comments and even ones given in jest may be taken to heart.*

- Encourage small positive steps that can improve self-image. For example, a parent can provide a variety of outdoor activities to help an overweight child get more exercise. *Small changes in behavior followed by praise or other positive reinforcement can build a new life pattern.*

- Develop a plan of care with the caregiver to obtain assistance with household chores, mental health care for the entire family, and support groups that might provide emotional care. *These steps can assist the family in identifying coping mechanisms and availability of support.*

- Discuss with the family the need to lower expectations and be flexible about future goals. *Often holding on to impossible goals and expectations can complicate coping with the reality of the situation.*

- Assist the family in the grief process once goals are adjusted. *Unrealized expectations often elicit feelings of grief.*

- Assist the child in finding alternative methods of communicating such as pen and pencil or flash cards. *Children with thought process disorders often need to find different ways of expressing thoughts and ideas.*

- Always speak slowly and clearly when addressing the child. *Role modeling is a way of teaching the child to communicate properly.*

- Refer to mental health professionals and speech therapists as needed. *Collaborative activities will facilitate improvement for the child with a thought process disorder.*

EVALUATING

To evaluate the outcomes for the child with psychological disorders, the nurse must develop and maintain a trusting relationship that encourages the child to verbalize thoughts and feelings in a safe environment. Evaluation must include questioning the caregiver about his or her level of strain and coping mechanisms. It will be important to immediately report any thoughts of self-inflicted harm or suicide to the nursing supervisor.

Anorexia Nervosa and Bulimia

Anorexia nervosa is an eating disorder characterized by weight loss, emaciation, and an exaggerated fear of gaining weight. Clients lose weight either by excessive dieting or by eating and then purging by inducing vomiting and diarrhea. A closely related condition is **bulimia**, which is characterized by binge eating and purging. **Purging** is self-induced vomiting, abusing laxatives or diuretics, or both. The typical client is a white female, between 13 and 18 years of age, in a middle- to upper-middle-class family; however, the condition can also affect males.

Many authorities view anorexia nervosa as a family problem. Often the parents are overly controlling and perfectionistic. The adolescent's eating disorder is an attempt to

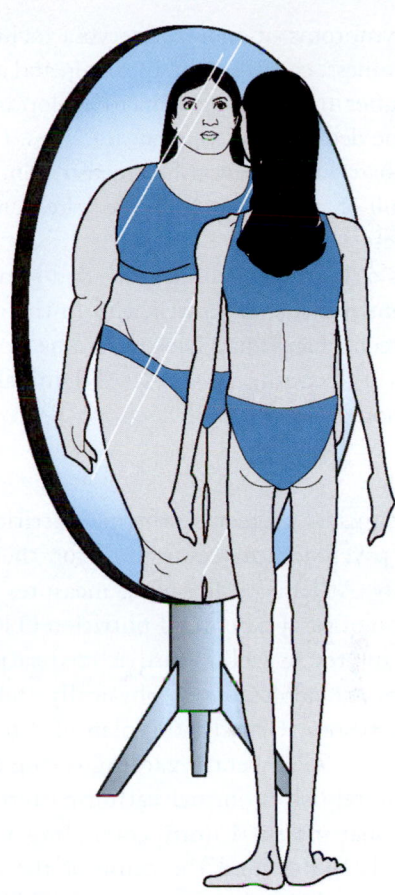

Figure 27-2. ■ Body image is the sum of a person's conscious and unconscious attitudes about his or her body. This illustration shows a disturbance in body image.

achieve independence and resolve psychological conflicts. Society's preoccupation with being thin may contribute to the adolescent's view of his or her body shape and the fear of becoming fat (Figure 27-2 ■). The teen may also have a history of abuse. Families of bulimics may live in chaos and lack emotional connection.

Manifestations

Anorexia nervosa is characterized by body weight less than 85% of the expected weight. For example, if the expected body weight is 120 lb, a weight of 102 lb could indicate a problem. To lose weight, the adolescent may not only decrease caloric intake, but also indulge in strenuous exercise programs. Other symptoms include preoccupation with food and preparing elaborate meals for others, while actually consuming very few calories. Individuals with anorexia may cut food and push it around on the plate. They act like they are eating, but they are not. Teens may cry frequently, feel depressed and lonely, and consider suicide. Anxiety and OCD may accompany other symptoms. The fear of becoming fat does not disappear with weight loss. Over time, the adolescent becomes emaciated. Malnutrition accompanied by fluid and electrolyte imbalance results in life-threatening cardiac arrhythmias.

Physical symptoms of anorexia nervosa include cold intolerance, dizziness, constipation, bloating, and amenorrhea. Teens who suffer from anorexia may develop osteoporosis, decreased bone density, and frequent fractures. *Lanugo* (fine, downy body hair) and bradycardia are also seen. Death may occur as a result of a weakened immune system, renal failure, or cardiac arrest.

Symptoms of bulimia include tooth and gum decay due to the frequent presence of gastric acid in the mouth. The back of the teen's hand may have abrasions from scraping the teeth during purging episodes. Abdominal distention may also be noted.

Treatment

Treatment begins by correcting the malnutrition and continues with psychological counseling for the adolescent and the family. At times, life-saving measures such as the administration of total parenteral nutrition (TPN), IV fluids, and electrolytes, as well as cardiac medications, are the priority. Once the adolescent is physically stable, intense counseling is begun. Usually, the plan of care includes a contract with the adolescent regarding eating habits. The goal is to re-establish a normal eating pattern with adequate nutritional intake. Family counseling is needed to help the family understand the cause of the adolescent's eating disorder and to take steps toward a higher level of family functioning.

Nursing Considerations

Hospitalization is required for teens who have lost significant weight, have severe electrolyte imbalances, or need constant psychological intervention. The teen with anorexia may resist treatment. The nurse must firmly enforce prescribed treatments. Because these teens have altered perceptions of themselves and are likely to have been concealing their condition, they are masters at deception. Manipulative behaviors are common and must be identified by the nurse.

It is also important that the nurse obtain accurate weight measurements on the schedule that is ordered. (Daily weights may be avoided because of the teen's preoccupation with weight.) Intake and output measurements will also be necessary. Lab values must be closely monitored to detect complications.

NURSING CARE

PRIORITIES IN NURSING CARE

When caring for adolescents with eating disorders, the nurse must implement nursing interventions to prevent nutritional and fluid and electrolyte deficits. Another priority nursing strategy is developing a trusting relationship with the client. This effective nurse/client relationship will assist the nurse to enforce prescribed treatments and open lines of communication to address the issues of disturbed body image.

ASSESSING

The child suffering from an eating disorder must have an accurate body weight. Some physicians order the weights to be done with the client's back to the scale to discourage focusing on weight. The nurse must also obtain a nutritional history of the child's daily intake, including beverages and their meal patterns as a baseline. A 24-hour diet recall can be helpful in obtaining this information. Determine the child's exercise habits, including type of exercise and frequency. If the child has gone through puberty, obtain a menstrual history.

DIAGNOSING, PLANNING, AND IMPLEMENTING

Nursing diagnoses for children with eating disorders might include:

- Imbalanced Nutrition: More than Body Requirements, related to overeating
- Imbalanced Nutrition: Less than Body Requirements, related to induced vomiting or inadequate intake and excessive exercise
- Deficient Fluid Volume, related to abuse of laxatives
- Disturbed Body Image, related to distorted perception of appearance
- Activity Intolerance, related to sedentary lifestyle (obesity) or fatigue (anorexia nervosa).

Some outcomes for children with eating disorders might include:

- Child will meet weight and BMI goal (decreased for obesity and increased for anorexia nervosa and bulimia).
- Child will maintain expected fluid volume.
- Child will view body size realistically.
- Child will be able to complete activities of daily living without fatigue.

The nurse's role in providing support to these clients would include the following:

- Establish a trusting relationship with the child/teen. *This relationship is essential so the child/teen will listen to instructions and comply.*
- Communicate clear and simple expectations for food intake and the amount of exercise prescribed. *Compliance with the medical regime is improved with clear instructions. The child/teen suffering from obesity needs to have obtainable goals that will allow him or her to see progress. The child/teen suffering from anorexia nervosa or bulimia is both goal oriented and manipulative, so clear expectations are necessary.*

- The child/teen with an eating disorder needs to be monitored. *Monitoring can help the child/teen avoid overeating or self-induced vomiting.*
- Assist the child/teen in learning how to make appropriate food choices. *Appropriate food choices can allow the child to achieve optimal nutrition and not gain excessive weight.*
- Teach the child/teen and family about the physical risks associated with obesity and anorexia nervosa and bulimia. *Knowledge of the risks will increase compliance with the medical regime.*
- Take weight measurements on the schedule ordered by the physician. Weight needs to be as accurate as possible. This can be accomplished by weighing the child/teen consistently at the same time, with the same amount of clothing. Document carefully. *Monitoring weight gain or weight loss needs to be consistent to make necessary changes in the plan of care.*
- Carefully monitor hydration status by performing skin turgor test, observing mucous membranes, palpating pulses bilaterally, calculating intake and output, and monitoring laboratory values. *Fluid imbalances can shift quickly and cause serious risks to the child's/teen's health. These imbalances need to be reported promptly.*
- Encourage the child/teen to talk about his or her body perceptions. If necessary, have the child/teen draw his or her body image. *The nurse must understand the child's/teen's true feelings in order to deal with him or her appropriately.*
- Provide respect and privacy when giving care to this child/teen. *This will give the child/teen a sense that his or her body is worth respecting.*
- Schedule rest periods throughout the day. *Rest will help the child/teen avoid fatigue and promote conservation of energy for important activities.*
- Assist the child/teen with activities of daily living. *Until proper nutritional status is restored, the child/teen may need assistance to conserve energy.*

EVALUATING

Outcomes will be evaluated based on the child's weight, daily intake and output, the child's perception of his or her body size, and the child's ability to perform activities of daily living without fatigue. Because variations in fluid balance and nutrition can cause serious risks, it is important for the LPN/LVN to report significant changes immediately to the supervising nurse.

NURSING PROCESS CARE PLAN
Client with Anorexia Nervosa

Meghan, a 14-year-old white female, is brought to the family physician's office by her mother. Meghan's mother reports that Meghan had been losing weight and has been tired and irritable for months. Meghan states that it is important to her to be thin and attractive. She states, "I'd do anything to avoid being fat like I am now. I really do not like the way I look and want to change it." Her weight today is 92 lb. She states that her last menstrual period was 6 months ago. Her hair is dry and brittle, and her skin is lacking moisture.

Assessment
- "I'd do anything to avoid being fat like I am now."
- States desire to be thin and attractive
- Recent weight loss
- "I really do not like the way I look and want to change it."

Nursing Diagnosis. The following important nursing diagnosis (among others) is established for this client:
- Disturbed Body Image, related to difficulty coping with maturation

Expected Outcomes. Expected outcomes for Meghan are that:
- She will express a positive body image.
- She will be able to manage her weight in an appropriate manner.

Planning and Implementation
- Assess client's self-concept and body image. *Knowing exactly what the client believes will assist the nurse in developing a specific plan.*
- Assess the family structure and stressors in the client's life. *It is important to identify aspects of the client's life that may have contributed to her condition.*
- Assist the client in differentiating between thin and healthy body size. *The client may have a distorted view of what is a normal body weight and may not understand the health hazards associated with extreme weight loss.*
- Assist the client in developing a realistic body image and nutritional intake. *Recovery is facilitated when the client is involved in planning her care.*
- Refer client to an adolescent support group. *Adolescents respond well to peer counseling.*

Evaluation. Consistent care and follow-up with the client and family will restore a positive body image, and she will develop appropriate skills to cope with her stressors.

Critical Thinking in The Nursing Process

1. What societal aspects may contribute to an unrealistic body image in the adolescent?
2. What type of family support will most likely help Meghan?
3. How could Meghan's friends assist with her recovery?

Note: Discussion of Critical Thinking questions appears in Appendix I.

Abuse and Family Violence

Child abuse is a crime punishable in all states. It can occur as physical abuse, emotional abuse or neglect, and sexual abuse. Unfortunately, child abuse can occur in any household, with any race or religion, with males or females, and in children of any age (Box 27-3 ■). Caring for children is difficult even in the best of situations. There will be many times in the rearing of children when parental frustration and anger occur. Parents who are not equipped to channel this frustration and anger properly are at risk for abusing their children.

Many parents who abuse their children were also abused as children. They learned a pattern of discipline and child rearing from their parents and tend to implement the same forms of punishment. They may have never been shown love and nurturing. Because they did not develop a healthy sense of trust, it is difficult, without intervention, for them to pass a sense of security and love on to their children.

Lack of knowledge about normal growth and development of the child may create unrealistic expectations of the child. When these expectations are not met, frustration develops. Parents may be socially isolated and not have a support system that could teach them proper parenting techniques. Child abusers often abuse alcohol and other substances. These substances impair judgment and are associated with poor decision making.

Parents who choose to abuse their children may view them as different. There is a higher incidence of abuse among children born with birth defects or who were born prematurely. These situations may keep infants and parents separated for periods of time following birth and complicate efforts to bond. These situations are also stressful to the parents physically, emotionally, and financially. Child abuse is more likely to occur during periods of stress. The Health Promotion Issue on pages 804 and 805 cites one type of situation in which abuse may occur.

BOX 27-3   **CULTURAL PULSE POINTS**

Discipline in Appalachian Culture

The Appalachian mountain range spans 13 states—Alabama, Mississippi, Georgia, Virginia, West Virginia, North and South Carolina, Kentucky, Tennessee, Ohio, Maryland, New York, and Pennsylvania.

Families are usually large, and a strict work ethic is enforced. Corporal and physical punishment is frequently used to discipline children.

If child abuse is suspected in a family from this region, consider that they *may* not perceive their forms of discipline as abusive and may not accept counsel from health care professionals.

REPORTING ABUSE

The nurse must report any suspicion of child abuse to local or state child protective services or law enforcement authorities. Agency policy will dictate the method of reporting but requires notification of the nursing supervisor in all situations. The report must also be made immediately when symptoms are recognized to prevent further danger to the child. Most child protective services have the authority to hold the child in their custody until a proper investigation can be implemented.

Documentation is a vital part of the report of child abuse. The nurse must be careful to clearly chart physical symptoms, as well as subjective data, gathered from the child and the parent. When charting physical findings, the nurse needs to be specific as to the location and size of the injury. Obtaining color pictures of the injury may be essential to proving abuse in a court of law.

State laws provide protection for the nurse from prosecution for reporting abuse. Although not required, it is advisable to notify the parents that a report of child abuse has been submitted. Although this can evoke anger on the part of the parent, it allows the health care personnel to communicate a rationale for holding the child in custody. If, however, the nurse fails to report suspected child abuse, a fine can be levied or the nurse's license could be revoked. Refer to Chapter 2 ⚭ for more information on the legal aspects of nursing.

PHYSICAL ABUSE

Physical abuse of a child is inflicting pain and injury in a deliberate manner. Injury may be inflicted on a child by hitting, burning, biting, choking, shaking, or throwing a child. The perpetrator may use his or her hands, fists, head, teeth, knees, or feet and legs. In addition, weapons, such as electrical cords, ropes, sticks, baseball bats, or cigarette lighters, may be used. Physical abuse also includes administering excessive doses of medication or withholding needed medications.

Manifestations

Clinical manifestation of physical child abuse include bruises, burns (see Figure 24-14 ⚭), rope or cord marks (usually on the back of the body), multiple fractures, shortness of breath, sedation from medication, or exacerbation of a chronic illness from withholding medications.

The nurse must be able to chart the color of the bruise objectively. Findings should be discussed with the physician and supervising nurse. A bruise that is less than 1 day old is red, blue, or bright purple with distinct margins (Figure 27-3 ■). A bruise that is 1 to 2 days old is bluish-brown to dark purple. A 3- to 5-day-old bruise is yellow-green to brown, while one that is 5 to 7 days old is fading to yellow without distinct borders. Finally, a bruise that is older than 1 week has only slight yellow-brown discolorations. The nurse must also carefully chart the subjective statements

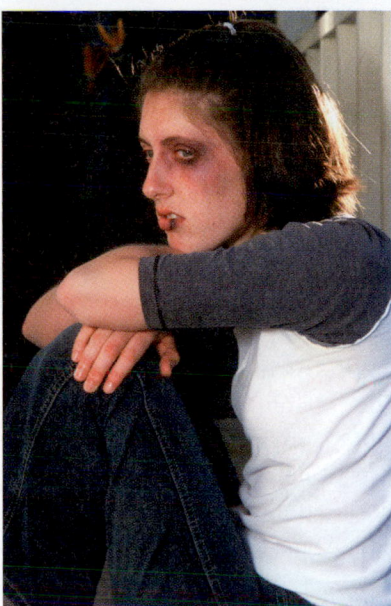

Figure 27-3. ■ The timing of physical abuse can be assessed by the color of bruises in soft tissue.
(Bill Aron/PhotoEdit, Inc.)

given by the parents regarding how the child became bruised. Box 27-4 ■ highlights some signs of abuse.

Treatment

Caring for a child who has been physically abused will require teamwork. The team will consist of physicians, nurses, social workers, school counselors and teachers, mental health professionals, and family. These team members will work to ensure the child's physical safety and recovery from inflicted injuries. Once abuse is reported, the child is removed from the environment in which the abuse occurred. Mental health professionals will assist the child in emotionally recovering from the abuse. They can use a variety of therapies. See the next section for a further description. The social worker develops a plan to provide the child a home environment free of abuse.

SHAKEN BABY SYNDROME

A serious form of physical abuse against the infant is **shaken baby syndrome.** The infant is particularly susceptible to head injuries because the head is large and the neck muscles are weak. If the caregiver shakes the infant, the jarring motion causes tearing of the nerve fibers in the brain, subdural hematoma, cerebral edema, and retinal hemorrhages.

The infant who has this type of head injury may experience seizures, vomiting, lethargy, and respiratory difficulties. The infant may also present with failure to thrive. One-third of infants die from this injury, while another one-third have permanent damage. Permanent damage may include

---

BOX 27-4	ASSESSMENT

Manifestations of Abuse

Child's Behavior

- Shows sudden changes in behavior or school performance
- Has not received help for physical or medical problems brought to the parents' attention
- Has learning problems (or difficulty concentrating) that cannot be attributed to specific physical or psychological causes
- Is always watchful, as though preparing for something bad to happen
- Lacks adult supervision
- Is overly compliant, passive, or withdrawn
- Comes to school or other activities early, stays late, and does not want to go home

Parent's Behavior

- Shows little concern for the child
- Denies the existence of—or blames the child for—the child's problems in school or at home
- Asks teachers or other caregivers to use harsh physical discipline if the child misbehaves
- Sees the child as entirely bad, worthless, or burdensome
- Demands a level of physical or academic performance the child cannot achieve
- Looks primarily to the child for care, attention, and satisfaction of emotional needs

Parent and Child's Behavior

- Rarely touch or look at each other
- Consider their relationship entirely negative
- State that they do not like each other

---

mental retardation, vision or hearing impairment, seizures, paralysis, or developmental delays.

BULLYING

Bullying is a type of physical and emotional abuse. A recent survey (Glewe, 2005) says that 22% of school-age children experience this form of abuse. The child may be teased, threatened, hit, shoved, kicked, or pushed. Bullying most commonly occurs during school hours, but can also occur at community activities, on a school bus, in the neighborhood, at religious activities, or via the Internet.

Children who are bullied feel anxious, isolated, depressed, and possibly suicidal. They often complain of headaches, stomachaches, and other vague complaints in an effort to avoid situations where they may be bullied. They may also express their anger toward the bully in the form of aggression to siblings, parents, or friends. The victim's grades begin to suffer, and he or she no longer feels safe at school.

Teachers and parents must recognize the signs of physical and emotional threats to the child's safety. The primary
(*Text continues on p. 806.*)

HEALTH PROMOTION ISSUE

PREVENTING INFANT ABDUCTION

Janice Pope, a 29-year-old gravida 2, para 1, is touring the birthing facility prior to the birth of her second child. She is accompanied by her mother and her 5-year-old son, Cody. She indicates to the nurse conducting the tour that she is concerned about the safety of her newborn while he is hospitalized. Mrs. Pope and her husband are in the midst of a divorce and a custody battle. Her husband has threatened to steal the baby if she does not agree to give him custody of Cody. He also made the statement that he is not interested in having custody of the baby, but that he does not want her to have it either. Mrs. Pope has reason to believe her husband because he has a history of violent behavior. Mrs. Pope is visibly shaken by these threats to her newborn's safety. The nurse wants to respond appropriately to her concerns.

DISCUSSION

The Joint Commission on Accreditation of Healthcare Organizations (JCAHO) calls infant abduction a sentinel event or critical incident. A *sentinel event* is an occurrence where death or serious physical or psychological injury could occur. Infant abductions could take place at the hospital or in a family's home. The abductor could be a family member or a stranger. The typical abductor is a female with emotional difficulties related to her marriage or relationships or her reproductive life. She may have low self-esteem and exhibit compulsive behaviors. The National Center for Missing and Exploited Children lists the following as typical characteristics of abductions: The abductor acts alone, dresses as medical personnel, tells the mother that the baby needs medical attention, seeks to befriend the mother, usually calls her by name, creates a distraction just prior to the abduction such as spilling a drink in the hallway, and thinks of the baby as her own immediately following the abduction.

JCAHO requires health care facilities to seriously address possible infant abductions. The commission requires these plans to be developed by health care personnel from many different disciplines, such as medicine, nursing, security, social services, and public relations. The plan must include proper newborn identification, staff and parent education, and a physical environment that ensures newborn safety. Following is an example of a plan for prompt response to an infant abduction:

1. Prompt notification of assistive personnel to include unit and nursing supervisors, security, and hospital administration. Also, an overhead page is used to alert all hospital personnel.
2. Secure the area, especially the exits. Observe for suspicious behavior.
3. Attend to the needs of the family both during the event and afterward. Regardless of whether the infant is found, the family will experience stress.
4. Following the event, the staff must review the scenario. They will also need an opportunity to debrief.

PLANNING AND IMPLEMENTATION

The nurse discusses with Mrs. Pope the specific plan her hospital uses to keep newborns safe. Newborns are identified in several ways. Immediately after birth, hospital identification bands are placed on the infant's wrist and opposite ankle. These bands have a five-digit number that matches the mother's and also has the mother's name on it. The mother can choose one other family member to whom to give a matching identification band. Only the mother and this other individual may transport the baby to the nursery or receive the baby from the nursery. Also, in the delivery room, the baby

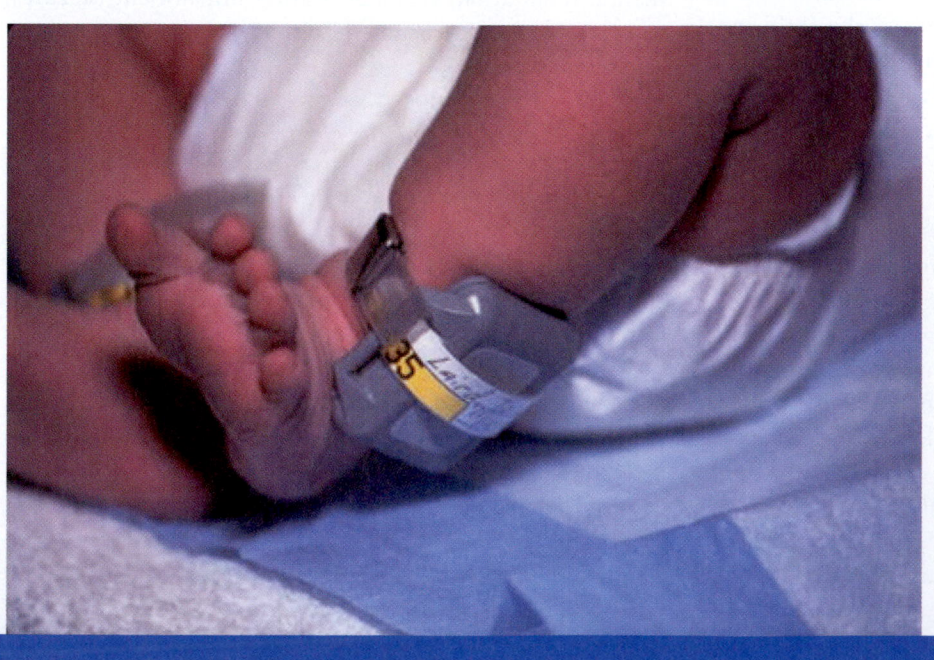

(Myrleen Ferguson Cate/PhotoEdit, Inc.)

will be footprinted. These footprints will be on the same page as a fingerprint from the mother's index finger. Shortly after birth, the baby is transported by nursing personnel to the nursery. If the baby's temperature is stable, the baby will receive his or her first bath. After the bath, the baby's picture is taken with a digital camera before he or she leaves the nursery. The pictures are printed for the mother and stored digitally for later retrieval, if necessary. These pictures can be placed on the hospital's website, but no last names are given. Mrs. Pope may decide not to place her baby's picture on the website.

The entire staff of the hospital is familiar with methods to avoid newborn abductions and safeguard the newborn while he or she is admitted to the hospital. The staff wears a unique style and color of scrubs that change weekly. All approved personnel have a picture identification badge. Babies are transported in their cribs, never in a nurse's arms. There will also be a daily security code that nurses are required to say when removing a baby from the mother's room. This security code word will be communicated to postpartum mothers at 7:30 each morning.

The nurse tells Mrs. Pope that all client identification is kept confidential and cannot be accessed by the public. She also tells Mrs. Pope about the policy for a confidential admission,

whereby her chart will be flagged to help staff be especially careful about her personal information. The infant may also be given a faux name to further conceal his or her identity. Security can also be alerted to the potential for danger, and extra surveillance can be arranged.

The nurse teaches Mrs. Pope to carefully study each nurse's identification badge when they remove the newborn from her room. She has the right to question anybody that seems suspicious and to accompany the newborn to any tests or examinations. The newborn should never be left unattended in the hospital room, even when Mrs. Pope needs to toilet or shower. The crib should not be placed next to the door.

Mrs. Pope should also understand that the women's unit is equipped with safety measures designed to prevent infant abductions. Each staff member wears an additional badge that allows him or her passage into the nursery and into the postpartum unit. These badges are signed out to each nurse and inventoried on a regular basis. The unit is also monitored by video cameras that are surveyed by security personnel. Signs are posted in the unit to alert the public that they are being monitored by video cameras.

When preparing for discharge, Mrs. Pope should consider the following safeguards. She should avoid any signs

or decorations that alert the public that there is a newborn in the home. The nurse must communicate to Mrs. Pope that the hospital does not have a postpartum home visit program, so health care personnel should not appear unannounced at her home. The nurse can also encourage Mrs. Pope to collect identification data about her infant. This data should include a color photograph, footprints, hair color, eye color, current length, current weight, date of birth, and a detailed description of any physical characteristics that might assist in identification.

SELF-REFLECTION

What safety measures have you observed in different health care facilities to prevent infant abductions? Which of these are most effective? Least effective? Think about your own practice of transporting infants within the health care facility. How could you improve this practice to ensure infant safety?

The fear of infant abduction creates fear and stress in both hospital personnel and new mothers. Describe these fears. What nursing interventions contribute to this fear? What nursing interventions help dispel this fear? Look at your practice. Are you contributing to fear or dispelling it?

SUGGESTED RESOURCES

For the Nurse

- Shogan, M.G. (2002). Emergency management plan for newborn abductions. *JOGNN, 31*(3), 340–346.
- Rabun, J., Jr. (2005). For Healthcare Professionals: Guidelines on Prevention of & Response to Infant Abductions. 8th ed. **www.missingkids.com** This document was created by the National Center for Missing and Exploited

Children and the Association of Women's Health, Obstetric and Neonatal Nurses. It provides a detailed plan to safeguard the newborn during hospitalization.

- **www.jointcommission.org** This Joint Commission on Accreditation of Healthcare Organizations website provides information about requirements of hospitals regarding newborn safety.

action is to remove the child from physical danger and to restore his or her emotional health.

EMOTIONAL ABUSE AND NEGLECT

Emotional abuse of a child includes attacks on a child's self-esteem. The perpetrator uses words to control and frighten the child. The child may be shamed, ridiculed, or embarrassed by the abuser (often an adult). Emotional abuse can also include acts of violence against someone or something that the child loves, such as a pet or favorite toy.

A child may also be neglected either physically or emotionally. Physical neglect of a child is the deliberate withholding of physical care or resources from the child. The perpetrator may withhold food, water, hygiene, shelter, or health care. Children who are emotionally abused do not have nurturing care. The perpetrator is cold and insensitive to the child's needs.

Clinical manifestations of emotional abuse or neglect include poor self-esteem, lack of friends, lack of trust in adults, and impaired communication. The child may be sick frequently and may present with failure to thrive. He or she often does not do well academically and presents with behavior problems at school. He or she may be depressed and think about suicide.

NONORGANIC FAILURE TO THRIVE

Nonorganic failure to thrive (NOFTT) is a disorder characterized by inadequate growth in height and weight. It usually occurs in infancy and early childhood. It occurs most commonly in children whose parents are depressed, abuse a variety of substances, are mentally retarded, or are psychotic. These parents are more likely to be poor, socially isolated, and have lower educational levels. Even if the parent has an education, he or she may not know the proper way to feed the child (e.g., formula preparation, methods of breastfeeding, or introducing solid foods).

Children with NOFTT will be below the third to fifth percentile on the growth charts for height and weight. They may have little if any subcutaneous fat and reduced muscle mass. They appear lifeless and apathetic. They avoid eye contact with the caregiver and have no expression in their face. They will also be irritable, difficult to soothe, and have poor sleeping habits. When they are held, children with NOFTT will not mold to the caregiver's body and quite frequently will arch the back in an effort not to be held. They have signs of neglect such as diaper rash; long, dirty fingernails; dirty clothes; and an unwashed body. They may have a foul odor. They also experience developmental delays.

Adequate nutritional support is the primary goal of treatment. The care of this child must also include promotion of bonding behaviors to help the parent and child attach. Parents who lack education must be taught about proper feeding methods and the need for physical interaction with the

---

Definitions Related to Sexual Abuse

- **Incest**—Sexual activity between family members.
- **Assault**—A sudden, violent physical attack on someone. Assault is an unlawful act.
- **Rape**—Sexual intercourse without consent that occurs as a result of threat or physical force.
- **Statutory rape**—Sexual intercourse that occurs between a minor and an adult. There is consent given by the minor.
- **Date rape**—Sexual intercourse during a social outing without consent, which occurs as a result of threat or physical force. The perpetrator is known socially by the victim.
- **Child molestation**—Sexual involvement other than intercourse with children. Child molestation includes oral-genital contact, genital fondling, and masturbation in the presence of children.
- **Child exploitation**—The unethical use of a child for one's own profit. Child exploitation may be in the form of prostitution or child pornography.
- **Child pornography**—The photography or visual representation of children nude and/or in sexual acts. These materials may be distributed in print media, in videos, or over the Internet.
- **Exhibitionism**—Exposing the genitals to strangers.
- **Pedophile**—A person who has a sexual interest in children.

---

child. A thorough evaluation of the home environment must be performed, and monitoring of this environment must be ongoing.

SEXUAL ABUSE

Sexual abuse can be defined as sexual acts that are imposed on children who cannot protect themselves due to their lack of emotional or cognitive development. Sexual abuse can happen in a variety of ways. Box 27-5 ■ provides definitions related to sexual abuse. Between 100,000 and 500,000 children in the United States are sexually abused each year (Ball & Bindler, 2006).

Most perpetrators are males. The victim may be male or female; however, more females are victims than males. Several risk factors have been identified for sexual abuse. These include a stepfather living in the home instead of the biologic father, poor parental relationships, a parent or caregiver who never finished high school, a parent or caregiver who has an annual income of less than $10,000, a mother employed outside the home, parental substance abuse, and a child with two or fewer friends.

Manifestations

Sexual abuse in children can be characterized by physical symptoms, mood changes, cognitive impairment, sexual symptoms, and lack of coping skills. Physical symptoms include vaginal discharge, possibly with a strong odor; vaginal or anal bleeding or bruising (underpants or diaper may be blood stained); genital irritation, such as redness, pain, itching, or burning; recurrent urinary tract infections; sexually transmitted infections; a positive pregnancy test, particularly at a young age; enuresis; and encopresis. The child may also complain frequently of a headache or stomachache when there is no physical indication for these symptoms. Mood changes associated with sexual abuse include depression, anxiety, withdrawal, hostility, irritability, fear of strangers and other phobias, and aggressive behavior. The child who has been sexually abused will be fearful of a physical examination and may become combative during the exam. Symptoms of cognitive impairment related to sexual abuse include sudden changes in school performance and school attendance; low self-esteem; frequent daydreaming; and nightmares or night terrors.

Children who have been sexually abused may demonstrate sexual symptoms such as promiscuous behavior. They may express confusion about their sexual identity and begin to masturbate frequently. Many children who have been sexually abused pursue prostitution as a form of income. It seems that the dissociation they developed to cope with the abuse also allows them to participate in prostitution.

These children may also demonstrate a lack of coping skills. They frequently abuse tobacco, alcohol, and drugs. They may run away from home. They may inflict pain on themselves and others. Sleeping and eating habits may change. The female victim of sexual abuse tends to act like a wife or mother to family members and/or friends.

Diagnosis and Treatment

History and physical evidence lead to the diagnosis of sexual abuse. However, the collection of forensic evidence is important to trace the perpetrator. Collection of body fluids and tissues needs to be done by trained experts so valuable evidence is not destroyed. Such experts are also trained to address the emotional issues of the child related to the examination. Referral to a mental health professional is necessary for the child who has been sexually abused. The child's physical safety must also be ensured.

Nursing Considerations

Due to the number of children who have been sexually abused, the nurse must explore the possibility of this type of abuse with all children. The following are questions that will assist the nurse in screening for sexual abuse:

- What sleeping arrangements do you have in your home?
- Tell me about bath time in your home?
- Do you keep secrets from anyone in your home? Who asked you to keep these secrets?
- Has anyone ever touched you when you did not want them to? Tell me where?
- Has anyone ever asked you to touch them when you did not want to? Tell me where?

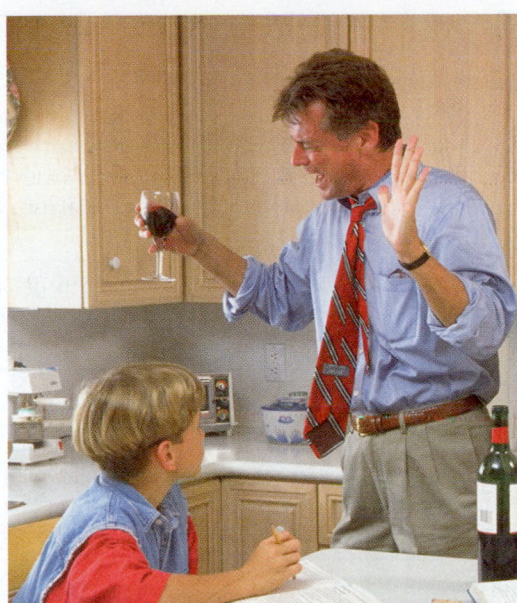

Figure 27-4. ■ Alcoholism runs in families because of a combination of genetic and environmental factors. (Tom and Dee Ann McCarthy/Corbis/Stock Market.)

- Would you tell me who has asked you to do these things? How often has it happened? Have you ever told anyone else about this? Who?

SUBSTANCE ABUSE

Crossing all socioeconomic boundaries, substance abuse affects children of all ages. The child is particularly vulnerable to the hazards of substance abuse due to his or her incomplete physical development. The adolescent, struggling for identity and independence, may experience periods of confusion and sadness. At these times, the teen is more vulnerable to substance abuse. Although some adolescents are exposed to addictive substances through peer contact, others witness their parents abusing substances and so believe using chemicals is the "adult" thing to do (Figure 27-4 ■). Flora (2006) found that 25% of children 18 and younger live with alcoholic parents. Some adolescents may experiment with only a few substances and then stop using them altogether, while others move from substance to substance until they become dependent on chemicals to "feel good." Table 27-2 ■ identifies the stages of substance abuse.

Substance abuse includes tobacco, alcohol, illegal drugs, and some over-the-counter chemicals. The younger adolescent with limited financial resources may experiment with household chemicals such as glue, cold medicine, or herbs. Common household chemicals that are inhaled include paint thinner, spray paint, nail polish remover, and helium. Methamphetamine is an extremely dangerous drug that can be manufactured with common household substances.

TABLE 27-2

Stages of Substance Abuse

STAGE	DESCRIPTION
0. Curiosity in a do drugs world	Occasional experimentation with alcohol or other drugs. Initial use may be unpleasant.
1. Learning the mood swing	With continued use, learns to "get high." Learns that some drugs work faster or better than others.
2. Seeking the mood swing	Wants the "high" more frequently, actively seeks alcohol or drugs.
3. Preoccupation with mood swing	Tolerance to substance builds with continued use. The majority of time is spent obtaining and using the drug.
4. Using drugs to feel normal	Physical and psychological dependence ensues. Signs of withdrawal occur without drug.

Children who live in households where this drug is manufactured and smoked are at risk for the effects of methamphetamine and for injuries such as burns due to chemical explosions. Methamphetamine causes hyperactivity, decreased appetite, a general sense of well-being, and possible agitation and violence. Long-term effects include a pattern of violent behavior, paranoia, auditory hallucinations, delusions, tooth decay, weight loss, and stroke.

Beer, wine, and other alcohol may also be available in the home. To purchase illegal drugs, the adolescent may work, steal, or indulge in prostitution. The most commonly abused drugs are identified in Table 27-3 ■.

Forms of tobacco abuse include cigarettes, cigars, and smokeless tobacco, including snuff and chewing tobacco. Imported cigarettes may appeal to children because they are typically less expensive; however, these forms of tobacco carry the same health risks. Examples of these imported cigarettes are *bidis* (fruit- or candy-flavored cigarettes) and *kretek* (clove cigarettes). Risks of tobacco abuse include oral or lung cancer, cardiovascular disease, chronic pulmonary

TABLE 27-3

Commonly Abused Drugs and Their Effects

DRUG	EFFECTS	SIGNS OF WITHDRAWAL	TREATMENT
Nicotine	Vasoconstriction, tachycardia, increased adrenalin, elevated blood pressure	Anxiety, mood swings, cravings, dizziness, insomnia, headache, difficulty concentrating, increased appetite	Smoking cessation programs
Narcotics Heroin Morphine Meperidine (Demerol)	Euphoria, drowsiness, pinpoint pupils, respiratory depression	Yawning, tearing eyes, gooseflesh, abdominal cramps	Narcotic antagonist naloxone (Narcan) Methodone (Dolophine)
Cocaine **Amphetamines**	CNS stimulation with marked euphoria and excitement	Depression, lethargy, psychosis, intense craving for drug	Frequent monitoring due to depression and fatigue Manipulate to get drug
Depressants Barbiturates (phenobarbital, secobarbital)	Sleepy, dizzy	Abdominal cramps, weakness, tremors	Withdrawal dangerous, must be done slowly, seizures could ensue
Hallucinogens LSD PCP Marijuana	Visual illusions, hallucinations, altered perceptions	No physical symptoms, psychotic episode, flashbacks	Monitor for psychosis
Alcohol	Euphoria, delayed reactions, unsteady gait	Hallucinations, tremors (delirium tremens or DTs), seizures	Monitor during withdrawal Antianxiety drugs to prevent DTs

obstructive disease, emphysema, and low-birth-weight babies. Even if the child does not smoke, living with family members who smoke puts him or her into the same risk category.

Manifestations

Symptoms of substance abuse vary, depending on the specific substance(s) being abused. Physical symptoms might include:

- Dilated or pinpoint pupils, bloodshot eyes
- Bruising or needle marks
- Runny nose
- Shaking hands
- Halitosis.

Psychological or cognitive symptoms might include:

- Inconsistent behavior
- Drowsiness
- Restlessness or increased energy, depending on whether stimulant or depressant
- Lack of concentration
- Agitation
- Decreased interest in school and/or decreased grades.

Diagnosis and Treatment

Toxicology studies can be done to determine if there are levels of harmful substances in the child's urine. Many schools are developing voluntary drug testing programs for students in an effort to promote positive peer pressure to avoid substance abuse. Treatment begins with removal of the abused substance. In many cases, sedative-hypnotics or major tranquilizers may be needed to ease the withdrawal symptoms. Withdrawal from some drugs is dangerous and requires hospitalization and frequent monitoring. Once the adolescent is stabilized, psychological therapy to understand and treat the underlying cause is necessary.

Nursing Considerations

The nurse caring for children and adolescents must give priority to assessing risk factors related to substance abuse. The child's social history and self-concept are a critical piece of this assessment. The nurse should also determine the child's knowledge about the hazards of substance abuse, including chronic illnesses. These hazards can be communicated to the pediatric client through peer counseling, posters, brochures, buttons, and formal presentations.

The nurse can encourage the child to participate in activities that will increase his or her self-esteem such as sports or scouting. Encourage the child to be future minded and goal oriented. Help him or her understand the negative impact that substance abuse may have on a future career and family life.

Family counseling allows both parents and siblings to understand and help the addicted adolescent. Support groups

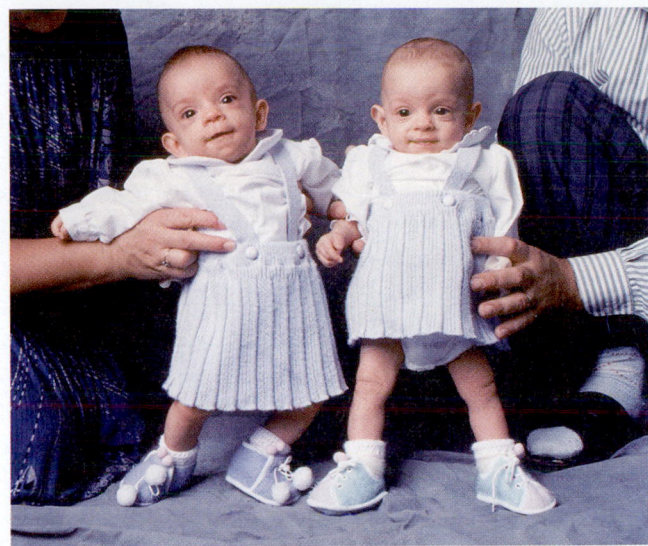

Figure 27-5. ■ Fetal alcohol syndrome is the result of a woman consuming alcohol during pregnancy, and it can have many severe effects on children. (George Steinmetz/San Francisco AIDS Foundation)

such as Ala-teen, NarcAnon, and Al-Anon are available in most communities.

FETAL ALCOHOL SYNDROME

Fetal alcohol syndrome (FAS) can occur if a pregnant woman consumes alcohol during pregnancy. No amount of alcohol intake during pregnancy has been determined safe. Obviously, the greater the consumption of alcohol, the greater the risks. Newborns with FAS have three types of characteristics: growth retardation, CNS abnormalities, and craniofacial abnormalities. Physically, they demonstrate growth retardation (Figure 27-5 ■). Most notably, this growth retardation is marked by decreased weight, height, and head circumference, as well as decreased adipose tissue. CNS abnormalities include developmental and cognitive delays and behavioral problems such as irritability and hyperactivity. Craniofacial abnormalities include microcephaly, small eyes, short palpebral fissures, thin upper lip, and a flattened maxillary area.

Immediate care of these newborns will focus on nutritional support. They are often fussy and poor eaters. The nurse will closely monitor their intake and output. For this child to thrive, the mother must be referred to an alcohol rehabilitation program and her care of the baby must be closely monitored. Also see Chapter 9 ⚭ for a discussion of FAS.

NURSING CARE

PRIORITIES IN NURSING CARE

Implementing nursing strategies to prevent abuse in all forms is a priority for the pediatric nurse. The nurse can provide parents and potential parents with teaching about the expected growth and development of children. Parents also need to be taught parenting techniques to promote nurturing and proper discipline. The pediatric nurse must also closely assess each client for signs and symptoms of abuse. If abuse is noted, prompt reporting and clear, objective documentation are essential. The nurse must also ensure that the victim of abuse is provided a safe environment where the child will be free from harm.

ASSESSING

Assessment for the children suffering from abuse and family violence includes a complete medical, family, and social history. The use of subjective data will avoid bias. The nurse must assist with a thorough physical examination, being sensitive to the child who has not been touched properly. For the child suspected of substance abuse, the nurse should ask direct, but nonjudgmental questions to determine the types of substances abused and how frequently they are used.

DIAGNOSING, PLANNING, AND IMPLEMENTING

Nursing diagnoses for children suffering from abuse and family violence might include:

- Deficient Knowledge, related to dangers of hazardous substances such as tobacco, alcohol, and illegal drugs
- Risk for Injury, related to forms of abuse, including substance, physical, emotional, and sexual
- Delayed Growth and Development, related to poor parenting
- Fear, related to past experience with abuse
- Anxiety, related to past experience with abuse or the unknown should the child be removed from the home environment.

Some outcomes for children suffering from abuse and family violence might include that the child will:

- Understand the risks associated with substance abuse
- Be free from evidence of injury from any form of abuse
- Demonstrate age-appropriate growth and developmental level
- Develop skills to overcome fear
- Be free of anxiety symptoms.

The nurse's role in providing support to these children would include the following:

- Provide teaching at the child's cognitive level about the hazards of substance abuse. *Factual information can change the child's behavior patterns.*
- Reinforce teaching with written materials and ask the child questions to validate understanding. *Evaluation of learning is important following teaching.*

- Parents and children should be taught how to recognize the symptoms of overdose. *Prompt action is necessary to restore health when the child has overdosed.*
- Report abuse promptly so the child who has been physically, emotionally, or sexually abused can be removed from the home where the abuse occurred. *Child abuse is a repetitive behavior, and the child will not be safe with the perpetrator.*
- Provide the child with delayed growth and development opportunities to interact with other children of appropriate growth and development. *The child may learn behaviors by watching other children act as role models.*
- Ensure that the child has age-appropriate toys and games. *This will promote appropriate growth and developmental levels.*
- For children with fear and anxiety as a result of abuse, the nurse must use a calm, soothing, nonjudgmental manner. *This approach will be reassuring and comforting to the child and assist the nurse in developing a trusting relationship.*
- Encourage the child to express his or her feelings of fear and anxiety. *The nurse will be able to assist the child in addressing these concerns and in correcting those that are not based in reality.*
- Provide consistency for the child, as well as comforting items such as a nightlight, favorite toy, or blanket. *Familiarity will help decrease fear and anxiety.*
- Provide positive reinforcement when the child is able to demonstrate coping behaviors and continue with activities of daily living despite expressed fears and anxiety. *Positive reinforcement will assist the child in replacing negative emotions with positive ones.*
- Teach the child self-calming behaviors such as breathing techniques, relaxation methods, and self-talk. *Helping the fearful, anxious child develop coping mechanisms will assist him or her in overcoming these negative emotions.*

EVALUATING

To evaluate outcomes, the nurse must interview the child to determine knowledge of the risks of substance abuse. Frequent follow-up visits may be necessary to evaluate future injury related to abuse, progress related to growth and developmental level, and symptoms of fear and anxiety. Ongoing accurate documentation will assist in the clinical treatment of these forms of abuse.

Traumatic Events

Children may experience trauma in their lives and be greatly affected. Children are exposed to violent crimes, sometimes in their neighborhood, on television, or in the movies. They may live through a natural disaster such as a flood, tornado, forest fire, mudslide, hurricane, or earthquake. Many will be involved in a motor vehicle crash.

Effects of Disasters on Children

- Infant: little to no effect
- Preschooler/toddler: regressive behavior; becomes clingy to trusted adults; difficulty sleeping; changes in eating habits; complains of aches and pains without obvious causes; disobedient behavior; hyperactivity; aggressive behavior; withdraws; tells exaggerated stories, particularly about the event
- School-age child: withdraws from friends; seeks to gain attention from parents; develops school phobia; sudden onset of poor school performance; aggressive behavior; difficulty concentrating; may begin acting childlike
- Adolescent: has vague physical complaints; shirks responsibility of chores, schoolwork, and extracurricular activities; competes for the attention of parents and other trusted adults; withdraws from friends; becomes resistant to authority; becomes disruptive in group settings, such as in class; experiments with risky situations, such as alcohol, drugs, and sex; feels helpless; feels guilty; may try to deny any emotions related to the traumatic event

Abuse of any kind is also considered to be a traumatic event. Children can have negative effects from a traumatic event whether they experience it personally or witness it.

Children may be affected mentally, emotionally, physically, or morally. As children try to understand the traumatic event, they feel frightened, confused, and insecure. They may feel anger, isolation, and anxiety. Box 27-6 ■ outlines the effects of disasters on children, depending on their age.

The nurse can play an instrumental role in helping children who have experienced a traumatic event deal with their emotions. Openly and honestly discuss the particulars of the event in a manner appropriate to the child's developmental level. Aid the parents of this child in understanding that the child needs to be protected from too much information about the event. Particularly if this is a national event, the child needs to be protected from too much media exposure. Graphic images, viewed repeatedly, become difficult for the child to rid from his or her mind.

The child needs reassurance, love, physical contact in the form of cuddling, and verbal support. The child needs to feel safe to ask any question and deserves to trust that he or she will receive a valid, honest answer. The child may be encouraged to express his or her emotions through drawing and painting.

Encourage parents to maintain a normal routine as much as possible. Exercise will assist the child in dealing with feelings of aggression and anger. Parents also need to relax their expectations for the child's behavior until the initial trauma has passed and the child has time to assimilate the event. The nurse should be aware of symptoms of anxiety, depression, suicidal behavior, or deviant behavior and be quick to seek professional counseling for the child.

Therapies to Assist the Child with Psychosocial Disorders

The child with a psychosocial disorder will most likely be cared for in an outpatient setting. Therapies involve the child and his or her caregivers. The nurse can assist physicians and mental health professionals to administer these therapies. If the psychosocial disorder is in an acute phase, hospitalization may be necessary. In the hospital, a psychiatric unit can provide the necessary treatment. There are also free-standing facilities that provide care to the child with substance abuse or thought process disorders.

PLAY THERAPY

Most children are comfortable playing at some level. Play allows the child to express his or her emotions through a nonthreatening media (Figure 27-6 ■). The mental health professional may encourage the child to play with dolls, toys, or clay to express anxiety, stress, and fears. The play is used to determine the child's feelings and to teach him or her appropriate methods of dealing with these negative emotions.

GROUP THERAPY

The teenager is especially receptive to group therapy. Because the teen is more responsive to his or her peers and not an authority figure, this type of therapy can assist in verbalizing the teen's feelings. Appropriate suggestions from the peer group can be accepted more readily than those from a therapist or parent. One hazard of this type of therapy is the lack of control the therapist has over the direction of the conversation and suggested resolutions.

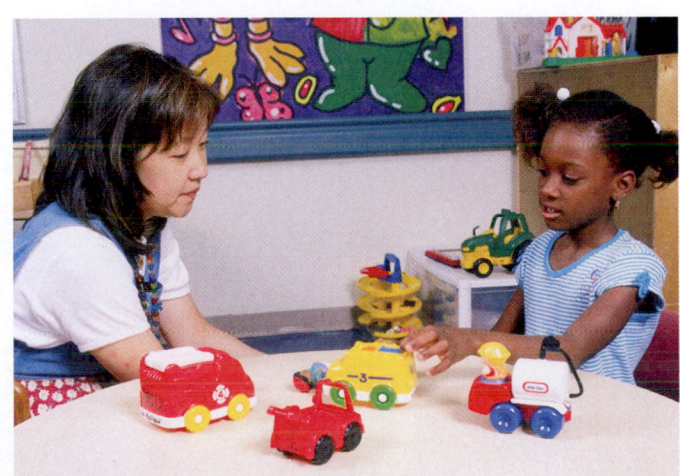

Figure 27-6. ■ The psychologist uses play therapy to help this girl re-enact a car crash. This helps her gain control over the event so it is not so frightening.

FAMILY THERAPY

Rarely is a problem within a family caused by only one member. Difficulties and the manifestations of them are typically due to the strength or weaknesses of the family unit. Family therapy seeks to build strong relationships that will promote healing of the child and future healthy relationships.

ART THERAPY

In art therapy, the child is given paper, colored pens, paint, scissors (if they are not dangerous), and glue and asked to create something that depicts what they feel inside. The therapist is then able to use this drawing to discuss the child's feelings and help the child develop methods of managing negative emotions. Art may also be used to discover hidden events of abuse or violence that the child is not able to verbalize.

BEHAVIOR THERAPY

Behavior therapy is a technique used to encourage the child to replace negative, unwanted behaviors with more positive, desirable behaviors. Rewards are used to reinforce the positive behaviors. This type of therapy works best when the therapist and family members use it consistently.

COGNITIVE THERAPY

In cognitive therapy, the child is taught to quickly recognize negative emotions such as anxiety. The child is also taught why it is detrimental to continue in these negative emotions and the benefits of avoiding them. In cognitive therapy, the mental health professional teaches the child mental activities such as breathing and relaxation techniques to counteract negative emotions.

Note: The references and resources for this and all chapters have been compiled at the back of the book.

Chapter Review

 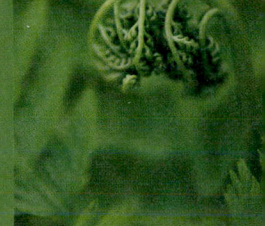

KEY TERMS by Topic

Use the audio glossary feature of either the CD-ROM or the Companion Website to hear the correct pronunciation of the following key terms.

Introduction
psychosocial health

Brief Assessment Overview
holistic health

Psychological Disorders and Associated Manifestations
Diagnostic and Statistical Manual of Mental Disorders, Fourth Edition; autism; Asperger's syndrome; echolalia; stereotypy; encopresis; generalized anxiety disorder (GAD); separation anxiety disorder (SAD); obsessive-compulsive disorder (OCD); tics; coprolalia; copropraxia; depression; bipolar disorder; suicide; obesity; bariatric surgery

Anorexia Nervosa and Bulimia
anorexia nervosa, bulimia, purging

Abuse and Family Violence
shaken baby syndrome, nonorganic failure to thrive, sexual abuse, incest, assault, rape, statutory rape, date rape, child molestation, child exploitation, child pornography, exhibitionism, pedophile

KEY Points

- Psychosocial health includes mental, emotional, social, and spiritual stability. Alterations in psychosocial health affect both the child and the entire family.

- The *Diagnostic and Statistical Manual of Mental Disorders, Fourth Edition* (DSM-IV) serves as the main diagnostic reference of mental health professionals in the United States.

- Children with autism have difficulty with verbal and nonverbal communication, social interactions, and leisure or play activities.

- Ensuring safety is a priority due to repetitive behaviors such as head banging.

- The child with ADD has difficulty finishing tasks, is easily distracted, and may move from topic to topic. The child with ADHD also fidgets, may become loud, and disrupts others. Both ADD and ADHD children have difficulty maintaining social relationships.

- Anxiety is subjective feelings of worry, helplessness, insecurity, and apprehension. The nurse can teach the child coping skills and relaxation techniques.

- Characteristics of depression vary from child to child and include declining school performance, irritability, withdrawal from social activities, sleep disorders (either unable to sleep or sleeping excessively), appetite disturbance (either overeating or anorexia), headache, stomachache, difficulty concentrating, and difficulty making decisions.

- Anorexia nervosa is a serious disorder and may require hospitalization.

- The nurse is legally obligated to report any suspicion of child abuse to local or state child protective services or law enforcement authorities.

- Physical abuse of a child is inflicting pain and injury in a deliberate manner. Emotional abuse of a child includes attacks on his or her self-esteem, as well as efforts to control, frighten, and embarrass the child.

- Sexual abuse can be defined as sexual acts that are imposed on children who cannot protect themselves due to their lack of emotional or cognitive development.

- Children and teens are vulnerable to the hazards of substance abuse due to their developmental levels.

- The nurse must be able to recognize the physical, psychological, or cognitive symptoms of substance abuse.

EXPLORE MediaLink

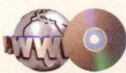

Additional interactive resources for this chapter can be found on the Companion Website at www.prenhall.com/towle.

Click on Chapter 27 and "Begin" to select the activities for this chapter.

For chapter-related NCLEX-style questions and an audio glossary, access the accompanying CD-ROM in this book.

Animations

What is autism?

Anorexia

Identifying child abuse

Children and overweight

ADD and ADHD

FOR FURTHER Study

For additional information on assessing fines and the revoking of the nursing license, see Chapter 2.

See Chapter 9 for a discussion on fetal alcohol syndrome.

See Chapter 16 for a further discussion of cognitive disorders.

For more information on enuresis, see Chapter 23.

Critical Thinking Care Map

Caring for a Client with Attention Deficit/Hyperactivity Disorder

NCLEX-PN® Focus Area: Psychosocial Integrity

Case Study: Jackson, age 6, is in first grade. Since the beginning of school, he has not been able to complete his coursework in the expected time frame and is frequently isolated from his peers during lunch and recess in an effort to get his work done.

Jackson did test positive for ADHD and has begun daily treatment with Adderall. Jackson's mother is concerned that Jackson does not have any friends because of his hyperactive behavior. She is seeking assistance for this concern.

Nursing Diagnosis: Impaired Social Interaction, related to altered thought processes (i.e., hyperactivity)

COLLECT DATA

Subjective

_____
_____
_____
_____
_____
_____
_____

Objective

_____
_____
_____
_____
_____
_____
_____

Would you report this? Yes/No

If yes, to: _____

Nursing Care

_____
_____
_____
_____
_____
_____
_____
_____
_____

How would you document this? _____
_____
_____
_____

Compare your documentation to the sample provided in Appendix I.

Data Collected
(use those that apply)

- Mother reports lack of peer interaction.
- "I couldn't sleep last night."
- Teacher states that Jackson is better able to do his coursework since he has been on Adderall.
- Jackson expresses a desire to earn an A on his math test.
- Jackson is observed attempting to talk to a group of boys in the lunchroom without success.
- Teacher reports lack of peer interaction.
- Jackson states that he has no friends.
- Jackson plays alone on the monkey bars at the playground.
- "I'm not hungry for lunch right now."
- Jackson completes his English assignment during the allotted time.
- Jackson brings his teacher a basket of apples.
- When buddies are picked for a class activity, Jackson is not picked.
- In PE class, Jackson is observed completing the obstacle course in the shortest amount of time.

Nursing Interventions
(use those that apply; list in priority order)

- Involve Jackson's parents and his teacher in developing a plan to improve social interactions between Jackson and his peers.
- Teach Jackson and his mother about the side effects of Adderall.
- Use role-play to observe the social interaction between Jackson and his peers.
- Plan an opportunity to observe Jackson in a social interaction during school hours.
- Refer Jackson to a tutoring program to enhance his schoolwork.
- Assist Jackson in developing social skills such as respect for others' privacy, and interpreting reactions from peers honestly.
- Develop a plan to reward Jackson for appropriate social interaction.
- Develop a plan for self-administration of Adderall during the school day.
- Help develop a plan for additional ways for Jackson to interact socially with other children.

NCLEX-PN® Exam Preparation

1 The nurse is assigned to care for a 4-year-old child with autism who has an upper respiratory infection. The nurse observes the following behavior and knows this is a clinical manifestation of autism:

1. conversing with others without shyness
2. displaying repetitive behaviors such as rocking back and forth
3. being able to work difficult math problems without assistance
4. playing with other children but not being able to share

2 The parents of a newly diagnosed 2-year-old with autism are having difficulty with the child's diagnosis. The nurse has just finished talking with the parents and answering their questions. She realizes additional information is needed when the mother states:

1. "I realize that with the proper care and medication our child will be cured."
2. "We understand we have to work with our child on behavior modification."
3. "I realize that we have to supervise our child constantly."
4. "We realize that when we talk with our son we must maintain eye contact and be consistent."

3 The nurse is caring for an infant born with fetal alcohol syndrome (FAS). The nurse knows that infants with FAS display the following characteristics:

1. hepatosplenomegaly, intussuception, and dysphagia.
2. hepatotoxemia, portal hypertension, and jejunoileitis.
3. growth retardation, CNS abnormalities, and craniofacial abnormalities.
4. club foot, hemophilia, and hepatitis.

4 A nursing student is asked to identify the characteristics of drug abuse. The nursing instructor steps in to correct the student when the student identifies which incorrect characteristic of drug abuse?

1. dilated or pinpoint pupils, bloodshot eyes
2. bruising or needle marks
3. runny nose
4. psoriasis

5 The nurse is observing a child with ADD. The child has been taking Adderall (amphetamine sulfate) and is exhibiting irritability and restlessness. Based on these observations, the nurse's initial response would be:

1. call the physician because these are abnormal side effects of the drug.
2. prepare for a code situation because the child is in a serious situation.
3. do nothing because these are common side effects of the drug.
4. call the drug manufacturer and report these abnormal side effects.

6 An emergency department nurse is collecting data on a child with suspected sexual abuse. What data would most likely key the nurse into suspecting sexual abuse and indicate the need for further investigation?

1. anorexia nervosa
2. vaginal redness, pain, and bloody discharge
3. fear of authority figures
4. severe diarrhea

7 A nursing student is caring for a client with anorexia nervosa and developing a plan of care. The nursing instructor speaks with the nursing student about which of the following entries as an incorrect nursing intervention for this disorder?

1. Observe strenuous exercise activities.
2. Monitor food intake.
3. Monitor fluid and electrolyte levels.
4. Observe for binge eating and purging.

8 The nurse answers the phone in the crisis center. The call is from the mother of a 16-year-old female who has told her mother that she "doesn't want to live any longer." The nurse's most appropriate response to the mother would be:

1. "Don't worry, all teens go through this stage."
2. "Please stay with your daughter and bring her in for a consult with our psychologist."
3. "Have your daughter lie down and check on her in the morning."
4. "Why would she say such a thing!?"

9 The nurse is collecting data on a severely obese 16-year-old female in the physician's office who states she wants bariatric surgery to correct her obesity. Select all criteria required before an adolescent can be considered for this surgery.

1. must have tried weight management techniques for longer than 6 months and failed
2. must be physiologically mature
3. must weigh over 150 lb
4. must agree to a psychological evaluation before surgery
5. must agree to a psychological evaluation after surgery
6. must avoid pregnancy for more than 1 year postoperatively

10 A nurse is preparing to admit an infant to the hospital with a diagnosis of shaken baby syndrome. Choose the correct statements about this syndrome.

1. Infants are susceptible to this injury because their neck muscles are weak.
2. Jarring motion causes tearing of the nerve fibers in the brain.
3. This type of injury always leads to death within 1 month.
4. After this injury infants may have seizures, lethargy, and respiratory difficulties.
5. Vision impairment or loss of hearing may result from this injury.

Answers for Review Questions, as well as discussion of Care Plan and Critical Thinking Care Map questions, appear in Appendix I.

Chapter 28

Care of the Family with a Dying Child

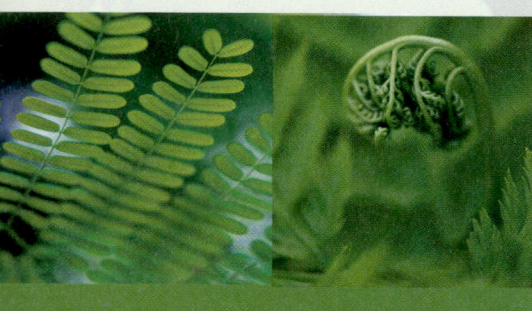

HEALTH PROMOTION ISSUE:
Pediatric Organ Donation

NURSING PROCESS CARE PLAN:
Care of a Child Dying at Home

CRITICAL THINKING CARE MAP:
Care of Mother with Anticipatory Grieving

BRIEF Outline

Grief Process
Anticipated Loss
Family of the Dying Child
Nurses' Grief
Culture and Grief
Caring for the Dying Child

Legalities Related to Death
Nursing Care
Signs of Impending Death
Care After Death
Death-Related Religious and
Cultural Practices

LEARNING Outcomes

After completing this chapter, you will be able to:

• Describe the stages of grief.
• Describe the signs of impending death.
• Describe the role of the LPN/LVN in caring for dying children and their families.
• Discuss the process of organ donation.

Threats to a child's life may be expected—as in a chronic illness or a progressively disabling condition—or be unexpected—as in a premature birth or accident. How the child, parents, and siblings cope with the threat will depend on the circumstances surrounding the event and the child's condition. If the child dies from a chronic, terminal disease such as muscular dystrophy, the child and family have time to adjust to the impending death. The parents and siblings who become involved in the care of the child who is terminally ill can feel that they have contributed to making the dying child as comfortable as possible. However, when an acute illness or unexpected injury threatens the life of a child, the parents and siblings are thrust into the unfamiliar environment of an emergency room or intensive care unit. The parents and siblings, unable to assist with care, may be totally unprepared to cope with the loss.

Nursing care of children with chronic disorders is discussed in Chapter 14 ⚮. This chapter focuses on helping the family through the grief process, making preparation for death, and providing care after death.

Grief Process

Much research has been done since the mid-1960s about the grief process. Five stages of loss or grief have been identified (Kübler-Ross, 1969) and described in detail in many nursing textbooks. These stages are reviewed and applied to the real or anticipated loss of a child.

Loss, either real or perceived, is experienced when something is removed from the body or the environment. The loss could be tangible such as misplacing a favorite toy, the amputation of a limb, or the death of a pet. The loss could be intangible such as the loss one's job, health, or respect. **Grief** is a feeling of extreme sadness resulting from a loss. At times, circumstances are such that we anticipate the loss before it actually occurs. In these cases, the stages of grief will be experienced twice: once when the loss is initially anticipated, and again when the loss actually occurs. It is important to note that individuals move through the stages of grief at different rates. The five stages are shown in Figure 28-1 ■.

Stage 1: Shock	*No! I don't believe it!*
Stage 2: Anger	IT'S NOT FAIR! I DON'T DESERVE THIS!
Stage 3: Bargaining	If you just make me better, I'll …
Stage 4: Depression	Leave me alone.
Stage 5: Acceptance	I AM READY NOW.

Figure 28-1. ■ Five stages of grief have been identified, but clients do not always experience all five stages. They may only experience some of the stages or move back and forth from one stage to another.

STAGE 1: SHOCK AND DISBELIEF

The initial reaction to a loss is one of shock and disbelief. The conscious mind is trying to process what is happening. Sensory perceptions may be altered. Time seems to stand still. It may take several minutes for the parent to understand what is being said. It may be several hours or days before the complete impact of the situation has "sunk in." Often parents describe their feelings during this time as being disconnected, in a daze, or "out of it." For most parents, the period of intense shock passes in about 24 hours. During this time, they grope for answers and explanations. They may think that the situation is just a bad dream and that they will wake up. They may make statements such as "this can't be happening" or "this isn't real." Because of their emotional state, information may need to be repeated several times. The nurse must be gentle in explaining and reinforcing the reality of the situation.

Parents display a wide range of behaviors upon hearing bad news. The parent may scream, cry, or collapse to the floor. They may remain in control, strike out at the nearest object, or try to run away. They may yell at the person who is telling them the news. The nurse must anticipate any of these reactions and be ready to provide support. Parents should not be alone at this time. If they try to run away, it is important for someone to go with them. Running away in an extreme emotional state puts the parent at risk for injury to themselves and others.

STAGE 2: ANGER

As the reality of the situation begins to penetrate the conscious mind, anger begins to surface. The parents may direct the anger at themselves in the form of guilt, or it may be directed toward the spouse, health care providers, other children, others involved in the situation, or God. In their anger, parents frequently make accusing or threatening comments. They may physically try to assault the person they believe is responsible for the child's death. It is important for the nurse to maintain objectivity, defuse the situation, and help the grieving parent work through the anger in a positive manner.

STAGE 3: BARGAINING

To bargain means to make a deal. For example, if I do something for you, then you can do something for me. The bargaining stage of grief is similar. In anticipation of the death of their child, parents may bargain with doctors, nurses, or God. Comments such as "I'll do anything, just save my child's life" indicate the parent is bargaining to prevent the loss. When death has occurred, parents may make statements such as, "I would do anything just to have one more day with my child." The nurse must understand these comments and support the parents as they come to the realization that there is nothing that can be done to change the inevitability of death.

STAGE 4: DEPRESSION

Depression is a state of persistent sadness. The depressed person lacks energy and enthusiasm to perform all daily activities. They may experience persistent hopelessness, tearfulness, and a sense of worthlessness. The times of sadness seem to come in waves. They are interspersed with times of relative calm as they remember happy experiences. Although this depressed state may last for up to a year, the parent should begin to have longer periods of happiness and shorter periods of extreme sadness. If depression prevents the parent from performing daily activities and interacting socially, professional help may be needed. The nurse can be instrumental in helping the parent explore and understand his or her feelings. Because of the seriousness of depressed states, early recognition and referral is important.

STAGE 5: ACCEPTANCE

The loss of a child is the most difficult experience a parent endures. When the birth of a child is expected, parents begin to dream and plan for the future. When the child dies or has a life-threatening illness or injury, the parents not only lose the child, but they also lose the dream. Over time the parents come to accept the loss. They are able to make new dreams and plans for the future. To keep the memory of the lost child alive, parents need to be encouraged to reminisce about the happy times. Keeping some pictures around the house, keeping in contact with the child's friends, or helping other grieving families may help the parents find some good out of their loss.

Anticipated Loss

Anticipated loss occurs during a life-threatening illness or injury. Anticipated loss begins when the parent first hears the diagnosis of the life-threatening illness (Figure 28-2 ■). If parents are present at the time of injury, they begin to make judgments about the extent of injury and possible prognosis. If they are not present at the time of injury, the anticipated

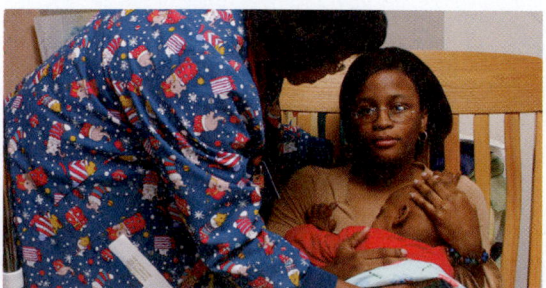

Figure 28-2. ■ This 3½-year-old's condition has deteriorated rapidly, and death is expected within 2 to 3 days. The nurse's role is to keep the child as comfortable as possible and to support the family.

loss begins the moment they are notified of the injury. When the child's condition is uncertain, the parents begin to anticipate death, permanent damage, or disfigurement. They imagine how their life will be changed if the child does not recover fully. They experience sadness at the thought of losing the lifestyle they have known and the hardships ahead.

As the child's condition stabilizes and improves, the parents adjust and make plans for transfer or discharge. If the child's condition is terminal, parents remain in the emotional turmoil of grief. If the child's illness involves periods of remission and exacerbation, the parents will have periods of calm acceptance and periods of emotional stress. As the child's condition deteriorates, the parents will need to make plans for terminal care. Following the child's death, the parents will again move through the grief process.

Family of the Dying Child

DYING CHILD

Care of the dying child is one of the most challenging experiences of nursing, requiring great sensitivity and compassion for the child and for the entire family. The age and developmental stage of the child who is ill influences his or her reaction to impending death. Table 28-1 ■ identifies children's understanding of and reaction to death at each stage of development.

The infant has no concept of illness or death but will develop separation anxiety when the parents or primary care provider are out of sight. The toddler responds to the anxiety of the parent. In a strange environment, they fear body mutilation and the possibility of pain. Even 5-year-olds can tell the seriousness of illness. They are aware of death but may not have a concept of its permanence. Young children can see their body deteriorate and feel the effects of toxic chemicals as the disease progresses. They may realize they are dying based on their own body changes and seeing other children who are undergoing treatment. Although the young child may not be able to express anxiety over death, he or she does express fear of body mutilation. Even when not told they are dying, children know their condition is worsening.

Children often keep their fears of dying to themselves. They are aware of the stress their family is undergoing, and they do not want to contribute to it. They fear the family will abandon them if they express anger over their illness and impending death. Because of their own fears and feelings of hopelessness, parents may not recognize the child's emotional needs and fears.

Adolescents are old enough to understand death and what is happening to them. However, due to their stage of development, adolescents have additional challenges. Adolescents struggle for independence and their own identity. They are preoccupied with their body image at a time when terminal illness may result in disfigurement. Dying teens

TABLE 28-1

Children's Understanding of Death

CHILD'S AGE	CONCEPT OF DEATH	BEHAVIOR
Infant	Has no concept of death. May react to caregiver stress.	Crying, fussy, eats less, may sleep more than usual.
Toddler	Has no true concept of death. Aware someone is missing but unable to tell temporary separation from permanent loss.	Separation anxiety, clinging to parents, biting, hitting, and refusing to eat or sleep.
Preschooler	May have beginning understanding of death of pets. Believes death is temporary and magic can cause death or return life.	Shows aggression, throws things, hits, hyperactive. Fears going to sleep due to nightmares. Asks a lot of questions about death.
School-Age	Understands that death is permanent. Understands that death will happen to everyone.	Tries to act "grown up" and not cry, tries to help with household chores, may develop stomachache or headache.
Adolescent	Understands death is associated with illness and trauma. Fear of death conflicts with feeling invincible. Recognizes effects of death on parents and others.	May develop severe depression, including suicide attempts. May exhibit risk-taking behaviors.

may feel isolated from their friends at a time when peers are an important part of their development. As death nears, adolescents should be allowed as much control over events as their condition allows.

The nurse must be diligent in providing care to the child who is terminally ill, while promoting a normal growth and development pattern and supporting the family and peers. Whether in the hospital or at home, helping the ill child maintain contact with peers will reduce the feeling of isolation (Figure 28-3 ■).

The biggest challenges to nursing care come not from the physical needs but from the emotional needs. The nurse must be sensitive to both the verbal and the nonverbal communication. By providing opportunities for fantasy play, storytelling, and art projects, the nurse encourages the child to express feelings for which he or she may not have words. Box 28-1 ■ identifies strategies for communicating with the dying child.

BOX 28-1	NURSING CARE CHECKLIST

Communicating with Dying Child

☑ Be flexible.

☑ Recognize that some children communicate best through nonverbal means (i.e., art, music). The child may be willing to talk through a puppet or a stuffed animal.

☑ Respect the child's need to be alone and the desire to share. Allow communication, but do not force it.

☑ Be receptive when children initiate conversation.

☑ Be specific and literal in explaining death.

☑ Acknowledge that the child's life can be complete, even if it is brief. Let dying children know that they will always be loved and remembered. Help children find a sense of accomplishment and purpose in the lives they have led.

☑ Empower children as much as possible in circumstances concerning their deaths. Reassure them of continued love and physical closeness.

Source: Adapted from London M., Ladewig P., Ball J., & Bindler R. (2003). *Maternal–newborn & child nursing.* Upper Saddle River, NJ: Prentice Hall.

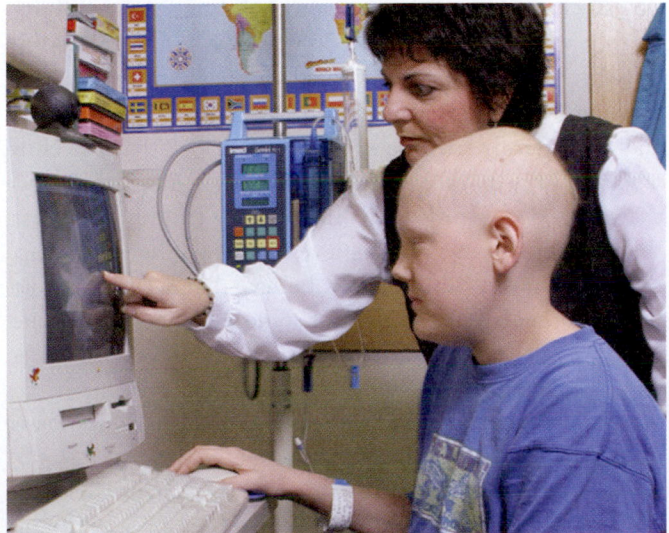

Figure 28-3. ■ This teenager and his mother are exploring computer chat rooms of terminally ill children receiving palliative care.

TABLE 28-2

Answering Children's Questions About Death

QUESTION	ANSWER
What will death be like?	"I think it will be peaceful. What do you think?"
What will happen to me when I die?	"What have your parents told you about what will happen to you?"
Will I be punished for the bad things I have done?	"Do you think you will be punished?"
When will I be with (person closest to child) again?	"I think (person) will be with you when he or she dies."
Will my parents be all right?	"Your parents will miss you because they love you, but they will be all right."
Will I experience pain?	"We will try to keep the pain away. Let us know if you hurt, okay?"

At times, the parents request that the child not be told about the prognosis. This can be emotionally conflicting for the nurse if the child asks about the condition. Table 28-2 ■ identifies questions commonly asked by children who are terminally ill. In such a situation, the nurse should tell the parents about the child's questions. Parents may feel unprepared to talk with the child and answer questions about dying. The nurse can anticipate the child's questions and give the parent developmentally appropriate words to use in discussing death. The family may benefit from a referral to a professional who has experience in bereavement and in counseling children and families.

PARENTS OF THE DYING CHILD

The death of a child is the most painful experience a parent will have to endure. When the death is sudden and unexpected, such as following an accident, the parent has little time to adjust to the shock. At times, due to resuscitation efforts, the parents may not be able to stay with the child. A private room should be provided for them. If possible, one spokesperson from the medical team should keep the family informed of the child's condition. When death appears inevitable, the spokesperson should provide time for the parents to absorb information of the child's worsening condition.

Federal regulations require the family to be given the option of donating the child's organs for research or transplant. Nurses with special education in organ procurement should be called to talk with the family and obtain informed consent. If organ donation is being considered, the physician should be notified immediately because the decision may alter use of some life support medications. The

Health Promotion Issue on pages 822 and 823 discusses organ donation.

Family, friends, and clergy should be called at the parents' request. Avoid giving news of death over the telephone. Instead, notify the family that the child has been seriously injured in an accident. Ask them to come to the hospital immediately. Bad news should be given in a private area. Assure parents and family that everything possible was done for the child. Prepare the child's body before allowing the parents to view their child.

When the child is dying of a chronic illness, the parents have more time to prepare for the loss. In most cases of chronic terminal illness, the child gradually deteriorates over a few hours or days. Parents usually have enough time to call family and friends to be with them. After months or years of watching their child struggle for life, parents may wish for the child's death. Parents will grieve, but they will also experience relief that the child is finally at peace. Being happy for the death of their child may bring feelings of guilt. At this time, parents need to be encouraged to talk about their feelings. They should be told that it is okay to let go of the child and be relieved that the suffering is over.

Over time, parents will work through the grief process and come to accept the loss of their child. However, there will continue to be times when an event, birthday, or anniversary will restimulate the grief process. These new periods of sadness may last only a few hours, or they may last for days. They are likely to become less frequent over time but will probably be with the parents forever.

SIBLINGS OF THE DYING CHILD

The reaction of siblings to the terminal illness and death of a child is as individual as the reaction of adults. Many factors, including age, development, birth order, and length of the illness, can influence the reaction of siblings. As stated previously, very young children do not have an understanding of death, so they may not know why their brother or sister is no longer present. Reacting to the stress of their parents and other family members, they may realize that the child who was ill is no longer present, but they may forget once they are gone for some time. If the dying child is the eldest, the younger siblings may believe that when they "grow up" they too will die. Siblings may believe that the loss of a sister or brother is punishment for something they have done, or that somehow the death was their fault. Some children may be jealous of the attention the child who is ill receives and then feel guilty once he or she dies. Many children have difficulty sleeping for fear they will not wake up.

Siblings need support and compassion. The nurse needs to explain what is occurring in age-appropriate language (Figure 28-4 ■). If the child is dying from a chronic illness, the siblings should be allowed to participate in care as much as possible.

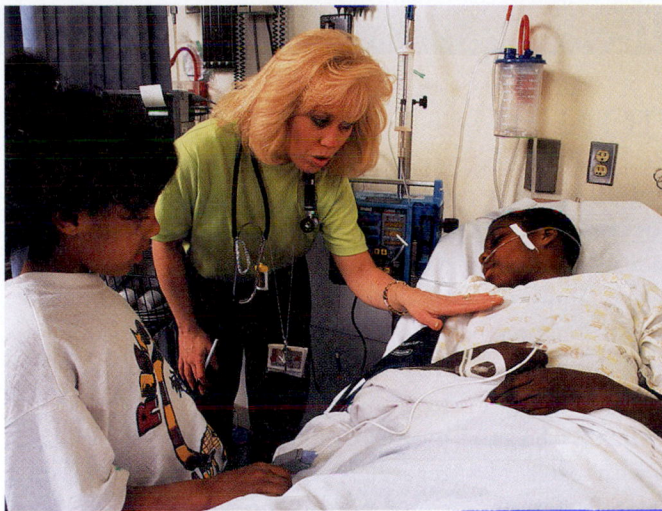

Figure 28-4. ■ When siblings visit the dying child, be prepared to answer questions honestly and in a manner that they can understand.

Encouraging and helping the siblings to make cards, posters, or gifts will help them as well as the child who is ill. When death does occur, the nurse should make statements such as "His heart stopped beating, and it will never start again" or "She will never be in pain again." Such statements help the siblings understand the finality of death. Siblings need to understand that their parents are grieving and may not be able to respond to their needs as usual. Friends and family members are invaluable to assist with routine household chores and to provide as much stability in the home as possible.

GRANDPARENTS OF THE DYING CHILD

The grief of grandparents is unique. When a parent becomes a grandparent, a special bond develops with the grandchild. Grandparents develop a feeling of pride in their own children and fulfillment that their family heritage will continue. When a child dies, a part of that family heritage dies, too. The grandparent grieves the loss. When a child dies, the grandparents also feel intense pain for their own child's loss. Having to watch their adult child in pain and being unable to relieve that pain, the grandparents experience helplessness and guilt. As they try to be strong for their child, the grandparents may find that their needs go unrecognized and unmet.

The nurse can offer support by encouraging the grandparents to express their feelings. By acknowledging the grandparents' loss and feelings of helplessness, the nurse communicates empathy for them. This opens a therapeutic relationship with the nurse that allows the grandparents to feel comfortable talking about their loss.

Nurses' Grief

Nurses also grieve the loss of their clients. Most enter the nursing profession to be of help to others. When a client dies, the nurse may believe that he or she failed to provide

quality care. When the client is a child, the nurse may feel he or she has failed the client, the parents, and the family.

When caring for a child who is terminally ill, the nurse develops a close relationship with the child and family. To remain objective and professional, many nurses begin to withdraw from the relationship prior to the death. When the nurse has children or grandchildren the same age as the dying child, the nurse may have more difficulty maintaining a professional relationship. The nurse may have difficulty identifying the child's and family's needs due to his or her own defenses against the feeling of hopelessness and helplessness. When the nurse realizes the inevitability of a child's death, he or she experiences feelings of anger, frustration, sadness, and powerlessness. These feelings can interfere with the nurse's decision making and good judgment.

It is important for nurses in these circumstances to share their grief with other health care professionals (Figure 28-5 ■). Nurses who work frequently with the dying child and his or her family must learn to cope with grief while maintaining their objectivity, empathy, and compassion. The employing agency must acknowledge the nurse's stress. By providing employee support groups and debriefing sessions with mental health professionals, the agency helps the nurse to manage his or her feelings.

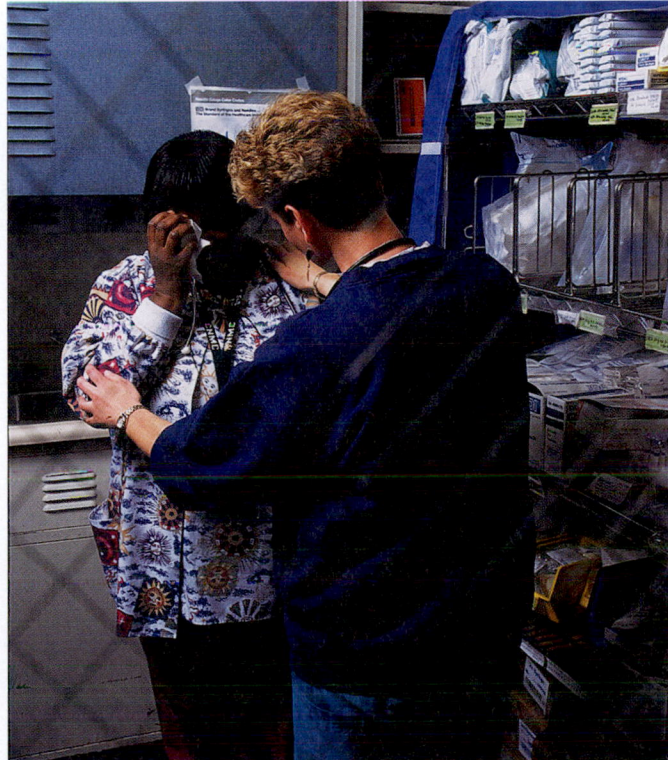

Figure 28-5. ■ Nurses who work with the dying need to express their own grief in a supportive environment after a child's death. Nurses who do not share their sadness and grief with colleagues may be unable to provide supportive care to the next family who needs compassionate care.

(Text continues on p. 825.)

HEALTH PROMOTION ISSUE

PEDIATRIC ORGAN DONATION

Delores and Juan Reyes rushed to the emergency room when their 2-year-old daughter Sandra climbed onto a porch railing and fell on her head to the concrete patio below. Sandra had been taken to the emergency department by ambulance. Upon arrival at the hospital, Sandra was comatose, her breathing was very slow and shallow, and her pulse was irregular. Within minutes, her pupils became fixed and dilated. The toddler did not regain consciousness. The child remained on life support while the doctor talked with the parents in a separate room. Both parents were distraught and stated that they "cannot believe their baby is gone." The charge nurse who was staying with or near the parents has the responsibility of discussing the possibility of organ donation with them. The nurse needs knowledge and compassion to discuss this topic with parents who are emotionally distraught. However, this discussion is not only a legal requirement, but it must also take place in a timely manner to ensure that the organs are preserved for successful transplantation.

DISCUSSION

In recent years, organ transplantation has become an acceptable treatment for clients with organ failure. The primary problem facing organ transplant teams is not the advanced technology required for successful transplantation, but a lack of donor organs, especially for pediatric populations. Annually more than 2,000 children younger than the age of 17 are on a waiting list for donor organs. Sadly, 30% to 50% of children younger than 2 years of age will die while waiting for various organs. Three reasons for this

shortage have been identified: Families are not being asked about organ donation, health care professionals do not pursue potential donors, and families fail to give consent for organ donation.

The process of obtaining donor organs usually begins with health care professionals who treat children who are critically ill. Any person with severe head trauma should be considered a candidate to donate organs. Most donors have suffered spontaneous intracranial bleeding, gunshot to the head, brain tumors, cerebral anoxia, or drug overdose.

Once a possible donor has been identified, signs of brain death must be recognized and evaluated. In the early 1980s, physicians were reluctant to apply brain death criteria to young children. Following years of research and dialog, however, it is now agreed that standard brain death criteria can be applied to all children with the exception of the premature infant (see Box 28-4).

Although medical personnel understand the diagnosis of brain death, families and the general public are

often confused by it. This is especially true when the brain dead individual is a child. Often, parents, in shock from grief, may not fully understand that their child will not recover. Parents may deny that their child is dead. They may not accept that all life support measures can and will be discontinued regardless of whether they give permission for organ donation. Organs cannot be removed until the client is declared brain dead and the parents or legal guardians give consent.

In 1998, the Health Care Financing Administration (HCFA) instituted a requirement that all hospitals notify the Organ Procurement Organization (OPO) of any death or impending death. This requirement is further supported by the federal law titled "Required Request." Federal policies require any hospital receiving Medicare and Medicaid reimbursements to establish a program for organ donation. The Joint Commission for the Accreditation of Healthcare Organizations (JCAHO) has a similar requirement.

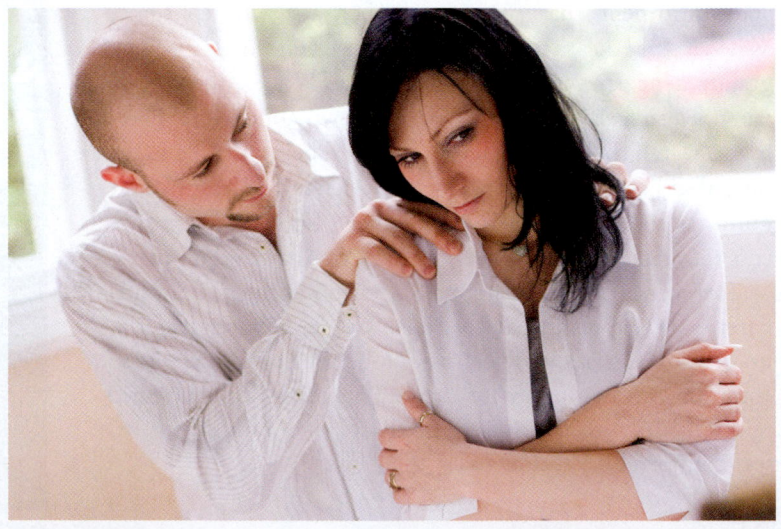

(Chris Rout/Alamy)

The OPO evaluates the potential donor's medical and social history for any issue that would rule out organ donation. If the OPO supports the organ donation, the next step is to discuss the idea with the family. This is a very delicate subject to discuss at an already emotional time. Many experts believe that the physician who determines the child to be brain dead should be the person to discuss organ donation with parents. Some physicians, however, believe that this could be viewed as conflict of interest and suggest someone else would be better suited. As part of the plan required by the 1998 Health Care Financing Administration recommendations, hospitals have designated, trained individuals, who work in collaboration with OPO, to meet with the family.

Timing of the discussion with the family is critical. The family must be given time to fully understand the meaning of "brain dead," to move past the shock and disbelief of their loss, and to have their questions answered. Then the topic of organ donation can be discussed. Many families are grateful for the opportunity to donate their child's organs and to know that "something good will come out of this tragedy." Other parents express discomfort with the discussion before having time to adjust to their loss. Some families believe that the discussion is hasty and callous. When families are treated with respect and compassion, they will be more open to discussing organ donation.

Donor families rely on health care professionals for comfort, support, and accurate information. Donor families should understand that the cost of organ donation is the responsibility of OPO and not of the donor families. Funeral ceremonies are usually not delayed or altered because of organ donation.

It takes time for recipients to be identified and contacted and for transplant teams to be prepared. Recovering or harvesting donated organs is a highly technical and specialized surgical procedure. Specially trained surgeons, anesthesiologists, nurses, and technicians may need to travel to the donor. During this time, the child's stability and organ function must be maintained. This includes maintaining normal cardiac output and tissue perfusion, ensuring adequate ventilation, preventing infection, maintaining adequate urinary output, maintaining fluid and electrolyte balance, and regulating body temperature. OPO personnel coordinate these activities.

PLANNING AND IMPLEMENTING

All children in critical condition with a brain injury or disease should be assessed by health care professionals for the possibility of becoming an organ donor. The function of all body systems must be assessed frequently. Signs of decreased function should be reported promptly and intervention begun to stabilize the child's condition.

Initially, the child's condition may not warrant a call to OPO or talking with the family. However, the nurse must anticipate that if the child's condition deteriorates, organ donation may become an issue. The nurse must be knowledgeable of the requirement of discussing organ donation and be aware of facility policy. The nurse needs to remember that whatever the family's decision, it will be a good one if they have been given information in a caring manner.

Emphasis needs to be placed on public awareness of organ donation. Families should talk about donation and share their decision with other family members and their primary health care provider. The nurse has the role of discussing the option of organ donation with families, including their own.

SELF-REFLECTION

What are your own thoughts about organ donation at death? Do you have any religious or cultural opposition to the idea? Are you in favor of the idea? What effect could your own opinion have when you are dealing with parents who must make this decision for their child?

SUGGESTED RESOURCES

For the Nurse

- Koch D'Agostino, C. (1998, September). Issues in pediatric organ donation. *Jacksonville Medicine/Northeast Florida Medicine.*

- www.optn.org Organ Procurement and Transplantation Network.
- www.unos.org United Network for Organ Sharing.

TABLE 28-3

Cultural Traditions in Mourning and After-Death Rites

RELIGIOUS GROUP	POSSIBLE RITUALS	ORGAN DONATION OR AUTOPSY BELIEFS
Native American	Beliefs and practices vary widely Navajo do not touch the deceased or their belongings Mourning is done in private	Varies among tribes
Baha'i	No embalming or cremation; must be buried within an hour's travel distance of place of death Body washed and wrapped in shroud Prayer for the Dead recited	Decision left to individual
Buddhism	Last-rite chanting at bedside Cremation common Prayers weekly for 49 days to help soul in its transformation and possible rebirth	Organ donation considered act of mercy, autopsy individual choice
Catholicism	Sacrament of the sick Obligated to take ordinary but not extraordinary means to prolong life Burial preferred (in Catholic cemeteries) Cremation allowed, but remains must be interred, not scattered	Autopsy, organ donation acceptable
Christian Science	Unlikely to seek medical help to prolong life Disposal of body and parts decided by family	Individual decides about organ donation
Hinduism	No restrictions to right-to-die issue Religious prayers chanted before and after death Body washed, wrapped in white cloth, laid in coffin Cremation common Men and women display outward grief, do not take part in any rituals for length of mourning period Thread tied around wrist signifies a blessing; do not remove No embalming	Autopsy, organ donation acceptable
Islam	Attempts to shorten life prohibited Body is washed only by Muslims of same gender and wrapped in a plain cloth (*kafan*) Only burial is permitted by Islamic law (*Shari'ah*) Prayer for forgiveness recited	Organ donation acceptable Autopsy only for medical or legal reasons
Jehovah's Witness	Use of extraordinary means to prolong life is individual choice Burial determined by family preference	Autopsy if required by law Organ donation forbidden
Judaism	If death is inevitable, no new procedure needed, but must continue those ongoing Body ritually washed Burial as soon as possible, all body parts must be buried together Seven-day mourning period	Autopsy permitted in certain circumstances, organ donation is a complex issue
Mennonite	Do not believe life must be continued at all cost	Autopsy, organ donation acceptable
Mormonism	If death inevitable, promote a peaceful and dignified death Burial in temple clothes Burial preferred to cremation ("dust to dust")	Autopsy permitted with permission of next of kin, organ donation is permitted
Protestantism	Burial or cremation is individual decision	Autopsy, organ donation are individual decisions
Seventh-Day Adventist	Follow ethic of prolonging life Disposal of body and burial are individual decisions	Autopsy, organ donation acceptable

Data from Spector, R. E. (2000). *Cultural diversity in health and illness* (5th ed.). Upper Saddle River, NJ: Prentice Hall Health, pp. 137–138, 144–149; Death and dying. (1997). *Hinduism Today.* Published by Hindu Press International; Funeral rites and customs. (2000). Microsoft Encarta Encyclopedia.

The nurse must also remember that he or she is human, and humans grieve. The family wants a nurse who provides care with compassion. If the nurse sheds a tear at times, the family will not see the nurse as weak and unprofessional, but as a person who cares about them and their child. This sharing of human emotion speaks more than words.

Culture and Grief

The nurse should work closely with the family of a dying child. To be most helpful, the nurse must understand the family's culture. There are many culturally influenced rites and rituals surrounding death. Table 28-3 ■ identifies some common cultural traditions regarding mourning and after-death care.

A nurse may sometimes work with a family whose culture is not familiar. In this situation, the nurse must ask the family questions. Statements such as "What are your traditions when a child dies?" can be helpful. Box 28-2 ■ provides some insight into cultural approaches to illness. The most important aspect of care for the child and family is to provide care with compassion and understanding of the extreme stress the family is undergoing. Many times, a gentle touch or sitting quietly with the family is the best intervention at the time.

DYSFUNCTIONAL GRIEF

Dysfunctional grief occurs when an individual is unable to accept what has occurred and move on with life. "Forgetting" the lost child is never a goal. However, being able to work through the pain and continue with other activities is a sign of healthy grieving. The individual who is unable to

---

| BOX 28-2 | **CULTURAL PULSE POINTS** |

Respecting Cultural Practices Related to Illness and Death

At death, cultural practices and patterns generally surface, even if people have drifted from many cultural habits in daily life. Problems may arise if a health care team does not understand behavior that is normal or expected within a culture. For example, a Southeast Asian may use "coining" (rubbing coins) as a way to try to heal a person who is ill. A person from the Caribbean might look to a witch or *shaman* (medicine man) to help regain health. After death, some Native Americans cleanse the body, drum, and then open the window to release the person's spirit. These behaviors might seem bizarre to a nurse who does not understand them or who believes that they somehow "break the rules."

When a family presents an idea that is foreign, the nurse should ask questions and try to understand what the practice means to the family in the context of their culture. If possible, a "cultural translator" should be asked to participate, to explain the meaning of the behavior and customs, and to help the staff accommodate these rituals as much as they can.

Source: Adapted from Eby, L. (2005). *Mental health nursing care.* Upper Saddle River, NJ: Prentice Hall.

---

continue with activities of daily living needs professional assistance. Signs of dysfunctional grieving might include:

- Continuous crying
- Sleep disturbances, including being unable to sleep or wanting to sleep all the time
- Eating disturbances, including overeating or undereating
- Being unable to manage household activities, or an obsession with household activities to the point that other things are omitted
- Being unable to work or participate in social activities within 3 to 6 months of the death
- Being unable to dispose of any of the child's belongings
- Being unable to show signs of sadness (no crying, no emotional response).

The LPN/LVN who sees these signs should inform the RN or physician. A referral to a counselor and, for some, antidepressant medication may be needed.

Caring for the Dying Child

PALLIATIVE CARE

As the child's condition deteriorates, decisions about palliative care must be made. The term **palliative care** or **palliative management** involves a shift in treatment goals from curative toward providing relief from suffering. Relief of suffering in dying clients goes beyond identifying and treating physical symptoms. The emotional, spiritual, and existential components of suffering and pain must also be addressed. It is important to note that palliative management can occur even in a hospital setting. The following are the major principles of palliative care:

- The overall goal of treatment is to optimize quality of life; that is, the hopes and desires of the dying person are fulfilled as much as possible.
- Death is regarded as a natural process, to be neither hastened nor prolonged.
- Diagnostic tests and other invasive procedures are minimized, unless they are likely to alleviate symptoms.
- Use of "heroic" treatment measures is discouraged.
- When using narcotic analgesics, the right dose is the dose that provides pain relief without unacceptable side effects.
- The client is the "expert" on whether pain and symptoms have been adequately relieved.
- Clients eat if they are hungry, drink if they are thirsty; feeding and fluids are not forced.
- Care is individualized and based on the goals of the client and family.

HOSPICE CARE

Hospice care is based on the holistic concepts of palliative care that emphasize care to improve the quality of life rather than to cure. The hospice movement was founded by the physician Cecily Saunders in London, England, in 1967 and was later

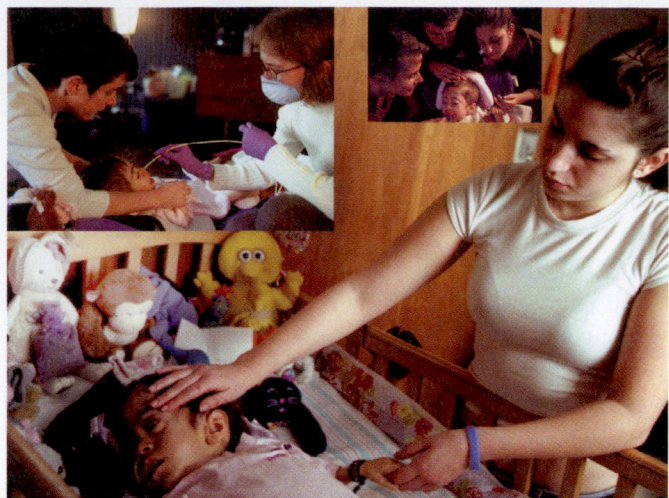

Figure 28-6. ■ Hospices like Pathways KIDS work with the client and family to provide quality of life for the dying child. Comfort measures and attention to emotional, psychological, and spiritual concerns are the priorities. (Photos courtesy of Sophia's Garden Foundation. © 2002–2005 Karen Schreiber.)

extended to the United States. It grew rapidly after the enactment of the Medicare Hospice Benefit in 1983. The Medicare benefit systematically outlines who can provide care, at what time, and in what way. Another facet of the Medicare program is to provide the client with durable medical equipment, such as oxygen and a hospital bed. Like palliative care, the principles of hospice care can be carried out in a variety of settings. However, the most common settings are the client's home or extended care facilities. Autonomous hospice and hospital-based palliative care units are also becoming more available.

Hospice services can range from being comprehensive to focusing on selected specialties such as symptom control and pain management services (Figure 28-6 ■). Hospice care is always delivered by a team of health care professionals, regardless of the setting, in order to ensure a holistic approach to care. The team members generally consist of the dying one, family and caregivers, physicians, nurses, aides, chaplains, social workers, and volunteers.

Entrance or admission into a hospice program requires a physician referral that can occur several ways. The referral may be initiated by the physician who finds at some point that curative treatment is no longer an option. The Medicare guideline governing admission is a prognosis of 6 months or less of life expectancy. Obviously, this has to be an educated guess, and clients should not be denied claims if they live longer than 6 months. Typically, the referring physician discusses the referral with the client and family and either contacts the hospice team or contacts the discharge planner or social worker to assist with the transition.

COMFORT MEASURES

Comfort measures are important for the dying child and for the family. By assisting with providing comfort, family members feel useful because they are contributing to their child's care. Comfort measures include:

- Frequent position changes. *The weak child may be unable to turn him- or herself. Frequent position changes relieve pressure on bony prominences, facilitate drainage of respiratory secretions, and ease breathing.*
- Frequent oral care, including swabbing mucous membranes with applicators and water and applying ointment to lips. *Mouth breathing dries mucus membranes and lips. If a child is unable to swallow, oral fluids should not be given.*
- Liquid tears. *Liquid tears may be needed if the child does not blink often enough to prevent drying of the cornea.*
- Pain medication as ordered. *Pain medication is frequently ordered "as needed." Pain medication should be administered to the dying child to maintain the blood level.*
- Alternative methods of reducing pain whenever possible (Box 28-3 ■). *Alternative methods such as distraction or biofeedback can be helpful in coping with pain.*

Legalities Related to Death

The nurse's roles in legal issues related to death are determined by the laws of the region and the policies of the health care institution. For example, in some states, a nasogastric feeding tube cannot be removed from a person in a persistent vegetative state without a prior directive from the client. In other states, the removal is allowed at the family's request or at a physician's order. Many of these legal issues stimulate strong ethical concerns. The nurse may need support from other team members in understanding and providing appropriate care to clients facing death.

ADVANCE DIRECTIVES

The Patient Self-Determination Act, implemented in 1991, requires all health care facilities receiving Medicare and Medicaid reimbursement to do the following:

- Recognize advance directives.
- Ask clients whether they have advance directives.
- Provide educational materials advising clients of their rights to declare their personal desires regarding treatment decisions, including the right to refuse medical treatment.

There are two types of advance medical directives: the living will and the health care proxy or surrogate. The living will provides specific instructions about what medical treatment the client chooses to omit or refuse (e.g., cardiopulmonary resuscitation [CPR], intubation, ventilatory support) in the event that the client is unable to make those decisions.

BOX 28-3	**COMPLEMENTARY THERAPIES**

Comforting a Dying Child

Providing comfort is a primary concern for the dying child. Pain management is an important nursing intervention. When medical interventions cannot control pain, the nurse looks to alternative methods to reduce or remove pain.

Biofeedback

With biofeedback, a client uses special machines to control such body functions as heart rate, blood pressure, and muscle tension. Biofeedback is sometimes used with people who have cancer to help them cope with pain and reduce anxiety.

Distraction

Distraction means turning your attention to something other than the pain. Distraction may actually work better than medicine when pain is sudden and intense or brief (lasting 5–45 minutes). It can be useful while waiting for pain medicine to start working. Distraction may be all that a person needs if pain is mild. It can even be a powerful way of relieving even the most intense pain temporarily. Some people think that a person who can be distracted from pain does not have severe pain. This is not necessarily true.

Skin Stimulation

Skin stimulation is the use of sensations (pressure, friction, temperature change, or chemicals) to excite the nerve endings in the skin. By providing a strong sensation that is not pain, we are able to lessen or block the pain sensation. Skin stimulation also alters the flow of blood to the affected area, which can reduce or

remove pain. *Note:* Skin stimulation should not be used on areas of skin receiving radiation therapy because it may increase trauma to the skin.

Pressure

Pressure is a method of relieving pain in some instances. Pressure can be applied with the entire hand, the heel of the hand, the fingertips, the knuckles, or the ball of the thumb, or with both hands. Pressure can be applied for about 10 seconds to 1 minute over or near the pain. Pressure is usually most effective if it is applied as firmly as possible without causing pain.

Vibration

Vibration over or near the area of pain may bring temporary relief. The scalp attachment of a handheld vibrator often relieves a headache. A vibrator placed at the small of the back may help low back pain.

Cold or Heat

Heat often relieves sore muscles; cold lessens pain sensations by numbing the affected area. Preference for heat or cold may be very individualized.

Menthol Preparations

Menthol preparations for pain are available in creams, lotions, liniments, or gels. When rubbed into the skin, they increase blood circulation to the affected area and produce a soothing feeling that lasts for several hours.

The *health care proxy,* also referred to as durable power of attorney for health care, is a written statement appointing someone else (e.g., a relative or trusted friend) to manage health care treatment decisions when the client is unable to do so. For example, it is often used for specific clients who are in a coma, are having life-sustaining procedures, or are receiving artificial nutrition or hydration.

In most cases, parents are the decision makers for their children. However, in some states, children as young as 15 years may sign informed consent forms. They may also determine whether they want to be organ donors and whether they want to terminate life-sustaining treatment. (See more on legal and ethical nursing issues in Chapter 2 ⬭.)

Nurses should learn the law regarding client self-determination for the state in which they practice. They are also responsible for knowing the policy and procedures for implementation in the institutions where they work. The legally binding nature and specific requirements of advance medical directives are determined by individual state legislation.

In most states, advance directives must be witnessed by two people but do not require review by an attorney or notarization. Some states do not permit relatives, heirs, or

physicians to witness advance directives. Again, it is important for nurses to be informed of their state and institutional policies and procedures.

DO NOT RESUSCITATE ORDERS

Physicians may order "no code" or do not resuscitate (DNR) for clients who are in a stage of terminal, irreversible illness or expected death. A DNR order is generally written when the client or surrogate has expressed the desire for no resuscitation in the event of a respiratory or cardiac arrest. Many physicians are reluctant to write such an order if there is any conflict between the client and family members. A "**comfort measures only**" order is written to indicate that the goal of treatment is a comfortable, dignified death and that further life-sustaining measures are not indicated. Many states permit clients living at home to arrange special orders so emergency technicians called to the home in the event of a cardiopulmonary arrest will respect the client's desire not to be resuscitated. Nurses should be familiar with the federal and state or provincial laws and the policies of their institution concerning withholding life-sustaining measures.

EUTHANASIA

Euthanasia is the act of compassionately putting to death a person suffering from incurable or distressing disease. It is sometimes referred to as "mercy killing." Regardless of compassion, good intentions, or moral convictions, euthanasia is illegal in both Canada and the United States. It can lead to criminal charges of homicide or to a civil lawsuit for withholding treatment or providing an unacceptable standard of care.

Voluntary euthanasia, or **assisted suicide,** refers to situations in which the dying individual desires some control over the time and manner of death. All forms of euthanasia are illegal, except in Oregon, where a physician-assisted suicide statute was passed in 1994. That statute permits physicians to prescribe lethal doses of medications to clients who request them and meet certain criteria. Since Oregon's action, several other states have proposed similar laws. Legal challenges and ethical debates continue.

NURSING CARE

PRIORITIES IN NURSING CARE

When death cannot be avoided, the priorities of care for the child and family include:

- Assisting with comfort measures for the child
- Preparing the child and family by making a plan for after-death activities (notifying family and friends, funeral arrangements, etc.)
- Providing emotional support.

Psychosocial issues will have greater impact in this situation than in other acute situations (e.g., care of a broken leg). Cultural competency will be important because pivotal decisions about life events (mourning and burial or cremation, organ donation) will need to be made. The nurse will need to encourage expression of grief.

ASSESSING

Because everyone progresses through the grief process individually, the nurse must continually assess each member of the family to determine the degree of coping and need for support. The child's needs are the priority, especially pain relief, comfort measures, and listening. Therapeutic listening is an important aspect of nursing care for the dying child and his or her family.

DIAGNOSING, PLANNING, AND IMPLEMENTING

Nursing diagnoses related to the dying child often include:

- Ineffective Coping
- Anticipatory Grieving
- Complicated Grieving.

Anticipated outcomes for these nursing diagnoses might be:

- Parents request presence of religious minister.

- Parents express need to seek support of other parents who have lost children.
- Child expresses anger that he or she is dying.
- Parent accepts appointment with grief counselor.

The role of the LPN/LVN in providing care for the child who is terminally ill and the family is one of an assistant. Often, the physical care of the child is routine, including hygiene, nutrition, elimination, and special treatment of the specific disease. Providing this care is generally in the scope of practice of the practical nurse. Techniques of therapeutic communication are important when working with the child and family. The nurse can help the child express feelings through drawings and play therapy (see Table 14-1 ⚭). When the LPN/LVN identifies signs that the child or any member of the family is having difficulty expressing his or her loss, either anticipated or actual, the registered nurse should be contacted.

The plan of care for a dying child and his or her family should include the following nursing interventions:

- Provide measures to keep the child as comfortable as possible. *Comfort measures help relieve the child's suffering and thereby provide psychological comfort to the family as well.*
- Encourage each member of the family to express his or her feelings. *Talking about their loss helps individuals move through the stages of grief toward acceptance. When they express their feelings, the nurse can determine if they are grieving in the usual manner, or if they are becoming dysfunctional in their grief.*
- Adapt interventions to the age and developmental stage of the individual (see Chapter 11 ⚭). *By adapting interventions to the developmental stage of the individual, the nurse allows the child to express his or her feelings and understanding of the events taking place. The nurse can also help the child understand the situation better.*
- Identify resources available to the family and assist in accessing support systems. *It is helpful to understand that others have had similar experiences and have come to acceptance. Families and individuals who exhibit signs of dysfunction will need professional help.*
- Attend professional support groups designed to help the nurse through the grief process. *In this kind of situation, the nurse can only be therapeutic when his or her own emotional needs are met.*

EVALUATING

In evaluating the dying child, family, and care providers, it is important for them to verbalize their feelings. Grief takes a minimum of a year for the family to resolve, so they should be evaluated several times. Besides listening closely to their comments, the evaluator should also observe their behavior, including dress, grooming, and crying. These data will be important to determine if the individual is moving through the process or is stuck in one of the stages.

NURSING PROCESS CARE PLAN
Care of a Child Dying at Home

Timmy, a 4-year-old in the end stage of a malignant brain tumor, is dying at home. Besides his parents, his 6-year-old brother, 2½-year-old sister, and maternal grandparents are with him.

Assessment. Vital signs: T 99.8 (O), P 92, R 28. Timmy's respirations are irregular, with moist breath sounds. He sleeps most of the time. Timmy is oriented when he is awake. He moans when turned. Timmy's mother and grandmother sit at his bedside constantly. Timmy's mother is crying. His father and grandfather have left the house to run errands. His brother and sister are playing around the house.

Nursing Diagnosis. The following important nursing diagnosis (among others) has been established for this client:

■ Pain, related to brain tumor and death process

The following important nursing diagnosis (among others) has been established for the client's mother:

■ Anticipatory Grieving, related to upcoming death of child

Expected Outcomes. The following expected outcomes have been identified:

■ Timmy is resting comfortably.
■ Timmy's mother will verbalize her feelings.

Planning and Implementation

■ Medicate for pain as ordered. *Keeping the child comfortable will decrease suffering.*
■ Turn and massage bony prominences every 1 to 2 hours. *Turning and massage increase circulation to skin and muscles and decrease discomfort.*
■ Play soft music, and light aromatic candles. *Soft music and pleasant aromas induce relaxation.*
■ Provide emotional support to mother and grandmother through touch, hugs, and encouraging verbalization. *At this time, the mother should be allowed and encouraged to grieve.*

Evaluation. Be alert for nonverbal cues of discomfort. Respirations may decrease with pain medication. This should be documented, but because it is expected during the dying process, there is no need to notify the RN or physician. Timmy's mother and grandmother should express feelings.

Critical Thinking in the Nursing Process

1. Should Timmy be medicated for pain if his respirations slow to 12 and he continues to moan?
2. Timmy's mother asks, "How much longer will this go on?" How should the nurse reply?
3. What support should Timmy's grandmother receive?

Note: Discussion of Critical Thinking questions appears in Appendix I.

Signs of Impending Death

Although the exact time of death cannot be predicted, physical changes in the child can indicate that death is approaching. If death occurs rapidly, like with a cardiac arrest from an allergic reaction, the signs may not be present. If death occurs slowly from a terminal illness, the signs will probably be present. The changes may take place over a few hours to a few days.

As a terminal illness progresses, the heart becomes less efficient in pumping blood. Initially, the pulse increases as the heart tries to meet the body's need for oxygen and nutrients. The heart muscle, receiving its oxygen between beats, becomes hypoxic when there is only a few hundredths of a second between beats. The hypoxic heart becomes irregular and eventually slows. In response to the failing heart, peripheral blood vessels constrict in order to shunt the blood to the vital organs: brain, heart, lungs, liver, and kidneys. The blood pressure drops, the skin becomes **mottled** (a bluish or purplish marbled appearance), and brain function slows. The child may become less responsive and slip into a coma. Reflexes such as cough and blink become absent. The kidneys, sensitive to the low blood pressure, slow and then stop production of urine. Peristalsis slows. Due to the slowing of circulation, blood pools in the pulmonary blood vessels, resulting in pulmonary edema and moist noisy respirations, at times referred to as a "death rattle." The respirations are usually through the mouth and become **Cheyne-Stokes breathing** (a period of progressive depth of breathing followed by a period of apnea). The periods of apnea become longer until respirations cease and the heart stops.

Care After Death

The LPN/LVN can provide postmortem care, including making the necessary phone calls and completing documentation. Facility policy will determine whether the LPN/LVN can pronounce the child's death.

PROVIDING POSTMORTEM CARE

After death, some characteristic physical changes occur. **Rigor mortis** is the stiffening of the body that occurs about 2 to 4 hours after death. It results from a lack of adenosine triphosphate (ATP), which is not synthesized because of a lack of glycogen in the body. ATP is necessary for muscle fiber relaxation. Its lack causes the muscles to contract, which in turn immobilizes the joints. Rigor mortis starts in the involuntary muscles (heart, bladder, etc.); then progresses to the head, neck, and trunk; and finally reaches the extremities. Rigor mortis usually leaves the body about 96 hours after death.

Algor mortis is the gradual decrease of the body's temperature after death. When blood circulation terminates and the hypothalamus ceases to function, body temperature falls about 1.8°F (1°C) per hour until it reaches room temperature. Simultaneously, the skin loses its elasticity and can easily be broken when removing dressings and adhesive tape.

After blood circulation has ceased, the red blood cells break down, releasing hemoglobin, which discolors the surrounding tissues. This discoloration, referred to as **livor mortis,** appears in the lowermost or dependent areas of the body.

Tissues after death become soft and eventually liquefy due to bacterial fermentation. The hotter the temperature, the more rapid the change. Therefore, bodies are often stored in cool places to delay this process. Embalming prevents the process through injection of chemicals into the body to destroy the bacteria.

After-death (*postmortem*) care may vary somewhat from area to area and culture to culture. However, there are some general principles that can be used as a guide.

CERTIFICATION OF DEATH

The formal determination, or *pronouncement*, of death must be performed by a physician, coroner, or nurse. In some areas, police officers or paramedics are also permitted to pronounce death. Again, the granting of the authority to nurses to pronounce death is regulated by the state or province. It may be limited to nurses in long-term care, home health, and hospice agencies, or to advanced practice nurses. By law, a death certificate must be made out when a person dies. It is usually signed by the attending physician and filed with a local health or other government office. The family is usually given a copy to use for legal matters, such as insurance claims. (Box 28-4 ■ lists criteria for diagnosing brain death.)

CARE OF THE BODY

Nursing personnel may be responsible for care of a body after death. Postmortem care should be carried out according to the policy of the institution. Because care of the body may be influenced by religious law, the nurse should check the client's religion and make every attempt to comply with the family's wishes.

If the deceased's family or friends want to view the body, it is important to make the environment as clean and pleasant as possible and to make the body appear natural and comfortable. All equipment, soiled linen, and supplies should be removed from the bedside. Some institutions require that all tubes in the body remain in place; in other institutions, tubes may be cut to within 1 in. (2.5 cm) of the skin

---

BOX 28-4	ASSESSMENT

Criteria for Brain Death

Clinical Signs

- Irreversible condition
- Apnea with arterial CO_2 level (P_{CO_2}) of at least 60 mm Hg
- No response to deep stimuli
- No spontaneous movement (some spinal cord reflexes may be present)
- No gag or corneal reflex
- No oculocephalic or oculovestibular reflex
- Absence of toxic or metabolic disorders

Confirmatory Tests

- Cerebral blood flow study
- Electroencephalogram

Source: LeMone, P., & Burke, K. (2004). *Medical surgical nursing: Critical thinking in client care* (3rd ed.). Upper Saddle River, NJ: Pearson Education.

---

and taped in place; and in others, all tubes may be removed. The nurse should be familiar with the institutional policies and procedures.

Normally, the body is placed in a supine position with the arms either at the sides, palms down, or across the abdomen. One or two pillows are placed under the head and shoulders, or the head of the bed is elevated 30 degrees, to prevent blood from discoloring the face by settling in it. The eyelids are closed and held in place for a few seconds. Often, the eyes and mouth do not remain closed and require a mortician's intervention.

Soiled areas of the body are washed. However, a complete bath is not necessary because the body will be washed by the *mortician* (also referred to as an undertaker or funeral director), a person trained in care of the dead. Absorbent pads are placed under the buttocks to capture any feces and urine released due to relaxation of the sphincter muscles. A clean gown is placed on the client, and the hair is brushed and combed. All jewelry is removed. The top bed linens are adjusted neatly to cover the client to the shoulders. Soft lighting and chairs should be provided for the family to make the surroundings as peaceful as possible.

LABELING OF THE DECEASED

Nurses have a duty to handle the deceased with dignity and respect and to label the body appropriately. Mishandling can cause emotional distress to survivors. Mislabeling can also create legal problems if the body is inappropriately identified and prepared incorrectly for funeral services. In the hospital, the deceased's wrist identification tag is left on, and another tag is tied to the client's ankle or toe, in case one of the tags becomes detached. A third tag is attached to the shroud. All identification tags should include the client's name, hospital number, and physician's name, which in most hospitals is provided via the addressograph plate or hospital card (which already has the appropriate information on it).

VIEWING BY PARENTS

If the parents were not present at the time of death, as is common in the emergency department, they should be allowed to be with the child. It is important to make the child's body presentable before the parents' viewing. When the parents see the lifeless body of their child, the reality of the death comes as a great shock. The nurse should stay with the parents to provide support.

CALLING THE MORTUARY

The nurse is responsible for notifying the mortuary selected by the parents. Mortuary staff will either come to the bedside or to the facility morgue to remove the body. All required paperwork must be completed before the child's body is removed. Personal belongings can either be given to the parents or sent with the body, but documentation must be made about their disposition.

AUTOPSY

An **autopsy** or **postmortem examination** is an examination of the body after death to determine more details about the cause of death, to learn more about a disease, or to assist in the accumulation of statistical data. It is performed only in certain cases. The law and the institutional policies and procedures describe under what circumstances an autopsy must be performed, such as when death is sudden and unexpected or when it occurs within 48 hours of admission to a hospital.

It is the responsibility of the physician or, in some instances, of a designated person in the hospital to obtain consent for autopsy. Consent must be given by the individual in a legal document before death or by the next of kin. Laws in many states and provinces prioritize the family members who can provide consent as follows: surviving spouse, adult children, parents, and siblings. After autopsy, hospitals cannot retain any tissues or organs without the permission of the person who consented to the autopsy.

INQUEST

An *inquest* is a legal inquiry into the cause or manner of death. When a death is the result of an accident, for example, an inquest is held into the circumstances of the accident to determine if there is any blame. The inquest is conducted under the jurisdiction of a coroner or medical examiner. A *coroner* is a public official, not necessarily a physician, appointed or elected to inquire into the causes of death, when appropriate.

A *medical examiner* is a physician and usually has advanced education in pathology or forensic medicine. Agency or institutional policy dictates who is responsible for reporting deaths to the coroner or medical examiner.

Death-Related Religious and Cultural Practices

The various cultural and religious traditions and practices associated with death, dying, and the grieving process help people cope with these experiences and give comfort to survivors. Nurses are often present throughout the dying process and at the moment of death. Knowledge of the client's religious and cultural beliefs helps nurses provide individualized care to clients and their families, even though they may not participate in the same rituals.

Beliefs about preparation of the body, autopsy, organ donation, cremation, and prolonging life can be related to the person's religion. Autopsy, for example, may be prohibited, opposed, or discouraged by Eastern Orthodox religions, Muslims, Jehovah's Witnesses, and Orthodox Jews. Some religions prohibit the removal of body parts and dictate that all body parts be given appropriate burial. Organ donation is prohibited by Jehovah's Witnesses. In contrast to this, Buddhists in America consider it an act of mercy and encourage it. Cremation is discouraged, opposed, or prohibited by the Mormon, Eastern Orthodox, Islamic, and Jewish faiths. Hindus, in contrast, prefer cremation and cast the ashes in a holy river. Prolongation of life is generally encouraged; however, some religions, such as Christian Science, are unlikely to use medical means to prolong life, and the Jewish faith generally opposes prolonging life after irreversible brain damage. In hopeless illness, Buddhists may permit euthanasia.

Nurses also need to be knowledgeable about the client's death-related rituals, such as last rites, administration of Holy Communion, chanting at the bedside, and other rituals, such as special procedures for washing, dressing, positioning, and shrouding the dead. For example, certain immigrants may want to retain their native customs, in which family members of the same gender wash and prepare the body for burial and cremation. Muslims also customarily turn the body toward Mecca. Nurses need to ask family members about their preferences and verify who will carry out these activities. The nurse must ensure that any ritual items present in the institution be given to the family or to the funeral home at the time of death to prevent lost items.

Note: The references and resources for this and all chapters have been compiled at the back of the book.

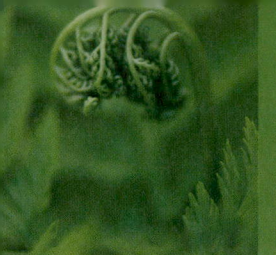

Chapter Review

 **KEY TERMS** by Topic

Use the audio glossary feature of either the CD-ROM or the Companion Website to hear the correct pronunciation of the following key terms.

Grief Process
loss, grief

Culture and Grief
dysfunctional grief

Caring for the Dying Child
palliative care, palliative management, hospice care

Legalities Related to Death
comfort measures only, euthanasia, assisted suicide

Signs of Impending Death
mottled, Cheyne-Stokes breathing

Care After Death
rigor mortis, algor mortis, livor mortis, autopsy, postmortem examination

KEY Points

- Five stages of grief have been identified with any major loss. Not everyone goes through all stages, and some people experience a stage more than once. It is helpful for the nurse to know the stages in order to communicate effectively with the client.

- The nurse must provide emotional support or resources for emotional support to the dying child as well as every member of the family.

- The nurse, caring for a dying child, must take time to regain his or her own emotional stability.

- As the child deteriorates, the plan should change from curative care to palliative care.

- The older child and parents should be encouraged to communicate their desires about advanced directives and DNR orders.

- Facility policy must be followed in providing postmortem care, including providing the death certificate, notifying the family, and contacting the mortuary.

- In the case of unexpected death, the family should receive the option of organ donation.

- Family religious and cultural practices related to death should be asked about and honored.

 **EXPLORE Media**Link

Additional interactive resources for this chapter can be found on the Companion Website at www.prenhall.com/towle.

Click on Chapter 28 and "Begin" to select the activities for this chapter.

For chapter-related NCLEX-style questions and an audio glossary, access the accompanying CD-ROM in this book.

FOR FURTHER Study

See Chapter 2 for information about legalities in the care of children.

Development of children is discussed in depth in Chapter 11.

Nursing care of children with specific chronic disorders is discussed in Chapter 14. Table 14-1 list some forms of therapeutic play.

Critical Thinking Care Map

Care of Mother with Anticipatory Grieving
NCLEX-PN® Focus Area: Psychosocial Integerity

Case Study: Teresa, age 4, has been fighting a malignant brain tumor for more than a year. She is now terminal. Her doctor has told the family that it is just a matter of time before she will die. The family has decided to have her death take place in the home. Teresa is comatose, her breathing is irregular, and she is beginning to show mottling in her legs. Teresa's mother is at the bedside. An LPN/LVN has been assigned to remain in the home with Teresa and her family.

Nursing Diagnosis: Anticipatory Grieving of Mother

COLLECT DATA

Subjective	Objective
_____	_____
_____	_____
_____	_____
_____	_____
_____	_____
_____	_____

Would you report this? Yes/No

If yes, to: _____

Nursing Care

_____
_____
_____
_____
_____
_____
_____
_____
_____
_____
_____

How would you document this? _____
_____
_____
_____

Compare your documentation to the sample provided in Appendix I.

Data Collected
(use only those that apply)

- Crying quietly
- Tells Teresa they will go to the beach next week
- States Teresa will recover from the brain tumor
- States she will be relieved when Teresa is gone
- Asks "how much longer?" every 10 minutes
- Identifies signs of impending death
- States Teresa will not die

Nursing Interventions
(use only those that apply;
list in priority order)

- Ask mother to help turn Teresa.
- Ask mother to leave during Teresa's routine care.
- Ask mother if other family should be called.
- Ask mother if clergy should be called.
- Agree with mother that Teresa will get better.
- Tell mother not to cry.
- Encourage mother to express feelings.
- Tell mother it will probably be several more days.

NCLEX-PN® Exam Preparation

1 Which of the following concepts should the nurse be aware of when interacting with parents of a child who died suddenly?

1. The parents had time to engage in anticipatory grief.
2. The parents may feel guilty for not engaging in special activities with the deceased child.
3. The parents feel immediate detachment.
4. The parents may experience an uncomplicated grief response.

2 A 5-year-old with leukemia asks the nurse, "Am I going to die?" The nurse should respond:

1. "Everyone will die sometime."
2. "Of course not, only old people die."
3. "Have you asked your parents that question?"
4. "We can ask the doctor when he arrives."

3 The adolescent who is terminally ill states to the nurse, "I'm just not ready to go." The most appropriate response by the nurse would be:

1. "Tell me more about what you mean when you say that you are not ready."
2. "You're not ready to go where?"
3. "Dying is a natural process, you have nothing to fear."
4. "Yes, I know. Most people don't want to die."

4 In providing support for parents following the death of their child, the nurse needs to be aware that grieving is:

1. best carried out alone.
2. socially unacceptable in today's American culture.
3. essential for good mental health after a loss.
4. detrimental to emotional health.

5 A 14-year-old girl is having her leg amputated tomorrow due to bone cancer. She has been grieving since she was told about the amputation last week. Which of the following best describes the grief she is experiencing?

1. complicated grief
2. perceived grief
3. bereavement
4. anticipatory grief

6 In which age group does the child first have a concept that death is permanent?

1. 4–5 years
2. 8–9 years
3. 11–12 years
4. 14–15 years

7 A 17-year-old is terminal with muscular dystrophy. He states, "When my time comes, I do not want any heroic measures." The nurse informs him that a living will:

1. allows health care workers to withhold fluids and medication.
2. allows the individual to express his or her desires regarding care.
3. is legally binding in all 50 states.
4. allows the courts to decide when care can be given.

8 Common symptoms of approaching death are (select all that apply):

1. loss of control of bowel and bladder
2. increased secretions in the throat
3. increase in blood pressure
4. increased awareness in surroundings
5. rapid respirations with periods of apnea
6. mottling

9 After a woman has delivered a 35-week-old stillborn baby, the nurse should tell the parents:

1. "Just go home and get on with your life."
2. "Hold the baby as long as you wish. I will get hair samples and hand- and footprints for your baby book later."
3. "You are young and can have other children."
4. "Can you make your wife stop crying while I get the room cleaned up?"

10 An 8-year-old has just died at home following a long illness. Place the following interventions in priority order:

1. Call the mortician.
2. Clean the body for viewing.
3. Complete the charting.
4. Call the nursing supervisor and physician.
5. Hold the parents and allow them to cry.

Answers for Review Questions, as well as discussion of Care Plan and Critical Thinking Care Map questions, appear in Appendix I.

Thinking Strategically About ...

You are employed by a pediatrician. Your responsibilities include obtaining client health histories, taking vital signs, weighing and measuring clients, vision and hearing screening, obtaining lab specimens, administering medications, assisting in procedures, and providing client teaching and discharge instructions. Today, there are 18 children scheduled.

CASE 1 SCENARIO

The first client of the day is Jeremy. He is 12 years old. He weighs 120 lb and is 5 ft tall. His vital signs are T 98.6, P 62, R 16, BP 106/76. Jeremy's mother relates that he is frequently fatigued. He is thirsty all the time, even during the night. He is also urinating many times a day and is always hungry. A review of the family history reveals that Jeremy's father has type I diabetes mellitus.

After conferring with the physician, you obtain a urine specimen and a blood specimen. A reagent strip is used to test the urine for glucose. The urine test is positive for glucose. Blood glucose reveals 210 mg/dL.

CRITICAL THINKING

1 The physician orders further testing to confirm the diagnosis of diabetes mellitus. What tests would you expect to obtain? What client teaching is necessary?

2 The test results reveal that Jeremy does have diabetes mellitus. You are responsible for teaching Jeremy to self-administer his insulin, but he is afraid of "shots." What measures could you take to minimize the pain of injections?

COLLABORATIVE CARE

1 Jeremy and his parents will need to adjust his diet in order to manage his disease appropriately. Describe the report of Jeremy's condition you will give when you contact the nutritionist.

2 Jeremy's mother is concerned about how she will manage Jeremy's care and keep him healthy. What resources would you want to suggest to Jeremy's mother?

CASE 2 SCENARIO

Jackson, 4 years old, is admitted to the pediatric unit with a diagnosis of gastroenteritis. For the past 48 hours, Jackson has been vomiting and having diarrhea. He has been unable to keep any food or beverage down. Over the last few hours, he has been irritable and sleepy. You take his vital signs and review his admission orders. The physician orders an electrolyte profile, complete blood count, and urinalysis. He also orders an IV of D5 ½ NS to infuse at 1,000 mL in 8 hours,

daily weight, and full liquid diet. Phenergan 12.5 mg, rectal suppository every 4 hours is ordered for nausea.

DATA COLLECTED

Jackson's admission vital signs are T 99.9, P 110, R 18, BP 90/60. Skin turgor is poor. Hematocrit is increased. Urine-specific gravity is increased. Current weight: 45 lb.

DELEGATING

Which of the previous orders could be delegated to the certified nursing assistant?

MANAGEMENT OF CARE

Calculate the infusion rate for the previous order using a drop factor of 10 drops/mL.

COMMUNICATION AND CLIENT TEACHING

Jackson improves and is ready for discharge. His mother asks the nurse what foods are appropriate if Jackson should have a stomach virus again. Develop a teaching plan to provide this nutritional information.

CASE 3 SCENARIO

Janice is a 17-year-old who is admitted to the emergency room following a motor vehicle crash. Janice has facial abrasions and a fractured right clavicle. She is being evaluated for an abdominal injury due to the impact of the seatbelt.

DATA COLLECTED

Janice is oriented to person, time, and place. She complains of shoulder and abdominal pain, 6 on a scale of 10. She is able to move the fingers of her right hand. The abrasions are not actively bleeding. Vital signs include T 98.6, P 110 and thready, R 14, BP 100/70. Her skin is pale and moist. Her bowel sounds are decreased in all four quadrants.

TIME MANAGEMENT AND PRIORITIES IN NURSING CARE

List in order the nursing interventions that need to be implemented for Janice.

DOCUMENTING AND REPORTING

What findings about Janice are important to document? Which are important to report to the physician?

CULTURAL CARE STRATEGIES

Janice's admission information reveals she is a Jehovah's Witness. How will this affect care management? What strategies are appropriate if she needs blood replacement?

Appendix I
Answers and Critical Thinking Discussion

Chapter 1

NCLEX-PN® ANSWERS

(1) 1—Primary nursing care encompasses prevention activities such as nutritional counseling to prevent gestational diabetes. (2) 4—Tertiary care is the management of chronic, long-term health care problems such as clients with permanent tracheostomies. (3) 1, 2, 3—Although the role of the LPN/LVN varies from state to state, generally administering PO meds, supervising UAP, and collecting data are allowable; usually, administering blood and developing the nursing diagnosis are not. (4) 3—Application of a fetal scalp electrode is a clinical skill not taught in a basic nursing education course. In many states, it is not an allowable skill for the LPN. Reporting to the RN is the best response. Response 4 is rude and does not promote collaborative care. (5) The LPN—Even though the supervising, LPN was not the one who provided care, he or she had ultimate responsibility and accountability for the nursing care provided. (6) 5—Right supervision includes the tasks of monitoring, evaluating, intervening when necessary, and providing feedback if appropriate. (7) 4—Delegation is transferring to a competent individual with authority to perform a nursing task. Only the CNA with experience meets this criteria. (8) 3—Insulin is a drug that is regulated by some nurse practice acts to be a task designated for the registered nurse. The UAP should never give medications or directly contact the physician without notification of the LPN. The client's husband, in an acute-care setting, should not be given the task of administering medication. (9) 2—The CNA has incorrectly instructed the client regarding collection of a 24-hour urine specimen. It is the responsibility of the supervising LPN to review the procedure with him or her to ensure that it is performed correctly the next time. (10) 1, 2, 3, 4, 5, 6, 7—These individuals may contribute to the health care provided to the client, and their specific care will be augmented by each discipline.

CARE PLAN HINTS

1. Parents may object to immunizations due to philosophical or religious reasons. They may also have some concerns about governmental control over their health. They may believe that immunizations are not safe, or they may desire to have an all-natural approach to their health care.
2. In the 1900s, polio was epidemic and frequently resulted in paralysis or death. A vaccine for polio was introduced in 1951. By 1967, polio was reduced by 99% and, by 1991, it was eradicated from the Western Hemisphere.
3. Once proper teaching has been done, the decision to vaccinate is in the parents' hands. If the family refuses immunizations, the nurse would need to provide additional teaching on disease recognition and reporting. The family should be treated with respect.

CRITICAL THINKING CARE MAP

Subjective Data   Mother states Andrew rarely hungry.

Objective Data   Decreased urine output (four diapers daily when typical should be six to eight); dry mucous membranes; lethargy; intake of 5 oz every 5 hours.

Report   Yes, to the registered nurse.

Interventions   Obtain vital signs every 1 to 2 hours; contact the registered nurse to report findings; teach parents to obtain and record vital signs; teach parents the importance of adequate fluid intake during the use of the BiliBlanket; teach parents the symptoms of dehydration, closely monitor vital signs, provide fluid replacement per order.

Documentation   (date) 12:00 4-day-old male infant, lethargic, dry mucous membranes. Mother reports four wet diapers daily. States oral intake 5 oz formula, every 5 to 6 hours. Mother states infant is rarely hungry. VS: T 99, P 150, R 42. Report called to supervising registered nurse. S. Smith, LPN

Chapter 2

NCLEX-PN® ANSWERS

(1) 4—Reporting possible child abuse is a legal obligation of health care professionals. (2) 3—It is vital for the nurse to provide nonjudgmental care. Her opinion of the situation cannot affect her nursing care. (3) 3—Discussing health care issues with health care personnel involved in the direct care of a client is allowable. (4) 2—In many states, reproductive rights of minors dictate that they may receive contraceptive information without parental consent. (5) 2—Life and death decisions should be made by the family with support from health care professionals. (6) 4—Giving Patty control in aspects of her health care is important. However, choosing whether to have an IV and where to place it is not an issue Patty can control. Instead, she can choose to take a familiar object into the surgical suite with her. (7) 2—Informed consent is essential for participation in medical research. (8) 1, 2, 5—Health care

personnel can expect families and clients to provide adequate information, seek knowledge, and participate actively in treatment. (9) If there is suspicion of intoxication, the nurse is legally bound not to allow the client to drive, because harm could occur to herself and others. The nurse must safeguard the public. (10) 1—Identifying information on the crib card is visible to the public and may compromise client privacy.

CARE PLAN HINTS

1. Typically, most states recognize the rights of parents to make health care decisions for minor children, unless the child is emancipated.
2. The nurse should discuss with Jean the importance of disclosing this information to her parents and create a safe environment where this communication can occur.
3. The family should fully understand the illness and prescribed treatment as well as the prognosis. Spiritual counseling would be helpful if desired by the family. Support groups of families who are experiencing long-term illnesses may be of assistance.

CRITICAL THINKING CARE MAP

Subjective Data   States lack of sleep times 3 days; 24-hour diet recall: six soft drinks; states unable to care for a baby; states family incapable of financially supporting another family member; my boyfriend says I have to abort the baby or he will not have anything to do with me; concerned father will be physically abusive if he finds out she is pregnant.

Objective Data   Crying; no eye contact with nurse.

Report   Yes, to the supervising nurse.

Interventions   Encourage client to express feelings and concerns openly; address client in a nonjudgmental fashion; explore options available to this client and the pros and cons of each; encourage client to engage parents in decision-making process; explore client's past successes in difficult circumstances; encourage client to explore personal strengths.

Documentation   (date) 08:30 G1, 15-year-old white female reported to school health nurse, crying. States 12 weeks pregnant. States parents do not know of pregnancy and she is unsure what to do. Feels there is no solution to this dilemma and has no hope. States fearful of father's reaction to the news of pregnancy, specifically concerned about his physical reaction. States boyfriend is encouraging her to abort the baby. States no sleep times 3 days. 24-hour diet recall: six soft drinks. Data reported to supervising RN. S. Metcalf, LPN

Chapter 3

NCLEX-PN® ANSWERS

(1) 2—A genogram is a diagram that identifies the members of a family and their relationship to each other. (2) An ecomap is a diagram used to demonstrate the interactions of a family within the community. (3) 2—The nurse chooses an intervention that demonstrates she is providing culturally sensitive care. Lack of eye contact is a sign of respect among the Chinese. (4) 1, 2, 5—An environmental assessment includes data about the physical aspects of the environment that would affect a family's health. The color of the house and number of televisions would have no direct effect on a family's health. (5) 3—The nurse appropriately responds with a question that shows he or she supports the client's spiritual beliefs. (6) 2—A client's culture and religious beliefs affect their health, and nursing care should be planned to support these aspects. (7) 2—The client mentions family. The nurse correctly determines that family support contributes to a family's ability to cope. (8) 3—Notifying the RN is an appropriate nursing action when family stress is assessed. (9) 2—The nurse has a responsibility to determine aspects of family functioning that might affect health. This is an honest response. (10) 3, 5—Contacting social services and consulting with the RN will result in reliable local resources. The other methods may not produce local resources that can be trusted.

CARE PLAN HINTS

1. The ecomap should include Jean's parents' workplaces, their professional organizations, the families' civic affiliations, their religious affiliations, Jean's school, extended family, and sports activities.
2. With Jean's amputation, access to the home and safety hazards should be assessed.
3. It would be important to assess Jean's school for access. The nurse could also look for a support group of young amputees. Jean's parents may benefit from a support group of others who have experienced traumatic events.

CRITICAL THINKING CARE MAP

Subjective Data   Refuses to go to school; parents recently divorced; parental relationship strained; some days spent with mother, some spent with father; father has new female relationship; complaint of daily stomachache.

Objective Data   Sam's responses barely audible; dark circles under eyes.

Report   Yes, to the registered nurse.

Interventions   Evaluate family strengths and weaknesses; encourage Sam and his mother to express concerns and fears; explore negative feelings of anger, worry, sorrow, etc.; encourage each family member to try to understand the other's feelings; assist the family in setting realistic goals; refer to community resources as needed.

Documentation   (date) 10:00 7-year-old male for office visit accompanied by mother who reports complaints of lack of appetite, excessive sleeping, frequent stomachaches, and refusal to go to school. Mother also reports the family has recently gone through a divorce, there is unrest in the family, and new living arrangements and new caregivers have been introduced to the child. Dark circles noted under the child's eyes bilaterally. Verbal responses to questions barely audible. D. Adams, LPN

UNIT I Thinking Strategically About …

CRITICAL THINKING

- The need for any alterations to permit access to and through Juan's house (e.g., need for ramps to be installed, doorways to be enlarged to accommodate wheelchair, hand railings to the tub and toilet, pathways to be cleared).
- How does Marie feel about the responsibility of the baby? What coping strategies does she plan to use in times of stress? To what resources does Marie have access?

COLLABORATIVE CARE

- Marie should be referred to WIC (Women, Infants and Children), a federal program that provides nutritious foods and education to low-income pregnant, postpartum, and lactating women and to infants and children up to age 5.

MANAGEMENT OF CARE AND PRIORITIES

- Visit Marie first, then Juan, and finally complete the environmental assessment on Juan's house.
- Visiting Marie would be the first priority because she is unsure of her ability to care for the infant and could accidentally harm or neglect him. Jenny is stable and has parents or CNA providing care. They could summon help if needed. An environmental assessment of Juan's house must be completed by afternoon.

DELEGATING

- When assessing Jenny, the LPN would identify areas of poor care, such as lack of hygiene, odor, or body position not in alignment. If there is evidence of poor care, further instruction in proper technique and follow-up supervision of the CNA would be warranted.

COMMUNICATION AND CLIENT TEACHING

- The LPN would talk with the CNA regarding the needed care and watch the CNA perform the care. If the CNA's technique is not appropriate, further instruction and supervision would be needed.
- Juan's family should be instructed in how to get the wheelchair up and down ramps, and in the importance of keeping clutter off the floor.

DOCUMENTING AND REPORTING

- If you believe Marie is at a high risk for neglecting the infant, you should stay in the house and call your supervising RN on the telephone.

CULTURAL STRATEGIES

- In Hispanic households, the male is usually the head of the house and would make the decisions regarding health care. Hispanic families should be assessed for the use of *curanderos* (healers), as well as for use of herbs or home remedies that may interfere with medical treatment.

Chapter 4

NCLEX-PN® ANSWERS

(1) 2—Fertilization could occur anywhere in the female reproductive system, but the most common place is in the distal one-third of the fallopian tube. (2) An "X" is placed over the testes (see Figure 4-9). (3) 1—Sperm contain either an X or a y chromosome. All ova contain an X chromosome. When an X sperm fertilizes an ovum, the result will be a female infant. When a y sperm fertilizes the ovum, a male infant will develop. (4) 3—The distal end of the fallopian tube is not attached to the ovary but opens into the pelvic cavity. (5) 3—Ovulation usually occurs halfway through the menstrual cycle. (6) 1—Milk is produced on an as-needed basis. When the breast is emptied, more milk will be produced. (7) 2—Female infants are born with all the ova they will ever produce. (8) 1, 2, 5—Part of a sexual history involves identifying the client's usual menstrual cycle. Because a yellow odorous discharge could indicate an infection, it is important to determine if she has sexual partners who could also be infected. Although birth control may be important to teach, it does not directly affect the symptoms of this client. Bowel movements and the number of children do not pertain to this client's problem. (9) 3, 4—Removing the prostate either destroys or alters the ejaculatory duct, making it difficult for sperm to leave the body. Prostatic fluid is necessary for sperm mobility. Any sperm that may be able to leave the body will be unable to swim through the female system. (10) 3—Hormones from both the pituitary gland and ovaries are necessary to regulate the menstrual cycle. The uterus does not produce hormones.

CARE PLAN HINTS

1. Ovarian complications are rare following a spontaneous ruptured ovarian cyst or surgery, and the ovary continues to function normally. If the cyst ruptures, blood and other fluid cause inflammation, but this usually resolves in a few days. Sometimes excessive bleeding could cause a surgical emergency.

2. At the beginning of laparoscopic abdominal surgery, carbon dioxide is instilled into the abdominal cavity to allow for visualization of the abdominal/pelvic organs. Following surgery, most of the CO_2 is removed. The remaining CO_2 forms bubbles that rise to the top of the abdominal cavity when the client sits or stands. The pressure of the CO_2 next to the diaphragm causes the pain the client feels in the right upper quadrant and the referred pain in the right shoulder.

3. Because ovarian cysts are caused by improper ovulation and formation of the corpus luteum, some doctors will prescribe birth control pills to prevent ovulation. The pros and cons of this preventive treatment should be discussed thoroughly with the client.

CRITICAL THINKING CARE MAP

Subjective Data States unprotected sexual intercourse with several women over the past few weeks; states "I hope this will not affect my being able to get an erection."

Objective Data Voice shaky; avoids eye contact.

Report Yes, to charge nurse or primary care provider. Client's lack of knowledge regarding sexuality, sexual function, and infection indicates a need for client teaching.

Interventions Encourage client to discuss sexuality; teach client about normal physiology of erection and infection of reproductive system; teach client about the need for protection from infection during sexual intercourse.

Documentation (date/time) Client states concerns over being able to have future erections. Encouraged to express feelings regarding sexuality. Provided instruction of normal physiology of erections and infection of reproductive system. Reported data to J. Smith, Nurse Practioner. C. Bragg, LPN

Chapter 5

NCLEX-PN® ANSWERS

(1) 2—Adolescents engage in premarital sexual intercourse due to feelings of invincibility, peer pressure, elevation of sex hormones, and increased sex drives. (2) 1, 2, 3, 5—Transmission of HIV can occur through homosexual or heterosexual relationships, and through genital sex, oral sex, or rectal sex. (3) 1, 2, 3, 4—It is important for the client to validate the presence of the string daily for a week and then following menses thereafter. She must also report promptly any signs of infection or pregnancy. (4) 3—The client is expressing feelings of anger and resentment that need to be explored further in order to assist her in resolving these feelings. (5) 3—A couple is diagnosed as infertile following 1 year of unprotected intercourse without achieving pregnancy. (6) 1—Monozygotic or identical twins occur from one fertilized egg that divides into separate embryos. (7) 2—An incomplete abortion is passage of the fetus but not the placenta. (8) 4—The nurse caring for the birth mother should provide emotional support. The birth mother and adoptive mother make decisions about visitation of the infant, not the nurse. (9) 4—Showering or bathing may wash away vital evidence and should be delayed until such evidence can be gathered in the appropriate manner. (10) 1—A therapeutic abortion is the termination of the pregnancy to save the life and preserve the health of the mother or when the fetus has a serious disorder or when the pregnancy is a result of rape or incest.

CARE PLAN HINTS

1. Ms. Kelly should be asked to describe the specific events of the attack. If possible, a law enforcement officer should be present. The nurse should remain nonjudgmental and empathetic. All subjective responses should be documented in the client's precise words.

2. It is important for Ms. Kelly to feel safe. Suggested personal protection devices include extra door locks, burglar alarms, mace or other legal weapons, or hiring a personal bodyguard.

3. Acts of violence can cause long-lasting effects. Professional counseling is recommended for Ms. Kelly and her family. She needs to have opportunities to verbalize her feelings, fears, and anxieties. Support people and professional counselors need to observe closely for signs and symptoms of denial and depression.

CRITICAL THINKING CARE MAP

Subjective Data Headache pain level 4; states vaginal spotting has occurred for 4 days; states has had three sexual partners in 3 months; LMP (record month/day/year).

Objective Data Small amount of dark red vaginal discharge noted; multiple cervical lesions measuring $\frac{1}{2}$ to 1 cm in diameter; labia with diffuse redness.

Report Yes, to MD. Would report vaginal spotting; sexual history; vaginal discharge, lesions, and condition of labia.

Interventions Assess characteristics of the lesion; teach the importance of informing all sexual partners; teach the importance of regular Pap smears; teach the client about cryotherapy treatment.

Documentation (date/time) Client reports headache—pain level 4—and vaginal spotting times 4 days. Small amount of dark, red vaginal discharge noted. LMP (mo/day/yr). States three sexual partners in 3 months. Multiple cervical vesicles measuring $\frac{1}{2}$ to 1 cm in diameter, with diffuse labia redness noted following cervical examination by nurse practitioner. Physician given verbal report. K. Smartt, LPN

Chapter 6

NCLEX-PN® ANSWERS

(1) 4—The fertilized egg travels through the fallopian tube and divides rapidly to form a mass that reaches the uterus in 4 to 5 days, at which time it is formed into a two-layered ball. The outer layer develops finger-like projections called villi to secure the blastocyst to the uterus. It is these villi that begin producing human chorionic gonadotropin 8 to 10 days after fertilization. (2) 3—The placenta produces the hormone progesterone to do several things, including prevention of uterine contractions. Relaxin causes softening in the collagen connective tissue of the symphysis pubis and sacroiliac joints. HPL helps the mother's body prepare for lactation; hCG maintains the corpus luteum. (3) 4, 5—The umbilical cord does contain two arteries and one vein. Maternal and fetal blood do not mix; nutrients and waste are exchanged in the placenta. The fetal respiratory system is not functioning *in utero* as it is in the process of developing. The ductus arteriosus is outside the fetal heart, and the blood exchange between placenta and fetus is via the two arteries and one vein. (4) 2—The expectant mother should, even if eating a well-balanced diet, add 300 kcal a day. This can be covered by the addition of two milk and one meat servings, which also meets the need for increased calcium and protein. (5) 4—The mother should be encouraged to sleep on her side to prevent hypotension; lying supine can cause supine hypotensive syndrome. (6) 3—The fetal heartbeat can be heard with a Doppler by 10 to 12 weeks. (7) 3—Naegele's rule involves taking the first day of the last menstrual period, subtracting 3 months and adding 7 days so the correct date using this rule would be February 13. (8) 3—The nurse should help the client explore options for the pregnancy. The nurse cannot impose his or her ideas and bias on the client by telling her that she "should have thought about that." By telling the client what to do or making decisions (appointment for abortion) for her, therapeutic communication is blocked. (9) 2, 4, 3, 5, 1—The first priority is to assess the mother's vital signs to establish a baseline. Then assess the fetal heart rate. If they are within normal range, then continue to assess the mother. If you take the FHT first and it is not normal, the stress will increase the mother's blood pressure and you will not know if the elevation is from the stress, hypertension, or both. All information would be reported to the physician. (10) 2—These symptoms could indicate a complication of pregnancy (pregnancy-induced hypertension) and need to be evaluated as soon as possible. Due to the late hour, it would be best for her to go to the hospital for the evaluation. She should not wait to be evaluated because her condition could get worse quite rapidly. The doctor will want her to be evaluated, so waiting to talk with the doctor will just waste time.

CARE PLAN HINTS

1. By 22 weeks, Mrs. Taylor's abdomen will be enlarging. Safety issues to discuss at this time include walking up and down stairs holding the hand rail, wearing low-heeled shoes, and getting in and out of shower/bath tub.
2. At the next visit, Mrs. Taylor will be 26 weeks pregnant. Signs of preterm labor must be discussed. It is also time to begin discussion regarding pain control during labor and preparation for breastfeeding.
3. The role of the LPN/LVN in providing care in the office is to collect data, answer questions, and support client decisions. The physician should be informed of all signs of complications. The RN or physician should approve all printed material prior to giving it to the client.

CRITICAL THINKING CARE MAP

Subjective Data   Money only for rent and food.

Objective Data   Wt 135 lb, vital signs WNL; urine negative for protein; pale, thin.

Report   Yes, report to the health care provider the information regarding living situation and referral to WIC. Report the pale, thin appearance and nurse's concern regarding nutritional stats.

Interventions   Refer to WIC program. *The WIC program can provide food vouchers to help ensure proper nutrition during pregnancy and for several years afterward.* Teach need for increased protein and lower carbohydrates in diet. *Eating adequate protein decreases risk of PIH.* Teach need for prenatal vitamins. *Helps ensure adequate nutrition.* Teach need for milk products. *Calcium and phosphosus are important for fetal development.* Although a therapist may be needed to treat depression, this intervention does not relate to the nursing diagnosis.

Documentation   (date) 04:30 17-year-old single female admitted to clinic with 10-week pregnancy. VS are WNL. Wt 135 lb. Skin pale. Urine negative for protein. Appears thin. Crying. States she does not know what to do about pregnancy. State she barely has enough money to meet current expenses. Information provided regarding diet, prenatal vitamins, and WIC program. N. Cooper, LPN

Chapter 7

NCLEX-PN® ANSWERS

(1) 1—Fetal cortisol production increases as the fetus matures, and when sufficient, decreases the placental production of progesterone. As progesterone decreases, the estrogen levels in the placenta rise. Estrogen increases sensitivity of myometrium to oxytocin, which is produced by the pituitary gland of the mother, and it is this oxytocin that causes the uterus to contract. (2) 1—"Lightening" refers to the fetus

having descended into the pelvis. The fetus's moving downward relieves pressure on the diaphragm, allowing the mother to breathe easier and thus feel "lighter"; however, there is now more pressure on the lower pelvis, which causes an increase in venous stasis, resulting in lower extremity edema, bladder pressure, and urge to void, and increased back pain. (3) 3, 4, 6—A prolapsed cord is an emergency situation and necessitates emergency C-section. The Trendelenburg position relieves pressure of the fetal head on the umbilical cord. It is important to document fetal heart rate as fetal oxygenation is compromised. (4) 4—A vertex position is the occiput presenting first. (5) 3—When the mother lies on her side, the contractions are less frequent but of greater intensity. (6) 2—The latent phase of the first stage of labor is from the onset of contraction until the cervix is dilated at 4 cm. (7) 4—The average length of active labor (active phase of first stage) is 4 to 6 hours for the primagravida client. (8) 3, 5, 6—It is normal for the client to become irritable and sometimes angry at this stage of labor. It is important to teach the client simple relaxation and breathing. Warm soaks provide relief via muscle relaxation and diversion from contractions. The lateral position facilitates maternal-fetal circulation and relieves the stress on the back. The client should not actively push until fully dilated at 10 cm. (9) 2—Engagement occurs when the presenting part (usually the fetal head) enters the true pelvis. At this time, the presenting part is even with or below the ischial spines, and the fetus is no longer ballotable. (10) 1—Any bleeding in excess of one pad saturated per hour in the fourth stage of labor/birth is abnormal. Any deviation from normal range should be reported to the registered nurse and physician. The fundus may need to be massaged and clots removed.

CARE PLAN HINTS

1. The first priority is pain control. The second priority is frequent monitoring of labor progression and maternal-fetal well-being. *When the client and fetus are stable, the highest priority is pain control. Fetal heart rate, maternal vital signs, and evaluating contractions should be done every 30 to 60 minutes.*

2. Yes, Jane should be offered a whirlpool bath. *A warm whirlpool bath can help the client relax, easing discomfort and shortening labor. There are no symptoms presented that would indicate complications that would prevent a whirlpool bath.*

3. How rapidly Jane is progressing in labor should be considered before narcotics are administered. Most primigravida mothers can have narcotics when they are 8 to 9 cm dilated. *Narcotic analgesics will have an effect for at least 1 hour and may cause respiratory depression in the newborn. The second stage of labor for most primigravida mothers*

is 1 to 3 hours. Narcotics therefore can be safely administered at 8 to 9 cm.

CRITICAL THINKING CARE MAP

Subjective Data   Obviously uncomfortable; having difficulty maintaining control.

Objective Data   Cervix 8 cm dilated, 100% effaced; station +2, BP 142/90; contractions every 3 minutes, lasting 90 seconds; fetal heart rate 110; clear fluid draining from vagina.

Report   Yes, supervising nurse; the LPN needs assistance when delivery is near.

Interventions   Position on left side to prevent compressing of uterine arteries. Encourage to breathe with each contraction because breathing helps with relaxation and prevents pushing until cervix is dilated. Prepare sterile field for delivery. Because this is Alyce's second delivery, it is best to prepare early. She is in transition and is expected to delivery fairly rapidly.

Documentation   (date) 06:30 G2P1 presented by wheelchair to L&D. BP 142/90, FHT 110–120 bpm. Contractions q3min, lasting 90 sec. Sterile vaginal exam done per RN. Cervix 8 cm dilated, 100% effaced. Fetus cephalic, at 2+ station. SROM 0600 clear fluid. Having difficulty keeping relaxed. J. Marshall, LPN

Chapter 8

NCLEX-PN® ANSWERS

(1) 4—CBC is the number of blood cells of the client. APTT is used to evaluate the coagulation of the blood. HCG is the hormone produced by the embryo. (2) 3—A client in shock would experience an increase in pulse and a decrease in blood pressure. The fetus would initially have an increase in pulse. A decrease in FHR would indicate fetal distress, but at 16 weeks' gestation, the health of the mother would have a higher priority. (3) 2—Erythroblastosis fetalis occurs when Rh-negative blood from the mother has been sensitized with Rh-positive blood. The mother's blood attacks the fetal blood. PG and LS ratio indicate fetal lung maturity. (4) 2—A major side effect of terbutaline is tachycardia. After initial stabilization, constant fetal monitoring and strict bed rest are not necessary. (5) 1—Epigastric pain is a sign of worsening pre-eclampsia. A blood pressure of 138/90 and some dependent edema are not signs of worsening condition. (6) 4—This client needs to be evaluated in a quiet, controlled environment. She is experiencing severe pre-eclampsia and is at risk for further complications and emergency treatment. Other rooms would not provide her with necessary observation. (7) 1, 2, 3, 4—The nurse should use personal protective equipment when contacting any body

fluids. Vaginal secretions and amniotic fluid can be present in the bath water. The newborn is considered to be contaminated with vaginal secretions and amniotic fluid until bathed. (8) 1—The first priority is to assess the mother and fetal well-being. The second priority would be to assess the amount of bleeding and then to prepare for medical intervention. (9) 4—Three days after delivery the client could be experiencing postpartum blues, but further assessment is needed. Options 1, 2, and 3 block therapeutic communication. (10) 3—The client's statements indicate emotional stress. The nurse must determine the risk to herself and her baby. The other comments block therapeutic communication.

CARE PLAN HINTS

1. The nurse could suggest reading a novel the client has always wanted to read, working on a self-directed study course for college credit, journaling about the pregnancy experience, writing family and friends, visiting with family and friends over the phone, doing crafts such as embroidery or knitting, or having phone calls with other pregnant women who are on bed rest.
2. Home tocolytic or uterine monitoring allows the physician to determine if the treatment for preterm labor is successful. This monitoring works the same as uterine monitoring in the hospital. Abdominal belts and monitors detect uterine contractions and translate the data to graph paper. Some home tocolytic companies have the capacity to translate the data via the telephone to the physician.
3. Symptoms of preterm labor that need to be reported include regular uterine contractions, regular backache, rupture of membranes, loss of mucous plug, and decreased fetal movement. Vaginal bleeding and fever (first signs of infection) must also be reported.

CRITICAL THINKING CARE MAP

Subjective Data   States she doesn't feel happy; states she can't get over baby's death.

Objective Data   Crying, breasts expressing small amount milk; wearing maternity clothes; delivered a stillborn 3 weeks ago; hair neatly combed.

Report   Yes, to primary care provider.

Interventions   Ask her if she has family or friends who are helpful. Ask what she has been doing to overcome her grief. Give her a list of support groups.

Chapter 9

NCLEX-PN® ANSWERS

(1) 4—Although the mother needs instruction on the risk of propping the bottle, more assessment is needed about the rea-son for propping the bottle. (2) Gonorrhea and chlamydia—Antibiotic ointment or solution is used to prevent eye infection from gonorrhea and chlamydia. (3) Irregular; 32 to 48; normal respirations may be irregular and are 32 to 48 per minute. (4) 2—Jaundice in the newborn appearing 24 hours after birth is physiologic in origin. It should be documented but does not have to be reported. (5) 1—Newborns frequently have blue hands and feet at birth due to slow circulation. The condition may last a few hours to a few days. (6) 2—The father needs some time to adjust to his son's spinal anomaly. Simple answers to questions at this point are the best response. More in-depth information will be given once the doctor has determined the extent of the defect. (7) 2—Flaring nostrils, grunting respirations, and retractions are early signs of respiratory distress. Cyanosis indicates hypoxia. (8) 3—The baby needs to take the entire areola into the mouth in order to release the milk from the mammary ducts properly and to prevent sore nipples. (9) 1—The penis needs to be cleaned with plain water. Alcohol will cause pain and will irritate the incision line. (10) 1—Generally, triple diapers are used for several months, so the nurse should suspect the father has not understood information. The nurse first needs to explore the father's understanding.

CARE PLAN HINTS

1. The nurse should provide the same teaching for Jeremy's parents as for any other new parent, including skin care, umbilical cord care, and nutrition. If his mother wants to breast feed, she may be taught to nurse in the NICU if Jeremy is stable enough. Otherwise, she will be taught to pump her breasts for a few days until Jeremy is strong enough to nurse.
2. Besides the routine discharge teaching of a newborn, the parents should be taught to care for his incision and to administer medications, including actions and side effects.
3. The role of the LPN/LVN in providing care in the NICU is one of assisting the RN and other health care professionals. Because the LPN/LVN may be providing care at the bedside, parent teaching is often of an informal nature, answering questions and demonstrating procedures.

CRITICAL THINKING CARE MAP

Subjective Data   None. *Subjective data are what the client tells the nurse. The newborn cannot verbalize complaints.*

Objective Data   Respiration 64/min, temperature 97.2°F (36.2°C), mother received morphine sulfate 2 hours ago, flaring nostrils, grunting respirations.

Report   Yes, report to the charge nurse. If the newborn's condition does not improve within a few minutes or retractions become apparent, the primary care provider should be notified.

Interventions Suction airway. Mucus in the airway can cause respiratory distress. Place under radiant warmer. Hypothermia can cause respiratory distress in the newborn. Administer Narcan (naloxone hydrochloride). *The newborn may have respiratory depression from the morphine sulfate the mother received during labor. The facility policy and doctor's order should be followed.* Apply pulse oximeter. *Data from pulse oximeter is helpful in monitoring the degree of respiratory distress.* Monitor vital signs every hour. *The condition of the newborn should be evaluated at least every hour. More frequent monitoring may be warranted to evaluate the effectiveness of treatment.*

Documentation (date/time) T 97.2, R 64. Nasal flaring and grunting respirations noted. Airway suctioned with bulb syringe. Small amount clear mucus obtained. Placed under radiant warmer, temperature probe applied to abdomen. Pulse oximeter applied to R foot. O_2 Sat 93%. Charge nurse notified. O. Shaud, LPN

Chapter 10

NCLEX-PN® ANSWERS

(1) 1, 2, 3, 5—A contracted uterus is firm and midline, and there will only be a scant amount of vaginal discharge. When the uterus is not contracted, it will be soft or boggy on palpation and may be displaced to the right or left. Vaginal bleeding will be increased with clots possible. (2) 1—The fundus should decrease about 1 cm/day until it is located below the symphysis pubis. This is a normal finding for the second day postpartum. (3) 2—A precipitous birth generally causes more birth trauma to maternal tissues and delays healing. (4) 3—Lochia alba is the term used for the creamy white or pale yellow discharge that occurs 2 to 3 weeks following birth. (5) 3—Barrier methods are preferred for breastfeeding mothers. Hormonal methods may interfere with breast milk production. Although ovulation may be altered during breastfeeding, it is not a reliable way to prevent pregnancy. (6) 2, 4, 5—It may take a while for peristalsis to return following birth, resulting in constipation. Exercise, increased fluids, and a diet high in fiber may assist in relieving constipation. (7) 3—Asian, Mexican, and African women will often avoid cold following birth; therefore, the ice pack would be refused. (8) 1—Temperature over 100.4°F after the first 24-hour period could indicate infection. The nurse should assess the wound for signs of infection. She could assess for abdominal tenderness. These symptoms should be reported. (9) 4—Before the milk comes in, the breast contains colostrum, which drains from the breast and looks like a thin, yellow fluid. (10) 250 mg (total dose) divided by 100-mg tablet (dose on hand) = 2.5 tablets.

Care Plan Hints

1. The nurse should first address the client's pain and seek to manage it. Once the pain is effectively managed, the nurse discusses the risks of immobility to seek compliance. Assist the client with movement to minimize discomfort.
2. The nurse should discuss with the client's husband the risks of deep vein thrombosis and how mobility can effectively prevent it.
3. Although it is important for the TED hose to remain in place to prevent deep vein thrombosis, the nurse must also assist the client with hygiene. Frequent assessment of the TED is important, especially in the postpartum client due to vaginal discharge. The TED hose should be removed daily and the legs assessed, bathed, and dried thoroughly before replacing them.

CRITICAL THINKING CARE MAP

Subjective Data No prenatal care; states leave the child in the nursery; asks will the nurses change the baby's diapers, I don't ever want to do that.

Objective Data Positive drug screen; did not make eye contact with baby.

Report Yes, report to the RN.

Interventions Continue to assess mother-child interaction. Inquire about the child's name. Teach the client about caring for a newborn. Report to the charge nurse behaviors that indicate impaired bonding. Take the newborn into the client's room, even if she has not requested him.

Documentation (date) 12:15 19-year-old G1P1 transferred to room 315 via stretcher from labor and delivery following vaginal birth of viable male with second-degree episiotomy at 10:50. States leave the baby in the nursery and asks will the nurses change the baby's diapers? I don't ever want to do that. No eye contact noted between client and newborn. Newborn transferred to nursery. Charge nurse notified of client's questions and statement. N. Nance, LVN

UNIT II Thinking Strategically About …

CRITICAL THINKING

- Newborns should stool within 24 hours of birth. Failure to stool within 24 hours of birth can indicate a bowel obstruction.
- Baby Philip is nursing enough. Newborns should nurse 5 to 8 minutes per breast in the first 24 hours and gradually increase to 15 minutes per breast. Signs of poor nutrition in the newborn include fewer than eight wet diapers per day, sunken fontanels, and not regaining the birth weight in 2 weeks.

COLLABORATIVE CARE

- Miss McQuire has had complications of pregnancy (PIH) and should be followed closely for several weeks. Being a single mother, she may also need assistance with the baby, including emotional and financial support.

PRIORITIES IN NURSING CARE

- Miss McQuire and her baby should be seen first, then Mrs. Chung, and finally Mrs. Owens and her baby. The initial contact will be an assessment of each client. With Miss McQuire needing close monitoring, the LPN cannot be tied up in other rooms providing lengthy care. Therefore, other care may need to wait until the RN returns from the delivery room, and then the LPN and RN can work as a team to provide care and teaching.

- Because Miss McQuire has PIH and IV magnesium, she must be monitored closely and should be seen first. Mrs. Chung may have cultural and language issues that must be accounted for. An induction is not a high priority and may need to wait until the RN is available. Mrs. Owens and her baby are stable; therefore, they can safely be seen last.

MANAGEMENT OF CARE

- Miss McQuire should be monitored a minimum of every 1 hour.
- If time allows, the LPN can begin subjective data collection with Mrs. Peters and apply the fetal monitoring equipment. Other aspects of induction may need to wait until the RN is available.

DELEGATING

- A CNA could obtain vital signs on the mothers, pass out breakfast and lunch trays, and help mothers to the bathroom. They can also change babies' diapers.

COMMUNICATION AND CLIENT TEACHING

- Mrs. Chung should be told that the induction will be started as soon as possible, but until the RN is available to assist, the administration of Pitocin cannot be started.
- Mrs. Owens should be taught to care for herself, including hygiene, nutrition and fluids, and exercise. She should be taught cord and circumcision care.

DOCUMENTING AND REPORTING

- Report an increase in blood pressure, an increase in reflexes and clonus. Because the RN is in the delivery area, the LPN should call the RN on another unit and request assistance.
- Sample documentation: (date/time) Instructed to clean circumcision with water with each diaper change. Instructed to watch for signs of infection and bleeding. Mother verbalized understanding of circumcision care. J. Keefer, LPN

CULTURAL CARE STRATEGIES

- Due to Mrs. Chung's limited English, it is important to assess her understanding of instructions, relaxation techniques, pain control, self-care, and infant care. Ask about Mrs. Chung's cultural practices regarding birth and postpartum care because they may differ from what you expect. An interpreter may be required.

Chapter 11

NCLEX-PN® ANSWERS

(1) 4—Autonomy is being self-sufficient. Helping toddlers complete tasks will not help them learn. Although it is important to teach right and wrong, as well as social skills in playing with other children, these responses do not answer the question. (2) 3—Reading books and watching TV are passive activities. Paint by numbers is messy for a hospital room and above the development of a 5-year-old. Playing with puppets can help develop cognitive skills and express feelings. (3) 1—Children of this age often engage in imaginative play and magical thinking. The other answers all relate to older children. (4) 4—The 2-year-old is beginning to gain some improved balance and coordination and can balance on one foot for a few seconds. The other answers relate to skills developed at later stages. (5) 3—Sports at this age are a good idea, but they should be geared to the child's abilities and interests. Response 1 is incorrect. Encourage parents to stress the value of sports for learning skills and teamwork. (6) Peers—An adolescent is most influenced by peers at this stage of development. (7) 2—The first action a nurse takes is assessment. Before strategies can be developed to resolve the problem, the nurse must talk with the child to determine the problem. (8) Empty nest syndrome occurs when children have moved out of the family home and the mother no longer is required to give daily attention to her children. (9) 4—Explanations should be given to a young child just before the procedure to prevent worry. Preoperative preparation involves more than medication, so 2 and 3 do not answer the question. (10) 2—The client in this situation is the 18-year-old grandson. This response acknowledges the client's feelings and opens the door to further exploration. Responses 1, 3, and 4 make some assumptions that may not be correct.

CARE PLAN HINTS

1. The nurse should ask the mother the following: Has Jim seen a doctor since his birth? Has she tried to offer him solid foods? Does he cry between feedings, or does he appear hungry after a bottle? Does she have any support with his care (emotional or physical)? Has anyone talked about normal activity and diet for a 9-month-old?

2. It would help to know if she lives alone and if she has the ability to obtain health care and proper nutrition for the baby. The nurse should also wonder why the first well-baby check is at 9 months.

3. With a birth weight of 7 lb, Jim should have doubled his weight by 5 to 6 months. His nutrition is inadequate. He is not reaching normal developmental milestones in a timely manner, and it appears that he has little stimulation and limited opportunities for socialization. Social services need to be notified for child protection; at the very least, the mother needs assistance with some parenting classes.

CRITICAL THINKING CARE MAP

Subjective Data Mother states turns front to back, puts toys in mouth.

Objective Data 4 months old; VS 98-120-30; Wt 15 lb; Ht 22½ in.; head 16 in.

Report No; data are within normal limits.

Interventions Teach need for close supervision because the child is becoming mobile. Instruct mother on toys for age of the child. Instruct mother to begin solid foods. Teach parent to avoid foods that could cause choking (raisins, peanuts, whole grapes). Instruct mother to keep syrup of ipecac in the first aid kit.

Documentation (date/time) 4-month-old infant, well-developed weight and length within normal limits; developmental milestones appropriate for age. Mother reports that child is rolling over. While in examining room, mother stepped away from exam table, leaving child unprotected. Mother cautioned about leaving child unattended now that she is rolling over. N. Geiber, LVN

Chapter 12

NCLEX-PN® ANSWERS

(1) 0.5 mL. (2) 1—Primary prevention interventions are those that keep the client from developing health problems. Immunizations prevent childhood diseases. (3) 2—Secondary prevention are interventions to detect health problems early in the process. Pap smears are necessary for sexually active females to detect some STIs and cervical cancer. (4) 2—Tertiary prevention includes treatments to keep the disease from getting worse and from developing complications. Administering antibiotics for otitis media is tertiary prevention. (5) 4—Choking and suffocation are safety hazards for the newborn. Also, a newborn cannot grasp and hold toys. Music is an appropriate choice to stimulate the newborn. (6) 1, 4, 5—Only soft, easy-to-swallow and easily digestible foods are appropriate for the infant. Purees and rice cereal are good choices. These foods should not cause choking. (7) 4—The nurse

should document date of injection, name and dosage of vaccine, lot number and expiration date, and site and route of administration. It is unnecessary to chart vital signs as they relate to vaccination. (8) 2—When cessation of smoking is unlikely, the nurse should clearly, but in a nonjudgmental manner, encourage the client to reduce the amount of cigarettes smoked daily. The nicotine patch may have the same harmful effects as smoking. (9) 1—Obesity is linked with family overeating, poor body image, stress, depression, and lack of parental attention. (10) 1—Narcotics cause pinpoint pupils, drowsiness, euphoria, and respiratory depression.

CARE PLAN HINTS

1. Corrosive cleaners, insect and rodent poisons, fertilizers, and cat litter.

2. Hazardous substances should be placed in a locked cabinet out of reach of children. Children can be taught how to recognize hazardous substances by placing Mr. Yuk stickers on them. Parental supervision at all times is vital in areas where these substances are stored.

3. The parent is likely to experience guilt and sorrow that the child was injured. The parent may blame him- or herself for not watching the child more closely or not properly storing the hazardous substances. The parent may also fear that the child will become injured again.

CRITICAL THINKING CARE MAP

Subjective Data Skips breakfast; chips and cola for lunch; chicken fingers, fries, and sweet tea for dinner.

Objective Data Current weight 100 lb; previous weight 110 lb.

Report Yes, to the supervising nurse.

Interventions Explain importance of nutrition during adolescence. Use the food pyramid to discuss essential nutrients. Present a sample daily meal plan. Discuss ways to overcome difficulties related to food preparation and food acquisition. Refer to a dietician prn.

Documentation (date) 15:00 14-year-old female to school clinic for initial assessment. Weight 100 lb. Previous records show weight 110 lb. States does not eat breakfast, has chips and cola for lunch, and has chicken fingers, fries, and sweet tea for dinner. States this is a typical diet. Discussed findings with supervising nurse. Plan of care developed to improve nutritional status. A. White, LPN

Chapter 13

NCLEX-PN® ANSWERS

(1) 1, 2, 4, 5—Head circumference may be routinely measured until age 36 months. (2) 3—An infant is unable to control urine output; therefore, to accurately assess the volume

of urine, a urine bag is the most appropriate method. (3) 1—Inside the tent, condensation is created. This creates moisture and makes the linen damp. Toys should be made of plastic so they will not become damp. The tent should be kept closed as much as possible to provide the client with the dosage of oxygen ordered. The air inside an oxygen tent is usually cool; therefore, a fan would not be necessary. (4) 4—The vastus lateralis is the preferred site for an intramuscular injection for an infant. Muscles are not fully developed in the other sites. (5) 1—To remove secretions properly, the nurse's first action is to use a bulb syringe and suction the mouth first, then the nose. (6) 2, 4, 5—Restraints should be used as a last resort and only temporarily. (7) 3—Suppositories in infants are inserted with the index or little finger and only ½ in. to avoid perforating the anus. (8) 1—Normal pulse for a 2-year-old is 80 to 140 and normal respirations are 20 to 40. (9) 1—Normal pulse for the adolescent is 50 to 90, and normal blood pressure is 120/80. (10) 4—Because the assessment can cause additional pain and create a change in the child's vital signs, it is important to assess the painful area last.

CARE PLAN HINTS

1. Keri can be allowed to say "ouch" or "that hurts" when the nurse is giving an injection. Music is appropriate for Keri. She also can play with stuffed animals or dolls. Watching nonviolent cartoons will allow Keri to be distracted from her pain.

2. The nurse should anticipate this question and discuss the possible answers with her father. It is important to be honest with Keri without giving her too many details. If possible, once Keri and her mom are stable, the nurse could arrange a visit.

3. Discuss with Keri's father what terms are typically used for injuries, such as "boo-boo" or "ouchy." Use these with Keri in discussing her pain. Pain in the toddler can be expressed by crying, aggressive behavior, grinding teeth, or rubbing the affected site. Some children may demonstrate regressive behavior.

CRITICAL THINKING CARE MAP

Subjective Data   Yelling no, no, no.

Objective Data   Crying, kicking and screaming, face red, carotid pulse 120 bpm.

Report   Yes, to the physician in order to obtain an order for mummy restraints.

Interventions   Obtain physician's order for mummy restraints; enlist assistance of a colleague during procedure; assess restraints every 15 minutes; provide emotional care during and after procedure; remove restraints immediately after procedure.

Documentation   (date) 08:00 18-month-old male crying, kicking, and screaming no, no, no. Face noted to be red. Dr. notified of child's anxiety and that safety was compromised. Order received for mummy restraints. S. Smith, LPN (date) 08:30 Mummy restraints applied per protocol with assistance from M. Jones, LPN. Nasogastric tube inserted without difficulty. Carotid pulse 120 bpm. S. Smith, LPN (date) 08:55 Mummy restraints removed. Carotid pulse 120 bpm. Emotional care provided. Transported client to father's arms. S. Smith, LPN

Chapter 14

NCLEX-PN® ANSWERS

(1) 2—A 10-month-old is unsure of new environments and unfamiliar people. They are beginning to develop separation anxiety and fear of strangers. It will be several months before the negativism of the toddler becomes apparent. There is nothing in the questions to indicate hostility or jealousy. (2) 1—The question is about a mist tent at night. The size of the child's room must be evaluated to be sure the equipment will fit in the room. Provisions for the mist tent must be made before the child is discharged in order to have continuity of care. Although the other choices might be important, they do not pertain to this question. (3) 3—As long as the child is not contagious, she should be allowed to attend school. Skipping or altering the time of administration of antibiotics can affect their effectiveness. The school personnel can be taught to safely administer medication. (4) Home routine—The 3-year-old needs as much stability as possible in an unfamiliar environment. Keeping the routine similar to the home environment provides stability. (5) 2—Allowing for the family's request promotes culturally sensitive care. It is important that the rituals do not interfere with the rights of other clients. (6) 3—The nurse must assess Joan's mother's condition to determine if she is experiencing caregiver strain. Help may be needed to provide a safe environment for Joan if her mother is too tired to care for her. (7) 4, 3, 2, 1—The first priority is for safety in case of an emergency. Next is to ensure the safe transfer from bed to wheelchair. Although bathing is important, several possibilities exist and therefore it is a lower priority at this time. Kindergarten is the lowest priority now. (8) 1—The safest way to transport a 9-month-old is in a crib with the side rails up. There is the possibility the child can fall with the other methods. (9) 1—A private room would be required to allow for the equipment that will be needed to care for this totally dependent child. A sitter may be required 24 hours a day, and extra room will be needed. A private room will also prevent the child from disturbing other residents. A room close to the nurses' station would be best

for client safety. (10) 4—The 16-year-old should be allowed privacy during questioning. Any use of illicit drugs could interfere with anesthesia and pain medication and therefore is a priority to assess.

CARE PLAN HINTS

1. The nurse should tell the child that he should feel better every day. It will be up to the doctor to say when he can play T ball again, but it will be several weeks. Showing him a calendar will help him have a better idea of the time frame.
2. It is unlikely that the umbilical hernia will recur as long as the surgical repair heals well.
3. If Timmy exhibits signs of an infection (fever, elevated WBC count, nausea and vomiting), there is a possibility that surgery will be postponed.

CRITICAL THINKING CARE MAP

Subjective Data   Does not like school, enjoys reading fiction stories, states pain in both hips, states he misses playing football.

Objective Data   Is in fourth grade.

Report   Yes, to the RN planning care; these are important observations related to his cognitive development.

Interventions   Orient to environment and facility routine. *Orientation to the environment and routine will help decrease fear and let client know what is expected of him.* Tell him he must attend classes to keep up with his schoolwork. *Even though he does not like school, getting behind will make school more difficult.* Insist he performs ADLs with minimal assistance. *Insisting that he do everything he can for himself will help prevent regression to a lower level of development.*

Documentation   (date/time) 10-year-old Andrew Paulson admitted to room 24 of the rehabilitation unit. Oriented to room, bathroom, dining room, and physical therapy department. Oriented to facility routine, including meals, physical therapy times, school activities, and visiting hours. States he does not like school but likes to read fiction stories. Informed that he will be able to read for pleasure after his schoolwork is completed daily. D. Jones, RN, notified of likes and dislikes. P. Stromberg, LPN

Chapter 15

NCLEX-PN® ANSWERS

(1) 3—Normal HCT for a 2-year-old child is 29% to 40%. (2) 1—Common symptoms of hypernatremia are thirst and neurologic symptoms. (3) 1—Potassium imbalances have the potential to affect cardiac and respiratory status. The child's pulse and respiratory rate and rhythm must be monitored diligently by the nurse. (4) Muscle weakness—

Weakness is a sign that the child's condition is worsening. (5) 3—The child is already weak, which can be a precursor for decreased LOC in children with hypercalcemia. (6) 1—Vomiting is a recordable output and is important to record in clients with dehydration. It should be part of the parent's instruction about methods of fluid loss. (7) 4—The nurse must monitor carefully the administration of oral and IV fluids as ordered. (8) 2—Respiratory alkalosis is characterized by decreased PCO_2. (9) 3—A weak, thready pulse is indicative of dehydration. (10) 3.2%. Convert weight in pounds and ounces to a decimal by dividing ounces by 16:

$$7 \text{ lb } 12 \text{ oz} = 7 \text{ 12/16 lb} = 7.75 \text{ lb}$$
$$7 \text{ lb } 8 \text{ oz} = 7 \text{ 8/16 lb} = 7.5 \text{ lb}$$

Subtract the current weight from the previous weight:

$$\begin{array}{r} 7.75 \text{ lb} \\ - \ 7.50 \text{ lb} \\ \hline 0.25 \text{ lb} \end{array}$$

Divide the weight lost by the previous weight to obtain the percent of weight lost.

$$0.25 \text{ lb}/7.75 = 3.2\%$$

CARE PLAN HINTS

1. Hypovolemic shock is recognized by confusion progressing to stupor or coma; tachypnea progressing to apnea; oliguria progressing to anuria; poor capillary refill progressing to weak, thready pulse; and hypotension.
2. Infants can have intolerance to formulas. However, this intolerance is not exhibited with symptoms of lethargy and irritability. The most common symptoms for formula intolerance are diarrhea, flatus, abdominal pain shortly after feeding, and mucus in the stools. Wesley may need to receive only oral rehydration solutions for 24 hours and then his normal formula could be resumed.
3. The harmful organism causing diarrhea can be found on toys, clothing, and furniture. After changing diapers and handling soiled linens and clothing, Wesley's mother and other caregivers should wash their hands thoroughly. During periods of illness, toys should not be shared and cleaned thoroughly.

CRITICAL THINKING CARE MAP

Subjective Data   LPN states, "This rate is twice the rate ordered by the physician."

Objective Data   Generalized edema, moist lung sounds, pulse 110 bpm and bounding, hematocrit, 40%, urine-specific gravity 1.000, sodium 133 mEq/L.

Report Yes, this condition needs to be reported immediately, first to the supervising RN and then to the physician.

Interventions Monitor intravenous fluid rate, monitor and document intake and output, monitor lab values and report imbalances, monitor vital signs, weigh the infant daily and document, observe for edema of the extremities, face and neck, observe closely for symptoms of pulmonary edema including restlessness, tachypnea, labored breathing, a full and bounding pulse or a weak and thready pulse, possible crackles on lung auscultation, and profuse diaphoresis. Position the child to facilitate breathing and notify the physician immediately if symptoms are present.

Documentation (date/time) 72-hour-old, term female infant lying prone under Bili lights. Eye protection in place. IV to right wrist infusing LR at 30 mL/hr per pump. IV rate ordered at 15 mL/hr. Pulse 110 bpm, bounding. Generalized edema noted. Lungs sounds, moist bilaterally to auscultation, IV rate decreased to 15 mL/hr and nursing supervisor notified. L.wiley, LVN

Chapter 16

NCLEX-PN® ANSWERS

(1) 2—The restraints are in place to protect the child. If the restraints are removed, an adult must be present to prevent the child from dislodging the IV. If the aunt is planning to leave the child unattended, the restraint must be replaced. (2) 7.5 mL—Order is 240 mg. Supply is 160 mg/5 mL. If there are 160 mg in 5 mL and you need 240 mg, how many milliliter will you need?

$$\text{Calculation: } \frac{160 \text{ mg}}{5 \text{ mL}} = \frac{240 \text{ mg}}{X \text{ mL}}$$

Cross-multiply: 160X = 1,200

X = 1,200 divided by 160

Solution: X = 7.5 mL needed to supply 240 mg of medication

(3) 2—The father needs some time to adjust to his son's spinal anomaly. Simple answers to questions at this point are the best responses. More in-depth information will be given once the doctor has determined the extent of the defect. (4) 1, 3, 5—The nurse must look for physiologic responses to pain because the infant is unable to verbally express pain. (5) Convert pounds to kilogram. 7 lb 5 oz = 7 5/16 lb = 7.31 lb. Divide pounds by 2.2 (number of pounds in 1 kg). 7.31/2.2 = 3.32 kg. Multiply infant's weight in kilogram by dose ordered in milligram. 3.32 × 20 = 66.4 mg. Calculate dosage: 66.4 mg divided by available concentration of 30 mg/mL = 2.2 mL dose to provide 20 mg. (6) 4—Visual acuity in any age is tested with the right eye, with the left eye covered, and the left eye is tested with the right eye covered. Then both eyes are tested together. Visual acuity is measured with the client standing or being held 20 ft away from the chart. The test can be done with or without corrective lenses. (7) 2—Reye's syndrome has been linked to the use of salicylates when caring for cold and flu symptoms. Products that do not contain salicylates should be used for these conditions. (8) 3—The client is placed in a lateral position, the knees flexed to the abdomen and the back bowed or arched at the edge of the examination table or bed with the chin resting on the chest. The nurse positions the client and maintains position stability during the procedure to prevent injury. (9) 2—Seizure precautions are instituted for clients with closed head injuries and suspected concussions. Specific seizure precautions vary slightly from one agency to another, but they, in general, have a common theme. Airway, oxygen, and suctioning equipment is kept at the bedside. The side rails are padded to prevent injury from seizure activity. An IV access should be in place already from the ER to administer antiseizure medications. Use of padded tongue blades is highly controversial and should never be taped to the bed of a pediatric client. (10) 4—CP is a chronic disability caused by an abnormality in the pyramidal or extrapyramidal motor system. The client with CP has difficulty with muscle control as a result of this abnormality.

CARE PLAN HINTS

1. Cerebral palsy clients may have difficulty speaking and communicating. Ambulation may be difficult and require ambulation aids.
2. Students may not have had any experience with clients with cerebral palsy. They may not understand the disorder and may make unkind comments. It may be difficult for Daniel to make friends.
3. Before school starts, the school nurse could have Daniel meet fellow students who have similar disabilities. Students without disabilities who have previously exhibited empathy could also meet with Daniel before school. The school nurse could also monitor Daniel's interactions with students and quickly address negative interactions.

CRITICAL THINKING CARE MAP

Subjective Data Mom states several children in her class at day care are sick with the same thing. Mom states child is very irritable.

Objective Data VS: T 101.4, P 70, R 12, BP 90/60; Wt 29 lb; emesis: 30 mL green vomitus × 1.

Report Yes, to the physician or charge nurse.

Interventions Monitor vital signs for subtle changes. Monitor CBC values for signs of infection. Review immunization record. Teach mom signs and symptoms of infection and when to seek medical attention. Discuss ways to prevent transmission of bacteria, including hand washing techniques and isolating child from other children who are sick.

Documentation (date) 09:00 4-year-old female presented to the office with T 101.4, tympanic; P 70, regular; R 12, even and unlabored; BP 90/60, right arm. Mother states the child has not had an appetite, has had several episodes of vomiting, and complains of neck pain. 30 mL green emesis noted. B. Razell, LPN

Chapter 17

NCLEX-PN® ANSWERS

(1) 2—The brace must be worn 23 hours a day in order to be effective. The real issue here is the child's feelings. Only response 2 acknowledges her feelings and enourages her to address the issue. (2) 3—Osteosarcoma is found in the femur, tibia, and humerus and characterized by pain, swelling, and ambulation difficulties. (3) 3—Teenagers who have had a limb amputated may develop signs of disturbed body image, such as hiding or overexposing of the limb, refusing to look at or touch the limb, or exhibiting preoccupation with loss of limb. (4) 1—Generally, triple diapers are used for several months, so the nurse should suspect the father has not comprehended the information. The nurse first needs to explore the father's understanding. (5) 4—Synthetic casts are preferred because they dry more quickly and allow for greater mobility than a plaster cast. Synthetic casts are weaker than plaster casts. (6) Resistance or hip click— The physician assesses the infant's hips while performing the Ortolani-Barlow maneuver for resistance, or a clicking sound, which indicates hip dislocation. (7) 2— Nothing should be placed on the traction ropes because of the risk of disrupting the traction. The other options are all correct actions that should be taken by the nurse. (8) 1— When assessing for capillary refill, the normal findings are the compressed nail bed returns to normal color in less than 3 seconds. This finding is within normal limits. (9) 1, 2, 3, 4, 5—The use of powder inside the cast is not recommended because it can cause skin irritation. (10) 1—The Milwaukee brace should be worn for 23 hours a day. The rest of the comments are appropriate.

CARE PLAN HINTS

1. Many individuals play all types of sports with a prosthesis. Running, team sports such as baseball, and golf are possible. Jake should be encouraged to try whatever he wants to try.
2. A balanced diet is essential to Jake's energy level. His diet should be high in protein and low in sugar. It should contain adequate whole foods such as fruits and vegeta-

bles. He should also have an adequate intake of water. Energy conservation is essential as well. His room and living quarters should be arranged to allow him to decrease excess walking. Exercising the major muscle groups will also increase endurance.

3. The nurse could respond by saying, "Tell me more about your fears about having people stare. (Allow Jake to respond.) Are you afraid they will say mean things or laugh at you? Remember that people in general are far from perfect and usually stare because they don't understand what you've been through." Another response is, "I guess it would be scary to see people's heads turning as you walk by. They could be thinking 'My, what an amazing young man that is!' It also would be okay if you look them directly in the eye and smile. You could even ask them if they'd like to hear you're amazing story of survival. You do have a great story to tell."

CRITICAL THINKING CARE MAP

Subjective Data States, it hurts real bad.

Objective Data Crying, nonweightbearing, ankle swollen and bruised, pedal pulses present.

Report Yes, to the physician.

Interventions Instruct to support cast on pillows until dry. Instruct not to put anything inside cast. Instruct regarding signs of impaired circulation. Ice pack to ankle; teach crutch walking.

Documentation (date) 08:00 States fell while roller blading and ankle hurts real bad. Nonweightbearing on left leg upon admission. Left ankle swollen and bruised. Pedal pulses present. Dr. notified. Provided written and verbal instruction in cast care prior to discharge. M. Fowler, LPN

Chapter 18

NCLEX-PN® ANSWERS

(1) 4—The nurse must ensure that respiratory pathogens are not transmitted from the infant with RSV to the general population. Sterile gloves and double bagging diapers would not prevent the spread of respiratory virus. The baby should not be allowed go to the play room. Respiratory pathogens are transmitted through the air; therefore, the person feeding the infant should wear a mask. When burping the infant, respiratory secretions can be mixed with formula, contaminating the nurse's hands and uniform. (2) 1— When a mist tent is used to administer oxygen, the bedding and clothing become moist from condensation. The bedding and clothing must be kept dry to prevent chilling the child. (3) 2—A fish is the best choice. Cat and dog dander, as well as bird feathers, can cause allergic asthma. (4) 1— The purpose of postural drainage is to drain mucus from the

lungs. When the mucus is removed, the lungs are better able to fully expand. Some bacteria will be removed with the mucus, but antibiotics will be necessary to treat the lung infection. (5) 2—Epiglottitis can result in airway obstruction. Anticipating this possible emergency situation, the nurse should plan ahead and have tracheostomy equipment available. (6) 1—Halitosis is common following a tonsillectomy until the scab comes off. Increased pulse and restlessness are signs of bleeding. Crying could cause bleeding from the surgical site. (7) 4—Orange juice is acidic and could irritate the throat, causing pain and bleeding. (8) 3, 1, 4, 5, 2—It is important for the nurse to stay with the client with breathing difficulty to relieve anxiety and to be available if the child's condition deteriorates. Inhalers are frequently ordered to treat asthma, so the client needs instruction on their use. While the child is in the hospital, the parents should identify possible allergy triggers and try to eliminate them from the home. The child and parents need to know that a good warm-up may prevent an asthma attack. The child will need follow-up care following discharge. (9) 4—Using a plastic syringe (without a needle) is the most accurate measurement, as well as allowing parent control in giving the liquid to the child. Small amounts can be squirted into the child's mouth. Having the child drink the medication from a cup could result in spillage. (10) Order is for 0.2 mg/kg. Convert pounds to kilogram. 43 lb divided by 2.2 lb/kg = 19.5 kg. Multiply 0.2 mg times 19.5 kg = 3.9 mg per dose for this child. Available medication supply 2 mg/5 mL.

$$\frac{2\ mg}{5\ mL} = \frac{3.9\ mg}{X\ mL}$$

Cross-multiply: 2X = 19.5. Divide 19.5 by 2 = 9.75 mL needed to provide 0.2 mg/kg (3.9 mg) of medication.

CARE PLAN HINTS

1. Blowing on a pinwheel, blowing bubbles, and blowing up balloons.
2. What were you doing prior to the asthma attack? Do you have any animals in the home? Are there any blooming plants in or around the house? What kind of pillows do you use? Have you eaten any new foods today?
3. While playing with dolls, the nurse can play the role of a sick child. The nurse's doll can say how she might feel and ask Jimmy to tell how he feels.

CRITICAL THINKING CARE MAP

Subjective Data   Withdrawn; sleepy.

Objective Data   Crying; T 103.2, P 148, R 40; nonproductive cough; labored breathing; lung sounds wheezy; circumoral cyanosis; weight gain.

Report   Yes, to RN in charge.

Interventions   Suction airway prn. *Maintaining the airway is always high priority.* Administer IV medication as ordered. *May not be LPN function in some states, but LPN is responsible for notifying RN that it must be done.* Offer 1,000 mL clear liquids. *Increased fluids help thin secretions. Milk and milk products increase mucus production.* Provide a mist tent. *Cool mist decreases bronchial swelling and thins respiratory secretions.* Administer expectorant cough syrup as ordered. *Expectorants thin secretions.* Provide droplet precautions. *Droplet precautions should be instituted to prevent spread of infection to others until cultures are obtained.*

Documentation   (date/time) Client admitted to room 402 with mother at bedside. VS: T 103.2, P 148, R 40. Lung sounds wheezy. Respirations labored. Circumoral cyanosis present. Airway suctioned of small amount white mucus. Expectorant given as ordered. Explained droplet precautions to mother. Charge nurse notified of client condition. M. Jones, LPN

Chapter 19

NCLEX-PN® ANSWERS

(1) 3—If the child vomits the diuretic, the parents should report this to the physician and not randomly give another tablet because another dose of medication can cause severe potassium deficits in the child. The other responses are all appropriate. (2) 4—Kawasaki disease is an acute systemic inflammatory disease also known as mucocutaneous lymph node syndrome. (3) 2—All of the above can be manifest in Kawasaki disease, but in the subacute phase, the client has sloughing off of the skin on the lips, hands, and feet. (4) 1—Rheumatic fever is confirmed by the presence of antistreptolysin O titer. (5) 3—Crackles heard on auscultation indicate an accumulation of fluid in the lungs. The others are not signs of fluid accumulation. (6) 3—Tetralogy of Fallot includes four defects: right ventricular hypertrophy, pulmonary stenosis, ventricular septal defect, and overriding aorta. (7) 4—Strong, bounding pulses in the upper extremities and thready, weak pulses in the legs, along with CHF are possible in the client with coarctation of the aorta. (8) 1— Prostaglandin E1 is given temporarily to increase cardiac output and oxygen saturation. The other options have nothing to do with transposition of the great arteries. (9) 1—Aspirin is given to decrease fever and inflammation, and IV immunoglobulin is given to decrease the occurrence of lesions and aneurysms that can form in Kawasaki disease. (10) 1, 3, 4, 6—All answers, except the pain medications and anticoagulants, are correct for hyperlipidemia.

CARE PLAN HINTS

1. Encourage the use of salt substitutes. Avoid smoked or cured meats. Avoid salted snack foods. Most cheese and peanut butters contain excessive sodium. Frozen vegetables contain less sodium than canned varieties. Sodas are typically high in sodium.

2. Encourage Branson's family to purchase an automatic blood pressure cuff. Give them guidelines for choosing the right size. Calibrate the cuff with a manual sphygmomanometer. Demonstrate to Branson the proper method of obtaining a blood pressure reading. Have Branson return the demonstration to verify his understanding. Teach Branson to take his blood pressure daily, prior to administering his blood pressure medication. Provide Branson with a documentation record to keep track of his daily blood pressure. Teach him when to report elevated blood pressure readings.

3. Encourage Branson and his parents to pursue allergy testing to determine the exact cause of his symptoms. Once the allergens have been identified, diligence in avoiding these allergens may allow Branson to reduce his intake of antihistamines.

CRITICAL THINKING CARE MAP

Subjective Data I am just not hungry. Nothing tastes good. The medication caused diarrhea, and we did not finish the prescription. Reports joint pain of 6 on a scale of 10; takes Tylenol every 4 to 6 hours for joint pain.

Objective Data Right wrist enlarged; winces when wrist and elbow are moved; VS: T 101.1, P 110, R 12, BP 110/60.

Report Yes, report promptly to the supervising nurse or, depending on the degree of pain, report directly to the physician.

Interventions Thoroughly assess the child's pain. Include location, characteristics, onset/duration, frequency, quality, intensity, precipitating factors, and relief methods. Teach the child and parent nonpharmacologic methods of pain relief such as gentle joint massage, ROM exercises, application of heat, control of environmental factors (lighting, noise, room temperature), and relaxation techniques. Teach the child and parent the proper administration of prescribed pharmacologic agents to include route, dosage, side effects, reportable symptoms, and drug interactions. Develop a plan to re-evaluate the child's pain.

Documentation (date) 09:00 Parent of 10-year-old female client called to report symptoms of rash, T 101°F, and sore and painful wrists and elbows. Recent medical history includes positive strep culture (date), treated with prescription for penicillin. Instructed parent to bring client to office for 11:00 A.M. appointment. G. Hoover, LPN

Chapter 20

NCLEX-PN® ANSWERS

(1) 1—Sickle cell anemia is caused by a recessive trait that primarily affects African Americans. (2) 1—Iron deficiency is a symptom of iron-deficiency anemia. The others listed are symptoms of a sickle cell crisis. (3) 4—Children of Mediterranean descent, those from the Middle East, Asia, or Africa, are most likely to have beta or alpha thalassemia. (4) 4—In sickle cell anemia, the blood values reveal decreased Hgb and increased reticulocyte counts. (5) 3—Symptoms of Hodgkin's disease include nontender, firm enlarged lymph nodes, usually in the cervical and supraclavicular areas. (6) 1—Chemotherapy can deplete the white blood cells, which can make the child susceptible to infections. (7) 2—ALL is the overproduction of immature lymphocytes. The other statements describe other blood dyscrasias. (8) 1, 2, 3, 5—All answers are correct for the child with hemophilia except avoiding carbonated beverages. (9) 4—Laboratory data for the child with ITP includes decreased platelet count, decreased antiplatelet antibodies, presence of antinuclear antibodies, and positive direct Coombs' test. (10) 1, 2, 4, 6, 7—All answers are correct except glass and anchovies.

CARE PLAN HINTS

1. This crisis may have been triggered by the stress surrounding preparations for the family trip. It may also have been triggered if Yolanda caught the cold virus from her brother.

2. The client's pain must be the focus. The nurse can provide interventions when pain is at a low level. When position changes are necessary, the nurse can try to perform more than one task that involves movement at the same time.

3. Warm compresses can provide a measure of relief. Massage may be useful. Distraction can be a good tool with this age group.

CRITICAL THINKING CARE MAP

Subjective Data States wants to see her friends as soon as possible and go to the movies. "The doctor said I could go about my normal life." Mother reports that Mandy's best friend has the flu.

Objective Data VS: T 99.0, P 59, R 12, BP 120/80; WBC count 5,000 mm³.

Report Yes, to the registered nurse.

Interventions Teach good hand washing techniques; screen visitors for those who may be ill. Avoid large crowds. Monitor white blood cell count; encourage well-balanced diet high in protein; teach client to monitor for symptoms of infection such as fever, redness, cold symptoms, etc.

Documentation (date) 15:00 15-year-old Black female for follow-up appointment after chemotherapy. Client states the doctor told her she could live a normal life, and she wants to go to the movies with her friends. Client's mother is concerned because client's best friend has the flu. VS: T 99.0, P 59, R 12, BP 120/80. Labs drawn. WBC count 5,000 mm^3. Vital signs and WBC reported to RN. Discussed methods of infection control with client and mother. A. Washington, LPN

Chapter 21

NCLEX-PN® ANSWERS

(1) 2, 4, 6—Clients who have sensitivities/allergies to bananas, avocados, potatoes, chestnuts, and tropical fruits can be at risk for developing an allergy to latex. The possible cause for this is a cross-reaction between the food and the latex allergen. (2) 4—Immunizations provide acquired immunity from diseases by causing the formation of specific antibodies. No immunization protects against all diseases; natural immunity is the condition present at birth and is part of acquired immunity. (3) 2—Mothers who are HIV positive must avoid breastfeeding. The other statements are indications of understanding about HIV precautions and transmission. (4) 4—Rhinitis is not associated with JRA. Responses 1 through 3 are associated with JRA. (5) 3—Medical tests used to confirm brain death are cerebral blood flow studies and electroencephalogram. These tests are usually performed after clinical signs and symptoms have been documented. (6) 1—Urinary dysfunction and fluid and electrolyte imbalances are indicators of potential problems in the kidney transplant recipient. The other choices are not correct. (7) 3—The symptoms described and results of the examination point toward HIV. Of course, further evaluation will be needed. The other choices are incorrect. (8) 1—Nursing interventions for the child with HIV are avoidance of contact with persons with infections, colds, flu, etc., and proper nutrition. The other choices are not specific nursing interventions for children with HIV. (9) 3—Humoral immunity destroys bacteria, viruses, parasites, allergens, and other foreign substances. The other choices are not correct. (10) 1, 2, 4, 6—If a client has a known latex allergy, only nonlatex items may be used, whether invasive or noninvasive. Regular blood pressure cuffs have latex, so specialized cuffs should be used. The latex-free cart should be kept available near the client.

CARE PLAN HINTS

1. Motor skills for a 4-year-old include hopping and skipping on one foot, catching and throwing a ball overhand, walking downstairs, using scissors, lacing shoes, copying a square, and adding three parts to a stick figure. Riley's parents can spend time daily demonstrating hopping and skipping and getting Riley to try these skills. They can also allot time daily to play catch with a ball. Paper and scissor activities would be another appropriate activity.

2. Language skills for a 4-year-old include a vocabulary of more than 1,500 words, using sentences of four or five words, asking frequent questions, singing simple songs, and naming one or more colors. Riley's parents should encourage her to use new words to express herself. They can play children's CDs while riding in the car. Flash cards can be used to help Riley learn her colors.

3. Toys that would assist Riley include a medium-size, lightweight ball; a rope for her to jump over; a craft kit to include scissors, paper, chunky crayons, and tracing paper; a collection of CDs with simple children's songs; and homemade or purchased flash cards depicting colors.

CRITICAL THINKING CARE MAP

Subjective Data I feel really tired. I would feel like a nerd if I wore that mask to school. My best friend has the flu.

Objective Data Vital signs; lab results to include CBC, blood or wound cultures; serum protein and albumin; and skin assessment for wounds and wound drainage.

Report Yes. The nurse needs to report these findings because they further compromise Joe's condition, and interventions need to be planned and implemented to assist Joe in preventing infection.

Interventions Instruct Joe in hand washing and other techniques to avoid contamination with harmful bacteria or viruses. Review immunization schedule and recommend required immunizations as appropriate. Teach Joe and his parents to recognize symptoms of infections, colds, and flu in themselves, family members, friends, or others with whom they may come in contact. Make sure Joe and his parents understand the proper handling, storage, and preparation of food. Make frequent follow-up appointments with Joe to monitor lab values.

Documentation (date/time) 15-year-old male with positive HIV test. VS: T 99.2, P 66, R 14, BP 110/74. CBC drawn, awaiting results. Skin warm, dry, pink, and without lesions. States "I'm really tired all the time." Teaching done regarding infection prevention and therapeutic regime, and information given about HIV and AIDS and the consequences. Following teaching, states "I'd feel like a nerd if I wore that mask to school" and "My best friend has the flu." Understanding of teaching is in question. Report given to charge nurse. Teaching plan revised. K. Anderson, LPN

Chapter 22

NCLEX-PN® ANSWERS

(1) 3—This response not only provides reassurance that Timmy will be okay, but also provides teaching because there is no guarantee that Timmy will never have another

bowel obstruction. (2) 1—The child with rickets needs extra calcium in the diet. Milk products are high in calcium and fortified with vitamin D. (3) 3—All of these can be seen with pyloric stenosis, but projectile vomiting is the highest priority because of the risk of dehydration and aspiration. (4) Hard objects—Following surgery for cleft palate, placing any hard object into the mouth could traumatize the incision and must be avoided. (5) 4—In this disease, the colon has a segment with limited nerve supply preventing movement. The other choices are not accurate. (6) 2—By positioning the infant upright after eating, gravity will help keep gastric contents from entering the esophagus. (7) 3—Passage of brown stool is common in the early stage of intussusception. The child will still need the barium enema for accurate diagnosis. (8) 2—Infants need a nurturing family that can independently provide care. The baby should gain weight while hospitalized. Developmental milestones will take time to change. (9) 1—Knowing what was taken and what treatment was provided is important for follow-up medical treatment. It is important to determine drug allergies, but emergency drugs rarely cause allergy, so this is not the highest priority. (10) 2—The nurse must assess before calling the doctor or parents. Giving a laxative or applying heat are contraindicated if appendicitis is the cause of the pain.

CARE PLAN HINTS

1. Although some pain medication can cause drowsiness and upset the stomach when taken without food, John will take formula better when there is less discomfort. It is important to observe John's reaction to medication and to adjust feeding and medication schedules as needed.

2. John can be fed with a cup. Place a small amount of formula (or breast milk) in a paper cup. Tip the cup slowly to encourage him to drink a little at a time.

3. He will have six to eight wet diapers a day. His mucous membranes will be moist. His anterior fontanel will be flat. His weight will be within normal limits.

CRITICAL THINKING CARE MAP

Subjective Data   Mother reports no fluid or solid intake in the past 48 hours. Mother reports infant is lethargic.

Objective Data   Current weight: 12 lb; previous weight: 16 lb; mucous membranes pale; vomiting ×6/day; diarrhea ×10/day; hyperactive bowels sounds in all four quadrants.

Report   Yes, to the pediatrician.

Interventions   Obtain a thorough nutrition history. Assess for possible causes of vomiting and diarrhea. Assess for signs and symptoms of dehydration. Develop a plan with the parents for nutritional and fluid replacement. Administer antiemetics as ordered. Monitor lab values carefully. Weigh daily.

Documentation   (date) 09:00 Mother of 7-month-old male infant calls the office to report vomiting and diarrhea of her child ×2 days. She states he has not had any fluid and is lethargic. Appointment made for 10:00. Report given to Dr. Smithson. K. Young, LPN

Chapter 23

NCLEX-PN® ANSWERS

(1) 3—Urine will be blood tinged following surgical repair of epispadias. The other responses are not appropriate responses. (2) 4—Infants with hypospadias are not circumcised right away to preserve the foreskin to use for surgical repair. The other responses are not correct for this condition. (3) 1—Symptoms of UTI are fever, nausea and vomiting, anorexia, strong-smelling urine, abdominal pain, dysuria, and hematuria. The other responses are not correct. (4) 3—Organisms related to the diagnosis of glomerulonephritis are group A beta-hemolytic *Streptococcus, Staphylococcus, Pneumococcus,* and coxsackievirus. (5) 4—Uremic syndrome occurs in end-stage renal disease, in which all body systems become affected when waste is not eliminated. The other responses do not have these symptoms. (6) 4—Due to the highly metastatic nature of Wilms' tumors, the abdomen should not be palpated in a client with this condition. (7) 3—The bladder is exposed to the outside in bladder exstrophy. The highest *priority* diagnosis with this condition is impaired tissue integrity, which is related to the exposed bladder tissue. The other responses are considered in this condition, but response 3 is the priority among those listed. (8) 3—Bladder exstrophy is a condition in which the bladder extrudes to the outside of the abdomen through a lower abdominal wall defect. (9) 1, 2, 3, 5, 6—All of the above, except answer 4, uremic frost, can be found on assessment of nephrotic syndrome. (10) 1, 2, 3, 4—All of the responses, except avoiding the use of disposable diapers, are appropriate for the child with a diagnosis of UTI.

CARE PLAN HINTS

1. Fluid-filled edematous tissue is at greater risk for impaired skin integrity. Turning James will reduce pressure on the tissue and prevent dependent edema.

2. An objective measurement of urine output is necessary to document a balance or imbalance of intake and output. When a child is unable to urinate in a measured container, the nurse may record weights of the diaper to document output.

3. The nurse should carefully assess whether the family understands James' medical condition and treatment. Their physical comfort during hospitalization is important. The nurse should also provide them an opportunity to express fears and concerns about James' condition.

CRITICAL THINKING CARE MAP

Subjective Data   Mother states, Casey has had sex and that's why she has these symptoms. Client states, I have not ever had sex with anyone.

Objective Data   Intact hymen; Mrs. Freidman is waving arms and pacing in examination room.

Report   Yes, the data gathered need to be reported to the supervising nurse. The mother's misunderstanding could result in ineffective treatment for her daughter's vaginitis, and it could damage their interpersonal relationship.

Interventions   Assess Mrs. Freidman's knowledge level regarding vaginitis. Explain the physiology and causes of vaginitis. Describe the signs and symptoms of vaginitis. Explain medical treatment of vaginitis. Describe methods of preventing vaginitis. Present teaching in a nonjudgmental manner.

Documentation   (date/time) 14-year-old female accompanied by mother to clinic with report of vulvar pain, edema, and pruritus. Mother states, "I'm sure she had sex. What am I going to do about that?" Client denies sexual intercourse. Procedure for pelvic examination described to client, who voiced understanding. Dr. Lewis assisted with pelvic examination and vaginal specimen obtained. Specimen sent to lab. H. Gregg, LVN

Chapter 24

NCLEX-PN® ANSWERS

(1) 1, 3, 5—The following instructions should be given: Swab oral mucosa with oral nystatin, disinfect all toys, and report rash in the diaper area. Bottle nipples should be cleaned in boiling water for 20 minutes. (2) 1—Lymphangitis indicates the infection is spreading and could lead to septicemia. (3) 2—Port-wine stains do not blanch. (4) Humid—The temperature should be kept cool with constant humidity levels. Helps prevent dry skin. (5) 1—Family history of asthma has been linked to children with eczema. (6) 2—Yellow, scaly patches on scalp and forehead are indicative of seborrheic dermatitis. (7) 3—Treatments may be needed for 3 months to see improvement. Sunscreen is necessary because some medications may cause skin sensitivity. (8) 4—Crust should be washed and removed several times a day. (9) 2, 4, 5—Prevention methods for melanoma include applying sunscreen of SPF 15 or greater, reporting moles that are black with irregular borders, and wearing long-sleeve cotton clothing when outside. (10) 1—Shower shoes should be worn at all times in public showers and locker rooms.

CARE PLAN HINTS

1. The wound has become infected and is spreading. Cellulitis is bacterial infection of the dermis and subcutaneous tissue. Cellulitis could lead to septicemia.

2. The nurse may respond by saying, "Lucy, the medication in your IV is stronger and will help fight the infection in your leg to keep it from spreading."

3. The nurse could respond by saying, "Lucy will be more comfortable if she rests her leg and elevates it on some pillows. You could apply warm compresses to her leg to increase circulation and promote healing. Lucy might also enjoy having a friend over to watch TV because cellulitis is not contagious."

CRITICAL THINKING CARE MAP

Subjective Data   Mother states they have had a lot of fish over the last week. Stopped attending youth group with friends. Mother states child is now wearing a small amount of makeup. Child reports her skin itches, and the sores leak fluid more during the winter. Child states she likes milk and cookies. Mother states the child does not shower after swimming.

Objective Data   Lesions on neck dry and scaly; ruptured papules with yellow crust behind knees.

Report   Yes, to the pediatrician.

Interventions   Apply wet compresses to lesions that are crusted. Hydrate skin with lotions and creams. Encourage showering after swimming. Administer oral antihistamines. Obtain a thorough nutrition history. Keep environmental temperatures cool. Instruct to keep fingernails short. Encourage child to wear loose-fitting clothing.

Documentation   (date) 13:30 Mother of 12-year-old female calls the pediatrician's office reporting skin on neck and behind knees is red and has crusted open lesions that itch $\times 3$ days. She states she is unable to rest and is scratching the areas constantly. Appointment made for 16:00. Report given to Dr. Peterson. S. Vargus, LPN

Chapter 25

NCLEX-PN® ANSWERS

(1) 2—When children are more active, they need more calories to supply the needed energy. Lack of calories will result in hypoglycemia. It is easier to maintain the blood glucose level with dietary changes than to alter the insulin dose. (2) 3—The adolescent is developing a sense of body image, the ability to think abstractly, and develop an image of self. Allowing and encouraging the adolescent to make decisions about the management of his or her diabetes fosters healthy development. (3) 4—Ketoacidosis is a life-threatening complication that should not occur when diabetes is diagnosed and brought under control in a timely manner. Because it is a life-threatening complication, diabetic ketoacidosis must be treated in the hospital. (4) 1—The insulin must be given at the time ordered. If the client is unable to

give the injection, the nurse must administer the drug, and allow her to practice injecting an orange or mannequin and try again the next time. (5) 1—Corticosteroids cause weight gain, delayed growth, delayed puberty, fat deposits, and moon face. (6) 3, 2, 5, 4, 1—Symptoms indicate hyperglycemia. However, the first step is always assessment. Therefore, the blood glucose level must be obtained in order to know how much insulin to give. Because the client has increased urine output, there will be a need for increased fluid intake. Assessing the intake and output record is needed before the intervention of increasing fluid intake is begun. The primary care provider needs to be made aware of the change in the client's condition. (7) 3— The age at which puberty begins is often similar to their parents. This question is necessary to assess familial traits. (8) Hypocalcemia—When the thyroid is removed, the parathyroid glands can inadvertently be removed or traumatized. Because the parathyroid glands work with the thyroid to regulate blood calcium, removal or trauma can result in hypocalcemia. (9) 1—Diabetes insipidus should be suspected when the child's specific gravity is below 1.005. This value should be reported because further testing is needed. (10) 4—Oral hypoglycemic medication does not replace insulin. If type II diabetes mellitus is not controlled with oral medication, insulin may be necessary.

CARE PLAN HINTS

1. The nurse can teach about a well-balanced diet that is high in calcium. Calcium will be needed for bone growth. Also, active exercise daily will promote bone growth.
2. Yes, because she has grown since birth, she would be expected to continue to grow at a rate slower than normal.
3. Allow her to make some choices and have some control. Suggest she choose the injection site. Place a Band-Aid of her choice on the site. Have her give a "shot" to her doll.

CRITICAL THINKING CARE MAP

Subjective Data   Hungry; irritable.

Objective Data   Sweating; tremors; pulse 102.

Report   Yes, to the health care provider.

Interventions   Give orange juice with one packet of sugar added. *Orange is high in sugar, adding more simple sugar will elevate the child's blood glucose (BG) within minutes. If BG can be elevated with fluids, it is better than starting an IV. If client is unable to take oral liquids, an IV would be necessary.* Monitor blood glucose every 1 hour. *Frequent monitoring of BG is necessary to evaluate effectiveness of treatment. BG should return to normal within 30 minutes. If condition worsens, more frequent monitoring and additional treatment will be necessary.* Obtain a thorough nutrition history. *This is necessary to determine cause of this episode of hypoglycemia and to determine knowledge deficit.* Review

causes, signs, and treatment of hypoglycemia. *Because client is a newly diagnosed diabetic, a review of content is necessary to ensure understanding of the disorder, the signs of complications, and what the client can do to prevent or alleviate the problem.*

Documentation   (date/time) 11-year-old admitted with irritability and hunger. VS: T 98, P 102, R 24, BP 102/66. Skin pale and diaphoretic. States he became weak and sweaty during soccer practice. States he did not have a snack before practice. BG 48 mg/dL. 240 mL orange juice with one packet of sugar given. Dietary intake included breakfast of eggs, toast, and banana; lunch of sandwich meat and lettuce salad. Signs, causes, and treatment of hypoglycemia reviewed. Report given to D. Wildman, CNP. A. Allen, LPN

Chapter 26

NCLEX-PN® ANSWERS

(1) 1—Passive immunity offers short-term protection from some organisms and is passed from the mother to the infant through the placenta. The other options are correct statements. (2) 1—By age 1, children have adult levels of immunoglobulin M antibodies. The other options are not correct. (3) 2—Infants who were exposed to the varicella virus during pregnancy may be born with congenital varicella syndrome. This syndrome is characterized by IUGR, skin scarring, limb hypoplasia (underdevelopment), eye defects, brain defects, and death. The other options are incorrect for this condition. (4) 4—An approved ice pack (not ice directly on the child's skin) should be applied to an injection site for relief of redness and swelling. The other options are not correct. (5) 3—The MMR vaccine contains very small amounts of neomycin, and anyone with a documented allergy to neomycin should not be given the MMR vaccine. The other options are not correct. (6) 3—The cause of roseola is unknown, but contact with respiratory secretions is suspected. The other options are incorrect. (7) 4—The parents need to know that they are to notify the physician if abdominal pain, left upper quadrant pain, or left shoulder pain occurs because this may indicate impending or complete splenic rupture. (8) 4—The avian flu, also called the bird flu or H5N1, is caused by influenza viruses that occur naturally among wild birds. H5N1 is deadly to domestic birds. It can be transmitted from birds to humans. Currently, there is no human immunity and no vaccine available. (9) 1, 2, 3, 4—Transmission-based precautions include standard precautions plus airborne precautions, droplet precautions, or contact precautions. (10) 1, 2, 3, 5, 6—It is advisable for health care workers to have the HBV vaccine series, but it is not part of standard precautions.

CARE PLAN HINTS

1. Aunt Betty should be informed about the routes of transmission of chickenpox and the period of communicability. She should understand that in order to prevent infection, she must not come in contact with Molly until her most recent outbreak of lesions have begun to crust over. Aunt Betty should also understand that the risks associated with transmission to the fetus in the first 20 weeks of pregnancy include intrauterine growth retardation (IUGR), skin scarring, limb hypoplasia (underdevelopment), eye defects, brain defects, and death.

2. The nurse must initially recognize this parental behavior as dangerous to the child. The child would be incapable of getting out of bed to go to the bathroom or to escape in case of fire. This is considered child abuse. The nurse must report this parental action to the supervising nurse or physician who will then report this act of child abuse to the proper state officials.

3. Chickenpox lesions that become infected develop tenderness, erythema, and purulent drainage. Cellulitis has a sudden onset. Symptoms include edema and erythema of the area. It is warm to the touch. The child may also have a fever, chills, and malaise.

CRITICAL THINKING CARE MAP

Subjective Data   Screaming loudly; crying inconsolably.

Objective Data   Clutches stuffed toy frog while sobbing loudly; clenched fists; tightened jaw; immediately hides head in mother's lap when nurse with mask approaches.

Report   Yes, to the supervising nurse.

Interventions   Stand further than 3 ft away from Wendy, remove the mask, and greet Wendy pleasantly each time the nurse enters the room. Replace mask. Repeat several times prior to moving closer to the child. Provide Wendy with a surgical mask to try on. Provide Wendy with a mask to put on her frog. Avoid approaching Wendy or touching her unless she is being held by her adoptive mother or father. Provide Wendy with age-appropriate diversional activities such as blocks.

Documentation   (date/time) 2-year-old female, recently adopted from Russia, diagnosed with diphtheria. Placed in private room, on droplet precautions. Adoptive mother and father at bedside. Immediate reaction to masked nurse entering the room witnessed. Screaming loudly. Crying inconsolably. Fists clenched and jaw tightened. Reported behaviors to supervising nurse. Developed plan of care to relieve fear. S. Shipman, LVN

Chapter 27

NCLEX-PN® ANSWERS

(1) 2—Autism is marked in the child by the presence of repetitive behaviors such as hand movements or rocking.

The other choices are not clinical manifestations of autism. (2) 1—There is no cure for autism, but with intensive interventions prior to age 5, behavior modification may be possible. (3) 3—Newborns with FAS have three types of characteristics: growth retardation, CNS abnormalities, and craniofacial abnormalities. The other choices are not linked to FAS. (4) 4—Symptoms of substance abuse vary, depending on the specific substance(s) being abused. Physical symptoms might include dilated or pinpoint pupils, bloodshot eyes, bruising or needle marks, runny nose, and shaking hands. As a rule, psoriasis is not a symptom of drug/substance abuse. (5) 3—Common side effects of Adderall are irritability, euphoria, palpitations, insomnia, and restlessness. The other options are incorrect responses for this situation. (6) 2—Sexual abuse in children can be characterized by physical symptoms, mood changes, cognitive impairment, sexual symptoms, and lack of coping skills. Physical symptoms include a vaginal discharge, possibly with a strong odor; vaginal or anal bleeding or bruising (underpants or diaper may be blood stained); genital irritation such as redness, pain, itching, or burning; recurrent urinary tract infections; sexually transmitted infections and a positive pregnancy test, particularly at a young age; enuresis; and encopresis. (7) 4— Bulimia is characterized by binge eating and purging. With anorexia nervosa, the adolescent may not only decrease the caloric intake, but also indulge in strenuous exercise programs in order to lose weight. Often, because of malnutrition, the client's fluid and electrolyte levels are unbalanced, which can lead to life-threatening arrhythmias. (8) 2—The teen should not be left alone and should be referred immediately to a qualified professional. Using therapeutic communication skills, the nurse should question the teen about depression and thoughts of suicide. If the teen admits suicidal thoughts, the plan for suicide should be explored, including method and opportunity. The more lethal the method and the more realistic the opportunity, the higher the probability the teen will attempt suicide. (9) 1, 2, 4, 5, 6—No weight criterion has been set for bariatric surgery, but the client must be severely obese (plus frame and height are also taken into consideration). (10) 1, 2, 4, 5—One-third of infants with shaken-baby syndrome die from their injuries.

CARE PLAN HINTS

1. The media, including printed advertisements and television, present thinness as the most desirable body type. Clothing is displayed on thin models. Makeover programs include body restructuring to a state of thinness. The diet industry is one of the most lucrative in the United States. These aspects give the impression that body types other than thin are less than desirable.

2. The family must provide consistent, sometimes firm, support. They need to consider themselves part of both the problem and the solution. Family counseling is suggested.
3. Meghan's friends may contribute to the problem if they, too, are focused on staying thin. Including them in counseling, discussing the hazards of extreme weight loss, and encouraging them to develop healthy nutritional habits could assist Meghan in her recovery.

CRITICAL THINKING CARE MAP

Subjective Data Mother's report of lack of peer interaction; teacher's report of lack of peer interaction; Jackson states that he has no friends, "The boys in my class run away when I come close to them."

Objective Data Jackson plays alone on the monkey bars on the playground. When buddies are picked for a class activity, Jackson is not picked. Jackson is observed attempting to talk to a group of boys in the lunchroom without success.

Report Yes, difficulties in social interactions can lead to social isolation if not managed properly. The supervising nurse would receive this report.

Nursing Interventions Involve Jackson's parents and his teacher in developing a plan to improve social interactions between Jackson and his peers. Use role-play. Plan an opportunity to observe Jackson during school hours. Assist Jackson in developing social skills such as appropriate verbal and nonverbal communication, respect for other's privacy, and interpreting reactions from peers honestly. Develop a plan for positive feedback that rewards Jackson for appropriate social interaction. Help Jackson's mother develop a plan for additional opportunities to interact socially with other children, such as sporting or scouting activities.

Documentation (date 1) 15:00 6-year-old male and mother in for follow-up visit after initial ADHD evaluation (date 2). Discussed adaptation to medication and resolution of previous problems identified. Mother states that child is not interacting socially with peers at school, and this is concerning to her. Report given to supervising nurse, and plan of care developed to assist child in improving social interaction. Follow-up visit scheduled in 4 weeks. O. Ames, LPN

Chapter 28

NCLEX-PN® ANSWERS

(1) 2—The sudden death of a child leaves many unresolved issues for the parents. Among these, parents are likely to feel guilty about things they have not done. (2) 3—When a child asks questions, it is important to determine whether the family has provided answers. The child's questions cue the nurse to ask the family what has been discussed with the dying child. The family may need suggestions from the nurse about how to discuss death. (3) 1—The nurse needs to assess the client's emotional status regarding death. This answer fosters therapeutic communication. The other responses block communication. (4) 3—Grief promotes a return to healthy mental functioning. Unresolved grief can lead to severe depression. The nurse can encourage activities that will foster healthy grieving. (5) 4—Because the amputation has not yet occurred, the client's reactions are due to anticipating the loss. Once the amputation occurs, she will again progress through the stages of grief. (6) 2—Prior to the school-age years, death is seen as temporary. The school-age child develops a concept that death is permanent through talking with friends, parents, and relatives, and by having pets die. (7) 2—The purpose of a living will is to allow the individual to express his or her desires regarding terminal care at a time when he or she is mentally clear and able to communicate. At 17, this client is encouraged to help family prepare for his death. (8) 1, 2, 5, 6—The client loses awareness of surrounding. The blood pressure will go down instead of up. The other choices occur during the death process. (9) 2—Fosters therapeutic communication, shows empathy, and supports the grieving parents. The other choices are cold and block communication. (10) 5, 4, 2, 1, 3— Once death has occurred, the parents become the focus of nursing care. Holding them and allowing them to cry provides needed emotional support. The nursing supervisor and physician should be notified as soon as parents are in control. The child's body will need to be prepared for viewing by cleansing the face, combing the hair, removing tubes if policy allows, and padding the perineum. The mortician should be notified when the family is ready for the body to be removed. All charting must be completed before the body is removed.

CARE PLAN HINTS

1. Timmy should be medicated for pain even if his respirations slow. Although prescribed medication may continue to slow his respirations and speed up the dying process, maintaining therapeutic blood levels of pain medication is important to provide comfort and alleviate suffering.
2. "I don't know. I know this is very difficult. Can you share with me how you are feeling?"
3. Timmy's grandmother should be encouraged to share her feelings about the loss of her grandson and the pain her daughter is experiencing.

CRITICAL THINKING CARE MAP

Subjective Data States she will be relieved when Teresa is gone; asking every 10 minutes how much longer?

Objective Data Crying quietly; identifies signs of impending death.

Reported No, they are signs of healthy grieving.

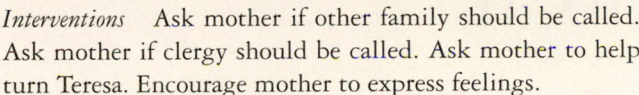

Interventions Ask mother if other family should be called. Ask mother if clergy should be called. Ask mother to help turn Teresa. Encourage mother to express feelings.

Documentation (date/time) Unresponsive to verbal or tactile stimuli. Resp. irregular. Legs mottling. Mother at beside, crying quietly. Mother identifies signs of impending death, and questions how much longer? Mother states she will be glad when this is over. Offered to call family and clergy. Mother encouraged to express feelings. Mother assisted with morning care. K. Shewmaker, LPN

UNIT III Thinking Strategically About …

CASE 1 SCENARIO

CRITICAL THINKING

1. The physician orders a fasting blood sugar. The parents and child are taught that the child must remain NPO for 12 hours before the test, except for water.
2. To minimize the pain of the injections, warm the insulin to room temperature (once open, it can be stored at room temperature); remove all air bubbles from the syringe prior to injection; allow alcohol to dry completely prior to the injection; assist the child in learning how to relax the muscle group to be used for the injection; praise him for his participation; observe the needle carefully for burrs; insert the needle swiftly in one motion; and hold the needle steady once it has penetrated the skin.

COLLABORATIVE CARE

1. The nutritionist will need Jeremy's complete health history, including all labs. To provide Jeremy and his family with an appropriate diet plan, the nutritionist will need to know Jeremy's height and weight, his typical diet, his likes and dislikes, what amount of exercise he engages in on a daily basis, and what medication regimen the physician has ordered.
2. The LPN should give Jeremy's mother reading material to reinforce teaching. Support groups can offer opportunities for exchange of information and assistance in problem solving.

CASE 2 SCENARIO

DELEGATING

The following orders could be delegated to the certified nursing assistant: vital signs, daily weight, and assistance with diet.

MANAGEMENT OF CARE

To find the infusion rate for an order D5 ½ NS to infuse at 1,000 mL in 8 hours using a drop factor of 10 drops/mL, convert 8 hours to minutes (480 minutes). Find the total number of drops in 1,000 mL (10,000). Divide the total number of drops by the total number of minutes to find the number of drops per minute.

$$\frac{10,000 \text{ drops/mL}}{480 \text{ minutes}} = 21 \text{ drops/minute}$$

COMMUNICATION AND CLIENT TEACHING

Develop a teaching plan to provide nutritional information. The LPN can teach Jackson's mother to progress the diet slowly. Once vomiting has slowed, small sips of water can be offered to Jackson. Gelatin and clear broth can be added next. Once Jackson can keep these liquids down, his mother can offer him bland carbohydrates such as plain toast, rice, or crackers. Small bites of banana or spoonfuls of applesauce can be offered next.

CASE 3 SCENARIO

TIME MANAGEMENT AND PRIORITIES IN NURSING CARE

Nursing interventions should be implemented for Janice in the following order: Assess carefully for symptoms of shock to include decreased blood pressure; rapid, thready pulse; rapid, shallow respirations; cool, pale, moist skin; thirst; restlessness; and changes in level of consciousness. Keep Janice's trunk and head flat with legs slightly elevated. Keep her warm with blankets. Do not give Janice anything to eat or drink. Provide emotional support.

DOCUMENTING AND REPORTING

All information gathered is important to document. Symptoms of shock must be reported promptly to the physician.

CULTURAL CARE STRATEGIES

Some followers of the Jehovah's Witness religion cannot accept blood or blood products. It is important to discuss the possibility of the need for blood replacement with the physician, nursing supervisor, and Janice's parents. If the parents will not give consent for the replacement, it is important that they understand the consequences if Janice does not receive the blood replacement. Some institutions may pursue a court order to be able to administer the blood without parental consent.

Appendix II

Newborn Rating Scales, Growth Charts, and Immunization Schedules

---

NEWBORN MATURITY RATING & CLASSIFICATION

ESTIMATION OF GESTATIONAL AGE BY MATURITY RATING
Symbols: X - 1st Exam O - 2nd Exam

NEUROMUSCULAR MATURITY

	–1	0	1	2	3	4	5
Posture							
Square Window (wrist)	>90°	90°	60°	45°	30°	0°	
Arm Recoil		180°	140°–180°	110°–140°	90°–110°	<90°	
Popliteal Angle	180°	160°	140°	120°	100°	90°	<90°
Scarf Sign							
Heel to Ear							

Gestation by Dates _____ wks

Birth Date _____ Hour _____ am pm

APGAR _____ 1 min _____ 5 min

MATURITY RATING

score	weeks
–10	20
–5	22
0	24
5	26
10	28
15	30
20	32
25	34
30	36
35	38
40	40
45	42
50	44

PHYSICAL MATURITY

Skin	sticky friable transparent	gelatinous red, translucent	smooth pink, visible veins	superficial peeling &/or rash, few veins	cracking pale areas rare veins	parchment deep cracking no vessels	leathery cracked wrinkled
Lanugo	none	sparse	abundant	thinning	bald areas	mostly bald	
Plantar Surface	heel-toe 40–50 mm:–1 <40 mm:–2	>50 mm no crease	faint red marks	anterior transverse crease only	creases ant. 2/3	creases over entire sole	
Breast	imperceptible	barely perceptible	flat areola no bud	stippled areola 1–2 mm bud	raised areola 3–4 mm bud	full areola 5–10 mm bud	
Eye/Ear	lids fused loosely:–1 tightly:–2	lids open pinna flat stays folded	sl. curved pinna; soft; slow recoil	well curved pinna; soft but ready recoil	formed & firm instant recoil	thick cartilage ear stiff	
Genitals male	scrotum flat, smooth	scrotum empty faint rugae	testes in upper canal rare rugae	testes descending few rugae	testes down good rugae	testes pendulous deep rugae	
Genitals female	clitoris prominent labia flat	prominent clitoris small labia minora	prominent clitoris enlarging minora	majora & minora equally prominent	majora large minora small	majora cover clitoris & minora	

SCORING SECTION

	1st Exam = X	2nd Exam = O
Estimating Gest Age by Maturity Rating	_____Weeks	_____Weeks
Time of Exam	Date _____ Hour _____ am pm	Date _____ Hour _____ am pm
Age at Exam	_____ Hours	_____ Hours
Signature of Examiner	_____ M.D.	_____ M.D.

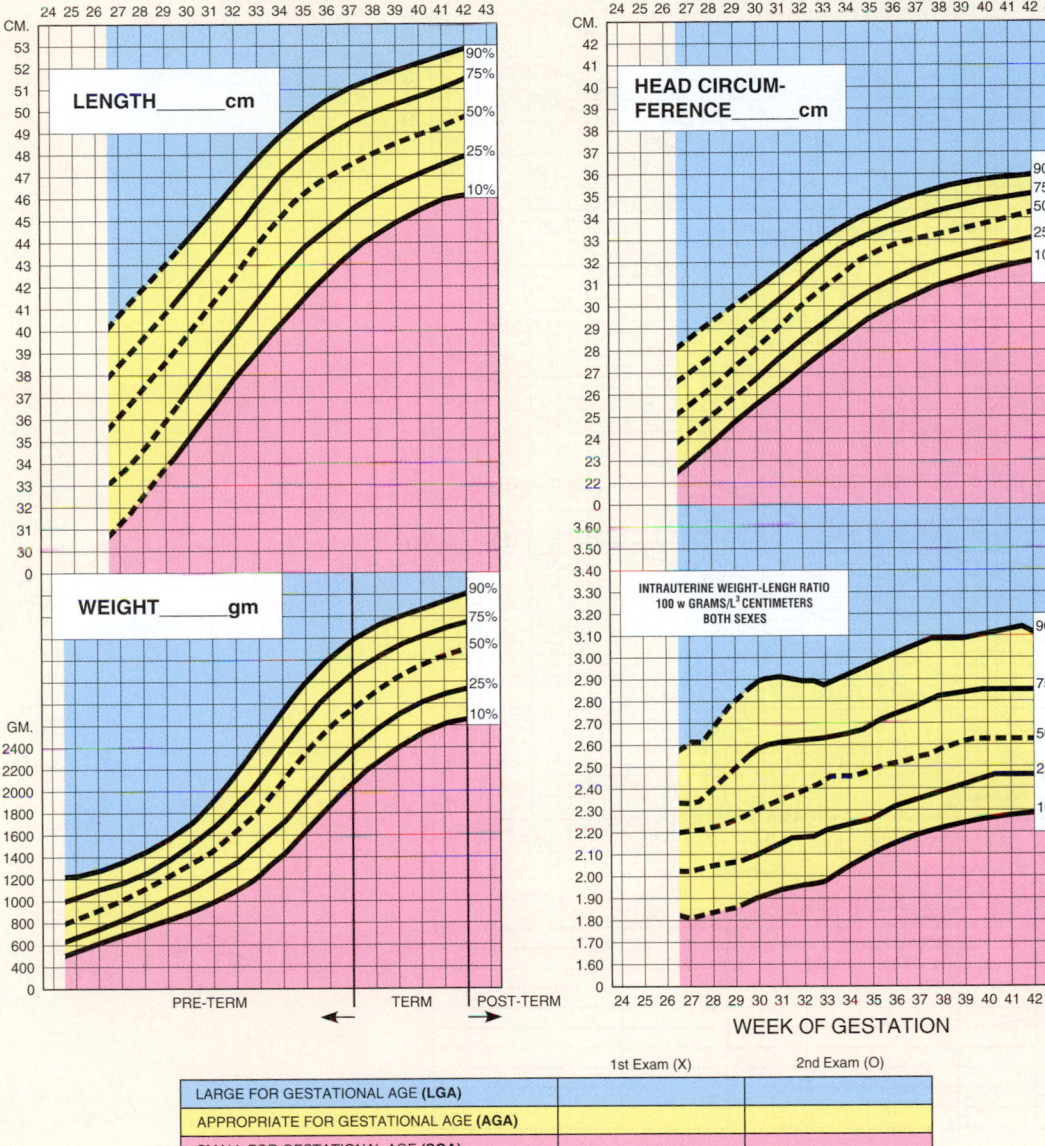

CLASSIFICATION OF NEWBORNS—
BASED ON MATURITY AND INTRAUTERINE GROWTH

Symbols: X-1st Exam O-2nd Exam

WEEK OF GESTATION

LENGTH_____cm

WEIGHT_____gm

PRE-TERM   ←   TERM   POST-TERM   →

WEEK OF GESTATION

HEAD CIRCUM-
FERENCE_____cm

INTRAUTERINE WEIGHT-LENGH RATIO
100 w GRAMS/L³ CENTIMETERS
BOTH SEXES

WEEK OF GESTATION

	1st Exam (X)	2nd Exam (O)
LARGE FOR GESTATIONAL AGE **(LGA)**		
APPROPRIATE FOR GESTATIONAL AGE **(AGA)**		
SMALL FOR GESTATIONAL AGE **(SGA)**		
Age at Exam	hrs	hrs
Signature of Examiner	M.D.	M.D.

Figure A-1. ■ Classification of newborns based on maturity and intrauterine growth. *Sources:* Adapted from Lubchenco, L. O., Hansman, C., & Boyd, E., (1966). Intrauterine growth in length and head circumference as estimated from live births at gestational ages from 26 to 42 weeks. *Pediatrics,* 37, 403–408; Battaglia, F. C., & Lubchenco, L. D. (1967). A practical classification of newborn infants by weight and gestational age. *Journal of Pediatrics,* 71, 159.

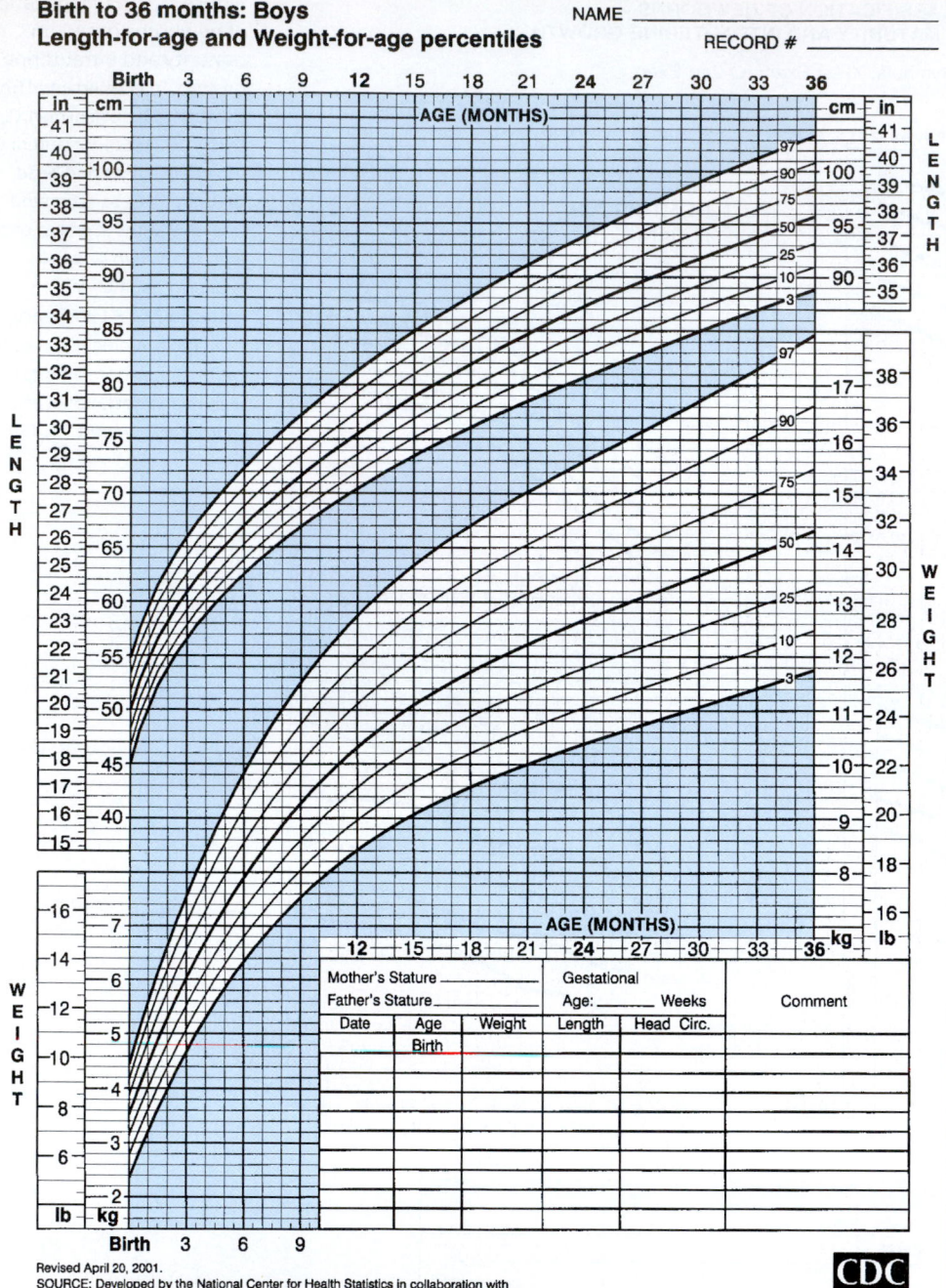

Birth to 36 months: Boys
Length-for-age and Weight-for-age percentiles

NAME _____

RECORD # _____

Revised April 20, 2001.
SOURCE: Developed by the National Center for Health Statistics in collaboration with
the National Center for Chronic Disease Prevention and Health Promotion (2000).
http://www.cdc.gov/growthcharts

CDC

Figure A-2. ■ Physical growth percentiles for length and weight—boys: birth to 36 months. From CDC, 2001. www.cdc.gov/growthcharts

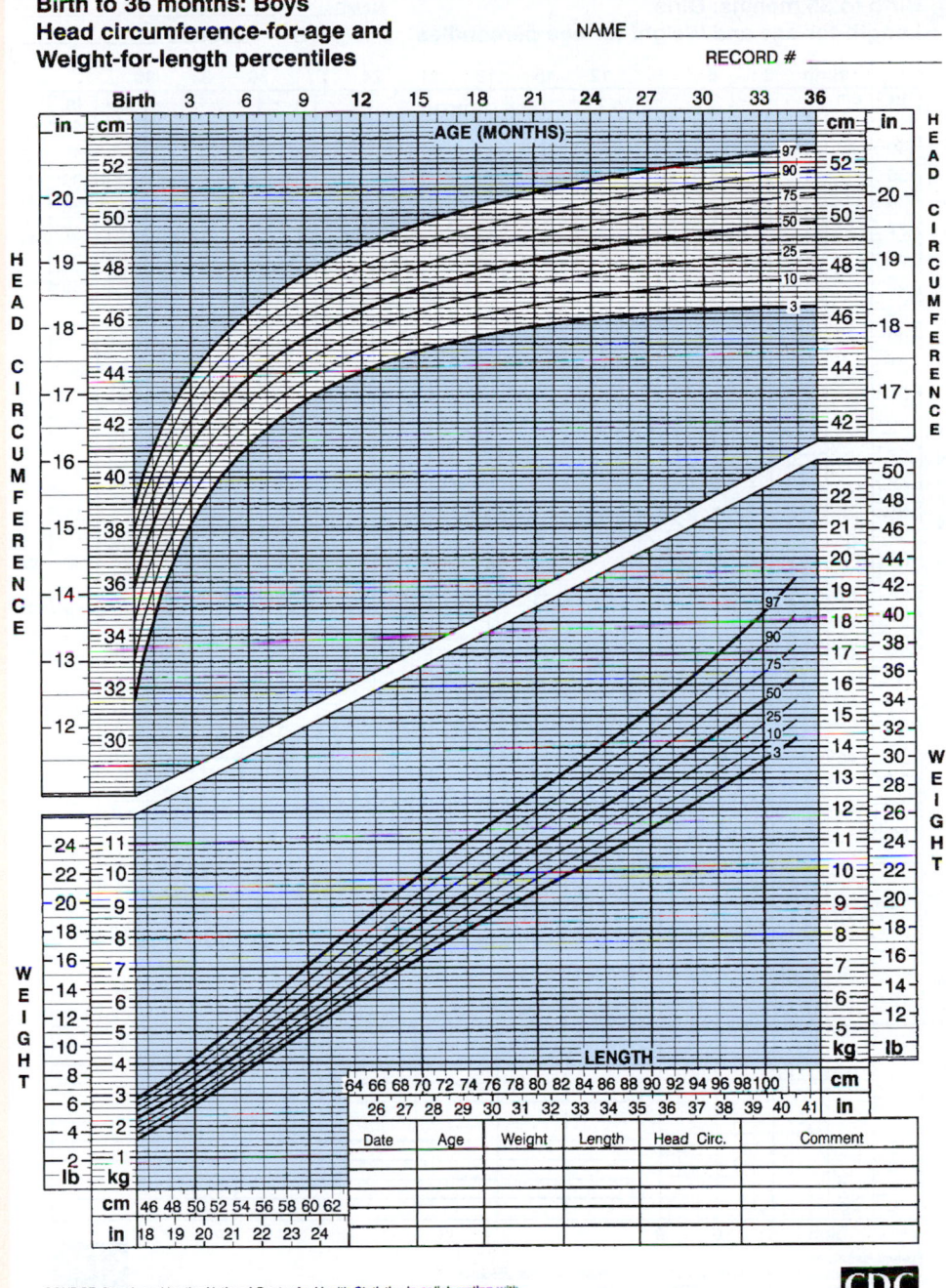

Birth to 36 months: Boys
Head circumference-for-age and
Weight-for-length percentiles

NAME _____

RECORD # _____

SOURCE: Developed by the National Center for Health Statistics in collaboration with the National Center for Chronic Disease Prevention and Health Promotion (2000).
http://www.cdc.gov/growthcharts

Figure A-3. ■ Physical growth percentiles for head circumference, weight for length—boys: birth to 36 months. From CDC, 2001. www.cdc.gov/growthcharts

Figure A-4. ■ Physical growth percentiles for length and weight—girls: birth to 36 months. From CDC, 2001. www.cdc.gov/growthcharts

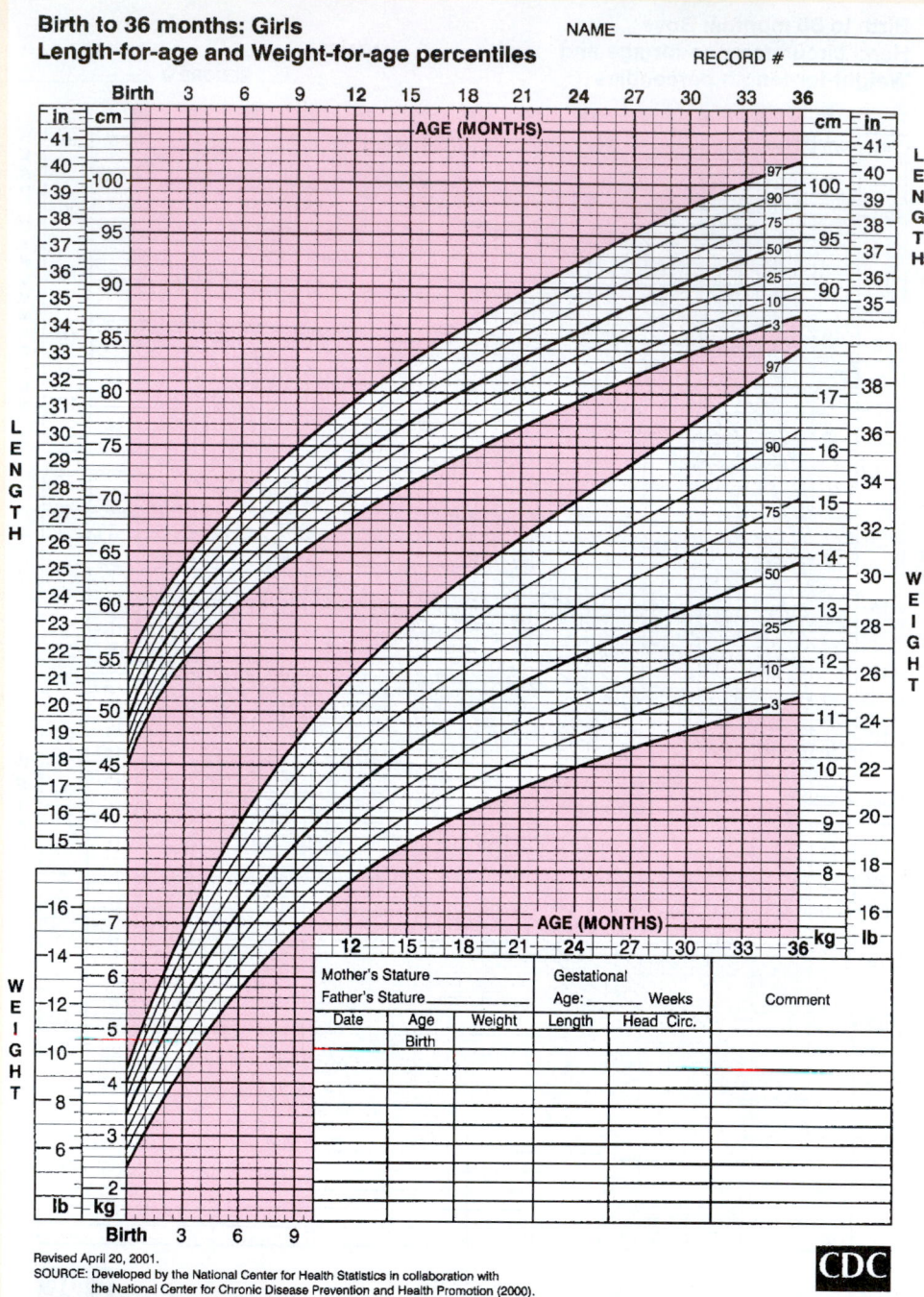

Birth to 36 months: Girls
Length-for-age and Weight-for-age percentiles

NAME _____

RECORD # _____

Mother's Stature _____
Father's Stature _____

Gestational
Age: _____ Weeks

Date	Age	Weight	Length	Head Circ.	Comment
	Birth				

Revised April 20, 2001.
SOURCE: Developed by the National Center for Health Statistics in collaboration with the National Center for Chronic Disease Prevention and Health Promotion (2000).
http://www.cdc.gov/growthcharts

CDC

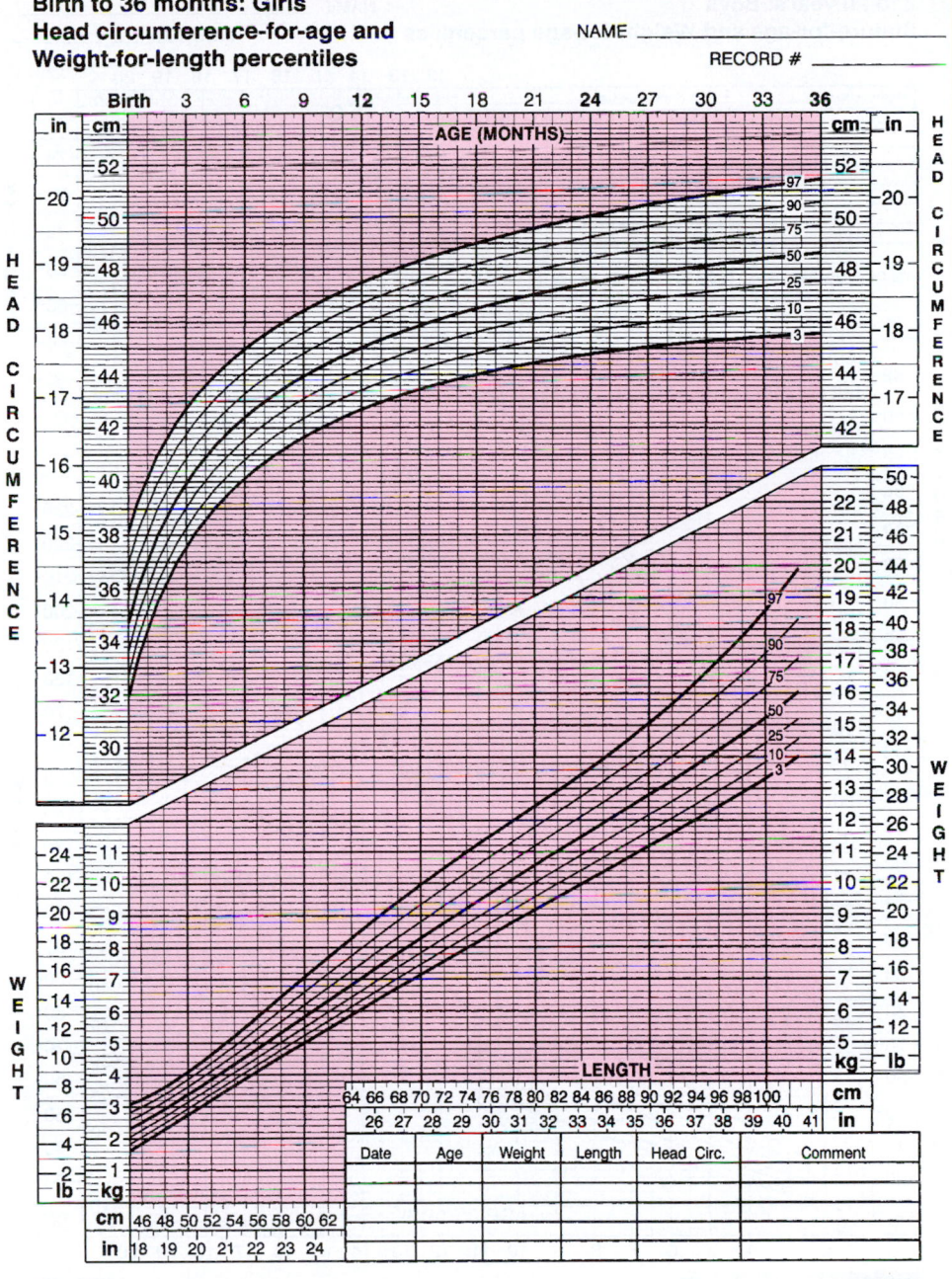

Birth to 36 months: Girls
Head circumference-for-age and
Weight-for-length percentiles

NAME _____

RECORD # _____

Figure A-5. ■ Physical growth percentiles for head circumference, weight for length—girls: birth to 36 months. From CDC, 2001. www.cdc.gov/growthcharts

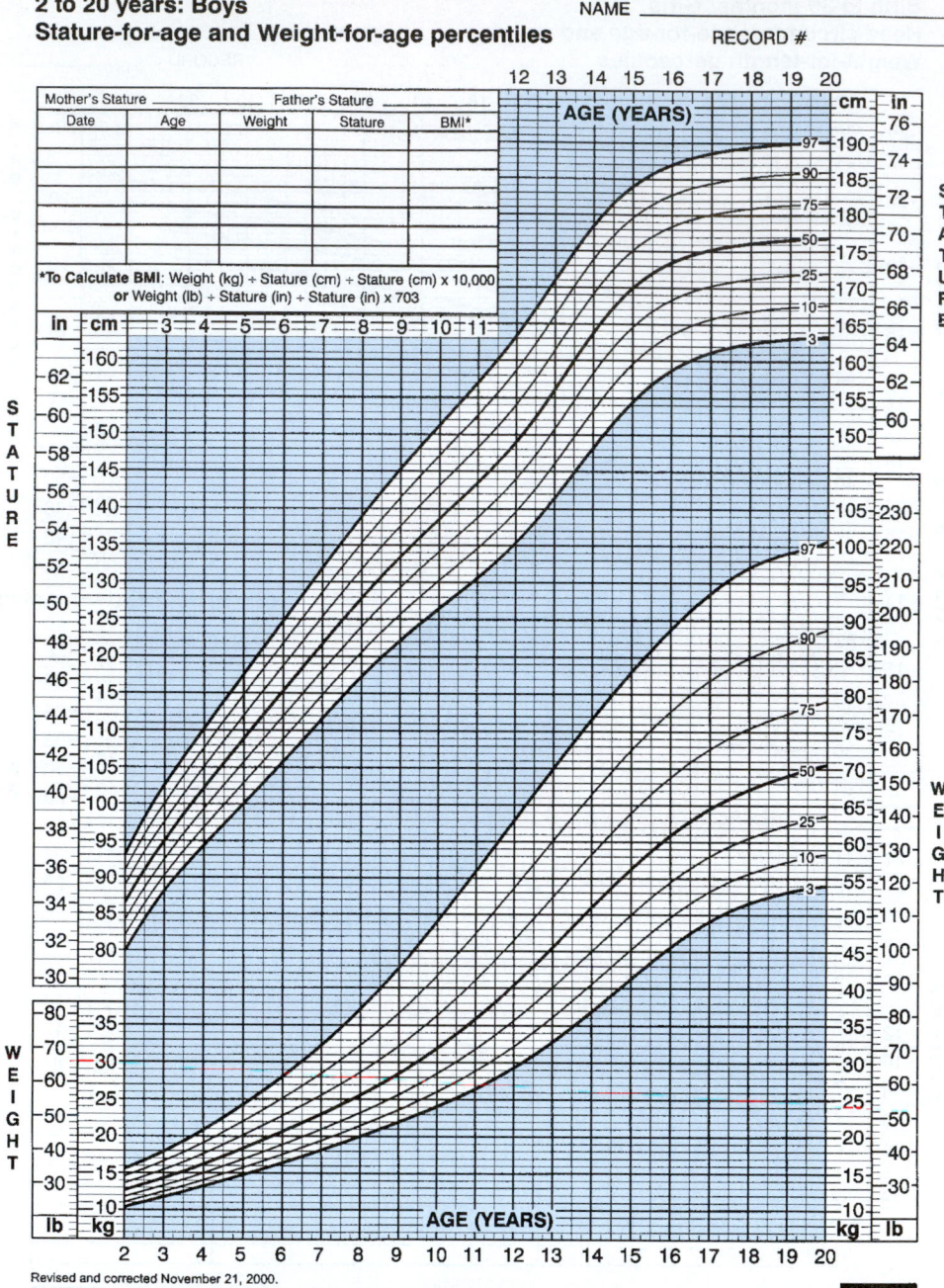

2 to 20 years: Boys
Stature-for-age and Weight-for-age percentiles

NAME _____

RECORD # _____

Revised and corrected November 21, 2000.
SOURCE: Developed by the National Center for Health Statistics in collaboration with
the National Center for Chronic Disease Prevention and Health Promotion (2000).
http://www.cdc.gov/growthcharts

CDC

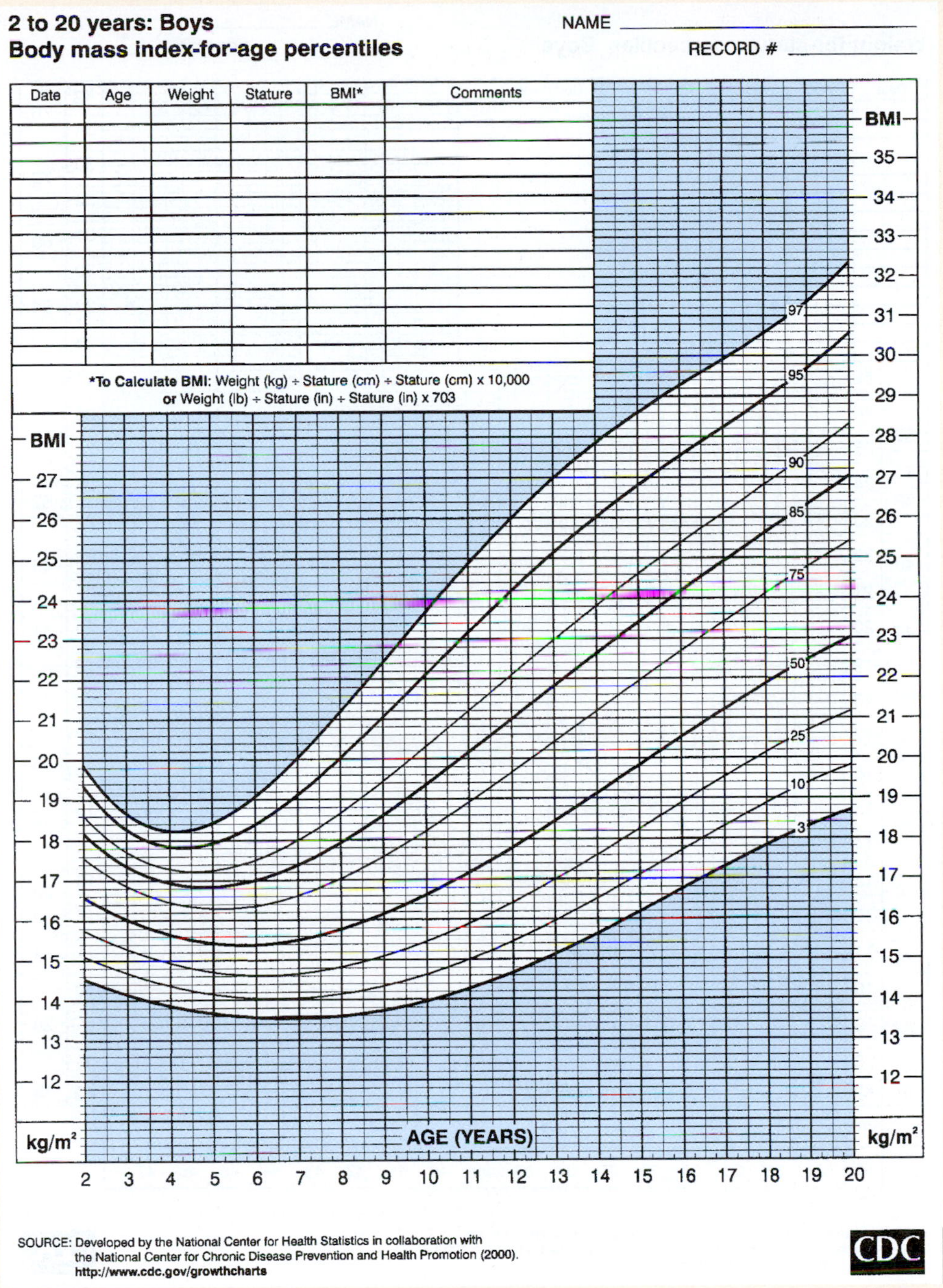

2 to 20 years: Boys
Body mass index-for-age percentiles
NAME
RECORD #
Date
Age
Weight
Stature
BMI*
Comments
*To Calculate BMI: Weight (kg) ÷ Stature (cm) ÷ Stature (cm) x 10,000
or Weight (lb) ÷ Stature (in) ÷ Stature (in) x 703
BMI
35
34
33
32
31
30
29
28
27
26
25
24
23
22
21
20
19
18
17
16
15
14
13
12
97
95
90
85
75
50
25
10
3
kg/m²
AGE (YEARS)
2
3
4
5
6
7
8
9
10
11
12
13
14
15
16
17
18
19
20
SOURCE: Developed by the National Center for Health Statistics in collaboration with
the National Center for Chronic Disease Prevention and Health Promotion (2000).
http://www.cdc.gov/growthcharts
CDC

Figure A-7. ■ Physical growth percentiles for body mass index according to age—boys: 2 to 20 years. From CDC, 2001. www.cdc.gov/growthcharts

Weight-for-stature percentiles: Boys

NAME _____

RECORD # _____

Date	Age	Weight	Stature	Comments

STATURE

SOURCE: Developed by the National Center for Health Statistics in collaboration with the National Center for Chronic Disease Prevention and Health Promotion (2000). http://www.cdc.gov/growthcharts

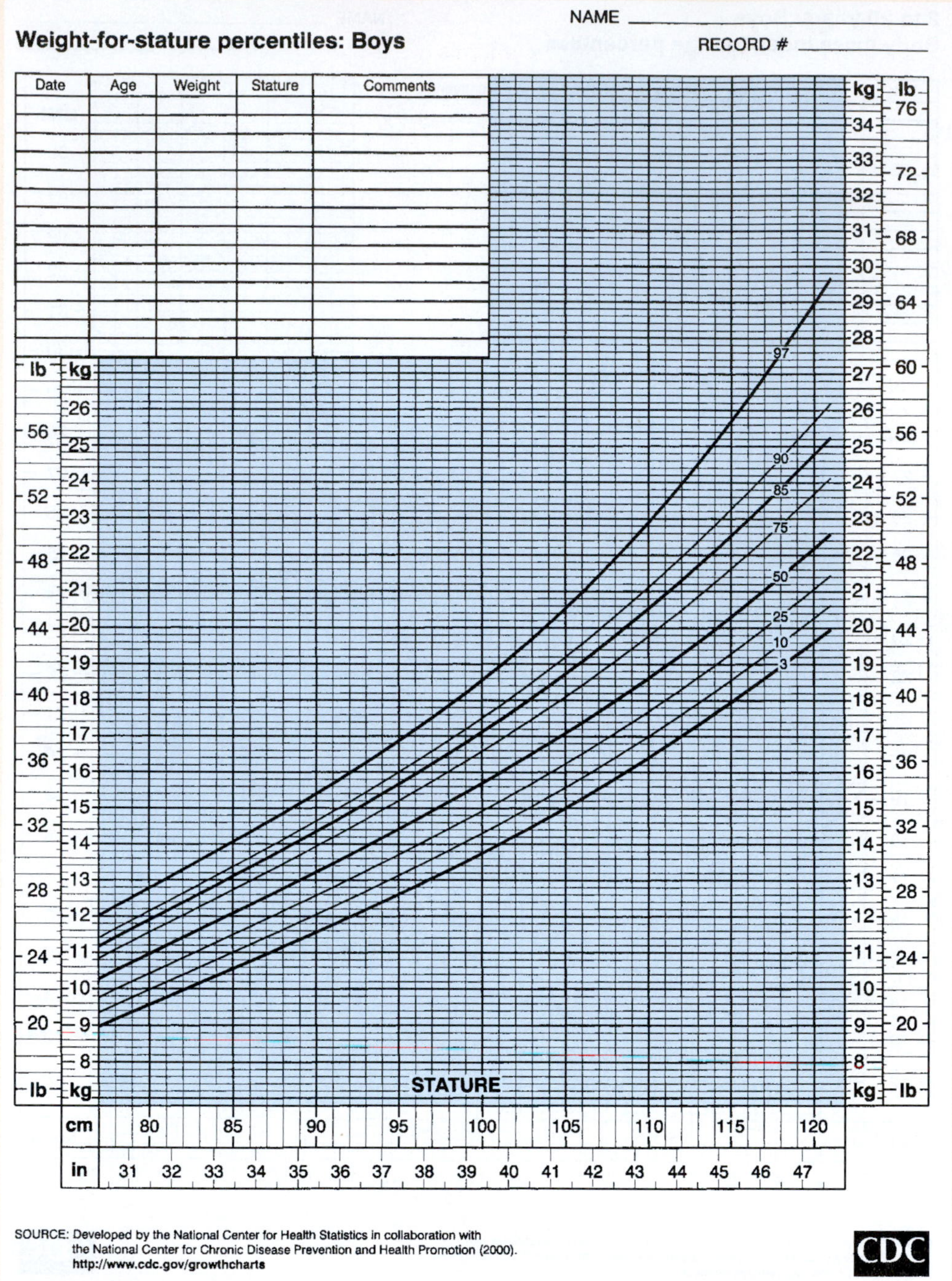

CDC

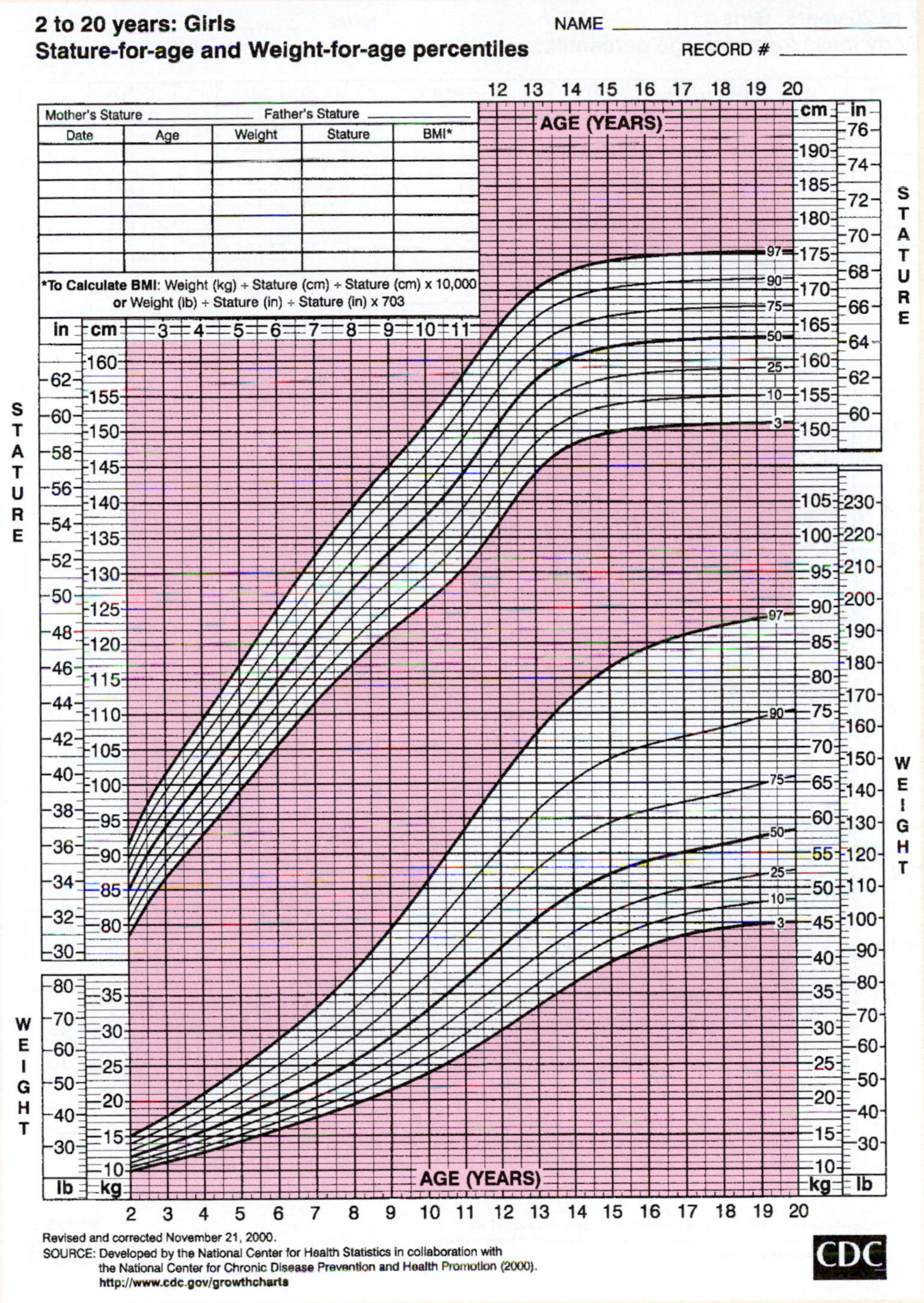

Figure A-9. ■ Physical growth percentiles for stature and weight according to age—girls: 2 to 20 years. From CDC, 2001. www.cdc.gov/growthcharts

Figure A-10. ■ Physical growth percentiles for body mass index according to age—girls: 2 to 20 years. From CDC, 2001. www.cdc.gov/growthcharts

2 to 20 years: Girls
Body mass index-for-age percentiles

NAME _____

RECORD # _____

Date	Age	Weight	Stature	BMI*	Comments

*To Calculate BMI: Weight (kg) ÷ Stature (cm) ÷ Stature (cm) x 10,000
or Weight (lb) ÷ Stature (in) ÷ Stature (in) x 703

BMI — 35
34
33
32
31
30
29
28
27
26
25
24
23
22
21
20
19
18
17
16
15
14
13
12

97
95
90
85
75
50
25
10
3

BMI
27
26
25
24
23
22
21
20
19
18
17
16
15
14
13
12

kg/m² | AGE (YEARS) | kg/m²

2 3 4 5 6 7 8 9 10 11 12 13 14 15 16 17 18 19 20

SOURCE: Developed by the National Center for Health Statistics in collaboration with
the National Center for Chronic Disease Prevention and Health Promotion (2000).
http://www.cdc.gov/growthcharts

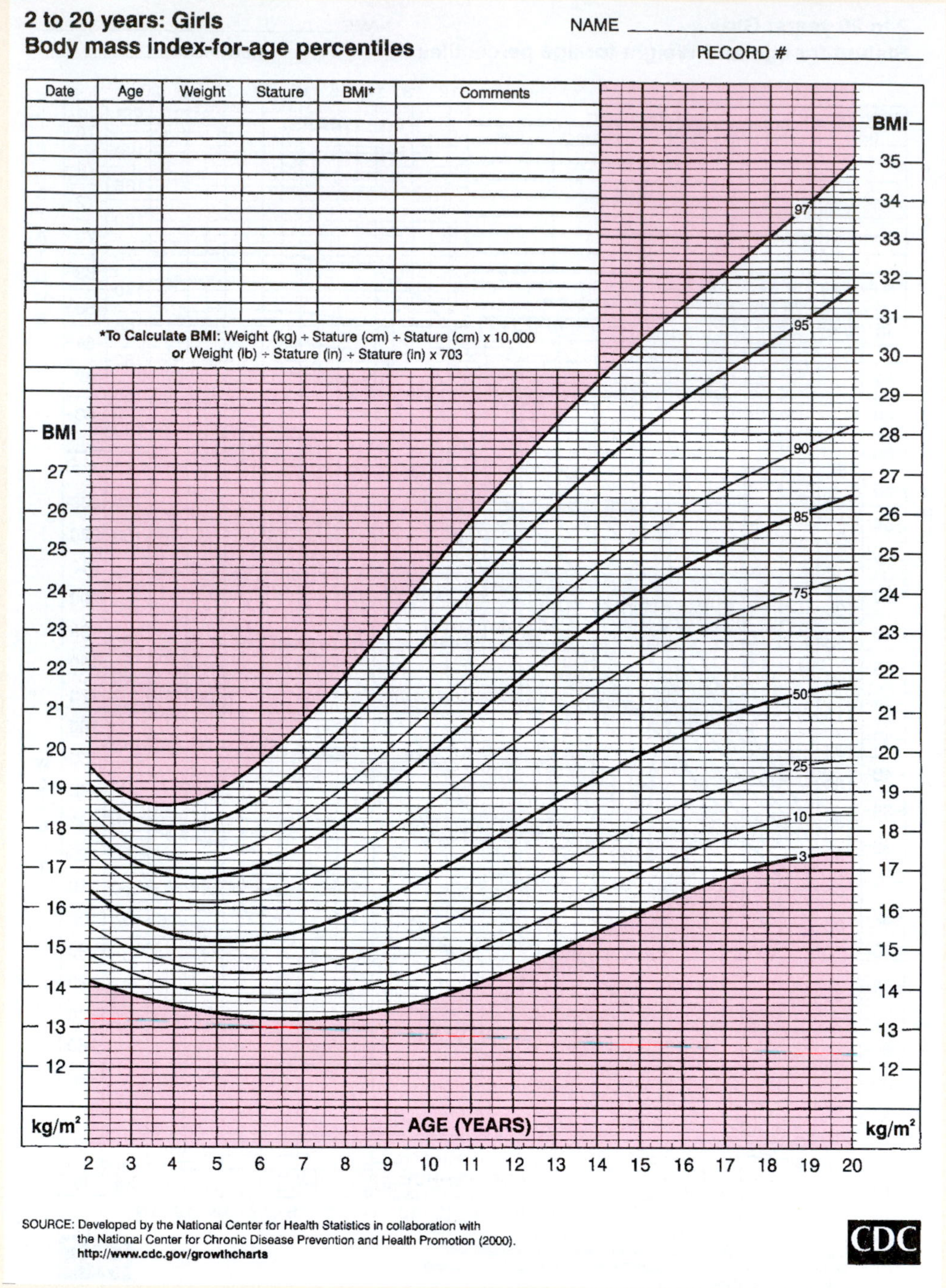

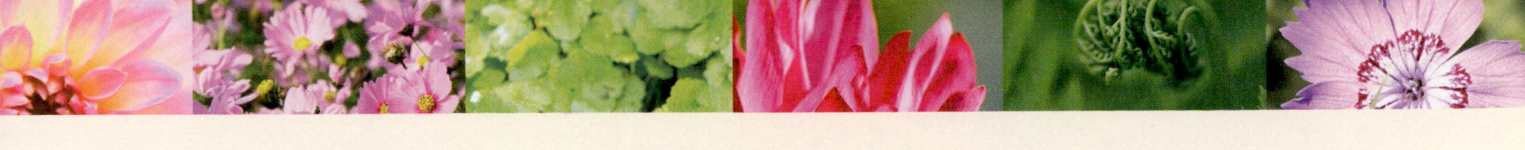

Figure A-11. ■ Physical growth percentiles for weight for stature— girls: 2 to 20 years. From CDC, 2001. www.cdc.gov/growthcharts

Weight-for-stature percentiles: Girls

NAME _____

RECORD # _____

Date	Age	Weight	Stature	Comments

97

90

85

75

50

25

10

3

lb — kg

56 — 26

25

52 — 24

23

48 — 22

21

44 — 20

19

40 — 18

17

36 — 16

15

32 — 14

13

28 — 12

24 — 11

10

20 — 9

8

lb — kg

kg — lb

34 — 76

33 — 72

32

31 — 68

30

29 — 64

28

27 — 60

26 — 56

25

24 — 52

23

22 — 48

21

20 — 44

19

18 — 40

17

16 — 36

15

14 — 32

13 — 28

12

11 — 24

10

9 — 20

8

kg — lb

STATURE

cm	80	85	90	95	100	105	110	115	120

| in | 31 | 32 | 33 | 34 | 35 | 36 | 37 | 38 | 39 | 40 | 41 | 42 | 43 | 44 | 45 | 46 | 47 |

SOURCE: Developed by the National Center for Health Statistics in collaboration with the National Center for Chronic Disease Prevention and Health Promotion (2000).
http://www.cdc.gov/growthcharts

CDC

DEPARTMENT OF HEALTH AND HUMAN SERVICES • CENTERS FOR DISEASE CONTROL AND PREVENTION

Recommended Childhood and Adolescent Immunization Schedule UNITED STATES • 2006

Vaccine ▼ Age ►	Birth	1 month	2 months	4 months	6 months	12 months	15 months	18 months	24 months	4–6 years	11–12 years	13–14 years	15 years	16–18 years
Hepatitis B[1]	HepB	HepB	HepB	*HepB[1]*	HepB						HepB Series			
Diphtheria, Tetanus, Pertussis[2]			DTaP	DTaP	DTaP		DTaP	DTaP		DTaP	Tdap		Tdap	
Haemophilus influenzae type b[3]			Hib	Hib	*Hib[3]*	Hib	Hib							
Inactivated Poliovirus			IPV	IPV	IPV		IPV	IPV		IPV				
Measles, Mumps, Rubella[4]						MMR	MMR			MMR		MMR		
Varicella[5]						Varicella	Varicella	Varicella			Varicella			
Meningococcal[6]									MPSV4	MPSV4	MCV4		MCV4	MCV4
Pneumococcal[7]			PCV	PCV	PCV	PCV	PCV		PCV	PCV	PPV			
Influenza[8]					Influenza (Yearly)	Influenza (Yearly)	Influenza (Yearly)		Influenza (Yearly)	Influenza (Yearly)	Influenza (Yearly)			
Hepatitis A[9]									HepA Series	HepA Series				

Vaccines within broken line are for selected populations

Legend:
- ▮ **Range of recommended ages**
- ▮ **Catch-up immunization**
- ▮ **11–12 year old assessment**

This schedule indicates the recommended ages for routine administration of currently licensed childhood vaccines, as of December 1, 2005, for children through age 18 years. Any dose not administered at the recommended age should be administered at any subsequent visit when indicated and feasible. ▮ Indicates age groups that warrant special effort to administer those vaccines not previously administered. Additional vaccines may be licensed and recommended during the year. Licensed combination vaccines may be used whenever any components of the combination are indicated and other components of the vaccine are not contraindicated and if approved by the Food and Drug Administration for that dose of the series. Providers should consult the respective ACIP statement for detailed recommendations. Clinically significant adverse events that follow immunization should be reported to the Vaccine Adverse Event Reporting System (VAERS). Guidance about how to obtain and complete a VAERS form is available at www.vaers.hhs.gov or by telephone, 800-822-7967.

Appendix III

NANDA-Approved Nursing Diagnoses

Activity Intolerance
Activity Intolerance, Risk for
Adaptive Capacity: Intracranial, Decreased
Adjustment, Impaired
Airway Clearance, Ineffective
Allergy, Latex Response
Allergy, Latex Response, Risk for
Anxiety
Anxiety, Death
Aspiration, Risk for
Attachment, Parent/Infant/Child, Risk for Impaired
Blood Glucose, Risk for Unstable
Body Image, Disturbed
Body Temperature: Imbalanced, Risk for
Bowel Incontinence
Breastfeeding, Effective
Breastfeeding, Ineffective
Breastfeeding, Interrupted
Breathing Pattern, Ineffective
Cardiac Output, Decreased
Caregiver Role Strain
Caregiver Role Strain, Risk for
Comfort, Readiness for Enhanced
Communication, Readiness for Enhanced
Communication: Verbal, Impaired
Confusion, Acute
Confusion, Chronic
Confusion, Risk for Acute
Constipation
Constipation, Perceived
Constipation, Risk for
Contamination
Contamination, Risk for
Coping: Community, Ineffective
Coping: Community, Readiness for Enhanced
Coping: Defensive
Coping: Family, Compromised
Coping: Family, Disabled
Coping: Family, Readiness for Enhanced
Coping (Individual), Readiness for Enhanced
Coping, Ineffective
Decision Making, Readiness for Enhanced
Decisional Conflict (Specify)
Denial, Ineffective
Dentition, Impaired
Development: Delayed, Risk for
Diarrhea
Disuse Syndrome, Risk for

Diversional Activity, Deficient
Dysreflexia, Autonomic
Dysreflexia, Autonomic, Risk for
Energy Field Disturbance
Environmental Interpretation Syndrome, Impaired
Failure to Thrive, Adult
Falls, Risk for
Family Processes, Dysfunctional: Alcoholism
Family Processes, Interrupted
Family Processes, Readiness for Enhanced
Fatigue
Fear
Fluid Balance, Readiness for Enhanced
Fluid Volume, Deficient
Fluid Volume, Deficient, Risk for
Fluid Volume, Excess
Fluid Volume, Imbalanced, Risk for
Gas Exchange, Impaired
Grieving
Grieving, Anticipatory
Grieving, Complicated
Grieving, Risk for Complicated
Growth, Disproportionate, Risk for
Growth and Development, Delayed
Health Behavior, Risk-Prone
Health Seeking Behaviors (Specify)
Home Maintenance, Impaired
Hope, Readiness for Enhanced
Hopelessness
Human Dignity, Risk for Compromised
Hyperthermia
Hypothermia
Identity: Personal, Disturbed
Immunization Status, Readiness for Enhanced
Infant Behavior, Disorganized
Infant Behavior: Disorganized, Risk for
Infant Behavior: Organized, Readiness for Enhanced
Infant Feeding Pattern, Ineffective
Infection, Risk for
Injury, Risk for
Insomnia
Knowledge, Deficient (Specify)
Knowledge (Specify), Readiness for Enhanced
Lifestyle, Sedentary
Liver Function, Risk for Impaired
Loneliness, Risk for
Memory, Impaired
Mobility: Bed, Impaired

Mobility: Physical, Impaired
Mobility: Wheelchair, Impaired
Moral Distress
Nausea
Neurovascular Dysfunction: Peripheral, Risk for
Noncompliance (Specify)
Nutrition, Imbalanced: Less than Body Requirements
Nutrition, Imbalanced: More than Body Requirements
Nutrition, Imbalanced: More than Body Requirements, Risk for
Nutrition, Readiness for Enhanced
Oral Mucous Membrane, Impaired
Pain, Acute
Pain, Chronic
Parenting, Impaired
Parenting, Readiness for Enhanced
Parenting, Risk for Impaired
Perioperative Positioning Injury, Risk for
Poisoning, Risk for
Post-Trauma Syndrome
Post-Trauma Syndrome, Risk for
Power, Readiness for Enhanced
Powerlessness
Powerlessness, Risk for
Protection, Ineffective
Rape-Trauma Syndrome
Rape-Trauma Syndrome: Compound Reaction
Rape-Trauma Syndrome: Silent Reaction
Religiosity, Impaired
Religiosity, Readiness for Enhanced
Religiosity, Risk for Impaired
Relocation Stress Syndrome
Relocation Stress Syndrome, Risk for
Role Conflict, Parental
Role Performance, Ineffective
Self-Care, Readiness for Enhanced
Self-Care Deficit: Bathing/Hygiene
Self-Care Deficit: Dressing/Grooming
Self-Care Deficit: Feeding
Self-Care Deficit: Toileting
Self-Concept, Readiness for Enhanced
Self-Esteem, Chronic Low
Self-Esteem, Situational Low
Self-Esteem, Risk for Situational Low
Self-Mutilation
Self-Mutilation, Risk for
Sensory Perception, Disturbed (Specify: Visual, Auditory, Kinesthetic, Gustatory, Tactile, Olfactory)
Sexual Dysfunction
Sexuality Patterns, Ineffective

Skin Integrity, Impaired
Skin Integrity, Risk for Impaired
Sleep Deprivation
Sleep Pattern, Disturbed
Sleep, Readiness for Enhanced
Social Interaction, Impaired
Social Isolation
Sorrow, Chronic
Spiritual Distress
Spiritual Distress, Risk for
Spiritual Well-Being, Readiness for Enhanced
Spontaneous Ventilation, Impaired
Stress Overload
Sudden Infant Death Syndrome, Risk for
Suffocation, Risk for
Suicide, Risk for
Surgical Recovery, Delayed
Swallowing, Impaired
Therapeutic Regimen Management: Community, Ineffective
Therapeutic Regimen Management, Effective
Therapeutic Regimen Management: Family, Ineffective
Therapeutic Regimen Management, Ineffective
Therapeutic Regimen Management, Readiness for Enhanced
Thermoregulation, Ineffective
Thought Processes, Disturbed
Tissue Integrity, Impaired
Tissue Perfusion, Ineffective (Specify: Renal, Cerebral, Cardiopulmonary, Gastrointestinal, Peripheral)
Tissue Perfusion, Ineffective (Peripheral)
Transfer Ability, Impaired
Trauma, Risk for
Unilateral Neglect
Urinary Elimination, Impaired
Urinary Elimination, Readiness for Enhanced
Urinary Incontinence, Functional
Urinary Incontinence, Overflow
Urinary Incontinence, Reflex
Urinary Incontinence, Stress
Urinary Incontinence, Total
Urinary Incontinence, Urge
Urinary Incontinence, Risk for Urge
Urinary Retention
Ventilation, Impaired Spontaneous
Ventilatory Weaning Response, Dysfunctional
Violence: Other-Directed, Risk for
Violence: Self-Directed, Risk for
Walking, Impaired
Wandering

Appendix IV

Denver Developmental Screening

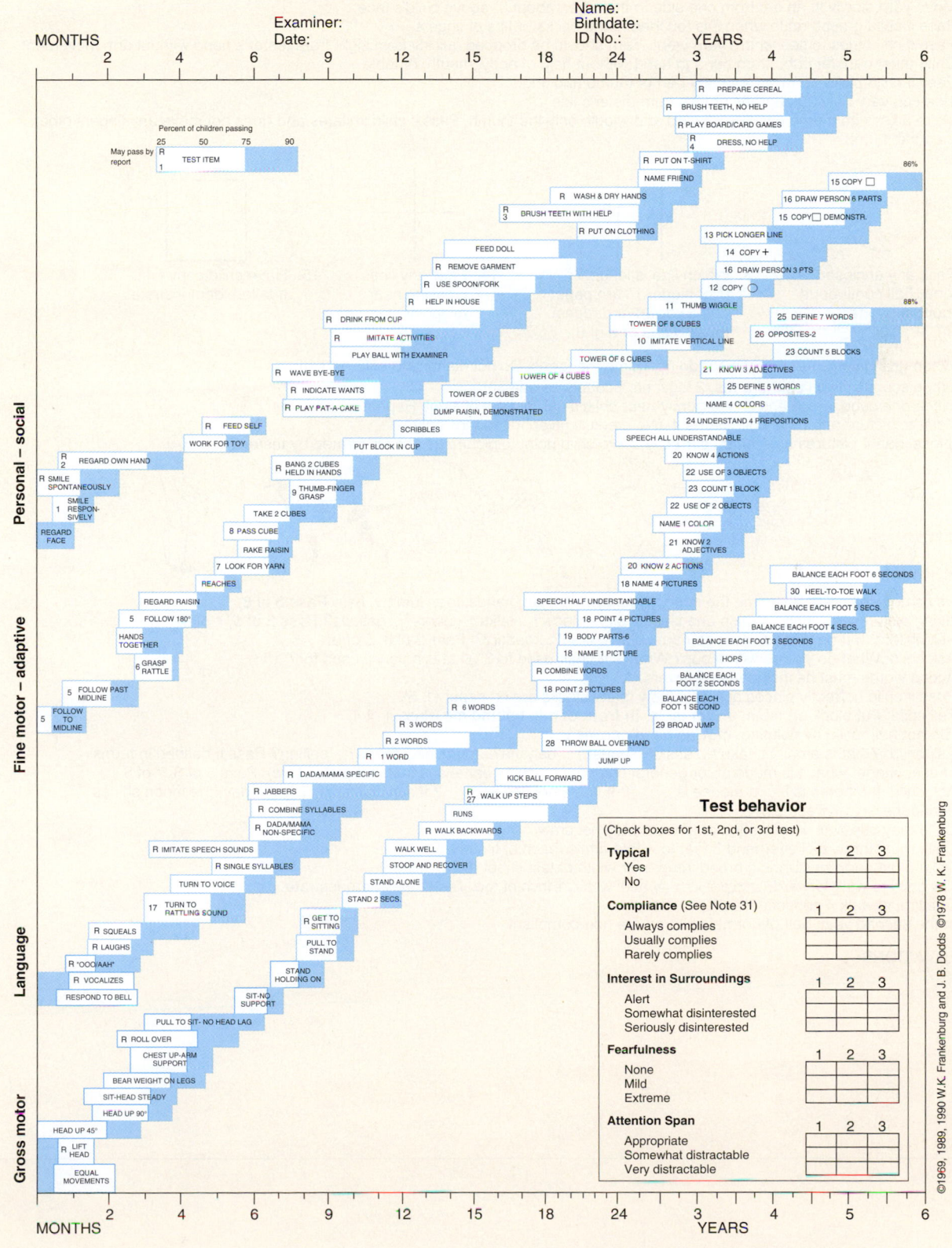

1. Try to get child to smile by smiling, talking or waving. Do not touch him/her.
2. Child must stare at hand several seconds.
3. Parent may help guide toothbrush and put toothpaste on brush.
4. Child does not have to be able to tie shoes or button/zip in the back.
5. Move yarn slowly in an arc from one side to the other, about 8" above child's face.
6. Pass if child grasps rattle when it is touched to the backs or tips of fingers.
7. Pass if child tries to see where yarn went. Yarn should be dropped quickly from sight from tester's hand without arm movement.
8. Child must transfer cube from hand to hand without help of body, mouth, or table.
9. Pass if child picks up raisin with any part of thumb and finger.
10. Line can vary only 30 degrees or less from tester's line.
11. Make a fist with thumb pointing upward and wiggle only the thumb. Pass if child imitates and does not move any fingers other than the thumb.

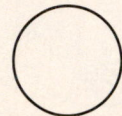 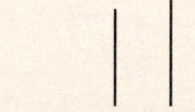 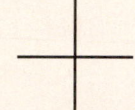 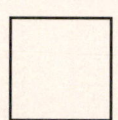

12. Pass any enclosed form. Fail continuous round motions.
13. Which line is longer? (Not bigger.) Turn paper upside down and repeat. (pass 3 of 3 or 5 of 6).
14. Pass any lines crossing near midpoint.
15. Have child copy first. If failed, demonstrate.

When giving items 12, 14, and 15, do not name the forms. Do not demonstrate 12 and 14.

16. When scoring, each pair (2 arms, 2 legs, etc.) counts as one part.
17. Place one cube in cup and shake gently near child's ear, but out of sight. Repeat for other ear.
18. Point to picture and have child name it. (No credit is given for sounds only.)
    If less than 4 pictures are named correctly, have child point to picture as each is named by tester.

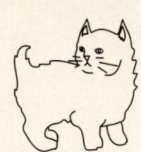 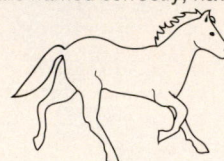 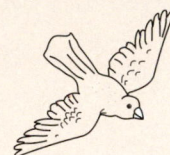 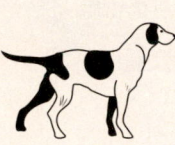 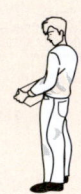

19. Using doll, tell child: Show me the nose, eyes, ears, mouth, hands, feet, tummy, hair. Pass 6 of 8.
20. Using pictures, ask child: Which one flies?... says meow?... talks?... barks?... gallops? Pass 2 of 5, 4 of 5.
21. Ask child: What do you do when you are cold?... tired?... hungry? Pass 2 of 3, 3 of 3.
22. Ask child: What do you do with a cup? What is a chair used for? What is a pencil used for?
    Action words must be included in answers.
23. Pass if child correctly places <u>and</u> says how many blocks are on paper (1, 5).
24. Tell child: Put block **on** table, **under** table, **in front of** me, **behind** me. Pass 4 of 4.
    (Do not help child by pointing, moving head or eyes.)
25. Ask child: What is a ball?... lake?... desk?... house?... banana?... curtain?... fence?... ceiling? Pass if defined in terms of use, shape, what it is made of, or general category (such as banana is fruit, not just yellow). Pass 5 of 8, 7 of 8.
26. Ask child: If a horse is big, a mouse is_____? If fire is hot, ice is_____? If sun shines during the day, the moon shines during the _____? Pass 2 of 3.
27. Child may use wall or rail only, not person. May not crawl.
28. Child must throw ball overhand 3 feet to within arm's reach of tester.
29. Child must perform standing broad jump over width of test sheet (8 1/2 inches).
30. Tell child to walk forward, ⌒⌒⌒⌒⌒ ➝ heel within 1 inch of toe. Tester may demonstrate.
    Child must walk 4 consecutive steps.
31. In the second year, half of normal children are non-compliant.

OBSERVATIONS:

Appendix V

Common Conversions and Lab Values

Pregnant and Nonpregnant Laboratory Values

TEST	PREGNANT VALUES	NONPREGNANT VALUES
Hematocrit (%)	32–42	37–47
Hemoglobin (g/dL)	10–14	12–16
Platelets (mm³)	Significant increase 3–5 days after birth	150,000–350,000
White blood cells (mm³)	5,000–15,000	4,500–10,000
Fibrinogen (mg/dL)	Up to 600	175–400
Serum glucose (mg/dL)	65 (fasting) less than 140 (2 hours PP)	70–80
Sodium (mEq/L)	135–145	135–145
Potassium (mEq/L)	3.5–5.1	3.5–5.1
Chloride (mEq/L)	100–108	100–108
Bicarbonate (mEq/L)	22–26	22–26
Calcium (mg/dL)	Falls 10% by term	8.5–10.5

Apgar Score

SIGN	SCORE 0	SCORE 1	SCORE 2
Heart rate	Absent	Slow—less than 100	Over 100
Respiratory rate	Absent	Slow—irregular	Good crying
Muscle tone	Flaccid	Some flexing of extremities	Active motion
Reflex irritability	None	Grimace	Vigorous cry
Color	Pale blue	Body pink, extremities blue	Completely pink (if light skinned); absence of cyanosis (if dark skinned)

Score: 0–4 requires resuscitation efforts; 4–7 requires administration of oxygen and rubbing the back to stimulate breathing; 8–10 requires no special attention.

Selected Common Conversions Between English and Metric Measurements

1 g = 1 mL (used when weighing diaper to determine fluid output)

1 grain = 60 mg

15 grains = 1 g

1 oz = 30 mL

1.2 lb = 1 kg (used when recording in metric or computing body mass index [BMI])

1 in. = 2.5 cm (used when recording in metric)

39 in. = 1 yd 3 in.

= 1 m (used when recording in metric)

Conversion Formulas for Temperature Readings

CELSIUS TO FAHRENHEIT:

From °C up to °F:

$$°F = 1.8 \times °C + 32$$

First **multiply** °C by 1.8; then **add** 32.

FAHRENHEIT TO CELSIUS:

From °F down to °C:

$$°C = (°F - 32) \text{ divided by } 1.8$$

First **subtract** 32 from °F; then **divide** by 1.8.

Normal Vital Sign Ranges by Age

AGE	TEMPERATURE IN DEGREES CELSIUS/ FAHRENHEIT	PULSE (AVERAGE AND RANGE)	RESPIRATIONS (AVERAGE AND RANGE)	BLOOD PRESSURE (mm HG)
Newborns	36.8 (axillary)	130 (80–180)	35 (30–80)	73/55
1–3 years	37.7 (rectal)	120 (80–140)	30 (20–40)	90/55
6–8 years	37 (oral)	100 (75–120)	20 (15–25)	95/57
10 years	37 (oral)	70 (50–90)	19 (15–25)	102/62
Teen years	37 (oral)	70 (50–90)	18 (15–20)	120/80
Adult	37 (oral)	80 (60–100)	16 (12–20)	120/80
Older adult (greater than 70 years)	36 (oral)	80 (60–100)	16 (15–20)	Possible increased diastolic

Typical Laboratory Results for Infants and Children

COMPONENT TESTED	NORMAL LABORATORY VALUES
Hematocrit	Newborn: 44–65%; 1–3 years old: 29–40%; 4–10 years old: 31–43%
Urine specific gravity	Newborn: 1.001–1.020; Child: 1.005–1.030
Blood urea nitrogen	Infant: 5–15 mg/dL; Child: 5–20 mg/dL
Potassium	Infant: 3.6–5.8 mEq/L; Child: 3.5–5.5 mEq/L
Sodium	Infant: 134–150 mEq/L; Child: 135–145 mEq/L
Calcium	Newborn: 3.7–7.0 mEq/L or 7.4–14.0 mg/dL; Infant: 5.0–6.0 mEq/L or 10–12 mg/dL; Child: 4.5–5.8 mEq/L or 9–11.5 mg/dL

Blood Gases
  pH
  $Paco_2$
  HCO_3
	
	Child: 7.36–7.44
	Child: 35–45 mm Hg
	Child: 22–26 mEq/L

Note: Lab values may vary. Consult the laboratory at your health care agency.

Pediatric Lab Values for Oxygen Saturation

Normal	95–98%
Mild hypoxemia	90–95%
Moderate hypoxemia	85–90%
Severe hypoxemia	85% or lower

Laboratory Values for Cholesterol

TEST	NORMAL	BORDERLINE LEVELS	HIGH LEVELS
Total cholesterol	Less than 170 mg/dL	170–199 mg/dL	More than 200 mg/dL
Low-density lipoproteins	Less than 110 mg/dL	110–129 mg/dL	More than 130 mg/dL
Triglycerides	100 mg/dL	100–150 mg/dL	More than 150 mg/dL
High-density lipoproteins	More than 35 mg/dL	Less than 35 mg/dL	

Lab Values for Urinalysis

CHARACTERISTIC	NORMAL VALUE
Bacteria	None to few organisms present
pH	4.50–8.0
Color	Clear, straw colored, amber
Odor	Slight, nonoffensive odor
Glucose	Negative
Protein	Negative
Red blood cells	Negative on gross examination; 0–5 per high-powered field
White blood cells	Negative; less than 2 per high-powered field
Specific gravity	Newborn: 1.001–1.020; Child: 1.005–1.030
Ketones	Negative

Lab Values for Children with Renal Failure

LAB	NORMAL	FINDING IN RENAL FAILURE
Blood urea nitrogen	Infant: 5–15 mg/dL	Increased
	Child: 5–20 mg/dL	Increased
Serum creatinine	Newborn: 0.8–1.4 mg/dL	Increased
	Infant: 0.7–1.7 mg/dL	Increased
	2–6 years old: 0.3–0.6 mg/dL	Increased
	Greater than 6 years old: 0.4–1.2 mg/dL	Increased
Serum potassium	Infant: 3.6–5.8 mEq/L	Increased
	Child: 3.5–5.5 mEq/L	Increased
Serum sodium	Infant: 134–150 mEq/L	Increased or decreased
	Child: 135–145 mEq/L	Increased or decreased
Bicarbonate (HCO_3)	24–28 mEq/L	Decreased

Appendix VI

Sign Language for Healthcare Professionals

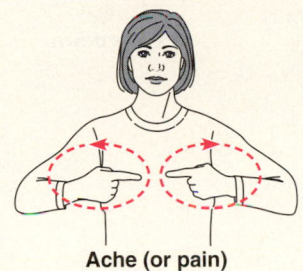

Ache (or pain)

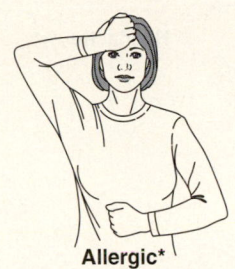

Allergic*

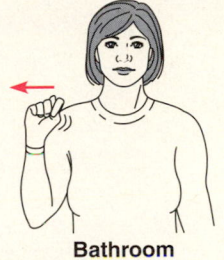

Bathroom

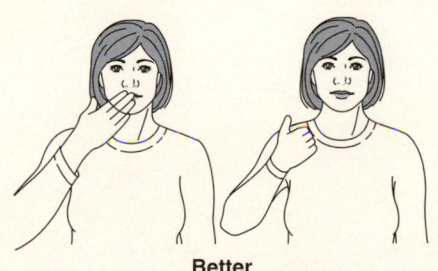

Better

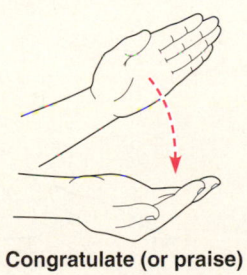

Congratulate (or praise)

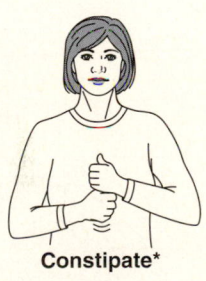

Constipate*

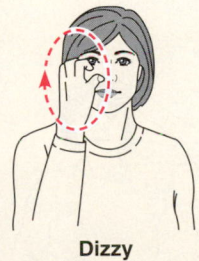

Dizzy

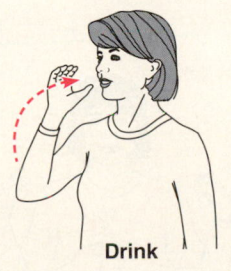

Drink

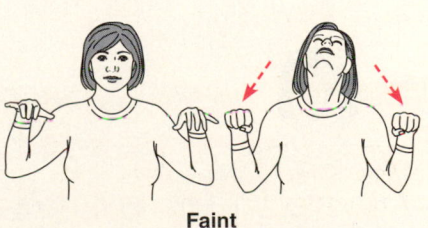

Faint

* Indicates signs that are in manually signed English. Those without an asterisk are American Sign Language.

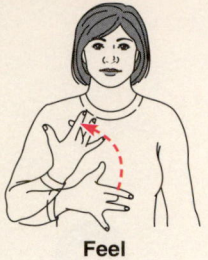

Feel

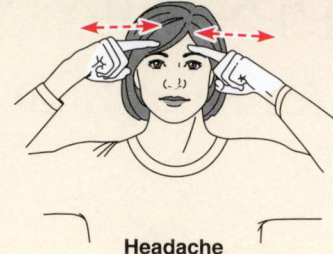

Headache

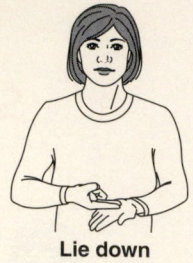

Lie down

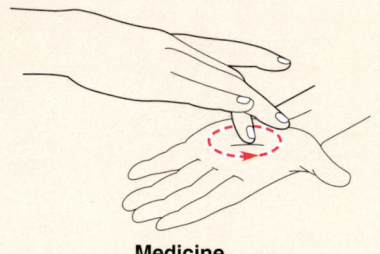

Medicine

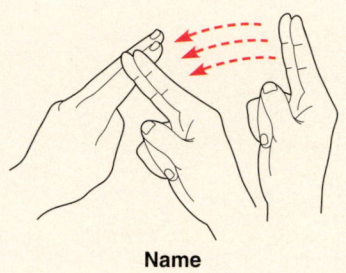

Name

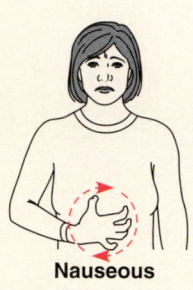

Nauseous

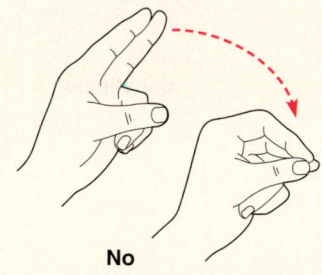

No

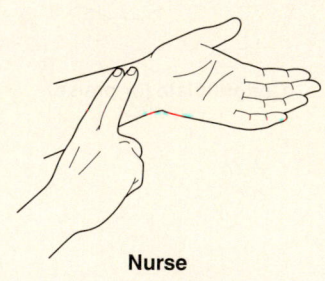

Nurse

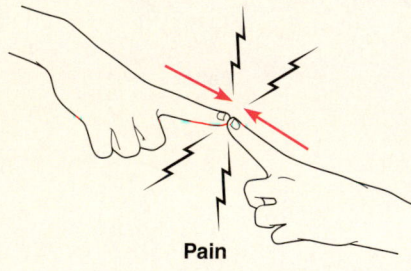

Pain

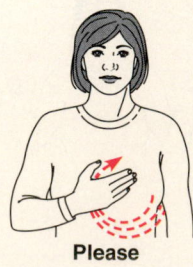

Please

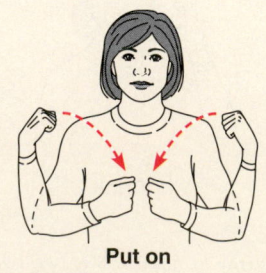

Put on

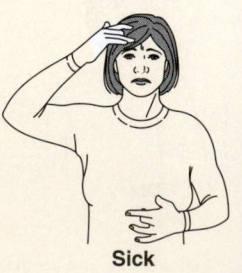

Sick

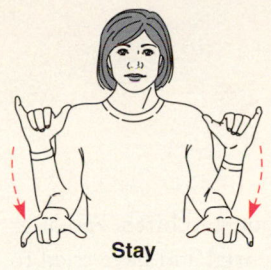

Stay

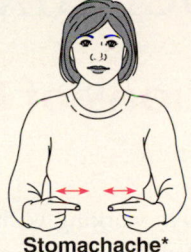

Stomachache*

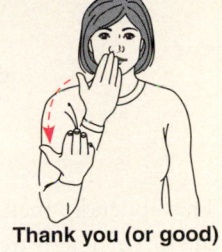

Thank you (or good)

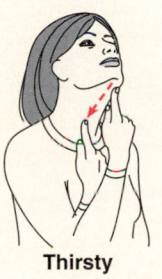

Thirsty

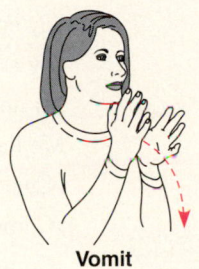

Vomit

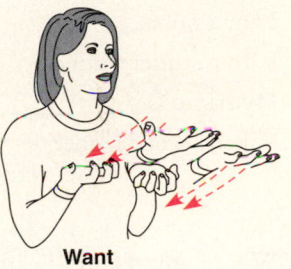

Want

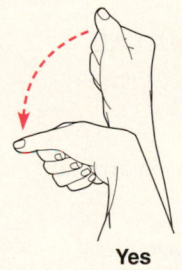

Yes

Appendix VII

Spanish Translations of English Phrases*

This appendix includes phrases you might find helpful in working with families during pregnancy, labor, and birth, and after the birth. There are many ways to phrase questions. We have chosen some statements we consider essential and have tried to phrase them in a straightforward way. The phrases are designed to help you in situations in which translation is not possible at the moment.

This list begins with introductory statements, which are presented in a logical conversational flow. The remaining phrases are arranged according to the phases of pregnancy and birth during which they are most applicable.

ESSENTIAL INTRODUCTORY PHRASES

Hello

I am a nurse.

I am a student nurse.

My name is _____.

What is your name?

What name should I call you?

Thank you

Please

Is someone here with you?

Does he (she) speak English?

Goodbye

FRASES INTRODUCTORAS ESENCIALES

Hola

Soy enfermera (enfermero).†

Soy estudiante de enfermería.

Mi nombre es _____.

Me llamo _____.

¿Cuál es su nombre?

¿Cómo se llama?

¿Cómo quiere que la llamemos?

¿Cómo quiere ser llamada?

Gracias

Por favor

¿Hay alquien aquí con usted?

¿Habla él (ella) inglés?

Adiós.

PHRASES FOR THE ANTEPARTAL PERIOD

Are you taking any medications now?

Show me the medicine bottles please.

Have you ever had trouble with your blood pressure?

When was the first day of your last period?

Have you had any spotting or bleeding since your last period?

Have you been on birth control pills?

When did you stop taking them?

Do you have an intrauterine device (IUD)?

How many times have you been pregnant?

Are you having any problems with your pregnancy?

Is there anything that is worrying you?

I would like to take your blood pressure.

I would like to take your pulse.

I would like to take your temperature.

I would like to listen to your heart and lungs.

FRASES PARA EL PERIODO PRENATAL

¿Está tomando algunas medicinas ahora?

Por favor, muéstreme los frascos.

¿Ha tenido problemas alguna vez con la presión arterial?

¿Cuál fue el primer día de su última regla?

¿Cuál fue el primer día de su última menstruación?

¿Ha sangrado o ha tenido manchas de sangre desde su última regla?

¿Ha estado tomando píldoras anticonceptivas?

¿Cuándo dejó de tomarlas?

¿Usa un aparato intrauterino?

¿Cuántas veces ha estado usted embarazada?

¿Tiene problemas con su embarazo?

¿Hay algo o alguna cosa que la preocupe?

Quisiera tomarle la presió arterial.

Quisiera tomarle el pulso.

Quisiera tomarle la temperatura.

Quisiera escucharle el corazon y los pulmones.

I would like to check your uterus.

Please urinate in this cup and leave it in the bathroom.

Please stand up.

Please sit down.

Please lie down.

PHRASES RELATED TO CLIENT SAFETY

I would like to talk to you alone.

Are you safe at home?

Are you afraid of your partner?

During your pregnancy has your partner hit, slapped, kicked, or punched you?

How many times?

Do you have someone for support?

QUESTIONS THE MOTHER OR FATHER MAY ASK

How big is my baby?

How much does the baby weigh now?

When will I feel my baby move?

PHRASES FOR THE INTRAPARTAL PERIOD

Note: Review the essential introductory phrases for beginning a conversation.

Are you having labor pains?

Are you having contractions?

Are you having pain?

Do you need medicine for pain?

Do you need to urinate?

This is a bedpan to urinate in.

Can I help you to the bathroom?

Do you need to have a bowel movement?

Has your bag of water broken?

Have you had any bright-red bleeding during your pregnancy?

How many births have you had?

I need to do a vaginal examination.

I will help you.

I will stay with you.

Please pant. I will show you how.

Do not push now.

Push now.

FRASES RELACIONADAS CON LA SEGURIDAD DEL CLIENTE

Quisiera examinarle el útero.

Puede orinar en este vaso y dejarlo en el baño.

Por favor, levántese.

Por favor, siéntese.

Por favor, acuéstese.

Quisiera hablar a solas con usted.

¿Sufre de peligros en casa?

¿Le tiene miedo a su compañero?

Durante su embarazo, ¿la ha golpeado?

¿la ha abofeteado?

¿la ha pateado? o

¿le ha dado puñetazos?

¿Cuántas veces?

¿Cuénta con alguien que la pueda ayudar?

POSIBLES PREGUNTAS QUE MADRES O PADRES HACEN

¿De qué tamaño es el (la) bebé?

¿Cuánto pesa el bebé ahora?

¿Cuándo lo (la) voy a sentir moverse?

FRASES DURANTE EL PARTO

Nota: Repase las frases introductoras para comenzar una conversación.

¿Tiene dolores de parto?

¿Tiene contracciones?

¿Tiene dolores?

¿Necesita medicina para el dolor?

¿Necesita orinar?

Aquí tiene el bacín (la chata) (el pato) para orinar.

¿La ayudo a ir al baño?

¿Necesita mover el vientre (obrar)? Necesita "Hacer caca"— coloquial

¿Se le ha roto la bolsa de agua(s)?

¿Ha tenido algún sangramiento de color rojo durante su embarazo?

¿Cuántos niños le han nacido?

Necesito hacerle un examen vaginal.

La voy a ayudar.

Me quedaré con usted.

Por favor, jadee. Le voy a mostrar cómo.

No puje ahora.

Puje ahora.

Stop pushing.	Pare de pujar.
	No puje más.
The doctor needs to do a cesarean birth.	El doctor le va a hacer una operación cesárea.
This is medicine for your pain. You will feel better soon.	Esta medicina es para el dolor. Va a sentirse mejor pronto.
When is your baby supposed to be born?	¿Cuando está supuesto a nacer el bebé?
January	enero
February	febrero
March	marzo
April	abril
May	mayo
June	junio
July	julio
August	agosto
September	septiembre
October	octubre
November	noviembre
December	diciembre
What is your doctor's name?	¿Cuál es el nombre de su doctor?
What is your midwife's name?	¿Cuál es el nombre de su comadrona (partera)?
Your baby is having some trouble now.	El bebé está pasando por algunos problemas.
	El bebé está sufriendo algunas dificultades.
I need to put this oxygen mask on you. It will help your baby. It may smell funny, but it is OK.	Le voy a poner esta máscara de oxígeno. Va a ayudar al bebé. Huele extraño, pero no hay problemas.
Please turn on your left side.	Por favor voltéese al lado izquierdo.
Please turn on your right side.	Por favor voltéese al lado derecho.
Your baby is OK.	El bebé está bien.

PHRASES FOR THE POSTPARTAL PERIOD AND THE NEWBORN AREA

FRASES PARA EL PERIODO DESPUES DEL PARTO Y EL AREA DEL RECIEN NACIDO

Note: Review the essential introductory phrases for beginning a conversation.	*Nota:* Repase las frases introductoras para comenzar una conversación.
Are you hungry?	¿Tiene hambre?
Are you thirsty?	¿Tiene sed?
Are you cold?	¿Tiene frío?
Are you tired?	¿Está cansada?
I am going to put antibiotic ointment in the baby's eyes.	Le voy a poner al bebé un ungüento antibiótico alrededor de los ojos.
It will help protect your baby from some infections.	Lo (la) va a proteger contra algunos infecciones.
I am going to take some blood from your baby's foot to check the blood sugar and hemocrit.	Le voy a sacar sangre del pie al bebé para determinar el azúcar de la sangre y el hematocrítico.
If your baby begins to spit up, please turn him (her) on his (her) side.	Si el bebé comienza a vomitar, colóquelo (colóquela) de costado.
It may help to position your baby like this.	Lo (la) ayudará— si lo coloca así.
	Lo (la) ayudaría—si lo colocara así.
I would like to suggest that you clean your nipples this way before you breastfeed your baby.	Es bueno que se lave los pezones de esta manera antes de darle el pecho al bebé.

It is better that you clean your baby's cord this way.	Es mejor para el bebé que le lave el ombligo de esta manera.
It is better that you bathe your baby this way.	Es mejor que lo (la) bañe de esta manera.
It is better that you clean your baby's penis this way.	Es mejor que le limpie el pene así.
I would like to suggest that you fold the diaper this way.	Le sugiero que doble el pañal así.
I would like to suggest that you fasten the diaper this way.	Le sugiero que asegure el pañal así.
Take the baby's temperature this way.	Tómele la temperatura así.
I need to check (your breasts, your uterus, your flow, your stitches, your legs and feet).	Necesito examinarle (los pechos, el útero, el flujo, los puntos, las piernas y los pies).
I need to feel your uterus.	Necesito examinarle el útero.
I need to massage your uterus.	Necesito darle un masaje en la región del útero.
Place your baby on its side.	Coloque al bebé de costado.
Place the baby's used diapers here.	Coloque aquí los pañales usados.
Please rub your uterus every half hour to keep it firm. I will show you how.	Necesita darse un masaje en la región del útero cada media hora para mantenerlo firme. Le voy a mostrar cómo.
Would you like to see your baby now?	¿Quiere ver a su bebé ahora?
Would you like me to help you feed your baby?	¿Quiere que le ayude a alimentarlo (la)?
Your baby needs a car seat to go home in.	El (la) bebé necesita un asiento para bebé en el automóvil.

SPECIAL NEONATAL NEEDS

NECESIDADES DEL RECIEN NACIDO

We are giving your baby oxygen.	Le vamos a dar oxígeno al (a la) bebé.
Your baby is having problems breathing.	El (la) bebé tiene problemas al respirar.
Your baby needs extra help.	El (la) bebé necesita ayuda especial.
Your baby needs to go to a special care nursery.	El (la) bebé necesita ir a la sala de cuidados especiales para bebés.

[*]Prepared by Elizabeth Medina, Ph.D. Associate Professor of Spanish, Regis University, Denver, Colorado.

[†]In Spanish, nouns that end in *a* indicate female gender; nouns that end in *o* indicate male gender.

Appendix VIII

Standard Precautions for Infection Control

Excerpted from *Guideline for Isolation Precautions in Hospitals* (January 1996)

Background

Standard Precautions synthesize Blood/Body Fluid Precautions and guidelines for body substance isolation and apply them to all clients regardless of their diagnosis or presumed infection status. Standard Precautions apply to 1) blood; 2) all body fluids, secretions, and excretions except sweat, regardless of whether or not they contain visible blood; 3) nonintact skin; and 4) mucous membranes. Standard Precautions are designed to reduce the risk of transmission of microorganisms from both recognized and unrecognized sources of infection in hospitals.

II. Standard Precautions

A. *Handwashing*

Wash hands after touching blood, body fluids, secretions, excretions, and contaminated items, whether or not gloves are worn. Wash hands immediately after gloves are removed, between client contacts. Use an antimicrobial agent or a waterless antiseptic agent for specific circumstances (e.g., when hands are not visibly soiled, for control of outbreaks, etc.).

B. *Gloves*

Wear gloves (clean, nonsterile gloves are adequate) when touching blood, body fluids, secretions, excretions, and contaminated items. Put on clean gloves just before touching mucous membranes and nonintact skin. Change gloves between tasks and procedures on the same client after contact with material that may contain a high concentration of microorganisms. Remove gloves promptly after use and wash hands immediately to avoid transfer of microorganisms.

C. *Mask, Eye Protection, Face Shield*

Wear a mask and eye protection or a face shield to protect mucous membranes of the eyes, nose, and mouth during procedures that are likely to generate splashes or sprays of blood, body fluids, secretions, and excretions.

D. *Gown*

Wear a gown (a clean, nonsterile gown is adequate) to protect skin and to prevent soiling of clothing during procedures and client-care activities that are likely to generate splashes or sprays of blood, body fluids, secretions, or excretions.

E. *Client-Care Equipment*

Handle soiled equipment so as to prevent personal contamination of clothing and transfer of microorganisms. Ensure that reusable equipment is not used for the care of another client until it has been cleaned and reprocessed appropriately. Ensure that single-use items are discarded properly.

F. *Environmental Control*

Ensure that hospital procedures for the routine care, cleaning, and disinfection of environmental surfaces, beds, bedrails, bedside equipment, and other frequently touched surfaces are being followed.

G. *Linen*

Handle, transport, and process used linen soiled with blood, body fluids, secretions, and excretions in a manner that prevents skin and mucous membrane exposures and contamination of clothing, and that avoids transfer of microorganisms.

H. *Occupational Health and Bloodborne Pathogens*

1. Take care to prevent injuries when using needles, scalpels, and other sharp instruments or devices. Never recap used needles using both hands, or use any other technique that involves directing the point of a needle toward any part of the body; rather, use either a one-handed "scoop" technique or a mechanical device designed for holding the needle sheath. Do not remove used needles from disposable syringes by hand, and do not bend, break, or manipulate used needles by hand. Place all sharp items in appropriate puncture-resistant containers. Use mouthpieces, resuscitation bags, or other ventilation devices as an alternative to mouth-to-mouth resuscitation methods.

I. *Client Placement*

Place client who contaminates the environment or who does not (or cannot be expected to) assist in maintaining appropriate hygiene or environmental control in a private room.

Date last modified: April 1, 2005

Source: Department of Health and Human Services, Centers for Disease Control and Prevention.

Standard Precautions†, ‡

Use Standard Precautions for the care of all patients

Airborne Precautions

In addition to Standard Precautions, use Airborne Precautions for patients known or suspected to have serious illnesses transmitted by airborne droplet nuclei. Examples of such illnesses include:

- Measles
- Varicella (including disseminated zoster)†
- Tuberculosis‡

Droplet Precautions

In addition to Standard Precautions, use Droplet Precautions for patients known or suspected to have serious illnesses transmitted by large particle droplets. Examples of such illnesses include:

- Invasive *Haemophilus influenzae* type b disease, including meningitis, pneumonia, epiglottitis, and sepsis
- Invasive Neisseria *meningitidis* disease, including meningitis, pneumonia, and sepsis

Other serious bacterial respiratory infections spread by droplet transmission, including:

- Diphtheria (pharyngeal)
- Mycoplasma pneumonia
- Pertussis
- Pneumonic plague
- Streptococcal (group A) pharyngitis, pneumonia, or scarlet fever in infants and young children

Serious viral infections spread by droplet transmission, including:

- Adenovirus†
- Influenza
- Mumps
- Parvovirus B19
- Rubella

Contact Precautions

In addition to Standard Precautions, use Contact Precautions for patients known or suspected to have serious illnesses easily transmitted by direct patient contact or by contact with items in the patient's environment. Examples of such illnesses include:

Gastrointestinal, respiratory, skin, or wound infections or colonization with multidrug-resistant bacteria judged by the infection control program, based on current state, regional, or national recommendations, to be of special clinical and epidemiologic significance

Enteric infections with a low infectious dose or prolonged environmental survival, including:

- Clostridium difficile
- For diapered or incontinent patients: enterohemorrhagic Escherichia coli O157:H7, Shigella, hepatitis A, or rotavirus

Respiratory syncytial virus, parainfluenza virus, or enteroviral infections in infants and young children

Skin infections that are highly contagious or that may occur on dry skin, including:

- Diphtheria (cutaneous)
- Herpes simplex virus (neonatal or mucocutaneous)
- Impetigo
- Major (noncontained) abscesses, cellulitis, or decubiti
- Pediculosis
- Scabies
- Staphylococcal furunculosis in infants and young children
- Zoster (disseminated or in the immunocompromised host)†

Viral/hemorrhagic conjunctivitis

- Viral hemorrhagic infections (Ebola, Lassa, or Marburg)

Source: Centers for Disease Control and Prevention Fundamentals of Isolation Precautions, http://www.cdc.gov/ncidod/hip/ISOLAT/ isopart2.htm

† Certain infections require more than one type of precaution.

‡ See CDC "*Guidelines for Preventing the Transmission of Tuberculosis in Health-Care Facilities.*" (23)

Contents *These precautions last reviewed and updated by CDC, April 1, 2005.*

References and Resources

CHAPTER 1

American Nurses Association (ANA). (1980). *Nursing: A social policy statement*. Kansas City, MO: Author.

American Nurses Association (ANA). (1998). *Standards of clinical nursing practice* (2nd ed.). Washington, DC: American Nurses Publishing.

American Nurses Association (ANA). (1991). *Nursing's agenda for health care reform*. Washington, DC: Author.

American Nurses Association (ANA). (1991). *Standards of clinical nursing practice. (NP-79)*. Kansas City, MO: Author.

Brady-Fryer, B., Wiebe, N., & Lander, J. (2004). Pain relief for neonatal circumcision. *The Cochrane Library*, 4.

Centers for Disease Control and Prevention (CDC). (1995). Differences in maternal mortality among black and white women—United States, 1990. *Morbidity and Mortality Weekly Report*, January 13.

Clifford, P. A., String, M., Christensen, H., & Mountain, D. (2004). Pain assessment and intervention for term newborns. *Journal of Midwifery and Women's Health*, 49(6), 514–519.

Gennaro, S., Hodnett, E., & Kearney, M. (2001). Making evidence-based practice a reality in your institution: Evaluating the evidence and using the evidence to change clinical practice. *American Journal of Maternal/Child Nursing*, 26(5), 236–250.

Henry, P. R., Haubold, K., & Dobrzykowski, T. (2004). Pain in the healthy full-term neonate: Efficacy and safety of interventions. *Newborn Infant Nursing Review*, 4(2), 126–130.

Leininger, M., McFarland, M., McFarlane, M. (2002). *Transcultural nursing* (3rd ed.). New York: McGraw-Hill Professional.

National Council of State Boards of Nursing, Inc. (1995). *Delegation: Concepts and decision-making process*. Chicago: Author.

North American Nursing Diagnosis Association (NANDA). (2005). *NANDA nursing diagnoses: Definitions and classification, 2005–2006*. Philadelphia: Author.

Razmus, I., Dalton, M., & Wilson, D. (2004). Practice applications of research. Pain management for newborn circumcision. *Pediatric Nursing*, 30(5), 414–417.

Reuters News Service. *Maternal mortality in US remains static*. Sept 2003. Retrieved June 16, 2005, from http://personalMD.com

U.S. Department of Health and Human Services. (1991). *Healthy people 2000*. Washington, DC: U.S. Government Printing Office.

U.S. Department of Health and Human Services. (2000). *Healthy people 2010* (2nd ed.). Washington, DC: U.S. Government Printing Office.

U.S. Department of Health and Human Services, Centers for Disease Control and Prevention (CDC). (2006). *National Vital Statistics Reports*, 54(16), 5.

U.S. Department of Health and Human Services, National Center for Health Statistics. (2002). *Health, United States 1950–1999*. Hyattsville, MD: Author.

Venes, D., Thomas, C. L., & Taber, C. W. (Eds.). (2001). *Taber's cyclopedic medical dictionary* (19th ed.). Philadelphia: FA Davis.

Zotti, M. E., Brown, P., & Stotts, R. C. (1996). Community-based nursing versus community health nursing: What does it all mean? *Nursing Outlook*, 44, 211.

CHAPTER 2

American Association of Colleges of Nursing. (1999). *Nursing educational agenda for the 21st century*. Washington, DC: Author.

American Nurses Association (ANA). (1998). *Standards of clinical nursing practice* (2nd ed.). Silver Spring, MD: Author.

American Nurses Association (ANA). (2000). *New position statement adolescent health task force*. Washington, DC: Author.

Anderson, M. A. (2001). *Nursing leadership: Management and professional practice for the LPN/LVN* (2nd ed.). Philadelphia: FA Davis.

Centers for Disease Control and Prevention (CDC). (2000). Building data systems for monitoring and responding to violence against women: Recommendations from a workshop. *MMWR*, 49(RR-11), 1. Retrieved September 17, 2006, from http://www.cdc.gov/mmwr/PDF/rr/rr4911.pdf

Coty, E., Davis, J., & Angell, L. (2002). *Documentation: The language of nursing*. Upper Saddle River, NJ: Prentice Hall.

Joint Commission on Accreditation of Healthcare Organizations (JCAHO). (2000). *2000 accreditation manual for hospitals*. Chicago: Author.

National Association for Practical Nurse Education and Service. (1998). *Code of ethics for licensed practical/vocational nurses*. Silver Spring, MD: Author.

National Federation of Licensed Practical Nurses. (1998). *Nursing practice standards for the license practical/vocational nurse*. Garner, NC: Author.

Ramont, R., Niedringhaus, D., & Towle, M. (2006). *Comprehensive nursing care*. Upper Saddle River, NJ: Prentice Hall.

Simpson, R. L. (1994). Ensuring patient data privacy, confidentiality, and security. *Nursing Management*, 25(7), 18–20.

Thompson, J. B., & Thompson, H. O. (1981). *Ethics in nursing*. New York: Macmillan.

U.S. Department of Health and Human Services, Office of Disease Prevention and Health Promotion. (2000). *Healthy people 2010*. Rockville, MD: Author.

CHAPTER 3

Bernhardt, J., & Dorman, K. (2004). Pre-term birth risk assessment tools: Exploring fetal fibronectin and cervical length for validating risk. *Lifelines*, 8(1), 38–45.

Duvall, E. (1977). *Marriage and family development* (5th ed.). Philadelphia: Lippincott.

Friedman, M. (1992). *Family nursing theory and assessment*. New York: Appleton-Century-Crofts.

Giger, J., & Davidhizar, R. (Eds.). (1995). *Transcultural nursing: Assessment and interventions* (2nd ed.). St. Louis, MO: Mosby.

Moos, M. (2004). Understanding prematurity: Sorting fact from fiction. *Lifelines*, 8(1), 33–37.

Sears, W., Sears, R., Sears, J., & Sears, M. (2004). *The premature baby book: Everything you need to know about your premature baby from birth to age one*. New York: Little, Brown.

Ramont, R. P., Niedringhaus, D. M., & Towle, M. A. (2006). *Comprehensive nursing care*. Upper Saddle River, NJ: Prentice Hall.

CHAPTER 4

Masters, W., & Johnson, W. (1966). *Human sexual response*. Philadelphia: Lippincott Williams & Wilkins.

National Institutes of Health (NIH). (2005). *Ethical, legal and social implications (ELSI) research program overview*. Available at www.genome.gov

Ramont, R. P., Niedringhaus, D. M., & Towle, M. A. (2006). *Comprehensive nursing care*. Upper Saddle River, NJ: Pearson Education.

Thibodeau, G. A., & Patton, K. T. (1997). *The human body in health & disease* (2nd ed.). St. Louis, MO: Mosby.

U.S. Department of Energy. (2004). *Human Genome Project information: Frequently asked questions*. Available at www.ornl.gov/sci/techresources

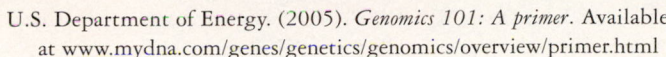

U.S. Department of Energy. (2005). *Genomics 101: A primer*. Available at www.mydna.com/genes/genetics/genomics/overview/primer.html

CHAPTER 5

Butts, J., & Hartman, S. (2002). Project BART: Effectiveness of a behavioral intervention to reduce HIV risk in adolescents. *American Journal of Maternal/Child Nursing, 27*, 163–170.

Centers for Disease Control and Prevention (CDC) website. Available at www.cdc.gov

Contraception Online website. Available at www.contraceptiononline.org

Girl Power! website. Available at www.girlpower.gov

Gravelle, K., Gravelle, J., & Palen, D. *The period book: Everything you don't want to ask (but need to know)*. New York: Walker & Company.

Hershberger, P. (1998). Smoking and pregnant teens: What nurses can do to help. *Lifelines, 2*, 26–31.

Kaufman, M. (2005). Morning-after pill study contradicts claim by foes: Easy access did not lead to riskier behavior. *Washington Post* (5 Jan 2005), p. A09.

Kitzinger, S. (1992). *Being born*. Grosset & Dunlap.

Madaras, L. *What's happening to my body? Book for girls*. New York: Newmarket Press.

The March of Dimes. *Teen pregnancy*. Retrieved September 17, 2006, from www.marchofdimes.com/professionals/681_1159.asp

Mayo Foundation for Medical and Educational Research. (2006). Morning-after pill: Emergency birth control. *Ask a Women's Health Specialist* (28 Aug 2006). Accessed at http://www.mayoclinic.com/health/morning-after-pill/AN00592.

McDowell, J. *How to help your child say "no" to sexual pressure*. Nashville, TN: Word Publishing.

The National Campaign to Prevent Teen Pregnancy website. Available at www.teenpregnancy.org

Piaget, J. (1969). The intellectual development of the adolescent. In G. Caplan & S. Lebovici (Eds.), *Adolescence: Psychological perspective*. New York: Basic Books.

Ramont, R., Niedringhaus, D., & Towle M. (2006). *Comprehensive nursing care*. Upper Saddle River, NJ: Prentice Hall.

U.S. Food and Drug Administration. (2006). Plan B: Questions and answers. Accessed at www.fda.gov/cder/drug/infopage/planB/planBQandA20060824.htm.

CHAPTER 6

American Pregnancy Association. (2006, August). *Natural herbs & vitamins and during pregnancy*. Available at www.americanpregnancy.org/pregnancyhealth/naturalherbsvitamins.html

Centers for Disease Control and Prevention (CDC), Division of Reproductive Health, National Center for Chronic Disease Prevention and Health Promotion, Division of Vital Statistics, National Center for Health Statistics. Washington, DC: U.S. Government Printing Office. Available at http://www.access.gpo.gov/

Choi, E. C. (1995). A contrast of mothering behaviors in women from Korea and the United States. *Journal of Obstetric, Gynecologic and Neonatal Nursing, 24*(4), 363–369.

DeJonge, C. J. (2000). Egg transport and fertilization. In J. J. Sciarra & T. J. Watkins (Eds.), *Gynecology and obstetrics* (Vol. 1, pp. 1–7). Philadelphia: Lippincott Williams & Wilkins.

Eisenberg, A., Murkoff, H., & Hathaway, S. (1986). *What to eat when you're expecting*. New York: Workman.

Fowles, E. (2004). Prenatal nutrition and birth outcomes. *Journal of Obstetric, Gynecologic, and Neonatal Nursing, 33*(6), 809–822.

Hardy, M. (2000). Herbs of special interest to women. *Journal of the American Pharmaceutical Association, 40*(2), 234–242.

Hood, M. Y., Moore, L. L., Sundarajan-Ramamurti, A., Singer, M., Cupples, L. A., & Ellison, R. C. (2000). Parental eating attitudes and the development of obesity in children. The Framingham Children's Study. *International Journal of Obesity Related Metabolic Disorders, 24*(10), 1319–1325.

Krieger/Elchai, L. (1996–1997). Herbs of special interest to women. *Herbs for a Healthy Balance*. © Creative Minds Unlimited. Available at www.create.org

London, M. L., Ladewig, P. W., Ball, J. W., & Bindler, R. C. (2003). *Maternal–newborn & child nursing*. Upper Saddle River, NJ: Prentice Hall.

Mattson, S. (1995). Culturally sensitive perinatal care for Southeast Asians. *Journal of Obstetric Gynecologic, and Neonatal Nursing, 24*(4), 335–341.

Moran, R. (1999). Evaluation and treatment of childhood obesity. *American Family Physician*, February 15.

Olds, S. B., London, M. L., Ladewig, P. A. W., & Davidson, M. R. (2004). *Maternal–newborn nursing & women's health care* (7th ed.). Upper Saddle River, NJ: Prentice Hall.

Roach, S. S., & Scherer, J. C. (2000). *Introductory clinical pharmacology* (6th ed.). Buffalo, NY: Lippincott.

Rogers, J., & Davis, B. (1995). How risky are hot tubs and saunas for pregnant women? *MCN, 20*(3), 137–140.

Somer, E. (2002). *Nutrition for a healthy pregnancy: The complete guide to eating before, during, and after your pregnancy*. New York: Owl Books.

Spector, R. E. (2000). *Cultural diversity in health and illness* (5th ed.). Upper Saddle River, NJ: Prentice-Hall Health.

CHAPTER 7

Adams, E., & Bianchi, A. (2004). Can a nurse and a doula exist in the same room? *International Journal of Childbirth Education, 19*(4), 12–15.

Adams, E. D., & Bianchi, A. L. (2005). *50 Ways to comfort a laboring woman*. Presented at the AWHONN 2005 convention, June 14, Salt Lake City, Utah.

Bianchi, A., & Adams, E. (2004). Doulas, labor support, and nurses. *International Journal of Childbirth Education, 19*(4), 24–30.

Callister, L. C. (2001). Culturally competent care of women and newborns: Knowledge, attitude and skills. *Journal of Obstetric, Gynecologic, & Neonatal Nursing, 30*, 209–215.

Doulas of North America website. Available at www.dona.org

Goetzl, L. M. (2002). ACOG practice bulletin. Obstetric analgesia and anesthesia. *Obstetrics & Gynecology, 100*, 177–191.

Hopper Deglin, J., & Hazard Vallerand, A. (2005). *Davis's drug guide for nurses* (9th ed.). Philadelphia: FA Davis.

International Childbirth Education Association website. Available at www.icea.org/

Miltner, R. (2002). More than support: Nursing interventions provided to women in labor. *Journal of Obstetric, Gynecologic and Neonatal Nursing, 31*(6), 753–761.

Olds, S. B., London, M. L., Ladewig, P. W., & Davidson, M. R. (2004). *Maternal–newborn nursing and women's health care* (7th ed.). Upper Saddle River, NJ: Prentice Hall.

Simkin, P., & Bolding, A. (2004). Update on nonpharmacologic approaches to relieve labor pain and prevent suffering. *Journal of Midwifery & Women's Health, 49*(6), 489–504.

St. Hill, P. F., Lipson, J. G., Ibrahim, A., & Meleis, A. F. (2003). *Nurse's drug guide: 2004*. Upper Saddle River, NJ: Prentice Hall.

CHAPTER 8

Beck Tatano, C. (1999). *Postpartum depression: Case studies, research and nursing care.* AWHONN.

Bennet, S., & Indman, P. *Beyond the blues: A guide to treating prenatal and postpartum depression.* San Jose, CA: Moodswings Press.

Burke, K., LeMone, P., & Mohn-Brown, E. (2003). *Medical surgical nursing care.* Upper Saddle River, NJ: Prentice Hall.

Johnson & Johnson. (2006). *The compendium of postpartum care.* AWHONN.

Placksin, S. (2000). *Mothering the new mother: Women's feelings and needs after childbirth a support and resource guide.* New York: Newmarket Press.

CHAPTER 9

American Academy of Pediatrics. (2006). Policy statements of the American Academy of Pediatrics. *Pediatrics, 117*(5), 1846–1847.

Ball, J., & Bindler, R. (2006). *Child health nursing.* Upper Saddle River, NJ: Prentice Hall.

Ballard, J. L., et al. (1991). New Ballard score, expanded to include extremely premature infants. *Journal of Pediatrics, 119*, 417.

Blackburn, S. T. (2003). *Maternal fetal & neonatal physiology: A clinical perspective.* (2nd ed.). St. Louis, MO: Saunders.

Committee on Bioethics. (1995). Informed consent, parental permission and assent in pediatric practice. *Pediatrics, 95*(2), 314–317.

Dougherty, G. (1998). When should a child be hospitalized? *Pediatrics, 101*(1), 6.

National Organization of Circumcision Information Resource Centers website. Available at www.nocirc.org

Olds, S. B., London, M. L., Ladewig, P. W., & Davidson, M. R. (2004). *Maternal–newborn nursing and women's health care* (7th ed.). Upper Saddle River, NJ: Prentice Hall.

Seidel, J. M., Ball, J. W., Dains, J., & Benedict, G. W. (2003). *Mosby's guide to physical examination* (5th ed.). St. Louis, MO: Mosby.

Tappero, E. P., & Honeyfield, M. E. (1996). *Physical assessment of the newborn* (2nd ed.). Petaluma, CA: NICU Ink.

CHAPTER 10

American Adoption Congress website. www.americanadoptioncongress.org

Concerned United Birth Parents website. www.cubirthparents.org

Cunningham, F. G., Grant, N. F., Leveno, K. J., Gilstrap, L. C., et al. (2001). *Williams obstetrics* (21st ed.). New York: McGraw-Hill.

Eby, L., & Brown, N. J. (2005). *Mental health nursing care.* Upper Saddle River, NJ: Prentice Hall.

International Soundex Reunion Registry website. Provides help to adopted children. www.isrr.net

Ladewig, P., London, M., & Davidson, M. (2006). *Contemporary maternal–newborn nursing care* (6th ed.). Upper Saddle River, NJ: Prentice Hall.

Olds, S. B., London, M. L., Ladewig, P. W., & Davidson, M. R. (2004). *Maternal–newborn nursing & women's health care* (7th ed.). Upper Saddle River, NJ: Prentice Hall.

Narad, C., & Mason, P. International adoption: Myths and realities. *Pediatric Nursing, 30*(6), 483–487.

National Adoption Information Clearinghouse website. www.naic.acf.hhs.gov

Ramont, R. P., Niedringhaus, D. M., & Towle, M. A. (2006). *Comprehensive nursing care.* Upper Saddle River, NJ: Prentice Hall.

Russell, M. (2004). *Adoption wisdom: A guide to the issues and feelings of adoption.* Lawrenceville, NJ: Tapestry Press.

Salladay, S. (2004). Ethical problems: Adoption dilemmas. *Nursing, 34*(12), 29.

Youngkin, E., & Davis, M. S. (1998). *Women's health: A primary care clinical guide* (2nd ed.). Upper Saddle River, NJ: Prentice Hall.

CHAPTER 11

Andrews, M. M., & Boyle, J. S. (2002). *Transcultural concepts in nursing care* (4th ed.). Philadelphia: Lippincott Williams & Wilkins.

Ball, J., & Bindler, R. (2003). *Pediatric nursing caring for children* (3rd ed.). Upper Saddle River, NJ: Prentice Hall.

Carter, B., & McGoldrick, M. (1999). *The expanded family life cycle—Individual, family, and social perspectives* (3rd ed.). Needham Heights, MA: Allyn & Bacon.

Cox, H., Hinz, M., Lubno, M. A., Scott-Tilley, D., Newfield, S., McCarthy Slater, M., & Sridaromont, K. (2002). *Clinical applications of nursing diagnosis: Adult, child, women's, psychiatric, gerontic, and home health considerations* (4th ed.). Philadelphia: FA Davis.

Eby, L. (2005). *Mental health nursing care.* Upper Saddle River, NJ: Prentice Hall.

Gralla, P. (2000). *The complete idiot's guide to internet privacy and security.* Indianapolis, IN: Alpha.

London, M. L., Ladewig, P. W., & Ball, J. W. (2003). *Maternal–newborn & child nursing: Family-centered care.* Upper Saddle River, NJ: Prentice Hall.

Marshall, W. A., & Tanner, J. M. (1969). Variations in the pattern of pubertal changes in girls. *Archives of Disease in Childhood, 445*(235), 291–303.

Marshall, W. A., & Tanner, J. M. (1970). Variations in the pattern of pubertal changes in boys. *Archives of Disease in Childhood, 45*(239), 13–23.

Olds, S. B., London, M. L., Ladewig, P. W., & Davidson, M. R. (2004). *Maternal–newborn nursing & women's health care* (7th ed.). Upper Saddle River, NJ: Prentice Hall.

Ramont, R. R., Niedringhause, D. M., & Towle, M. A. (2006). *Comprehensive nursing care.* Upper Saddle River, NJ: Prentice Hall.

Tanner, J. M. (1962). *Growth of adolescents.* Oxford: Blackwell.

Tanner, J. M. (1966). *Growth at adolescence.* New York: Appleton.

CHAPTER 12

Abraham, K. (2004). Recognizing and treating childhood obesity. *American Journal of Nurse Practitioners, 8*(9), 31–32, 3538.

Abrams, S. A. (2001). Calcium turnover and nutrition through the life cycle. *Proceedings of the Nutrition Society, 60*(2), 283–289.

American Academy of Pediatric Dentistry. (2003). *Clinical guidelines of fluoride therapy.* Chicago: Author.

American Academy of Pediatrics. (2001). The use and misuse of fruit juice in pediatrics. *Pediatrics, 107*(5), 1210–1213.

American Academy of Pediatrics. (2006). *Car safety seats: A guide for families.* Author.

Anderson, R. N., & Smith, B. L. (2005). *Deaths: Leading causes for 2002. National Vital Statistics Report* (Vol. 53, No. 17). Hyattsville, MD: National Center for Health Statistics.

Breastfeeding and the use of human milk. (2005). *Pediatrics, 115*(2), 496–506.

Consumer Product Safety Commission (CPSC). (2003). CPSC amends age guidelines. *CPSC Monitor*, April, 50.

Guidance for effective discipline. (2004). *Pediatrics, 114*(4), 1126.

Hay, W., Hayward, A., Levin, M., & Sondheimer, J. (2002). *Current pediatric diagnosis and treatment* (16th ed.). New York: McGraw-Hill.

Healthy people 2010. (2000). Rockville, MD: U.S. Department of Health and Human Services.

National Safety Council. (2004). *Child passenger safety: Fact sheet.* Washington, DC: Author.

O'Neil, J., Kelly, T., & Kirby, J. (1995). *350 Tested strategies to prevent crime: A resource for municipal agencies and community groups*. Washington, DC: National Crime Prevention Council.

Pediatric Nutrition Practice Group of the American Dietetic Association. (2003). *Infant feedings: Guidelines for preparation of formula and breast milk in health care facilities*. www.eatright.org/cps/rde/xchg/ada/hs.xsl/nutrition_1562_ENU_HTML.htm

U.S. Consumer Product Safety Commission. (2003). www.cpsc.gov

U.S. Department of Agriculture, Center for Nutrition Policy and Promotion. (2005, April). *My pyramid: Steps to a healthier you*. CNPP-15. Retrieved September 17, 2006, from www.mypyramid. gov/downloads/miniposter.pdf

U.S. Department of Health and Human Services. (1979). *Healthy people*. Washington, DC: U.S. Government Printing Office.

U.S. Department of Health and Human Services. (1980). *Promoting health/preventing illness: Objectives for the nation*. Washington, DC: U.S. Government Printing Office.

U.S. Department of Health and Human Services. (1991). *Healthy people 2000*. Washington, DC: U.S. Government Printing Office.

U.S. Department of Health and Human Services. (2000). *Healthy people 2010* (2nd ed.). Washington, DC: U.S. Government Printing Office.

Wilkinson, B. (1983). *The 7 laws of the learner: How to teach almost anything to practically anyone*. Sisters, OR: Multnomah Press.

CHAPTER 13

Bindler, R., & Howry, L. (2005). *Pediatric drug guide with nursing implications*. Upper Saddle River, NJ: Prentice Hall.

Bindler, R. C., Ball, J. W., London, M. L., & Ladewig, P. W. (2003). *Clinical skills manual for maternal–newborn and child nursing*. Upper Saddle River, NJ: Prentice Hall.

Blackwell, P., & Baker, B. (2002). Estimating communication competence of infants and toddlers. *Journal of Pediatric Health Care, 16*(1), 19–35.

Childbirth Graphics website. Available at www.childbirthgraphics.com

Humphries, J. (2002). The school health nurse and health education in the classroom. *Nursing Standard, 16*(17), 42–45.

Sydnor-Greenberg, N., & Dokken, D. (2001). Communication in healthcare: Thought on the child's perspective. *Journal of Child and Family Nursing, 4*(3), 225–230.

CHAPTER 14

Bindler, R., & Howry, L. (2005). *Pediatric drug guide with nursing implications*. Upper Saddle River, NJ: Prentice Hall.

Carney, K. L. (1998). *What is cancer anyway?* New York: Dragonfly.

McDaniel, L. (1993). *Let him live (one last wish)*. Boston: Laurel Leaf.

Newachek, P. A., McManus, M., Fix H. B., Hung, Y. Y., & Halfon, N. (2000). Access to health care for children with special health needs. *Pediatrics, 105*(4), 760–766.

Richmond, C. (1996). *Chemo Girl: Saving the world one treatment at a time*. New York: Jones & Bartlett.

CHAPTER 15

Atherly-John, Y., Cunningham, S., & Crain, E. (2002). A randomized trial of oral vs. intravenous rehydration in a pediatric emergency department. *Archives of Pediatric and Adolescent Medicine, 156*, 1240–1243.

Ball, J. W., & Bindler, R. C. (2003). *Pediatric nursing: Caring for children* (3rd ed.). Upper Saddle River, NJ: Prentice Hall.

Dale, J. (2004). Oral rehydration solutions in the management of acute gastroenteritis among children. *Journal of Pediatric Health Care, 18*(4), 211–212.

Fluid & electrolytes made incredibly easy. (2005). Philadelphia: Springhouse.

Hogan, M. A., & Wane, D. (2003). *Fluids, electrolytes, and acid–base balance, reviews and rationales*. Upper Saddle River, NJ: Prentice Hall.

Kee, J. (2005). *Laboratory and diagnostic tests with nursing implications* (7th ed.). Upper Saddle River, NJ: Prentice Hall.

Le, D., & Macnab, A. J. (2001). Self strangulation by hanging from cloth towel dispensers in Canadian schools. *Injury Prevention, 7*(3), 231–233.

Santosham, M. (2002). Oral rehydration therapy. *Archives of Pediatric and Adolescent Medicine, 156*, 1177–1179.

Shapiro, L. (2004). *The secret language of children: How to understand what your kids are really saying*. Naperville, IL: Sourcebooks.

Smith, S., Duell, D., & Martin, B. (2004). *Clinical nursing skills: Basic to advanced skills* (6th ed.). Upper Saddle River, NJ: Prentice Hall.

Wilson, B., Shannon, M., & Stang, C. (2006). *Nurses' drug guide*. Upper Saddle River, NJ: Prentice Hall.

CHAPTER 16

American Academy of Pediatrics, Committee on Fetus and Newborn & American College of Obstetricians and Gynecologists, Committee on Obstetrics. (2002). *Guidelines for perinatal care* (5th ed.). Evanston, IL: Author.

American Academy of Pediatrics, Committee on Quality Improvement, Subcommittee on Febrile Seizures. (1999). Practice parameter: Long-term treatment of the child with simple febrile seizures. *Pediatrics, 103*(6), 1307–1309.

American Association of Mental Retardation (AAMR). (2002). *The AAMR definition of mental retardation*. Available at www.aamr.org/Policies/pdf/definitionofMR.pdf

Ball, J. W., & Bindler, R. C. (2006). *Child health nursing: Partnering with children & families*. Upper Saddle River, NJ: Prentice Hall.

Crist, W. M. (2000). Neoplastic disease and tumors. In R. E. Behrman, R. M. Kliegman, & H. B. Jenson (Eds.), *Nelson textbook of pediatrics* (16th ed.). Philadelphia: WB Saunders.

D'Amico, D., & Barbarito, C. (2007). *Health and physical assessment in nursing*. Upper Saddle River, NJ: Prentice Hall.

Halloran, D. (2005). Hearing screening at well child visits. *Archives of Pediatric and Adolescent Medicine, 159*, 949–955.

Hospice and Palliative Nurses Association website. Available at www.hpna.org

The International Dyslexia Association. (2002). *Just the facts: Definition of dyslexia*. Available at www.interdys.org

Johnson, A. N. (2002). Update on newborn hearing screening programs. *Pediatric Nursing, 22*(3), 267–270.

Joseph, D. (2001). *Spina bifida association fact sheet: Urologic care and management*. Available at www.sbaa.org/site/PageServer?pagename=fs_managment

Kassin, S. (2001). *Psychology* (3rd ed.). Upper Saddle River, NJ: Prentice Hall.

Kee, J. (2005). *Laboratory and diagnostic tests with nursing implications* (7th ed.). Upper Saddle River, NJ: Prentice Hall.

LeMone, P., & Burke, K. (2004). *Medical-surgical nursing* (3rd ed.). Upper Saddle River, NJ: Prentice Hall.

Melzack, R., & Wall, P. (1965). Pain mechanisms: A new theory. *Science, 150*, 971–979.

The National Hospice and Palliative Care Organization website. Available at www.nhpco.org/templates/1/homepage.cfm

Niemala, M., Pihakari, O., Pokka, T., & Uhari, M. S. (2000). Pacifier as a risk factor for acute otitis media: A randomized, controlled trial of parental counseling. *Pediatrics, 106,* 483–488.

Olson, S. L. (1998). Bedside musical care: Applications in pregnancy, childbirth, and neonatal care. *JOGNN, 27*(5), 569–575.

Peck, P. (2005). Listen up: Cradle to grave, many Americans can't hear what is being said. *MedPage Today,* November 8.

Peck, P. (2005). Sound vs. silence may divide those with hearing loss. *MedPage Today,* November 8.

Pepino, M., & Mennella, J. (2005). Sucrose-induced analgesia is related to sweet preferences in children but not in adults. *Pain, 119,* 210–218.

Shachtman, T. (2006). Medical sleuth. *Smithsonian,* February, 23–30.

Smith, S., Duell, D., & Martin, B. (2004). *Clinical nursing skills: Basic to advanced skills* (6th ed.). Upper Saddle River, NJ: Prentice Hall.

Wilson, B., Shannon, M., & Stang, C. (2006). *Nurses' drug guide.* Upper Saddle River, NJ: Prentice Hall.

Wismer Fries, A., Ziegler, T., Kurian, J., Jacoris., S., & Pollack, S. (2005). Early experience in humans is associated with changes in neuropeptides critical for regulating social behavior. *Proceedings of the National Academy of Sciences, 103,* 17237–17240.

CHAPTER 17

American Academy of Pediatrics. (2001). Strength training by children and adolescents. *Pediatrics, 107*(6), 1470–1472.

American Association of Cheerleading Coaches and Advisors. (2000). *Position paper addressing the issue of cheerleading as a sport.* Accessed at www.aacca.org American College of Sports Medicine website. Available at www.acsm.org

Anrig, C. (2004). Relief versus wellness care in the family practice. *Dynamic Chiropractic, 22,* 7.

Anrig, C. (2005). The backpack dilemma: Function vs. fashion. *Dynamic Chiropractic, 23,* 18.

Ball, J., & Bindler, R. (2006). *Child health nursing: Partnering with children & families.* Upper Saddle River, NJ: Prentice Hall.

D'Amico, D., & Barbarito, C. (2007). *Health & physical assessment in nursing.* Upper Saddle River, NJ: Prentice Hall.

Fallon, J. M. (2004). The role of the chiropractic adjustment in the care and treatment of 332 children with otitis media. *Journal of Clinical Chiropractic Pediatrics, 2,* 167–183.

Hart, E. S. (2003, April 22). *Boston brace: The role of bracing in the treatment of idiopathic scoliosis.* Boston: Massachusetts General Hospital Orthopaedic Surgery.

Kee, J. (2005). *Laboratory and diagnostic tests with nursing implications* (7th ed.). Upper Saddle River, NJ: Prentice Hall.

Lee, A. C., Li, D. H., & Kemper, K. J. (2000). Chiropractic care for children. *Archives of Pediatric and Adolescent Medicine, 154,* 401–407.

Macias, B. R., Murthy, G., Chambers, H., & Hargens, A. (2005). High contact pressure beneath backpack straps of children contributes to pain. *Archives of Pediatrics and Adolescent Medicine, 159*(12), 1186–1187.

National Center for Health Statistics. (2001). *Sports-related injuries cause 2.6 million visits annually by children and young adults to emergency rooms.* Hyattsville, MD: Author.

National Clearinghouse on Child Abuse and Neglect Information (DHHS). (2003). Recognizing child abuse and neglect: Signs and symptoms. Washington, DC: Author.

Sheir-Neiss, G. I., Kruse, R. W., Rahman, T., et al. (2003). The association of backpack use and back pain in adolescents. *Spine, 28*(9), 922–930.

Shields, B., & Smith, G. (2006). Cheerleading related injuries to children 5 to 18 years of age: United States 1990–2002. *Pediatrics, 117,* 122–129.

Smith, S., Duell, D., & Martin, B. (2004). *Clinical nursing skills: Basic to advanced skills* (6th ed.). Upper Saddle River, NJ: Prentice Hall.

Wilkinson, J. (2000). *Nursing diagnosis handbook* (7th ed.). Upper Saddle River, NJ: Prentice Hall.

Wilson, B., Shannon, M., & Stang, C. (2006). *Nurses' drug guide.* Upper Saddle River, NJ: Prentice Hall.

CHAPTER 18

Aligne, C. A., Auinger, P., Byrd, R. S., & Weitzman, M. (2000). Risk factors for pediatric asthma. *American Journal of Respiratory and Critical Care Medicine, 162*(3), 873–877.

Baroi, M., Anderson, Y., & Mischler, E. (1997). Cystic fibrosis newborn screening: Impact of early screening results on parenting stress. *Pediatric Nursing, 23*(2), 143–151.

Bindler, R., & Howry, L. (2005). *Prentice Hall pediatric drug guide with nursing implications.* Upper Saddle River, NJ: Prentice Hall.

Clinical practice guideline: Diagnosis and management of childhood obstructive sleep apnea syndrome. (2002). *Pediatrics, 109*(4), 704–712.

Everydaykidz website. Available at www.Everydaykidz.com

Gutierrez, K., & Queener, S. F. (2003). *Pharmacology for nursing practice.* St. Louis, MO: Mosby.

Marcus, C. L., Chapman, D., Ward, S. D., McColley, S. A. (2003). Clinical practice guideline: Diagnosis and management of childhood obstructive sleep apnea syndrome. *Pediatrics, 109*(4), 704–712.

Paradise, J. L. (2002). Tonsillectomy and adenotonsillectomy for recurrent throat infection in moderately affected children. *Pediatrics, 110*(1), 7–15.

Ramilo, O., & Jafri, H. (2004). RSV can increase the risk of asthma. *Journal of Infectious Diseases, 189*(10), 1856–1865.

CHAPTER 19

Ball, J., & Bindler, R. (2006). *Child health nursing: Partnering with children & families.* Upper Saddle River, NJ: Prentice Hall.

Bernardini, R. (2003). *The truth about children's health: The comprehensive guide to understanding, preventing and reversing disease.* New York: Pri.

Connor, J. A. (2002). Alternations in cardiovascular function in children. In K. L. McCance & S. E. Huether (Eds.), *Pathophysiology: The biologic basis for disease in adults and children* (4th ed., pp. 1048–1081). St. Louis, MO: Mosby.

D'Amico, D., & Barbarito, C. (2007). *Health & physical assessment in nursing.* Upper Saddle River, NJ: Prentice Hall.

Grifka, R. G. (1999). Cyanotic congenital heart disease with increased blood flow. *Pediatric Clinics of North America, 46*(2), 420–4.

Kavey, R. E., Daniels, S. R., Lauer, R. M., Atkins, D. L., Hayman, L. L., & Taubert, K. (2003). American Heart Association guidelines for primary prevention of atherosclerotic cardiovascular disease beginning in childhood. *Circulation, 107*(11), 1562–1566.

Kee, J. (2005). *Laboratory and diagnostic tests with nursing implications* (7th ed.). Upper Saddle River, NJ: Prentice Hall.

Mussatto, K. A., & Tweddell, J. S. (2005). Quality of life following surgery for congenital cardiac malformations in neonates and infants. *Cardiology in the Young, 15*(suppl 1), 174–178.

Mussatto, K. A., & Wernovsky, G. (2005). Challenges facing the child, adolescent and young adult after the arterial switch surgery. *Cardiology in the Young, 15*(suppl 1), 111–121.

National High Blood Pressure Working Group on High Blood Pressure in Children and Adolescents. (2004). The fourth report on the diagnosis, evaluation, and treatment of high blood pressure in children and adolescents. *Pediatrics, 114*(2), 555–576.

Rempel, G. R. (2004). Technological advances in pediatrics: Challenges for parents and nurses. *Journal of Pediatric Nursing, 19*(1), 13–24.

Rempel, G. R., Cender, L. M., Lynam, M. J., Sandor, G. G., & Farquharson, D. (2004). Parents' perspectives on decision making after antenatal diagnosis of congenital heart disease. *Journal of Obstetric, Gynecologic, and Neonatal Nursing, 33*(1), 64–70.

Smith, S., Duell, D., & Martin, B. (2004). *Clinical nursing skills: Basic to advanced skills* (6th ed.). Upper Saddle River, NJ: Prentice Hall.

Soetenga, D., & Mussatto, K. A. (2004). Management of infants with hypoplastic left heart syndrome: Integrating research into nursing practice. *Critical Care Nurse, 24*(6), 46–66.

Sothern, M., & Almen, T. (2001). *Trim kids: The proven 12-week plan that has helped thousands of children achieve a healthier weight*. London: Harper Collins.

Taubert, K. (1994). Seven-year national survey of Kawasaki disease and acute rheumatic fever. *Pediatric Infectious Disease Journal, 13*, 704–708.

Wilkinson, J. (2000). *Nursing diagnosis handbook* (7th ed.). Upper Saddle River, NJ: Prentice Hall.

Wilson, B., Shannon, M., & Stang, C. (2006). *Nurses' drug guide*. Upper Saddle River, NJ: Prentice Hall.

CHAPTER 20

Ball, J. W., & Bindler, R. C. (2006). *Child health nursing: Partnering with children and families*. Upper Saddle River, NJ: Prentice Hall.

D'Amico, D., & Barbarito, C. (2007). *Health and physical assessment in nursing*. Upper Saddle River, NJ: Prentice Hall.

Kee, J. (2005). *Laboratory and diagnostic tests with nursing implications* (7th ed.). Upper Saddle River, NJ: Prentice Hall.

Lemone, P., & Burke, K. (2004). *Medical-surgical nursing: Critical thinking in client care* (3rd ed.). Upper Saddle River, NJ: Prentice Hall.

The Leukemia & Lymphoma Society website. Available at www.leukemia.org

National Cancer Institute website. Available at www.cancer.gov

Pui, C. H., Campana, D., & Evans, W. E. (2001). Childhood acute lymphoblastic leukaemia—Current status and future perspectives. *Lancet Oncology, 2*(10), 597–607.

Pui, C. H., Sandlund, J. T., Pei, D., et al. (2003). Results of therapy for acute lymphoblastic leukemia in black and white children. *JAMA, 290*(15), 2001–2007.

Smith, S., Duell, D., & Martin, B. (2004). *Clinical nursing skills: Basic to advanced skills* (6th ed.). Upper Saddle River, NJ: Prentice Hall.

Wilkinson, J. (2000). *Nursing diagnosis handbook* (7th ed.). Upper Saddle River, NJ: Prentice Hall.

Wilson, B., Shannon, M., & Stang, C. (2006). *Nurses' drug guide*. Upper Saddle River, NJ: Prentice Hall.

CHAPTER 21

AIDS Alliance for Children, Youth and Families website. Available at www.aids-alliance.org

Arthritis Foundation. Systemic lupus erythematosus (lupus) in children and adolescents. Retrieved November 22, 2006 from http://www.arthritis.org/conditions/DiseaseCenter/JLupus/intro.asp

Ball, J. W., & Bindler, R. C. (2006). *Child health nursing: Partnering with children and families*. Upper Saddle River, NJ: Prentice Hall.

D'Amico, D., & Barbarito, C. (2007). *Health and physical assessment in nursing*. Upper Saddle River, NJ: Prentice Hall.

Ignatavicius, D. D., Workman, M. L, & Mishler, M. A. (1995). *Medical-surgical nursing: A nursing process approach* (2nd ed.). Philadelphia: WB Saunders.

Kee, J. (2005). *Laboratory and diagnostic tests with nursing implications* (7th ed.). Upper Saddle River, NJ: Prentice Hall.

NANDA International. (2005). *NANDA nursing diagnoses: Definitions and classifications 2005–2006*. Philadelphia: Saunders.

Smith, S., Duell, D., & Martin, B. (2004). *Clinical nursing skills: Basic to advanced skills* (6th ed.). Upper Saddle River, NJ: Prentice Hall.

Stichweh, D., Arce, E., & Pascual, V. (2004). Update on pediatric systemic lupus erythematosus. *Current Opinion in Rheumatology, 16*, 577–587.

Wilkinson, J. (2000). *Nursing diagnosis handbook* (7th ed.). Upper Saddle River, NJ: Prentice Hall.

Wilson, B., Shannon, M., & Stang, C. (2006). *Nurses' drug guide*. Upper Saddle River, NJ: Prentice Hall.

CHAPTER 22

Ariza, A. J., Chen, E. H., Binns, H. J., Christoffel, K. K. (2004). Risk factors for overweight in five- to six-year-old Hispanic-American children: A pilot study. *Journal of Urban Health, 81,* 150–161.

Bindler, R., & Howry, L. (2005). *Pediatric drug guide with nursing implications*. Upper Saddle River, NJ: Prentice Hall.

Bowman, S., Gortmaker, S., Ebbeling, C., et al. (2004). Effects of fast-food consumption on energy intake and diet quality among children in a national household survey. *Pediatrics, 113*(1), 112–118.

Freeland-Graves, J., & Nitzke, S. (2002). Position of the American Dietetic Association: Total diet approach to communicating food and nutrition information. *Journal of the American Dietetic Association, 102*, 100–108.

Kalliomäki, M., Salminen, S., Poussa, T., Arvilommi, H., & Isolauri, E. (2003). Probiotics and prevention of atopic disease: 4 year follow-up of randomized placebo-controlled trial. *Lancet, 361*(9372), 1869–1871.

Nestle, M. (2002). *Food politics: How the food industry influences nutrition and health*. Berkeley: University of California Press.

Pick, M. (2006). *Probiotics—For life!* Portland, ME: Women to Women. Retrieved September 17, 2006, from www.womentowomen.com/digestionandgihealth/probiotics.asp

Taveras, E., Berkey, C., Rifas-Shiman, S., Ludwig, D., et al. (2005). Association of consumption of fried food away from home with body mass index and diet quality in older children and adolescents. *Pediatrics, 116*(4), e518–e524.

Wong, W. Y., Eskes, T. K., Kuihpers-Jagtman, A. M., Spauwen, P. H., Steegers, E. A., et al. (1999). Nonsyndromic orofacial clefts: Association with maternal hyperhomocysteinemia. *Teratology, 60*, 253–257.

Yuan, M., Konstantopoulos, N., Lee, J., Shulman, G. et al. (2001). Reversal of Obesity- and Diet-Induced Insulin Resistance with Salicylates or Targeted Disruption of Ikk^β *Science, 293,* 1673–1677.

CHAPTER 23

Ball, J. W., & Bindler, R. C. (2006). *Child health nursing: Partnering with children and families*. Upper Saddle River, NJ: Prentice Hall.

Campoy, S. (2005). Pharmacology and chronic kidney disease: How chronic kidney disease and its complications alter drug response. *American Journal of Nursing, 105*(9), 60–71.

Condon, M. (2004). *Women's health: Body, mind, spirit: An integrated approach to wellness and illness*. Upper Saddle River, NJ: Prentice Hall.

D'Amico, D., & Barbarito, C. (2007). *Health and physical assessment in nursing*. Upper Saddle River, NJ: Prentice Hall.

Greydanus, D. (2003). *American Academy of Pediatrics: Caring for your teenager*. New York: Bantam.

Greydanus, D. (2003). *American Academy of Pediatrics: Caring for your teenager*. New York: Bantam.

Kee, J. (2005). *Laboratory and diagnostic tests with nursing implications* (7th ed.). Upper Saddle River, NJ: Prentice Hall.

Legg, V. (2005). Complications of chronic kidney disease. *American Journal of Nursing, 105*(6), 40–49.

Lichtman, R. (2005). *Gynecology: Well-woman care* (2nd ed.). Upper Saddle River, NJ: Prentice Hall.

London, M. L., Ladewig, P. W., Ball, J. W., & Bindler, R. C. (2007). *Maternal & child nursing care* (2nd ed.). Upper Saddle River, NJ: Prentice Hall.

Lopez, R. I. (2003). *The teen health book: A parent's guide to adolescent health and well-being.* New York: WW Norton & Company.

Mercer, R. (2003). Dry at night: Treating nocturnal enuresis. *Advances for Nurse Practitioners*, February, 26–32.

National Kidney and Urologic Diseases Clearinghouse. *How can urinary tract infection be prevented?* Bethesda, MD: Author. Retrieved September 5, 2006, from www.niddk.nih.gov

National Women's Health Information Center. (2003). *A lifetime of good health: Your guide to staying healthy.* Washington, DC: U.S. Department of Health and Human Services.

The Pennsylvania State University Health Services. (2005, September 30). *What happens during a pelvic exam.* Retrieved September 17, 2006, from www.sa.psu.edu/uhs/womenshealth/pelvicexam.cfm

Reichert, G. (1998). Female circumcision: What you need to know about genital mutilation. *Lifelines, 2*(3), 28–34.

Reisser, P. (2002). *Teen health guide.* Colorado Springs, CO: Focus on the Family.

Smith, S., Duell, D., & Martin, B. (2004). *Clinical nursing skills: Basic to advanced skills* (6th ed.). Upper Saddle River, NJ: Prentice Hall.

Varney Burst, H. (2004). *Varney's midwifery* (4th ed.). Sudbury, MA: Jones and Bartlett.

WebMD. *A–Z health guide from WebMD: Medical tests.* Retrieved September 17, 2006, from www.webmd.com/hw/healthy_women/hw5266.asp

Wilkinson, J. (2000). *Nursing diagnosis handbook* (7th ed.). Upper Saddle River, NJ: Prentice Hall.

Wilson, B., Shannon, M., & Stang, C. (2006). *Nurses' drug guide.* Upper Saddle River, NJ: Prentice Hall.

Youngkin, E., & Davis, M. (2004). *Women's health: A primary care clinical guide* (3rd ed.). Upper Saddle River, NJ: Prentice Hall.

CHAPTER 24

American Academy of Dermatology, in cooperation with Federal Drug Administration. (1997, February 4). *The darker side of tanning.* Retrieved September 26, 2006, from www.fda.gov/cdrh/consumer/ tanning.html

Atherton, P. (1997). Aloe vera: Myth or medicine? *Positive Health 20.* Retrieved June 20, 2006 from www.positivehealth.com

Ball, J., & Bindler, R. (2006). *Child health nursing: Partnering with children & families.* Upper Saddle River, NJ: Prentice Hall.

Center for Young Women's Health, Children's Hospital Boston. (2006, August 1). *Body piercing: A guide for teens.* Retrieved September 26, 2006, from www.youngwomenshealth.org/body-piercing.html

Dillon, P. (2003). *Nursing health assessment: A critical thinking case studies approach.* Philadelphia: FA Davis.

Flinders, D., & De Schweinitz, P. (2004). Pediculosis and scabies. *American Family Physician, 69*, 341.

Hatfield, N. (2003). *Introductory pediatric nursing.* Philadelphia: Lippincott Williams & Wilkins.

Kemper, K., Gardiner, P., & Coles, D. (2001). The skinny on herbal remedies for dermatologic disorders. *Contemporary Pediatrics, 7*, 103.

International Aloe Science Council. (2002). The complete story of aloe vera. Retrieved June 20, 2006 from www.tasc.org.

La Leche League International. (2006, March 17). *FAQ on tattoos and breastfeeding.* Retrieved September 26, 2006, from www.lalecheleague. org/FAQ/tattoos.html

National Institute of Arthritis and Musculoskeletal and Skin Disorders (NIAMS). (2003, April). *Defining dermatitis.* Retrieved September 26, 2006, from www.niams.nih.gov/hi/topics/dermatitis/#link_a

National Institute of Arthritis and Musculoskeletal and Skin Disorders (NIAMS). (2003, April). *Handout on health: Atopic dermatitis.* Retrieved September 26, 2006, from www.niams.nih.gov/hi/topics/dermatitis/ index.html

Potts, N., & Mandleco, B. (2002). *Pediatric nursing caring for children and their families.* Albany: Delmar.

Skin Cancer Foundation Nursing. www.skincancer.org/artificial/ index.php

Stein, K. (2001). Piercing perils & tattoo taboo. *Dermatology Insights,* Fall, 14–15. Retrieved September 26, 2006, from www.aad.org/NR/ rdonlyres/529273A8-FD17-4C59-94FB-2097D436DBE4/0/ DIfall01.pdf#page=16

CHAPTER 25

American Academy of Pediatrics, Section on Endocrinology and Committee on Genetics. (2000). Technical report: Congenital adrenal hyperplasia. *Pediatrics, 106*(6), 1511–1518.

American Diabetes Association. (2000). Type 2 diabetes I children and adolescents. *Diabetes Care, 23*(3), 381–389.

Jacobson-Dickman, E., & Levitsky, L. (2005). Oral agents in managing diabetes mellitus in children and adolescents. *Pediatric Clinics of North America, 52*(6), 1689–1703.

Kidson, W. (1998). Polycystic ovary syndrome: A new direction in treatment. *Medical Journal of Australia, 169*, 537–540.

Largo, R. S., Gnatuk, C. L., Kunselman, A. R., & Dunaif, A. (2005). Change in glucose tolerance over time in women with polycystic ovarian syndrome: A controlled study. *Journal of Clinical Endocrinology and Metabolism, 90*(6), 3236–3242.

London, M. L., Ladewig, P. W., Ball, J. W., and Bindler, R. C. (2007). *Maternal and child nursing care* (2nd ed.). Upper Saddle River, NJ: Prentice Hall.

Robinson, D., & Drumm, L. (2001). Maple syrup urine disease: A standard of nursing care. *Pediatric Nursing, 27*(3), 255–264, 270.

Tay-Sach's disease. www.marchofdimes.com/professional 681_1227.asp

CHAPTER 26

Allen, P. (2006). Avian influenza pandemic: Not if, but when. *Pediatric Nursing, 32*(1), 76–81.

American Academy of Pediatrics. (2003). *Red book: Report of the Committee on Infectious Disease* (26th ed.). Elk Grove Village, IL: Author.

Ball, J., & Bindler, R. (2006). *Child health nursing: Partnering with children & families.* Upper Saddle River, NJ: Prentice Hall.

Bindler, R. M., & Howry, L. (2005). *Pediatric drugs with nursing implications.* Upper Saddle River, NJ: Prentice Hall.

D'Amico, D., & Barbarito, C. (2007). *Health & physical assessment in nursing.* Upper Saddle River, NJ: Prentice Hall.

Immunization Action Coalition. (2004). *Mosby's drug consult 2004.* St. Louis: Mosby.

Kee, J. (2005). *Laboratory and diagnostic tests with nursing implications* (7th ed.). Upper Saddle River, NJ: Prentice Hall.

Peck, P. (2006). FDA approves diarrhea vaccine for infants. *MedPage Today,* February 13.

Prymula, R. (2006). Pneumococcal capsular polysaccharides conjugated to protein D for prevention of acute otitis media caused by both *Streptococcus pneumoniae* and *Haemophilus influenza*: A randomized double-blind efficacy study. *Lancet, 367*(9509), 740–748.

Ray, M., & Walker-Jenkins, A. (2006). Confronting bird flu: Will pandemic avian flu be the next public health threat? *Lifelines, 10*(1), 21–29.

Rosenfeld, I. (2006, April 6). New vaccines that protect the young. *Parade Magazine,* p. 20.

Sheff, B. (2006). Avian influenza: Poised to launch a pandemic? *Nursing2006, 36*(1), 51–53.

Smith, S., Duell D., & Martin, B. (2004). *Clinical nursing skills: Basic to advanced skills* (6th ed.). Upper Saddle River, NJ: Prentice Hall.

Wilkinson, J. (2000). *Nursing diagnosis handbook* (7th ed.). Upper Saddle River, NJ: Prentice Hall.

Wilson, B., Shannon, M., & Stang, C. (2006). *Nurses' drug guide.* Upper Saddle River, NJ: Prentice Hall.

CHAPTER 27

Ball, J., & Bindler, R. (2006). *Child health nursing: Partnering with children & families.* Upper Saddle River, NJ: Prentice Hall.

D'Amico, D., & Barbarito, C. (2007). *Health & physical assessment in nursing.* Upper Saddle River, NJ: Prentice Hall.

Eby, E. (2005). Creativity and depression. Retrieved February 2, 2006 from http://ezinearticles.com/?expert=Doublas_Eby

Faraone, S., Sergeant, J., Gillberg, C., Biederman, J. (2003). The worldwide prevalence of ADHD: Is it an American condition? *World Psychiatry, 2*(2), 104–113.

Findling, R. L., et al. (2003). Combination lithium and divalproex sodium in pediatric bipolarity. *Journal of the American Academy of Child & Adolescent Psychiatry, 42*(8), 908–914.

Findling, R. L., McNamara, N. O'Riordan, M. A., Reed, M. D., et al. (2003, August). An open-label pilot study of St. John's wort in juvenile depression. *Journal of the American Academy of Child and Adolescent Psychiatry, 42,* 908–914.

Flora, D. (2006). Changes in drug use during young adulthood: The effects of parent alcoholism and transition into marriage. *Psychology of Addiction Behaviors, 19*(4), 18–20.

Glewe, G. (2005). Bullying, psychosocial adjustment, and academic performance in elementary school. *Archives of Pediatric and Adolescent Medicine, 159,* 1026–1031.

Inge, T. H., Krebs, N. F., Garcia, V. F., Skelton, J. A., Guice, K. S., Strauss, R. S., et al. (2004). Bariatric surgery for severely overweight adolescents: Concerns and recommendations. *Pediatrics, 114*(1), 217–223.

Joint Commission on Accreditation of Healthcare Organization (JCAHO). http://www.jointcommission.org

National Center for Missing and Exploited Children. (2005). *For healthcare professionals: guidelines on prevention of and response to infant abductions* (8th ed.). Retrieved September 26, 2006, from www.missingkids.com/en_US/publications/NC05.pdf

Office of Disease Prevention and Health Promotion, U.S. Department of Health and Human Services. (2006). *Healthy people 2010.* Washington, DC: Author. Retrieved September 26, 2006, from www.healthypeople.gov

Shogan, M. G. (2002). Emergency management plan for newborn abductions. *Journal of Obstetric, Gynecologic, and Neonatal Nursing, 31*(3), 340–346.

Vlam, S. (2006). Attention-deficit/hyperactivity disorder: Diagnostic assessment methods used by advanced practice registered nurses. *Pediatric Nursing, 32*(1), 18–24.

CHAPTER 28

Death and dying. (1997). *Hinduism Today.* Published by Hindu Press International; retrieved September 25, 2006 from www.hinduismtoday.com

Eby, L. (2005). *Mental health nursing care.* Upper Saddle River, NJ: Prentice Hall.

Farrell, M. M., & Levine, D. L. (1993). Brain death in the pediatric patient: Historical sociological, medical, religious, cultural, legal and ethical considerations. *Critical Care Medicine, 21*(12), 1951–1965.

Funeral rites and customs. (2000). *Microsoft Encarta Encyclopedia.*

Gootman, M. E. (1994). *When a friend dies: A book for teens about grieving and healing.* Minneapolis: Free Spirit.

Greenlee, S. (1992). *When someone dies.* Atlanta: Peachtree.

How to relieve pain without medicine. (2004, November 15). *Medical News Today.* Retrieved September 26, 2006, from http://www.medicalnewstoday.com/medicalnews.php?newsid=16373

Koch D'Agostino, C. (1998, September). Issues in pediatric organ donation. *Jacksonville Medicine/Northeast Florida Medicine.* Retrieved September 25, 2006 from

Kübler-Ross, E. (1969). *On death and dying.* New York: Macmillan.

LeMone, P., & Burke, K. (2004). *Medical surgical nursing critical thinking in client care* (3rd ed.). Upper Saddle River, NJ: Pearson Education.

London, Ladewig, Ball, & Bindler. (2003). *Maternal–newborn & child nursing.* Upper Saddle River, NJ: Prentice Hall.

National Association of School Psychologists (NASP). (2001, October 22). *Helping children cope with loss, death, and grief: Response to a national tragedy.* Retrieved September 26, 2006, from www.nasponline.org/NEAT/grief.html

Organ Procurement and Transplantation Network. www.optn.org Organ Procurement and Transplantation Network (OPTN) is the unified transplant network established by the United Network for Organ Sharing. www.unos.org This site provides information about living donation, collects and manages data about every transplant event occurring in the United States Congress under the National Organ Transplant Act (NOTA) of 1984.

Spector, R. E. (2000). *Cultural diversity in health and illness* (5th ed., pp. 137–138, 144–149). Upper Saddle River, NJ: Prentice Hall Health.

Wolfelt, A. (2001). *Healing your grieving heart for kids.* Ft. Collins, CO: Companion.

Worden, J. W. (1991). *Talking to children about death.* Paper presented at the 1991 ADEC annual meeting. www.Hospice.net

Worden, J. W. (1996). *Children and grief: When a parent dies.* New York: Gilford Press.

Glossary

(Note: Glossary terms may appear in several chapters. Boldface numbers after the glossary term indicate the chapter(s) in which the term is defined. Other words or terms that may require definitions are italicized in the text and are defined there.)

A

Abortifacients: abortion-inducing agents **(6)**

Abortion: the termination of a pregnancy before the fetus is viable **(5, 6)**

Acetone breath: breath with odor of nail polish remover or rotting apples, indicating diabetic ketoacidosis **(25)**

Acidosis: condition that develops when there is an increase of hydrogen ion concentration; body pH less than 7.36 **(15)**

Acquired immunity: immunity that is developed over a period of time after birth by exposure to foreign substances; developed through humoral immunity and cell-mediated immunity **(21)**

Acquired immunodeficiency syndrome (AIDS): a life-threatening, end-stage infection with HIV **(5)**

Acrocyanosis: bluish discoloration of the hands and feet common in neonates for several hours after delivery **(9)**

Acrosome: a specialized structure at the head of the sperm containing enzymes that can break down the covering of the ovum **(4)**

Active immunity: process in which the body reacts rapidly by producing a specific antibody to stop or slow the growth of an antigen until white blood cells can destroy it. The body will recognize and respond faster on future exposure to the antigen **(21, 26)**

Active phase: part of first stage of labor, from 4 to 8 cm of cervical dilatation, with moderate to strong contractions occurring every 3 to 5 minutes and lasting 60 to 90 seconds **(7)**

Active transport: movement of solutes across the cell membrane by means of metabolic activity and carrier cells **(15)**

Acute: having a rapid onset, severe symptoms, and a short course **(14)**

Acute conjunctivitis: (also known as *pinkeye*) inflammation of the conjunctiva caused by allergies, bacteria, or viruses **(16)**

Acute lymphoblastic leukemia (ALL): overproduction of immature lymphocytes **(20)**

Acute myelogenous leukemia (AML): condition that occurs when cancer cells develop in the bone marrow (*myeloid tissue*) **(20)**

Acute renal failure (ARF): sudden onset of diminished kidney function, resulting in the imbalance of fluids and electrolytes **(23)**

Adaptability: the ability to change when faced with problems **(3)**

Adoption: legal transfer of responsibility for raising a child from the birth mother to the adoptive parent(s) **(5)**

Adrenocorticotropic hormone (ACTH): hormone that stimulates the adrenal cortex to increase in size and to secrete larger amounts of its hormones, especially cortisol (hydrocortisone) **(25)**

Afterload: resistance against which the ventricles pump **(19)**

Afterpains: discomfort from uterine contraction after delivery **(10)**

Agglutination: after vasoconstriction, the clumping together of red blood cells **(20)**

Airborne transmission: transmission of harmful organisms suspended in the air **(26)**

Aldosterone: hormone that increases blood sodium and decreases potassium by influencing the renal tubule **(25)**

Algor mortis: gradual decrease of the body's temperature after death **(28)**

Alkalosis: condition that develops when there is a decrease of hydrogen ion concentration; body's pH more than 7.44 **(15)**

Allergy: altered reaction to an antigen or allergen **(21)**

Alveoli: glandular cells that are arranged in grapelike clusters, as in the lung **(4)**

Ambiguous genitalia: a rare condition in which determining the gender of the infant is difficult **(9)**

Amblyopia: (also known as *lazy eye*) reduction of vision in one eye **(16)**

Amenorrhea: absence of menses **(6)**

Amniocentesis: the withdrawal of amniotic fluid through a needle inserted into the abdomen and the uterus as a means of gathering data about the developing fetus **(6)**

Amnion: inner layer of the fetal membranes, originating from inside the blastocyst **(6)**

Amniotic fluid: fluid formed by the amnion, consisting of about 98% water, and containing glucose, proteins, urea, lanugo (fine fetal hair), and vernix caseosa **(6)**

Amniotomy: artificial rupturing of the fetal membranes **(7)**

Anaphylactic shock: systemic reaction to an allergen that occurs within minutes or up to 2 hours after exposure **(21)**

Androgens: steroid hormones, such as testosterone or androsterone, that control the development and maintenance of masculine characteristics; in females, they stimulate the female sex drive **(25)**

Anemia: decrease in the number of red blood cells and a decrease in hemoglobin or both **(20)**

Anions: negatively charged electrolytes **(15)**

Anomalies: abnormal development of an organ or structure **(6)**

Anorexia nervosa: eating disorder characterized by weight loss, emaciation, and an exaggerated fear of gaining weight **(27)**

Antibodies: protein substances produced in the blood or tissues in response to a specific antigen **(21)**

Antidiuretic hormone (ADH): hormone that accelerates the reabsorption of water from urine back into the blood in the renal tubules; important in preventing dehydration **(25)**

Antigenic drift: minor genetic changes that occur to the virus as it replicates within host cells **(26)**

Antigenic shift: abrupt or major change in a virus that makes it capable of infecting humans **(26)**

Antigens: foreign substances that when introduced into the body stimulate the production of an antibody **(21)**

Antrum: the cavity of a hollow organ or a sinus, as the *antrum* of the Graafian follicle **(4)**

Apgar score: rapid evaluation of an infant's adaptation to extrauterine life in five areas (by priority): heart rate, respiratory rate, muscle tone, reflex irritability, and color; each item is assigned a score from 0 to 2, and the scores are totaled **(7)**

Apnea: brief period of absence or cessation of breathing **(18)**

Apneic spells: periods without breathing **(9)**

Appendicitis: inflammation of the vermiform appendix, a small sac at the end of the cecum **(22)**

Areola: the colored ring around the nipple **(4)**

Arrector pili: an involuntary muscle that raises hair vertically in response to cold or fear **(24)**

Artificial insemination: process of artificially instilling sperm into the vagina or uterus **(5)**

Ascites: an abnormal accumulation of serous fluid in the abdominal cavity **(23)**

Asperger's syndrome: disorder similar to autism in which the child exhibits social isolation, communication difficulties, clumsiness, and a focused area of interest and attention **(27)**

Assault: sudden, violent physical attack on someone **(27)**

Assisted suicide: (also known as *voluntary euthanasia*) situations in which the dying individual desires control over the time and manner of death **(28)**

Associative play: learning to share and work together on a project **(12)**

Asthma: chronic inflammatory disorder of the tracheobronchial tree **(18)**

Astigmatism: uneven focusing of light resulting in blurred images **(16)**

Atelectasis: congenital condition characterized by the incomplete expansion of the lungs at birth **(18)**

Aura: recognizable sensation that signals a seizure is about to occur **(16)**

Autism: complex developmental disability that typically appears during the first 3 years of life and is the result of a neurologic disorder that affects the normal functioning of the brain, impacting development in the areas of social interaction and communication skills **(27)**

Autogenous graft: skin graft in which skin is transplanted from one site to another in the same recipient **(21)**

Autoimmune: immune response by the body against itself **(21)**

Autonomic reflexes: reflexes that control cardiac and smooth muscles and glands **(16)**

Autopsy: (also known as *postmortem examination*) examination of the body after death to determine more details about the cause of death, the disease, or other data **(28)**

Autosomes: chromosomes that are alike in males and females **(4)**

Avian flu: (also known as *bird flu* or *H5N1*) illness caused by influenza viruses that occur naturally among wild birds and are deadly to domestic birds, and which, if transmitted to humans, could spark a pandemic **(26)**

Axon: fiber carrying the impulse away from a nerve cell body **(16)**

B

Babinski's reflex: reflex elicited by stroking the lateral side of the foot from heel to toe; the big toe should dorsiflex and the other toes should flare; this reflex disappears before the infant begins to walk **(9)**

Bag of waters: the fetal membranes **(6)**

Balanoposthitis: inflammation or infection of the glans penis **(23)**

Balloon atrial septostomy: (also known as *Rashkind procedure*): procedure in which an enlargement of the existing opening in the cardiac septum is made, allowing better mixing of oxygenated blood from the lungs with the systemic blood **(19)**

Ballotable: able to be pushed away from the cervix **(7)**

Ballottement: a sharp upward pushing against the uterine wall with a finger inserted into the vagina; used for diagnosing pregnancy by feeling the return impact of the displaced fetus **(6)**

Bariatric surgery: surgery to reduce stomach size **(27)**

Barriers: devices, including male and female condoms, vaginal diaphragms, and cervical caps, placed in the vagina or over the penis to prevent sperm from entering the cervix **(5)**

Bartholin's glands: (also known as *greater vestibular glands*) glands whose ducts open onto the vestibule and secrete a thin mucus-like substance that provides lubrication during sexual intercourse **(4)**

Basal body temperature: body temperature in the morning before rising, moving about, or eating anything **(5)**

Benign prostatic hyperplasia (BPH): a prostate disorder in which the prostate gland enlarges in the center, compressing surrounding tissue and narrowing the urethra **(5)**

Biliary atresia: failure of the bile ducts outside the liver to form properly **(22)**

Biophysical profile: a test that assesses five variables: fetal breathing, fetal movement, fetal tone, amniotic fluid volume, and fetal reaction **(6)**

Bioterrorism: release of deadly infectious agents for the purpose of causing chaos and fear **(26)**

Bipolar disorder: (also known as *manic depression)* disorder involving mood swings between mania and depression **(27)**

Bladder exstrophy: a defect in which there is an absence of part of the abdominal wall and anterior wall of the bladder, causing the posterior wall of the bladder to protrude through the defect **(23)**

Blastocyst: stage of embryo formation in which cells have formed a two-layer ball **(6)**

Blended family: a family in which one or both spouses have had a previous marriage and children from that marriage **(3)**

Bloody show: release of the mucus plug from the cervix **(7)**

Body: the upper portion (of the uterus) **(4)**

Boggy: soft and spongy (reference to uterine fundus) **(10)**

Bonding: establishment of a strong emotional attachment between two unique individuals **(10)**

Braxton Hicks contractions: irregular, painless contractions occurring throughout pregnancy, also known as *false labor* **(6, 7)**

Breast reconstruction: mammoplasty **(5)**

Breech presentation: buttocks-down position of a fetus during birth **(7)**

Bronchiolitis: infection and inflammation of the smaller airways or bronchioles, results in wheezing from partial obstruction **(18)**

Bronchopulmonary dysplasia (BPD): chronic lung disease that affects infants with respiratory distress syndrome, congenital heart defects, meconium aspiration, or other conditions that result from assisted mechanical ventilation **(9, 18)**

Brushfield spots: white speckles on the edge of the iris **(16)**

Buccal space: area inside the cheek by the second molars **(22)**

Buffalo hump: fat deposits on the back between the shoulders **(25)**

Bulbourethral glands: (also known as *Cowper's glands*) either of two glands that discharge a component of seminal fluid into the urethra **(4)**

Bulimia: binge eating and purging **(27)**

Buphthalmos: enlargement of the eyeball **(16)**

C

Calcitonin: thyroid hormone that decreases the concentration of blood calcium by inhibiting the release of calcium from the bone; important to prevent a harmful excess of blood calcium (25)

Candidiasis: (also known as *Monilia* or *yeast infection*) a common organism causing vaginitis (5)

Caput succedaneum: edema of the scalp (9)

Cardiac output: total volume of blood forced out of the ventricles in 1 minute (19)

Cardiac region: area around the cardiac sphincter (22)

Cardiac sphincter: ring surrounding the opening between the esophagus and the stomach that prevents food and gastric acid from being pushed from the stomach into the esophagus (22)

Cardinal movements: (also called *mechanisms of labor*) the movements of a fetus changing positions as it moves through the pelvis (7)

Cardiomegaly: enlargement of the heart (19)

Carditis: inflammation of the heart (19)

Care plan: organized, prioritized plan for addressing nursing diagnoses and helping the client reach measurable, identified outcomes (or goals) (1)

Cataracts: opacities of the lens of one or both eyes (16)

Cations: positively charged electrolytes (15)

Celiac disease: gluten-sensitive enteropathy or sprue; a chronic malabsorption syndrome in which one is unable to digest gluten, a protein found in wheat, barley, rye, and oats (22)

Cell body: part of the cell that contains the nucleus and cytoplasm (16)

Cell-mediated immunity: immunity that provides protection against bacteria, viruses, fungi, and tumors; the process that causes rejection of organs that have been transplanted (21)

Cellulitis: bacterial infection of the dermis and subcutaneous tissue (24)

Cephalhematoma: accumulation of blood between the periosteum and the skull bone (9)

Cephalic presentation: head-down position of a fetus during birth (7)

Cephalocaudal: proceeding from head to toe (6, 11)

Cephalopelvic disproportion (CPD): condition in which the maternal pelvis is smaller than the fetal head (7)

Cervical dysplasia: abnormal changes in the tissue of the cervix (5)

Cervix: the narrow lower or outer end of the uterus (4)

Chadwick's sign: a bluish-purple discoloration of the cervix and vagina (6)

Chancre: painless open sore (5)

Chemical burns: burns caused by strong acids or alkaline, such as the chemical found in cleansers containing lye, toilet cleaners, or preparations used to open clogged drains (24)

Cheyne-Stokes breathing: period of deep breathing followed by period of apnea (18, 28)

Child exploitation: unethical use of a child for one's own profit (27)

Child life specialist: trained professional who plans therapeutic activities for the child who is ill or hospitalized (14)

Child molestation: sexual involvement other than intercourse with children (27)

Child pornography: photography or visual representation of children nude or in sexual acts (27)

Chlamydia: a sexually transmitted infection caused by *Chlamydia trachomatis* (5)

Chloasma: (also known as *mask of pregnancy*) darkening of the forehead, cheeks, and area around the eyes (6)

Choking: asphyxiation by a foreign object lodged in the respiratory tract (12)

Chordee: congenital anomaly that causes a ventral curvature of the penis, which is caused by fibrous tissues along the corpus spongiosum (23)

Chorea: involuntary, spasmodic movements of the limbs and face (19)

Chorion: outer layer of the membranes enclosing the embryo (6)

Chorionic villus sampling: test in which a sample of placental tissue is taken from a woman's abdomen and placental tissue is aspirated through a needle; the tissue, formed from the zygote, reflects the genetic makeup of the fetus (6)

Chromosomes: structures made of DNA (deoxyribonucleic acid) and protein that govern development of an organism (4)

Chronic: of long duration, with little change or slow progression (14)

Chronic renal failure (CRF): progressive, irreversible loss of kidney function (23)

Chyme: semiliquid substance of digestive acid and enzymes (22)

Cilia: minute hairlike structures (4)

Circumcision: surgical removal of the foreskin (*prepuce*) of the penis (4, 9)

Circumoral: around the mouth (9)

Circumoral cyanosis: bluish discoloration of the skin around the mouth (18)

Cleft lip: condition that results from failure of the upper lip to join medially; can be unilateral or bilateral (9)

Cleft palate: condition that results from failure of the medial nasal and maxillary processes to join, leaving an opening between the roof of the mouth and the floor of the nasal passage (9)

Clients: participants who obtain assistance from specialists (1)

Climacteric: menopause, the permanent cessation of menstruation (5)

Clitoris: a small elongated erectile organ at the anterior part of the vulva, homologous with the penis (4)

Clonus: spasms or seizures (7)

Closed head injury: result of head trauma, either from an external force such as a blow to the head or an internal force, such as shaking the infant hard enough for the brain to strike the inside of the skull (16)

Closed reduction: reduction of a fractured bone by manually moving the bones into alignment (17)

Clubbing: enlargement of the end of the fingers associated with disorders that cause cyanosis (19)

Coarctation: narrowing or constricting, especially of the aorta or of a blood vessel (19)

Cochlear implants: implanted devices that can help children who are deaf to hear (16)

Cognitive development: intellectual ability of an individual (11)

Cold stress: condition in newborns that occurs when excessive heat is lost; temperature change sufficient to cause the newborn to generate heat by nonshivering thermogenesis (9)

Colic: acute abdominal pain caused by spasmodic contractions of the intestines most commonly occurring during the first 3 months of life (22)

Colostrum: a translucent yellow fluid rich in protein, antibodies, and other substances to meet the needs of the newborn **(4)**

Comedones: whiteheads and blackheads **(24)**

Comfort measures only: order written to indicate that the goal of treatment is a comfortable, dignified death and that further life-sustaining measures are not indicated **(28)**

Communal family: a family that includes adults and children who may or may not be related **(3)**

Communicable diseases: diseases transmitted from one person to another by way of direct contact with body fluids **(26)**

Community-based nursing: philosophy of nursing that care should be provided to individuals, families, and groups wherever they are, including where they live, work, play, pray, or go to school **(1)**

Compartment syndrome: condition that occurs when increased pressure in a limited space compromises circulation and nerve innervation, possibly leading to necrosis **(17)**

Competent individual: person who has received training, including instruction and clinical practice, to perform certain tasks and who can demonstrate safe performance **(1)**

Complete abortion: results when all the fetal tissue is passed, the cervix closes, and minimal bleeding occurs **(5)**

Conception: uniting of ovum and sperm **(6)**

Conchae: three shelflike structures protruding into the nasal cavity from the sides **(18)**

Concrete operational: period in which child interacts primarily with the local environment **(11)**

Concussion: injury that causes temporary neurologic impairment but no permanent damage to brain tissue; may be caused by blunt injury to the head or by shaking an infant or child **(16)**

Confidentiality: ethical principle or legal right that a health professional will keep private any privileged information **(2)**

Congenital condition: condition present at birth **(14)**

Conization: removal of a cone-shaped wedge of tissue from the cervix **(5)**

Conjoined twins: (also known as *Siamese twins*) condition that results when the division of a fertilized egg occurs without complete separation or cleavage **(5)**

Conjunctival hyperemia: increased amount of blood in the conjunctiva **(19)**

Conscious sedation: the administration of IV medication to produce an impaired level of consciousness **(14)**

Consumers: purchasers of a service **(1)**

Contact dermatitis: dermatitis from allergens (poison ivy, poison oak, latex, and/or nickel) or repeated exposure to irritants (detergents, bleaches, soaps, lotions, urine, and stool) **(24)**

Contraception: prevention of pregnancy **(5)**

Contractility: ability of the ventricles to stretch **(19)**

Contractions: tightening of the uterus, beginning in the fundus; the result of shortening of muscle fibers **(7)**

Convalescent period: time frame from the beginning of the resolution of symptoms to restoration of wellness **(26)**

Cooperative play: organized play such as games at school or sports **(12)**

Coprolalia: uncontrollable use of obscene language **(27)**

Copropraxia: involuntary obscene gestures **(27)**

Corpus luteum: yellow endocrine tissue that forms in a ruptured Graafian follicle following the release of an ovum **(4)**

Coryza: (also known as *rhinitis* or *nasopharyngitis*) inflammation of the nasal mucosa, often caused by a viral infection such as the common cold **(18)**

Cotyledons: irregular sections of the maternal side of the placenta **(6)**

Cowper's glands: (also known as *bulbourethral glands*) either of two glands that discharge a component of seminal fluid into the urethra **(4)**

Crabs: pubic lice **(24)**

Crackles: course sounds in breathing; formerly called rales **(18)**

Craniofacial: relating to the head and face **(6)**

Cranium: bony structure surrounding the brain **(16)**

Critical thinking: process of analyzing one's own thinking and improving how one thinks or solves problems **(1)**

Crohn's disease: random inflammation of the entire gastrointestinal tract that involves all layers of bowel wall **(22)**

Croup: term used to represent a group of respiratory illnesses that result from inflammation and swelling of the larynx, trachea, and large bronchi; the causative agent can be either viral or bacterial **(18)**

Crowning: time in second-stage labor when the largest part of the fetal head is past the vulva and remains visible between contractions **(7)**

Cryotherapy: freezing with liquid nitrogen **(24)**

Cryptorchidism: a condition in which one or both of the testicles fail to descend into the scrotum **(23)**

Cult family: group in which a leader makes all decisions and controls the actions of all those who live there **(3)**

Cultural competence: set of skills, knowledge, and attitudes that includes awareness and acceptance of differences, awareness of one's own cultural values, understanding of the dynamics of difference, development of cultural knowledge, and ability to adapt practice skills to fit the cultural context of the client or patient **(1)**

Cultural proficiency: quality obtained when cultural competence components become second nature to the nurse **(1)**

Culture: a style of behavior patterns, beliefs, and products of human work of a given community or population **(3)**

Culture theory: factors of culture that should be considered when working with families **(3)**

Cushing's syndrome: hyperfunction of the adrenal cortex **(25)**

Cyst: fluid-filled sac **(5)**

Cystitis: bladder infection **(23)**

Cystocele: prolapse of the urinary bladder into the vagina **(5)**

D

Date rape: sexual intercourse during a social outing without consent, occuring as a result of threat or physical force **(27)**

Deciduas: tissue that lines the uterine wall during pregnancy **(10)**

Deductive reasoning: process of taking a generalized idea and figuring out what specifics to expect from it **(1)**

Deep sedation: controlled state of depressed consciousness or unconsciousness in which the child is unable to maintain protective reflexes **(14)**

Defense mechanisms: ways of protecting the ego from threatening impulses or painful realities of life experiences **(11)**

Delegation: transfer to a competent individual of the authority or right to perform selected nursing tasks in a selected situation **(1)**

Demandingness: a state relating to the demands that parents make on the children, their expectations for mature behavior, the discipline and supervision they provide, and their willingness to confront behavioral problems **(3)**

Dendrite: extension of a nerve cell that conducts the electrical impulses toward the cell body **(16)**

Depression: prolonged feeling of sadness or hopelessness that interferes with normal activities of life **(27)**

Dermatitis: inflammation of the dermis or skin **(24)**

Dermis: inner thicker layer of the skin that contains most of the associated structures **(24)**

Descent: movement in labor that begins with engagement and continues as the contractions push the fetus through the pelvis **(7)**

Desensitization: process of administering doses of medication in increasing increments in an effort to avoid the allergic reaction **(21)**

Desquamation: to shed, peel, or come off in scales, as in skin **(26)**

Development: process of maturation including the refinement of body systems, thought processes, and judgment **(11)**

Diabetes mellitus: disorder of carbohydrate, protein, and fat metabolism; the most common metabolic disorder in children **(25)**

Diabetic ketoacidosis: an increase in ketone bodies in the urine, caused by an increased rate of free fatty acid metabolism by the liver **(25)**

Diagnostic and Statistical Manual of Mental Disorders, Fourth Edition (DSM-IV): main diagnostic reference of mental health professionals in the United States **(27)**

Dialysis: mechanical process of removing wastes from blood or lymph through the processes of diffusion, osmosis, and ultrafiltration; once the blood or lymph is filtered, it is returned to the body **(23)**

Diaper dermatitis: dermatitis caused by irritation from urine and/or stool **(24)**

Diaphragm: large muscle dividing the chest and abdominal cavities **(18)**

Diaphysis: main section of a long bone, contains the medullary cavity **(17)**

Diastasis recti abdominis: separation of the abdominal muscle **(10)**

Diffusion: process in which solutes move across the cell membrane from an area of higher concentration to an area of lower concentration **(15)**

Dilatation: opening (as of the cervical opening or *os*) **(7)**

Dilatation stage: (also known as *first stage of labor*) begins with regular contractions and ends with complete effacement and dilatation of the cervix; usually the longest stage, it is divided into three phases: latent, active, and transition **(7)**

Disequilibrium syndrome: complication caused by cerebral edema; symptoms include fatigue, nausea, vomiting, tremors (which can progress to delirium), seizures, and coma **(23)**

Diverticulum: out-pouch in the ileum, usually near the ileocecal valve **(22)**

Doula: a supportive companion who accompanies the woman through birth, providing physical and emotional support and information, and advocating for the woman and the family **(6)**

Down syndrome: most common chromosomal abnormality, results from trisomy 21; signs include *microcephaly* (small head), wide short neck, epicanthal folds, and short broad hands with a simian line; associated with increased incidence of congenital heart defects, diabetes, and hearing loss **(9)**

Droplet method: indirect method of transmission of harmful organisms **(26)**

Drowning: loss of life within 24 hours following submersion in water or other liquid **(16)**

Ductus arteriosus: a blood vessel in a fetus that connects the pulmonary artery to the aorta **(6)**

Ductus deferens: (also known as *vas deferens*) the main duct through which semen is carried from the epididymis to the ejaculatory duct **(4)**

Ductus venosus: a vein passing through the liver and connecting the left umbilical vein with the inferior vena cava of the fetus **(6)**

Duncan mechanism: separation of the placenta with the maternal side out in third-stage labor **(7)**

Duration: time from the onset to the end of a contraction **(7)**

Dysfunctional grief: condition of grief in which an individual cannot accept what has happened or move on with life **(28)**

Dyslexia: specific, common learning disability that is neurologic in origin **(16)**

Dysmenorrhea: painful menses **(5)**

Dyspareunia: painful intercourse **(5)**

Dysphagia: difficulty swallowing **(18)**

Dysphonia: muffled or hoarse voice **(18)**

Dyspnea: difficulty breathing **(18)**

Dysuria: painful urination **(23)**

E

Ecchymosis: bruising **(9)**

Echolalia: words repeated over and over again **(27)**

Ecomap: a diagram of the interactions of family members to the immediate environment **(3)**

Ectopic: outside normal placement (as in pregnancy outside the uterus) **(5)**

Effacement: shortening and thinning of the cervix **(7)**

Effleurage: light stroking with the fingertips in a circular motion **(7)**

Ego: realistic part of the personality that searches for acceptable methods of meeting pleasure needs **(11)**

Ejaculatory duct: a part of the seminal duct formed by the duct from the seminal vesicle and the vas deferens; it passes through the prostate gland **(4)**

Elective abortion (EAB): abortion performed at the request of the mother but not for reason of maternal risk or fetal disease **(5)**

Electrical burns: burns caused by contact with exposed electric wires **(24)**

Electrolytes: solutes within the body fluid; also called minerals or salts **(15)**

Emancipated minors: those minors responsible for their own health care decisions and expenses **(2)**

Embryonic disc: the part of the inner cell mass of a blastocyst that will become the embryo **(6)**

Embryonic stage: (also known as *Stage II*) from weeks 3 through 8 of fetal development; stage in which all body systems are formed **(6)**

Encephalitis: inflammation of the brain, most often caused by a viral infection **(16)**

Encopresis: condition in which child delays defecation or experiences frequent soiling of feces **(27)**

Endometriosis: the presence of endometrium elsewhere than in the lining of the uterus; causes premenstrual pain and dysmenorrhea **(5)**

Endometrium: inner lining of the uterus **(4)**

End-stage renal disease (ESRD): condition in which kidney function is less than 10%; person requires dialysis or kidney transplantation to survive **(23)**

Engagement: point at which the presenting part (usually the fetal head) enters the true pelvis; the presenting part is even with or below the ischeal spines, and the fetus is no longer ballotable **(7)**

Engrossment: interest in and preoccupation with the infant after childbirth, manifested by holding, maintaining eye contact with, and talking to the infant **(10)**

Enuresis: urinary incontinence occurring in a child who is capable of obtaining bladder control **(23)**

Epidermis: outer thin layer of the skin consisting of several layers **(24)**

Epididymis: a single very tightly coiled tube in each testis, approximately 20 ft in length, which carries sperm to vas deferens **(4)**

Epididymitis: inflammation of the epididymis **(5)**

Epiglottitis: inflammation of the epiglottis caused by a bacterial infection of the pharynx and soft tissue of the larynx **(18)**

Epilepsy: chronic disorder characterized by repeated seizure activity **(16)**

Epinephrine (adrenalin): hormone that causes the body to be geared for strenuous activity ("fight-or-flight" reaction) **(25)**

Epiphora: watering of the eyes **(16)**

Epiphyseal plate: growth plate; remains open until late adolescence **(17)**

Epiphysis: attachment site for muscles; considered the site for ossification **(17)**

Episiotomy: surgical cutting of perineal tissue **(7)**

Epispadias: condition that occurs when the urethra opens on the dorsal (upper) surface of the penis **(9)**

Epistaxis: nose bleed **(18)**

Epstein's pearls: small white cysts present on palate of neonates that disappear in a few weeks **(9)**

Erectile dysfunction: (also known as *ED*, or *impotence*) the inability to achieve or maintain an erection that allows for satisfactory sexual intercourse **(5)**

Erythema marginatum: a red skin rash that sometimes occurs with rheumatic fever **(19)**

Erythema migrans: early symptom of Lyme disease; a red rash with a bull's eye appearance at the site of the bite **(26)**

Erythema toxicum neonatorum: raised pink papule with a light-colored center resembling a mosquito bite that appears suddenly on the chest, abdomen, and back 24 to 48 hours after birth; benign condition that disappears without treatment **(9)**

Erythroblastosis fetalis: a serious anemia, usually resulting from maternal antibodies to Rh-positive fetal blood **(6)**

Erythrocytes: red blood cells (RBCs) **(20)**

Erythropoiesis: formation or production of red blood cells **(20)**

Eschar: dead matter that is sloughed off the surface of the skin, especially after a burn **(24)**

Esophageal atresia: a potentially life-threatening defect in which the esophagus ends in a blind pouch before reaching the stomach **(9)**

Esotropia: turning of the eye inward **(16)**

Estrogen: a general term for female steroid sex hormones that are secreted by the ovary and are responsible for typical female sexual characteristics **(4)**

Ethics: system of values and ideas that shape a sense of right and wrong **(2)**

Ethnicity: a group with a common ancestry, race, religion, and culture **(3)**

Eupnea: normal breathing pattern **(18)**

Euthanasia: act of compassionately putting to death a person suffering from incurable or distressing disease **(28)**

Exfoliation: shedding of the outer layer **(10)**

Exhibitionism: exposing the genitals to strangers **(27)**

Exophthalmos: prominent or bulging eyes **(25)**

Exotropia: turning outward of the eye **(16)**

Expiratory grunting: grunting sound on exhalation that is a sign of respiratory distress in a newborn **(9)**

Expulsion: delivery of the rest of the fetus after restitution **(7)**

Exstrophy of bladder: rare condition in which the abdominal wall fails to fuse, allowing the urinary bladder to protrude to the outside **(9)**

Extended family: a network of relatives and/or close friends who take an active role in the emotional support of the family **(3)**

Extension: condition that occurs when the fetus extends its head, pushing its occiput against the maternal symphysis pubis and causing the fetal head to emerge through the vaginal opening **(7)**

External rotation: rotation of the fetus until the shoulders are in an anterior/posterior position **(7)**

F

Failure to thrive (FTT): general term used to describe the child who fails to gain weight or loses weight for unknown reasons **(22)**

Fallopian tubes: (also known as *uterine tubes* or *oviducts*) structures that serve to transport the ovum from the ovary toward the uterus **(4)**

False labor: (also known as *Braxton Hicks contractions*) pains resembling those of normal labor but occurring at irregular intervals and without dilation of the cervix **(7)**

Family: two or more individuals who come together for the purpose of nurturing **(3)**

Family assessment: an ongoing process of examining relationships and functioning of members of the family **(3)**

Family development theory: analytical description of the changes the family undergoes over time **(3)**

Family systems theory: analysis of family systems and boundaries between the family and the world **(3)**

Family-centered care: treatment to a designated client with recognition that the family system or unit may also need intervention **(3)**

Ferguson's reflex: spontaneous urge to push during labor that occurs when the presenting part reaches the pelvic floor; may occur without full cervical effacement **(7)**

Fertility awareness: family planning based on the assumption that ovulation takes place at the same time each month **(5)**

Fertilization: uniting of ovum and sperm **(6)**

Fetal alcohol syndrome (FAS): series of malformations found in infants whose mothers drank large quantities of alcohol during pregnancy; includes facial anomalies, microcephaly, central nervous system dysfunction, mental retardation, and hyperactivity **(9)**

Fetal attitude: relationship of fetal body parts to one another **(7)**

Fetal heart tones (FHTs): the fetal heartbeat **(6)**

Fetal lie: relationship of the long axis (head-to-foot or *cephalocaudal* axis) of the fetus to the long axis of the mother **(7)**

Fetal membranes: (also known as the *bag of waters*) any membrane that functions for the protection or nourishment of respiration or excretion of a developing fetus **(6)**

Fetal position: relationship of the presenting part of the fetus to the four quadrants of the maternal pelvis; the fetal landmarks are identified in the right or left, anterior or posterior quadrants of the mother's pelvis **(7)**

Fetal presentation: body part of the fetus that is closest to the cervix **(7)**

Fetal stage: Stage III from weeks 9 through 38 to 40; during this stage, all body systems are refined and begin to function **(6)**

Fibroadenoma: a freely movable rounded mass with well-defined borders and a solid rubbery texture **(5)**

Fibrocyst: fluid-filled mass **(5)**

Fibromyalgia: disorder characterized by widespread musculoskeletal pain and fatigue **(16)**

Fibrosis: replacement of inflamed or damaged tissue with connective or scar tissue **(5)**

Filtration: process by which solvents and solutes are pushed across a cell membrane from an area of higher pressure to an area of lower pressure **(15)**

Fimbriae: finger-like projections at the opening of the fallopian tubes **(4)**

First stage of labor: (also known as the *dilatation stage*) stage that begins with regular contractions and ends with complete effacement and dilatation of the cervix; usually the longest stage; divided into three phases: latent, active, and transition **(7)**

Fissures: cracks or lines present on skin tissues **(19)**

Flexion: describes the attitude the fetus assumes in relation to its own body parts; ideal flexion is positive, with head flexed onto the chest, arms flexed across the chest, and legs flexed across the abdomen **(7)**

Focal seizures: seizures caused by abnormal electrical activity in a specific area of the brain, most commonly in the temporal, frontal, or parietal lobes of the cerebrum **(16)**

Follicle-stimulating hormone (FSH): hormone of the anterior pituitary gland that stimulates the Graafian follicles and assists in follicular maturation and in the secretion of estradiol **(4)**

Fomites: inanimate objects that transmit harmful bacteria indirectly **(26)**

Fontanels: (also known as *soft spots*) any of the soft membranous gaps between the incompletely formed cranial bones of a fetus or an infant that prevent undue pressure on the fetal brain **(7)**

Foramen ovale: an opening in the septum between the right atrium and left atrium **(6)**

Foreskin: (also known as *prepuce*) loose-fitting retractable skin that covers the glans of the penis **(4)**

Formal operations: period when the child gradually completes intellectual development necessary to function as an adult **(11)**

Fourth stage of labor: first hour after delivery during which the mother's body begins to return to a nonpregnant state **(7)**

Fracture: condition that results from an injury and causes the continuity of the bone to be altered **(17)**

Fraternal twins: twins that occur from two eggs fertilized by two sperm; they generally have two separate placentas, amnions, chorions, and could be different genders; dizygotic twins **(5)**

Frequency: the time from the onset of one contraction to the onset of the next contraction **(7)**

Frostbite: skin and tissue damage caused by overexposure to low environmental temperatures **(24)**

Fulminating hepatitis: progressive, total destruction of the liver **(22)**

Fundus: rounded top of an organ, such as the uterus or the stomach **(4)**

Funic soufflé: sound occurring at the fetal heart rate, caused by fetal blood flowing through the umbilical cord **(6)**

G

Gamete: sex cell **(4)**

Gametogenesis: sex cell formation **(4)**

Ganglia: groups of nerve cell bodies located in the PNS **(16)**

Gastroenteritis: inflammation of the stomach, may be caused by bacteria, such as *Escherichia coli* or salmonella; virus, such as rotavirus; as well as toxins and allergies **(22)**

Gastroesophageal reflux disease (GERD): condition caused by a relaxation of the cardiac sphincter **(22)**

Generalized anxiety disorder (GAD): (also known as *overanxious disorder*) disorder in which the child is prone to excessive worry about the future **(27)**

Generalized seizures: seizures that result from diffuse electrical activity that begins in one area of the brain and spreads to involve the entire cerebral cortex and brainstem **(16)**

Genital warts: (also known as *condylomata acuminatum*) a sexually transmitted infection with human papilloma virus **(5)**

Genitourinary system: consists of structures of the urinary system and the reproductive system **(23)**

Genogram: a diagram of relationships of members of the family **(3)**

Genome: an organism's complete set of DNA **(4)**

Genu valgum: (also known as *knock knees*) inward slant of the thigh **(17)**

Genu varum: (also known as *bowlegs*) legs bowed outward at the knee (or below the knee) **(17)**

Gestation: fetal development **(6)**

Gingival: mucous membrane covering the front of the mouth and the inside of the lips **(22)**

Glans: the enlarged distal end of the penis **(4)**

Glaucoma: condition caused by increased intraocular pressure (IOP) due to inadequate drainage of the aqueous humor **(16)**

Glomerulonephritis: inflammation of the glomeruli **(23)**

Glucagons: hormone that increases the blood glucose by stimulating glycogenolysis in the liver **(25)**

Glucocorticoids: any of a group of steroid hormones, such as cortisone, produced by the adrenal cortex and involved in carbohydrate, protein, and fat metabolism, and having anti-inflammatory properties **(25)**

Gluconeogenesis: conversion of amino acids and fatty acids to glucose in the liver **(25)**

Glucosuria: excretion of glucose in the urine **(25)**

Glycogenolysis: chemical process of changing stored glycogen into glucose **(25)**

Goiter: painless enlargement of thyroid gland **(25)**

Goniotomy: surgical technique by which the flow of aqueous humor is increased from the anterior chamber **(16)**

Gonorrhea: a sexually transmitted infection caused by *Neisseria gonorrhoeae* (**5**)

Goodell's sign: an indication of pregnancy in which the cervix and vagina soften (**6**)

GP/TPAL: an abbreviation for gravida, para/term, preterm, abortion, live birth (**6**)

Graafian follicles: mature follicles (**4**)

Granulosa cells: layer of cells surrounding the oocyte (**4**)

Grave's disease: autoimmune disorder in which antibodies attack the thyroid gland (**25**)

Gravida: the number of pregnancies a woman has had (**6**)

Greater curvature: outer curved area of the stomach (**22**)

Greater vestibular gland: (also known as *Bartholin's glands*) glands opening onto the vestibule that secrete a thin mucus-like substance that provides lubrication during sexual intercourse (**4**)

Greenstick fracture: fracture in which one side of the bone is broken and the other side is bent (**17**)

Grief: feeling of extreme sadness resulting from a loss (**28**)

Growth: process of increasing in physical size (**11**)

Growth hormone (GH): hormone that promotes normal growth by speeding the movement of amino acids from the blood into cells (**25**)

Growth hormone deficiency (GHD): decrease in growth hormone that results from injury or disease of the hypothalamus or pituitary gland, inheritance, or genetic mutation (**25**)

Guillain–Barré syndrome: (also known as *postinfectious polyneuritis*) relatively rare disorder characterized by ascending and then descending paralysis (**16**)

H

Health: sense of physical, psychological, emotional, and spiritual well-being, not just the absence of disease (**12**)

Health promotion: encouraging lifestyle changes that result in the individual's becoming healthier (**12**)

Hegar's sign: softening of the lower uterine segment, present by the 8th week of pregnancy (**6**)

Hematology: study of blood and blood-forming tissues (**20**)

Hematoma: accumulation of blood under the skin (**10**)

Hematopoiesis: process in which blood cells are produced in the bone marrow (**17, 20**)

Hematuria: blood in the urine (**23**)

Hemolysis: destruction or dissolution of red blood cells, with subsequent release of hemoglobin (**20**)

Hemophilia: rare hereditary gender-linked disorder causing a deficiency in a specific blood clotting factor (**20**)

Hemoptysis: bloody sputum (**5**)

Hemosiderosis: iron overload; the buildup of iron in tissues and organs (**20**)

Hemothorax: the presence of body fluid in the chest cavity (**18**)

Hepatitis: inflammation of the liver caused by a viral infection (**22**)

Hepatomegaly: enlarged liver (**21**)

Hereditary condition: condition caused by genetic characteristic transmitted from parent to child (**14**)

Hernia: protrusion of intestines through a weakness in the abdominal or pelvic muscles (**9**)

Hip spica cast: cast covering the upper thighs and lower torso (**17**)

Hirschsprung's disease: (also known as *megacolon*) a condition in which the autonomic parasympathetic ganglion that normally causes peristalsis in the intestine is absent (**22**)

Hirsuitism: excessive hair growth (**5**)

Holistic: inclusive of the physical, psychological, and spiritual aspects of the person (**1**)

Holistic health: concept that approaches an individual's health as an integrated system rather than divided into various parts (**27**)

Homeostasis: state of balance of fluids and electrolytes within the body (**15**)

Hormonal contraceptives: contraceptives, usually a combination of estrogen and progesterone, which are available in a variety of forms (**5**)

Hormones: main regulators of growth and development, metabolism, and reproduction (**25**)

Hospice care: movement of care based on the holistic concepts of palliative care that emphasize quality of life rather than cure (**28**)

Human chorionic gonadotropin (hCG): a hormone produced by the placenta that maintains the corpus luteum during pregnancy; the chemical that pregnancy kits identify in order to determine pregnancy (**6**)

Human immunodeficiency virus (HIV): a retrovirus that attacks and destroys the body's immune system (**5**)

Human placental lactogen (hPL): hormone that stimulates changes in maternal metabolism during pregnancy (**6**)

Humoral immunity: immunity that destroys bacteria, viruses, parasites, allergens, and other foreign substances by producing antibodies called immunoglobulins (**21**)

Hydrocele: fluid in the scrotal sac (**5**)

Hydronephrosis: distension of the renal pelvis caused by increased pressure due to urinary backup (**23**)

Hydrophobia: in rabies, a reflex contraction at the sight of liquid accompanied by painful contractures in the muscles used for swallowing (**26**)

Hymen: a thin membrane that partially covers the vaginal orifice (**4**)

Hyperbilirubinemia: abnormally high concentration of bilirubin in the blood (**9**)

Hypercalcemia: condition characterized by an increase in serum calcium above normal levels (**15**)

Hyperemesis gravidarum: prolonged vomiting related to pregnancy (**6**)

Hyperkalemia: condition that occurs when there is an increase above normal range in serum potassium levels (**15**)

Hyperlipidemia: condition characterized by increased total cholesterol, low-density lipoproteins, and triglycerides accompanied by decreased high-density lipoproteins (**19**)

Hypernatremia: state of sodium excess related to the body's water (**15**)

Hyperopia: farsightedness (**16**)

Hyperplasia: excessive proliferation of normal cells (**5**)

Hypertonic dehydration: fluid and sodium loss in which relatively more fluid than sodium is lost (as in diabetes) (**15**)

Hypertropia: (also known as *anoopsia*) vertical deviation of one of the eyes (**16**)

Hyperventilation: deep, rapid respirations (**18**)

Hypervolemia: abnormally increased volume of blood; fluid volume excess (FVE); occurs with retention of fluid and sometimes sodium in the extracellular compartment **(15)**

Hyphema: hemorrhage into the anterior chamber of the eye **(16)**

Hypoalbuminemia: abnormally low level of albumin in the blood **(23)**

Hypocalcemia: condition characterized by serum calcium levels below normal levels **(15)**

Hypokalemia: condition that occurs when there is a decrease below normal range in serum potassium levels **(15)**

Hyponatremia: state of sodium deficit related to the body's water **(15)**

Hypopituitarism: condition in which there is a decreased function of the pituitary gland resulting in GHD **(25)**

Hypospadias: condition that occurs when the urethra opens on the ventral (lower) surface of the penis **(9)**

Hypotonic dehydration: fluid and sodium loss in which relatively more sodium than fluid is lost (as, for example, in renal disease) **(15)**

Hypoventilation: slow, shallow respirations **(18)**

Hypovolemia: abnormally decreased volume of blood **(15)**

Hysterectomy: removal of the uterus **(5)**

I

Id: basic energy that drives the individual to seek pleasure **(11)**

Idiopathic thrombocytopenic purpura (ITP): bleeding disorder of unknown cause that leads to a decrease in the number of platelets **(20)**

Illness: state of disease or sickness; may be physical or psychological; may be acute, chronic, or terminal **(14)**

Illness prevention: specific behaviors that can prevent illness and limit injury **(12)**

Immune response: bodily defense reaction that recognizes an antigen and produces antibodies specific against that antigen **(21)**

Immunization: process of inducing resistance to communicable diseases **(26)**

Immunoglobulins: any of a group of large glycoproteins that are secreted by plasma cells and that function as antibodies in the immune response by binding with specific antigens **(21)**

Imperforate anus: condition that results when the connecting tissue fails to break down and the opening of the colon does not develop **(9)**

Impetigo: superficial skin infection that appears on the face, hands, neck, or extremities, caused by streptococci or staphylococci **(24)**

Implantation: embedding of the blastocyst into the endometrium **(6)**

Incest: sexual intercourse between close blood relatives that may or may not be consensual **(5, 27)**

Incomplete abortion: abortion that occurs when the fetus is passed but the placenta is retained in the uterus **(5)**

Incubation period: time between the entry of a pathogen into a reservoir and the onset of clinical signs and symptoms **(26)**

Individualized education plan (IEP): plan for meeting educational requirements of a child with special needs **(14)**

Inductive reasoning: process of making generalized statements from a limited set of facts **(1)**

Inevitable abortion: abortion that occurs when the cervix dilates and part of the placenta detaches from the uterus resulting in moderate to heavy bleeding **(5)**

Infertility: inability to achieve pregnancy after a year or more of unprotected intercourse **(5)**

Informed consent: written approval for a treatment or procedure, following explanation of pros and cons by the physician or other professional who is performing the procedure **(2)**

Inotropic: affecting the contraction of muscle, especially heart muscle **(19)**

Insulin: only hormone that decreases blood glucose by accelerating movement of glucose out of the blood and into the cells **(25)**

Insulin resistance: condition in which the body produces enough insulin but is unable to use it effectively **(25)**

Intensity: the strength of the contraction at its peak **(7)**

Intercostal: between the ribs **(9)**

Intercostal muscles: muscles between the ribs **(18)**

Internal rotation: when the fetus turns to an anterior position (OA), the fetal occiput is next to the maternal symphysis pubis; may take place prior to labor, but most commonly occurs during the first or second stages of labor **(7)**

Interstitial: relation to spaces within a structure, such as the spaces within a tissue or organ **(15)**

Interstitial cells: spaces within a tissue or organ, excluding body cavities or potential space **(4)**

Interventions: nursing actions to assist the client toward an improvement in health **(1)**

Intraductal papillomas: tumors growing in a mammary duct, most commonly occurring during menopause **(5)**

Intrauterine device (IUD): a small T-shaped piece of metal covered with copper or levonorgestrel that is placed in the uterus to prevent pregnancy **(5)**

Intraventricular hemorrhage: hemorrhage within the cerebral ventricles of the brain **(9)**

Intussusception: condition that occurs when one portion of the intestine telescopes into another portion **(22)**

In vitro fertilization: process of uniting eggs and sperm in a test tube in the laboratory **(5)**

Involution: return of uterus to nonpregnant state **(10)**

Iron-deficiency anemia: condition that results when the demand for stored iron is greater than what the body can supply **(20)**

Irritant: source of irritation as a foreign substance **(24)**

Isotonic dehydration: loss of fluid and sodium in equal proportions (as from vomiting); common dehydration in children **(15)**

J

Jaundice: condition that occurs because the infant's liver is immature and cannot conjugate the amount of bilirubin released by the destruction of the RBCs **(9)**

K

Karyotype: a picture analysis of the chromosomes **(5)**

Ketoacidosis: occurs when glucose storage is depleted and fat storage must be used for energy needs **(15)**

Koplik's spots: small, irregular red spots with a bluish-white center appearing on the buccal mucosa in association with measles **(26)**

Kussmaul: (respiration) rapid and deep, labored breathing **(15)**

Kwashiorkor: deficiency in protein in the diet resulting in muscle wasting **(22)**

Kyphosis: (also known as *hunchback*) excessive convex curvature of the thoracic spine **(17)**

L

Labia majora: the two outer folds of the vulva **(4)**

Labia minora: the two inner folds of the vulva **(4)**

Labor: a process, or sequence of events, that begins with uterine contractions and ends 1 hour after delivery of the placenta **(7)**

Lactiferous ducts: the milk-carrying ducts of the mammary gland that open on the nipple **(4)**

Lactogenesis: milk production **(4)**

Lactogenic hormone: (also known as *prolactin*) hormone secreted during pregnancy that stimulates breast development and milk production (lactation) **(25)**

Lactose intolerant: congenital or acquired disorder in which the child fails to produce lactase, an enzyme needed in the digestion of lactose **(22)**

Lanugo: fine fetal hair **(6)**

Latch-key children: school-age children who come home from school to an empty house and may remain unsupervised until parents return from work **(12)**

Latent phase: during the first stage of labor, the phase from the onset of contractions until the cervix is dilated 4 cm **(7)**

Leopold's maneuver: maneuver that helps caregivers determine the position of the fetus **(7)**

Lesser curvature: inner curved area of the stomach **(22)**

Let-down reflex: release of milk after delivery **(6)**

Leukemia: cancer of the blood-forming organs **(20)**

Leukocytes: white blood cells (WBCs) **(20)**

Libido: sexual drive **(5)**

Ligation: obstructing a vessel or duct using suture or wire ligature **(19)**

Lightening: sensation a pregnant woman feels when descent of the fetus into the pelvis relieves pressure on the diaphragm, allowing her to breathe more easily and to "feel lighter" **(7)**

Linea nigra: a dark line on the abdomen from the umbilicus to the pubis **(6)**

Lingual frenulum: thin membrane that attaches the tongue to the floor of the mouth **(22)**

Livor mortis: discoloration that results after blood circulation has ceased and red blood cells break down, releasing hemoglobin; appears in the lowest or dependent areas of the body **(28)**

Lochia: discarded uterine blood, mucus, and tissue **(10)**

Lochia alba: creamy white or pale yellow lochia that consists of the last pieces of decidua, white blood cells, mucus, and bacteria **(10)**

Lochia rubra: dark red lochia that contains epithelial cells, red blood cells, pieces of decidua, and sometimes meconium, lanugo, and vernix caseosa **(10)**

Lochia serosa: pinkish lochia that is present from days 4 to 10 and contains serous exudate, red blood cells, mucous, and many bacteria **(10)**

Logan clamp: metal bow taped to both sides of the suture line **(22)**

Lordosis: (also known as *sway back*) excessive concave curvature of the lumbar spine **(17)**

Loss: feeling, either real or perceived, that is experienced when something important is removed from the body or the environment **(28)**

Lumpectomy: removal of a lump (usually cancerous) from a woman's breast **(5)**

Luteinizing hormone (LH): hormone that stimulates the ovary to ripen and release ova; in males, stimulates the production of sperm; stimulates the interstitial cells in the testes to secrete testosterone; sometimes called a *sex steroid* **(25)**

Lymphadenopathy: enlarged lymph nodes **(21)**

M

Mammography: imaging exam of the breast with x-rays, ultrasound, or nuclear magnetic resonance **(5)**

Mammoplasty: breast reconstruction **(5)**

Mantoux test: tuberculin test in which a small amount of tuberculin is injected under the skin **(18)**

Mastectomy: removal of the breast **(5)**

Maternal–child nursing: care of women through pregnancy, childbirth, and postpartum; also care of the child from birth through the teenage years **(1)**

Maturation: process of becoming fully developed **(11)**

Mature Minor Act: an act that permits adolescents age 14 or 15 to make decisions about their treatment **(2)**

Mechanisms of labor: (also known as *cardinal movements*) movements of a fetus changing positions as it moves through the pelvis **(7)**

Meconium: the first fetal stool **(6)**

Meconium aspiration: aspiration of amniotic fluid contaminated with meconium by a fetus in hypoxic distress **(9)**

Medical diagnoses: statements about a disease process or disorder **(1)**

Megacolon: (also known as *Hirschsprung's disease*) a condition in which the autonomic parasympathetic ganglion that normally causes peristalsis in the intestine is absent **(22)**

Melanin: pigment that adds color to the skin **(24)**

Melanocytes: pigment-producing cells **(24)**

Melatonin: principal hormone produced by the pineal gland; it regulates body cycles (e.g., sleep/wake cycle) and inhibits *gonadotropic* (sex organ-promoting) hormones **(25)**

Menarche: the first menstrual period, usually during puberty **(4)**

Meningitis: inflammation of the meninges by either a bacteria or a virus **(16)**

Meningocele: herniation of the meninges through the vertebral defect **(9)**

Meningomyelocele: herniation of the spinal nerves and the meninges through the vertebral defect **(9)**

Menopause: the period marked by the natural and permanent cessation of menstruation, occurring between the ages of 35 and 58 **(4)**

Menorrhagia: excessive menstruation in volume or number of days **(5)**

Menorrhalgia: (also known as *dysmenorrhea*) painful menses **(5)**

Menses: the monthly flow of blood and cellular debris from the uterus that begins at puberty and ceases at menopause **(4)**

Mental retardation (MR): disability characterized by significant limitations both in intellectual functioning and in adaptive behavior as expressed in conceptual, social, and practical adaptive skills **(16)**

Mentum: chin **(7)**

Metabolic acidosis: condition involving an excess of acids in the body **(15)**

Metabolic alkalosis: condition that results from a loss of metabolic acid or an excess of bicarbonate **(15)**

Metaphysis: zone of growth between the epiphysis and diaphysis during development of a bone, responsible for converting new cartilage into bone **(17)**

Metrorrhagia: bleeding between periods **(5)**

Milia: white pinpoint spots on a newborn that resemble whiteheads **(9)**

Mineralocorticoids: hormones that control the blood levels of minerals, mainly sodium chloride **(25)**

Miscarriage: (also known as *spontaneous abortion*) nonelective abortion that occurs within the first 20 weeks of pregnancy **(5)**

Missed abortion: condition in which the fetus dies, but spontaneous abortion does not occur **(5)**

Mittelschmerz: abdominal pain with ovulation **(5)**

Molding: shaping of the fetal head to the bones of the maternal pelvis **(7)**

Mongolian spot: dark discolored area found over the lower back and sacrum of infants of Black, Hispanic, Indian, or Oriental descent; over time, skin tones darken to become the same color as the Mongolian spot **(9)**

Monilia: (also known as *candidiasis* or *yeast infection*) a common organism causing vaginitis **(5)**

Monozygotic twins: (also known as *identical twins*) twins that result when one fertilized egg divides into separate embryos **(5)**

Mons pubis: the skin-covered fat pad over the symphysis pubis **(4)**

Moon face: round cheeks and double chin associated with Cushing's syndrome **(25)**

Morbidity: prevalence of a specific disease or disorder in the population at a specific period of time **(1)**

Moro reflex: (also known as *startle reflex*) reflex that occurs when newborns have a sense of falling, in which newborn quickly extends (abducts) the arms with fingers flared and thumb and first finger forming a "C," then adducts in an embracing motion; the lower extremities may extend and flex; a slight tremor may be noted **(9)**

Mortality: number of deaths over a given period of time for a given population **(1)**

Morula: mulberry-shaped mass of blastomeres that forms when the zygote splits; develops into the blastula **(6)**

Motility disorders: conditions that prevent gastrointestinal contents from moving through the system in a normal manner **(22)**

Mottled: bluish or purplish marbled appearance of the skin **(28)**

Multifetal pregnancy: a pregnancy with more than one fetus **(5)**

Multigravida: woman who has been pregnant two or more times **(6)**

Multipara: woman who has delivered two or more times after 24 weeks' gestation **(6)**

Multiple pregnancy: multifetal pregnancy **(5)**

Muscular dystrophy (MD): group of inherited diseases that cause muscle degeneration and wasting **(17)**

Myelin sheath: lipoprotein covering of the axon **(16)**

Myomectomy: removal of tumor and surrounding myometrium **(5)**

Myometrium: the muscular layer of the wall of the uterus **(4)**

Myopia: nearsightedness **(16)**

Myringotomy: surgical procedure in which a small plastic tube is inserted through the tympanic membrane to facilitate drainage of fluid and ventilation of the middle ear **(16)**

N

Naegele's rule: a method used to determine date of birth taking the first day of the last menstrual period (LMP), subtracting 3 months, and adding 7 days **(6)**

Nasal flaring: outward movement of the nostrils, earliest sign of respiratory distress in a newborn **(9)**

Nasopharyngitis: (also known as *rhinitis* or *coryza*) inflammation of the nasal mucosa, often caused by a viral infection such as the common cold **(18)**

Natural childbirth: labor and birth without medical interventions or pain medication **(7)**

Natural immunity: immunity that is present at birth and lasts about 3 to 6 months **(21)**

NCLEX-PN® focus area: 1 of 11 areas of Client Needs around which the NCLEX-PN® test is constructed **(1)**

Near-drowning: suffocation from submersion in liquid that is survived in the first 24 hours following the incident; most often associated with asphyxia and aspiration **(16)**

Negative feedback: mechanism in blood levels of most hormones where high levels of a hormone in the blood inhibit (switch off) hormone production and low levels trigger (switch on) hormone production **(25)**

Neonatal respiratory distress syndrome (RDS): severe impairment of respiratory function in a preterm newborn, caused by immaturity of the lungs **(18)**

Nephroblastoma: (also known as *Wilms' tumor*) highly metastatic cancerous tumor of the kidney **(23)**

Nephrolithiasis: kidney stones **(23)**

Nephrotic syndrome: clinical state characterized by edema, proteinuria, hypoalbuminemia, hyperlipidemia, and altered immunity **(23)**

Neural tube: fetal tissue that develops into the central nervous system **(16)**

Neurons: nerve cells that transmit impulses from one part of the body to another **(16)**

Newborn: infant from delivery through the first month of life **(9)**

Nits: louse eggs **(24)**

Nociceptor: sensory receptor that detects and differentiates pain sensation **(16)**

Nocturia: the need to void frequently at night **(5)**

Nonorganic failure to thrive (NOFTT): disorder characterized by inadequate growth in height and weight **(27)**

Nonshivering thermogenesis: production of heat in a neonate by moving and crying, which raises metabolism and burns stores of brown fat to increase body temperature **(9)**

Nonstress test (NST): a test used to assess fetal movement and fetal heart rate **(6)**

Norepinephrine (noradrenalin): hormone that causes the body to be geared for strenuous activity ("fight-or-flight" reaction) **(25)**

Nuclear family: members of a single-family unit **(3)**

Nulligravida: woman who has never been pregnant **(6)**

Nullipara: woman who has never delivered an infant after 24 weeks' gestation **(6)**

Nursing diagnoses: names for client conditions that nurses are qualified and trained to treat independently; they have been defined and developed by the North American Nursing Diagnosis Association (NANDA) **(1)**

Nystagmus: involuntary movement of the eyes **(16)**

O

Obesity: excessive weight and accumulation of body fat **(27)**

Objective data: data that can be observed and measured by the senses or by mechanical instruments **(1)**

Obsessive-compulsive disorder (OCD): disorder characterized by ritualistic thoughts or actions that interfere with activities of daily living **(27)**

Obstructive uropathy: condition in which the structure or function of the urinary system is altered, resulting in obstruction of urine flow **(23)**

Occiput: back of head **(7)**

Omphalocele: congenital malformation of the abdominal wall allowing the abdominal contents to herniate into the umbilical cord **(9)**

Oocyte: an immature sex cell from which an egg or ovum develops by meiosis; a female gametocyte **(4)**

Oogenesis: the development of the female gamete or ovum, resulting from the process of meiosis **(4)**

Oophorectomy: surgical removal of one or both ovaries **(5)**

Open reduction: reduction of a fractured bone by surgically aligning the bone and stabilizing the ends with nails, plates, or screws **(17)**

Ophthalmia neonatorum: inflammation of the eyes of the newborn, resulting from contact with gonorrhea or chlamydia during the birth process **(9)**

Opisthotonos: rigid hyperextension of the entire body **(26)**

Oral candidiasis: (also known as *thrush*) chronic condition caused most commonly by the fungus *Candida albicans* **(21)**

Orchiectomy: removal of one testis and spermatic cord **(5)**

Orchitis: inflammation of the testes **(5)**

Ordinal position: order of birth in the family **(11)**

Organogenesis: formation of organs, days 15 to 60 of pregnancy **(16)**

Orthopnea: dyspnea or difficulty breathing that is relieved by sitting or standing **(18)**

Orthoptics: eye exercises **(16)**

Osmosis: movement of fluid (the solvent) across the cell membrane from an area of lesser solute concentration to an area of greater solute concentration; causes the concentration of solutes on both sides of the cell membrane to become equal **(15)**

Ossification: the hardening or calcification of soft tissue into a bonelike material, marking the transition from embryo to fetus **(6)**

Otalgia: ear pain **(16)**

Otitis media: inflammation of the middle ear that may be accompanied by fluid in the middle ear **(16)**

Outcome: client goal that relates to a specific nursing diagnosis **(1)**

Ovarian cancer: the most lethal of female reproductive cancers, remains asymptomatic until the cancer has spread to surrounding tissue or has been transported by the lymphatic system to other parts of the body; risk factors include older age, early menarche, late menopause, history of infertility, treatment of infertility with Colomid (clomiphene), and history of breast or ovarian cancer **(5)**

Ovarian follicle: a cavity in the ovary containing a maturing ovum surrounded by its encasing cells **(4)**

Ovum: the female reproductive cell or gamete; egg **(4)**

Oxytocin: hormone produced by the posterior pituitary gland; stimulates uterine contractions **(6)**

P

Palliative care: (also known as *palliative management*) care in which the goal is relief from suffering, not cure **(28)**

Palliative management: (also known as *palliative care*) care that involves a shift in treatment goals from cure to providing relief from suffering **(28)**

Palmar grasp reflex: reflex that occurs when a finger or small object is placed in the newborn's hand; newborns grasp the finger tight enough to be lifted from the bed; reflex disappears after 4 months **(9)**

Pandemic flu: global outbreak of virulent human flu **(26)**

Papillae: small, raised bumps covering the tongue **(22)**

Para: the number of deliveries after 24 weeks' gestation **(6)**

Parallel play: side-by-side play, typical of toddlers **(12)**

Paraphimosis: inability to return the foreskin over the glans, causing constriction of the penis **(23)**

Parasympathetic nervous system: part of the autonomic nervous system that controls bodily processes in nonstressful situations; clinical manifestations include constriction of pupils, decreased heart rate, constriction of bronchioles, and increased peristalsis **(16)**

Parathyroid hormone (PTH): hormone that increases the concentration of blood calcium by stimulating the breakdown of hard bone matrix, thus releasing the calcium into the blood; works with calcitonin to maintain normal blood calcium level **(25)**

Parenchymal: functional part of an organ **(22)**

Parotid gland: largest of the salivary glands, located below and in front of the ears at the angle of the jaw **(22)**

Passage: maternal structures through which the fetus must travel **(7)**

Passenger: fetus **(7)**

Passive immunity: immunity provided by administering immunoglobulins to protect children against diseases to which they may have been exposed already **(21)**

Pathogens: harmful organisms **(26)**

Patients: ill people who need care and decisions to be made by others for their benefit **(1)**

PCA pump: patient-controlled analgesia device, which allows the client to control the amount and timing of medication up to a preset amount **(14)**

Pediatrics: the medical science related to diagnosis and treatment of childhood illness **(1)**

Pediculosis: infestation with parasites (lice) that live on the outside of a human host **(24)**

Pedophile: person who has sexual interest in children **(27)**

Peer pressure: influencing a person to follow the desire or behavior of the group **(5)**

Penis: the male organ of copulation or sexual intercourse **(4)**

Percentile: measure of what portion of the overall population is the same **(11)**

Percutaneous umbilical cord sampling: a test similar to amniocentesis done in the second and third trimesters in which the physician locates the fetal parts, identifies the placenta and umbilical cord by ultrasound, and aspirates fetal blood for analysis of chemical content; the test is useful in diagnosing inherited blood disorders, detecting fetal infection, and determining acid-base balance **(6)**

Periorbital edema: edema around the eyes **(23)**

Peristalsis: wavelike contraction of the smooth muscle that lies underneath the mucous membrane **(22)**

PERRLA: pupils equally round and react to light and accommodation **(16)**

Petechiae: pinpoint hemorrhages **(9)**

Pheochromocytoma: adrenal tumor, most commonly benign and curable **(25)**

Phimosis: condition that occurs when the opening of the foreskin is small and unable to be retracted over the glans **(9)**

Photophobia: sensitivity to light **(16)**

Phototherapy: exposure of the newborn to high-intensity light **(9)**

Phenylketonuria (PKU): congenital disorder that results in toxic accumulation of phenylalanine and its metabolites; can lead to mental retardation and/or brain damage **(22)**

Physiologic anemia of pregnancy: drop in iron that results from hemodilution, as evidenced by a hematocrit of 34% to 40%; the number of white blood cells increases beginning in the second trimester **(6)**

Pica: ingestion of nonfood material **(22)**

Placenta: a highly vascular organ connecting the mother and the fetus **(6)**

Plantar grasp reflex: reflex that occurs when the sole of the foot is touched; toes curl under as if newborns are trying to "grasp" with their feet **(9)**

Plasma: clear, fluid portion of circulating blood **(15)**

Pneumonia: inflammation or infection of the bronchioles and alveoli in the lung **(18)**

Pneumothorax: air in the chest cavity that can result from chest trauma or spontaneous rupturing of alveoli **(18)**

Point of maximal impulse (PMI): site where the heart rate can be best heard **(13)**

Poisoning: ingestion of a toxic substance **(22)**

Polar body: a small cell containing little cytoplasm that is produced along with the oocyte and later discarded **(4)**

Polycystic kidney: condition in which one or both kidneys are enlarged and contain fluid-filled cysts **(23)**

Polycystic ovary syndrome (PCOS): condition that results from numerous follicular cysts **(5)**

Polydactyly: presence of more than five fingers per hand or toes per foot **(9)**

Polydipsia: excessive thirst **(25)**

Polyphagia: excessive hunger **(25)**

Polyuria: excessive urine output **(25)**

Portal of entry: method in which a harmful organism enters a new host **(26)**

Portal of exit: method in which a harmful organism leaves the reservoir **(26)**

Positive feedback: mechanism in which increase in one substance causes an increased response until some major event occurs that causes a decrease in the substance **(25)**

Postictal: following a seizure **(16)**

Postinfectious polyneuritis: (Guillain–Barré syndrome) relatively rare disorder characterized by ascending and then descending paralysis **(16)**

Postmortem examination: (also known as *autopsy*) examination of the body after death to determine more details about the cause of death, the disease, or other statistical data **(28)**

Postpartal chills: uncontrolled shaking or chills as a physiologic response to labor and a result of the rapid weight loss at delivery **(7)**

Postpartum: period that begins immediately after birth of the baby and continues for 6 weeks or until the woman's body has nearly returned to a prepregnant state **(10)**

Postpartum blues: transient period of mild depression that often occurs in the early postpartum period **(10)**

Postterm: delivery after 42 weeks' gestation **(6)**

Precocious puberty: the presence of any secondary sex characteristics before the age of 8 in girls and before the age of 9 in boys **(25)**

Pre-embryonic stage: (also known as *Stage I*) from fertilization through 14 days or 2 weeks; the time when the fertilized ovum travels through the fallopian tube, differentiates into trophoblast and embryonic disc, and attaches to the endometrium **(6)**

Pregnancy: process of uniting two sex cells into one, and the carrying of the resulting offspring in the uterus **(6)**

Preload: volume of blood in the ventricles at the end of diastole **(19)**

Premature rupture of membranes (PROM): occurs when the membranes rupture before the 38th week of gestation **(7)**

Premenstrual syndrome (PMS): a group of symptoms resulting from an imbalance of estrogen and progesterone, as well as increased prolactin and aldosterone levels **(5)**

Preoperational: level at which the child learns to interact with members in the environment **(11)**

Prepuce: (also known as *foreskin*) loose-fitting retractable skin that covers the glans of the penis **(4)**

Presbycusis: loss of hearing **(11)**

Presbyopia: farsightedness **(11)**

Presumptive signs: subjective signs the mother experiences during pregnancy **(6)**

Preterm: delivery after the 24th week, but before the 38th **(6)**

Primigravida: first pregnancy **(6)**

Primapara: first delivery after 24 weeks' gestation **(6)**

Primary care: care that includes preventive activities such as immunizations, well-child checkups, and routine physical examinations **(1)**

Primary immune response: body's first response to antigens **(21)**

Primary prevention: keeping health problems from beginning **(12)**

Primary spermatocyte: a diploid spermatocyte that has not yet undergone meiosis **(4)**

Probiotics: foods or supplements containing live, beneficial organisms **(22)**

Prodromal period: stage of an infectious process that occurs just prior to the onset of clinical symptoms **(26)**

Progesterone: a steroid hormone produced in the ovary; it prepares and maintains the uterus for pregnancy and stimulates thickening and vascularization of the endometrium **(4)**

Prolactin: (also known as *lactogenic hormone*) hormone secreted during pregnancy that stimulates breast development and milk production (lactation) **(25)**

Prolapsed umbilical cord: condition that occurs when the infant's body (usually the head) compresses the cord against the pelvis, obstructing blood flow through the umbilical cord; results in an obstetric emergency **(7)**

Proliferative phase: phase of the menstrual cycle that begins around day 3 when follicle-stimulating hormone (FSH) secretion form and the anterior pituitary gland begins to increase **(4)**

Prostaglandin: any of a group of potent hormone-like substances that mediate physiologic functions such as control of blood pressure, contraction of smooth muscle, and modulation of inflammation **(25)**

Prostate cancer: leading type of cancer in men; it rarely occurs before the age of 40; usually begins in the posterior region of the prostate and may spread into the seminiferous tubules or bladder **(5)**

Prostate gland: a doughnut-shaped gland located just below the urinary bladder that controls release of urine from the bladder and secretes a fluid that is a major constituent of semen **(4)**

Prostatitis: inflammation of the prostate **(5)**

Proteinuria: protein in the urine **(23)**

Proximodistal: from the center of the body to the periphery and from general to specific **(11)**

Pruritis: itching **(22)**

Ps affecting labor: five variables that affect: passage, passenger, powers, position, and psyche **(7)**

Pseudohermaphroditism: (also known as *ambiguous genitalia*) rare condition in which determining the gender of the child is difficult **(23, 25)**

Pseudomenstruation: mucus or slightly bloody vaginal discharge from female newborn related to the influence of maternal hormones; disappears in a few days **(9)**

Pseudopregnancy: false pregnancy **(6)**

Psyche: mother's emotional status during labor **(7)**

Psychosexual: related to emotional, mental, physiologic, and behavioral components of sex or sexual development **(11)**

Psychosocial health: aspects of health, including mental, emotional, social, and spiritual stability **(27)**

Puberty: a period of transition and sexual maturation **(4)**

Puerperium: (also known as *postpartum*) period that begins immediately after birth of the baby and continues for 6 weeks or until the woman's body has nearly returned to a prepregnant state **(10)**

Pulmonary stenosis: narrowing of the pulmonary valve **(19)**

Purging: induction of vomiting, abuse of laxatives or diuretics, or both **(27)**

Purpura: rash in which blood cells leak into the skin **(20)**

Pyelonephritis: kidney infection **(23)**

Pyeloplasty: removal of the obstructed ureter segment and replacement into the renal pelvis **(23)**

Pyloric sphincter: ring of smooth muscle fibers around the opening of the stomach into the duodenum **(22)**

Pyloric stenosis: progressive hypertrophy of the pyloric sphincter resulting in obstruction **(9)**

Pyloroplasty: surgical widening of the pyloric canal to facilitate emptying of gastric contents into the duodenum **(22)**

Pylorus: passage at the lower end of the stomach that opens into the duodenum **(22)**

Q

Quickening: the first fetal movements felt by the mother **(6)**

R

Race: biologic deviations as shown in physical features **(3)**

Radiation burns: burns caused by exposure to radiation, the most common type being sunburn **(24)**

Rape: forced sexual intercourse, including vaginal, anal, or oral penetration **(5)**

Rashkind procedure: (also known as *balloon atrial septostomy*) procedure in which an enlargement of the existing opening in the cardiac septum is made, allowing better mixing of oxygenated blood from the lungs with the systemic blood **(19)**

Reanastomosis: reconnection of a divided vessel **(22)**

Rebound tenderness: following palpation, the increase in discomfort when abdominal pressure is released **(22)**

Rectocele: develops when the anterior rectal wall protrudes into the vagina **(5)**

Reduction mammoplasty: reduction in the size of the breast by removing fat tissue with an attempt to leave the mammary glands intact **(5)**

Regional blocks: regional anesthetics administered by the physician, anesthesiologist, or nurse anesthetist **(7)**

Relaxin: a hormone produced by the placenta that causes softening in the collagen connective tissue of the symphysis pubis and sacroiliac joints **(6)**

Religion: the belief in a superhuman power recognized as creator and governor of the universe **(3)**

Remission: lack of evidence of any clinical symptoms of a disorder **(20)**

Renal failure: inability of the kidneys to remove liquid waste from the blood **(23)**

Reportable disease: disease that poses a public health hazard **(2)**

Reservoir: site where harmful organisms grow and reproduce **(26)**

Residual volume: (of food) amount of the feeding that remains in the client's stomach **(13)**

Respiratory acidosis: an accumulation of carbon dioxide caused by states of hypoventilation, altered perfusion, or inadequate respiratory diffusion **(15)**

Respiratory alkalosis: condition characterized by a low level of carbon dioxide in the blood **(15)**

Respiratory syncytial virus (RSV): RNA-containing virus that causes bronchiolitis and bronchopneumonia in children **(18)**

Responsiveness: relates to how much parents foster individuality, self-assertion, and self-regulation and how responsive they are to special needs and demands **(3)**

Restitution: turning of the fetal head to be in normal alignment with the shoulders **(7)**

Retractions: inward movement of the tissue over the sternum and intercostal muscles **(9)**

Reverse isolation: precaution used for individuals who are immunocompromised to protect them from harmful organisms that may be brought in from outside **(26)**

Reye's syndrome: acute encephalitis characterized by an onset of symptoms 1 to 3 weeks following a viral infection **(16)**

Rhinitis: (also known as *nasopharyngitis* or *coryza*) inflammation of the nasal mucosa, often caused by a viral infection such as the common cold; classic symptoms include redness and swelling of the nasal and pharyngeal mucosa **(18)**

RhoGAM blood stick: test to identify incompatibility of mother's and infant's Rh factor **(10)**

Rhonchi: coarse rattling sounds, usually caused by secretion in a bronchial tube, common in the child with respiratory disorders **(18)**

Rickets: condition caused by a vitamin D deficiency preventing the proper absorption and utilization of calcium and phosphorus **(22)**

Rigor mortis: stiffening of the body that occurs about 2 to 4 hours after death **(28)**

Ringworm: (also known as *tinea*) group of fungal infections of the skin that are transmitted from human to human or from animals to human **(24)**

Role: expectations or behaviors associated with position in the family (e.g., mother, father, grandparent, child) **(3)**

Rooting reflex: reflex that occurs when the newborn's cheek is stroked and the infant turns the head in that direction; disappears between 3 and 4 months **(9)**

Rugae: a fold, crease, or wrinkle, as in the lining of the mucus membranes in the vagina **(4)**

S

Salpingitis: infection of the fallopian tubes **(6)**

Salpingo-oophorectomy: removal of the uterus and both ovaries **(5)**

Scabies: infestation caused by the mite *Sarcoptes scabiei* **(24)**

Scarf sign: sign indicating prematurity, in which the neonate's elbow can pass the midline when the arm is moved in front of the neck **(9)**

Schultze mechanism: expulsion of the placenta with the maternal side in **(7)**

Scrotum: a skin-covered pouch that protects the testicles and is suspended from the groin **(4)**

Scurvy: condition caused by a lack of vitamin C in the diet **(22)**

Seasonal flu: (also known as *common flu*) respiratory illness that can be transmitted from person to person, generally caused by influenza A or B **(26)**

Seborrheic dermatitis: "cradle cap" in babies may be a result of changes in sebaceous glands **(24)**

Second stage of labor: stage of labor that begins when the cervix is completely dilated and ends with birth **(7)**

Secondary health care: care that refers to relatively serious or complicated care **(1)**

Secondary immune response: body's response to a second exposure to an antigen **(21)**

Secondary prevention: early detection and screening for health problems **(12)**

Secretory phase: the second half of the menstrual cycle after ovulation during which the corpus luteum secretes progesterone that prepares the endometrium for the implantation of an embryo; if fertilization does not occur, then menstrual flow begins **(4)**

Seizures: periods of sudden discharge of electrical activity in the brain that cause involuntary muscle activity, change in level of consciousness (LOC), or altered behavior and sensory manifestation **(16)**

Semen: (also known as *seminal fluid*) the mixture of sperm and fluid from the reproductive glands **(4)**

Seminal fluid: (also known as *semen*) the mixture of sperm and fluid from the reproductive glands **(4)**

Seminal vesicle: part of male reproductive tract that produces a thick, yellowish fluid rich in fructose, which provides energy for the highly mobile sperm **(4)**

Seminiferous tubules: long narrow coiled tubes in each lobule of the testis in which spermatozoa develop **(4)**

Sensorimotor: first level of cognitive development in which baby and young child begin interaction with the environment by reflex response, from birth to 2 years of age **(11)**

Separation anxiety: feelings of anger, fear, grief, and revenge in association with a closely related person **(11)**

Separation anxiety disorder (SAD): (also known as *anaclitic depression*) fear of separation from individuals or locations **(27)**

Septum: wall **(19)**

Sexual abuse: sexual acts that are imposed on children who cannot protect themselves due to their lack of emotional or cognitive development **(27)**

Shaken-baby syndrome: syndrome in infants in which brain injury is caused by shaking of such violence that the child's brain rebounds against the skull **(27)**

Sickle cell anemia: hereditary disorder affecting the formation of hemoglobin **(20)**

Sickle cell crisis: acute episode of severe symptoms of sickle cell anemia **(20)**

Simian crease: horizontal crease extending across the entire palm **(16)**

Sinciput: forehead or brow **(7)**

Single-parent family: either a mother or a father who raises the children alone **(3)**

Smegma: secretion consisting of epithelial cells found around the external genitalia that may be present in the labial folds of a newborn **(9)**

Solute: substance dissolved in a solution or fluid **(15)**

Solution: substance formed when one or more solutes are dissolved in a solvent **(15)**

Solvent: liquid in which a substance or solute is dissolved **(15)**

Somatic reflexes: reflexes that control skeletal muscle contractions **(16)**

Spanking: one or two flat-handed swats on a child's wrist or buttocks **(12)**

Spermatic cord: a structure resembling a cord that suspends the testis within the scrotum and contains the vas deferens and other vessels and nerves **(4)**

Spermatids: any of the four haploid cells formed by meiosis in a male that develop into spermatozoa **(4)**

Spermatogenesis: sperm production, which begins at puberty **(4)**

Spermatogonia: sperm precursor or stem cells **(4)**

Spermatozoa: sperm cells **(4)**

Spermicides: chemicals in the form of creams, foams, jellies, or suppositories that are inserted into the vagina prior to sexual intercourse in order to prevent conception **(5)**

Spina bifida: incomplete closure of the vertebra and neural tube **(9)**

Spinnbarkeit: the stringy, elastic character of cervical mucus during the ovulatory period **(5)**

Splenomegaly: enlarged spleen **(21)**

Spontaneous abortion: (also known as *miscarriage*) nonelective abortion that occurs within the first 20 weeks of pregnancy **(5)**

Spontaneous rupture of the membranes (SROM): disruption of the integrity of the placenta, usually occurs after labor begins **(7)**

Sprain: condition that occurs when the ligament associated with a joint is torn following trauma to the joint **(17)**

St. Vitus's dance: chorea occurring chiefly in children and associated with rheumatic fever **(19)**

Staging: process of naming the extent of the spread of cancer **(20)**

Standard precautions: combination of universal precautions and body substance isolation techniques that apply to all clients in a hospital **(26)**

Startle reflex: *See* Moro reflex **(9)**

Stasis: pooling of urine or other body fluids **(23)**

Station: relationship between the fetus and the maternal ischeal spines **(7)**

Status epilepticus: continuous seizure for more than 30 minutes accompanied by loss of consciousness **(16)**

Statutory rape: sexual intercourse that occurs between a minor and an adult with consent given by the minor **(27)**

Steatorrhea: fat in the stool **(22)**

Stepping reflex: reflex obtained by holding newborns with the feet touching the table; newborns will step as if walking **(9)**

Stereotyping: not allowing for individual or group diversity **(3)**

Stereotypy: rigid and obsessive behaviors **(27)**

Stork bites: (also known as *telangiectactic nevi*) dark red spots on the eyelids, forehead, or nape of the neck, that usually fade in time **(9)**

Strabismus: lack of coordination of the visual axes of the eye; eyes do not stay parallel to each other but may diverge in any direction **(9)**

Strain: minor injury to the muscle or tendon **(17)**

Striae gravidarum: (also known as *stretch marks*) marks that occur when the underlying connective tissue separates during periods of rapid growth **(6)**

Stridor: high-pitched inspiratory crowing sound caused by severely narrowed airways **(18)**

Stroke volume: amount of blood forced out by the ventricles during a heart contraction **(19)**

Subcostal: below the ribs **(9)**

Subjective data: knowledge gained from an understanding of the client's or group's subjective or personal experience **(1)**

Sublingual glands: glands that open into the floor of the mouth **(22)**

Submandibular glands: glands that lie behind the mandible and secrete saliva into the submandibular ducts **(22)**

Substernal: below the sternum **(9)**

Sucking reflex: sucking movements of an infant's lips elicited when the newborn's lips are touched; disappears by 10 months **(9)**

Suicide: taking of one's own life **(27)**

Superego: moral system that contains learned values and conscience **(11)**

Supervision: the act of giving directions to workers and inspecting the tasks performed **(1)**

Supine hypotensive syndrome: reduction in blood pressure that occurs when the mother lies supine; the heavy uterus presses on the inferior vena cava, resulting in reduced blood flow back to the right atrium **(6)**

Supraclavicular: above the clavicles **(9)**

Suprasternal: above the sternum **(9)**

Surfactant: a substance that decreases the surface tension of fluid inside the alveoli, allowing the lungs to expand **(6)**

Surgical sterilization: (also known as *vasectomy* or *tubal ligation*) the tying and cutting of the vas deferens or fallopian tubes **(5)**

Susceptible host: individual at risk for contracting the disease caused by the harmful organism **(26)**

Sutures: line of junction of the skull bones **(7)**

Sympathetic nervous system: part of the autonomic nervous system that provides assistance to a person in a stressful or life-threatening situation, causing physical changes that allow the person to respond quickly to danger **(16)**

Syndactyly: fusion of two or more digits **(9)**

Syphilis: sexually transmitted infection caused by *Treponema pallidum* **(5)**

T

Taking-hold stage: period of time after childbirth when a mother is taking control of the activities of caring for herself and her newborn **(10)**

Taking-in stage: period of time after childbirth when a mother is absorbing information about her baby, recalling the experience of delivery, and storing this information in her memory **(10)**

Talipes: (also known as *clubfoot*) a congenital unilateral or bilateral twisting of the foot, usually inward **(17)**

Telangiectactic nevi: (also known as *stork bites*) dark red spots on the eyelids, forehead, or nape of the neck; usually fade in time **(9)**

Tenesmus: painful straining to defecate **(5)**

Teratogen: chemical that can cause abnormal fetal development **(6)**

Term: delivery between 38 and 42 weeks **(6)**

Terminal: final, fatal **(14)**

Tertiary care: management of chronic, terminal, complicated, long-term health care problems **(1)**

Tertiary prevention: disease treatment to prevent further health problems **(12)**

Testicular cancer: cancer that grows within the testicle, eventually replacing all normal tissue **(5)**

Testis: male reproductive gland, occurring paired in an external scrotum **(4)**

Testosterone: a hormone produced in the interstitial cells that causes development of the male accessory organs, greater muscle mass and strength, and masculine characteristics such as a deep voice and body hair **(4)**

Therapeutic abortion (TAB): the termination of the pregnancy to save the life and preserve the health of the mother or when the fetus has a serious developmental or hereditary disorder **(5)**

Therapeutic play: play that allows the individual to deal with fears associated with the health care experience **(14)**

Thermal burns: burns caused by flame or hot objects such as coffee, grease, or stoves **(24)**

Thermoregulation: maintenance of a constant internal body temperature independent of the environmental temperature **(9)**

Third stage of labor: stage of labor that begins with delivery of the fetus and ends with delivery of the placenta **(7)**

Threatened abortion: vaginal spotting noted with a closed cervix **(5)**

Thrombocyte: (also known as *platelet*) assists the body's clotting mechanism **(20)**

Thromboembolism: blood clot moving within the blood vessels **(10)**

Thrombosis: formation of clots in blood vessels **(10)**

Thrush: (also known as *oral candidiasis*) fungal infection of the mouth that is caused by *Candida albicans* **(21, 24)**

Thymosin: group of hormones that play an important role in body's immune system **(25)**

Thyroid-stimulating hormone (TSH): hormone that stimulates the thyroid gland to increase secretion of thyroid hormones **(25)**

Thyroxine (T$_4$): iodine-containing hormone produced by the thyroid gland that increases the rate of cell metabolism and regulates growth **(25)**

Tics: sudden, rapid, involuntary movements of head, eyes, and upper body **(27)**

Tinea capitis: scalp fungus **(24)**

Tinea corporis: fungal infection that creates a circular reddened patch on the skin with raised borders **(24)**

Tinea cruris: (also known as *jock itch*) fungal infection that causes the skin in the groin area to become red and scaly, with raised papules or vesicles forming a circular rash **(24)**

Tinea pedis: (also known as *athlete's foot*) fungal infection that causes the skin between the toes and on the soles of the feet to become red, with deep scaly fissures that are painful and itchy **(24)**

Tinnitus: ringing or other sound in the ears **(16)**

Tonic neck reflex: reflex demonstrated by placing newborns supine on a firm surface; when the head is turned to one side, newborns will extend the arm and leg on that side and the opposite arm and leg will flex **(9)**

Tonometer: instrument used to measure intraocular pressure (IOP) **(16)**

Tonsillectomy: surgical removal of the tonsils **(18)**

Tonsillitis: inflammation of the palatine and pharyngeal tonsils **(18)**

Torticollis: tilt of the head caused by rotation of the cervical spine; also known as wry neck **(17)**

Tracheoesophageal fistula: potentially life-threatening defect when a connection between the trachea and esophagus is present **(9)**

Transition phase: period of first-stage labor during which the cervix widens from 8 to 10 cm **(7)**

Transmission: means by which an infectious agent travels from a portal of exit to a portal of entry **(26)**

Transmission-based precautions: precautions that include standard precautions *plus* airborne precautions, droplet precautions, or contact precautions **(26)**

Transposition of the great arteries (TGA): condition in which the aorta is attached to the right ventricle, and the pulmonary artery is attached to the left ventricle, causing the blood to be insufficiently oxygenated **(19)**

Transposons: jumping DNA **(4)**

Transverse lie: condition of the fetus when the long axis of the fetus and mother are at right angles **(7)**

Trichomoniasis: a sexually transmitted infection caused by *Trichomonas vaginalis* **(5)**

Triiodothyronine (T$_3$): thyroid hormone similar to thyroxine but more potent **(25)**

Trimester: 3-month blocks of time that describe the progression of pregnancy **(6)**

Triplets: pregnancy that occurs from three separate eggs, from two eggs (one of which divides), or from one egg that divides into three embryos **(5)**

Tripod position: position with person sitting upright, leaning forward with the chin thrust forward, mouth open, and tongue protruding **(18)**

Trisomy: the condition of having three copies of a given chromosome in each somatic cell rather than the normal number of two **(5)**

Trisomy 21: three chromosomes at position 21 **(9)**

Trophic hormones: hormones that stimulate other endocrine glands **(25)**

Trophoblast: the outermost layer of cells of the blastocyst that attaches the fertilized ovum to the uterine wall and that becomes the placenta and fetal membranes **(6)**

True perineum: the area between the vaginal opening and the anus **(4)**

Tuberculosis (TB): infection of the respiratory system by the acid-fast bacillus *Mycobacterium tuberculosis* **(18)**

Tunica albuginea: covering on the outside of the testes that forms the septum between the many sections or lobules **(4)**

Tunica vaginalis testis: a pouch of serous membrane covering the testis and derived from the peritoneum **(4)**

U

Ulcerative colitis: inflammation with sloughing of the mucosa of large intestine **(22)**

Ultrasound: a diagnostic test used to outline the shape and determine the consistency of various organs and diagnose pregnancy; it can also be used to determine the exact position, size, and gender of the fetus and to identify some developmental anomalies **(6)**

Umbilical arteries: two arteries in which blood flows from the internal iliac arteries in the fetus to the placenta **(6)**

Umbilical cord: cord that connects the fetus to the placenta **(6)**

Umbilical vein: vessel that brings clean, oxygenated fetal blood and nutrients back to the fetus from the placenta **(6)**

Universal precautions: set of precautions designed to prevent transmission of bloodborne pathogens when providing first aid or health care **(26)**

Uremic frost: urea crystals deposited on the skin **(23)**

Uremic syndrome: condition that develops in end-stage renal disease characterized by nausea, vomiting, anorexia, uremic breath odor, anemia, uremic frost, pruritis, malaise, headache, confusion, tremors, pulmonary edema, dyspnea, and congestive heart failure **(23)**

Urethra: the canal through which urine is discharged from the bladder and through which semen is discharged in the male **(4)**

Urinary meatus: surface opening through which urine is released **(4)**

Uterine prolapse: condition in which ligaments supporting the uterus in the pelvic cavity are stretched or damaged **(5)**

Uterine soufflé: sound occurring at the same rate as the maternal pulse and caused by increased maternal blood flow to the uterus **(6)**

Uterine tubes: (also known as *fallopian tubes* or *oviducts*) structures that serve to transport the ovum from the ovary toward the uterus **(4)**

Uterus: a hollow muscular organ in the pelvic cavity of females that contains the developing fetus **(4)**

V

Vaccines: product containing killed, live, recombinant, or conjugated micro-organisms that is administered parenterally to induce immunity **(26)**

Vacutainer®: hollow, plastic device with a shielded or blunted needle on one end and a sharp needle on the other end that enters the vein; the device facilitates the collection of blood specimens **(13)**

Vagina: a 4-in.-long tube that connects the cervix to the outside of the body, composed mainly of smooth muscle and lined with a mucous membrane; the site of deposition of sperm and the passageway for the delivery of the infant **(4)**

Vaginitis: inflammation of the vagina that may be accompanied by vulvar pain, foul odor, pruritus, and vaginal discharge or bleeding **(23)**

Valve ablation: removal of a faulty valve **(23)**

Vas deferens: (also known as *ductus deferens*) the main duct through which semen is carried from the epididymis to the ejaculatory duct **(4)**

Vaso-occlusion: sickle cells obstructing circulation **(20)**

Vernix caseosa: a white, cheesy substance covering the fetus's skin to protect it from the amniotic fluid **(6)**

Vertex presentation: fetal presentation when the occiput or crown presents first; fetal head is in complete flexion **(7)**

Vesicoureteral reflux: defect of the vesicoureteral valve **(23)**

Vestibule: the area between the labia minora containing the orifice of the urethra **(4)**

Viability: ability to live outside the uterus, usually 24 weeks **(6)**

Villi: (singular, *villus*) finger-like projections **(6)**

Volvulus: abnormal twisting of the intestine causing obstruction **(22)**

W

Webbing: skin between two or more digits **(9)**

Wharton's jelly: white gelatinous tissue making up the umbilical cord **(6)**

Wilms' tumor: (also known as *nephroblastoma*) highly metastatic cancerous tumor of the kidney **(23)**

Witches' milk: milk resembling colostrum sometimes secreted from the breasts of newborns of either gender 3 to 4 days after birth and lasting no longer than 2 weeks **(9)**

X

Xenograft: organ or tissue obtained from an animal for transplantation into a human **(21)**

Y

Yeast infection: (also known as *candidiasis* or *monilia*) a common organism causing vaginitis **(5)**

Yolk sac: a membranous sac attached to an embryo, providing early nourishment and functioning as the circulatory system of the embryo before internal circulation begins **(6)**

Z

Zygote: fertilized egg **(6)**

Index

(*Note:* Figures and tables, denoted by *f* and *t,* are generally cited only when they appear outside the text discussion.)

A

AAP (American Academy of Pediatrics). *See* American Academy of Pediatrics (AAP)
ABCDE (asymmetry, border, color, diameter, elevation) mnemonic, for skin lesions, 714
ABCs (airway, breathing, circulation)
 burn victims, 730
 newborns, 195–196
Abdomen
 auscultation, 661
 enlargement as sign of pregnancy, 137
 girth, measuring, 411
 hernias, and peritoneal dialysis, 696
 newborns, characteristics of, 272–273
 postpartum assessment, 311–315, 311*f,* 312*f,* 313*f*
 postpartum muscle changes, 303–304, 303*f*
 Wilms' tumor, 697, 698
Abduction of infants, 197, 278, 804–805
ABO incompatibility
 high-risk pregnancies, 233–234
 newborns, high-risk, 291
Abortifacients, 148, 149
Abortion
 prenatal care health history, 146, 147*t*
 reproductive issues, 118–119, 118*f*
 spontaneous (miscarriage), 118, 118*f,* 147, 222–223, 223*f*
Abruptio placentae, 224–225, 225*f*
Abt, Isaac, 4*t*
Abuse
 burns, 729, 729*f*
 cupping appearing as bruising, 785
 family violence, 802–809, 803*f,* 807*f,* 808*t,* 809*f*
 legal and ethical issues, 28*f,* 32
 musculoskeletal trauma, 561, 561*f*
 potential, assessment of, 55, 58
 preventing further, 32
 reporting, 5*t,* 59, 802
 sexual, 706, 806–807
Acceleration of fetal heart rate, 240
Acceptance, in grief process, 817*f,* 818
Accomodator learning, 362, 363
Accuracy, in informed consent terminology, 30
Accutane (isotretinoin), 720
Acel-Immune (DTaP, Tripedia), 365*t,* 771*t*
Acetaminophen (Tylenol)
 communicable diseases, 785
 newborn male circumcision, 12
 poisonings, 680*t*
 postpartum, 321*t*
 tonsillitis, 578
Acetazolamide, 501
Acetone (fruity) breath, 755, 756*t*
Acid-base disorders. *See also* fluid, electrolyte, and acid-base disorders
 diabetic ketoacidosis, 756
 Health Promotion Issue, 502–503
 metabolic acidosis, 501, 501*f*

metabolic alkalosis, 501, 504
 nursing care, 504
 principles related to, 498–499, 498*f*
 respiratory acidosis, 499–500, 500*f*
 respiratory alkalosis, 500
Acidosis, 498
Acids, as poisons, 680*t*
Acne vulgaris, 720, 720*f,* 721
Acquired heart diseases
 congestive heart failure, 608, 608*f*
 heart health in children, promoting, 610–611
 hyperlipidemia, 609, 612, 612*t*
 hypertension, systemic, 608–609, 609*t*
 Kawasaki syndrome, 612–613, 612*f*
 rheumatic fever, acute, 613–614
Acquired hypogammaglobulinemia (common variable immunodeficiency), 642
Acquired immunity, 640
Acquired immunodeficiency syndrome (AIDS). *See also* human immunodeficiency virus (HIV)
 family planning issues, 106
 high-risk pregnancies, 232–233, 233*t*
 immune disorders, 642, 646
Acrocyanosis, 268, 270*f*
Acrosomes, 72, 72*f,* 128*f*
ACTH (adrenocorticotropic hormone), 743*t,* 745
Activated charcoal, 680, 680*t,* 681*t*
Active immunity, 640, 641*f,* 767
Active phase of first stage of labor, 181*f,* 189*f,* 190
Active transport of solutes, 481–482, 483*f*
Activity. *See also* exercise
 diabetes, managing during illness, 757
 fluid and electrolyte status, 484*t*
 newborns, high-risk, 290
 pregnancy, during, 162
 rheumatic fever, following, 614
Acute and chronic renal failure, 694–697, 695*f,* 695*t,* 697*f*
Acute illness, home care for, 455
Acute lymphoblastic leukemia, 630–631, 630*f*
Acute myelogenous leukemia, 630–631
Acute postinfectious glomerulonephritis, 692–693, 693*f*
Acyclovir (Zovirax), 231*t,* 232, 233*t*
Adapalene (Differin), 720
Adaptability, in family systems theory, 47
ADD (attention deficit disorder), 794–795, 795*t*
Adderall (amphetamine sulfate), 794, 795*t*
Addison's disease (adrenal insufficiency), 752
Adenine, 68
Adenosine triphosphate (ATP), 829
Adenovirus infections, 524
ADH (antidiuretic hormone). *See* antidiuretic hormone (ADH)
ADHD. *See* attention deficit/hyperactivity disorder (ADHD)
Admission to hospital
 admission forms, pediatric, 455, 456*f*
 process of, 460, 461*t,* 462*f*
Adolescence stage of psychosocial development, 336*t,* 337
Adolescents
 disasters, effects on, 811
 dying, care of, 818–819, 819*f,* 819*t*

families with, 50*t*
 health promotion, 384
 hospitalization, preparation for, 460
 intramuscular injection volumes, 443*t*
 medication routes, 441*t*
 nervous system assessment, 513, 514, 514*t*
 nutrition, 374*t,* 385, 386*f*
 physical growth and development, 348–350, 349*t,* 350*f,* 350*t*
 prenatal teaching, 156, 156*f*
 psychosocial health, 384–385, 385*f*
 sexuality and pregnancy, 114–115, 115*f,* 116–117, 118
 sexuality and teenage pregnancy, 114–115, 115*f,* 118
Adoption, 119, 305, 306–307
Adrenal glands
 adrenal crisis, 752
 cortex, 743–744*t,* 745–746
 disorders, 751–753
 location, secretions, and effects, 742*f,* 743–744*t,* 745–746
 medulla, 743*t,* 744*t,* 745, 756
Adrenal insufficiency (Addison's disease), 752
Adrenalin. *See* epinephrine (adrenalin)
Adrenocortical hyperplasia (congenital adrenal hyperplasia), 752
Adrenocorticotropic hormone (ACTH), 743*t,* 745
Adriamycin, 629*t*
Adults, older
 physical growth and development, 351
 psychosocial development, 336*t,* 337
 stages of family development, 50*t*
Adults, physical growth and development of, 350–351, 350*f*
Advance directives
 care of dying child, 826–827
 Patient Self-Determination Act, 32, 33*f*
 Patient's Bill of Rights, 31
Aerosol medications, 440
African heritage, people with
 bone density, 550
 cleft lip and cleft palate, 664
 cultural and ethical issues, 40
 cultural considerations during pregnancy, 158*t*
 dark skin, and assessing cyanosis, 603
 diabetes mellitus type II, 757
 female circumcision, 703
 HIV and AIDS in women, 232
 infant mortality rates, 9, 9*t*
 major cultural groups and traits, 51
 maternal mortality rates, 10*t*
 phenylketonuria, 677
 prenatal care, 146b
 prostate cancer, 103
 sickle cell anemia, 625–626
 systemic lupus erythematosus, 647
 thalassemia, 628
African sleeping sickness, 767
Afterload, cardiovascular, 603
Age
 gestational, 265, 266*f,* 267–268, 267*f,* 268*f,* 269*f*
 maternal, 10*t,* 218

Celiac disease (gluten-sensitive enteropathy, sprue), 671–672
Cell bodies of neurons, 509
Cell-mediated immunity, 640–641, 642f
Cellulitis, 724–725, 725f
Celsius conversion to Fahrenheit, 395
Centers for Disease Control and Prevention (CDC)
    avian and pandemic influenza, 768, 769
    immunization schedule for children, 771
    newborn immunizations, 280
    prenatal HIV screening, 642
    universal precautions, 767
Central abruptio placentae, 225, 225f
Central nervous system (CNS)
    anatomy and physiology, 509–511, 509f, 510f, 511f
    fetal alcohol syndrome, 126, 809
    newborns, 299
Central obesity, 760
Cephalic presentation, 174, 174f
Cephalocaudal axis of the fetus, 173
Cephalocaudal fetal development, 134, 333, 333f
Cephalohematoma, 271, 271f
Cephalopelvic disproportion
    dystocia, 242
    passage for labor, 171
Cerclage (Shirodkar procedure), 223, 223f
Cerebellar astrocytoma, 528, 529t
Cerebral palsy, 522–523, 522f
Cerebrospinal fluid, 524
Cervical caps, 107t, 108–109
Cervical dysplasia, 98
Cervix
    cancer, 98, 98f, 704
    changes in, during labor, 169, 170f
    dilatation and effacement, 189f
    dysplasia, 98
    false versus true labor, 170t
    female reproductive system, 75, 75f, 76f
    maternal changes during pregnancy, 139
Cesarean section deliveries
    anesthesia, general, 188
    high-risk labor and delivery, 244, 244f, 245–246f, 247
    postpartum complications, 310t
    postpartum diet, 304
    postpartum self-care after discharge, 324
Chadwick's sign, 138
Chain of infection, communicable diseases, 766, 766f
Chamomile, Roman, 149
Chancres, 104, 106f
Chaste tree berry, 149
Cheerleading, 561
Chelation therapy, 680t, 681
Chemical burns, 729
Chemical digestion, 660–661
Chemical thermometers, 397f, 398
Chest circumference
    measuring, 410, 410f, 411
    neonatal measurements, 197, 198f, 272
Chest physiotherapy (postural drainage), 583–584, 585f
Chest tubes, 594
Chests, newborns, 272
Cheyne–Stokes respirations, 576, 829
Chiari II malformations, 517
Chickenpox, 786
Chifong, 681

Child Health Assessment Program, 6
Child life specialists, 457, 457f
Child molestation, defined, 806
Child pornography, defined, 806
Childbirth education classes
    labor, discomfort during, 187
    pregnancy, during, 162
Childproofing homes, 375, 376f
Children
    foreign body airway obstruction, 581f, 582
    height, measuring, 407, 407f
    legal and ethical issues affecting, 29–32
    sputum specimen collection, 419–420, 420f
Children's Bureau, 4t
Chinese heritage, people with
    birthing practices, 181
    pregnancy, 158t
    traditional medicine, 23
Chiropractic
    health promotion teaching, 22–23
    scoliosis, 556
Chlamydia infections
    family planning issues, 104, 105t
    ophthalmic ointment for newborns, 277
    prenatal testing, 127
Chlamydia trachomatis, 104, 105t, 231t
Chloasma ("mask of pregnancy"), 141
Chloride levels
    cystic fibrosis, 583t
    electrolytes, 482
    pregnancy, during, 148t
Chlorinated lime solution, 3t
Choking
    injury and safety, guidelines for, 371
    self-asphyxiation, 502
    toddlers, 377
Cholesterol levels
    cardiovascular disorders, 609, 612t
    metabolic syndrome, 760
Chordee, 689
Chorea, 613
Chorion, 128, 130f
Chorionic villi sampling
    fetal status, tests of, 142–143, 144f
    genetic screening, 5t
Christian Scientists
    death-related issues, 831
    mourning and after-death rites, 824t
    organ donation, 649, 824t
Chromosomes. See also genetics
    newborns, high-risk, 293
    reproductive anatomy and physiology, 67–70, 68f
Chronic hypertension, 226, 227
Chronic illness. See also hospitalized and chronically ill children
    exacerbation of, with possible abuse, 802
    fluid and electrolyte status, 484t
    home care, 455
Chronic renal failure, 694. See also acute and chronic renal failure
Chyme, 659, 660
Cigarette burns, 729
Cimicifuga racemosa (black cohosh), 97, 149
Circulation
    burn victims, 730
    neonates, 196

Circulatory system. See also cardiovascular system
    blood vessels, fetal development of, 131t
    children, 602–603, 602f
    fetal, 134–135, 134f
    neonate, delivery room care of, 196
Circumcision
    advantages and disadvantages, 279, 280–281
    cultural considerations, 279
    female, 77, 703
    male reproductive system, 73
    newborn discharge teaching, 286
    newborns, healthy, 279–281, 279t, 282f
    phimosis, 702
    without anesthesia, 12–13
Circumoral cyanosis
    cardiovascular disorders, 614
    newborns, high-risk, 291
    respiratory system assessment, 576
Clavicle straps, 563f
Cleanliness, home assessment, 54f
Cleft lip and palate, 293, 661, 664–665, 664f
Client and family teaching
    disease transmission, 773
    family development, stages of, 49–50t
    fractures, 562
    illness and health promotion, 360–361, 362–363
    postpartum care, 321–326, 322f, 323f, 324f
    thinking strategically, 64, 330, 835
Client Teaching
    bottle-propping, 370
    diabetes insipidus, 750
    diabetic ketoacidosis, 757
    emotional and physical care, importance of, 511
    enuresis alarms, 699
    fire safety, 381
    health promotion topics during pregnancy, 156
    home care of child with HIV, 646
    infant massage, 287
    pedestrian travel by school-age children, 382
    physical injury and safety guidelines, 371
    postoperative signs of infection, 700
    postpartum emergencies, 325
    postpartum self-care after discharge, 324–325
    rabid animals, 784
    rheumatic fever, discharge teaching for, 614
    school-age children with braces, 555
    strains and backpacks, 560
    toilet training, 378
    toy safety, 379
Clients
    condition of, in prioritizing care plans, 18
    parents as, 6
    response to nursing measures, 48
Climacteric. See menopause (climacteric)
Clinical Alerts
    abdominal distension in newborns, 272
    Accutane, teratogenic effects of, 720
    antibiotics for procedures following rheumatic fever, 614
    axillary temperatures, 395
    ballottement false positive tests, 138
    birth control and breastfeeding, 303
    blood pressure, newborns, 264
    blood pressure elevation, 310
    blood pressure increase during pregnancy, 139
    carotid pulse, bilateral measurement of, 400

SINGLE PC LICENSE AGREEMENT AND LIMITED WARRANTY

Guide to Special Features

 CLIENT TEACHING

 CRITICAL THINKING CARE MAPS

 CULTURAL PULSE POINTS

Guide to Special Features

HEALTH PROMOTION ISSUES

NURSING CARE CHECKLISTS

NURSING PROCESS CARE PLANS

PROCEDURES